Textbook of
Adult and Pediatric Echocardiography and Doppler

Textbook of
Adult and Pediatric Echocardiography and Doppler

MARTIN ST. JOHN SUTTON, M.B., M.R.C.P., F.A.C.C.
Director of the Noninvasive Cardiac Laboratory, Brigham and Women's Hospital, Associate Professor of Medicine, Harvard Medical School, Boston, Massachusetts

PAUL JOHN OLDERSHAW, M.A., M.R.C.P.
Consultant Cardiologist, Brompton Hospital, London, England

Blackwell Scientific Publications
BOSTON OXFORD LONDON EDINBURGH MELBOURNE

Blackwell Scientific Publications
Editorial Offices:
   Three Cambridge Center, Cambridge,
   Massachusetts 02142, USA
   Osney Mead, Oxford OX2 0EL, England
   8 John Street, London WC1N 2 ES, England
   23 Ainslie Place, Edinburgh EH3 6AJ, Scotland
   107 Barry Street, Carlton, Victoria 3053, Australia

Distributors:
USA and Canada
   Year Book Medical Publishers, Inc.
   200 North LaSalle Street
   Chicago, Illinois 60601
Australia
   Blackwell Scientific Publications (Australia), Pty., Ltd.
   107 Barry Street
   Carlton, Victoria 3053, Australia
Outside North America and Australia
   Blackwell Scientific Publications, Ltd.
   Osney Mead
   Oxford OX2 0EL, England

Typset by The William Byrd Press.
Text printed by Winthrop Printing Company.
Color inserts by Eastern Press.
Bound by Maple Press.

Blackwell Scientific Publications, Inc.
© 1989 by Blackwell Scientific Publications, Inc.
Printed in the United States of America
89 90 91 92 5 4 3 2 1

Library of Congress Cataloging-in-Publication Data
Textbook of adult and pediatric echocardiography and doppler.

  Includes index.
  1. Echocardiography.   2. Doppler echo-
cardiography.   3. Pediatric cardiology.
I. St. John Sutton, Martin G., 1945–
II. Oldershaw, Paul.
RC683.5.U5T49   1989   616.1′207543   89-236
ISBN 0-86542-032-7

To Evelyne Magali and Claire-Helene St. John Sutton
and to Alexander and Jonathan Oldershaw

Contents

CARDIAC MASSES, EXTRACARDIAC VASCULAR ABNORMALITIES, AND THE TRANSPLANTED HEART

ECHOPHONOCARDIOGRAPHY, CONTRAST ECHOCARDIOGRAPHY AND COMPUTER PROCESSING OF ECHOCARDIOGRAPHIC IMAGES

Contributors

LINDSEY D. ALLAN, M.D., F.R.C.P.
Senior Lecturer in Paediatric Cardiology, British Heart Foundation Research Centre for Perinatal Cardiology, London, England.

ROBERT H. ANDERSON, B.Sc., M.D., F.R.C.Path.
Joseph Levy Professor in Paediatric Cardiac Morphology, supported by the British Heart Foundation; Department of Paediatrics, Cardiothoracic Institute, Brompton Hospital, London, England.

SATINDER J.S. BHATIA, M.D.
Cardiovascular Medical Group of Southern California, Beverly Hills, California.

KENNETH M. BOROW, M.D.
Professor of Medicine and Pediatrics, The University of Chicago Medical Center, Chicago, Illinois.

REX DAWSON, M.B., M.R.C.P.
Senior Registrar in Cardiology, Brompton Hospital, London, England.

PAMELA S. DOUGLAS, M.D.
Assistant Professor of Medicine and Cardiology, Hospital of the University of Pennsylvania, University of Pennsylvania School of Medicine, Philadelphia, Pennsylvania.

RODNEY FOALE, M.B.B.S., M.R.C.P., F.A.C.C.
Consultant Cardiologist, St. Mary's Hospital; Honorary Consultant Cardiologist and Senior Lecturer in Cardiovascular Diseases, Hammersmith Hospital, London, England.

JOHN T. FUNAI, M.D.
Assistant Professor of Medicine, Medical College of Virginia, Co-Director, Cardiac Noninvasive Laboratory, VA Medical Center, Richmond, Virginia.

EDWARD ANTHONY GEISER, M.D.
Associate Professor of Medicine, Division of Cardiology, University of Florida College of Medicine, Gainesville, Florida.

MICHAEL H. GEWITZ, M.D.
Associate Professor of Pediatrics, Director of Pediatric Cardiology, New York Medical College, Valhalla, New York.

DEREK G. GIBSON, M.B., F.R.C.P.
Consultant Cardiologist, Brompton Hospital, London, England.

ANTHONY P. GOLDMAN, M.D.
Cardiovascular Consultant, Tampa, Florida.

DONALD J. HAGLER, M.D.
Professor of Pediatrics, Mayo Medical School; Consultant, Section of Pediatric Cardiology and Division of Cardiovascular Diseases and Internal Medicine, Rochester, Minnesota.

LIV HATLE, M.D.
University Hospital, Trondheim, Norway.

SIEW YEN HO, B.Sc., Ph.D.
Department of Paediatric Cardiac Morphology, Cardiothoracic Institute, Brompton Hospital, London, England.

JOHN KENNY, M.D., M.R.C.P.I.
Consultant Cardiologist, Bon Secours Hospital, Cork, Ireland.

MORRIS N. KOTLER, M.D., F.R.C.P. (Edin.)
Chief of Cardiology, Albert Einstein Medical Center; Professor of Medicine, Temple University, Philadelphia, Pennsylvania.

AUBREY G. LEATHAM, M.D., F.R.C.P.
Honorary Consultant Cardiologist, St. George's and National Heart Hospitals, London, England.

RICHARD M. LEE, B.S.
Director, Research and Development, Diasonics Corporation, Milpitas, California.

GRAHAM J. LEECH, M.A.
Senior Lecturer, St. George's Hospital Medical School, London, England.

PETER G. MILLS, M.D., F.R.C.P.
Consultant Cardiologist, Department of Cardiology, The London Hospital, London, England.

GARY S. MINTZ, M.D.
Professor of Medicine; Director, Cardiac Ultrasound Laboratory, Hahnemann University Hospital, Philadelphia, Pennsylvania.

PAUL JOHN OLDERSHAW, M.A., M.R.C.P.
Consultant Cardiologist, Brompton Hospital, London, England.

NATESA G. PANDIAN, M.D.
Director, Noninvasive Cardiac Laboratory, New England Medical Center Hospitals; Associate Professor of Medicine and Radiology, Tufts University School of Medicine, Boston, Massachusetts.

IOANNIS P. PANIDIS, M.D.
Associate Professor of Medicine, Director of the Noninvasive Cardiac Laboratory, Temple University, Philadelphia, Pennsylvania.

WAYNE R. PARRY, B.S.
Senior Technologist, Noninvasive Cardiac Laboratory, Albert Einstein Medical Center, Philadelphia, Pennsylvania.

TED PLAPPERT, C.V.T.
Senior Technologist, Noninvasive Cardiac Laboratory, Brigham and Women's Hospital, Harvard Medical School, Boston, Massachusetts.

CHARLES POLLICK, M.B., Ch.B., M.R.C.P.(UK), F.R.C.P.(C), F.A.C.C.
Director of Echocardiography Laboratory, Toronto Western Hospital; Assistant Professor, University of Toronto, Toronto, Ontario, Canada.

JOEL S. RAICHLEN, M.D.
Assistant Professor of Medicine, Director, Noninvasive Cardiac Laboratory, Thomas Jefferson University Hospital, Philadelphia, Pennsylvania.

MICHAEL L. RIGBY, M.D., Ch.B., M.R.C.P.
Consultant Paediatric Cardiologist, Department of Pediatrics, Cardiothoracic Institute, Brompton Hospital, London, England.

DEEB N. SALEM, M.D.
Professor of Medicine, Chief, Cardiology Division, New England Medical Center Hospitals, Tufts University School of Medicine, Boston, Massachusetts.

NORMAN HENRY SILVERMAN, D.Sc., M.D.
Professor of Pediatrics and Radiology (Cardiology), Director of Pediatric Echocardiography Laboratory, University of California, San Francisco, California.

JEFFREY FORSTER SMALLHORN, M.B.B.S., F.R.A.C.P., F.R.C.P.(C)
Associate Professor of Paediatrics, University of Toronto; Staff Paediatric Cardiologist, The Hospital for Sick Children, Toronto, Ontario, Canada.

MARTIN G. ST. JOHN SUTTON, M.B., M.R.C.P., F.A.C.C.
Director of the Noninvasive Cardiac Laboratory, Brigham and Women's Hospital; Associate Professor of Medicine, Harvard Medical School, Boston, Massachusetts.

SHAN SHEN WANG, M.D.
Research Fellow, Noninvasive Cardiac Laboratory, New England Medical Center Hospitals, Tufts University School of Medicine, Boston, Massachusetts.

Preface

The importance of diagnostic ultrasound has grown to overwhelming proportions since its introduction 25 years ago. It is no longer possible to practice modern cardiology without a comprehensive knowledge of Doppler echocardiography. Advances in ultrasound imaging and Doppler assessment of hemodynamics have made major contributions to the understanding of both congenital and acquired heart disease which are currently the greatest cause of morbidity and mortality in the western world.

The cardiac chambers, great arteries and great veins can all be visualized in multiple tomographic planes by two dimensional echocardiography and right and left ventricular functions accurately quantitated. Intracardiac blood flow velocities, cardiac output, valve gradients and orifice areas and the severity of valvular regurgitation can be calculated from Doppler signals. Doppler echocardiography also plays an increasingly important role in the cardiac catheterization laboratory in assessing complex congenital heart disease, the results of thrombolysis, coronary angioplasty, valvuloplasty and catheter closure of intracardiac shunts.

The aims of this textbook are to provide a comprehensive description of acquired and congenital heart disease for adult and pediatric cardiologists, cardiology fellows, general internists and echocardiographic technologists. The book is arranged in two parts—adult acquired heart disease and congenital heart disease. In both parts, new material is presented in a step-wise fashion to progressively build upon a secure knowledge of cardiac anatomy and an understanding of the physical principles and applications of Doppler echocardiographic techniques. The text is fully illustrated throughout with high quality M-mode and two dimensional echocardiograms; pulsed, continuous wave and color flow Doppler velocity recordings. Line diagrams have been avoided where possible since the objective of Doppler echocardiography is to record high quality image and velocity information to unequivocally establish the correct diagnosis. In addition the chapters describing complex congenital heart disease include pathoanatomic sections oriented to correspond with the two dimensional echocardiographic images.

The initial chapters detail the physical principles of ultrasound, the formation of echocardiographic images and Doppler velocity information, waveform analysis and technical considerations important in instrumentation. The normal Doppler echocardiographic examination provides detailed "how to" methodology which enables the novice to obtain complete integrated M mode, 2D and Doppler assessment of the heart and great vessels. This chapter explains how image quality can be optimized in the presence of abnormal cardiac position and abnormal chest geometry. The examination is followed by an overview of the clinical applications of Doppler in a wide spectrum of cardiac diseases.

The chapters on right and left ventricular systolic and diastolic function and ventricular interdependence emphasize a physiological approach to the assessment of the normal heart and right and left sided pressure and volume overload states. Doppler echocardiographic assessment of atrioventricular, semilunar and prosthetic valve disease, myocardial and pericardial disease, cardiac masses, disease of the aorta, and description of the transplanted heart are presented in detail, with plentiful representative echocardiographic images, pulsed and continuous wave and color flow Doppler velocity recordings. Detailed accounts of phonocardiography, contrast echocardiography and computer analysis of M mode, 2D echocardiograms and tissue characterization are provided and their place in current clinical cardiology emphasized.

The second part of the text outlines a method of classifying complex congenital heart disease using 2D echocardiography. This methodology relies on determination of atrial situs from the position of the abdominal aorta and vena cava with respect to the spine, and performing a sequential chamber analysis to elucidate the atrioventricular and ventriculoarterial connections. This methodology is used throughout the section on congenital heart disease. The final chapter on fetal echocardiography describes the normal cardiac growth patterns and the importance of examining fetuses at high risk for congenital anomalies. Prenatal recognition of structural heart disease has proved useful in monitoring fetal viability and in the parental counselling.

—*Martin St. John Sutton*

Acknowledgments

I wish to thank my friend and colleague Ted Plappert with whom I have worked for the past nine years, Maureen Plappert, Christopher Lord, David Hsi, Kim McAndrew and Karen Robotham my technicians at the Brigham and Women's Hospital who have been of inestimable help in acquiring representative high quality echocardiographic images. I also thank the many medical students, residents and cardiology fellows with whom I have worked at Harvard Medical School who have been a major stimulus to me throughout.
—*Martin St. John Sutton*

I would like to thank colleagues who have helped and supported the concept of this book—particularly Dr. D. Gibson and Professor R.H. Anderson of the Brompton Hospital—and former research fellows and registrars who have collaborated in the reading of manuscripts and acquisition of high-quality echocardiograms. I would also like to give special thanks to my secretary Jill Gunn for her assistance at all stages of preparation of the text.
—*Paul John Oldershaw*

Notice

The indications and dosages of all drugs in this book have been recommended in the medical literature and conform to the practices of the general medical community. The medications described do not necessarily have specific approval by the Food and Drug Administration for use in the diseases and dosages for which they are recommended. The package insert for each drug should be consulted for use and dosages as approved by the FDA. Because standards for usage change, it is advisable to keep abreast of revised recommendations, particularly those concerning new drugs.

I
Adult Doppler Echocardiography

1

The Physical Principles of Echocardiography

Graham J. Leech

BASIC CONCEPTS

If a mechanical disturbance takes place in a medium whose constituent particles have some freedom of movement, energy is transmitted through the medium in the form of a compression wave. Initially, those particles adjacent to the source of the disturbance are displaced, but after traveling a short distance (depending on the density of the medium), they collide with their neighbors, passing on their energy and bouncing back toward their original positions. This process is repeated, propagating a wave of disturbance through the medium. There is a characteristic value for the propagation velocity in a given medium. In air, it is about 300 m/s; in bone, which is much denser, it is over 4000 m/s. For soft body tissues, such as muscle, fat and blood, the value is about the same and is usually taken to be 1540 m/s. The amount of energy the wave carries is determined by the amplitude of the local fluctuations in the density of the medium, which is in turn proportional to the amplitude of the particle vibrations.

If a succession of waves is generated by a vibrating source, a regular pattern of alternating pressure peaks and troughs is transmitted. The distance between successive peaks is the wavelength; the number of peaks passing a given point per second is the frequency. Propagation velocity, frequency, and wavelength are linked by an important relationship:

Propagation velocity = frequency × wavelength

Thus, at a frequency of 1000 Hertz (the unit of frequency equal to 1 wave per second) the wavelength in soft body tissues is about 154 cm. Such a large wavelength is unsuitable for obtaining detailed information about the structure of the heart, whose valve leaflets are less than 1 mm thick. Since the propagation velocity is fixed, it is necessary to use frequencies of over 2 million Hz (2 MHz) to obtain wavelengths of less than 1 mm.

The human ear detects pressure waves. Incoming waves are channeled via the eardrum to the cochlea, where the vibrations are converted to electrical impulses and passed to the brain for analysis. The resulting sensation is called sound. The ear is sensitive only to frequencies from about 30 Hz to 15 kHz, so it is necessary to use another term to describe frequencies outside this range. The word *ultrasound* has been coined for frequencies far above the human hearing limit.

It is simple to generate and to detect ultrasound waves by employing the piezo-electric properties of crystals. If thin metal foil electrodes are cemented to opposite faces of a slice of a suitable crystal and connected to a source of electric voltage, the resulting potential gradient stresses the crystal lattice and causes it to change shape. This disturbs the medium surrounding the crystal and propagates compression waves through it. It is convenient to think of the piezo-electric crystal as a bell and the electrical excitation as a hammer striking it. A decaying train of waves results, the frequency of which is determined by the dimensions of the crystal. By choosing a crystal of suitable size and shape, it is possible to generate waves of almost any frequency. The piezo-electric effect is reversible: waves striking the crystal deform it slightly, generating small electrical impulses that indicate their arrival. The same crystal can be used alternately as a transmitter and receiver, and acts as a transducer of electrical energy to pressure wave energy, and vice versa. Lead zirconate titanate exhibits strong piezo-

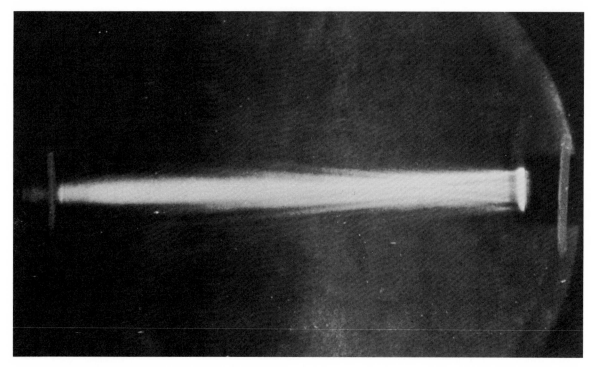

Figure 1.1. A photograph taken by the Schlieren technique, showing an ultrasound beam passing through water from a transducer at the left to a target at the right. Note the complex pattern of high and low intensity zones in the main beam close to the transducer (the near field) and the secondary side lobes.

electric properties and is used for most commercial echocardiographic transducers.

Since both light and sound are examples of wave motion, they share many physical properties. Thus, sound waves passing from one medium into another are partially reflected and partially transmitted, the path of the transmitted portion being deflected by refraction. Waves striking an extensive plane boundary are reflected in a specular (mirrorlike) manner such that the angles between the incident and reflected beams and the normal to the reflecting plane are equal. Waves can bend to a certain degree around a sharp edge by diffraction, and waves arising from separate but synchronized (coherent) sources summate to generate regions of alternating high and low intensity, a process called *interference.*

The apparent differences between light and sound arise mainly from their greatly differing wavelengths. An obstacle that is relatively small compared to a sound wavelength of 1000 mm is vast when compared to a light wavelength of less than 0.0001 mm. The wavelength of ultrasound used for echocardiography is approximately halfway between that of audible sound and light, and it exhibits corresponding properties. Unlike sound, ultrasound can be directed in a well-defined beam, but it cannot be focused as sharply as light (Fig. 1.1).

USING ULTRASOUND TO MAP CARDIAC STRUCTURES

Most of us have estimated the distance from the center of a storm by timing the delay between the instantaneous arrival of a lightning flash and the slower propagation velocity of its thunderclap. Similarly, if we stand in a large building like a cathedral and clap our hands, the waves reflected from the walls return a short time later as an echo. Provided the propagation velocity is known, the time delay can be converted into distance using the relationship:

Total distance = propagation velocity × time delay

This equation is the basis for echocardiographic imaging. A brief burst or pulse of ultrasonic waves is generated by a piezo-electric transducer placed in contact with the body surface. As the pulse passes through the body, it encounters different tissues: muscle, fat, blood, etc. At each interface between different tissues, some of the incident energy is reflected and the remainder is transmitted across the boundary. The relative intensity of the reflected and transmitted parts is determined by the densities of the two tissues. If these differ greatly, more is reflected and less transmitted. In practice, less than 1 percent of the incident energy is reflected at a typical soft-tissue interface, but this means that 99 percent is transmitted to penetrate to deeper structures. The reflected waves return to the

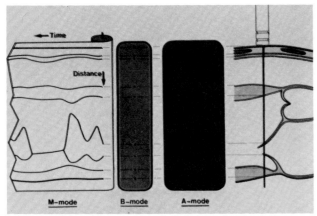

Figure 1.2. Diagram showing how echoes from cardiac structures can be displayed in A-mode, B-mode, and M-mode formats.

transducer only if the angle of incidence of the ultrasound pulse path to the interface is 90 degrees. This has important practical implications for echocardiography since access to the heart is limited by bone and lung tissues, both of which are almost impenetrable to ultrasound, the former because its much higher density reflects almost all incident energy, and the latter because its myriad air-tissue interfaces absorb ultrasound in a few mm. To obtain an echo, it is necessary not only to direct the ultrasound pulses at the chosen structure, but to do so in such a way that they strike it at right angles. A case in point is the tricuspid valve, which is the largest valve and nearest to the chest surface, but because it lies beneath the sternum it is often difficult to obtain echoes from it.

Returning echoes strike the piezo-electric crystal

and are converted into electrical impulses, which can be amplified and displayed on a cathode-ray tube (Fig. 1.2). When a pulse is transmitted, the light spot on the display begins to move downward at a velocity proportional to the ultrasound propagation. The returning signals can be used either to deflect the spot sideways (called A-mode) or to modulate its brightness (B-mode). Echoes from more distant interfaces take longer to return to the transducer, so they are represented as points further down the display screen, which is calibrated to represent centimeters of body tissue. When echoes from the furthest structure of interest have returned, the sequence is initiated again with transmission of another pulse. For a typical depth of 20 cm, the round-trip pulse journey takes 260 μs. It is thus possible to transmit up to 3860 pulses per second in a stream known as an ultrasound beam. Each pulse results in one traverse of the light spot across the display screen, but with such a large number per second, individual traces cannot be detected visually. Moving heart structures are detected by successive pulses at slightly different depths, and the resultant echo signals move up and down on the display. To register this movement for analysis, the cathode-ray tube used for the B-mode display has a special surface comprising millions of glass fibers, which conduct the light without defocusing it directly onto light-sensitive paper pulled across the tube face. The spots of light trace lines on the paper, resulting in a graphic representation, called an M-mode echocardiogram, of the reflecting interfaces and their motion patterns (Fig. 1.3).

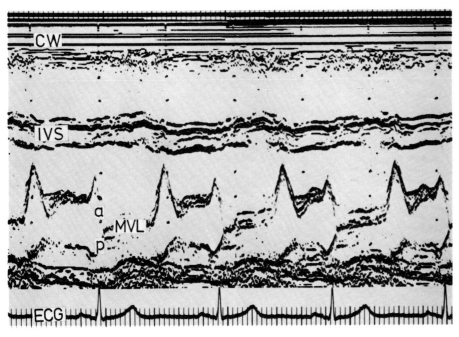

Figure 1.3. An example of an M-mode recording showing the mitral valve leaflets. Vertical columns of dots indicate 1-cm depth calibrations, and markers on the paper edges indicate 0.04-s time intervals. An electrocardiographic (ECG) trace is added. CW = chest wall; IVS = interventricular septum; MVL = mitral valve leaflets; a = anterior; p = posterior.

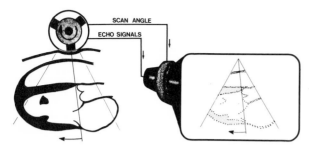

Figure 1.4. Diagram showing the principle of operation of a mechanical sector scanner of the rotating type, utilizing transducers.

Two-Dimensional (2-D or Cross-Sectional) Images

Because all the information-gathering capacity is concentrated along a single beam direction, M-mode echocardiography is a powerful tool for studying the motion patterns of individual cardiac structures and obtaining accurate measurements of chamber sizes and wall thicknesses. However, it does not provide any information on spatial inter-relationships of the parts of the heart and cannot, for example, indicate the shape of the left ventricle. To obtain spatial data, it is necessary to scan the ultrasound beam rapidly across a chosen plane of the heart. Because of the limited access available, all cardiac scanners are of the sector type, in which the transducer is positioned on the chest wall and the angle of the beam emanating from it is changed so that it traverses a sector of a circle, typically over an angle of 90 degrees. Sector scanners can be divided into two classes: mechanical scanners, in which the beam direction is changed by steering the transducer crystal, and electronic systems, in which the beam is scanned without physical motion of the crystal.

A mechanical scanner can use either an oscillating or a rotating scan head. In the rotating type (Fig. 1.4), several crystals are mounted on a wheel that spins in a small liquid-filled dome. As each crystal in turn passes over the heart, it transmits ultrasound pulses and receives echoes. The echo signals are displayed in B-mode form and signals from the scan head are used to steer the oscilloscope trace so that its direction corresponds to that of the ultrasound beam. The transducer thus acts like a lighthouse sweeping its light across the sea and illuminating objects in its path. Alternatively, a single crystal can be used, which is oscillated back and forth by a magnetic motor.

Electronically steered or *phased array* transducers contain a rectangular crystal about 20 × 10 mm, cut into 64 or more thin strips, each of which has its own electrical connections. These are excited in a rapid and precisely controlled sequence (Fig. 1.5). Because each element is narrow, the wave it generates is cylindrical. Immediately after the first element is excited, the

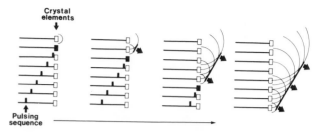

Figure 1.5. Diagram showing the principle of operation of an electronically steered (phased array) sector scanner. The transducer typically contains 64 elements, but only 8 are shown to aid clarity.

second is pulsed, and so on. The individual wavelets combine to form a single, compound wavefront that, because of the pulsing sequence, travels at an angle to the axis of the transducer. Varying the electrical excitation sequence allows the beam direction to be scanned in the same manner as the mechanical systems.

There is some controversy regarding the relative merits of mechanical versus electronic beam steering systems. Some of the differences between the two will be discussed later in this chapter, but for the basic purpose of forming a two-dimensional image of the heart, there is little difference between them.

Whichever method is used, the resultant image comprises a pattern of B-mode lines, as shown in Figure 1.6A. To convert the pattern of radial lines into one of parallel horizontal lines for television displays, a digital scan converter is used. The intensity of the echo signal along each B-mode scan line is sampled and expressed in numerical form [for example, on a scale of 0 (black) to 64 (white)]. This value is then stored in a matrix of electronic memory cells at an address corresponding to the spatial location of the point on the image. Once the memory has been filled, it is read out in the sequence required to form a television image. This process has the additional advantage of permitting manipulation of the image between the writing and reading phases. In particular, memory cells lying between the radial scan lines can be filled according to a predetermined formula (for example, each unassigned cell can be given a value equal to the average of the eight cells surrounding it). The gaps between the B-mode scan lines can be filled in and the resulting image is more aesthetically pleasing (Fig. 1.6B), although it does not contain any additional information. The final image is thus made up of a matrix of small squares, termed *pixels*, each of which has uniform intensity, like a printed picture in a newspaper is made up of a pattern of black ink dots.

Attenuation of Ultrasound

In water (a homogeneous medium whose molecules are closely spaced) ultrasound can travel several

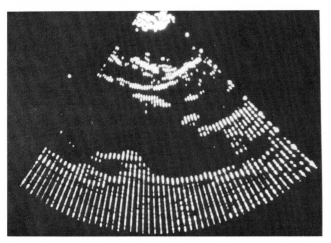 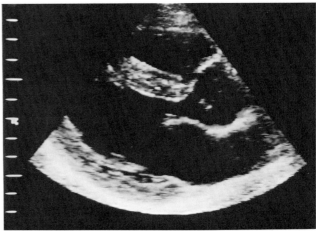

A   **B**

Figure 1.6. A single frame from an older type of mechanical sector scanner, showing the way in which the picture is built up of a number of radial B-mode lines (*A*), and a corresponding view from a machine with a scan converter (*B*).

meters, whereas in air it penetrates only a few millimeters. Body tissues are not homogeneous but contain many small structures whose dimensions are comparable to those of the ultrasound wavelength. These do not generate specular reflections; instead, they scatter incident energy in all directions, like the ripples formed when a pebble is thrown into a pond. Most of this energy is lost, although a proportion does return along the incident path to form small "grass" echoes, which are usually eliminated by the machine operator. The combined attenuation of an ultrasound beam from this and other causes depends on the frequency: at 1 MHz, about 50 percent is lost every 4 cm; at 2.5 MHz, 50 percent every 2 cm; and at 7 MHz, 50 percent attenuation occurs in just 0.5 cm. Although these values may not seem too great, the effect on an echo from a distant structure is profound. For example, consider a reflecting interface 20 cm from a transducer using a frequency of 2.5 MHz. After the first 2 cm, half the transmitted energy is lost; after a further 2 cm, half of the remainder, leaving only one-fourth of the original. By the time the target is reached, the energy has fallen to $\frac{1}{2}^{10}$, or 1/1024 of the transmitted power. For a typical soft-tissue interface, about 1 percent of the incident energy is reflected and this is then attenuated by a further factor of 1024 on the return journey. The echo that eventually arrives back at the transducer is thus $1/1024 \times 1/100 \times 1/1024$, or about 1/100,000,000 of the original! Not only is this a small signal indeed, requiring enormous amplification to bring it to a level suitable for driving the display system, but it is has only 1/250,000 the amplitude of an echo from an identical tissue interface 2 cm away from the transducer, which has undergone a total attenuation of $\frac{1}{2} \times 1/100 \times \frac{1}{2}$. To display both echoes correctly, some device that automatically increases the level of amplification of the distant echo is required. This is called *depth compensation*, or *time-gain compensation* (TGC). Each time a pulse is transmitted, the receiver amplification level is initially set to a low level, since the first echoes to return have been minimally attenuated. As later echoes return from more distant structures, the gain is progressively increased so that signals from similar interfaces have the same amplitude on the display, regardless of their distances from the transducer. Some degree of operator adjustment is usually provided in the form of a bank of sliding potentiometers, each of which adjusts the gain level for a depth band of 1 or 2 cm.

Multiple Reflection Artefacts

Referring to Figure 1.7, it has been assumed so far that an incident ultrasound pulse encountering two interfaces, P and Q, generates two echoes, but the echo from interface Q has to cross interface P on the return journey and is again partly reflected. By repeating this process, the spurious echo, Q′, is generated. Because Q′ travels further, it takes longer to return, and so the machine assumes that it has come from a structure further away than Q. Additional reflections can result in generation of multiple reverberation artefacts. However, these are not normally observed because the reflection at each interface is relatively weak and the secondary echo, which has had to undergo two additional reflections, has only about 0.01×0.01 the intensity of Q. In special circumstances, when the reflections are particularly strong (for example, from a heavily calcified or prosthetic valve), the higher order reflections may still have enough intensity to be detected (Fig. 1.8).

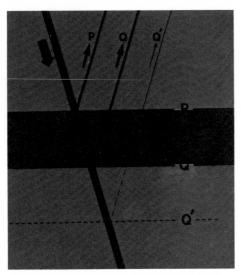

Figure 1.7. Diagram showing how multiple reverberation artefacts are produced. See text for explanation of nomenclature.

Gray Scale

The range of echo intensities detected by the transducer is great, the strongest having about 100,000 times the amplitude of the weakest. It is impossible to register this large dynamic range on any form of photographic image because the difference between the reflectance of the extreme white and black tones is surprisingly small, only about 20:1. Furthermore, the human eye can only differentiate between about 20 intermediate shades of gray within this range. If recorded intensity is related linearly to echo amplitude, all the higher amplitude echoes are registered as white and all those of lower amplitude as black, with only a narrow intensity range shown in any shade of gray. This problem can be alleviated by employing a nonlinear signal amplitude/recording intensity relationship, for example, allotting 25 percent of the available gray range to all high amplitude echoes, 25 percent to low amplitudes, and 50 percent to the midranges. Such manipulations are quite easy once the echo signals have been digitized, so commercial machines generally offer several processing curves, enabling the operator to select the one that generates the most pleasing images. The limited dynamic range of photographic images can be extended by using color. If high amplitude echoes are represented by hot colors (red and white) and low amplitudes by cold colors (green and blue), the dynamic range can be more than doubled.

Resolution of Echocardiographic Images

Resolution determines the degree of fine detail that can be seen in an image and is quantified by the minimum distance required between two objects for them to be shown as separate. In echocardiography, different factors determine axial resolution (in the direction of pulse propagation) and lateral resolution (at right angles to the beam path). For two-dimensional systems, lateral resolution is further divided into azimuthal (in the plane of the scan) and elevation (above and below the scan plane) components (Fig. 1.9).

Axial resolution is determined by the pulse duration. At a propagation velocity of 1500 m/s, a pulse lasting

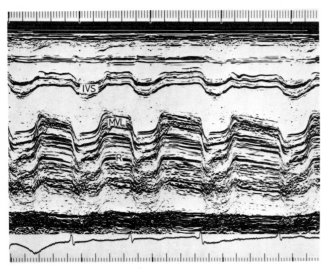

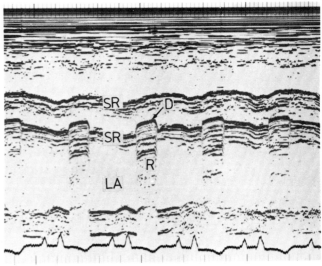

A

B

Figure 1.8. Multiple reverberation echoes from a heavily calcified mitral valve (*A*) and from a Björk-Shiley aortic prosthesis (*B*). IVS = interventricular septum; MVL = mitral valve leaflets; SR = prosthesis sewing ring; LA = left atrium; D = prosthetic disc; R = reverberation echoes.

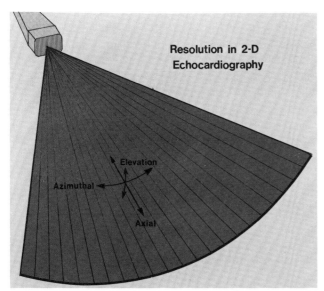

Figure 1.9. Diagram showing the terminology used to describe resolution of two-dimensional echocardiographic images.

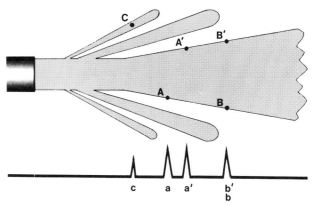

Figure 1.10. Diagram showing how lateral resolution is dependent on the width of the ultrasound beam. See text for explanation of nomenclature.

3 m/s is 1.5 mm long. If two tissue interfaces are less than this distance apart, the leading edge of the pulse arrives at the second interface before its trailing edge has finished crossing the first interface, and the machine cannot separate them. Axial resolution in practical echocardiographic systems is of the order of 1 mm. It can be improved by reducing pulse power (which reduces ringing of the transducer crystal and shortens the pulse duration) or by increasing the ultrasound frequency, since the same number of waves at a higher frequency takes up less time.

Lateral resolution is determined by the width of the ultrasound beam. As shown in Fig. 1.1, an ultrasound beam is not a laserlike probe but is more akin to a poorly focused flashlight. Its complex structure can be described broadly in terms of three main components. There is a central main beam, which comprises a *near field*, where the beam has approximately the same width as the transducer and there are regions of varying intensity, and a *far field*, in which the beam gradually diverges and its intensity decreases with increasing distance. Surrounding the main beam are a series of secondary, cone shaped beams, called *side lobes*.

Referring to Figure 1.10, both the objects A and A′ are illuminated by the ultrasound beam and each generates an echo. The machine indicates their different ranges because the echo from A′ takes slightly longer to return, but does not show that they lie on opposite sides of the beam axis. Objects B and B′, are on opposite sides of the beam, but happen to be the same distance from the transducer; their echoes arrive simultaneously and the machine cannot separate them.

Worse still, object C, illuminated by one of the side lobes, can generate an echo that appears on the display as though C were on the axis of the beam.

Lateral resolution artefacts can be troublesome. Figure 1.11 shows an M-mode recording of a patient with mild mitral stenosis and a Björk-Shiley aortic prosthesis. The ultrasound beam is directed at the mitral valve, but one of the side lobes is generating strong echoes from the prosthetic valve. These are shown superimposed on the mitral valve image to give the impression that the prosthesis has prolapsed into the left ventricle. Lateral resolution artefacts also affect two-dimensional images. Referring to Figure 1.12, as the beam scans across the heart, object A should be seen only when the beam is in position 4. However, the beam profile is such that it also generates echoes in positions 2, 3, 5, and 6, resulting in smearing of the image and sometimes the production of secondary images from echoes generated by the side lobes.

Lateral resolution can be improved by reducing the width of the main beam and the intensity of its side lobes. The former is done by fitting a plastic lens onto the transducer face. This works in the same way as an optical lens, but because of its dimensions relative to the ultrasound wavelength, it is far less effective. Further improvement can be obtained with electronically steered scanners by modifying the transducer pulsing sequence to generate a concave wavefront, the radius of which can be set to focus the beam at a chosen range. However, this only affects beam width in the plane of the scan (azimuthal plane). Even with optimal focusing, beam width at maximum image depth is typically 10 to 20 mm, making lateral resolution at least 10 times worse than axial resolution and the biggest single limitation to overall image quality.

Electronically steered systems can further improve resolution in the azimuthal plane by employing what is called *dynamic focusing*. Referring to Figure 1.13, the

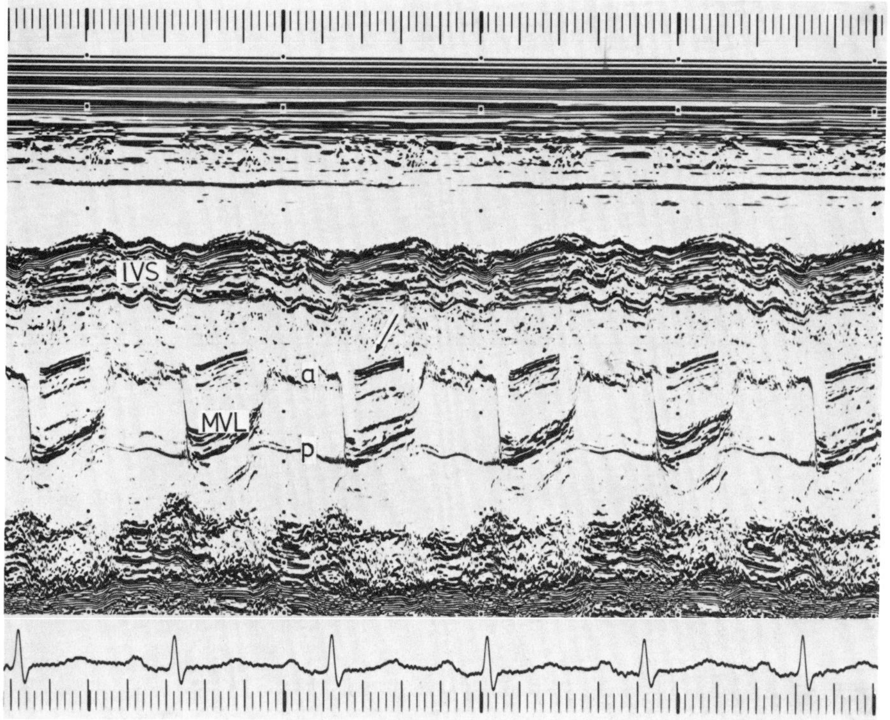

Figure 1.11. Lateral resolution artefact on an M-mode recording from a patient with mild rheumatic mitral valve disease and a Björk-Shiley aortic valve prosthesis. Reflections from the prosthesis generate echoes from the side lobes of the ultrasound beam that are strong enough to register on the recording (*arrow*). They appear superimposed on the mitral valve to give a false impression that the prosthesis has prolapsed into the left ventricle. IVS = interventricular septum; MVL = mitral valve leaflets; a = anterior; p = posterior.

wavefront of an echo returning from a particular target does not arrive at all the transducer elements simultaneously. The small electrical impulses it generates are thus out of phase but can be adjusted electronically so that, when the signals from all the elements are added together, those from a selected range reinforce each other, while those from other ranges or from off-axis targets are dispersed. The phase correction is adjusted as echoes from more distant targets return. A modern machine provides 10 or more of these focal zones. Because all echoes from off-axis targets are attenuated, the effect is to reduce unwanted side-lobe artefacts. This technique is analogous to that used when tracking a fast moving airplane with binoculars: as its range changes, the focus can be adjusted to keep the airplane's image sharp and other distracting objects defocused.

The ability to improve lateral resolution by electronic focusing is one of the most attractive features of the electronic beam steering technique and provides it with the potential to offer significantly better resolution than mechanically steered systems. However, this advantage tends to be offset by the larger transducer and the fact that the crystal is cut into a number of elements, which generate additional artefacts in the ultrasound beam called *grating lobes*. Furthermore, the transducer and its associated electronic circuitry are more expensive to manufacture.

During the 1970s, mechanical systems were generally superior, but the problems of the electronically steered systems have gradually been overcome and their theoretical advantages are now seen in practical terms. A possible exception is in neonatology, where the heart is only 1 to 2 cm from the transducer. The complex process by which the multiple crystal elements form a single beam tends to produce artefacts in the extreme near field that are not present when the beam is generated from a single crystal.

Detecting Small Targets

It is of clinical importance to know how small an object an ultrasound scanner can detect. Specular echoes are generated only if the extent of the reflecting surface is large compared to the wavelength of the ultrasound. As a target gets smaller, it scatters more and less of the energy returns along the beam axis to the transducer. Its echo eventually becomes so weak that it is lost in the background noise of the system. An object is easier to detect if it generates relatively strong echoes (for example, a catheter that is made of material having different physical characteristics from body tissues) and if it is surrounded by a relatively noise-free area of the image, such as in a blood-filled chamber, rather than embedded in the myocardium. An object's shape can also influence ease of detection. If its smallest dimension is in the direction of the ultrasound beam, the axial resolution of the system will aid detection, whereas if it lies along the beam, the relatively poor lateral resolution may not be able to separate it from its

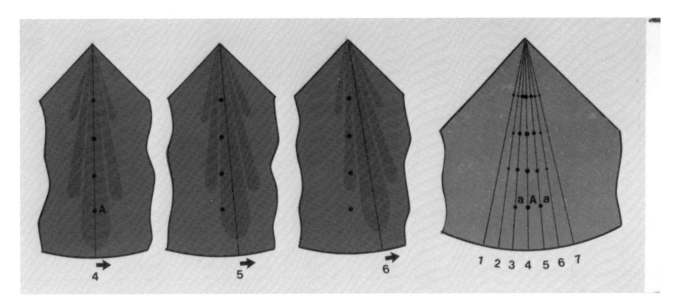

A

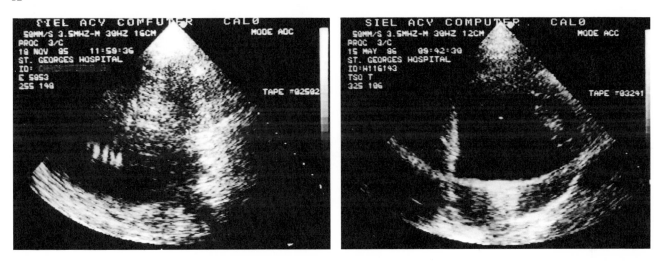

B

Figure 1.12. Diagram showing how side lobes can result in lateral smearing and side-lobe images on a two-dimensional recording (*A*). Apical four-chamber views showing multiple side-lobe artefacts from a single pacing wire (*B, left*) and lateral smearing from the cage mitral prosthesis (*B, right*).

surroundings. Finally, but most importantly, an object will be noticed more readily if it is moving relative to the structures around it, since this makes it much easier for the human observer to recognize the image. It is thus impossible to offer a simple quantitative measure of minimum detectable target size. As an approximate guide, 1 to 2 mm is a generally accepted figure (Fig. 1.14).

Image Size and Line Density

For a particular depth of image, the propagation velocity of ultrasound provides a fundamental limitation to the number of pulses that can be transmitted per second, since a pulse cannot be sent until all the echoes from the preceding one have returned. For a depth of 20 cm, and allowing time for the machine to switch from transmit to receive mode, a typical maximum pulse rate is 3600 per second. To study motions of rapidly moving cardiac structures, it is desirable to scan the heart as frequently as possible. For compatibility with television requirements, 30 scans per second is a suitable rate, which means that 120 pulses are available to form each image. For a scan angle of 90 degrees, the angle between two adjacent scan lines is 0.75 degrees and their separation in the azimuthal plane at maximum range is 0.25 mm. This is not

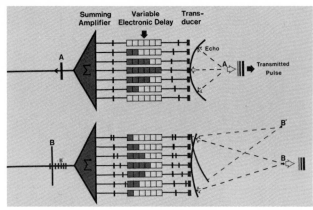

Figure 1.13.   Diagram showing the principle of dynamic focusing. The transducer normally has at least 32 elements, but only a few are shown for clarity. The electronic delay is first set to synchronize echoes received from object A, then readjusted by the time those from B return. Spurious echoes from B′ are not synchronized, lowering their intensity and thus reducing side-lobe artefact.

unacceptable but does require considerable "filling in" in the scan converter and clearly acts to limit detection of very small targets.

It is desirable to be able to record a sector image simultaneously with an M-mode recording, derived from a particular beam direction shown by a movable cursor on the display. Any attempt to do this with a mechanical scanner is severely handicapped because the transducer can only scan the beam across the image from one side to the other, and thus can generate only one M-mode line per scan, giving a total of only about 30 lines per second, which does not produce an acceptable M-mode recording. In an electronically steered system, the beam direction can be changed in

any desired sequence, and as many lines as required can be used to form one, or even two, M-mode recordings. It must be remembered, however, that the pulses used to form the M-modes come from the total pulses available, and either the scan rate or the line density of the two-dimensional image will suffer.

DOPPLER ULTRASOUND

The Doppler Effect

Ultrasound images are derived from large specular echoes, and small structures scatter incident wave energy in all directions, most being lost but some returning to form unwanted noise artefacts. An individual red blood cell could never generate a detectable echo, but the summated scattered energy from the millions of cells in a blood vessel is sufficient to be recorded. If the blood is moving relative to the direction of the ultrasound beam, the frequency of the returning echoes differs slightly from that of the transmitted waves as a consequence of the Doppler effect. This well-known phenomenon is generally associated with a moving wave source. When the source is moving toward an observer, its emitted waves are compressed, shortening the wavelength and increasing the frequency. When the source is receding, the wavelength is increased and frequency lowered. It was first described in 1842 by Christian Doppler, an Austrian mathematician who observed that the line spectra of distant stars are shifted slightly toward the red (longer wavelength) end of the spectrum, and deduced that the stars must be moving away from the solar system at enormous speeds. It does not matter whether the observer is moving toward the source or vice versa, as it is the

Figure 1.14.   The resolving capability of a modern two-dimensional system is illustrated by this parasternal short-axis recording of the coronary artery (*arrow*) in a 34-week premature infant. The artery is shown clearly because its orientation is such that the axial resolving power is used, rather than the lateral. The arterial lumen diameter can be appreciated by reference to the centimeter scale on the left.

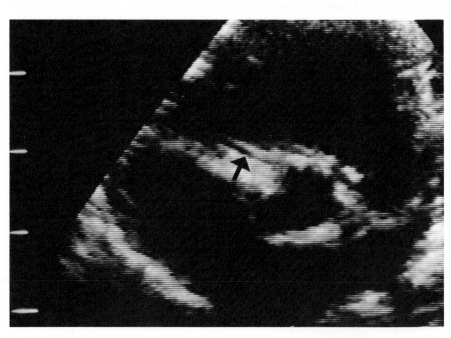

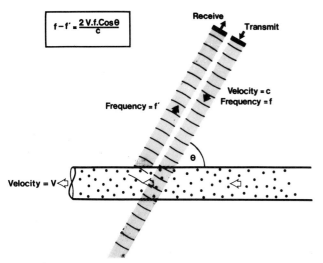

Figure 1.15. The Doppler equation. f and f′ = transmitted and received frequencies, respectively; c = ultrasound propagation velocity; v = blood flow velocity; θ = angle between ultrasound beam and direction of flow.

relative velocity that produces the frequency shift. To see how the Doppler effect applies to reflected waves, consider the reflecting object as a receiver, which then retransmits the waves. If the object moves toward the source, the frequency it receives is increased. Echoes arriving back at the source are further increased in frequency by the fact that the transmitter is moving toward it. The total frequency shift produced by a reflector is thus double that if it were either a transmitter or receiver alone. If the motion of the reflector is not along the axis of wave propagation, only that component of its velocity in the axial direction can modify the wave frequency. These properties are summarized in the Doppler equation shown in Figure 1.15. Two piezo-electric crystals are used: one transmits a continuous series of ultrasonic waves toward a moving bloodstream, and the other detects back-scattered echoes. The difference between transmitted frequency, f, and received frequency, f′, is given by:

$$f - f' = 2 \times v \times f \times \cos \theta / c$$

where v is the blood velocity, c the propagation velocity, and θ the angle between the beam axis and flow direction. The frequency shift (f − f′) is called the *Doppler frequency* and, if the other terms in the equation are kept constant, is directly proportional to the blood velocity. Thus, for many purposes, the terms can be treated as synonymous. This technique is called continuous wave (CW) Doppler. It can be seen from Figure 1.15 that there is a fundamental dichotomy between the requirements for imaging a blood vessel and for measuring the blood velocity. For the former, the ultrasound beam should strike it at right angles (θ = 90 degrees), but the blood flow has no velocity

component in this direction. To obtain the maximum flow signal, θ should be 0 degrees, but this makes it difficult to image the vessel due to the limited lateral resolution of the scanning system. For any intermediate angle, the value of θ must be known. Remember that one is generally dealing with a three-dimensional space and the two-dimensional images does not provide any information on the relative alignment of the beam and blood flow in the elevation plane. Despite the poorer imaging, it is almost always desirable to measure blood velocity with the ultrasound beam and the flow aligned as closely as possible. If the angle can be kept below 15 degrees, for which cos θ = 0.97, the error is negligible. Furthermore, if the angle is not exactly correct, an error of, say, ±10 degrees about a nominal zero value leads to a velocity measurement error of only 2 percent, whereas the same error about a nominal value of 30 degrees gives an error of about ±10 percent. Many commercial machines provide an *angle corrector*, a small cursor that can be rotated to align with the flow direction when the beam is not itself aligned and that adjusts the measured velocity. For the reasons given above, the use of such devices is not recommended.

Characteristics of Blood Flow

When liquid flows in a pipe, not all of it travels at the same velocity. Velocity is maximum in the center, and at the edges friction slows it down so that the layer in contact with the wall hardly moves at all. Several terms could be used to describe the velocity: the peak velocity is that in the center of the tube. The space-averaged mean is the average of all the velocities present and, for steady flow, is equal to the volume flowing per second divided by the cross-sectional area of the pipe. The total range of velocities present is called the velocity spectrum. In a wide pipe, friction at the edges affects only a small proportion of the flow, and the velocity profile across the pipe is flat. The peak and mean velocities are approximately the same, and there is a narrow velocity spectrum. In contrast, in a narrow pipe only the center is unaffected by wall friction; the peak velocity is higher than the mean and the velocity spectrum is broader.

For arteries, the above-mentioned considerations are further complicated by the fact that blood flow is pulsatile. Not only do the peak and mean velocities vary throughout the cardiac cycle, but the frictional effect varies as the blood is accelerated and decelerated. The velocity profile changes, being flatter (narrower spectrum) during acceleration and having a broader spectrum toward the end of systole.

In the nineteenth century, an English engineer, Pascal Reynolds, studied the flow of water in pipes, in which fine streams of dye were injected to demonstrate the flow patterns. He observed that, at relatively low velocities, the flow was stable or streamlined, but at high velocities, the flow became chaotic or turbulent. He found that turbulent flow occurred if Reynolds' number (equal to the product of liquid density, velocity, and pipe diameter, divided by the liquid viscosity) exceeded 2200. This analysis is inapplicable to blood flow in arteries because blood is not a true liquid, arterial walls are not smooth, and flow is not steady, but it is interesting to note that inserting approximate values for blood viscosity (10^{-2} Pascal seconds) and density (1.06×10^3 kg/m^3) yields a Reynolds' number of 530 for an artery 0.5 cm in diameter and blood velocity of 1 m/s. At the same velocity in the aorta, diameter 2.5 cm, it is 2650. This is in accord with the clinical experience that a small increase in flow velocity in major arteries due to pyrexia, anemia, or pregnancy frequently generates enough turbulence to produce an audible murmur.

Displaying and Recording Velocity Data

To provide the maximum potential clinical value, it is necessary to display information derived from Doppler frequency shifts caused by moving blood in such a way that all the flow characteristics referred to above can be analyzed. Because the blood cells are moving at different velocities, there is not one single Doppler frequency but rather a spectrum of frequencies corresponding to the velocity spectrum of the blood flow interrogated by the ultrasound beam. The complex mathematical analysis required to separate all the individual frequency components and to determine their relative magnitudes can now be undertaken at very high speed by specially designed microcircuits. Most commercial machines employ a fast Fourier transform (FFT) analyzer, named after a French mathematician who showed that it is possible to break down almost any complex wave into a series of constituents comprising a fundamental and a series of harmonics whose frequencies are integral multiples of that of the fundamental. In musical terms, a violin and an oboe playing the same note generate the same fundamental frequency, but because of their different construction, their harmonics have different amplitudes and this gives each its tonal characteristics. The waves arriving at the listener's eardrum are a complex mixture of the fundamental and the harmonics. Each constituent frequency excites different groups of sensory hairs in the cochlea, and the impulses conveyed to the brain indicate which instrument is being played. The FFT analyzer works in a similar way. It comprises a bank of filters (usually 64), each tuned to a different narrow frequency band. Over a brief period (typically 10 m/s), the incoming waves are passed through the filters and the amount of energy each detects is stored in memory cells, like a postman sorting a heap of letters. At the end of the analysis period, the contents of each cell are shown on the display as a vertical row of pixels, the density of each indicating the accumulated energy in the corresponding frequency band (Fig. 1.16). A horizontal line marks zero velocity. The pixel immediately above the line shows the amount of blood having the lowest Doppler frequency (corresponding to velocity) during the analysis period, the one above it shows the amount in the next velocity band, and so on.

Some filtering of the spectral signals is usually desirable. Cardiac structures such as the myocardium and valve leaflets generate very high amplitude signals but, since they are moving relatively slowly, their Doppler frequencies are low. Their effect on the recordings can therefore be minimized by using a high-pass filter, which attenuates them without affecting the higher Doppler frequencies from blood jets. This filter is often called a *wall motion artefact filter*. As will be shown below, it is important to be able to record correctly the highest velocity present in a blood jet. This generates the highest Doppler frequency, but its amplitude is usually low and it is often submerged in the electronic noise present in the recording system. Additional filters therefore are usually provided to enhance the high Doppler frequencies. Optimizing these filters represents one of the major elements of skill in equipment design.

The Doppler frequencies are also presented as an audible signal, usually in stereo with flow toward the transducer fed to one channel and flow away from it to the other. The velocity is represented by the pitch of the sound. Laminar flow is indicated by pure whistling tones and turbulence by much harsher noises. By harnessing the excellent tonal recognition qualities of the ear, the experienced operator can both assess the presence of abnormal flow patterns and ensure that the signal quality is free from artefact.

Applications of Continuous Wave Doppler

As will become apparent in the later chapters of this book, many of the clinical applications for Doppler in cardiology arise from two fundamental concepts: the ability to measure volumetric flow and the ability to derive from blood velocity the pressure gradient responsible for the flow.

On a recording of spectral flow data, such as Figure 1.16, the dimensions in the plane of the paper represent time on the abscissa and velocity on the ordinate. An area in the plane of the paper therefore has the dimensions of time multiplied by velocity, or distance. A useful application of this concept arises in the

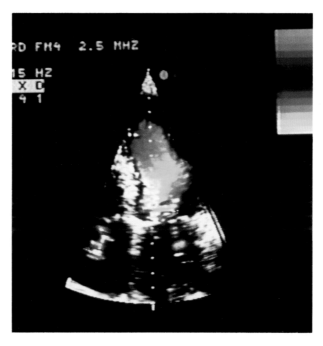

Figure 1.23. Apical four-chamber view with flow information superimposed in color. Red and yellow indicate
flow away from the transducer. In this systolic frame, there
is evidence of mild mitral and tricuspid regurgitation. The
major flow in the left ventricle is normal systolic ejection.
(Photograph courtesy of Hewlett-Packard.)

Plate I

Complex Doppler Frequency

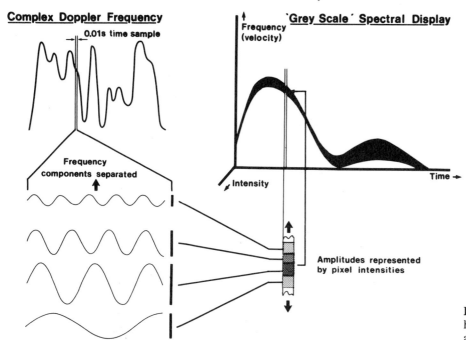

'Grey Scale' Spectral Display

Figure 1.16. Diagram showing how a digital scan converter generates a gray-scale display of blood flow velocity data.

measurement of stroke output (Fig. 1.17). A Doppler recording of blood velocity in the ascending aorta is made from the suprasternal notch. The area under the systolic ejection portion of the curve is called the *stroke distance* and, in physical terms, represents the distance that a particular layer of blood moves along the aorta during one cardiac cycle. If the cross-sectional area of the aorta is measured separately from an M-mode recording obtained from the parasternal region, the product of the two (aortic area × stroke distance) is the volume of the cylinder of blood ejected during one cycle, or the stroke volume. It is important

to emphasize that the boundary of the velocity curve used for this purpose should not be its outer edge, which corresponds to the instantaneous peak velocity, but the space-averaged mean velocity, which for laminar flow in a large artery is almost the same as the modal velocity (the most commonly occurring value). This is indicated on the spectral display by the region of greatest recording intensity. Some commercial machines provide a facility for displaying modal and/or mean velocity, either separately or superimposed on the spectral display. If the peak velocity contour is used for this calculation, significant overestimation of stroke volume will result.

If a heart valve is partially obstructed, blood velocity through it must increase to maintain the same rate of flow because blood is incompressible. For a unit volume of blood of density ρ, the change in kinetic energy when its velocity increases from V_1 to V_2 is given by:

$$\frac{1}{2} \times \rho \times (V_2{}^2 - V_1{}^2)$$

Provided there is no change in height (not always true in the heart), this energy is derived from the pressure gradient across the obstruction. Thus, referring to Figure 1.18, we have the important relationship:

$$P_1 - P_2 = \frac{1}{2} \times \rho \times (V_2{}^2 - V_1{}^2)$$

This is known as the Bernoulli equation. It is a statement of the conservation of energy and applies only to

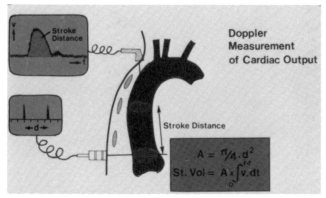

Figure 1.17. Calculation of stroke output from the product of stroke distance (the area under the systolic mean-velocity/time curve) and the aortic area, determined from an M-mode recording.

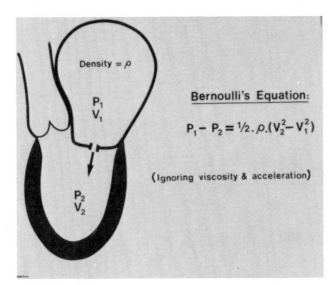

Figure 1.18. Application of a simplified form of Bernoulli's equation to determine the pressure gradient across a mitral valve. P_1, P_2 = pressures; V_1, V_2 = velocities.

incompressible, nonviscous fluids with steady, laminar flow. The additional terms needed to take into account energy used for viscous friction and acceleration can usually be ignored. The Bernoulli equation is used for many practical devices, perhaps the most important being the airplane, where increased velocity over the upper, more curved wing surface lowers pressure and provides the lift to raise its mass off the ground. For many, but not all, cardiac applications, the velocity upstream of the obstruction is very low and can be ignored. If the velocity is measured in meters per second and the pressure gradient in millimeters of mercury, the equation reduces to:

$$P_1 - P_2 = 4 \times V_2^2$$

The value of velocity used for this measurement is the peak velocity in the jet passing through the orifice.

Pulsed Wave Doppler

Continuous wave Doppler permits quantification of blood velocity, from which indexes of cardiac performance and pressure gradients across stenotic valves can be derived. However, because the waves are transmitted in a continuous stream, it is not possible to identify the time interval between transmission of a particular wave and arrival of its echo, and so continuous wave Doppler cannot provide any structural information. Is it then possible to extract Doppler information from returning echoes in an imaging system? Referring to Figure 1.19, two-dimensional and M-mode images are derived from large specular echoes, but between these are much lower intensity echoes, some of which arise from blood cells. If a small time aperture is positioned at a selected point along the beam path, the frequency of echoes returning from a chosen depth can be compared with that of the transmitted pulse and any Doppler shift used to indicate the the chosen point, which can be identified on the simultaneously generated image. The time aperture is called the *sample volume*, and its position is indicated on the display by a marker superimposed on the cursor used for deriving M-modes from the two-dimensional images. By positioning the sample volume appropri-

Figure 1.19. Derivation of M-mode and blood velocity recordings from a two-dimensional (2D) image using pulsed Doppler.

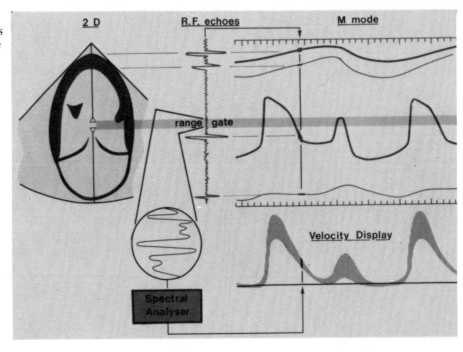

ately, blood velocity at any point within the heart and great vessels can be measured. It is important to remember, however, that the sample volume is a time-slice of the ultrasound beam and suffers from the same limitations of lateral resolution. It is three-dimensional and much larger than indicated, its size increasing with range. This method, called pulsed wave (PW) Doppler, overcomes the limitation of continuous wave by providing an image, but it introduces another difficulty, and to understand it, it is necessary to discuss some basic concepts of information theory.

Since the ultrasound beam now consists of a series of brief pulses, each a few microseconds long and separated by intervals of about 300 μs, the motion of the blood is being recorded as a series of very brief snapshots. A similar situation is found in a movie, where each opening of the camera shutter lasts for less than 1/100 second and the exposures are spaced at about 1/25 second intervals. In the familiar Western, as the stagecoach moves off, the spoked wheels rotate normally at first but as the speed increases, they suddenly appear to be rotating backward. With further increase in speed, the backward motion slows down, stops, and rotation again appears to be in the normal direction. To understand how this effect is produced, consider a wheel with a single radial spoke. If it rotates slowly, the angular displacement of the radial line between successive film shutter openings is small and no confusion concerning its motion arises. As it speeds up, the angle it turns through between successive exposures increases, until eventually it becomes exactly 180 degrees. At this point, one exposure occurs when the line is in the 12 o'clock position, the next at 6 o'clock, the next at 12 o'clock, and so on. The position of the spoke alternates between the two extremes, and there is no way the observer watching the film can identify the direction of rotation. With further increase in speed, the rotation between exposures becomes greater than 180 degrees. To the observer, the wheel appears to be rotating in the reverse direction, slowing down until, when it turns exactly 360 degrees per exposure, it appears to be stationary. Further increases in rotational speed repeat this entire process. This is an example of a phenomenon called *aliasing* and is represented graphically in Figure 1.20.

It will be seen from the above analysis that the wheel's rotational velocity is recorded correctly by the intermittent exposures of the movie camera only when it rotates less than 180 degrees per exposure (when at least two exposures are made per rotation). This is a fundamental principle of sampling theory, first stated by Nyquist: the maximum frequency that can be detected by intermittent sampling is equal to half the sampling rate. When applied to pulsed wave Doppler, it means that the maximum Doppler frequency that can

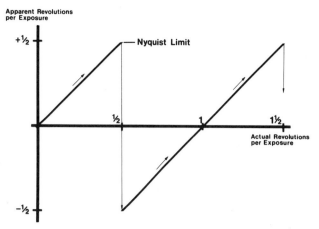

Figure 1.20. Graphic representation of aliasing associated with filming a rotating wheel (see text). Its speed and direction of rotation are shown correctly only below the Nyquist limit, when the revolution frequency is less than half the exposure frequency.

be detected without aliasing is equal to half the pulse repetition frequency (PRF). When the blood velocity exceeds this value, called the Nyquist limit, the high velocity portion of the spectral display is cut off and shown on the negative velocity portion of the display (Fig. 1.21). When the Doppler frequency is equal to the PRF, the velocity is shown as having zero value (corresponding to a 360 degrees wheel rotation per exposure). Up to this point, peak velocity can still be estimated by adding the two portions of the display (which can be achieved electronically by moving the baseline to the bottom of the scale), but if velocity exceeds this, there is complete wrap-around. In extreme cases, it can be difficult even to tell the direction of blood flow. Any degree of aliasing distorts computation of mean or modal velocity values.

Aliasing presents a real practical limitation to use of pulsed wave Doppler for quantification of blood velocity. For example, for a working depth of 10 cm, for which the roundtrip echo delay is 155 μs, the maximum possible pulse rate is 6450 per second. The maximum detectable Doppler frequency without aliasing is therefore 3225 Hz. Putting this value into the Doppler equation of Figure 1.15, for zero angular offset at an ultrasound frequency of 3.5 MHz, the maximum detectable blood velocity is 0.71 m/s, a value below that of normal aortic ejection velocity. There are three possible ways in which this limit can be extended. First, if the angle θ is deliberately increased, the maximum measurable velocity is increased by a factor of 1/cosine θ but, as pointed out previously, this introduces significant errors in any velocity measurement due to inability to know the exact angle. Second, the ultrasound frequency can be reduced. At 2.25 MHz, the velocity limit increases to 1.1 m/s, and at 1.5 MHz it

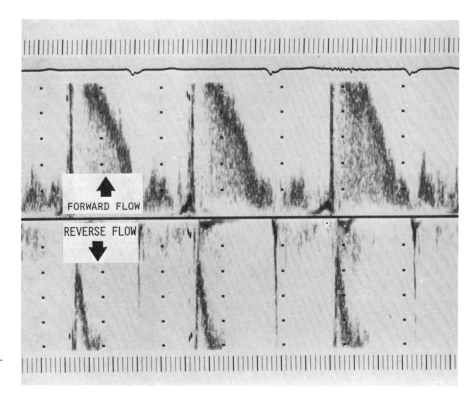

Figure 1.21. Pulsed wave recording of mitral valve flow velocity showing mild aliasing.

is 1.7 m/s. Lowering the frequency degrades image quality, but the Doppler information is better, and this is one reason why it is preferable to use low frequencies for Doppler studies. Finally, if depth can be reduced, the velocity limit increases because the pulse rate can be increased proportionally. This is often not possible in practice due to limitations of imaging windows and the need to align the ultrasound beam with blood flow. It does illustrate the principle that, because maximum measurable velocity is inversely proportional to pulse rate, and hence range, for each value of ultrasound frequency, there is a fixed value of (range × blood velocity) above which aliasing occurs. This is shown graphically in Figure 1.22.

In practice, pulsed wave Doppler is useful for any application involving detection of abnormal flow where the value of the blood velocity is not important, for example, diagnosis of mild aortic regurgitation. Where quantitative data are required, continuous wave is generally necessary to document high velocities.

Figure 1.22. Diagram showing the effect of increasing the pulse frequency on velocity and range information.

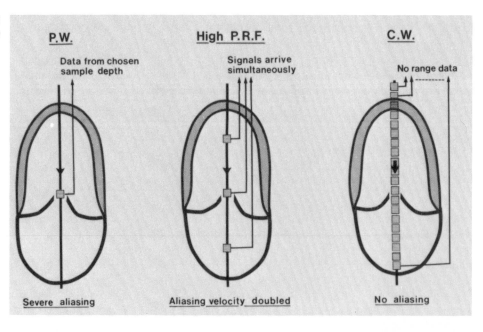

Extended Range or High Pulse Repetition Frequency Doppler

Extended range, or high PRF, Doppler is an ingenious way of partly overcoming the limitation imposed by aliasing on the measurement of high blood velocities by pulsed wave Doppler. To understand how it works, consider measurement of mitral valve velocity from an apical transducer position, as shown in Figure 1.22. Using normal pulsed wave Doppler, the sample volume is positioned in the mitral orifice. Echoes returning after a time delay appropriate to this range are analyzed to provide both structural information about the mitral valve and velocity information on flow through it. A second pulse can be sent immediately after these echoes have returned. The pulse rate is limited by the range of the mitral valve from the transducer, and the maximum measurable velocity can be calculated from the product (range × velocity) for the ultrasound frequency being used.

What happens if the pulse rate is doubled? At the moment an echo from a particular pulse returns to the transducer from the mitral valve, echoes from the next pulse arrive from a point halfway between the transducer and the valve. They, too, contain both structural and velocity information, which is superimposed on that obtained from the first pulse in the mitral orifice. In effect, two Doppler sample volumes are in use simultaneously. This could be confusing, but by careful choice of beam direction it is usually possible to ensure that velocity and structural data from the proximal sample is of relatively little importance, as is shown in the example where it is in the middle of the left ventricular cavity. This technique offers the advantage of doubling the total number of pulses passing through the mitral valve orifice, and therefore the aliasing velocity is doubled. Further extension by quadrupling the pulse rate is possible. It can be seen that increasing the PRF improves the quantification of velocity data but at the expense of introducing ambiguity in the spatial data. Taken to its extreme, if the number of pulses transmitted is increased to the point where the pulses merge together, all spatial data is lost, but there is now no problem with aliasing and we have returned to continuous wave operation. High PRF thus offers a compromise between continuous and pulsed wave Doppler. It shares both the advantages and disadvantages of each method.

Color Flow Mapping

Pulsed wave Doppler provides both structural and velocity data, and it is possible to analyze velocity from a chosen point on a two-dimensional image. However, to search the entire two-dimensional plane by positioning the sample at all possible sites on the image is tedious and often difficult, for example, in a restive child in whom a small ventricular septal defect is suspected. This problem could be overcome if it were possible to have hundreds of sample volumes spread all over the image plane, each analyzed continuously. This is the aim of color flow mapping. The technology is complex and beyond the scope of this chapter, but in essence it detects phase changes in all returning echo signals. The origin of the technique lies in radar, where it is important to be able to isolate and identify moving objects against a stationary background that otherwise would obscure them. The resulting flow information is presented in the form of a color overlay, superimposed on a two-dimensional image (Fig. 1.23, Plate I). Flow away from the transducer is represented by blue, and flow toward it by red. Local variations in velocity due to turbulence are indicated by additional colors, such as white and green. The amount of data to be processed in real-time puts a severe strain on current technology and significantly limits the frame rate if a wide-sector angle and large depth of view are required. Because it is essentially a pulsed wave technique, it is subject to aliasing, but early experience suggests that this is not a severe problem. A high velocity jet away from the transducer, which would normally be blue, may have a red (aliased) central core, but its blue penumbra still indicates the true flow direction. This technology presents an exciting prospect and is likely to replace single-sample pulsed wave Doppler completely.

2
Waveform Analysis and Technical Considerations in Doppler Instrumentation

Richard Lee

This chapter aims to provide an understanding of the applied physical principles and instrumentation in conventional pulsed and continuous wave Doppler as well as color flow-mapping technology and an insight into their diagnostic capabilities in cardiology. A brief review of some technical considerations regarding waveform analysis employed in instrumentation is important before examining some of the new developments in ultrasound technology.

TECHNICAL CONSIDERATIONS

All ultrasound information exists in the form of a returning signal or echo traversing from the tissue being interrogated. The tissue echo possesses several measurable characteristics including time of travel, amplitude, duration, wavelength, center frequency, bandwidth, frequency shift, and phase data. Each of these characteristics carries unique descriptive information about the tissues from which the echo was generated.

THE ORIGIN OF THE ECHO

Echocardiography is dependent upon heart structures reflecting fractions of broadcast sound pulses at their boundaries with other tissues. Within the density

ranges of biologic tissues, this reflectivity is dependent primarily on differential fluid ratios among neighboring tissues and, secondarily, on variations in collagen and calcium distribution among these same tissues.[1]

THE NATURE OF REFLECTIONS

The generation of an echo by a reflector is a three-stage process of encounter, absorption, and rebroadcast of a fraction of the sound energy originally emitted by the transducer. This process is illustrated in Figure 2.1. As the outgoing sound pulse meets a target, its boundary molecules, defined as those within one wavelength of the surface, absorb energy from the sound pulse (stage 1). This causes the boundary molecules to oscillate at the same frequency (sympathetically) as the parent sound pulse (stage 2). At the third stage the acquired energy is immediately dispersed by the target into its surrounding environment in the form of echo reflections as well as sound transmission deeper into tissue along the beam path.

Each echo reflector can be considered an active broadcaster or emitting source of sound energy. If the overall size of the reflecting anatomic structure exceeds approximately one wavelength of the interrogating sound, the energy emitted by the target is primarily unidirectional according to the law of refraction and

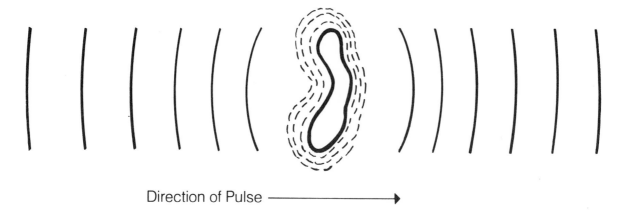

Direction of Pulse ⟶

Figure 2.1. A target blood cell is encountered by broadcast sound energy from the transducer. The cell absorbs energy from the pulse and then restores itself to equilibrium by broadcasting the stored energy. Because the target pictured here is small relative to the wavelength of the sound, the broadcast energy is distributed (scattered) in all directions across three dimensions. (Reproduced courtesy of Programs in Diagnostic Ultrasound (PIDU), all rights reserved.)

the law of incidence and reflection (see Chapter 1). However, if the target is smaller than a single wavelength—for example, a blood cell or even regional concentrations containing many thousands of blood cells—all the molecules become boundary molecules. The emitted sound tends to be dispersed in all directions, which greatly reduces the fraction of sound energy that is directed back toward the transducer (Chapter 1).

The returning signals that are of greatest interest in the study of blood flow arise from blood cells and hence, are the weakest, the ones most subject to noise interference at the receiver, and the ones most difficult to detect. These tiny targets are commonly referred to as scatterers of sound or point source reflectors.

FREQUENCY/WAVELENGTH

The wavelength and frequency components of an off-spring echo rebroadcast from a stationary target are identical to those of the parent sound pulse. This observation holds true in all circumstances except when either the scatterer or the receiver are in motion relative to one another.

AMPLITUDE

The amplitude of a single signal relates to the relative amount of sound energy contained within the echo during the time that it encounters the transducer crystal.

TRANSIT TIME EFFECTS

A blood cell moves slowly (<10 m/s) compared with a sound pulse (≈1540 m/s). When short duration Doppler sound pulses are emitted, any given blood cell is in

contact with each speeding sound pulse for a very short period of time, during which target motion must be detected. Also, when from 4000 to 25,000 sound pulses are emitted per second, the same blood cell will move a very short distance *between* interrogations. It is therefore optimal to expose the target to as many pulses over as long a period of time as is practical for accurate velocity identification and target localization. The amount of time that a scatterer is interrogated is an important determinant of the accuracy of Doppler velocity measurements.

SPATIAL TRANSIT EFFECTS

An important extraneous factor that influences echo amplitude is the sound broadcast power. Broadcast power distribution varies widely across the sound pathway: It is highest at the center of the beam and progressively decreases laterally toward its margins. Thus, moving blood cells encountered near the center of the beam will generate stronger signals than will blood cells encountered at the periphery of the beam.

DIFFRACTION EFFECTS

The laws of diffraction define the relationships between waveforms that interact with one another as they travel. Shifting diffraction patterns occur over time and across distance, and as the residue of the encounter between sound and tissue provide information about the tissue itself.

Diffraction effects are also referred to as interference patterns. In Figure 2.2 the relationships between two waveforms and their combined power values derived over time are demonstrated (1). The two waveforms in Figure 2.2A are described as interfering destructively, or out of phase. Because the amplitudes

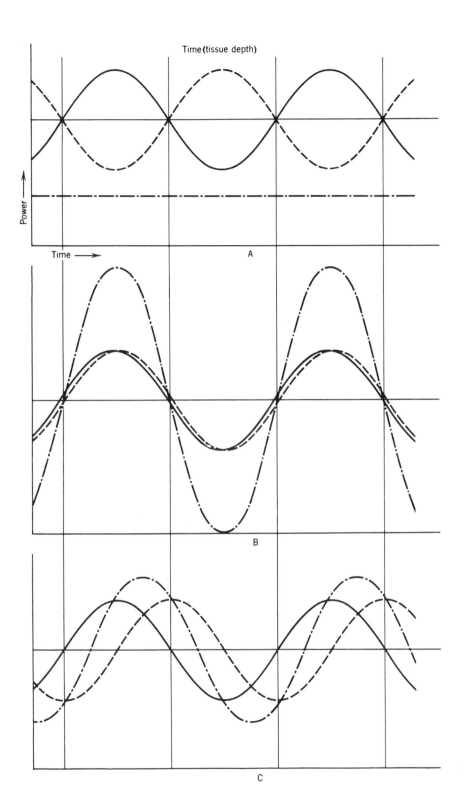

Figure 2.2. In panel (A) two waveforms of equal amplitude are precisely out of phase relative to one another. The result (– · – · – · –) is a net cancellation of amplitude values over time (power). In panel (B) the two waveforms are precisely in phase with one another. The diffraction result is a net summation of amplitudes. Panel (C) depicts that arbitrary relationships of waveforms produce diffraction patterns which, over time, are unique to those frequencies. (From Harrigan P, Lee R. Principles of Interpretation in Echocardiography. New York: John Wiley and Sons, 1985. Reproduced with permission.)

of each waveform are identical, each cancels the other so that there is a net amplitude of zero. By contrast the diffraction patterns in Figure 2.2B demonstrate constructive interference: The alignment of the two waveforms is such that the sum of their amplitudes over time results in a power level twice that of each waveform. These waveforms are described as in phase.

This figure illustrates what the echo machine "sees" in the Doppler study. The echo machine can measure only the amplitude of the tissue echo at any point in time. The amplitude of any Doppler signal is determined by the superimposition of two or more waveforms and is the sum of all the contributing waveforms at each instant in time. The frequencies of the wave-

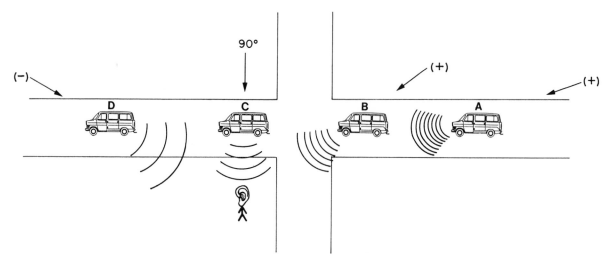

Figure 2.3.   Relative to a stationary observer, the direction of motion of a sound broadcaster affects the detected frequency. With the vehicle at position (A), where the direction of the sound source is almost directly toward the listener, wavelength is the shortest and perceived frequency is the highest. As the auto moves toward the subject, the angle between the direction of vehicular motion and the receiver of sound approaches the perpendicular and the *perceived* frequency becomes closer to the actual frequency. Once past the perpendicular, the opposite set of events occurs and as the angle between the path of the auto and the position of the pedestrian progressively departs from 90 degrees, wavelength increases and the frequency heard drops. At (C) heard frequency is near its lowest when the axial direction of the car is predominantly away from the listener. During this entire episode the *actual* frequencies emitted by the sound source remain unchanged. (Reproduced courtesy of PIDU.)

forms that contribute to the composite amplitude of a signal can only be determined later by spectral analysis.

COHERENCY/UNCHANGING PHASE

Two simultaneously generated waveforms of identical frequency traveling through the same medium should always remain in phase. In echocardiographic systems the frequency content of the outgoing pulse is determined by an oscillator modified by the acoustic behavior of the transducer crystal. Thus, a broadcast sound pulse should retain its frequency mix during its voyage out and back through stationary tissue and upon its return ($\pm$ 200 μs later) to the same transducer element still be in phase with the oscillator frequency.[2]

FREQUENCY SHIFTS

When the returning sound pulse is out of phase with the oscillator pulse, it is assumed that the difference is due to the traveling sound pulse having been rebroadcast from a moving target. The frequency of any detected periodic signal is shifted in a predictable fashion by the relative axial velocities either toward or away from the transducer. The velocity of the target can be determined as a function of the magnitude of frequency shift between the outgoing and returning waveforms when the transducer is stationary. This concept was first advanced in 1842 by Christiaan Doppler.

This phenomenon can be observed on any busy street corner. The frequency of the sound from an approaching vehicle which the ear interprets as pitch is always higher than when the vehicle is adjacent to or moving away from the observer (Fig. 2.3). Similarly, the frequency of the sound reflected or rebroadcast by a group of moving blood cells is shifted in proportion to their axial velocity.

The mechanism of frequency shift is illustrated in

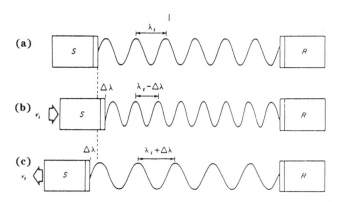

Figure 2.4.   In (a) the lack of axial target motion relative to the receiver has a null effect on perceived frequency. In (b) the motion of the sender (S) toward the transducer (R) compresses the wavelength and increases the frequency. In panel (c) the motion of the sender away from the transducer elongates the broadcast wavelength and decreases the detected frequency. (From Atkinson P, Woodcock JP. Doppler Ultrasound and Its Use in Clinical Measurement. London: Academic Press, 1982. Reproduced with permission.)

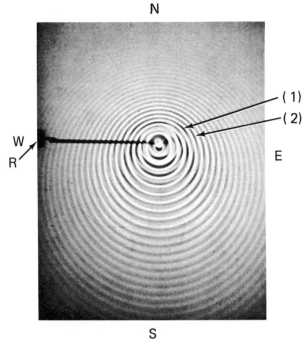

Figure 2.5. Experimental proof of the Doppler effect on wavelength and perceived frequency [at constant propagation velocity]. A vibrating rod (R) is angled to strike the surface of a fluid reservoir while moving in a northerly direction (N). Wavelength thereby becomes compressed toward the north, elongated toward the south (S), and remains unchanged perpendicular to the path of travel of the rod, i.e., east (E) and west (W). By tracking peaks (1) and (2) one can appreciate that wavelength progressively changes with variations in the angle between the direction of the emitting source and the receiver. (From Huggins E. Physics. Menlo Park, CA: Benjamin/Cummings Publishing Co., 1968. Reproduced with permission.)

Figures 2.4 and 2.5. When the direction of motion of the scatterer is toward the transducer, the wavelength of the emitting sound is compressed (Fig. 2.4B) (2). In contrast, when the direction of movement of the scatterer is away from the transducer, the rebroadcast wavelength is elongated (Fig. 2.4C).

When the reflected sound arrives at the transducer and excites the element, the wavelength changes are perceived as frequency shifts. The velocity of sound on a round trip through soft tissues is assumed to be constant and is related to the frequency and wavelength as $v = f/\lambda$, where v is the mean sound propagation velocity through soft tissue, λ is the wavelength, and f is the frequency of a signal.

Frequency shifts create progressive changes in the diffraction patterns of noncoherent transmitted and received waveforms. From these changing diffraction patterns, signal amplitude variations arise in the receiver to form the basis of Doppler information. Figure 2.6 illustrates this event in which two waveforms of differing frequencies are superimposed. During this time diffraction effects change the amplitude of the combination of the two waveforms. Furthermore, the amplitude of the resultant waveform will vary predictably over time, provided that the constituent frequencies do not change.

The derived amplitude plot in Figure 2.6 has a Gaussian distribution of frequencies, which is an important assumption made in spectral analysis. A Gaussian distribution of frequencies in the derived signal must exist over any period of time that any two frequencies maintain an unchanging wavelength relationship to one another. This holds true except when the constituent waveforms interfere precisely destructively or when the waveforms interfere precisely constructively.

ANGULAR DEPENDENCE

The frequency of the sound from an approaching vehicle increases progressively as the vehicle approaches the observer and decreases as the vehicle travels away. This pertains even when the velocity of the vehicle remains constant.

Figures 2.3 and 2.5 illustrate the relationship between the perceived frequency and the angle between the sound source and the sound receiver. The proportion of total frequency shift perceived at any point in time by a stationary observer varies as the cosine of the angle between that observer and the true direction of motion of the sound pulse.[3]

Unless the angle between the ultrasound beam is close to zero (cosine of 0 degrees = 1.0), the measured velocities will systematically underestimate the actual velocities. Thus, at all angles to the transducer, except directly toward or directly away, the measured velocity will always be less than the actual velocity. Angular dependence applies to all Doppler velocity measurement. A complicating factor in many clinical Doppler applications is that the true direction of motion of the reflecting blood cells in the cardiovascular system is not accurately known, and thus there is a potential risk of underestimating the true blood flow velocities. Cosine θ effects cannot be reliably compensated, even with angle correction.[4]

THE COMPARATOR/DEMODULATION

To modulate a signal is to change it in some way from its original form. For example, an FM radio station, which is identified by a basic frequency that it broadcasts—for example, 98.5 (MHz) on the radio dial—causes variations in the frequency content of broadcast signals that are unscrambled by the radio receiver into a program. These variations around a central frequency are a type of code that carries information for later

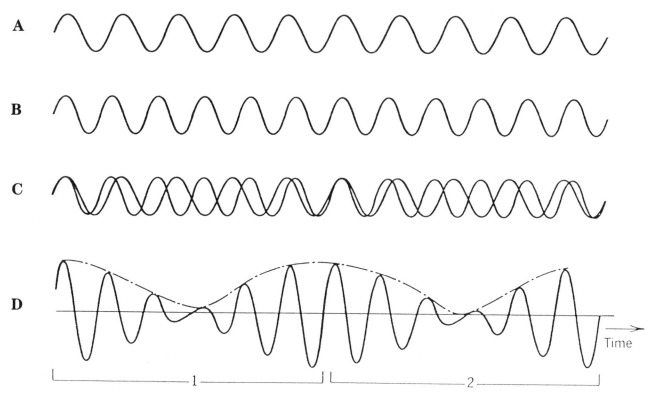

Figure 2.6. Derivation of the "difference", or Doppler, signal by the process of waveform comparison. Signal (A) containing ten cycles is superimposed upon signal (B) containing twelve cycles. In (C) the waveforms are compared (beat) and are seen to exist alternately in and out of phase. A third waveform, represented in (D), (– · – · – – · – · – ·) derived from the combined amplitude values of (A) and (B) contains two cycles peak to peak and represents the difference in frequency between the original two waveforms. (From Harrigan P, Lee R. Principles of Interpretation in Echocardiography. New York: John Wiley and Sons, 1985. Reproduced with permission.)

decoding and interpretation. The central frequency is referred to as the carrier frequency. In changing the wavelength of a broadcast sound pulse, a moving blood cell modulates the frequency mix and thereby encodes velocity information onto it. This information is then carried back to the transducer by the returning tissue echo.

Demodulation is the process of extracting the encoded information from the returning signal by separating it from the frequencies contained in the carrier wave. An FM radio demodulates the broadcast signal into music in a fashion similar to the method by which a Doppler system extracts frequency shift information from the tissue echoes.

Demodulation is accomplished by the comparator, a circuit that is responsible for deriving the "difference" signal from the outgoing pulse and the incoming echoes. The process is referred to as demodulation, or "beating" two waveforms together.[5]

The term "difference signal" in Doppler applications represents the difference between the frequency mix of the transmitted signal compared with the frequency mix of the tissue echo. A comparator circuit compares

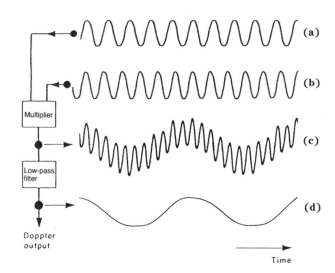

Figure 2.7. Phase sensitive detection (coherent demodulation): (a) reference signal (frequency f_o); (b) Doppler shifted echo frequency ($f_o + f_d$); (c) Product waveform [frequencies ($f_o + f_d$) $-f_o$ and ($f_o + f_d$) $+ f_o$]; (d) Doppler difference signal (frequency f). (From Atkinson P, Woodcock JP. Doppler Ultrasound and Its Use in Clinical Measurement. London: Academic Press, 1982. Reproduced with permission.)

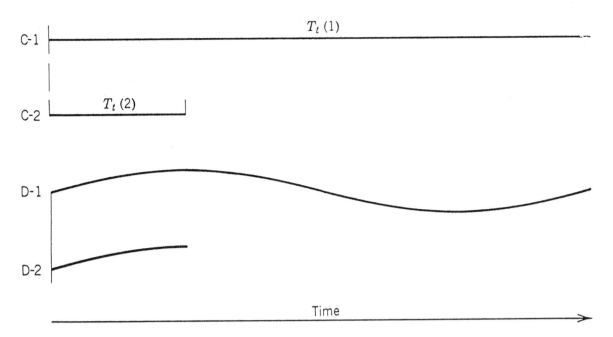

Figure 2.8. The transit time effect on frequency resolution. A frequency can only be sampled during the time that it exists, which is partly a function of the duration of the encounter between target and pulse. Doppler frequencies D-1 and D-2 are identical. Available comparison time (C-1), equal to the transit time (Tt1), is sufficient to derive an entire cycle of the Doppler signal. Comparison time (C-2) made available by transit time Tt2 is not of sufficient duration for a single cycle of the Doppler signal to be derived. This results in an uncertainty or less than a sharp definition of that frequency in spectral analysis of the Doppler signals. (From Harrigan P, Lee R. Principles of Interpretation in Echocardiography. New York: John Wiley and Sons, 1985. Reproduced with permission.)

the frequency content of the oscillator pulse with the frequency mix of the tissue echo (Fig. 2.7). From this process a third or difference signal is derived as a result of rhythmic variations in interference patterns between the waveforms, which is the Doppler shift signal. The output of the comparator is a periodic variation in derived signal amplitude, as shown in Figure 2.7. Over time this output defines the power aspects of the difference signal without its frequency components.

Thus, diffraction effects are the mechanism by which the Doppler signal is created. Figures 2.6 and 2.7 exaggerate the frequency values that exist in echocardiographic applications. Nevertheless Figure 2.6 demonstrates how a waveform containing 12 cycles beat with one containing 10 cycles yields a difference waveform or Doppler signal of 2 cycles. In clinical echocardiography, frequency shifts are very small so that the Doppler signal represents only a thousandth part of the transmitted and received frequencies. Fortunately several critical but unrelated factors (e.g., ultrasound frequencies that penetrate tissue well, cardiac flow velocities, and the frequency range of human hearing) will permit audio as well as visual presentation of Doppler data.

The compatibility of conventional Doppler technology with imaging requirements is severely restricted as illustrated in Figure 2.8. The primary problem is that Doppler information requires prolonged transit times, or pulse lengths, which limits axial resolution in imaging. This constraint dictates that the scatterer must be interrogated over such a long period of time in order to generate an identifiable Doppler waveform that spatial resolution requirements for imaging are negated.

This may represent a paradox because systems appear to perform imaging and Doppler studies simultaneously. However, the velocity of the sound pulse is such that many thousands of them can be sent each second without any of them—or their returning signals—interfering with one another. Because each sound pulse is an independent entity, most can be sent optimized for Doppler, interspersed occasionally with groups of short duration sound pulses suitable for the acquisition of imaging data. Systems vary in terms of their ratios of imaging to Doppler pulses, but the overall effect is the same: rapid alternation between two modalities at a rate that "fools" the senses into perceiving they are being performed simultaneously.

For the present it is necessary only to understand that frequency shifts must be derived over comparatively long intervals using a single long pulse (continuous wave Doppler) or multiple short pulses distributed over some minimum of time (pulsed Doppler).

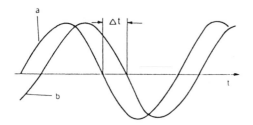

Figure 2.9. Two waveforms that exist with a time difference (out of phase) with respect to one another. (From Omoto R, ed. Color Atlas of Real-Time Two-Dimensional Echocardiography. Tokyo: Shindan-To-Chiro, Ltd., 1984. Reproduced with permission.)

CONVERSION OF FREQUENCY SHIFT TO VELOCITY

The Doppler formula is:

$$v = \frac{c}{2f_o} \cdot \frac{f_d}{\cos \theta}$$

where f_o is the center frequency of the transducer, f_d is the shift in frequency, $\cos \theta$ is the cosine of the angle between the beam and the direction of flow, v is the velocity of the targets, and c is the velocity of sound through tissue. The Doppler formula is a statement of the relationship between what is measured by the echo machine and the derived data that the echocardiographer requires for diagnosis. The theoretical basis and validity of the application of Doppler techniques to clinical problems has been demonstrated elsewhere (3–5).

A relationship exists between the frequency of the sound broadcast from the transducer that encounters the blood cells, the magnitude of frequency shift, and the velocity of the blood cells. That relationship is:

$$f_d = \frac{(2f_o)(v \cdot \cos \theta)}{c}$$

which derives approximately to: 1.3 kHZ (of shift) per 1.0 MHz (of transducer frequency) per 1.0 m/s (of flow velocity). For example, using a 1.0-MHz transducer, a 1.3-kHz shift translates to 1.0 m/s of blood flow; a 2.6-kHz shift to 2.0 m/s of flow; a 5.2-kHz shift to 3.3 m/s of flow (5.2/1.3), and so on. With a 2.0-MHz transducer, the same 5.2-kHz shift yields a flow velocity of only 2.0 m/s (5.2/2.6). However, with pulsed Doppler it is more useful to work this equation backward. For example, a 5.0-m/s flow velocity generates a 6.5-kHz shift from a 1.0-MHz pulse (5.0 × 1.3) and a 13.0-kHz shift at 2.0 MHz of transducer frequency (5.0 × 2.6). Thus, for any given flow velocity, the higher the center frequency of the transducer, the higher the frequency shift derived. However very low frequencies are not used for Doppler studies because they are not compatible with imaging, which precludes the use of the same transducer for imaging and Doppler alternatively.

Of equal importance is the fact that higher frequencies carry shorter wavelengths so that a greater number of cycles can be fit into a given sample volume compared with a lower frequency pulse. Thus, at a fixed sample volume size, the higher frequency pulse delivers more cycles to the comparator and improves frequency resolution.

PHASE SHIFTS

The concepts of frequency shift and phase shift are similar, although waveforms of the same frequency can be out of phase, as illustrated in Figure 2.9. The definition of frequency is the rate of phase change. Progressive changes in phase relationships between waveforms are the raw material from which frequency shifts produce amplitude variations (difference waveforms) in the comparator.

Phase analysis describes the physical or spatial relationships of one waveform to another. Figure 2.9 shows that waveform b is displaced somewhat ahead

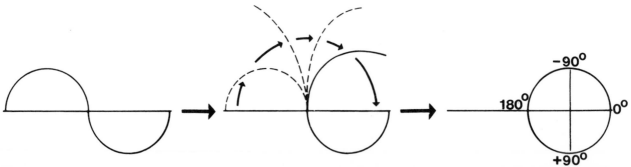

Figure 2.10. The vector designation model facilitates mathematical and verbal description of waveform relationships. Phase is described as degrees of a circle representing the carrier wave. Interference pattern is indicated by the vectors of the circle and frequency mismatch is referenced by the rate at which the indicator vector rotates in either direction around the carrier. (Courtesy PIDU, reproduced with permission.)

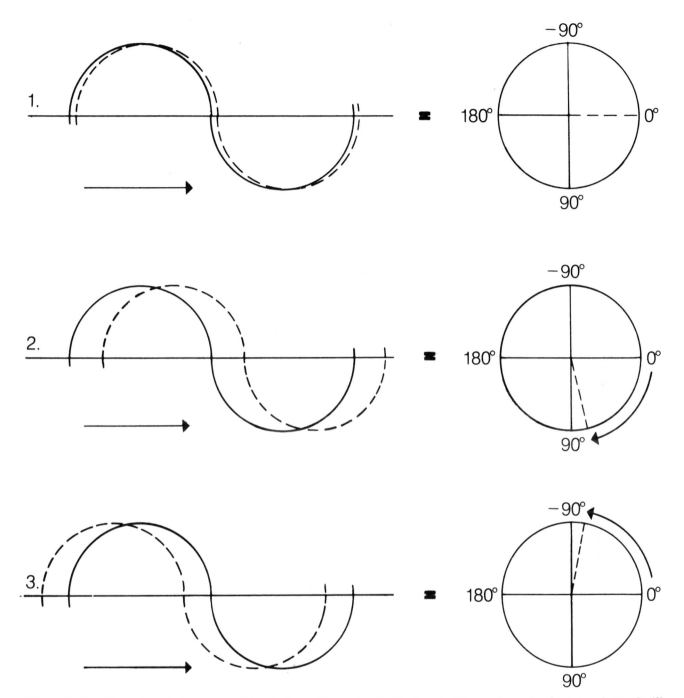

Figure 2.11.   Examples of phase mismatches indicated by vector designation. In (1) waveforms in phase are shown. In (2) a waveform shifted 1/4λ ahead of the carrier would be designated as +90 degrees. In (3) a waveform shifted 1/4λ behind the carrier is designated as −90 degrees. Perfectly destructive interference is indicated as 180-degree rotation of the received signal against the carrier. (Courtesy PIDU, reproduced with permission.)

of waveform a. However, "somewhat ahead" is too imprecise a definition in either imaging or Doppler. Thus, the vector indication is used.

If one takes the line as representing a single waveform, straightens it, and then connects the ends, a circle is formed, the vectors of which can be used to indicate precisely a relationship with any other waveform (Fig. 2.10). Phase relationships are designated by

the degrees of this circle (Fig. 2.11). Compared waveforms are assigned to the four quadrants of the circle according to their interference relationship (Fig. 2.11).

The traditional compass heading of 270 degrees is replaced by the designation of −90 degrees. Therefore, the nonperfectly constructive (not in phase, or 0 degrees) and nonperfectly destructive categories (not out of phase, or 180 degrees) of waveform interference patterns can be described within the positive and negative quadrants of a circle representing the carrier wave. The second category in Figure 2.11 defines waveforms arising from targets moving away from the transducer that are displaced forward or ahead of the carrier frequency. The designations for all waveforms in this category are reconciled to +90 degrees, usually referred to as 90 degrees. The third grouping defines waveforms that are displaced backward or behind the carrier wave (Fig. 2.11). The designations for all waveforms in this category are taken to −90 degrees. Within the region from 90 to 180 degrees lies an area of velocity and directional ambiguity that is addressed in the section on waveform sampling.

It is important to examine the interference dynamics of waveforms of slightly different frequencies that slowly drift, or slide, past one another over time. Figure 2.12 replicates Figure 2.6 except that the higher frequency wave is a dotted line for easier visual differentiation. Waveform B (dotted line), which contains 12 cycles as the received waveform, begins in phase (0-degree shift) with waveform A (solid line). By the next cycle B has moved behind A (−90-degree rotation) and eventually moves more than halfway behind A (↓) and begins to catch up ahead of the next cycle, ultimately to move back again into phase with A. Waveforms A and B do not necessarily have to be together or even in the same location. Waveform B could be returning through a tissue with a transmission velocity equal to the machine calibration while waveform A is "stored" within the oscillator of the echo machine.[6] As long as B encounters no moving targets, the two waveforms, which were generated in phase,

should still be in phase when they reach the comparator of the ultrasound machine. If waveform B becomes rebroadcast from a target moving axially to the receiver, and both waveforms started in phase its wave length will be altered and it will begin to slide past waveform A, the oscillator pulse. When both waveforms meet in the comparator and are beat together, a measurable shift will be detected by the comparator in the form of a difference waveform or Doppler signal.

The shifted waveform may be described as rotating around the broadcast frequency. This makes use of the vector designation model in the description of frequency shift dynamics. Figure 2.12 is an exaggeration, for illustrative purposes, of the rotational rates for a comparison between frequencies that have been selected for their ability to penetrate tissue well and shifts that are generated by blood flow velocities. For example, of a 2.0-kHz shift from a 2.0-MHz pulse (i.e., a blood flow velocity of 2.6 m/s) 1000 cycles of the transmitted and received waveforms would have to be compared to derive 1 cycle of the Doppler waveform (360-degree rotation). Thus, in the real-life example, the shifted signal would rotate on the order of only one-third of a degree from cycle to cycle in the comparator rather than the ±60 degrees per cycle shown in the figure.[7]

DIRECTION

The forward and backward rotation of the received waveform relative to the carrier indicates the direction of flow (Fig. 2.13). Waveforms shifted forward toward +90 degrees are presumed to have arisen from targets

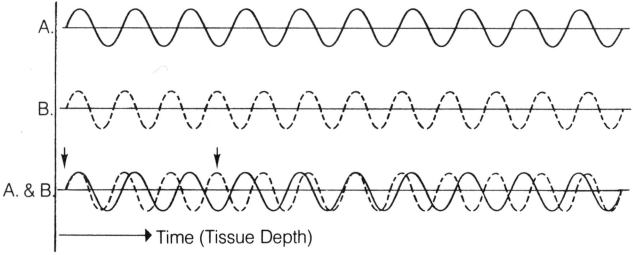

Figure 2.12.   Phase (frequency) shift is a dynamic process that continues over time exactly like waves on the ocean that constantly change their interference patterns as they travel past one another. In cardiology velocity and direction are obtained from these patterns which imposes strict requirements on sampling times to avoid artifact. If, for example, following waveform generation, samples were undertaken at the times indicated by the arrows, one would not know whether the received waveform was rotated 180 degrees ahead or 180 degrees behind the carrier by the time of the second sample. This is the aliasing threshold where directional ambiguity in the data results. (Courtesy PIDU, reproduced with permission.)

traveling away from the transducer. Waveforms rotated toward −90 degrees behind the carrier wave indicate flow toward the transducer.

QUADRATURE PHASE DETECTION

Bidirectional discrimination is more complicated than is indicated in Figure 2.13, so a simple explanation is necessary. The heterodyne demodulation function is one in which an artifactual, lower center frequency is beat against the returning waveform, so that both positive and negative sidebands are derived as positive. The degree of positive phase shift becomes the basis for the assignment of waveforms to one of two quadrature channels, indicating flow forward or away, respectively. The term *quadrature* refers to the vector designation model wherein interference patterns are classified by the four quadrants of a circle representing the carrier wave. Thus, the quadrature phase detector is an electronic function that assigns directionality to an incoming signal on the basis of its diffraction pattern with the carrier signal at any instant in time.

MOVING TARGET INDICATOR/ FIXED TARGET CANCELLER

The moving target indicator detects motion the same way the human eye does: by observing a moving object over a period of time. Imagine an outfielder attempting to catch a baseball in flight. A quick glance at the ball in the air would be insufficient time to gather information necessary to calculate direction and velocity and thereby arrive at an estimate of intersection of ball and glove. The more time available to study the flight of the ball, the greater the likelihood of a successful catch. This relationship would be particularly important if wind changed the course of the ball in midflight.

This latter example bears on the study of blood flow velocities in disease states. Cardiac lesions may result in turbulent rather than laminar blood flow, in which reflective targets often change velocity and direction, which affects Doppler shift data. To continue the baseball analogy, if the outfielder could look at the ball continuously, constantly noting its changes in position and direction, the probability of a catch would be high. In reality, the fielder must run to a calculated spot at which the ball is predicted to arrive, which means that tracking time is only periodic because attention must also be focused on running. The accuracy of noncontinuous ranging and tracking is less likely to result in a successful catch.

The enormous disparity in velocity between sound pulse and blood cell means that the target moves only the tiniest distance during the encounter time. Therefore, the distance the wavelength is offset (i.e., the extent to which frequency and phase are shifted and amplitude is altered in the comparator) is too small for velocity quantitation because the period of interrogation by a *single* typically short pulse duration used for imaging is not sufficiently long (1–3, 6). Accordingly, multiple interrogations of each site are required for flow *imaging*.

DELAY LINES

Combined imaging and Doppler flow velocity analysis are not possible without the use of an electric delay circuit. A delay circuit alters the progression of an electric waveform while preserving its diffraction pattern with other waveforms. Delay circuitry is capable of delaying an impulse by discrete increments of time, which are necessary for conventional phased array imaging techniques (1) and color flow mapping (5).

Figure 2.14 indicates the placement of delay circuits in a chain of signal-processing functions in phase analysis. The layout shows the delay circuits following the quadrature phase detector in order to preserve directional information. Delay circuits are used in each range gate on the color flow map to collect signals from successive sound pulses interrogating that gate. These phase shifted signals are then compared and summated

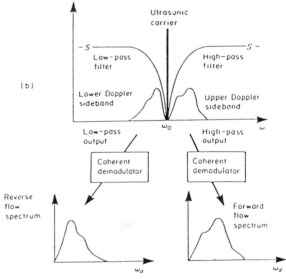

Figure 2.13. Separation of the complex tissue echo into its quadrature components in order to extract directional information. Frequencies above (toward velocities) and below (away velocities) the carrier are directed along separate pathways to the comparator where they beat with the center frequency generating positive and negative frequency spectra. The spectra rotate in opposite directions so that when fed alternatively to the spectrum analyzer, the spectra retain their directional tags. (From Atkinson P, Woodcock JP. Doppler Ultrasound and Its Use in Clinical Measurement. London: Academic Press, 1982. Reproduced with permission.)

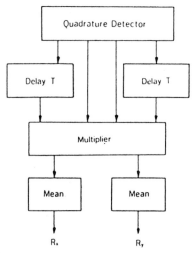

Figure 2.14. The location of delay circuits in the processing chain in order to align in time returning signals from successive pulses. With this strategy, directionality (quadrature channel outputs) is preserved and a mean velocity value is derived over the period of multiple tissue interrogations. (From Omoto R, ed. Color Atlas of Real-Time Two-Dimensional Echocardiography. Tokyo: Shindan-To-Chiro, Ltd., 1984. Reproduced with permission.)

in order to extract flow parameters at a useful signal to noise level. Figures 2.15 and 2.16 detail the effect of this circuit which in Doppler allows a short-duration interrogatory pulse to generate a level of frequency shift associated only with a lengthy period of waveform comparison.

TIME AS A DISTANCE: RESOLUTION AND THE COMPROMISES IN ECHO

One of the central principles in echocardiographic imaging is that what the interpreter sees as tissue depth the machine measures as time. The measurement capabilities of an echo system extend to only two variables: 1) the time delays between the transmission of a sound pulse and the progressive reception of echoes, and 2) the instantaneous amplitude of any tissue echo as it excites the crystal. All images and other clinical information produced by the echo machine must be calculated (or estimated in the case of certain Doppler data) from only these two fundamental values.

Instrument calibration for sound transmission velocity through lean, soft tissue is similar for all commercial instruments and is centered around 1540 m/s, although velocity varies slightly from one tissue to another. In biologic tissue sound travels 1.0 cm every 6.5 μs. A round trip of 1 cm takes 1.3 μs. Figure 2.17 illustrates the time/distance relationships across typical dimensions in the human heart.

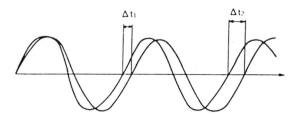

Figure 2.15. Two waveforms of different frequency "slide" past one another at a rate that is dependent on the frequency difference. In the simple case of two waveforms, frequency differences can be identified using a zero crossing detector according progressive changes in zero crossing times (t1) (From Omoto R, ed. Color Atlas of Real-Time Two-Dimensional Echocardiography. Tokyo: Shindan-To-Chiro Ltd., 1984. Reproduced with permission.)

PULSE LENGTH/IMAGING RESOLUTION VERSUS FREQUENCY/SAMPLE VOLUME SIZE

The previous chapter indicated that a broadcast sound pulse intended for imaging is restricted in length to optimize axial resolution. The clinical goals of frequency accuracy in conventional Doppler measurements mandates a lengthy sound pulse due to transit time requirements. Of all of the disparate requirements for imaging and conventional Doppler, none is more absolute than the dependence of each on radically different sample volume sizes.

The terms *pulse* applied to imaging and *sample volume* applied to Doppler are synonymous. The short-duration imaging pulse may be defined as a sample volume equally as well as a lengthy continuous wave Doppler signal train. In neither case can the system determine from where within the pulse the echo originated (i.e., axial resolution limits). In flow imaging range gates are defined as successive regions of anatomy encompassed by the sample volume at progressive instants in time as it propagates through tissue. The sample *volume* has fixed lateral characteristics determined by beam width and variable axial traits defined by pulse length.

Additional factors that diminish high-quality combined echo imaging and Doppler flow velocity determinations include pulse bandwidth, transducer construction, and damping functions. The aggregate effect of these factors on quality has induced many manufacturers to offer separate imaging and Doppler transducers or transducers that automatically change from Doppler to imaging by pin encoding at the connector.

SAMPLE VOLUME SIZE/SENSITIVITY

Sensitivity is the most critical performance factor in Doppler, whereas spatial resolution is the main criterion for excellence in echo imaging.

Sensitivity is the ability of the system to sieve information from noninformation or noise. To some

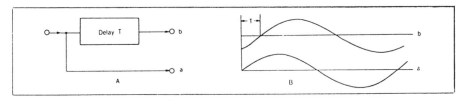

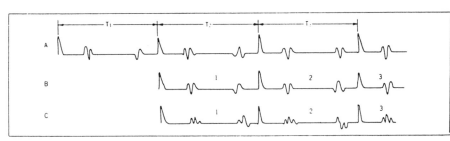

Figure 2.16. The use of a delay line to identify signals that otherwise would be regarded as identical (indistinguishable). Wave (b) is delayed relative to wave (a). In the comparator the effects on amplitude can be seen. (From Omoto R, ed. Color Atlas of Real-Time Two-Dimensional Echocardiography, Tokyo: Shindan-To-Chiro, Ltd., 1984. Reproduced with permission.)

degree sensitivity is determined by the signal-to-noise ratio. An excellent signal-to-noise ratio can be obtained by restricting the dynamic range of the instrument so that only the strongest signals pass the receiver. Thus, low amplitude signals, including noise, are reduced to virtually zero compared with signals strong enough to qualify for display. Such a design strategy is not ideal for clinical purposes because information is contained in the low-level scattered signals that make up Doppler information and in the fine, gray speckling within such structures as the myocardium in imaging. Therefore, to obtain high sensitivity, signals must be reliably separated in the presence of an extended dynamic range

that acts to decrease signal-to-noise ratio. A major effort in Doppler system design involves expanding dynamic range while maintaining the integrity of the data.

One method of increasing Doppler sensitivity without changing the signal-to-noise ratio is to enlarge the size of the sample volume. A larger sample volume interrogates more blood cell reflectors than a smaller sample volume. With more targets, more sound is broadcast back to the transducer, producing an increase in signal amplitude while electronic noise remains constant. Thus, signal-to-noise ratio and the dynamic range can be expanded to include even smaller

Figure 2.17. Distance (depth of tissue) and time are identical to the echo machine. With a fixed calibration for sound travel velocity, each time increment indexes a specific depth of tissue with an accuracy (axial/range resolution) limited only by the length/duration of the sound pulse. (Courtesy PIDU, reproduced with permission.)

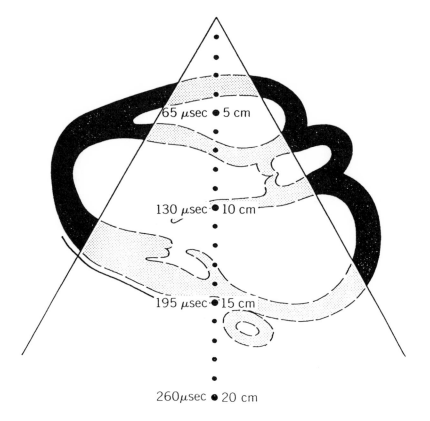

clinically significant signals. Enhancement of signal-to-noise ratio is evident in pulsed wave Doppler exams where flow signals are invariably louder relative to the background noise, when large rather than small sample volumes are employed by the examiner.

RANGE RESOLUTION

There can be no more than one sound pulse at a time in the examination field if an image is to be obtained. Figure 2.17 illustrates the difficulties that arise if this rule is not followed. If the machine pulses every 60 μs (5.0 cm), the first pulse will not have cleared the heart before the second is broadcast. Echoes constantly stream back to the transducer while *any* sound pulse and returning signals are still in the tissue (as long as 260 μs). In Figure 2.17 a 60 μs pulse spacing would leave three pulses in the examination field. The system would be unable to differentiate echoes from separate pulses that arrived simultaneously, a situation referred to as range ambiguity.

Increasing the sample volume size to enhance frequency resolution and sensitivity induces a form of range ambiguity. The extreme cases in range resolution are when 1) the imaging sound pulse is too short for frequency identification and lacks low-level sensitivity (e.g., blood cell reflections are rarely seen on the image), and 2) the continuous wave Doppler pulse is devoid of range resolution and imaging capabilities.

Range resolution is a prerequisite to any mapping technique including conventional gray scale cross-sectional imaging as well as color flow mapping. Thus, certain compromises must be made in cardiac ultrasound. For example, the depth of tissue interrogated by the examiner limits the pulse repetition frequency of the instrument in the interests of range resolution. Reduced pulse rate adversely affects temporal resolution in M mode, line density and frame rate in cross-sectional imaging, and the detection of higher velocity flows in Doppler and flow imaging studies. Also, because range resolution varies indirectly with sample volume size, imaging requirements compromise frequency accuracy and sensitivity of the Doppler study.

SAMPLING RATE

Imaging with a digital system is a process of reconstructing the whole from an incomplete number of parts. A signal is sampled for the purpose of extracting information from it—a process known as demodulation. How often the signal needs to be sampled depends on the type of information required. In echo imaging, tissue signals are amplitude modulated with tissue depth in a progressive fashion according to variations in tissue compressibility. Thus, as the imaging pulse speeds through tissue, a high rate of sampling

or digitization of the returning echoes is desirable to produce an M-mode or cross-sectional image without visible gaps or missing information. Following sampling, the echo machine must display data accumulated over successive time increments. The minimum time (tissue depth or range resolution) relates to the length of the sound pulse and the period required for it to pass a target. At 3.5 MHz a typical three-cycle imaging sound pulse spans a 1.2-mm sample volume axially and requires 0.78 μs to transit a perpendicular membranous interface. All data gathered across that sample volume at any location will be enveloped over that time by the echo machine and displayed as a video dot representing 1.2 mm of distance along the scan line. Thus, the imager may be regarded as "taking" one complete sample of the returning signal every 0.78 μs with an optimal possible axial resolution of 1.2 mm at 3.5 mHz.

Doppler sampling requirements are less rigorous because the longer duration sound pulse results in a larger sample volume that integrates data acquired over longer periods of time (tissue depth). Doppler sampling means detecting the voltage output of the comparator as the Doppler signal is created. What the machine "sees" from this process is a sample and hold waveform that duplicates the zero crossing characteristics of the analog Doppler wave in a series of voltage steps (Figure 2.18). The purpose of sampling is to demodulate a signal, and as signals become more complex, sampling requirements become more rigorous.

THE NYQUIST LIMIT/ALIASING

In a system that pulses and receives constantly (i.e., continuous wave Doppler), the comparison between two waveforms can be performed continuously, giving rise to an uninterrupted Doppler signal available for sampling. Continuous receiving of echoes is not possible in a Doppler system with any degree of range resolution (i.e., pulsed Doppler). For example, if the region of blood flow of interest is 10 cm (or 130 μs) from the transducer, as in Figure 2.17, the returning signals from 10 cm would exist only every 130 μs with a single gate pulsed Doppler system. This imposes a limit on the rate at which the tissue echo at that depth can be sampled for Doppler shifts. The availability of signals for sampling (i.e., the sampling rate) must, therefore, equal the pulse repetition frequency (PRF) of the instrument. When pulse repetition frequency is reduced to preserve range resolution to deeper tissue depths, the sampling rate is necessarily reduced as well. This means that there will be large gaps in the comparison process while the machine waits for each pulse to travel to the range gate positioned by the operator and for echoes to return from that depth. In

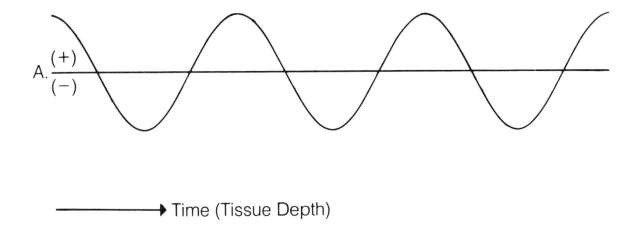

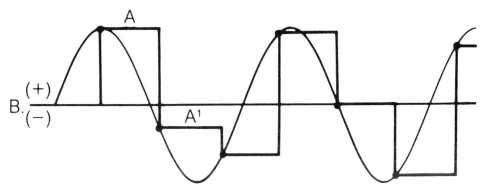

Figure 2.18.   A sample and hold waveform represents the digital reproduction of the analog signal returning from tissue. Each sample consists of a voltage measurement which is retained until the next sample. One sample per zero crossing (or two per cycle) is necessary to reproduce the directional characteristics (positive and negative quadrants) of the Doppler signal. (Courtesy PIDU, reproduced with permission.)

this example, of 10 cm, sampling would be limited to only once every 130 μs.

By contrast, with continuous sampling, signals are constantly returning from 10 cm of tissue depth as well as from every other tissue depth. This permits uninterrupted demodulation of the tissue signal in increments suitable for accurate frequency identification.

There is a potential risk as the targets continue to move and the transmitted and received waveforms continue to rotate against one another. The combination of a sufficiently rapid sliding rate (i.e., high-frequency shift) combined with long gaps in the comparison process (i.e., low PRF) with a pulsed system could result in as much as an entire cycle of the Doppler signal passing undetected. Thus, the time between samples exceeds the time required for a 360-degree rotation because of rapid rotation rate (high-frequency shift), or long gaps between pulses (sampling opportunities), or both.

The situation is still more precarious because vector indication allots 180 degrees of rotation each to forward and reverse flows. Therefore, if a half cycle passes undetected, the data become directionally am-

biguous. One sample of the Doppler waveform must take place during each positive and negative phase to reproduce that signal digitally. Therefore, any waveform of any given frequency mandates sampling at least twice for each cycle in order for it to be identified with the correct frequency and directional information. Failure to do so generates a signal that is a combination of frequency and sampling rate that is uninterpretable. This is described as an aliased signal.

An alternative way of expressing the same concept is shown in Figure 2.19 in which a single cycle of the Doppler waveform is shown peak to peak. Two crossings of the zero value baseline are involved in this one cycle. Accurate identification of the frequency of this one waveform requires a sample for each of the zero crossings. The Doppler frequency which equals 50 percent of the sampling rate/PRF in a pulsed Doppler system is referred to as the Nyquist frequency.

AVERAGING AND SMOOTHING

Data averaging is commonly used in modern digital electronics and is achieved by dividing time into a finite

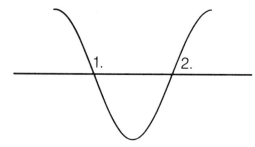

Figure 2.19. A single cycle of a waveform. If time (t) is 0.0001 s, for example, then the frequency of this wave is 1.0 kHz. Each cycle contains two crossings of the zero value baseline. The positive and negative components of the wave each indicate 180 degrees of rotation in opposite directions which indexes directionality. (Courtesy PIDU, reproduced with permission.)

number of sampling intervals and reconstructing the whole from less than the total sum of the parts.

This is illustrated in Figures 2.20 and 2.21 which plots velocity against time. The figure has been constructed so that velocity fluctuates widely and rapidly over time, similar to a Doppler difference signal derived from a region of flow turbulence. If the digital system samples velocity only at point A or point B and assumes either sample to represent amplitude over the represented time period the velocity might be either under- or overestimated.

The amplitude sampled at point C would correspond more closely to mean amplitude over the period s to f. However, with a random signal one cannot know in advance when to sample to derive a representative result. A sampling rate sufficient to generate samples A, B, and C consecutively would derive results that could be averaged together to yield a mean value. The greater the number of samples, the higher the probability that aberrant data will cancel out on averaging.

There are potential trade-offs in Doppler. Pulsed Doppler sampling is dependent upon pulse repetition frequency, which in turn is dependent upon the depth of the tissue of interest, and the velocity of sound. An effort to retain range resolution using pulsed wave Doppler reduces the sampling rate, which forces an increased reliance on the assumption that blood flow is unchanged in the 250 μs between pulses. The physical properties of blood (4) and the similarity of pulsed and continuous wave Doppler tracings demonstrate that this assumption is valid. The display process in spectral analysis combines many samples into outputs of 5.0 msec to 10.0 msec of time called the Doppler calculation time. This represents data gathered from 25 to 50 pulses at a 5-kHz pulse repetition frequency. Compared with enveloping of that magnitude, 250 μs or so between individual pulses is inconsequential.

Averaging has two beneficial effects on the display of ultrasound information. First, it has a smoothing effect

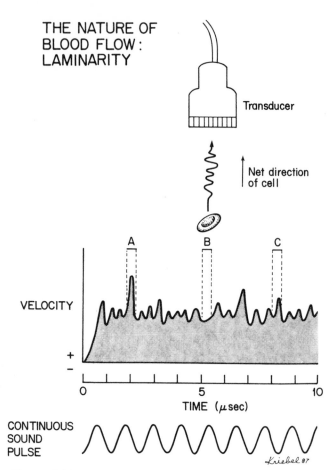

Figure 2.20. A plot of laminar blood flow velocity and directional traits within a single Doppler gate. Over a short time period (<10 ms) flow direction and flow velocity (multiplied by cos θ) vary unpredictably. A random, single sample (A), (B) or (C) would be statistically unlikely to yield a value representing the mean velocity over the displayed time period. (Courtesy PIDU, reproduced with permission.)

on video and audio data by blurring sharp boundaries between adjacent samples. Second, in conjunction with a high sampling rate it improves the signal to noise ratio (1, 3, 4, 7, 8).

The addition of signal can be accomplished only by using signal from previous samples that has been stored somewhere. In most cases, past data are combined by averaging with current signals on a weighted basis, favoring recently acquired over old information. However, there are limits to the degree of smoothing beyond which the fidelity of the clinical data deteriorates. In every instance great efforts are made to validate statistically the application of smoothing routines, based on sampling rate and knowledge of target characteristics and behavior.

POWER AND FREQUENCY SPECTRA

Thus far, the Doppler signal has been regarded as consisting of a single frequency derived from an en-

THE NATURE OF BLOOD FLOW: TURBULENCE

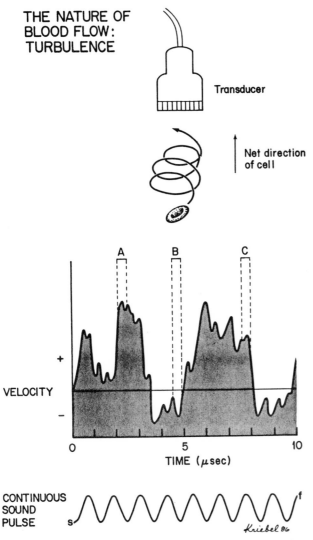

Figure 2.21. A plot of turbulent blood flow directional and velocity traits within a single Doppler gate. Multiple samples over time yield a wide spread of values. (Courtesy PIDU, reproduced with permission.)

quencies, each with an independent amplitude representing the numerous velocities encountered across the width of the beam at each successive depth of tissue.

The purpose of Doppler systems is to describe blood flow velocity as accurately as possible. If the system dealt only with single transmitted and received frequencies, the task would be straightforward in that a zero crossing counter could be used for analysis. With the magnitude of

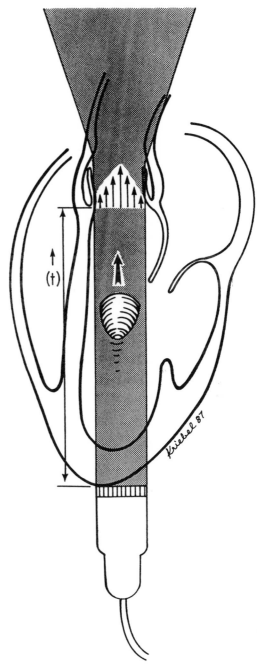

counter with a single velocity within a flow. This is an oversimplification as shown in Figure 2.22. The width of the ultrasound beam is variable. Blood cells are tiny echo targets and are minute compared with the width of the typical ultrasound beam. Therefore, at any given depth of tissue, multiple targets are available for rebroadcast.

A further complication in Doppler is that flow characteristics may vary regionally, giving rise to the possibility that at any instant in time (i.e., at any tissue depth) multiple reflective targets with different velocities and directional characteristics may be encountered simultaneously. Even in laminar flow, velocities vary with the distance from the blood vessel walls; they are close to zero near the containment structure and highest in the center of the flow stream. Thus, the returning signal in Doppler echocardiography will contain a variety of fre-

Figure 2.22. Any sample volume is likely to encounter multiple velocities during the sampling period. Additionally, the sample volume is three-dimensional, incorporating pulse length and beam width factors. (Courtesy PIDU, reproduced with permission.)

simultaneous incoming frequencies and amplitudes that represent the real situation in Doppler, the rate of zero crossings approaches infinity, and other methods must be used to provide rapid estimates of the frequency and power content of the Doppler signal.

SPECTRAL ANALYSIS/ TRANSFORM FUNCTIONS

Spectral analysis is a technique for *estimating* the frequency content of a complex signal. The complexity of the incoming frequency mix precludes the use of zero crossing techniques on a real-time basis. Fast Fourier transforms or chirp Z form the mathematical foundation for this transform function, which cancels similar angular frequencies in the incoming and outgoing signal mixes, leaving only the difference or Doppler frequencies.

The validity of a spectral analysis approach to Doppler is dependent upon several assumptions, one of which is that the independent complex motion of a number of targets generates multiple shifts of the carrier frequency at any given depth of tissue. It is assumed that because blood flow is dynamic, velocity characteristics at any given depth of tissue will change over time. A sound pulse passing through the heart chamber would constantly encounter blood cells and generate returning signals continuously. Additionally, a sound pulse broadcast 2 μs later will encounter a different set of velocity profiles as it travels the same pathway.

In continuous wave Doppler systems, the electronics continuously compare acquired data with incoming data, upgrading the display at a rate appropriate for the physiologic changes. A common interval for commercial devices is every 5.0 msec. Thus, all information collected over that period is averaged (Figs. 2.20, 2.21). Because blood flow is dynamic, velocity traits at any given location will change over time. The sampling rate for the system to describe the physiology adequately requires the assumption that the velocity profile at this location be sufficiently constant to generate negligible error in the velocity estimate over the sampling period.

In continuous wave Doppler instruments, the sampling duration is sufficiently long to average aberrant flow values that might otherwise contaminate a frequency estimated on a short sampling interval as in Figures 2.20 and 2.21. Alternatively, a short sample, the flow values of which are taken as representative of the period of time until the next pulse, may misrepresent flows over that time (Fig. 2.21).

Therefore, in pulsed systems some minimum sampling duration (pulse length) and rate (pulse repetition frequency) are required to ensure 1) the accurate frequency identification of the waveforms being sampled, and 2) that the derived values represent average frequency content during the time until the next pulse.

Pulse repetition frequency is the easiest variable to monitor because it is always known and the instrument can be calibrated to display the Nyquist limit for any given repetition frequency. As regards pulse duration, it has been proposed that a pulse of seven cycles or more meets accuracy requirements at 2.0 MHz for commonly encountered blood flow velocities (3). Such a pulse will generate phase shifted echoes of the same seven-cycle length, which is too short for the comparator to derive a single cycle of the difference or Doppler waveform (Fig. 2.8.) Therefore it must be assumed that the frequencies surrounding the center frequency have a Gaussian distribution. Thus, from a segment of the spectrum the frequency envelope can be completed and transform algorithms applied to estimate frequency content.

THE DOPPLER DISPLAY

Figure 2.23 is an example of a conventional Doppler tracing from a patient with aortic stenosis and aortic insufficiency. Many characteristics of a typical Doppler trace are shown in this figure, which was obtained from an apical transducer position in the continuous wave mode. Time is displayed on the horizontal X axis, frequency shift—or its velocity conversion—is measured on the Y axis, and amplitude is displayed on the Z axis as gray scale gradations.

Blood flow velocity away from the transducer is displayed as a downward deflection from the zero value baseline. Flow toward the transducer is indicated as an upward deflection from the baseline. An expanded view of the Doppler display (Fig. 2.23) reveals that it is comprised of a series of boxes arranged in vertical columns. The columns are traditionally referred to as bins, which are alternately emptied and filled according to the frequency content of the spectral analyzer output over time. Each box, or frequency category, is called a point.

Data presented by a digital system have, by definition, finite start and end points: duration and amplitude. This necessitates two assumptions in spectral analysis that 1) blood flow velocities remain constant over the sampling interval, and 2) a mean velocity value is statistically relevant over that interval. Most spectral analyzers output frequency information in 5.0 msec to 10.0 msec blocks of time occupied by the width of each bin. This represents a temporal accuracy limit because the transient changes in frequency content of a signal, which persist less than the duration of a display interval, will be averaged across that entire interval.

Each point in each of the bins represents a frequency range as written in the vertical axis. This imposes minor limits on frequency resolution. Borderline frequency groupings are often "bumped" upward or

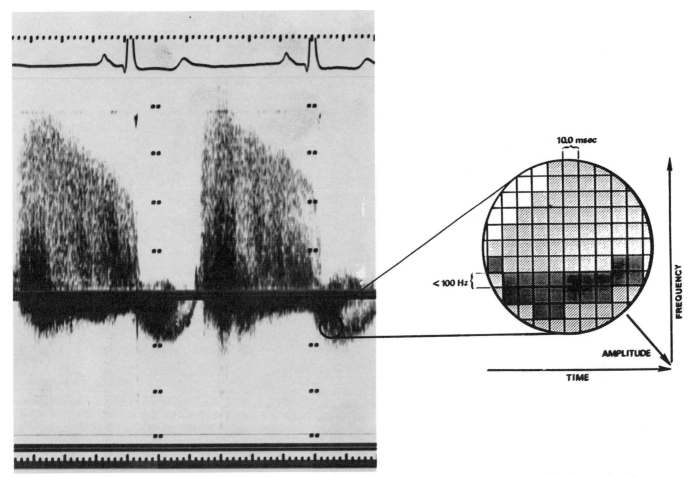

Figure 2.23. A "blow-up" of the Doppler display. Time is displayed on the horizontal axis and amplitude is indexed on the Z axis as gray scale variations. Directionality and velocity are indicated on the vertical axis. Flows toward the transducer are displayed above the zero value baseline while flows away from the transducer are written below the baseline. Frequency shift, which is converted to velocity, increases as the vertical distance from the baseline in both directions. (Courtesy PIDU, reproduced with permission.)

downward to the nearest category, creating negligible distortion of the frequency content of the data. Commercial machines differ in terms of the display intervals and numbers of frequency categories. The typical system has 10-ms sampling intervals and 128 frequency points within each bin. Half of the frequency points are allocated to the display of flow toward the transducer and half to the display of flow away from the transducer. The entire frequency content of the Doppler signal accumulated the Doppler calculation time must be allocated among the available frequency points.

TYPES OF CONVENTIONAL (NONMAPPING) DOPPLER SYSTEMS

Continuous Wave Doppler Systems

The distinguishing feature of continuous wave Doppler is the use of two transducer elements, one for transmission and one for reception of ultrasound. Figure

2.24 shows a typical beam configuration from a single crystal split into halves, each with its own electric connections. The elements are slightly angled toward one another, thereby creating an elongated common sound pathway in tissue. This is necessary because the transmitting crystal, which is constantly excited by the oscillator, is incapable of simultaneously receiving the tiny scattered reflections from blood cells without overwhelming them with the outgoing signals.

Doppler and imaging with continuous wave systems provide the visual impression of simultaneity; this is actually achieved by rapid switching between the Doppler and imaging functions several times per second. In these systems Doppler interrogation is interrupted periodically to update the image, but it is sufficiently "continuous" during flow interrogation to fulfill the advantages of continuous wave in sensitivity and frequency. The transmission velocity of sound compared with the velocity of blood ensures that each target is

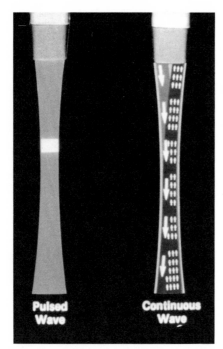

Figure 2.24. The continuous wave transducer contains two elements angled along intersecting pathways in order that outgoing and incoming pulses do not interfere with one another. (From the Johnson & Johnson Library, reproduced with permission.)

insonated with many cycles of sound every millisecond (2000 cycles at 2.0 MHz). Because approximately seven cycles (3) are needed to provide acceptable frequency accuracy, plenty of time exists within each second to perform imaging and Doppler functions reliably.

Simultaneous imaging and Doppler result in significant deterioration of the image and Doppler quality (Fig. 2.25). Because of the need to acquire ±100 real data lines per picture, imaging robs its companion procedure of time to a much greater degree than vice versa. Time spent imaging leaves large gaps in the Doppler data. Many manufacturers attempt to fill those gaps using high-speed signal trending techniques. Even with these circuits, however, quality is never fully restored, and the highest data quality is obtained only when the instrument is allowed to devote full time to either modality.

Single-Gate Pulsed Doppler Systems

Flow interrogation at a single point in the examination field is most commonly referred to as pulsed Doppler. Usually the operator is provided with a visual guide to the position of the Doppler sample location (or gate) on the cross-sectional image.

The major advantage of pulsed Doppler is its range resolution, which allows measurement of blood flow velocities at selected sites of interest. The limitations

of pulsed wave Doppler include the small size of the sample volume, which decreases sensitivity as well as signal-to-noise ratio, and the tendency to generate aliased data at low sampling rates and high velocities.

Unlike the continuous wave system, pulsed Doppler uses the same crystal for imaging and Doppler. Therefore, the reflected echoes follow the same pathway as the broadcast signals but at different *times*, because range resolution requires that all echoes be home before the next pulse is sent.

Sensitivity/Variable Gate Size

At constant broadcast sound power levels per square centimeter of tissue and at constant hematocrit, the size of the sample volume influences the number of reflectors encountered by the insonating beam and, hence, the amount of signal contained in the echo. Range (axial) resolution improves as the sample volume is reduced. Small gates are often desirable when interrogating blood flow in small areas and in children or neonates in whom different anatomic structures are juxtaposed.

Most instruments provide the capability for enlarging the size of the sample volume, which reduces the certainty of flow location but which may have a profound effect on signal detection. From frequency accuracy and sensitivity viewpoints, each location should

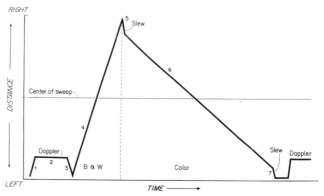

Figure 2.25. In "simultaneous" modes all data is derived on a time-share basis. A plot of scan line screen display position is along the vertical axis. At step (1) the sound beam is moved to the scan line selected by the operator for Doppler data acquisition. During step (2) Doppler data is acquired. The duration of step (2) varies with the operator setting of a mode priority control. At step (3) the beam position is moved to the edge of the display preparatory to generating a complete cross-sectional image. During step (4) two-dimensional imaging is performed and no Doppler data is acquired. Steps (5), (6) and (7) illustrate that adding flow-mapping tasks to the system duties further limits the time available for the machine to acquire conventional Doppler data. (Diagram concept from Kjell Kristofferson, VingMed Sound, Horten, Norway. Figure supplied courtesy of PIDU, reproduced with permission.)

be interrogated with the largest sample volume available in pulsed Doppler.

Sensitivity/Time Gain Compensation/Gain/Reject

Echoes intended for frequency analysis are not different from those used for imaging, except that they are several orders of magnitude weaker. Both are attenuated with increasing tissue depth and require amplification. Time gain compensation (TGC) is usually automated in Doppler systems, although at least one commercial device permits operator interaction. Additionally, variable overall gain and reject functions permit the operator to optimize signal characteristics.

The Alias-Baseline Shift

The indication of the direction of flow by Doppler systems can be clinically important. Directionality is extracted from the returning echo by feeding forward and reverse shifted signals through separate quadrature channels to the comparator as in Figure 2.14.

A processing feature of the spectral analyzer is its ability to reconstruct the Doppler trace to 1.0 times the Nyquist value. Thus, the velocity display range of Doppler data following spectral analysis can equal the Nyquist limit in both directions.

However, a display convention adopted by many laboratories is to position the zero velocity baseline halfway, or in the center of the picture as in Figure 2.26. This divides in half the velocity display range for flows in either direction (Fig. 2.26) which increases the tendency for higher velocities to be displayed in the opposite directional display range. This is often referred to as aliasing as indicated by (A) (Fig. 2.26.)

By shifting the baseline upward or downward, as in Figure 2.27, the display can be unwrapped to avail greater velocity ranges in either direction than with the baseline positioned in the middle of the trace. Shifting the baseline maximally in either direction takes advantage of the waveform reconstruction feature of the spectral analyzer and makes 1.0 times a Nyquist value velocity range available in both directions.

Multigate Pulsed Doppler

Recently there has been interest in developing approaches which combine some of the benefits of continuous wave Doppler and two-dimensional echocardiographic imaging. One solution involves the use of signal trending circuits (MSE), which allow rapid switching between Doppler and imaging modalities at a rate that suggests simultaneity. The disadvantage is that the quality of the continuous wave Doppler data decreases in proportion to the time "stolen" to make the echo image.

An alternative solution is to send multiple, evenly spaced pulses during the Doppler interrogation time between 2-D image updates. This increases sampling opportunities for signals from any tissue depth of interest. In Figure 2.17 the area of interest for flow examination might be 15 cm (195 μs) from the transducer. If the machine pulsed every 65 μs, a pulse would arrive at the 15-cm tissue depth every 65 μs, and an echo would reach the transducer from the depth of interest every 65 μs. This would guarantee the coexistence of incoming and outgoing pulses necessary for comparison at a higher pulse repetition frequency than if the system pulsed every 260 μs for imaging purposes. This strategy places more than one sample volume in the exam field at a time and introduces a condition of partial range ambiguity in that the gate at which a shift is derived cannot be determined.

Theoretically, there can be as few or as many sample volumes as required according to the velocities to be measured and the range resolution required at any instance. If one wished to measure higher velocities than would be allowed by the sampling opportunities in Figure 2.17, then the pulse interval could be decreased to 32.5 μs, for example, which would provide higher velocity resolution and more sampling opportunities because the echoes from 15 cm would arrive at the transducer every 32.5 μs. This strategy would displace eight sample volumes across the field of view to the detriment of range resolution. The system will have pulsed eight times before the first pulse will have cleared the entire field of view and will no longer be sending echoes back to the transducer.

With the image of the heart as a guide, the operator seldom has difficulty identifying which sample volume is responsible for the highest velocity flows; it is usually the one closest to a value orifice or obstruction. Most multigate pulsed systems allow the operator to slide the set of gates along the scan line until one volume or another is within the region of interest. The machine keeps track of appropriate pulse spacing to sample consistently at the same depths.

The multigate pulsed Doppler approaches are most useful in examining flows close to the transducer using the most proximal range gates. This is because incoming echoes from the more distal gates tend to be interfered with by outgoing pulses which, unlike the single gate Doppler, are traveling along the sound pathway at the same *time*. In continuous wave Doppler, incoming and outgoing signals follow slightly different paths in order to avoid mutual interference.

In circumstances where two lesions are in very close proximity along the same scan line, and the Nyquist limit is not exceeded, the multigate approach is useful in assessing each site independently. In combined idiopathic hypertrophic subaortic stenosis and aortic steno-

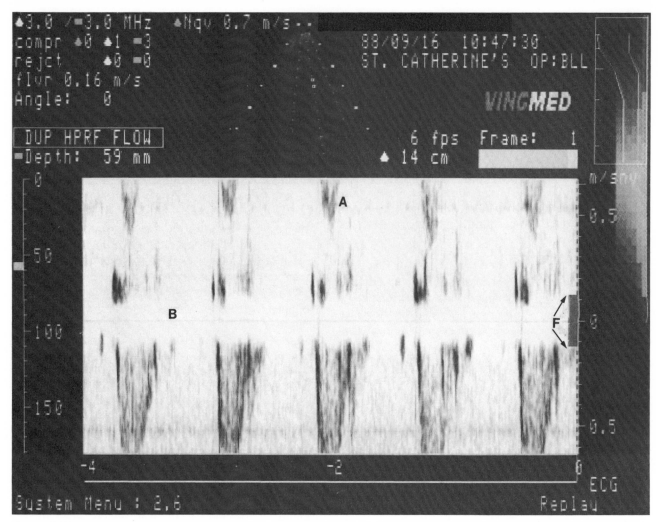

Figure 2.26.   At any velocity range setting on the Doppler display that is equal to or below the Nyquist limit, velocity displays can wrap around to the opposite directional display field when flow velocities exceed display or Nyquist limits. In this case of pulmonary artery flow from a parasternal transducer position, the operator has chosen to limit the velocity range directional display fields to 0.5 times the Nyquist limit. This is accomplished by positioning the baseline (B) at the center of the picture. Thus detected flow appears in both directional display fields which is often referred to as aliasing. F = velocities eliminated from the display by the operator-selected wall filter setting. (Courtesy PIDU, reproduced with permission.)

sis, for example, it is the sum of the two obstructive gradients (provided that flow has relaminarized between them) that increases left ventricular workload. Continuous wave Doppler from the cardiac apex would superimpose the two spectra, yielding a peak velocity from the greater obstruction and ignore the hemodynamic influence of the lesser obstruction. In cases where the frequency shifts exceed the Nyquist limit for single-gate pulsed Doppler, the multigate approach may be useful.

Stand-Alone Doppler

A 10-mm, nonimaging Doppler probe containing a single fixed element with a center frequency of around 2.0 MHz is usually available on cardiac Doppler ma-

chines. This transducer is intended for Doppler studies alone and on some machines is limited to continuous wave exams only. Other systems permit its split crystal to be phased coherently to perform pulsed Doppler and crude M-mode echocardiograms. These transducers are incapable of performing two-dimensional imaging. There are four advantages to the use of these stand-alone probes to collect Doppler data. The small size of these probes facilitates Doppler exams under space-limited transducer positions such as the suprasternal notch, right supraclavicular fossa, right parasternum or even the cardiac apex in a patient rotated left lateral decubitus. A second advantage of these probes is that the center frequency can be kept low since image quality is not a consideration with their use. Accordingly,

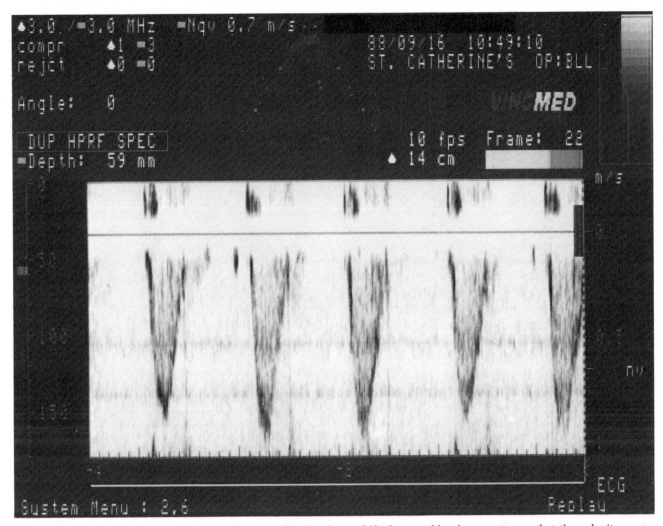

Figure 2.27. As compared to Figure 2.26 the baseline has been shifted upward by the operator so that the velocity range display field for flows away from the transducer is increased at the expense of velocity for flows in the opposite direction. This allows all of the velocities present in the profile of flows away from the transducer to be seen in the negative velocity display field. (Courtesy PIDU, reproduced with permission.)

patient penetration is increased at the longer wavelengths. Additionally, the Nyquist value is higher at the lower frequencies.

A third benefit of these transducers may be the most clinically significant: enhanced signal-to-noise ratio based on increased sound power to the patient. Live tissue dosage of sound energy is expressed in terms of power (mW) measured per area (cm) per second. Invariably, the highest power measurements are found at the onset of the focal zone of the sound pathway. Food and Drug Administration (FDA) regulations place a clearly stated upper limit on sound dosage for a variety of ultrasound exams on live humans. A more tightly focused sound pathway improves lateral resolution in imaging but also concentrates broadcast energy at the focal point so that FDA limits are reached with less *total* energy emitted by the transducer. Owing to their reduced aperture, the stand-alone Doppler

probes have poorer focusing traits than larger diameter imaging/Doppler transducers. With less concentration of sound energy at a focal point, *more total power* can be emitted by these probes before the FDA limits are reached at any single point in the examination field.

A major factor affecting Doppler sensitivity in cardiac studies is the size of the population of blood cells that aggregates individual reflections into an echo. The poorly focused beam of the stand-alone Doppler transducer insonates more targets within the blood pool producing a composite Doppler signal of higher amplitude than would a focused beam interrogating a smaller number of cells at the same power limits. Since noise tends to be independent of focus, the stand-alone transducers yield an enhanced signal to the background noise than do transducers with tighter focal traits.

The fourth advantage of stand-alone probes in Doppler is relatively minor. Part of the noise on the Doppler trace arises from within the machine itself as circuits pick-up stray signals shed from the electronics involved in image processing. In the stand-alone Doppler mode, the instrument is not acquiring and processing images and so a substantial portion of the system electronics are eliminated. This decreases the component of background noise on the Doppler trace generated by the ultrasound system and improves the signal to noise performance.

DOPPLER COLOR FLOW MAPPING

Color flow mapping displays the characteristics of blood flow in various hues and intensities of color. In reality, it is not so different from image mapping in that the information extracted from the returning signal is displayed in an M-mode or cross-sectional format. In the case of imaging, the system gleans variations in signal *amplitude* from the echo, converts the data to gray scale, and writes it into the display according to tissue depth in the case of the M mode or axially and laterally in the two-dimensional image.

The flow mapper performs a similar task in that it writes velocity information, obtained by phase analysis, into an image format.

CURRENT ISSUES IN COLOR FLOW MAPPING: SYSTEM TYPES

In terms of frequency or velocity accuracy, the capabilities and limitations of the two existing phased array approaches—anular and linear—are almost identical. Each is plagued by a pair of spectral broadening effects that introduce minor errors into the flow data as illustrated in Figs. 2.28 and 2.29. However, these errors are predictable and can be corrected. Over the near future both transducer approaches are likely to continue to be equally suitable for flow mapping. During this time the newer anular array technologies will continue to develop. It remains to be determined whether the large receive aperture of the anular phased array combined with its ability to sculpt beam focal patterns in all lateral planes will allow the design to become predominant.

Color Assignments

Color is a parameter that current video recording and display technology allows us to exploit. Lacking a better alternative, Doppler flow-mapping data are displayed in color despite widespread variations in color perception within the general population.[8] Doppler color flow mapping encodes three basic features of flow—namely direction, velocity and quality (lamina-

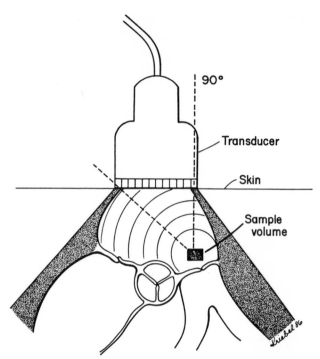

Figure 2.28. The receiving of Doppler signals across the elements of a stationary linear array at any angle other than the perpendicular causes a variable broadening of the spectral estimate which must be corrected by receive delays. Additionally, as scan lines depart from the perpendicular, the receive aperture offered by the transducer face progressively decreases which creates an uneven distribution of sensitivity across the diffraction field being worst toward the edges. Both anomalies relate to a single cause; the transducer remains stationary while the positions of the scan lines vary during the generation of a single sweep. (Courtesy PIDU, reproduced with permission.)

rity and turbulence). The following sections describe how the color flow images in this particular chapter are encoded (Fig. 2.31, Plates II, III).

Sub-Nyquist Flows

Laminar flow toward the transducer is described with variations in the "hot" colors of orange and red. Dark red depicts the lowest "toward" velocities, whereas progressively lighter shades of red indicate increasing "toward" velocities. Flows away from the transducer are depicted in the "cold" colors of blue and white. Dark blue identifies the lowest "away" velocities, whereas increasing lighter blue shades indicate higher "away" velocities. In some color presentations of flow-mapping data, the Z axis, or intensity, of the display represents the amplitude of the returning signal, which is presumed to vary according to the average number of reflectors in the beam during a sampling interval.

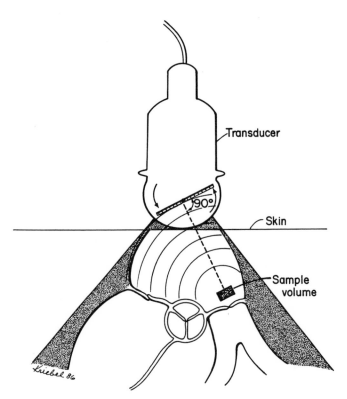

Figure 2.29. The motion of the transducer element in a mechanical system—which includes all annular phased arrays—causes a broadening of the spectral estimate of all incoming Doppler data. However, the center frequency remains unchanged. Additionally, since the crystal is moved so as to always be perpendicular to every scan at the time that it is generated, sensitivity variations based on the area of the receive aperture are not seen. (Courtesy PIDU, reproduced with permission.)

Flows above the Nyquist Limit

At an aliasing threshold of 0.7 m/s to 0.9 m/s, some normal mean velocities cannot be presented by flow mapping without frequency artefact. In disease states such as valvular stenoses the carrier and received frequencies may alias repeatedly between samples taken at a rate dictated by the requirements of flow mapping.

Therefore reading the color assignment as an absolute indicator of direction and velocity must be interpreted with caution. The color encoding imparts limited information of interest; for example, it enables differentiation of adjacent flows of different velocities. Additionally, the colors do map the area of flow at some yet to be determined level of accuracy, which may prove useful in valvular regurgitation. Finally, the flow mapper does fulfill its initial promise as a device to indicate the spatial properties of flows at an acceptable level of accuracy and sensitivity.

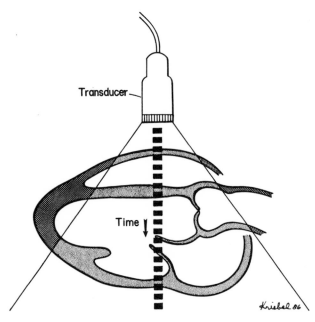

Figure 2.30. Each scan line of the color flow-mapping image is occupied by multiple gates (or sampling sites). In instruments with variably sized gates, the sample sites may actually overlap. Each gate on each line is sampled multiple times in rapid succession during the flow-mapping process. (Courtesy PIDU, reproduced with permission.)

Line Scan Rate: Temporal Resolution

How fast a device generates data indicates the temporal resolution of a machine, a particularly relevant factor in physiology. This section concerns the "time accuracy" of the flow-mapping process and whether additional "costs" are incurred in resolution to obtain the flow map. Existing echo techniques serve as reference standards of temporal resolution necessary for examining events in the cardiac cycle. At a pulse repetition frequency of 1000, M mode is considered reliable for the most critical of time determinations. Cross-sectional echocardiography with a frame generation rate of 30 per second has marginal time resolution relative to the rate at which cardiac events occur. Assessing the temporal resolution of a flow mapper requires an understanding of how the device acquires information.

Multiple Range Gates

Each scan line of the color flow image must be spanned by multiple range gates representing time increments (tissue depths) during which returning signals are acquired along each sound transmission line in sequence. Figure 2.30 illustrates that each scan line of the flow map image is occupied by numerous gates. Following the broadcast sound pulse, signals from progressively more distal gates are sampled for phase information.

Resolution: Sensitivity

The number of range gates may become an issue of clinical diagnostic importance. Large sample volumes are advantageous in gathering Doppler data because of their increased sensitivity to flow. However, the larger each range gate, the fewer there can be over any given depth of tissue. Alternatively, the smaller the sample volumes, the greater the population that can contribute to a visual display, which therefore appears more finely detailed. However, small sample volumes lack sensitivity and may result in discrepancies between data detected by continuous wave and that seen on the flow map.

Some subjects are easy to echo and make few demands on sensitivity of the instrument. At the other end of the spectrum, there are patients in whom one becomes willing to make great sacrifices to obtain any data at all. In the first instance small sample volumes are suitable, whereas in the second large sample volumes are necessary. Smaller sample volumes can produce a more detailed flow map. Whether such a visually pleasing display is more descriptive of physiology is an issue deserving investigation.

In flow mapping the operator has the option of changing the sample volume size and population to optimize the sensitivity requirements in any given patient. At present a range of selections between 32 and 128 sample volumes seems appropriate for tissue depths typically used during examination of the heart in adults.

Multiple Samples

In structural imaging modes each scan line of each picture need be scanned only once per frame to produce an accurate image of cardiac anatomy. By contrast, flow imaging modes require that each scan line must be sampled more than once in order: 1) to detect the lower velocity constituents of a flow profile, 2) to enhance signal-to-noise ratio and 3) to produce a more statistically reliable overall flow velocity profile.

The most commonly used color flow mode is really an image of the distribution of flow *velocities* superimposed on a gray scale M-mode or two-dimensional echocardiographic image (see Figure 2.25).

It is in the detection of lower velocity flows that the flow imager encounters its greatest technical difficulties and requires the most compromises. Basically, the *time* required to detect flow is in an inverse relationship to its velocity. The hands of an analog clock are an everyday example. A quick glance at the clock-face is sufficient for the observer to detect the motion of the second hand because it moves fast. More patience and study are required to observe the movement of the minute hand while only heroic concentration will permit one eventually to visualize any motion of the hour hand.

The basic principle is clear. An object must move some *minimal* distance in order to be perceived as moving. The greater the *time* taken by an object to move that minimum perceptible distance, the longer must be the observation *time*.

The clock analogy can be carried further. One could infer movement of the slower hands by noting their initial position and then returning at some later time to note that the position of the hands had changed. This is similar to what the flow imager does by sending a series of individual pulses along a scan line. Pulse spacing must allow each sample volume to clear the field of view before the next is sent which is a *time* consuming process. The time required to perform these operations for every scan line of a cross-sectional image significantly reduces the overall scan rate for the instrument. It is not unusual to find frame rates of 9, 10 or 11 in adult cardiology which is the minimum required for visual integration of physiology by the eye of the observer.

It follows that the flow imager is inherently superior at detecting high velocity flows than those moving at low speeds. Since flow velocities tend to be higher in the heart and great vessels than elsewhere in the body, flow imaging has developed more readily in cardiology than in other clinical services.

A second reason for multiple samples of each scan line in flow imaging is the improvement in the signal-to-noise ratio when digital data is summated against constant background noise levels.

The final reason for repetitive sampling of each line of data is to improve the statistical validity of the flow data. This is so because at any given location within the heart flow traits may be variable. Figure 2.21 is a graph of hypothetical changes of turbulent flow direction and velocity at a single location (range gate) within the heart. Because of the short duration pulse requirements for acceptable axial resolution of the imaging part of flow mapping, flow sampling is transit time limited as indicated by periods A, B and C in Figure 2.21. If the direction and velocity traits detected at this arrow were taken to represent flow behavior over the illustrated time, then serious discrepancies in the data would result. The best way to restore the "averaging effect" of the long sampling period (transit time) associated with the long sound pulse is to sample each gate multiple times in rapid succession and thereby to track the scatterer over a time equivalent to that of a longer wave train. This concept has previously been

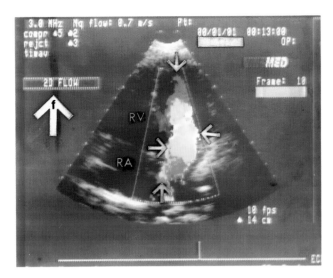

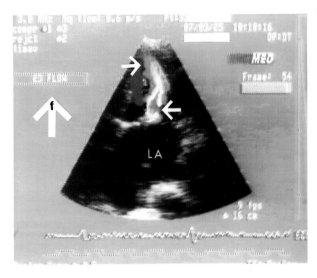

A

B

Figure 2.31. (*A*) Color flow map of mitral valve inflow in a normal subject from the cardiac apex. The Nyquist limit, which is determined by the depth of tissue selections, is 0.7 m/s. The normal mean flow velocities do not exceed the Nyquist limit. Hue indicates regional CHANGES in velocity. In diastole, blood within the left atrium moves at a low velocity toward the mitral valve (↑). These low velocities are encoded with a deep red hue. As blood accelerates toward the mitral valve its color assignment becomes progressively lighter and eventually registers as orange (→). Around the mitral valve, where flow velocities are the highest, the color encoding is seen to be bright yellow (←) which also indicates a moderate spectral broadening of flow. Within the left ventricle flow velocities decrease as indicated by the color encoding which passes through orange to deep red at the apex (↓). Since flow direction (f) is primarily axial in this plane, hue variations can be ascribed to velocity changes rather than cos φ effects. (*B*) Color flow map of diastolic flow velocities in mitral stenosis. The transducer is at the apex. An area of blue encoded, aliased, forward flow is seen (←) with dark blue indicating the highest velocity in the center. A contour of yellow encoded, nonaliased, forward velocity is seen around the central high velocity core. An outer contour of low velocity forward flow (→) is indicated in various red shades with the deepest red (lowest velocity) at the apex (↓). f = average flow direction in this plane; LA = left atrium.

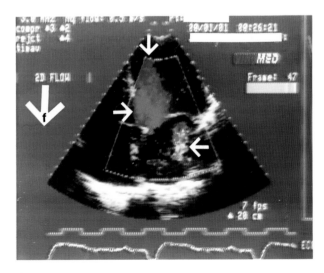

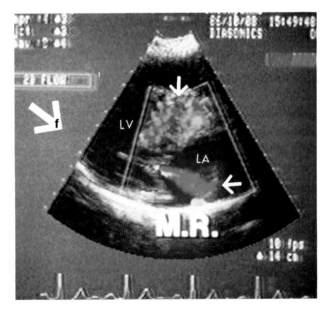

C

D

Figure 2.31, continued. (*C*) Color flow map of mitral regurgitation. Velocity contours of the left ventricular outflow are clear, with the lowest velocities most distant from the aorta encoded deep blue (↓). As flow accelerates the blue hue becomes progressively lighter (→). The pattern of mitral regurgitation (←) indicates aliasing due to turbulent flow. The regurgitant jet is multicolored, including green and yellow, which indicate flow turbulence. f = average direction of regurgitant flow within this imaging plane. (*D*) Color flow map of mitral regurgitation from the parasternal position. A minority of patients will best present mitral and aortic flow events from this position. The regurgitant flow is blue encoded (←). Higher velocities (lighter hues) are closest to the mitral valve. Aortic ejection is seen as red in this plane (↓). f = direction of regurgitant jet.

Plate II

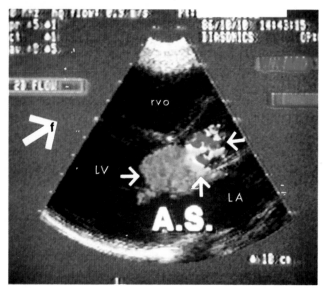

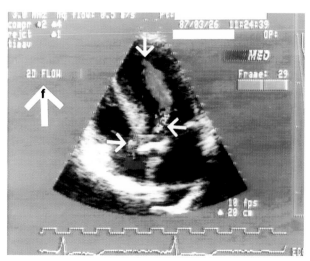

E   F

Figure 2.31, continued. (*E*) Color flow map of aortic stenosis with high velocities and turbulence in the parasternal long axis view. The lowest velocity flows (→) most distant from the aorta are encoded deepest red. Subvalvular acceleration is seen as a band of yellow (↑); above the valve flows are aliased with a multicolor assignment (←). f = flow direction (*F*) Color flow map of aortic insufficiency. The transducer is at the apex. A region of turbulent and aliased flow (←) is seen below the aortic valve. The flow stabilizes and slows toward the apex (↓), indicated by progressively darker shades of red. (→) = a small glimpse of tricuspid inflow.

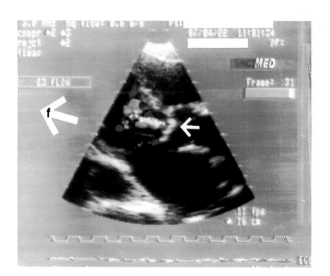

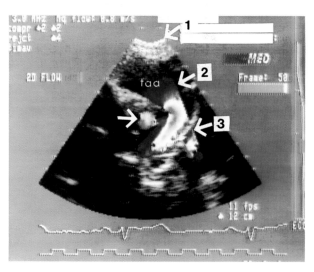

G   H

Figure 2.31, continued. (*G*) Color flow map of aortic insufficiency. Some flows are better seen from the parasternal position. Two coapted, stenotic aortic cusps are visualized (←) below which a blue encoded diastolic jet is seen. f = average direction of aortic insufficiency flow. (*H*) Reverberation artefacts in color flow mapping. The transducer is in the suprasternal notch (arrow 1) showing the transverse aortic arch (taa). Strong flow signals are derived from the descending aorta with an aliased central jet toward the wall of tightest curvature. Blue encoded low velocity "away flows" are seen toward the margins of the descending aorta. Color reduplication occurs outside the posterior wall of the aorta (arrow 3). Arrow 2 marks high amplitude Doppler signals returning from a location close to the transducer. The "flow patterns" at arrow 3 indicate a second-time-around trip for the echo reflections. Color flow reverberations are associated with moving, high amplitude reflectors such as nonbiological prostheses and sewing rings, PA lines and unattenuated blood cell reflections as in this figure. (→) = right pulmonary arterial flow.

Plate III

stated using a baseball analogy and is made possible by the enormous disparity in velocity between sound pulse and blood cell, a fact that insures that the targets have not moved much between one interrogation and the next.

It follows that each scan line of the flow map sector image will be scanned numerous times in quick succession. In order to improve temporal resolution something must be compromised: 1) frame rate must decline from the 30 frames per second used in structural imaging, 2) scan lines will have to become shorter, thus requiring less time to complete, 3) there must be fewer of them, or 4) the scan angle must decrease. Historically, there has been a reluctance to reduce the depth of visualizable tissue that is inherent in sacrifice number (2). Therefore, reducing the scan rate and the number of scan lines as well as narrowing the angle of the flow image are the choices which appear to least compromise clinical objectives.

From a time-accuracy standpoint, decreased frame rate can cause color flow data from different phases of the heart cycle to appear in successive frames at operator selected wide sector angles or deeper range settings.

Accordingly, the accuracy with which the flow mapper documents the temporal aspect of events can be compromised by the fact that multiple samples of each line are required to compensate for the limited sampling duration resulting from a short sound pulse necessary to fulfill the imaging part of flow mapping requirements.

Variance

The purpose of the flow mapper is to define accurately as many aspects of blood flow physiology as possible. One factor to emerge from Doppler analysis of blood flow is variance. Variance is a sampling term and relates to the differences in velocity and directional information (i.e., increased bandwidth of the Doppler signal) obtained across the multiple samples of each gate on each line of the flow map.

Variance contains information about the quality of flow, its state of laminarity (flow smoothness) or turbulence. The detection of turbulence is of interest because it indicates a wasting of cardiac pump power as energy "stored" in the form of flow momentum becomes dissipated at elevated Reynolds numbers.[9]

Figure 2.20 indicates that when blood flow is laminar, successful rapid samples at the same location in the heart will yield similar directional and velocity information, even if the velocity signals are aliased. By contrast, in turbulent flow repetitive samples at the same location yield variable values of these factors, a situation described as variance (Fig. 2.21).

The lack of variance in a sample indicates laminar flow, especially in regions of the heart where velocities would be expected to generate shifts below the Nyquist limit. For example, diastolic flows across the normal tricuspid valve in the adult are often at a sub-Nyquist velocity in color flow mapping so that from a parasternal or an apical transducer position they are displayed as a homogenous region of reds and oranges. Conversely, increased bandwidth, in the form of variance in the returning signal, might indicate turbulence within the heart where velocities would be expected to generate shifts below the Nyquist limit.

Where velocities are increased above the 0.7 to 0.9 m/s aliasing limit typical of color flow-mapping applications in adult cardiology, the clinical implication of variance is uncertain, although flow turbulence would be one cause. However, a unidirectional flow might contain higher velocity flows at the center and lower velocity flows at the edges, adjacent to walls, anuli, or leaflets. Aliasing would then cause those velocities that exceeded the Nyquist limit to be registered in the opposite directional color, while the sub-Nyquist velocities would be encoded in the correct directional colors. A mosaic pattern of colors would then be created.

This uncertainty has been overcome by reserving the use of certain colors, usually yellow and green, to indicate variance within individual sample volumes or between adjacent sample volumes. Thus, yellow and green appear only under limited conditions. Accordingly, in "mixed Nyquist" types of flow patterns containing laminar velocities above and below the alias threshold, an overall blue and red "checkerboard" image might be perceived, indicating consistency of the estimate over time at individual sampling locations. In cases where each sample volume produced variable flow values over time (increased bandwidth), yellow or green would be the colors encoded in each location.

Compensating Studies: A Balance of Capabilities

Sacrifices in frequency and temporal resolution are the costs to be borne in obtaining spatial resolution of the Doppler data sufficient to construct an image or flow map. The temporal accuracy of either pulsed or continuous wave Doppler is adequate for timing events in diagnostic cardiology. Additionally, the frequency uncertainty of flow mapping is compensated by the continuous wave approach, a process made easier by the fact that the color flow map can act as a guide to the placement of the Doppler cursor.

From a technical standpoint, flow mapping will not supplant other noninvasive procedures currently used in diagnostic cardiology. Rather, it is complementary and adds a dimension of spatial resolution to conventional Doppler studies.

END NOTES

1. Sound propagation involves the cyclic compression and rarefaction of the molecules of a conductant medium such as blood or myocardium. Fluid, collagen and calcium content, as the major determinants of tissue *compressibility*, heavily influence the acoustic impedance value of any tissue. It is the *difference* in acoustic impedance (or impedance mismatch) that determines the total amount of sound reflected from any tissue interface. The proportion of total reflected sound that is directed back toward the transducer in the form of an echo is a function of the size of the interface and its degree of perpendicularity to the sound pathway.
2. Frequency dependent attenuation in tissue is not a shift in the frequency mix of a pulse. The energy to compress and rarefy the molecules of a medium must come from the sound pulse itself. Higher frequency components of the pulse perform these functions more often and are depleted of energy more rapidly than the low frequencies. This affects the *calculation* of center (or median) frequency which is based on relative amplitudes but does not alter the actual frequency content of the pulse nor create a phase shift.
3. Usually expressed as the cosine of the angle θ.
4. Angle correction is standard examination protocol for velocity estimates in peripheral vascular imaging which accounts for the universality of the feature on imaging/Doppler machines.
5. The term *waveform beating* relates to the phenomena of musical beats which arise from the rhythmic interaction of similar frequency tones within the range of human hearing. A common engineering reference to the Doppler signal is the "beat frequency."
6. In both pulsed and continuous wave Doppler, the oscillator frequency is stepped down in amplitude and fed directly to the comparator for multiplication with incoming signals when they appear. This assumes that the crystal both rings and receives "true."
7. If the scatterers are moving away from the transducer so that the 2.0-kHz shift is downward (to 1.998 MHz) then from 12.0-cm the

shift will rotate less than -90 degrees against the broadcast signal.
8. Some major impediments to advancements in ultrasound involve lack of display technology. For example, given the "slow" rate at which cardiac events occur relative to the "fast" capabilities of ultrasound to track them, three-dimensional echocardiography is entirely feasible. The methods of storing and displaying the information in three dimensions in a widely available format are currently under investigation.
9. Reynolds number—a dimensionless value which describes a threshold at which the viscosity, or cohesiveness, of a nonsolid medium is "overcome" by an external force applied to it so that molecular momentum becomes directionally random, a condition which dissipates propulsive energy.

REFERENCES

1. Harrigan P, Lee R. Principles of Interpretation in Echocardiography. New York: John Wiley and Sons, 1985.
2. Atkinson P, Woodcock JP. Doppler Ultrasound and Its Use in Clinical Measurement. London: Academic Press, 1982.
3. Hatle L, Angelsen B. Doppler Ultrasound in Cardiology, Physical Principles and Applications. Philadelphia: Lea & Febiger, 1982.
4. Hatle L, Angelsen B. Doppler Ultrasound in Cardiology, Physical Principles and Applications, 2nd ed. Philadelphia: Lea & Febiger, 1985. Pp. 4, 34, 42, 174.
5. Omoto R, ed. Color Atlas of Real-Time Two-Dimensional Echocardiography. Tokyo: Shindan-To-Chiro Co., Ltd.,1984. Pp. 1–44.
6. Shrader WW. MTI Radar. In Skolnik ML, ed. Radar Handbook. New York: McGraw-Hill, 1972.
7. Huggins E. Physics. Menlo Park, CA: Benjamin/Cummings Publishing Co., 1968.
8. Hoffman EA. Rittman, EL., Intracardiac Cycle Constancy of Total Heart Volume. Dynamic Cardiovascular Imaging 1987; 1(3): 199–205.

Drawings by Nancy Kriebel, Kriebel Arts, Arlington, MA.

3

Normal Doppler Echocardiographic Examination

Martin St. John Sutton
Ted Plappert
Paul Oldershaw

INTRODUCTION

The aims of M-mode, two-dimensional, and Doppler echocardiography are to obtain the highest quality cardiac images and blood flow velocity information for clinically accurate diagnosis and reliable measurements of cardiac chamber dimensions, hemodynamics, and function. Acquisition of high-quality Doppler echocardiographic information depends on reliable ultrasound recording equipment and on the combination of a number of different factors, each of which deserve careful consideration in the examination of every patient. These factors include patient comfort and cooperation, patient position, selection of the transducer that maximizes both penetration and resolution, transducer placement for the best ultrasound access to the heart and great vessels, and optimal use of the gain and reject controls.

M-mode echocardiography was the first noninvasive means of identifying intracardiac structures. M-mode echocardiography is now rarely used alone because 1) it lacks lateral resolution, 2) the region imaged may not be representative of the heart as a whole, and 3) high-quality images are obtainable in only three-quarters of all patients examined. However, the higher pulse repetition frequency of M-mode (1000 cycles/s) compared with two-dimensional echo (30 cycles/s) provides better temporal resolution and good interface definition. For this reason, the most accurate measurements of cardiac chamber dimensions are obtained with two-dimensionally guided M-mode echocardiography. Two-dimensional guidance of the M-mode beam ensures that diameters and not chords of the great vessels and cardiac chambers are obtained. Electrocardiograms from the limb leads should always be recorded simultaneously with M-mode, two-dimensional, and Doppler echocardiograms for accurate timing of cardiac events.

TOPOGRAPHIC ANATOMY OF THE HEART

Precise knowledge of the position of the normal heart and its anatomic relations within the thorax and abdomen is important for optimal echocardiographic imaging. There are minor variations in the position of the heart that relate to body habitus—in aesthenic subjects, the heart is more vertical than in endomorphic subjects, in whom the heart tends to be more horizontal. However, there are some easily identifiable topographic landmarks that describe the long axis of the left ventricle in the majority of subjects. In the frontal or coronal plane, the long axis of the left ventricle is defined by a line connecting the point of maximal impulse at the apex of the heart, usually located in the fifth left intercostal space close to the midclavicular line, to the junction of the medial and middle thirds of the right clavicle (Fig. 3.1). The long axis of the left ventricle in the anteroposterior or parasagittal plane is described by a line from the point of maximum impulse at the apex of the heart (fifth left intercostal space at the

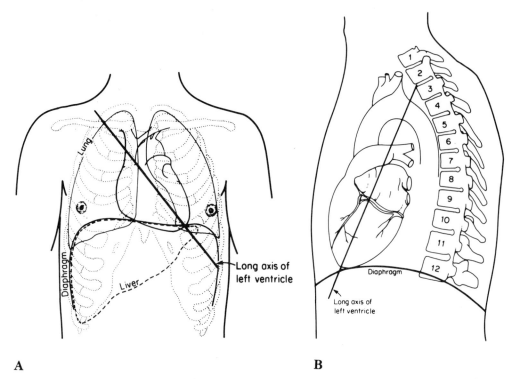

A   **B**

Figure 3.1.   The long axis of the left ventricle in the frontal or coronal plane is shown running from the apex of the heart to the junction of the middle and the medial thirds of the right clavicle (*A*). Long axis of the left ventricle in the lateral or parasagittal plane is shown running from the cardiac apex to the intervertebral disc space between the second and third vertebral bodies (*B*).

midclavicular line) to the disc space between the second and third thoracic vertebrae (Fig. 3.1). The interventricular septum is oriented between 30 and 45 degrees to the true sagittal plane of the body, so that the right heart chambers are positioned not only rightward but also anteriorly. The inferoposterior surface of the heart is in contact with the central tendon and left leaf of the diaphragm, with the liver immediately subjacent.

In addition to the orientation of the left ventricle within the chest, a working knowledge of the surface markings of the semilunar and atrioventricular valves provides the echocardiographer with information to reconstruct in three-dimensional space the positions of the cardiac chambers, the great arteries, and the great veins (Fig. 3.2). The pulmonary valve lies to the left of the midline at the level of the third sternocostal joint (Fig. 3.2). The aortic valve is positioned inferomedially to the pulmonary valve at the level of the fourth sternocostal joint and is posterior to the pulmonary valve in the sagittal plane. The mitral valve is contiguous with the aortic valve but inferiorly placed in the fourth left intercostal space at the left sternal border. The tricuspid valve is retrosternal and almost in the midline at the level of the sixth or seventh sternocostal joints, immediately to the left of the sternal articulation. There is no continuity between the right-sided atrioventricular and semilunar valves, as there is in the

left heart, because the infundibulum is interposed between the tricuspid and pulmonary valves. The immediate anatomic relations of the heart and great vessels to the intrathoracic and intra-abdominal viscera are not only important in understanding the

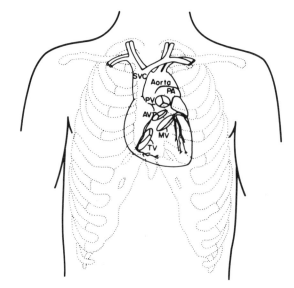

Figure 3.2.   The position of the heart and its anatomic relations to the lungs, diaphragm, and liver in the frontal plane, showing the location of the mitral (MV), tricuspid (TV), aortic (AV), and pulmonary (PV) valves.

orientation of cardiac images obtained from the conventional transducer positions, but are also important for the classification of congenital heart disease by sequential chamber analysis (see Chapter 22).

PATIENT COOPERATION

Before beginning any echocardiographic examination in either children or adults, it is important to obtain the patient's full cooperation because this often bears a direct relationship to the quality of images obtained. Cooperation is achieved most easily first, by ensuring that the patient is comfortable lying on the examination table and second, by explaining the nature and aims of the study and pointing out that no known damage has resulted from ultrasound examination of the heart. Once anxiety or apprehension regarding the echocardiographic examination have been alleviated, explain to the patient before and during the study that he or she should relax, keep as still as possible, and breathe normally except when requested to sustain end-expiration or end-inspiration.

High-quality ultrasound recordings in neonates and infants are easiest to obtain when performed with as little disturbance to the baby as possible. This is usually achieved by performing the study after feeding or while the infant is sleeping or positioned comfortably in the mother's arms. Crying greatly increases respiratory tidal volume and causes lung tissue to appear in front of the heart, which makes echocardiographic imaging technically difficult.

TRANSDUCER SELECTION

The size and frequency of the optimal echocardiographic transducer depends greatly on the patient's body habitus. Low-frequency transducers have greater body or tissue penetration than high-frequency transducers, but their resolution is limited by the wavelength of the ultrasound transmitted and therefore is less than that of the high-frequency transducers. The transducer selected is the one that combines the best balance between penetration and resolution. In a 65-kg male with normal body habitus, the most commonly used transducer is the 2.25 MHz. In children and neonates, penetration is almost never a problem. Unequivocal resolution of small intracardiac structures, for which 3.5-MHz transducers are used most commonly, is of critical importance, and 5.0-MHz transducers are used in small or premature babies and fetuses.

An important consideration in transducer selection, independent of either penetration or resolution, is the size of the ultrasound emitting crystal within the transducer scanhead. The larger the crystal, the more parallel the ultrasound beam; the smaller the crystal,

the earlier the ultrasound beam diverges. There are practical limitations with regard to the transducer scanhead size, however, because transmission of ultrasound into the chest is dependent on contact between the whole area of the crystal transducer (footprint) and the skin in the intercostal spaces. If the scanhead is too large to fit between the ribs and does not maintain continuous skin contact in the intercostal spaces, the echo image quality obtained will not be optimal.

The introduction of Doppler has further complicated transducer selection because the majority of commercially available ultrasound equipment provides range-gated Doppler and nonimaging continuous wave Doppler probes. Velocity amplitude determines the choice of transducer since the velocity signal will alias if it exceeds the Nyquist limit of the pulsed wave transducer (see Chapter 1), in which case a continuous-wave transducer will be required to measure high-velocity blood flow. Recently, transducers that allow combined imaging with continuous-wave Doppler sampling have been developed.

TRANSDUCER PLACEMENT AND PATIENT POSITION

Two-dimensional echocardiography enables imaging of the heart from the chest and abdomen in an almost infinite number of planes, and for this reason the American Society of Echocardiography (ASE) has for-

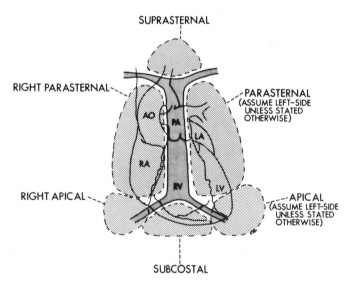

NOMENCLATURE FOR TRANSDUCER LOCATION

Figure 3.3. The transducer positions for routine two-dimensional echocardiographic image acquisition include the left and right parasternal, left and right apical, suprasternal, and subcostal locations. (Reproduced with permission of the American Society of Echocardiography. The report of the ASE committee on nomenclature and standards in two-dimensional echocardiography, August, 1980.)

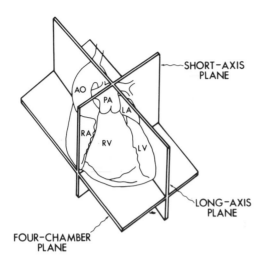

SHORT-AXIS
PLANE

LONG-AXIS
PLANE

FOUR-CHAMBER
PLANE

TWO-DIMENSIONAL ECHOCARDIOGRAPHIC
IMAGING PLANES

Figure 3.4. Cardiac images are conventionally oriented with respect to the three orthogonal axes of the left ventricle. The two orthogonal long axes of the left ventricle are visualized in the four-chamber and long-axis planes, respectively, from the apex of the heart, and the short axis of the LV is visualized in the parasternal position. (Reproduced with permission of the American Society of Echocardiography. The report of the ASE committee on nomenclature and standards in two-dimensional echocardiography, August, 1980.)

mulated recommendations regarding transducer placement, in an attempt to standardize echo image acquisition and orientation so that images from the same heart and from different hearts can be compared (1). The transducer locations recommended by the ASE for routine use include the left and right parasternal positions, the cardiac apex, the subcostal position, and the suprasternal positions (Fig. 3.3). From these positions, complete two-dimensional echocardiographic imaging of the heart can be achieved in three orthogonal planes (Fig. 3.4).

Echocardiographic examination begins with the patient lying comfortably on the left side, with the head and thorax elevated 30 degrees and electrocardiographic electrodes on each limb.

Echocardiographic images are acquired from the left parasternal position with the transducer in the second, third, or fourth intercostal space close to the sternum. Elevation of the left arm so that it rests on the bed above the patient's head separates the ribs in the left chest and opens up the intercostal spaces, providing better access for the transducer. Before two-dimensional echocardiographic imaging was available, M-mode echocardiograms were obtained with the transducer in this position. Rotation of the patient to the left lateral position enables delineation of the right and left sides of the septum by M-mode echo, but this is facilitated using two-dimensional imaging to direct the

M-mode ultrasound beam. Rotation of the patient from the supine of the left lateral position changes the plane through which the ultrasound beam transects the right ventricle, so that M-mode measurements of right ventricular dimension with the patient supine are consistently smaller than those obtained from the same patient in the left lateral position. This discrepancy can be minimized when the patient is rotated to the left lateral position and the M-mode beam is directed with two-dimensional imaging.

The left parasternal position is used to obtain images of the short-axis aorta; the short axis of the left ventricle at mitral valve, midcavity, and apical levels; the long axis of the left ventricle, and the right ventricular inflow and outflow tracts. Doppler interrogation of the tricuspid and pulmonic valves is also accomplished from this position.

Imaging of the heart from the apical region is performed with the patient rotated between 60 and 90 degrees to the left, with the transducer applied inferiorly, caudally and lateral to the point of maximum cardiac impulse. Two-chamber, four-chamber, and the long-axis views of the left ventricle should be obtained with the transducer at the apex. Blood flow velocity profiles in the left ventricular outflow tract and across the mitral and tricuspid valves are obtained from the apical transducer position.

Subcostal imaging is achieved with the patient lying supine and the transducer scanhead applied to the epigastrium in the angle between the xiphoid process and the left costal margin (or from the right subcostal region when imaging is performed with the ultrasound beam first passing through the liver). Manipulation of the transducer in the subcostal region may cause discomfort or apprehension, and this can be minimized by flexing the hips and knees to relax the rectus abdominus muscle, which runs in the midline from the costal margin superiorly to the pubis inferiorly. Imaging is best obtained with the patient sustaining end-inspiration and should include short-axis views of the aorta and left ventricle, the four-chamber view, the inferior vena cava and abdominal aorta, and blood flow velocity profiles from the pulmonary artery.

Echocardiographic images are aquired from the right intercostal space with the patient rotated 90 degrees to the right and the transducer applied close to the sternal border in the second to the fourth intercostal spaces. This transducer position is used to image the proximal ascending aorta in the normal heart, and for evaluating the blood flow velocity profiles across the aortic valve. This acoustic window is especially valuable in aortic stenosis, when Doppler flow velocity signals from the apex and suprasternal regions are inadequate. In addition, when left parasternal imaging is unsuccessful, parasternal long- and short-axis views of the left ventricle can occasionally be obtained from the right parasternal region. The right parasternal position is used routinely to obtain short- and long-axis views of the heart in patients with dextrocardia.

Two-dimensional echo images of the ascending aorta, aortic arch, brachiocephalic vessels, proximal descending thoracic aorta, right pulmonary artery, and superior vena cava, and Doppler blood flow velocity signals distal to the aortic valve are obtained with the transducer scanhead positioned in the suprasternal region. These are most easily obtained with the patient lying supine, a pillow placed under the scapulae, and the head extended and turned to the left to provide the best balance between patient comfort, relaxation of the cervical strap muscles, and optimal ultrasound access to the heart and great vessels.

Although these transducer placements and patient positions are the most frequently used and allow for complete imaging of the heart and great vessels in the majority of patients (2), they may not be optimal in patients with chest deformities due to pectus excavatum or carinatum, severe kyphoscoliosis, or barrel-shaped chests secondary to chronic obstructive lung disease, or in patients with displacement of the heart within a normally shaped chest, such as those with large pneumothorax or postpneumonectomy. Adherence to the conventional transducer placement positions in such patients may prove unrewarding and provide little or no useful images of the heart. The transducer should be used intelligently as an exploratory probe to first locate the heart within the thorax. The heart may vary greatly in position; for example, it may be in the paravertebral gutter in severe kyphoscoliosis. When the heart has been located, its orientation must be determined accurately so that the cardiac chambers can be imaged in their long and short axes and their respective dimensions measured appropriately. Sometimes when the heart is in the normal position, imaging is possible only from one transducer location. This is most frequent in patients with hyperinflated chests due to obstructive lung disease, in whom ultrasound access to the heart is possible only via the subcostal route. However, optimal imaging techniques employed with sound knowledge of cardiac anatomy will enable acquisition of diagnostic echocardiographic images in most of the conventional planes.

TWO-DIMENSIONAL ECHOCARDIOGRAPHIC EXAMINATION

The aim of this section is to describe an integrated, two-dimensional M-mode and Doppler echocardiographic examination of the heart and great vessels from each transducer placement rather than describe seriatim M-mode, two-dimensional ultrasound imaging

and Doppler assessment of blood flow velocity. The precise order in which two-dimensional echo images are obtained is a matter of personal preference. Whichever order is chosen, however, the echocardiographer should adopt a systematic approach and should adhere to it at all times so that no important information is omitted.

It is always helpful to obtain a succinct clinical history and perform a quick but careful clinical examination of the cardiovascular system before beginning the echocardiogram, not only to focus on the clinical questions raised by the referring physician, but also to ensure that no additional cardiac pathology is overlooked. In this way uninformed, repetitious, routine echocardiographic examinations are obviated, each examination remains interesting and different, and one can look for any known but clinically unsuspected associated abnormalities.

Whenever the transducer is placed on a patient's chest or abdomen, there must be air-free contact between the transducer and the skin to minimize dispersion of ultrasound by an air interface. This is achieved by liberal application of a coupling medium. The scan plane of the ultrasound emission should be known, and this is indi-

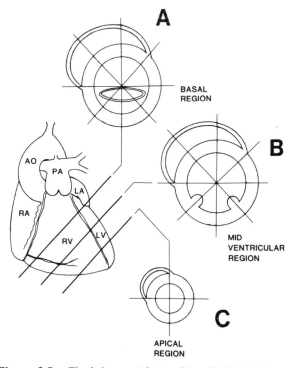

Figure 3.5. The left ventricle is arbitrarily divided into three equal parts along its long axis. The basal portion includes the mitral valve, the middle portion encloses the papillary muscles, and the apical portion is distal to the insertion of the papillary muscles into the left ventricular free wall. Short-axis images obtained at the mitral valve level (*A*), at papillary muscle level (*B*), and at the apex (*C*). (Reproduced with permission of the American Society of Echocardiography. The report of the ASE committee on nomenclature and standards: identification of myocardial wall segments, November, 1982.)

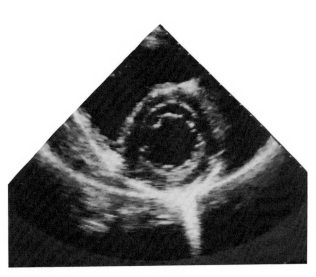

A

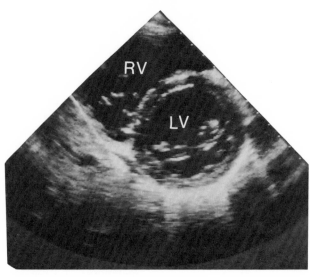

B

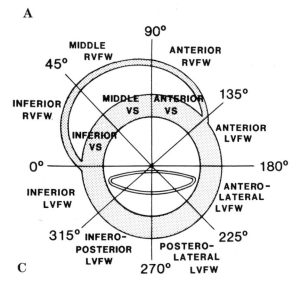

C

Figure 3.6. Two-dimensional echocardiogram of the short axis of the left ventricle through the basal segment, showing the mitral valve, which is open in diastole (*A*) and closed in systole (*B*). This short-axis section of the heart includes the septum and the left and right ventricular free walls, which are divided into regions as shown. (Reproduced with permission of the American Society of Echocardiography. The report of the ASE committee on nomenclature and standards: identification of myocardial wall segments, November, 1982.)

cated on all commercially available transducer scanheads by a knob or groove on the transducer housing.

Left Parasternal Position

Left Ventricular and Aortic Short-Axis Views

It is customary to begin two-dimensional echocardiographic imaging with the transducer in the left parasternal region with the patient rotated between 60 and 90 degrees to the left side. The transducer is first applied in the second to fourth intercostal space with the scanhead as close to the left sternal border as possible, with the scan plane at right angles to the left ventricular long axis (indicated by a line connecting the point of maximal cardiac impulse and the junction of the medial and middle thirds of the right clavicle).

The left ventricle is arbitrarily divided along its long axis into three equal parts: the basal, the middle, and the apical segments (Fig. 3.5). The basal region includes the mitral valve leaflets and extends from the mitral valve ring to the tips of the papillary muscles; the middle segment includes the papillary muscles from their tips, from which the chordae tendineae take origins, to their insertion into the left ventricular free walls; and the apical segment extends from the bases of the papillary muscles to the apex of the heart.

A useful starting point is to locate the mitral valve leaflets, which may involve moving the transducer up or down an interspace, occasionally moving it laterally from the sternal border, or rotating the patient from the left lateral to the left semilateral position to locate the optimal acoustic window. Once the anterior mitral valve leaflet is identified, the scanhead is angled toward the apex of the left ventricle so that both anterior and posterior leaflets are visualized simultaneously. By a combination of adjusting the angulation of the transducer along the long axis of the left ventricle and

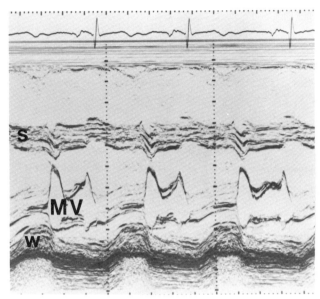

Figure 3.7. M-mode echocardiogram from a normal subject obtained through the basal region of the left ventricle, showing the septum (s) and the left ventricular cavity, with the anterior and posterior leaflets of the mitral valve (MV) and the posterior LV wall (w).

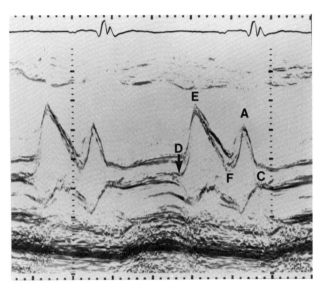

Figure 3.8. M-mode echocardiogram showing a normal mitral valve with anterior and posterior leaflets separating as the valve opens (D point) (*arrow*). The anterior cusp moves anteriorly to its peak excursion (E point), then drifts posteriorly (F point) before reopening with atrial systole, reaching a peak excursion (A), and finally coapting with the posterior leaflet as the valve closes (C point). The posterior mitral valve cusp excursion is less than the anterior cusp, but its motion pattern is similar.

rotating it clockwise or counterclockwise about its longitudinal axis, the left ventricle should appear circular. The short-axis echo image of the left ventricle obtained at the level of the mitral valve leaflets is termed the basal level or segment (Fig. 3.6). The left ventricular free wall and septum in short axis is divided into octants and each octant is specifically designated as anterolateral, posterolateral, etc., to avoid problems with nomenclature. Similarly, the right ventricular free wall is divided into three equal parts. In this scan plane, the septal and lateral commissures of the mitral valve are in apposition to the inferior and anterolateral left ventricular walls, respectively.

In real time the endocardial surfaces of the septum and left ventricular free wall move concentrically inward in systole as the myocardium shortens and thickens, and concentrically outward in diastole as the myocardium relaxes and thins. During diastole, the mitral valve leaflets move in opposite directions, the anterior leaflet moves anteriorly, and the posterior leaflet posteriorly, so that when they are fully open the mitral valve orifice area is between 4 and 6 cm^2 (Fig. 3.6). Once this short-axis view of the right ventricle and the left ventricle at mitral valve level is obtained, the gain, reject, and compression controls are adjusted to obtain clear and continuous epicardial and endocardial images throughout the cardiac cycle. The left ventricle at the level of the mitral valve should be circular in cross section; if it appears oval, it is invariably because

the left ventricle is imaged obliquely and not in true short axis, most often because the transducer is too low on the chest wall. Occasionally this can be remedied by slight corrective angulation or rotation of the

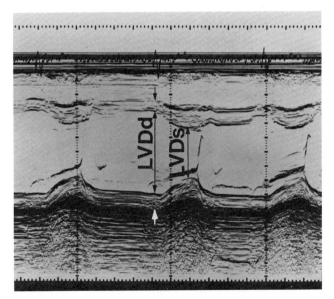

Figure 3.9. M-mode echocardiogram of the normal left ventricle at the tips of the mitral valve leaflets, showing end-diastolic dimension (LVDd), end-diastolic septal and posterior wall thicknesses, and left ventricular end-systolic dimension (LVDs). Note the similar excursion of the septum and posterior wall.

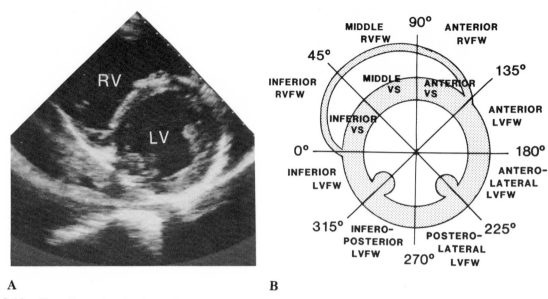

A   B

Figure 3.10. Two-dimensional echocardiogram of the short axis of the left ventricle in a normal subject at papillary muscle level. The papillary muscles are discrete structures that protrude into the cavity (A). The septum and left and right ventricular walls are divided into regions similar to those at the base (B). (Reproduced with permission of the American Society of Echocardiography. The report of the ASE committee on nomenclature and standards: identification of myocardial wall segments, November, 1982.)

transducer, without altering its position in the intercostal space. If this does not obtain an adequate short-axis view, however, the transducer should be moved up one interspace, or moved medially until optimal imaging is obtained. If the images are obscured by lung tissue in front of the heart, image quality may be greatly improved if the patient maintains expiration.

When the two-dimensional images of the basal short axis have been obtained, an M-mode echocardiogram can be recorded using two-dimensional guidance of the M-mode cursor (Fig. 3.7). With the transducer perpendicular to the chest wall, the M-mode beam passes consecutively through the right ventricular wall, the right ventricular outflow tract, the right and left endocardial surfaces of the septum and the left ventricular cavity, the mitral valve leaflets, and finally through the endocardial and epicardial surfaces of the posterior left ventricular wall. At the onset of diastole, the anterior and posterior mitral valve leaflets move rapidly in opposing directions from their closed position (see Fig. 3.8, D point) to their maximal separation (E point). Toward the end of the rapid diastolic filling phase, they drift toward the closed position (F point) and are subsequently reopened by atrial contraction (A point), following which the two leaflets come into apposition (C point) immediately before the onset of systole. The anterior and posterior mitral valve leaflets remain in apposition throughout ventricular systole; their closure line moves slightly anteriorly before the valve reopens with the onset of diastole, which occurs within 0 to 10 ms of the onset of peak posterior wall

thickness. The excursion of the septum is less than that of the posterior wall when both anterior and posterior mitral valve leaflets are visualized in the basal segment of the ventricle by M-mode echocardiography (Fig. 3.8).

Measurements of left ventricular chamber diameter and septal and posterior wall thicknesses are made at the level of the tips of the mitral valve leaflets, where their free edges insert into the chordae tendineae (Fig. 3.9). The two-dimensional transducer is angled slightly caudally and laterally so that the M-mode beam tran-

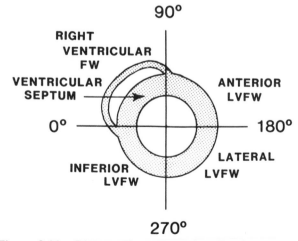

Figure 3.11. Diagramatic cross section of a short-axis section through the apex, showing the regional wall segments. (Reproduced with permission of the American Society of Echocardiography. The report of the ASE committee on nomenclature and standards: identification of myocardial wall segments, November, 1982.)

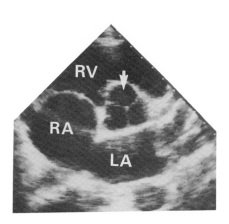
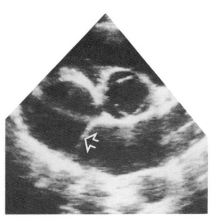

A   **B**

Figure 3.12. Two-dimensional echocardiogram of the short-axis view of the aorta at aortic valve level in diastole (*A*), showing the three aortic valve leaflets. The right coronary cusp is superior (*arrow*), the noncoronary cusp is on the left, and the left coronary cusp is on the right. The left atrium is posterior, the tricuspid valve is on the left, and the right ventricular outflow tract wraps around the aorta superiorly. The aortic leaflets are shown open during systole (*B*), and the interatrial septum is visualized running from the base of the noncoronary leaflet downward and to the left (*arrow*).

sects the left ventricle through its diameter. Left and right ventricular dimensions and septal and posterior left ventricular wall thicknesses are measured from M-mode echocardiograms using the leading edge methodology. That is, measurements are made from the leading edge of the initial echo boundary to the leading edge of the second echo boundary (3) (Fig. 3.9). Measurements are made at end diastole, using the point of the R wave on the simultaneously recorded EKG, and at end systole, defined echocardiographically as the most posterior excursion of the left side of the interventricular septum. The peak posterior excursion of the septum occurs earlier than peak posterior wall thickness and minimum left ventricular dimension (Fig. 3.9). The M-mode measurements of right and left ventricular chamber dimensions and septal and wall thicknesses at end diastole and at end systole have been normalized to unit body surface area in a large number of normal subjects of all ages, and these values are provided in the appendix.

Although the left ventricle can be imaged in multiple serial cross sections from the base to the apex by progressively angling the transducer caudally along the left ventricular long axis with the scan plane at right angles to it, short-axis sections of the left ventricle are obtained conventionally from three regions along its long axis: the basal, middle, and apical regions (Fig. 3.5).

Two-dimensional echo images of the short axis of the left ventricle at midcavity level are obtained by angling the transducer slightly caudally and laterally along the left ventricular long axis. The left ventricular free wall and septum at this level are also divided into octants similar to the basal segment (Fig. 3.10). The papillary muscles project into the left ventricular cavity and divide the free wall into the anterolateral and posterolateral regions, and into the inferior and inferoposterior regions, respectively. The papillary muscles may vary slightly in position, and infrequently, one may

appear larger in diameter than its counterpart, although this is usually due to improper rotation of the transducer. The septum is divided into three equal portions—inferior, middle, and anterior—similar to the right ventricular free wall. The left ventricle should appear circular in short axis, with uniform wall and septal thickness and concentric inward and outward wall motion in real time. If the ventricle at midcavity level is not circular in cross section, it may be necessary to move the transducer up an interspace to obtain a true short axis.

The short-axis echocardiographic images of the apical segments of the right and left ventricles are

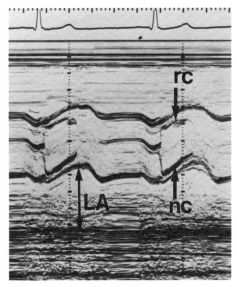

Figure 3.13. M-mode echocardiogram of the aorta, aortic valve, and left atrium from a normal subject. The aortic valve is seen between the anterior and posterior aortic roots with the right coronary cusp (rc), and the noncoronary cusp (nc) open widely in systole, almost in apposition with the aortic walls. The left atrium (LA) is posterior to the aorta and its dimension is measured at end ejection (*double arrows*).

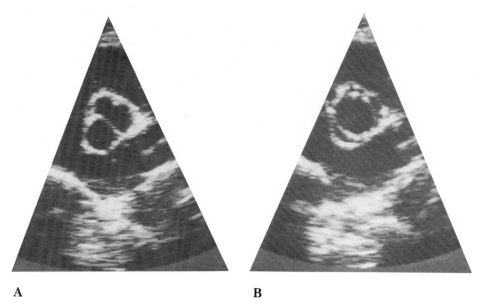

A   B

Figure 3.14.   Two-dimensional echocardiogram of the short axis of the aorta, showing a bicuspid aortic valve in diastole with a single commissure running obliquely from left to right, with almost equal sized cusps (*A*). In systole, the valve opens widely and is nonobstructive (*B*).

obtained by moving the transducer down one or two intercostal spaces, angling slightly toward the apex while keeping the scan plane at right angles to the long axis of the left ventricle. In this way the scan plane transects the left ventricle immediately below the level at which the papillary muscles take origin (Fig. 3.11). The left ventricular free wall and septum at this level are divided into quadrants. The septum and free right ventricular wall are visualized in the left upper quadrant. Left ventricular wall and septal thicknesses are uniform, and wall motion is concentric in systole and in diastole.

When the two-dimensional echo images of the short axis of the left ventricle at the basal, middle, and apical levels have been recorded, the transducer is returned to the position from which the mitral valve was imaged, and the scan plane is angled upward and medially to obtain a short-axis section of the aorta at aortic valve level (Fig. 3.12). If the valve leaflets are not well visualized, they can be brought into view by moving the transducer 1 to 2 cm laterally and angling more medially. The commissures of the three semilunar leaflets of the aortic valve run from the center of the aorta upward and leftward, upward and rightward, and ver-

Figure 3.15.   M-mode echocardiogram showing the pulmonic valve with the initial posterior deflection due to atrial systole (*arrows*), and then the brisk posterior motion as the valve opens.

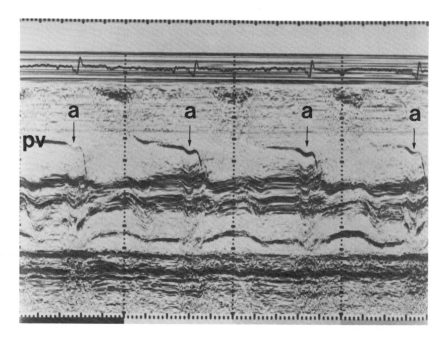

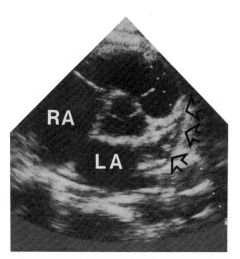

Figure 3.16. Two-dimensional echocardiogram showing the aorta and aortic valve in cross section with the pulmonary valve on the right. Note the left atrium posteriorly and the muscular trabeculations in the left atrial appendage (*arrows*).

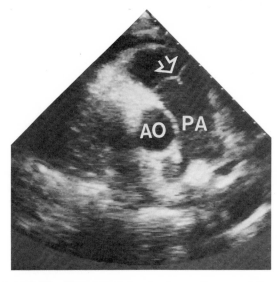

Figure 3.17. Two-dimensional echocardiogram of the right ventricular outflow tract and main pulmonary artery in long axis. The pulmonary valve is visualized (*arrow*), as is the bifurcation of the main pulmonary artery into its right and left branches.

tically downward (Fig. 3.12). The right coronary cusp is superior, the left coronary cusp is situated inferiorly and to the right, and the noncoronary cusp is positioned inferiorly and to the left.

When the two-dimensional images of the aortic valve and left atrium have been recorded, an M-mode echo can be obtained with two-dimensional echo guidance so that the M-mode beam passes through the right ventricular outflow tract, the aortic diameter at aortic valve cusp level, and the left atrium posteriorly (Fig. 3.13). The aortic valve leaflets on M-mode echo open rapidly with the onset of systolic ejection, during which the aorta moves anteriorly. The right coronary leaflet superiorly and the noncoronary leaflet inferiorly remain in the fully open position throughout systole, forming a boxlike configuration with the right coronary leaflet in apposition to the anterior aortic root and the noncoronary leaflet in apposition to the posterior aortic root (Fig. 3.13). The left coronary leaflet is not usually visualized by M-mode echo. The aortic leaflet closure line is usually in the middle of the aortic root. The whole aortic root moves anteriorly during left ventricular ejection and posteriorly in diastole. Measurement of left atrial dimension is made at end ejection. Aortic root dimension is measured at aortic valve opening, using the leading edge–to–leading edge technique recommended by the American Society of Echocardiography (Fig. 3.13). Between 0.8 and 1.0 percent of the normal population have a bicuspid aortic valve (4). Most commonly, the two cusps are almost the same size with a single commissure running obliquely from left to right (Fig. 3.14); however, a constellation of cusp sizes and commissural anatomy has been described. The anterior and septal leaflets of

the tricuspid valve are visible to the left of the aorta (Fig. 3.12). The interatrial septum is situated inferiorly and leftward of the noncoronary aortic cusp and runs obliquely posteriorly, so that the right atrium is to the left and the left atrium to the right, with the body of the left atrium inferoposterior to the aorta. In this plane the right ventricle is crescent-shaped, wrapping around the aorta from the tricuspid valve at left to the right ventricular outflow tract and the pulmonary valve to the right of the aorta. An M-mode echocardiogram can be obtained of the pulmonic valve by directing the

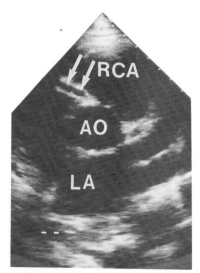

Figure 3.18. Two-dimensional echocardiogram of the aorta in short axis, angled to demonstrate the proximal right coronary artery (*arrows*). The ostia of the left coronary artery is also visible.

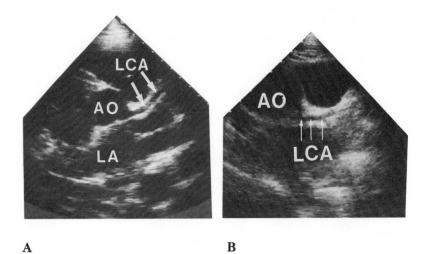

A   **B**

Figure 3.19. Two-dimensional echocardiogram of the aorta in short axis, angled to demonstrate the origin of the proximal course of the left main coronary artery (*A, arrow*). The proximal right coronary artery is also visible. The bifurcation of the left main coronary artery into left anterior descending and left circumflex branches can be seen in another patient (*B, arrows*).

cursor through it with two-dimensional imaging in this scan plane. The anterior position and characteristic abrupt posterior motion of the cusp of the pulmonary valve in systole is anteceded by a small dip posteriorly due to right atrial contraction (Fig. 3.15), which may disappear in pulmonary hypertension (5).

Slight angulation of the transducer scan plane enables visualization of the left atrial appendage with its narrow neck and trabeculated endocardial surface (Fig. 3.16). The atrial appendage extends laterally and superiorly almost to the commissure between the right and left coronary cusps, and overlies both the origin of the left main coronary artery and the main pulmonary trunk at the level of the pulmonary valve. The main pulmonary trunk courses vertically downward and may be imaged by superior and lateral angulation and 5- to 10-degree, counterclockwise rotation of the transducer. This demonstrates the main pulmonary artery bifurcation into left and right pulmonary arteries (Fig.

3.17). The proximal right pulmonary artery passes under the left atrium. This same scan plane transects the right coronary artery sinus above the right coronary leaflet of the aortic valve, so that the right coronary artery can be examined in its proximal course (Fig. 3.18), and sometimes as far as the origin of its acute marginal branch. The left main coronary artery can be visualized in a slightly different plane from the right coronary artery in its first 2 to 3 cm, and the origins of the left anterior descending and left circumflex branches can be imaged if the bifurcation occurs proximally (Fig. 3.19).

When the short-axis sections of the left ventricle and aorta have been recorded from the left parasternal position, the blood flow velocity profile in the right ventricular outflow tract and proximal main pulmonary artery should be assessed by pulsed wave Doppler. The main pulmonary trunk is first imaged in its long axis from the pulmonary valve to its primary bifurcation, so

Figure 3.20. Pulsed wave Doppler velocity signal obtained from the main pulmonary artery immediately distal to the pulmonary valve. Note the low peak velocity of 0.6 m/s.

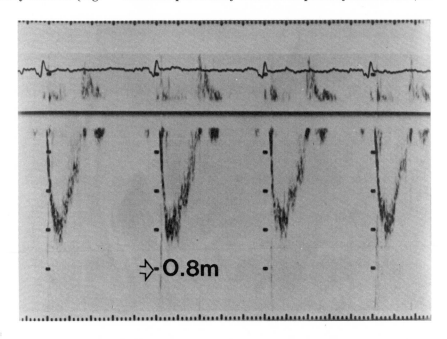

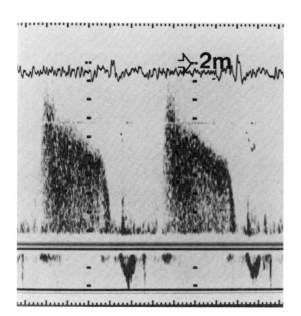

Figure 3.21. Pulsed wave Doppler velocity signal obtained from the right ventricular outflow tract immediately proximal to the pulmonary valve in a patient with pulmonary valve thickening and associated pulmonary regurgitation.

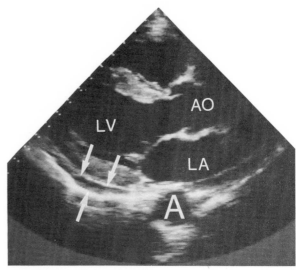

Figure 3.23. Two-dimensional echocardiogram of the left ventricular long axis from a patient with a small pericardial effusion, which is visible posteriorly (*arrows*). The fluid extends up to the atrioventricular groove, where the pericardium is reflected onto the pulmonary veins, and is anterior to the thoracic aorta (A). Its anterior relation to the thoracic aorta distinguishes pericardial from pleural effusions posterior to the heart.

that blood is flowing vertically downward in this imaging plane. It is important to ensure that the angle between the interrogating ultrasound beam and the direction of blood flow in the main pulmonary trunk is close to 0 degrees because the accuracy of the velocity

measurements are inversely proportional to the cosine of this angle (see Chapter 1). The Doppler sample volume is first positioned in the right ventricular outflow tract, approximately 1 cm proximal to the pulmonary valve. The direction of blood flow is away from

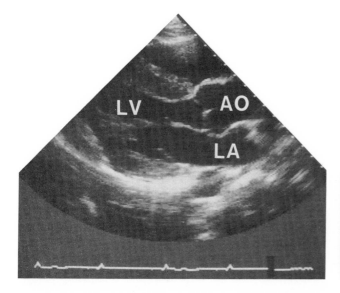

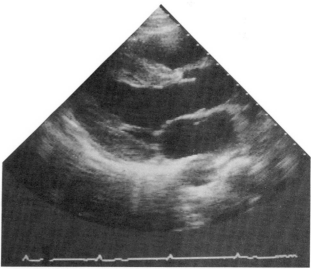

A   B

Figure 3.22. Two-dimensional echocardiogram of the long axis of the left ventricle in a normal subject in diastole (*A*), showing the aortic valve, the mitral leaflets and subvalve tensor apparatus, the septum, and the posterior LV wall. The thoracic aorta is visible posterior to the atrioventricular groove at the left ventricular–left atrial junction. In systole (*B*), the aortic valve leaflets open and are retracted into their respective sinuses of Valsalva; the mitral valve is in the closed position with the left atrium posterior to the aorta.

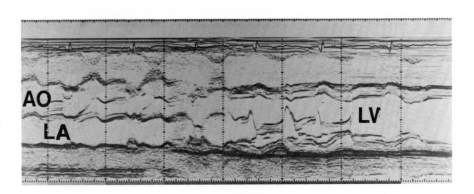

Figure 3.24. M-mode echocardiographic sweep from the aorta on the left to the left ventricular cavity on the right. The aortic root is continuous with the interventricular septum, and the posterior aortic root is continuous with the anterior mitral valve leaflet.

the transducer, and by convention is displayed as a negative signal on the lower register. The blood flow velocity spectral display recorded from the pulmonary artery and the right ventricular outflow tract in normal subjects consists of a thin velocity envelope indicating laminar flow, with acquisition of the peak velocity in midsystole (Fig. 3.20). The peak amplitude in normal subjects ranges from 0.4 to 0.7 m/s (6). A minor degree of pulmonary regurgitation has been reported by Doppler in almost one-third of normal subjects (7) as a short-duration signal early in diastole, displayed on the upper register and indicating regurgitant flow across the pulmonic valve toward the transducer (Fig. 3.21). The Doppler sample volume is then positioned 1 cm beyond the pulmonary valve and the blood flow velocity recorded. The blood flow velocity profile and the peak velocity are similar to those obtained in the right ventricular outflow tract.

Left Ventricular Long-Axis View

The transducer is angled to obtain the left ventricular short axis at mitral valve level and then rotated counterclockwise 90 degrees without changing its position on the skin, so that the scan plane is parallel to the left ventricular long axis (Fig. 3.22). This brings into view the posterior wall of the left ventricle from the atrioventricular groove to within about 3 cm of the apex; the interventricular septum from its membranous insertion into the anterior aortic root, almost to the apex of the left ventricle; the anterior and posterior mitral valve leaflets; the right coronary aortic valve leaflet (superiorly) and the noncoronary aortic valve leaflet (inferiorly), in their respective sinuses of Valsalva; the proximal 3 to 5 cm of the ascending aorta; the left atrium; the descending thoracic aorta; and right ventricular outflow tract. The left-sided ventriculoarterial connec-

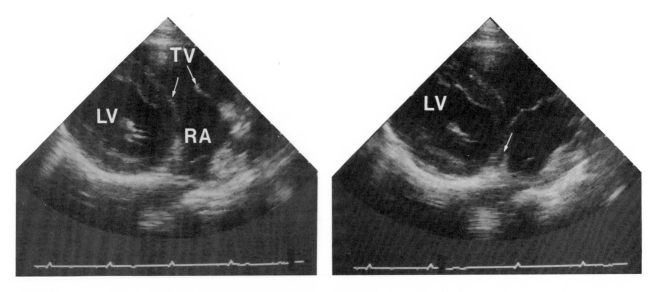

A   **B**

Figure 3.25. Two-dimensional echocardiogram of the right ventricular outflow tract, showing the anterior and septal tricuspid valve leaflets in diastole (*A, arrows*). The interventricular septum runs upward and to the left. The anterior and septal tricuspid valve leaflets are in apposition during systole (*B*), the coronary sinus is shown by the arrow.

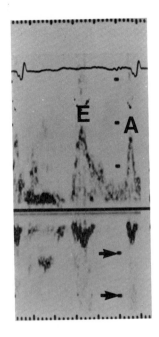

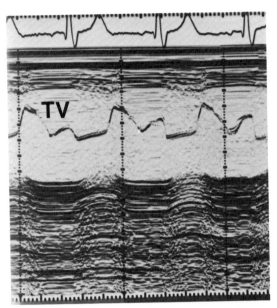

A   B

Figure 3.26. M-mode echocardiogram of the tricuspid valve, showing initial rapid anterior motion, followed by partial closure and reopening with atrial contraction (A). Pulsed wave Doppler velocity signal of transtricuspid blood flow (B) with a peak velocity of 0.4 m/s during the rapid filling wave (E wave), and the peak velocity during atriosystolic contraction (A wave) of 0.3 m/s. The transtricuspid valve velocities during rapid filling and atrial contraction are consistently lower than the peak E wave and A wave velocities of transmitral flow. The calibration marks represent 20 cm/s (*arrows*).

tions can be demonstrated in this view with the membranous intraventricular septum contiguous with the anterior aortic root and anterior mitral valve leaflet with the posterior aortic root. The transducer should be rotated and angled until the scan plane is correctly aligned with the left ventricular long axis, in which both the aortic valve leaflets and the mitral valve leaflets are seen opening and closing alternately in real time. In this scan plane the interventricular septum runs horizontally from the anterior aortic root; if the septum angles upward toward the apex, the transducer is too low on the chest wall. Slight oblique angulation of the scan plane from the long axis demonstrates the tensor apparatus of the posteromedial papillary muscle with its chordae tendineae running to both anterior and posterior mitral valve leaflets. The apex of the left ventricle is imaged only in the long axis from the parasternal position. When the scan plane is rotated off axis, the ultrasound beam transects the left ventricle obliquely truncating its long axis.

The two-dimensional long axis scan plane is invaluable in detecting pericardial effusions and in distinguishing them from left-sided pleural effusions. The pericardium is reflected onto the pulmonary veins at the posterior atrioventricular groove, and thus pericardial effusions do not accumulate behind the left atrium unless there are abnormal pericardial reflections (Fig. 3.23). Furthermore, pericardial effusions in the two-dimensional echo long view of the left ventricle are anterior to the thoracic aorta, while pleural effusions are posterior to the thoracic aorta.

An M-mode echocardiographic sweep can be re-corded by slowly angling the M-mode cursor with two-dimensional imaging from the aorta toward the apex of the left ventricular cavity, making sure that the cursor passes through the diameters of the aorta and left ventricular cavity. This demonstrates the left-sided ventriculoarterial and atrioventricular connections and is helpful in detecting posterior pericardial effusions (Fig. 3.24).

Right Ventricular Inflow Tract

The right ventricular inflow tract can be visualized from the left parasternal region by first obtaining a good long-axis view of the left ventricle then angling the transducer medially and caudally, and rotating the scan plane between 15 and 20 degrees counterclockwise (Fig. 3.25). Sometimes it may be necessary to move the transducer scanhead down one interspace. A foreshortened image of the right ventricle is obtained with its apex pointing upward and leftward, showing the trabeculated endocardial surface of the right ventricle. The motion of the septal and larger anterior leaflet of the tricuspid valve can be visualized well from this scan plane (Fig. 3.25). The leaflets drift into apposition at end diastole, following right atrial systole. The large anterior leaflet has a wide excursion, sweeping posteriorly to coapt with the septal and posterior leaflets such that the line of coaption is at right angles to the direction of blood flow, with the tips of the leaflets pointing toward the right ventricular apex (Fig. 3.25). The right atrium is inferior and rightward of the right ventricle, with the coronary venous sinus toward

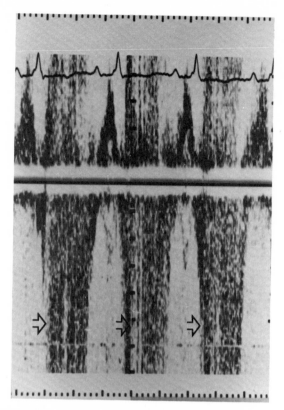

Figure 3.27. Pulsed wave Doppler recording from the right atrium showing high velocity systolic signals of retrograde blood flow due to tricuspid regurgitation. The velocity signal aliases and appears on the upper register. The pulsed wave sample volume is being used here, not to measure flow velocity but to detect the presence and location of abnormal flow. The calibration marks represent 20 cm/s (*arrows*).

the septal surface. The wide base of the right atrial appendix is contiguous with the atrioventricular groove proximal to the origin of the anterior tricuspid valve leaflet. This right ventricular inflow scan plane enables close inspection of the tricuspid leaflets and subvalve apparatus and Doppler assessment of blood flow velocity profiles across the tricuspid valve.

The pulsed wave Doppler sample volume is positioned in the middle of the right ventricular inflow tract 1 cm distal to the tricuspid valve, so that the ultrasound beam is parallel to the direction of blood flow and the maximum velocity profile recorded. Blood flow across the tricuspid valve in this plane is toward the transducer and will therefore be displayed by convention as a positive signal in the upper register (Fig. 3.26). The velocity profile in the right ventricular inflow tract in the normal heart has a thin spectral envelope consistent with laminar blood flow. There is an initial peak velocity occurring soon after tricuspid valve opening during rapid right ventricular filling, which is known as the E wave. This is followed by a fall in blood flow

velocity as the ventricle reaches 75 to 80 percent of its total end-diastolic volume. Toward the end of diastole, there is a second but smaller peak in the velocity profile, which is known as the A wave and results from the increase in blood flow velocity during right atrial contraction. The peak blood flow velocities across the tricuspid valve vary from 0.4 to 0.8 m/s (6). The ratio of the peak velocities during the E and A waves—the E/A ratio—may relate to right ventricular diastolic function similar to the mitral E/A ratio in the left heart. The mitral and tricuspid E/A velocity ratios vary with age, being less than unity in utero (8) and greater than unity after birth (9).

The right ventricular inflow tract scan plane is also useful for detecting regurgitant flow across the tricuspid valve. The direction of regurgitant flow into the right atrium is away from the transducer, so that it is represented as a negative signal and appears on the inferior register. However, regurgitant flow has a high velocity that exceeds the Nyquist limit and therefore aliases, and also appears on the upper or positive register, resulting in directional ambiguity (Fig. 3.27). Tricuspid regurgitation signals have been reported in between 20 and 44 percent of normal subjects (7), with a still greater frequency during pregnancy (10). When tricuspid regurgitation is detected, its severity should be evaluated by flow mapping of the right atrium as previously described (11), and graded from 1+ to 4+ in increasing order of severity (Fig. 3.28). Flow mapping entails positioning the ultrasound beam so that it is parallel to antegrade blood flow across the tricuspid valve. The right atrium is divided into four regions related to the tricuspid valve ring (Fig. 3.28). The Doppler sample volume is positioned in each slice and the sample volume is moved from one side of each slice to the other to detect the regurgitant jet. If the jet is detected only in the slice adjacent to the tricuspid valve, this is grade 1 (mild) tricuspid regurgitation; whereas if the regurgitant signal is detected throughout the right atrium, this is grade 4 (severe) tricuspid regurgitation. When tricuspid regurgitation is present, the peak velocity of the regurgitant jet should be measured with continuous wave Doppler (Fig. 3.29) (which is used to measure high velocities), and from this peak velocity a reliable indirect estimation of pulmonary artery systolic pressure can be obtained from the Bernoulli equation (12) (see Chapter 7).

Right Ventricular Outflow Tract

The right ventricular outflow tract can be imaged, with the transducer 2 to 3 cm lateral to the left sternal border in the third or fourth intercostal space, by cephalad angulation and clockwise rotation from the

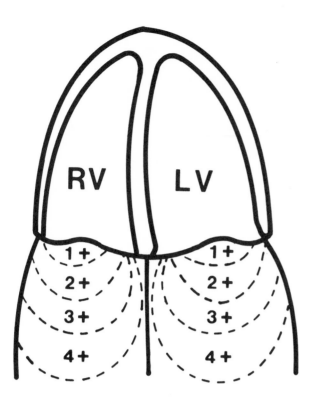

Figure 3.28.   Schematic demonstrating pulsed wave Doppler assessment of the severity of tricuspid regurgitation by flow mapping. The right atrium is arbitrarily divided into four regions. When the velocity signal is detectable only immediately proximal to the valve, this indicates mild, or 1+, tricuspid regurgitation. When the signal is detectable throughout the right atrium, the tricuspid regurgitation is severe, or 4+.

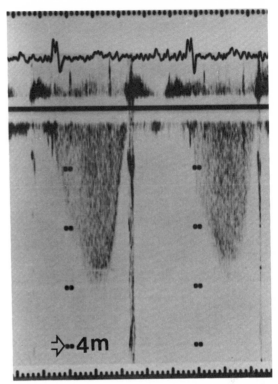

Figure 3.29.   Continuous wave Doppler velocity signal of tricuspid regurgitation, obtained from the apex, shows a holosystolic signal with a maximum velocity of 2.9 m/s occurring in midsystole. The right atrium–right ventricular systolic pressure gradient can be obtained from the Bernoulli equation [$P = 4v^2$, which equals $4(2.8)^2$ or 31]. Pulmonary artery systolic pressure can be calculated either by adding to this the clinical estimate of right atrial pressure, or by adding 14 mm Hg, which results in a PA systolic pressure of approximately 45 mm Hg (See Chapter 7).

position from which images of the right ventricular inflow tract were obtained. This brings into view the pulmonary valve leaflets, the right ventricular outflow tract, and the infundibulum and proximal interventricular septum. Posterior to the interventricular septum are the left ventricular outflow and inflow tracts juxtaposed, the mitral valve apparatus, and the left atrium (Fig. 3.30).

Left Parasternal Four-Chamber View

A limited view of the four cardiac chambers can be obtained from the left parasternal region, with the transducer in the third to fifth intercostal space, by angling and rotating the scan plane counterclockwise from the position used to obtain images of the normal left ventricular long axis. This scan plane transects the right and left ventricles, obliquely truncating their long axes so that neither of the apices are visible, but allows visualization of both atrioventricular valves, the tricuspid valve superiorly, and the mitral valve inferiorly (Fig. 3.31). The interventricular septum is imaged in

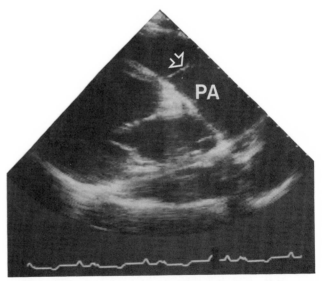

Figure 3.30.   Two-dimensional echocardiogram of the right ventricular outflow tract, showing the right ventricular infundibulum, pulmonary valve (*arrow*), and the main pulmonary artery.

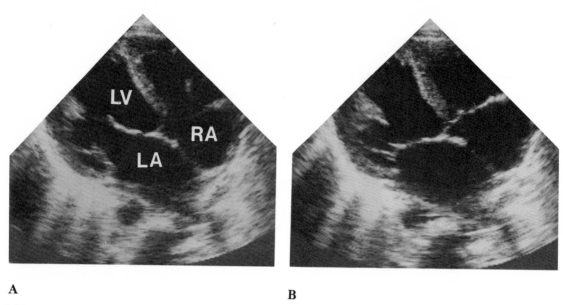

Figure 3.31.   Two-dimensional echocardiogram of the four cardiac chambers obtained from the left parasternal region in diastole (A) and in systole (B).

profile, running toward the apices of the two ventricles upward and leftward, with the trabeculated right-sided surface superiorly and the smooth left ventricular surface inferiorly. The transition of the interventricular septum from its distal muscular to its proximal membranous portion and the junction with the interatrial septum can be clearly visualized. The more apical origin of the septal leaflet of the tricuspid valve, and the more proximal origin of the septal leaflet of the mitral valve at the crux of the heart can be appreciated from this scan plane. The septum between the origins of the

right- and left-sided atrioventricular valves is the atrioventricular septum. The interatrial septum is visualized in profile in this view running from the crux of the heart to the fossa ovalis (which may appear thinned out or absent) to the roof of the atria, dividing them into left- and right-sided chambers. Evaluation of the crux of the heart and, in particular, the junction of the interventricular septum with the atrioventricular septum, the interatrial septum, and the origin of the right- and left-sided atrioventricular valve leaflets is of paramount importance in patients with malformations

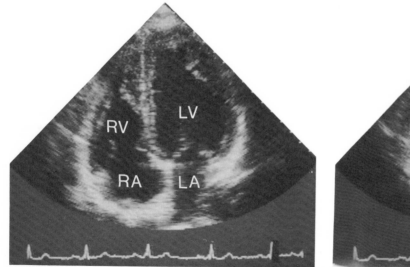

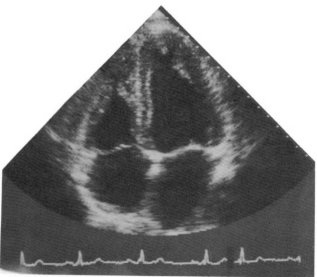

Figure 3.32.   Two-dimensional echocardiogram of the apical four-chamber view in diastole (A), showing the tricuspid and mitral valve leaflets open, respectively, and in systole (B), during which the atrioventricular valves are closed.

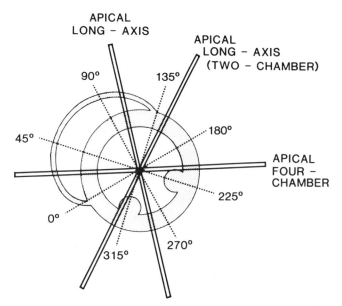

Figure 3.33. Schematic demonstrating the orientation of the apical four-chamber view of the LV short axis, the apical two-chamber view, and the apical LV long-axis view. (Reproduced with permission of the American Society of Echocardiography. The report of the ASE committee on nomenclature and standards: identification of myocardial wall segments, November, 1982.)

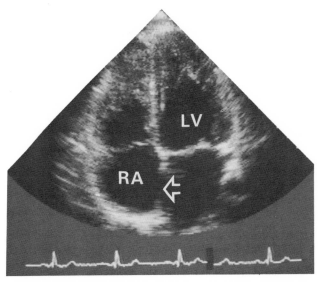

Figure 3.35. Two-dimensional echocardiogram of the apical four-chamber view, showing the echo dropout in the interatrial septum at the fossa ovalis (*arrow*).

and abnormal development of the endocardial cushions.

Apical Position

Four- and Five-Chamber Views

The point of maximal cardiac impulse is located with the index finger, with the patient supine and rotated 60 degrees to the left side. The transducer is applied slightly lateral and inferior to the point of maximal

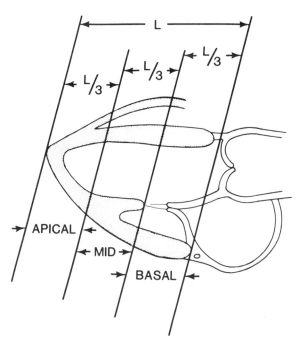

Figure 3.34. Schematic showing division of the left ventricle into three regions along its long axis. The basal third includes the mitral valve, the middle third includes the papillary muscles, and the apical third includes the apex of the ventricle. (Reproduced with permission of the American Society of Echocardiography. The report of the ASE committee on nomenclature and standards: identification of myocardial wall segments, November, 1982.)

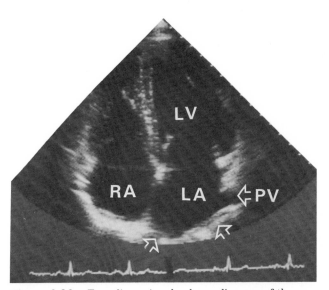

Figure 3.36. Two-dimensional echocardiogram of the apical four-chamber view in diastole, showing the positions of three of the four pulmonary veins draining into the left atrium (*arrows*). From left to right they are the right superior pulmonic vein, the left superior and the left inferior pulmonic veins.

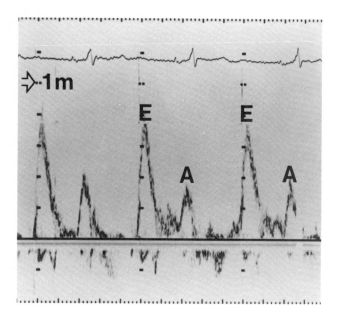

Figure 3.37. Pulsed wave Doppler flow velocity signals recorded across the mitral valve, with the sample volume positioned in the middle of the mitral valve anulus. There is an increase in velocity immediately following mitral valve opening (E wave), with a peak velocity of approximately 0.8 m/s during the rapid diastolic filling phase. Note the narrow velocity envelope indicating laminar flow. A second peak in the velocity signal of 0.4 m/s occurs during atriosystolic contraction (A wave).

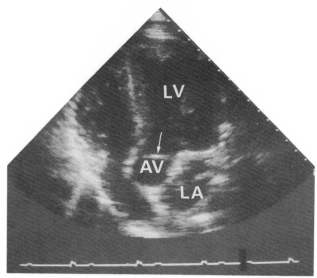

Figure 3.38. Two-dimensional echocardiogram obtained from the apex, showing the five-chamber view. The fifth chamber is the left ventricular outflow tract. The other four chambers include the right and left ventricles and right and left atria. The aortic valve (*arrow*) can be seen in the closed position.

cardiac impulse and directed toward the right shoulder, with the scan plane oriented at right angles to the interventricular septum. The images obtained from the apex with the scan plane in this orientation show the left ventricle on the right and the right ventricle on the left, with the interventricular septum visualized in profile, in its entirety, and running vertically from the crux to the apex of the heart (Fig. 3.32). The interventricular septum should be vertical in the apical four-chamber view. If it points upward and leftward, the transducer should be moved laterally; if it points upward and rightward, move the transducer medially on the chest wall.

The moderator band in the right ventricle takes origin from the apical third of the septum at an acute angle, carrying the specialized conducting tissue to the right ventricular free wall (Fig. 3.32). The right ventricular wall and the right ventricular surface of the interventricular septum are noticeably more trabeculated than the left ventricular wall and left side of the septum. This feature is used to determine ventricular morphology in patients with congenital heart disease. Care must be taken to avoid foreshortening the right and left ventricular and atrial chambers when recording images from the apex, which is a frequent mistake of the novice sonographer. When the correct orienta-

tion is obtained of the four cardiac chambers from the apex, the length of the normal left atrium is between one-half and one-third that of the left ventricular length. The left ventricular apex should be conical or bullet-shaped. The septal leaflet of the tricuspid valve takes its origin from the interventricular septum be

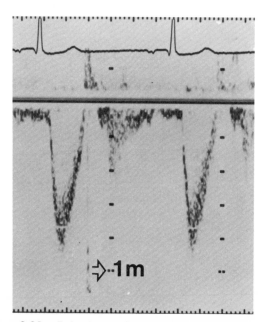

Figure 3.39. Pulsed wave Doppler blood flow velocity signal obtained from the left ventricular outflow tract, showing a peak velocity of 0.8 m/s, with acquisition of a maximum velocity in early systole.

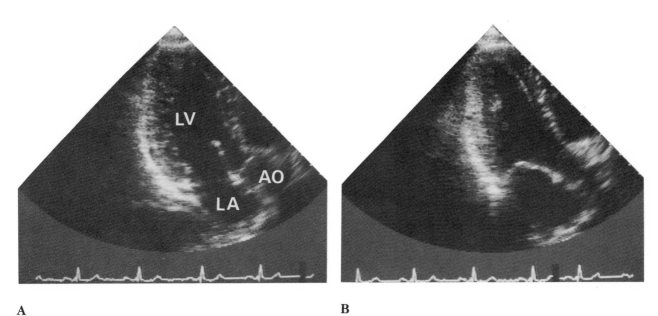

A   **B**

Figure 3.40.   Two-dimensional echocardiogram of the apical LV long-axis view in a normal subject in diastole (*A*) and systole (*B*).

tween 3 and 8 mm distal to the origin of the septal (anterior) leaflet of the mitral valve. In the normal heart, the different origins of the two atrioventricular valves at the crux of the heart are easily appreciated, but this relationship is altered in some congenital cardiac anomalies, such as complete atrioventricular canal and Ebstein's anomaly (see Chapters 25 and 28).

The walls of the left ventricle visualized in the apical four-chamber view are the posterior interventricular septum and the lateral wall (Fig. 3.33). This view is particularly important for studying regional wall motion abnormalities involving the septum and lateral wall in coronary artery disease. The lateral wall and septum are divided into the same three levels visualized in the short-axis views of the left ventricle (Fig. 3.34). No attempts should be made to measure left ventricular wall or septal thicknesses from the apical four-chamber view because endocardial definition is poor. This poor endocardial definition is due to the ultrasound beam being parallel to, rather than at the ideal 90-degree angle to, the left ventricular walls. Minor angulation of the scan plane from the apex demonstrates the papillary muscle and its tensor apparatus extending to the tips of both mitral valve leaflets. The mitral valve leaflets coapt at end diastole such that they form a line joining the septal and lateral aspects of the mitral valve anulus (Fig. 3.32). The anterior and posteroinferior walls are not visualized in this view.

The interatrial septum in the adult heart extends from the crux to the roof of the atria with the fossa ovalis located in the middle (Fig. 3.35). The fossa ovalis usually appears thinner than the rest of the intra-atrial septum, in which there is often adipose tissue between

the endocardial surfaces. The fossa ovalis may appear as an area of echo dropout, and the thin flaplike structure may not be appreciated. No attempts should be made to assess interatrial septal thickness from the apical four-chamber view. It appears thicker than it is in reality because the ultrasound beam begins to diverge the further it is from its source. The pulmonary veins are visualized entering the left atrium posterolaterally; the most frequently visualized are the right and left superior pulmonary veins and the inferior left pulmonary vein (Fig. 3.36).

When high-quality images of the apical four-chamber view of the heart have been recorded, the next objective is to assess the blood flow velocity profiles across the right ventricular and left ventricular inflow tracts. The apical four-chamber view is ideal for assessing these blood flow velocity profiles because the angle between the ultrasound beam and the direction of blood flow is close to zero. The pulsed wave Doppler sample volume is positioned in the respective ventricles, immediately subjacent to the mitral or tricuspid valve leaflets. The blood flow velocity signal across the mitral valve demonstrates an immediate increase in velocity following mitral valve opening, reaching a peak early during rapid left ventricular filling of between 0.6 and 1.0 m/s. This is termed the E wave (Fig. 3.37). Blood flow velocity diminishes during slow filling, and a second peak blood flow velocity, known as the A wave, occurs due to atrial contraction, and has a velocity of 0.4 to 0.8 m/s. The normal transmitral velocity profile has a thin spectral envelope, indicating laminar flow across the mitral valve orifice. The peak E wave velocity in normal subjects is greater than the

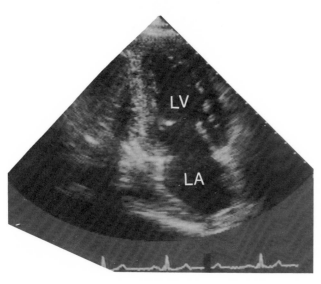

A

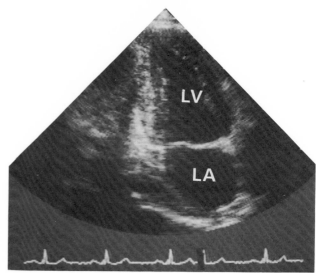

B

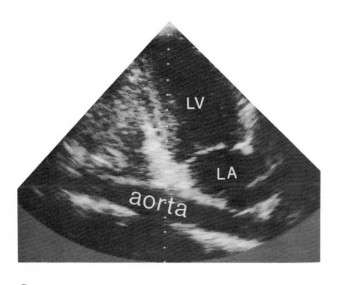

C

Figure 3.41.   Two-dimensional echocardiogram of the apical two-chamber view, showing the left ventricle and left atrium with the mitral valve open in diastole (*A*), and extending across the left ventricular outflow tract in systole, separating the two chambers (*B*). The descending thoracic aorta is visualized behind the left atrium in the two-chamber view by inferior and medial angulation of the transducer (*C*).

peak A wave velocity, and thus the E/A ratio is greater than 1.0, although this ratio varies with age, heart rate, and ventricular loading conditions (9). The transmitral blood flow velocity profile is altered by changes in left ventricular compliance; for example, in severe hypertrophy (13) and in coronary artery disease, the A wave velocity may increase and the E wave velocity decrease such that the E/A ratio is less than 1.0. The ratio of E/A wave velocities has thus been advocated as an index of diastolic function (14) and appears to correlate with left ventricular architecture expressed as the ratio of mass and volume (15).

Attempts have been made to assess volume flow across the mitral valve orifice in the normal heart as the product of the cross-sectional area of the mitral

valve orifice and the mitral blood flow velocity integral, which is the area under the blood flow velocity profile across the mitral valve (16). The mitral valve orifice area has been calculated by measuring the diameter of the mitral valve anulus in the apical four-chamber view and making three assumptions: 1) the mitral valve orifice is circular, 2) the mitral orifice area does not change in shape during diastole, and 3) the mitral valve area remains constant throughout diastole.

The Doppler sample volume is positioned in the left atrium to detect regurgitant flow across the mitral valve in systole, which has been reported in a small proportion of normal subjects but is usually of no hemodynamic consequence (7). The left atrium is divided into four equal regions in relation to the mitral

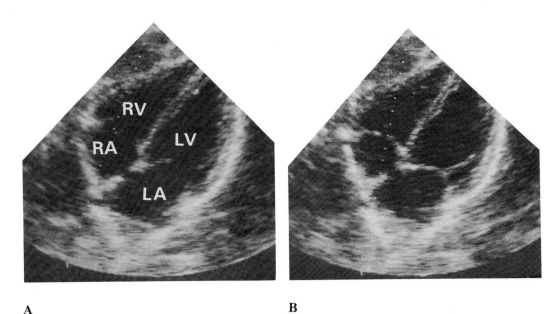

A   B

Figure 3.42.   Two-dimensional echocardiogram showing the four cardiac chambers from the subcostal root, with the interventricular septum running diagonally upward and to the right from the crux of the heart to the apex in diastole (*A*) and systole (*B*).

valve anulus. Each region is systematically scanned with the Doppler sample volume from the interatrial septum to the lateral left atrial wall to detect and semiquantitate the severity of mitral regurgitation (Fig. 3.28). If a regurgitant jet is detected only in the region adjacent to the mitral valve anulus, this is graded as mild or 1+ mitral regurgitation; whereas if the regurgitant signal is detectable throughout the four regions, this is graded severe or 4+ mitral regurgitation. This semiquantitative assessment of the severity of mitral regurgitation corresponds closely to the grades of severity assessed by left ventricular contrast angiography. Identification and semiquantitation of mitral and tricuspid regurgitation is facilitated by the use of Doppler color flow mapping (Chap. 7).

Blood flow velocity spectral envelopes are also obtained in the right heart chambers by positioning the sample volume first in the right ventricle immediately subjacent to the tricuspid valve to examine right ventricular inflow blood flow velocity profiles. Following this, the Doppler sample volume can be positioned in the right atrium in the middle of the tricuspid valve anulus to detect tricuspid regurgitation by flow mapping—if high-quality Doppler recordings have not been obtained in the right ventricular inflow tract view from the left parasternal position.

Apical Five-Chamber View

Superior angulation of the transducer by 10 to 20 degrees from the apical four-chamber view without any change in rotation opens up the left ventricular outflow

tract and brings into view the apical five-chamber view (Fig. 3.38). The fifth chamber is the complete left ventricular outflow tract, aortic valve, and 1 to 2 cm of the proximal ascending aorta. This scan plane may provide clinically important diagnostic information when the aortic valve leaflets cannot be imaged satisfactorily from the left parasternal or subcostal views. The apical five-chamber view is used routinely to examine the blood flow velocity profiles in the left ventricular outflow tract when the pulsed wave Dopp-

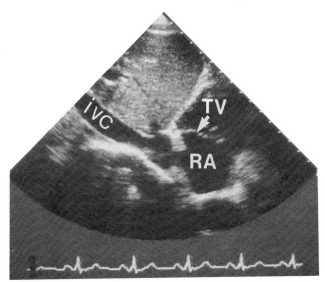

Figure 3.43.   Two-dimensional echocardiogram, obtained from the subcostal route, showing the inferior vena cava running into the right atrium, the tricuspid valve (*arrow*), the right ventricle, and the liver anteriorly and to the right.

Figure 3.44. Pulsed wave Doppler blood flow velocity signal obtained from the middle hepatic vein in a normal subject. The horizontal arrow (*top left*) equals zero velocity. Following the P wave on the electrocardiogram, there is a small positive wave (*arrow*) due to reversed blood flow during systole, which occurs because there are no valves between the right atrium and the cavae. The peak velocities of the two subsequent negative waves vary slightly with the respiratory cycle. The initial negative wave represents acceleration of blood toward the heart as the right ventricle contracts and the pericardial pressure falls. The second wave represents acceleration of blood into the right ventricle as the tricuspid valve opens at the beginning of diastolic filling.

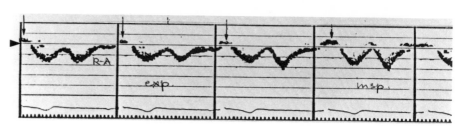

ler sample volume is positioned 1 cm proximal to the aortic valve leaflets. The blood flow velocity profile obtained in the normal heart shows a thin velocity envelope with acquisition of the peak velocity early in systole (Fig. 3.39), which varies in amplitude from 0.7 to 1.5 m/s (6). There should be no blood velocity signal in the left ventricular outflow tract in diastole in normal subjects, but in patients with aortic regurgitation, a high velocity signal greater than 2.0 m/s resulting in aliasing indicates the presence of regurgitant blood flowing toward the transducer. In patients with aortic regurgitation, the regurgitant jet of blood is detected by pulsed wave Doppler sampling in the apical five-chamber view or apical long-axis view (see Chapter 8). Doppler color flow mapping is especially helpful in characterizing the aortic regurgitant jet (see Chapter 8).

Apical Long-Axis View

In the apical four- and five-chamber views, the anterior and inferior left ventricular walls are not visible because they are in front of and behind these scan planes, respectively. By slow counterclockwise rotation of the transducer from the four-chamber view without changing the transducer angulation, the scan plan transects the left ventricle in long axis with the anterior septum on the right and the inferoposterior wall on the left, so that their wall motion can be evaluated. The left ventricular inflow tract and outflow tract are visualized adjacent to one another. The left atrium, both mitral valve leaflets, and the right and noncoronary aortic valve leaflets can also be seen (Fig. 3.40). As with the apical four-chamber view, care must be taken to avoid foreshortening of the left ventricular long axis. Doppler

Figure 3.45. Pulsed wave Doppler velocity signals recorded from the inferior vena cava showing the same wave form as recorded from the middle hepatic vein. There is flow reversal during atrial systole (*arrow*) and two consecutive negative velocity waves. The first of these occurs during right ventricular ejection, and the second when the tricuspid valve opens, initiating the rapid right ventricular filling phase. P refers to the P wave on EKG and 0 to zero velocity.

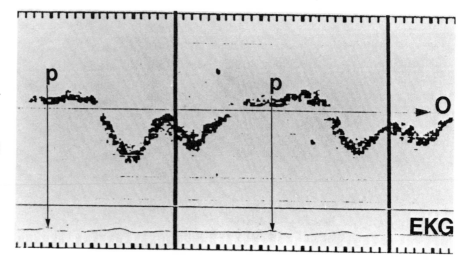

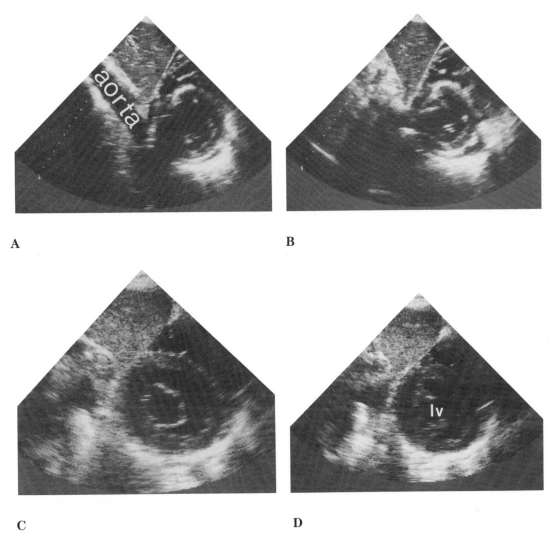

A   **B**

C   **D**

Figure 3.46.   Two-dimensional echocardiogram showing the short-axis view of the left ventricle from the subcostal route in diastole with the mitral valve open (*A* and *C*), in systole (*B* and *D*).

sampling of the left atrium for mitral regurgitation and the left ventricular inflow and outflow tracts can be accomplished from this scan plane. It is the plane of choice for Doppler examination of fixed and dynamic left ventricular outflow tract obstruction.

Apical Two-Chamber View

Clockwise rotation of the scan plane from the apical long-axis view of the left ventricle brings into view the apical two-chamber view of the left ventricle. The scan plane in this two-chamber view transects the anterior left ventricular wall on the right and the inferior left ventricular wall on the left (Fig. 3.41). The left ventricular apex points upward, the mitral valve extends all the way across the atrioventricular groove, and the left atrium is positioned inferiorly. The left ventricle is subdivided into three regions so that wall motion can be assessed and semiquantitated. The blood flow ve-

locity profile across the mitral valve and flow mapping of the left atrium can be examined by Doppler, as in the other apical views. Medial and inferior angulation of the transducer from the apical two-chamber view demonstrates the descending thoracic aorta (Fig. 3.41).

Subcostal Views

Images of the four cardiac chambers and great vessels can also be obtained from the subcostal route. This is of clinical importance, particularly in patients in whom echocardiographic images obtained from the left parasternal or apical transducer locations are suboptimal. In patients with chronic obstructive pulmonary disease, the diaphragm is usually depressed and the heart is more vertical, so that it is especially amenable to imaging from the subcostal region. The patient is placed supine, with the hips and knees flexed to relax the rectus abdominus muscle, which runs in the ante-

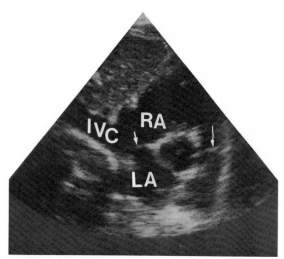

Figure 3.47. Two-dimensional echocardiogram obtained from the subcostal route, showing the short-axis aorta at aortic valve level in diastole with the trileaflet aortic valve and pulmonary valve closed (*long arrow*). The inferior vena cava is on the left and the interatrial septum runs horizontally from the inferior vena cava to the aorta (*short arrow*). The pulmonary artery is seen in long axis running vertically downward from the pulmonary valve.

rior abdominal wall from the lower costal margin to the symphysis pubis. Imaging from the subcostal route is facilitated when the patient sustains full inspiration. The transducer is positioned in the subxiphoid region and angled toward the left shoulder with the scan plane parallel to the precordium in the coronal plane. From this scan plane, a four-chamber view is obtained (Fig. 3.42) with the apex of the heart pointing upward and to the right, and the right heart chambers juxtaposed to

the diaphragm and liver, anterior and leftward to the left heart chambers. This four-chamber view is particularly useful for visualizing the tricuspid valve apparatus, the right atrium, and the right ventricle.

The interatrial septum and interventricular septum are both visualized in profile, running obliquely from left to right (Fig. 3.42). In this view, the interatrial septum can be inspected carefully from the roof of the atrial cavities to the foramen ovale, and from the foramen ovale to the crux of the heart. This is useful for excluding atrial septal defects, especially sinus venosus defects. The tricuspid valve leaflets and subvalve tensor apparatus can be assessed better in this scan plane than in the apical four-chamber view.

Angulation of the transducer to the right shoulder brings into view the tricuspid valve, the right atrium, the hepatic venous system, and, in particular, the middle hepatic vein and the inferior vena cava as it enters the right atrium (Fig. 3.43). The superior vena cava is rarely visualized from the subcostal route in adults. The blood flow velocity profiles in the systemic veins may be assessed by placing the Doppler sample volume in the middle hepatic vein, which runs vertically with an angle between the direction of blood flow and the Doppler beam of almost zero. Blood flow in the middle hepatic vein, inferior vena cava, and superior vena cava is laminar and pulsatile, with the velocities varying in amplitude with the respiratory cycle (Fig. 3.44). Flow in the inferior vena cava reverses temporarily during right atrial systole, but this is followed by two discrete waves of flow toward the heart, the first during right ventricular systole, and the second imme-

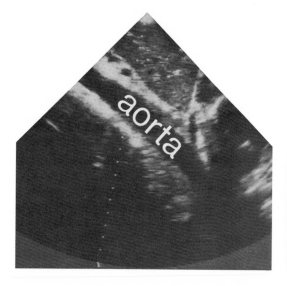

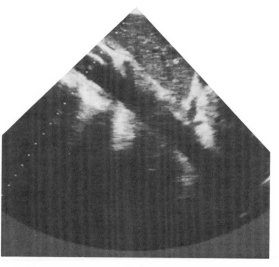

A   B

Figure 3.48. Two-dimensional echocardiogram of the subcostal route showing the thoracoabdominal aorta (*A*) with the celiac axis at top left (*B*). The celiac and superior mesenteric arteries are seen taking origin from the aorta anteriorly (*B*); the celiac artery is on the right.

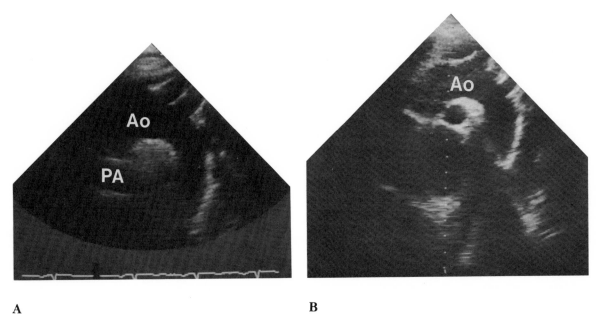

A   **B**

Figure 3.49. Two-dimensional echocardiogram obtained from the suprasternal notch, showing the aortic arch, the brachiocephalic branches, and the proximal descending thoracic aorta (*A*). The right pulmonary artery is seen in short axis passing under the aortic arch (*B*).

diately following tricuspid valve opening at the onset of the right ventricular rapid diastolic filling phase (Fig. 3.45).

When the four-chamber views have been acquired, the transducer is rotated clockwise so that the scan plane is directed sagittally but angled slightly toward the left shoulder. This scan plane brings into view the right ventricle and left ventricle in short axis (Fig. 3.46). Minor manipulation of the transducer is often necessary to obtain a true short axis, which shows the left ventricle as completely circular with concentric wall motion in real time. The short-axis section through the base of the left ventricle demonstrates both anterior and posterior mitral valve leaflets. The plane of the mitral commissures is shifted 30 to 60 degrees clock-

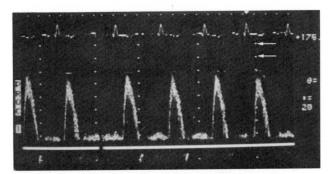

Figure 3.50. Pulsed wave Doppler velocity signal recorded from the ascending aorta with a maximum velocity of 1.0 m/s. 0 calibration markers equal 20 cm/s (*arrows*).

wise from the left ventricular short axis obtained from the left parasternal position (Fig. 3.46). The right ventricular cavity and free wall is anterior to the septum. To obtain short-axis views of the left ventricle at midcavity and apical levels, the transducer is angled progressively toward the left. Left ventricular wall motion can be assessed from the subcostal position in serial short-axis sections, but care must be taken to ensure that the left ventricle is circular in shape because regional wall motion abnormalities may be incorrectly diagnosed from off-axis or oblique images.

Progressive cephalad angulation of the transducer from the short axis at the base of the left ventricle, with the scan plane at right angles to the left ventricular long axis, brings into view the aorta in short axis at the level of the valve leaflets (Fig. 3.47) with the left atrium posteriorly. In this scan plane, the tricuspid valve is located superiorly and the interatrial septum extends leftward from the aorta, so that the right atrium is above and leftward of the left atrium. The right ventricular inflow tract, body, outflow tract, pulmonary valve, and main pulmonary artery to its bifurcation are visualized forming an arch around the aorta. The pulmonary valve is immediately lateral and rightward of the aortic valve, with the main pulmonary artery running vertically downward and the right pulmonary artery crossing under the left atrial appendage. This scan plane is useful for recording blood flow velocities in the right ventricular outflow tract and main pulmonary artery (if these data have not already been obtained satisfactorily from the left parasternal position) be-

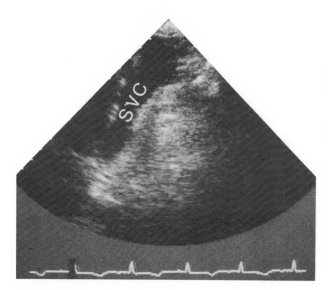

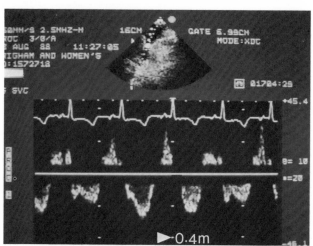

A   B

Figure 3.51.   Two-dimensional echocardiogram obtained from the right supraclavicular fossa showing the superior vena cava (*A*) with Doppler flow velocity recordings from it (*B*). Calibration markers equal 20 cm/s.

cause the angle of incidence between the ultrasound beam and the direction of blood flow is close to zero.

The entire abdominal aorta can be imaged from the subcostal route. This is achieved by directing the transducer scan plane at right angles to the axial skeleton and tilting the scan plane cephalad to image the aorta in short axis. From this scan plane, the aortic cross section is to the left of the bodies of the spinal vertebrae, with the inferior vena cava to the right and slightly anterior. The transducer is then rotated clockwise 90 degrees so that the long axis of the thoracoabdominal aorta can be visualized with the celiac axis at

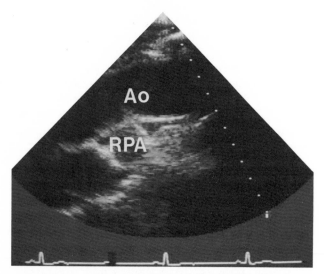

Figure 3.52.   Two-dimensional echocardiogram of the ascending aorta obtained from the right upper parasternal region, with a right pulmonary artery posterior to the lesser curvature of the ascending aorta.

the upper left (Fig. 3.48). The arterial pulsations of the aorta are usually obvious, but in patients with low cardiac outputs and no discernible pulsations, the high velocity blood flow and its direction can be determined by placing the Doppler sample volume within its lumen.

Suprasternal View

With the transducer positioned in the suprasternal notch, images can be obtained of the ascending aorta, aortic arch with its brachiocephalic vessels, and the proximal descending thoracic aorta for 2 to 5 cm distal to the origin of the left subclavian artery (Fig. 3.49). The optimal position for imaging from the suprasternal notch is when the patient is comfortable, lying supine with a pillow under the shoulders, and the head is extended and turned to the left. It is preferable to use a transducer with a small footprint, positioned in the suprasternal notch and oriented with the scan plane between 50 and 60 degrees to the coronal plane to bisect the aortic arch and thoracic ascending and descending aorta. Minor variation in the scan plane rotation opens up the aorta so that it is seen as a tubular structure extending from 2 to 3 cm distal to the aortic valve through the aortic arch, with the origins of the three brachiocephalic branches (the inominate, the left common carotid, and the left subclavian) and the proximal part of the descending thoracic aorta 2 to 3 cm distal to the ligamentum arteriosum (Fig. 3.49). The normal aorta has parallel walls with a uniform diameter between 2.5 and 3.5 cm throughout the ascending and descending portions. This scan plane is especially useful for detecting aneurysmal dilatation and dissections of the aorta involving the ascending, proximal descending, and arch of the thoracic aorta, and for detecting and assessing the hemodynamic severity of postductal coarctation and patent ductus arteriosus (see Chapter 14). Under the lesser curvature of the aortic arch, the right pulmonary artery is imaged in cross section passing into the hilum of the right lung.

In this scan plane the blood flow velocity profiles from the ascending and descending aorta can be examined by pulsed wave or continuous wave Doppler (Fig. 3.50). This is of particular importance in aortic stenosis, when blood flow distal to the aortic valve may be greatly increased. The scan plane is ideal for directing continuous wave Doppler, either blindly with acoustic guidance or with the continuous wave Doppler imaging probe. This route may be the optimal acoustic window when Doppler signals cannot be obtained in the right parasternal region, and it is the only window for assessing the increased peak velocity across coarctations of the aorta. Rotation of the transducer scan plane 90 degrees enables visualization of vascular anatomic relations of the aortic arch. In this scan plane, the aortic arch is seen in cross section, and the right pulmonary artery immediately subjacent is visualized in its long axis, which is perpendicular and to the right of the long-axis section of the superior vena cava. The superior vena cava can also be visualized in long axis if the transducer is moved from the suprasternal notch to the right supraclavicular fossa, with the scan plane oriented in the coronal section parallel to the front of the chest and aimed directly caudally (Fig. 3.51). Preliminary studies have shown that the blood flow velocity profiles in the superior vena cava are similar to those obtained in the inferior vena cava and middle hepatic vein interrogated from the subcostal root (Fig. 3.51).

Right Parasternal Region

The upper right parasternal region enables visualization of the ascending aorta, from the aortic valve to beyond the segment imaged from the left parasternal view, and proximal to the region of the ascending aorta visualized from the suprasternal notch (Fig. 3.52). The patient is rotated 90 degrees to the right side, and the transducer is positioned at right angles to the front of the chest, close to the sternum in the second or third intercostal spaces. In this view, the left ventricular long axis may be visualized. The aortic valve and the first 5 to 7 cm of the aorta may be clearly imaged with the left atrium posteriorly. This view is also useful in assessing blood flow velocity profiles across the aortic valve, particularly in patients with aortic stenosis, in whom apical and suprasternal imaging proves difficult.

REFERENCES

1. Henry WL, DeMaria A, Gramiak R, et al. Report of the American Society of Echocardiography committee on nomenclature and standards in two-dimensional echocardiography. Circulation 1980;62:212–217.
2. Bansal RC, Tajik AJ, Seward BJ, Gifford KP. Feasibility of detailed two-dimensional echocardiographic examination of adults. Prospective study of 200 patients. Mayo Clin Proc 1980;55:291–308.
3. Sahn DJ, DeMaria A, Kisslo J, Weyman A. The Committee on M-Mode Standardization of the American Society of Echocardiography. Recommendations regarding quantitation in M-mode echocardiographic measurements. Circulation 1978;58:1072–1082.
4. Roberts WC. The congenitally bicuspid aortic valve. A study of 85 autopsy cases. Am J Cardiol 1970;26:72–83.
5. Weyman AE, Dillon JC, Feigenbaum H, Chang S. Echocardiographic patterns of pulmonary valve motion in valvular pulmonary stenoses. Am J Cardiol 1974;34:644–651.
6. Hatle L. Doppler ultrasound in cardiology. In: Hatle L, Angelsen B, eds. Physical principles and applications. 2nd ed. Philadelphia: Lea & Febiger, 1985.
7. Kostucki W, Vandenbossche J-L, Friart A, Englert M. Pulsed Doppler regurgitant flow patterns of normal valves. Am J Cardiol 1986;58:309–313.
8. Kenny JF, Plappert T, Doubilet P, et al. Changes in intracardiac blood flow velocities and right and left ventricular stroke volumes with gestational age in the normal human fetus: A prospective Doppler echocardiographic study. Circulation 1986;74:1208–1216.
9. Miyatake K, Okamoto M, Kinoshita N, et al. Augmentation of atrial contribution to left ventricular inflow with aging as assessed by intracardiac Doppler flowmetry. Am J Cardiol 1984;53:586–589.
10. Limacher MC, Ware JA, O'Meara ME, Fernandez GC, Young JB. Tricuspid regurgitation during pregnancy: 2-dimensional and pulsed Doppler echocardiographic observations. Am J Cardiol 1985;54:1059–1062.
11. Abbasi AS, Allen MW, DeCristofaro D, Ungar I. Detection and estimation of the degree of mitral regurgitation by range-gated pulsed Doppler echocardiography. Circulation 1980;61:143–147.
12. Currie PJ, Seward JB, Chan K-L, et al. Continuous wave Doppler determination of right ventricular pressure: A simultaneous Doppler-catheterization study in 127 patients. J Am Coll Cardiol 1985;6:750–756.
13. Snider AR, Gidding SS, Rocchini AP, et al. Doppler evaluation of left ventricular diastolic filling in children with systemic hypertension. Am J Cardiol 1985;56:921–926.
14. Kitabatake A, Inoue M, Asao M, et al. Transmitral blood flow reflecting diastolic behaviour of the left ventricle in health and disease—a study by pulsed Doppler technique. Jpn Circ J 1982;46:92–102.
15. St. John Sutton MG, Plappert T. Relation between instantaneous Doppler velocity across the mitral valve and changes in left ventricular volume in normal, dilated and hypertrophied hearts, abstracted. J Am Coll Cardiol 1986;7(2):226A.
16. Rokey R, Kuo LC, Zoghbi WA, Limacher MC, Quinones MA. Determination of parameters of left ventricular diastolic filling with pulsed Doppler echocardiography: Comparison with cineangiography. Circulation 1985;71:543–550.

4

Clinical Use of Doppler Ultrasound

Liv Hatle

INTRODUCTION

Doppler ultrasound in cardiac lesions was first used to record wall and valve motions (1, 2); later, it was used to record the velocity of blood flow (3, 4). An early clinical application was pulsed wave Doppler combined with M-mode echocardiography as a diagnostic tool in patients with systolic murmurs (5). Combined with two-dimensional echocardiography (6, 7), Doppler became easier to use in positions other than those traditionally used with M-mode echocardiography. Doppler without imaging was used to record flow velocities in the descending and ascending aortas (8–10) and continuous wave (CW) Doppler to record the increased velocities present in many heart lesions (11, 12).

The combination of both pulsed wave and CW Doppler with two-dimensional echocardiography gives complementary hemodynamic and anatomic information. The recent development of two-dimensional Doppler is likely to improve further the recording and the understanding of abnormalities of blood flow in cardiac lesions (13–15).

The clinical uses of Doppler are estimation of flow and cardiac output, diagnosis and assessment of obstructions and regurgitations, and assessment of prosthetic valve function, abnormalities of filling and ejection, and pulmonary hypertension. The use of Doppler in evaluation of congenital lesions is described in Chapter 21.

TECHNIQUE OF DOPPLER RECORDING

In practical use, imaging helps to localize the area of interest for recording flow-velocity signals. The image may suggest the best direction for velocity recording, but it is only an approximation, and the Doppler signal itself must be used for this assessment. This becomes particularly important in recording narrow high-velocity jets.

Continuous wave Doppler is easiest to use when searching for flow signals and recording high velocities. Figure 4.1 shows how the audio signal is used to find the high jet velocities. With the beam across the jet, the frequencies become higher as the angle becomes smaller, and more of the highest frequencies will be recorded and shown as a concentrated band at the edges of the curve. Such a signal may also be obtained by recording across the beginning of a jet with a large angle, even if the frequencies then obtained are lower. To avoid underestimation of velocity, recording should be attempted from more than one direction.

The importance of using the Doppler signal to obtain maximal velocities is illustrated in Figure 4.2, where a minimal change in beam direction results in a significant change in the recorded velocity. Two-dimensional Doppler may become valuable as an alignment guide, while angle correction can still introduce errors both at larger angles and from diversion of jets.

Better Doppler signals can sometimes be obtained using a separate Doppler transducer; this is partly due to better access with a smaller transducer and to better sensitivity.

VOLUME FLOW

Aortic Flow Velocity

In the ascending aorta, velocity of flow is best recorded from the suprasternal notch or the upper right sternal border as well as across the aortic valve from the same positions or from the apex. Reproducibility is good (16–18). Changes in velocity with increase or decrease

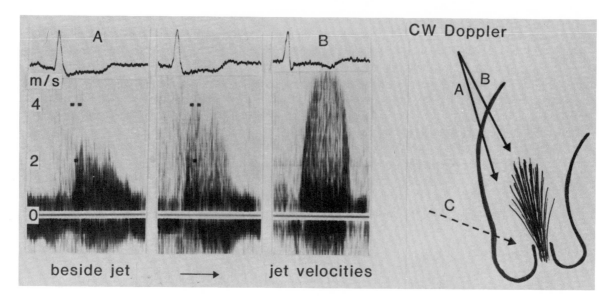

Figure 4.1.   In *A*, beam direction is beside the jet in aortic stenosis, and only low velocities are recorded. With a slight change in beam direction, higher velocities are recorded, and in *B*, a concentration of the highest velocities around the edges of the curve is seen. With a beam direction as indicated by *C*, recorded velocities would have been much lower, but a clear narrow-band signal would have been obtained due to a flat velocity profile and lack of disturbed flow at this level.

in flow are easily shown, and a change in cardiac output is likely to be detected.

Figure 4.3 shows the changes that occur in both velocity and acceleration with a premature beat in a normal subject. With disease, changes may occur in one or both, as well as in time to flow or duration of flow (i.e., pre-ejection and ejection times). In Figure 4.3B, where the low velocity and low cardiac output are due to reduced filling, the shape of the velocity curve is normal. In Figure 4.3C, where the velocity and cardiac output are within normal limits, the long pre-ejection period and late peak velocity are indicators of the marked systolic dysfunction present. In Figure 4.3D, where the velocity curve is characteristic of increased sympathetic tone, the increase in stroke volume after volume loading is easily seen.

The aortic flow velocity is used to assess a patient's response to treatment (19–21). Prior to pacemaker

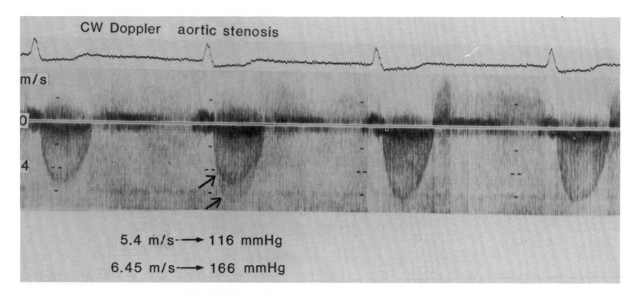

Figure 4.2.   Aortic stenosis and regurgitation recorded from the apex. With a minimal change in beam direction, a marked increase in velocity is seen from the first to the next beat. In the second beat, both contours are seen (*arrows*) with the calculated peak pressure drop for the two curves. Note also the change in the course of the velocity curve from the third to the fourth beat; the last would give the highest calculated mean pressure drop.

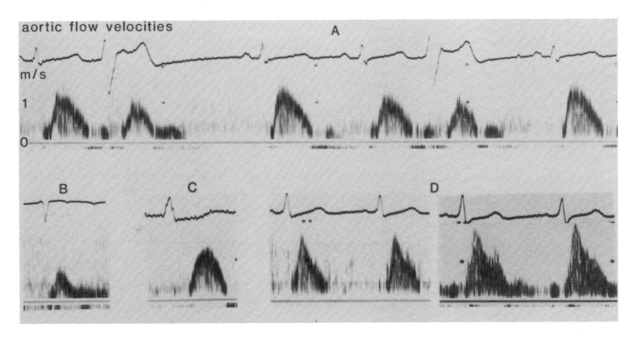

Figure 4.3. (*A*) The recording is from a normal subject and shows the variation in flow velocity caused by premature beats. (*B*) The reduced velocity of flow with low cardiac output in a patient with mitral stenosis. (*C*) Recorded from a patient with dilated cardiomyopathy, peak velocity is normal, but the shape of the curve is abnormal, and a long pre-ejection period is seen. (*D*) The recording from a patient in septic shock shows a rapid upstroke, early peak, and early rapid decrease in velocity. The second recording shows the change after volume replacement; an increase in stroke volume is shown by a larger area under the curve and a longer ejection time.

implantation, aortic flow velocity can be used to establish whether atrioventricular pacing will be an advantage in the individual patient (22); later, it can be used to assess optimal pacing rates.

Cardiac Output

Cardiac output is obtained mainly from the recorded velocity and the cross-sectional area of the ascending aorta (23, 24). Possible errors are underestimation of the velocity due to an excessive angle to flow and errors in diameter measurements, which will be more significant with small diameters. The largest error in adults is probably in the assumption that the recorded velocity represents the mean across that lumen. With an increase in diameter above the valve (Fig. 4.4), velocities just above the valve will not be equal across the lumen; there will be lower velocities to the sides and formation of eddies. This has led to the use of the highest velocity recorded across or above the valve together with the smallest diameter (25) or the velocity in the outflow tract and the diameter of the aortic annulus (26, 27).

In children and young adults, changes in diameter from the outflow tract to the ascending aorta are often minor. Higher up in the ascending aorta, marked variations in the velocity across the lumen have been shown also in normal subjects (28).

Flow Across Other Valves

In calculating flow in the pulmonary artery, diameter and velocity have been recorded in the main pulmonary artery (29, 30) or in the right ventricular (RV) outflow tract (26). Calculation of flow across the mitral (27, 31) and the tricuspid valves (32) has been reported. In one study, the measurement of flow across all four valves compared well in normal subjects, except for the mitral valve (33).

Recording the aortic flow velocity can be useful in assessment of acutely ill patients and in monitoring and assessing changes with therapy. The calculation of cardiac output, together with flow across other valves, can give estimates of shunt size (26, 29, 30), and it provides the potential for calculating valve areas and regurgitant fractions.

OBSTRUCTIONS TO FLOW

Calculation of Pressure Drop

In the presence of an obstruction, the pressure drop can be calculated from the increase in the maximal velocity across the obstruction using a modified Bernoulli equation (34):

$$P_1 - P_2 = 4 \times (V_2^2 - V_1^2) \text{ millimeters of mercury}$$

where $P_1 - P_2$ is the pressure drop, V_1 is the velocity prior to and V_2 the velocity past the obstruction. In

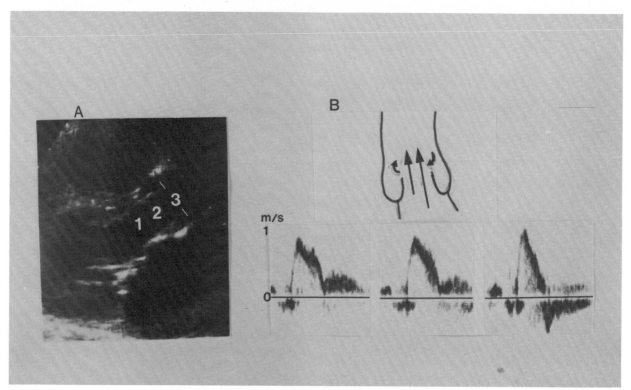

Figure 4.4.   (*A*) Flow velocities can be expected to be equal at the three levels and lower velocities and eddies to be present to the sides at the third level. Therefore, a velocity recorded at 3 will not represent the mean for the aorta at this level. (*B*) The aortic flow velocity curves recorded across the lumen just above the valve in a normal subject show the presence of eddies. To the left, more forward flow is recorded in late systole and early diastole, and at the same time, reversal of flow is seen in the recording to the right.

Figure 4.5, the formula is used to calculate the pressure drop in one patient with severe aortic stenosis and one with an aortic valve prosthesis. The maximal velocity gives the peak instantaneous pressure drop. By calculating the pressure drop for several points during systole, the mean pressure drop is obtained.

In most instances, the velocity prior to an obstruction is so low that it can be ignored. However, when this velocity exceeds 1 meter per second, it may be necessary to include it in the calculation in order to avoid overestimation, especially in mild obstructions. With severe lesions (as in Fig. 4.5B), the influence of V_1 becomes relatively small, even when V_1 is increased.

The applied formula only gives the part of the pressure drop that comes from the convective acceleration; inertia and viscous losses are neglected. Inertia causes a slight delay in the velocity curve (34). Viscous friction becomes important with small orifice sizes (35, 36) but so far has not been shown to be of importance in valvular obstructions.

Increased velocities can also be recorded in the absence of obstruction when there is increase in flow. Velocity will then be increased prior to the valve, but the increase at valve level can be more marked than with normal flow.

Aortic Stenosis

The best orientation to the jet in aortic stenosis is frequently from a high right parasternal position with the patient in a right lateral position. In other cases, the highest velocities can be obtained from the suprasternal notch at or lateral to the apex or occasionally from a subcostal or supraclavicular transducer position. From the apex, the image can be helpful for a more rapid localization, but since the direction of the jet cannot be assumed from the image, the audio signal is used to find the highest frequencies. From the other positions, access is usually better with a separate Doppler transducer.

With the ultrasound beam across the jet at the orifice, a narrow band signal with a concentration of the highest frequencies will be obtained even if there is a significant angle to the jet. Therefore, it is necessary to search from different directions in order to avoid underestimation of velocity (Fig. 4.6). Attention should also be paid to the timing of the flow signal as other high-velocity jets can be present and have a direction similar to an aortic jet. Mitral regurgitation may have a superior direction but is of longer duration than flow through the aortic valve and can be seen to continue past aortic valve closure (Fig. 4.7).

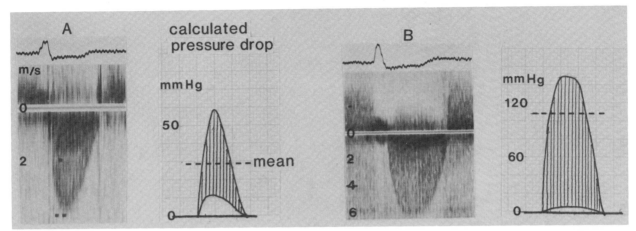

Figure 4.5. Aortic jet velocities recorded with CW Doppler ultrasound from the apex. (*A*) In a patient with a leaking aortic valve prosthesis. (*B*) In a patient with severe aortic stenosis. The pressure drop is calculated for several points during systole for both the maximal velocity and the velocity below the valve seen as a darker band within. The hatched areas show the pressure drop during systole and the dotted lines the mean. In (*A*), the increased velocity below the valve should be included in the calculation as shown; in (*B*), this makes less of a difference.

A peak or mean pressure drop calculated from Doppler compares well with the pressure drop obtained at catheterization (37–39). It should be noted that the peak velocity during systole gives the instantaneous peak pressure drop, which always differs from the peak-to-peak pressure drop often measured at catheterization. The latter compares peak left ventricular (LV) and peak aortic pressures, which occur at different times during systole. The mean pressure drop by the two methods can be directly compared and is a better indicator of severity.

With increasing severity, the velocity tends to stay high for a longer period of systole than in moderate obstructions when velocity is high due to increased flow (Fig. 4.5B). In assessing the importance of a calculated pressure drop, it is useful to consider both heart rate and the velocity below the valve or an estimate of flow across the valve.

An estimate of the aortic valve area can be obtained by recording velocity across the valve and the diameter and velocity in the LV outflow tract. Since the product of the velocity and flow area below the valve is equal to that across the valve, the flow area at the valve can be obtained (40). A similar approach using the pressure drop and estimates of flow from other valves in the Gorlin formula has been reported (41). The first approach (40) has the advantage that it can be used whether or not aortic regurgitation is present. Calculating the valve area is helpful to avoid underestimation of severity in patients with low pressure drops due to low cardiac output.

In aortic stenosis, the increase in velocity occurs

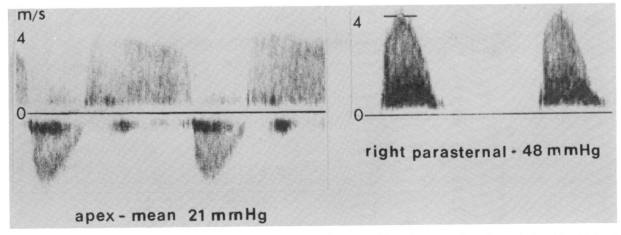

Figure 4.6. Aortic stenosis and regurgitation recorded from different positions in one patient. A good signal is obtained from the apex, but a clearly higher velocity with a later peak is recorded from the right parasternal position.

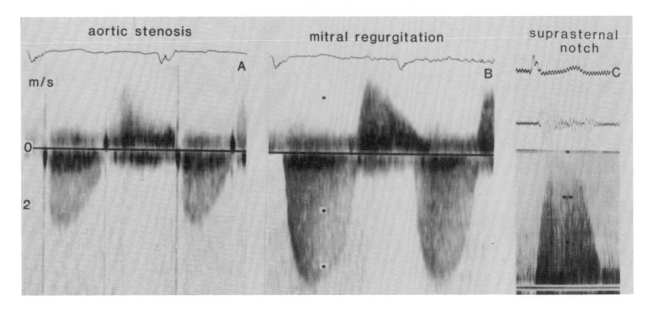

Figure 4.7. Mild aortic stenosis (*A*) and mitral regurgitation (*B*) recorded from the apex in one patient. In mitral regurgitation, the velocity is higher and the duration longer. The high-velocity jet toward the transducer (*C*) is recorded from another patient, and the early start and duration past aortic closure show that this is not an aortic jet. The signal is mitral regurgitation with a superior direction.

over a short distance (0.5 cm) at the level of the valve. With pulsed wave Doppler ultrasound, the increase in velocity can be shown to occur lower within the LV if the obstruction is subvalvular (42) or above the aortic valve if a supravalvular obstruction is present.

Continuous wave Doppler has proved useful in assessing the severity of aortic stenosis, its progression, and the results of surgery. The aortic jet can be reached in all patients and a good assessment of severity obtained if care is taken to search for a good signal

from different directions. The possibility of underestimating the velocity should still be taken into account. Recording changes in the mitral flow velocity curve or increases in mitral regurgitation can give additional information on the effect of the obstruction on the LV.

Mitral Stenosis

In mitral stenosis, the increased velocity is easily recorded. In most patients, it is best recorded from the

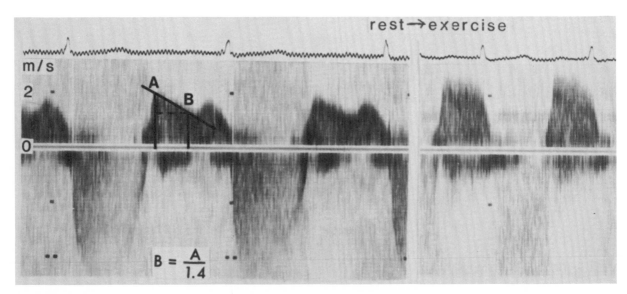

Figure 4.8. Mitral stenosis and regurgitation recorded at rest and during exercise. With increase in heart rate from 66 to 90, the calculated mean pressure drop increases from 11 to 27 mm Hg. The measurement of the pressure half-time (A to B) gives an estimated mitral valve area of 1.2 cm².

apex, but in some, it is recorded better from a more medial position. The mean pressure drop is obtained by calculating the pressure drop for several points during diastole. The calculated pressure drop corresponds well to that recorded at cardiac catheterization if the measurements are done simultaneously (11, 34). The pressure drop in mitral stenosis can vary greatly with heart rate and flow. Therefore, it is best considered together with the heart rate at which it is recorded.

The increase in velocity and pressure drop with exercise can easily be recorded (Fig. 4.8) and can help assess patients whose obstructions are considered significant but who are symptomatic.

With increasing obstruction, a slower decrease in velocity during diastole is seen. The rate of decrease can be expressed as the pressure half-time, which can be measured directly from the velocity curve (Fig. 4.8). In normal subjects, the pressure half-time is less than 60 ms, and in mitral stenosis, values from 100 up to 300 to 600 ms can be found (43, 44). An estimate of mitral valve area (MVA) can be obtained:

$$MVA = \frac{220}{\text{pressure half-time}} \text{ cm}^2$$

The number 220 is empirical. In Figure 4.9, valve area estimated using this formula is compared to valve area obtained at catheterization. Others have suggested that using the number 215 in the formula may be more accurate (45).

The pressure half-time is also influenced by flow, and on exercise, a slight decrease can be recorded in most patients. Other determinants are compliance of the left atrium (LA) and LV. The good correlation with MVA is therefore surprising. The measurements show the least variation in patients with severe obstruction; in these cases, obstruction may be the dominant factor. In patients with more moderate obstruction, beat-to-beat variations can be more marked, so a mean value should be obtained from several beats.

By calculating both the mean pressure drop and the valve area, underestimation of severity is avoided in patients with a low pressure drop due to low cardiac output. Likewise, overestimation of severity is avoided in patients in whom a high pressure drop is partly due to increased flow.

As in aortic stenosis, calculation of valve area from pressure drop and cardiac output is possible (46). Estimation of valve area from the pressure half-time has the advantage that it can be used also in patients with combined stenosis and regurgitation. Right heart pressures obtained by recording the maximal velocity of pulmonary and tricuspid regurgitation adds to the assessment.

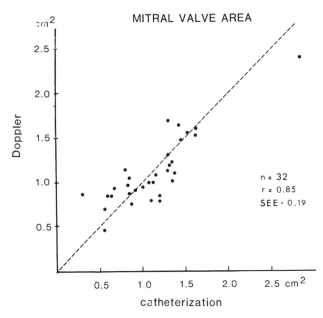

Figure 4.9. Mitral valve area obtained from the pressure half-time compared to that obtained at catheterization.

Tricuspid Stenosis

Tricuspid stenosis is easily diagnosed from the increased velocity across the tricuspid valve, and the pressure drop is calculated as it is in mitral stenosis. Figure 4.10 shows the increased velocity of forward tricuspid flow, tricuspid regurgitation, and right atrial (RA) and RV pressures. The pressure differences calculated from the velocity correspond to those recorded at cardiac catheterization during both diastole and systole. In tricuspid stenosis, a marked change in velocity at valvular level is seen. This differs from the increased velocity due to increased flow as in atrial septal defects, where the increased velocity can also be recorded in the RA and the change at valvular level is less marked.

Pulmonary Stenosis

In pulmonary stenosis, the position giving the best orientation to the jet can vary from a high to a low parasternal or a subcostal or infraclavicular position. The calculated pressure drop compares well with recorded pressures (47). The velocity can also be recorded during exercise. With the pulsed mode, it can be determined whether the obstruction is valvular or infundibular or if a combined lesion is present (48).

REGURGITATIONS

Aortic Regurgitation

The diagnosis of aortic regurgitation can be made by recording a diastolic high-velocity jet continuous with

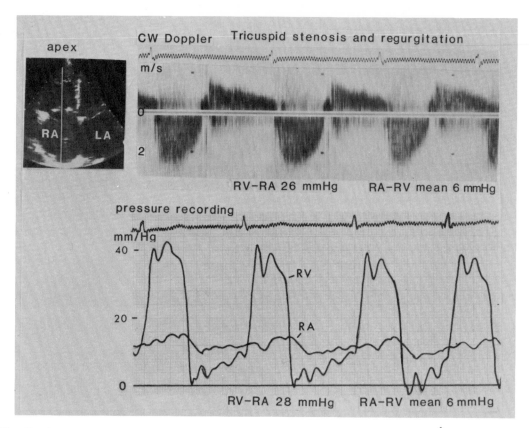

Figure 4.10.   Continuous wave Doppler recording of tricuspid flow velocities and pressure recording from the RV and RA in a patient with tricuspid stenosis and regurgitation. The calculated and recorded pressure drops are similar. (Reproduced by permission from Hatle L, Angelsen B. Doppler ultrasound in cardiology. 2nd ed. Philadelphia: Lea & Febiger, 1985.)

forward aortic flow but with opposite direction (Figs. 4.2 and 4.6). With the pulsed wave mode, reversal of flow is recorded at the aortic orifice and into the LV during diastole. High sensitivity and specificity have been shown (49–54). The sensitivity of Doppler in diagnosing regurgitations has shown that clinical diagnosis is less sensitive: Aortic regurgitation is not infrequently recorded when no diastolic murmur can be heard (53, 54). While most of these regurgitations are mild, occasionally more severe leaks are found with no diastolic murmur present.

There are several ways of assessing severity. With pulsed wave Doppler, the extension of the regurgitant jet into the LV can be recorded (50–52), and two-dimensional Doppler can show the area of reversed flow (15). With the CW mode, the intensity of the signal from the regurgitant jet can be helpful; with mild lesions, the intensity is low. The rate of decrease in the velocity of the regurgitation is useful in the more severe lesions. A rapid decrease shows a marked decrease in the pressure difference between the aorta and the LV during diastole and can indicate patients with high end-diastolic pressure (Fig. 4.11).

In aortic regurgitation, reversal of flow in the aorta and peripheral arteries can be recorded during dias-

tole. This is less sensitive for diagnosing mild lesions but is useful in assessing severity. The relation between forward and reverse flows recorded in the descending aorta has most commonly been used (55–57), but reversal of flow in the subclavian arteries has also been used (58). The pulsed wave mode should be used to avoid interference from nearby veins. Reversal of flow can be well recorded in the ascending aorta also, but assessing the degree can often be difficult due to marked variation in the flow velocity pattern across the lumen. This occurs in the descending aorta in some patients; in the subclavian arteries, a more homogeneous flow velocity pattern is regularly found (Fig. 4.11).

It is useful to assess the severity from a recording in the LV and from reversal of arterial flow since the recording of the extension may be influenced by whether the jet is central or directed toward one of the walls of the LV and the reversal in the arteries may be influenced by changes in vessel diameter and peripheral resistance. By using both approaches, a good assessment of severity can be obtained. Patients with severe aortic regurgitation and near equalization of end-diastolic pressures in the LV and the aorta who are in need of urgent surgery are rapidly identified. Assess-

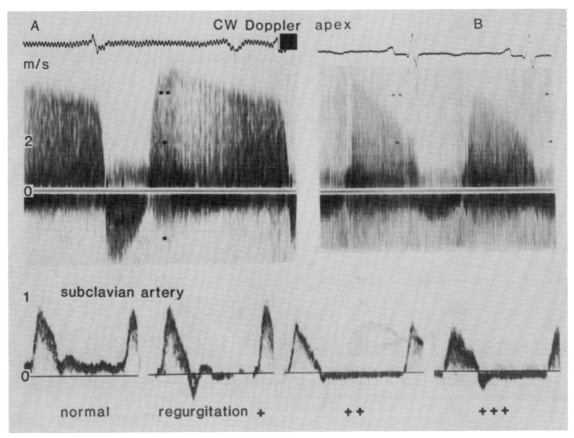

Figure 4.11. Aortic regurgitation recorded with CW Doppler from the apex in two patients. The rapid decrease of velocity in (*B*) is seen only with severe regurgitation, when pressures in the aorta and the LV tend to equalize during diastole. The velocity at end diastole in (*B*) gives a calculated pressure difference of 15 to 20 mm Hg, indicating a high end-diastolic pressure in the LV. In the subclavian artery, there is forward flow during diastole in the normal subject; with regurgitation, less forward and increasing reversal of diastolic flow is seen.

ment of severity is otherwise helpful in mixed lesions and for advice on follow-up.

Mitral Regurgitation

Mitral regurgitation is recorded as reversal of flow at the mitral orifice back into the LA during systole. It is often best recorded from the apex but, in some patients with mitral valve prolapse or flail leaflets, is better recorded from a parasternal position. In some, the regurgitant jet has a superior direction and can be well recorded toward the transducer from the suprasternal notch (Fig. 4.7). With two-dimensional Doppler ultrasound, the direction of the regurgitant jet is better visualized (15). The regurgitation starts at mitral valve closure, except in some patients with mitral valve prolapse when it starts later and in some patients with high end-diastolic pressure when the regurgitation may start before onset of systole. Regurgitation usually continues until the mitral valve opens again, but mild regurgitation can be well recorded only in early systole.

A high sensitivity and specificity are reported (59–

64). Mild regurgitation has been missed in some patients, but more than mild regurgitation has regularly been recorded. The sensitivity for detecting mild regurgitation, especially in large patients, may vary with the sensitivity of the Doppler used, the size of the sample volume, and whether both pulsed wave and CW Doppler are used. Severity has been assessed mainly from the extension of the regurgitant jet in the LA (61, 62). With large hearts where the mitral orifice is too far from the transducer to assess the extension in the LA, the range ambiguity of the pulsed wave Doppler can be used (65).

The intensity of the signal increases with increasing amounts of regurgitation (65). The aortic flow velocity curve shows less flow in late systole when the regurgitation is significant (66). Another method is to obtain the regurgitant fraction by comparing volume flow across the mitral valve with flow across a competent valve (67).

When regurgitation causes a marked systolic increase in LA pressure, the decreasing pressure difference between the ventricle and the atrium results in

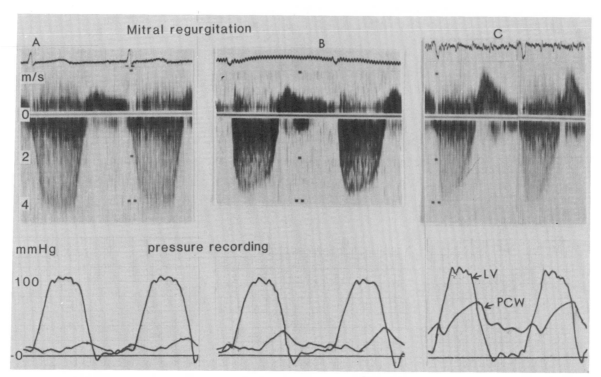

Figure 4.12.   Mitral regurgitation recorded with CW Doppler in three different patients. The recorded LV and pulmonary capillary wedge (PCW) pressures are seen. (*A*) The high velocity of the mitral regurgitation and the pressure difference are both maintained during systole. (*B*) Velocity decreases, and the pressure tracings show a moderate V wave and some reduction in the pressure difference during systole. (*C*) A large V wave reduces the pressure difference, and the maximal velocity in the regurgitation also decreases rapidly from early systole. The possible overestimation of a mitral valve gradient from a PCW pressure can also be seen. The pressure recording suggests significant obstruction, but both Doppler and echocardiography showed that there was no obstruction. (Reproduced by permission from Hatle L, Angelsen B. Doppler ultrasound in cardiology. 2nd ed. Philadelphia: Lea & Febiger, 1985.)

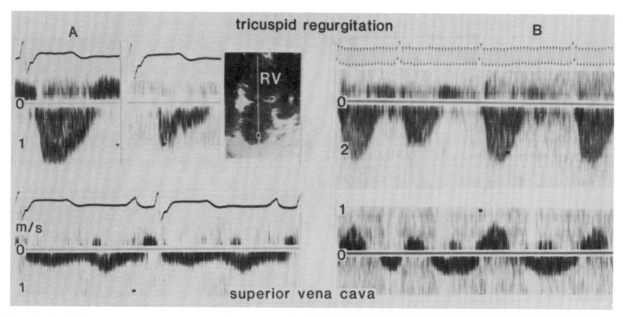

Figure 4.13.   Tricuspid regurgitation recorded from two patients, both with low velocity. A marked increase in jugular venous pressure (*B*) gave an estimated systolic pressure in the RV of 40 to 50 mm Hg and less than 20 mm Hg in (*A*), where venous pressure was normal. With pulsed wave Doppler in (*A*), the regurgitation was recorded throughout the RA; there was still only reduction in forward systolic flow in the superior vena cava. In (*B*) where RV function was markedly reduced, reversal of flow during systole was recorded.

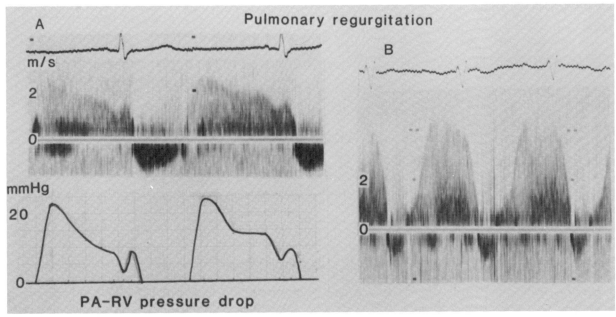

Figure 4.14.   Pulmonary regurgitation recorded with CW Doppler ultrasound in two patients, one without (A) and one with (B) pulmonary hypertension. The low velocity in (A) is barely higher than that recorded in normal subjects, and from the calculated pressure difference seen below, a practically normal diastolic pressure can be assumed provided there is no increase in jugular venous pressure. The decrease following atrial contraction corresponds to increase in pressure in the RV. This is less likely to show in (B), where the velocity is much higher. In (A), forward flow velocity is normal; in (B), the early peak and early decrease are indicators of increased pulmonary vascular resistance. PA = pulmonary artery.

decrease of the velocity of the regurgitation earlier in systole than when LA pressure is normal (Fig. 4.12).

The rate of increase in the maximal velocity of the regurgitation early in systole reflects the rate of rise of the pressure in the LV. By comparing the duration of mitral regurgitation and flow across the aortic valve, the isovolumetric phases are well defined (Fig. 4.7).

Tricuspid Regurgitation

Tricuspid regurgitation can frequently be recorded in patients both with and without pulmonary hypertension as well as in many normal subjects (68–70). Most of these regurgitations are mild, but Doppler has shown that more than mild lesions are frequently missed on clinical examination (68, 69). Recording these mild regurgitations gives useful information about right heart pressures.

From the maximal velocity in the regurgitation, the pressure difference to the RA can be calculated using the same formula as in obstructions (Fig. 4.10). The calculated pressure difference has been shown to correlate well with that recorded at catheterization, and RV systolic pressure can be obtained by adding an estimate of RA pressure from jugular venous filling (71, 72). The systolic pressure can thus be obtained in the majority of patients with heart lesions. However, to

record the maximal velocity of mild regurgitations, the sensitivity of the Doppler used is important.

Severity can be assessed from the extension in the RA and from systolic reversal of flow in jugular veins, the superior vena cava, or hepatic veins (73–79). Holosystolic reversal indicates that the regurgitation is more than moderate; with lesser degrees of regurgitation, reduction in forward flow during systole may be seen. A combined assessment is useful since the extension in the RA may be influenced by the pressure in the RV, while reduction in forward systolic venous flow may be influenced by RV function (76, 79). This may explain why some patients with significant regurgitation show reduction in forward systolic flow only when RV function is normal. With reduced ventricular function, forward systolic flow would already be reduced, and the same degree of regurgitation might result in systolic reversal of flow (Fig. 4.13).

Pulmonary Regurgitation

Pulmonary regurgitation can frequently be recorded in patients with heart lesions, and high sensitivity and specificity have been shown (69, 80). It can also be recorded frequently in normal subjects, especially children and young adults (70, 81).

In normal subjects, pulmonary regurgitation is very

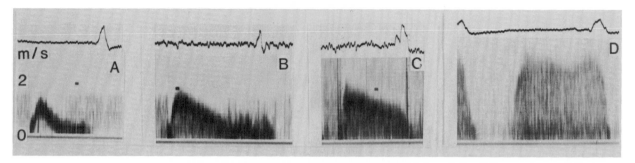

Figure 4.15. (*A*) Increased mitral flow across a normal valve. (*B*, *C*, and *D*) Mitral prostheses with normal function (*B*), moderate obstruction (*C*), and severe obstruction (*D*). Pressure half-times are 50, 120, 220, and 400 m/s in (*A*) to (*D*), respectively, with estimated valve areas of 1.85, 1.0, and 0.55 cm^2 in (*B*) to (*D*), respectively. The calculated mean pressure drops are 5 to 6, 12, and 36 mm Hg in (*B*) to (*D*), respectively.

localized and can usually be recorded less than 1 cm below the valve. With normal pulmonary artery pressure, the velocity of the regurgitation is low, at end diastole 1 m/s or less depending on the heart rate and corresponding to a pressure difference of 1 to 4 mm Hg to the RV. The velocity of the regurgitation decreases on inspiration due to the decrease in pulmonary artery pressure. In sinus rhythm, a decrease in the velocity following atrial contraction is seen (Fig. 4.14).

With pulmonary hypertension, the velocity of the pulmonary regurgitation increases (Fig. 4.14). The pressure difference between the pulmonary artery and the RV during diastole can be calculated, and in the absence of venous congestion this practically equals diastolic pressure in the pulmonary artery. With increased diastolic pressure in the ventricle, an estimate of this from jugular venous filling should be added to obtain actual pressure. The estimated pulmonary dias-

tolic pressure corresponds well to recorded pressures and is useful in assessing progression of pulmonary hypertension or reversal with treatment.

With significant pulmonary regurgitation as can be seen after valvulotomy, the velocity of the regurgitation decreases rapidly and may end before onset of systole, indicating equalization of pressures in the pulmonary artery and the RV.

When CW Doppler is used in order to obtain the maximal velocity of the pulmonary regurgitation, one should be aware of the small difference in direction toward the pulmonary and the mitral valves. The velocities across the mitral valve in mitral stenosis and in pulmonary regurgitation are usually in the same range, and it is possible to obtain a weak signal from mitral flow together with flow into the pulmonary artery. The pulmonary regurgitation can be shown with the pulsed wave mode in the outflow tract, and in sinus

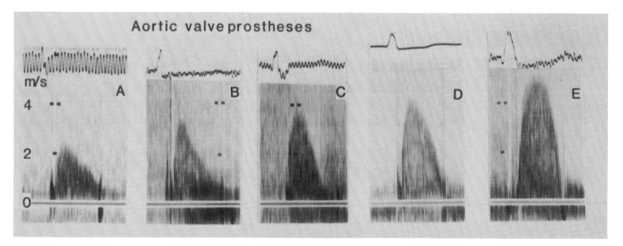

Figure 4.16. Flow velocities across aortic valve prostheses recorded with CW Doppler from the suprasternal notch or a right parasternal position in five patients. Velocity in (*B*) is higher than in (*A*), due to a smaller valve and a slower heart rate. In (*C*), recorded early after surgery, systole is shortened. The velocity in (*D*) is increased due to severe regurgitation and in (*E*) due to obstruction. The calculated pressure drops from (*A*) to (*E*) are 11, 17, 21, 36, and 68 mm Hg, respectively.

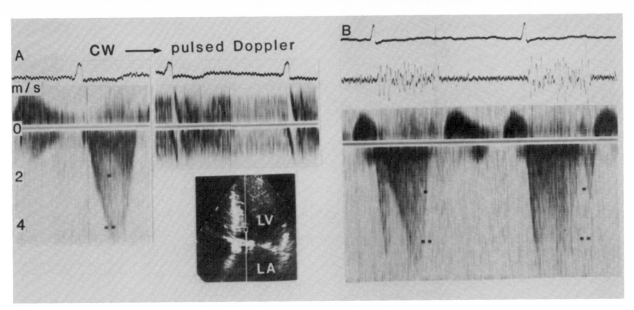

Figure 4.17. With CW Doppler, a high-velocity jet is recorded away from the transducer in systole (*A*), and with pulsed Doppler the increase in velocity is recorded within the LV as shown by the square in the image. The high velocity causes aliasing in the pulsed wave mode, but the contour of the increasing velocity can be seen to cross the zero line twice, showing that the velocity is at least 4 m/s. In (*B*) recorded from another patient, the high-velocity jets both from the intraventricular obstruction and the mitral regurgitation can be seen. The regurgitation starts earlier, shows a more rapid increase in velocity, and lasts until forward mitral flow starts again. The signal from the obstruction shows a more gradual increase in velocity and ends earlier, at aortic valve closure. Forward mitral flow shows a late start, slow decrease in velocity of early filling, and increased velocity at atrial contraction.

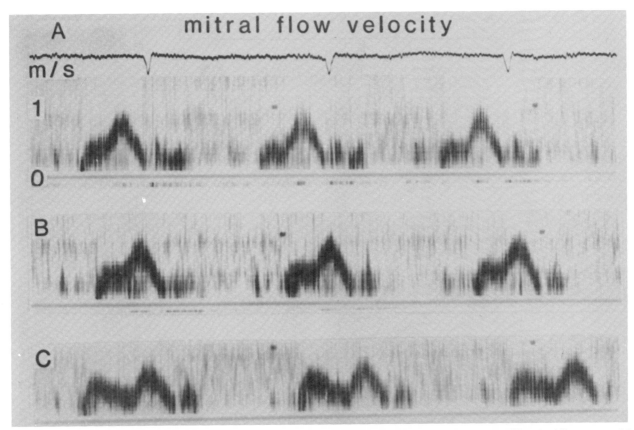

Figure 4.18. Aortic closure is seen as a small spike, start of mitral flow is delayed, and the main filling in (*A*) occurs with atrial contraction. (*B*) Recorded after one dose of verapamil (40 mg). (*C*) Recorded after a week on 120 mg verapamil daily. There is a slight increase in early peak velocity, but improved filling before atrial contraction is mainly due to the moderate reduction in heart rate.

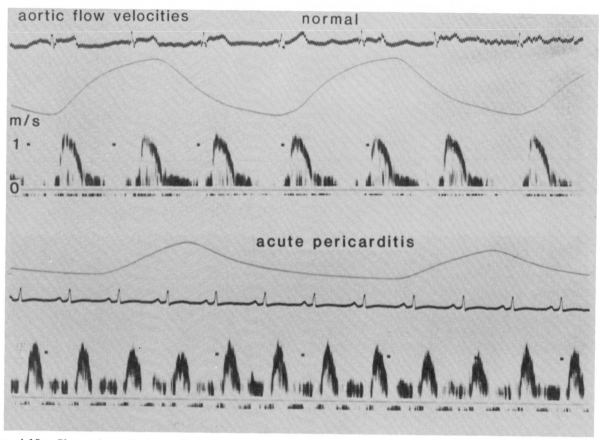

Figure 4.19.   Change in aortic flow velocity with respiration is minimal in a normal subject, but in a patient with pericardial effusion, a clear decrease on inspiration is seen. This disappeared after pericardiocentesis.

rhythm, there is decrease in velocity with atrial contraction while mitral flow at this time shows an increase in velocity.

PROSTHETIC VALVES

From the increase in the maximal velocity across prosthetic valves, the pressure drop can be calculated as it is for the native valves and has been shown to correlate well with invasive measurements (82, 83). Valvular areas can be estimated as they are for mitral and aortic stenosis. The degree of obstruction produced by a normally functioning prosthesis can thus be assessed in the individual patient. The increase in pressure drop with exercise can also be recorded.

To diagnose malfunction, one has to consider the type and size of prosthesis, the patient's heart rate and cardiac output, and presence and degree of regurgitation. Since some degree of regurgitation is normally present in some of the valves, it is necessary to assess the degree before diagnosing malfunction. Pulsed wave Doppler may show whether the regurgitation is recorded in a central position or at the valve ring,

suggesting a paravalvular leak. In both mitral and aortic prostheses, leaks may be present in the absence of a systolic or diastolic murmur, occasionally severe enough to require reoperation.

Figure 4.15 shows the increased velocity recorded across one normally functioning mitral valve prosthesis and two with obstruction (one moderately severe and one severe), with estimated valve areas of 1.85, 1.0, and 0.55 cm^2, respectively.

In Figure 4.16, the recordings across various aortic valve prostheses are shown. The pressure drop is low across a large-size prosthesis in Figure 4.16A. With a smaller size in Figure 4.16B, the pressure drop is higher, partly due to a lower heart rate giving a larger stroke volume. Early in the postoperative period with a hyperdynamic state, a high peak velocity and a shortened ejection time may be seen (Fig. 4.16C). This velocity curve differs from the increase seen due to significant regurgitation in Figure 4.16D and to obstruction in Figure 4.16E. In calculating the pressure drop across aortic valve prostheses, V_1 is routinely included in the calculation since the obstruction is moderate

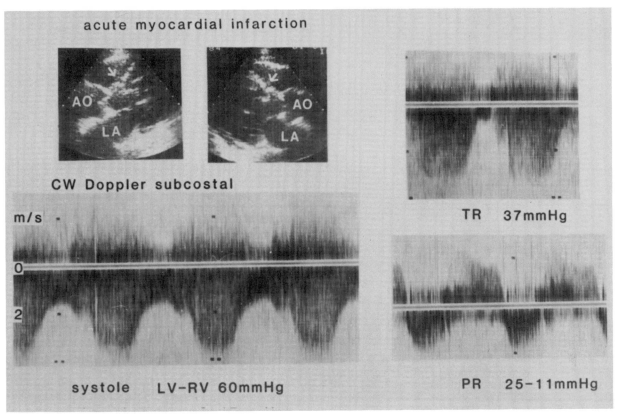

Figure 4.20. With the position shown in the image, flow through the defect was recorded toward the transducer into the RV, but the highest velocities were obtained from another position and away from the transducer. The velocity through the defect shows the higher pressure in the LV in both systole and diastole and the increase in pressure in the right heart in the regurgitations. PR = pulmonary regurgitation; TR = tricuspid regurgitation.

and the velocity below the prosthesis is increased in some patients (Fig. 4.5).

In the majority of patients, Doppler can show normal function of a prosthetic valve or a clear malfunction. In the few patients with borderline results, a closer fol-

low-up is indicated. The method has proved helpful in assessing conduit valve function (84–86), and progression of obstruction in tissue valves can be closely followed. After valve replacement, Doppler ultrasound is helpful in assessing progression of other valve

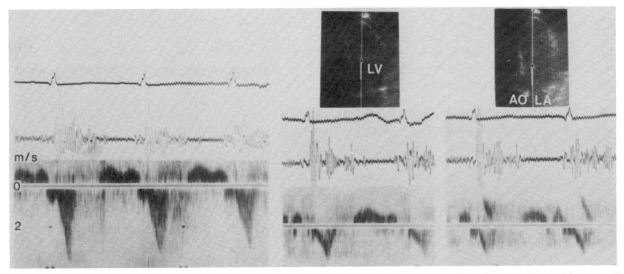

Figure 4.21. Increased velocity within the LV with cessation of flow in midsystole is recorded in a patient with a systolic murmur after coronary bypass surgery. Both murmur and velocity decreased after increased fluid and beta blockade.

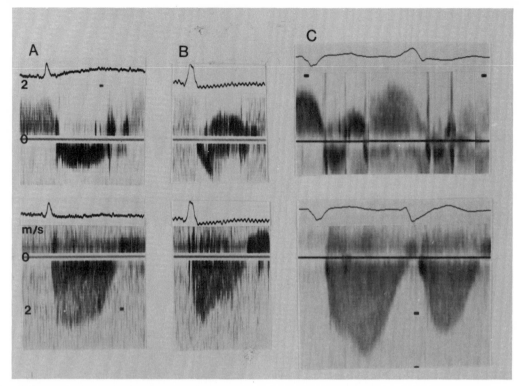

Figure 4.22.   Pulmonary flow velocity (above) and tricuspid regurgitation (below) recorded in three subjects. The pulmonary flow velocity curve is normal in (*A*) and abnormal in (*B*) and (*C*) with an early peak and reversal of flow in midsystole. The low velocity of the regurgitation in (*B*) (without venous congestion) shows there is no pulmonary hypertension, and the rapid rise and decrease of the velocity suggests increased sympathetic tone. The similar duration of pulmonary flow and tricuspid regurgitation also indicates normal pulmonary artery pressure. In (*C*), the pulmonary hypertension is shown by both the velocity of the tricuspid regurgitation and its duration and late tricuspid valve opening.

lesions and progression or reversal of pulmonary hypertension.

HYPERTROPHIC CARDIOMYOPATHY

In patients with hypertrophic cardiomyopathy, the presence of obstruction can be shown by recording increased velocity of flow within the LV in systole (86). The characteristic velocity curve shows first a gradual, then often a more abrupt, increase in velocity, with maximum toward end systole suggesting a dynamic obstruction. Since the velocity often exceeds the limits for the pulsed wave mode, it is best recorded with the CW mode. The pulsed wave mode is used as shown in Figure 4.17 to verify that the increased velocity occurs within the ventricle and to show the level of obstruction. In this way, it can be clearly distinguished from the mitral regurgitation that is frequently present. The direction of the two jets can be quite close with both partly within the beam, but they can usually be recorded separately by slight changes in beam direction. In most, they differ clearly both in duration and course as seen in Figure 4.17B.

The velocities recorded across the aortic valve are in the normal range or slightly higher. In the ascending aorta, the curve usually shows an early peak and less flow in late systole; the latter finding varies with the position of the sample volume and with the ejection time, which is often prolonged with obstruction and normal or short without it.

Changes in LV filling are easily seen in the mitral flow velocity curve; by recording in the RV outflow tract, right-sided obstructions can be diagnosed.

ABNORMALITIES OF FILLING AND EJECTION

Changes in ventricular filling are shown in the flow velocity across the atrioventricular valves. In patients with dyspnea on exercise and normal systolic function of the LV, changes in the mitral flow velocity as shown in Figure 4.18 are frequent findings. The change with therapy and the influence of heart rate are seen. Similar mitral flow velocity curves in patients with impaired LV function may indicate those most likely to benefit from reduction in heart rates. The tricuspid flow velocity curve shows similar changes with increased resistance to RV filling.

In pericardial constriction or effusion, a clear decrease in aortic flow velocity on inspiration is an early sign of increased pericardial pressure (Fig. 4.19).

Another useful application of Doppler is in the evaluation of systolic murmurs (87). In patients with acute myocardial infarction, a ventricular septal defect can be rapidly diagnosed, and Doppler can aid in localizing small defects (88, 89). In Figure 4.20, a continuous left-to-right shunt shows higher pressure in the LV in both systole and diastole, and pulmonary artery pressures are shown by the velocities of the regurgitations.

When systolic murmurs appear in acutely ill patients or postoperatively, a more frequent finding is a localized increase in velocity in the LV or sometimes the RV (Fig. 4.21). The increase occurs at the same level as seen in hypertrophic cardiomyopathy. Velocities corresponding to an intraventricular pressure drop of up to 50 to 60 mm Hg have been recorded and have disappeared together with the murmur with volume loading or beta-blocking agents.

In postoperative patients, the pulmonary flow velocity curve may show an early peak similar to that seen in pulmonary hypertension while the velocity of a tricuspid regurgitation shows a more rapid rise in velocity than usual, suggesting increased sympathetic tone (Fig. 4.22).

In other patients, the pulmonary flow velocity curve is a useful indicator of increased pulmonary vascular resistance (90–92), with the early decrease in velocity suggesting reflection waves and the rapid upstroke and systolic reversal of flow. A similar pattern can also be seen in idiopathic dilatation of the pulmonary artery (92), but as in postoperative patients, a low pulmonary artery pressure can be shown by a low velocity and short duration of a tricuspid regurgitation (Fig. 4.22B). The changes in the pulmonary flow velocity curve may become less marked when RV failure occurs. The flow velocity curve is especially useful in distinguishing pulmonary hypertension due to high flow from that due to increased resistance.

PITFALLS

The possibility of underestimating the velocity should be kept in mind, even with good Doppler signals (Fig. 4.6). The precaution is to record from different positions. Weak signals such as from mild regurgitations are more easily missed. When pulsed wave Doppler is used to localize a flow signal, range ambiguity may occur. With CW Doppler, more than one signal may be present within the beam. Misinterpretation of signals may occur whether or not Doppler ultrasound is used with imaging but can be avoided by recording flow across the four valves and by paying attention to the timing of flow (Fig. 4.7).

These pitfalls can be avoided with awareness, and Doppler can be of great help in the clinical diagnosis and assessment of a variety of heart lesions.

REFERENCES

1. Satomura S. Ultrasonic Doppler method for the inspection of cardiac functions. J Acoust Soc Am 1975;29:1181–5.
2. Yoshida T, Mori M, Nimura Y, et al. Analysis of heart motion with ultrasonic Doppler method and its clinical application. Am Heart J 1961;61:61–75.
3. Franklin DL, Schlegal WA, Rushmer RF. Blood flow measured by Doppler frequency shift of backscattered ultrasound. Science 1961;134:564–5.
4. Light LH. Non-injurious ultrasonic technique for observing flow in the human aorta. Nature 1969;224:1119–21.
5. Johnson SL, Baker DW, Lute RA, Dodge HT. Doppler echocardiography. The localization of cardiac murmurs. Circulation 1973;48:810–22.
6. Matsuo H, Kitabatake A, Hayashi T, et al. Intracardiac flow dynamics with bidirectional ultrasonic pulsed Doppler. Jpn Circ J 1977;41:515–28.
7. Griffith JM, Henry WL. An ultrasound system for combined cardiac imaging and Doppler blood flow measurement in man. Circulation 1978;57:925–30.
8. Huntsman LL, Gams E, Johnson CC, Fairbanks E. Transcutaneous determination of aortic blood-flow velocities in man. Am Heart J 1975;89:605–12.
9. Sequeira RF, Light LH, Cross G, Raftery EB. Transcutaneous aortovelography: a quantitative evaluation. Br Heart J 1976;38:443–50.
10. Angelsen BAJ, Brubakk AO. Transcutaneous measurement of blood flow velocity in the human aorta. Cardiovasc Res 1976;10:368–79.
11. Holen J, Aaslid R, Landmark K, Simonsen S. Determination of pressure gradient in mitral stenosis with a non-invasive ultrasound Doppler technique. Acta Med Scand 1976;199:455–60.
12. Hatle L, Angelsen B. Doppler ultrasound in cardiology. Philadelphia: Lea & Febiger, 1982.
13. Bommer W, Miller L. Real-time two-dimensional color-flow Doppler. Enhanced Doppler flow imaging in the diagnosis of cardiovascular diseases, abstracted. Am J Cardiol 1982;49:944.
14. Omoto R, Yokote Y, Takamoto S, et al. The development of real-time two-dimensional Doppler echocardiography and its clinical significance in acquired valvular diseases. Jpn Heart J 1984;25:325–40.
15. Miyatake K, Okamoto M, Kinoshita N, et al. Clinical applications of a new type of real-time two-dimensional Doppler flow imaging system. Am J Cardiol 1984;54:857–68.
16. Fraser CB, Light LH, Shinebourne EA, Buchtal A, Healy MJR, Beardshaw JA. Transcutaneous aortovelography: reproducibility in adults and children. Eur Heart J 1976;4:181–9.
17. Gisvold SE, Brubakk AO. Measurements of instantaneous blood-flow velocity in the human aorta using pulsed ultrasound. Cardiovasc Res 1982;16:26–33.
18. Gardin JM, Dabestani A, Matin K, Allfie A, Russell D, Henry WL. Reproducibility of Doppler aortic blood flow measurements: studies on intraobserver, interobserver and day-to-day variability in normal subjects. Am J Cardiol 1984;54:1092–8.
19. Buchtal A, Hanson C, Peisach AR. Transcutaneous aortovelography. Potentially useful technique in management of critically ill patients. Br Heart J 1976;38:451–6.
20. Gardin JM, Iseri LT, Elkayam U, et al. Evaluation of dilated cardiomyopathy by pulsed Doppler echocardiography. Am Heart J 1983;106:1057–65.
21. Elkayem U, Gardin JM, Berkley R, Hughes CA, Henry WL. The use of Doppler flow velocity measurement to assess the hemodynamic response to vasodilators in patients with heart failure. Circulation 1983;67:377–83.
22. Stewart WJ, Dicola VC, Harthorne JW, Gillam LD, Weyman A. Doppler ultrasound measurement of cardiac output in patients with physiologic pacemakers. Am J Cardiol 1984;54:308–12.
23. Magnin PA, Stewart JA, Myers S, von Ramm O, Kisslo JA. Combined Doppler and phased-array echocardiographic estimation of cardiac output. Circulation 1981;63:388–92.
24. Huntsman LL, Stewart DK, Barnes SR, Franklin SB, Colocousis

JS, Hessel EA. Noninvasive Doppler determination of cardiac output in man. Clinical validation. Circulation 1983;67:593–602.

25. Ihlen H, Amlie JP, Dale J, et al. Determination of cardiac output by Doppler echocardiography. Br Heart J 1984;51:54–60.

26. Kitabatake A, Inoue M, Asao M, et al. Noninvasive evaluation of the ratio of pulmonary to systemic flow in atrial septal defect by duplex Doppler echocardiography. Circulation 1984;69:73–9.

27. Lewis JF, Kuo JC, Nelson JG, Limacher MC, Quinones MA. Pulsed Doppler echocardiographic determination of stroke volume and cardiac output: clinical validation of two methods using the apical window. Circulation 1984;70:425–31.

28. Jenni R, Vieli A, Ruffmann K, Krayenbuehl HP, Anlilar M. A comparison between single gate and multigate ultrasonic Doppler measurements for the assessment of the velocity pattern in the human ascending aorta. Eur Heart J 1984;5:953–84.

29. Goldberg SJ, Sahn DJ, Allen HD, Valdes-Cruz LM, Hoenecke H, Carnahan Y. Evaluation of pulmonary and systemic blood flow by 2-dimensional Doppler echocardiography using fast Fourier transform spectral analysis. Am J Cardiol 1982;50:1394–400.

30. Sanders SP, Yeager S, Williams RG. Measurements of systemic and pulmonary blood flow and QP/QS ratio using Doppler and two-dimensional echocardiography. Am J Cardiol 1983;51:952–6.

31. Fischer DC, Sahn DJ, Friedman MJ, et al. The mitral valve orifice method for noninvasive two-dimensional echo-Doppler determination of cardiac output. Circulation 1983;67:872–7.

32. Meijbom EJ, Horowitz S, Valdes-Cruz LM, Sahn DJ, Larson DF, Lima CO. A Doppler echocardiographic method for calculating volume flow across the tricuspid valve: correlative laboratory and clinical studies. Circulation 1985;71:551–6.

33. Loeber CP, Goldberg SJ, Allen HD. Doppler echocardiographic comparison of flows distal to the four cardiac valves. J Am Coll Cardiol 1984;4:268–72.

34. Hatle L, Brubakk A, Tromsdal A, Angelsen B. Noninvasive assessment of pressure drop in mitral stenosis by Doppler ultrasound. Br Heart J 1978;40:131–40.

35. Holen J, Aaslid R, Landmark K, Simonsen S, Østrem T. Determination of effective orifice area in mitral stenosis from noninvasive ultrasound Doppler data and mitral flow rate. Acta Med Scand 1977;201:83–8.

36. Vasco SD, Goldberg SJ, Requarth JA, Allen HD. Factors affecting accuracy of in vitro valvar pressure gradient estimates by Doppler ultrasound. Am J Cardiol 1984;54:893–6.

37. Hegrenaes L, Hatle L. Aortic stenosis in adults. Assessment with continuous wave Doppler ultrasound. Br Heart J (in press).

38. Berger M, Berdoff RL, Gallerstein PE, Goldberg E. Evaluation of aortic stenosis by continuous wave ultrasound. J Am Coll Cardiol 1984;3:150–6.

39. Williams GA, Labivitz AJ, Nelson JG, Kennedy HL. Value of multiple echocardiographic views in the evaluation of aortic stenosis in adults by continuous wave Doppler. Am J Cardiol 1985;55:445–9.

40. Skjaerpe T, Hatle L, Hegrenaes L. Noninvasive estimation of valve area in aortic stenosis with Doppler ultrasound and echocardiography. Circulation (in press).

41. Kosturakis D, Allen HD, Goldberg SJ, Sahn DJ, Valdes-Cruz LM. Noninvasive quantification of semilunar valve areas by Doppler echocardiography. J Am Coll Cardiol 1984;3:1256–62.

42. Hatle L. Noninvasive assessment and differentiation of left ventricular outflow obstruction by Doppler ultrasound. Circulation 1981;64:381–7.

43. Hatle L, Angelsen B, Tromsdal A. Noninvasive assessment of atrioventricular pressure half-time by Doppler ultrasound. Circulation 1979;60:1096–104.

44. Stamm BR, Martin RP. Quantification of pressure gradients across stenotic valves by Doppler ultrasound. J Am Coll Cardiol 1984;2:707–18.

45. Dennig K, Rudolph W. Dopplerechokardiographische Bestimmung des Schweregrades der Mitralstenose. Herz 1984;9;222–30.

46. Robson DJ, Flaxman JC. Measurement of the end-diastolic pressure gradient and mitral valve area in mitral stenosis by Doppler ultrasound. Eur Heart J 1984;5:660–7.

47. Lima CO, Sahn DJ, Valdes-Cruz LM, et al. Noninvasive prediction of transvalvular pressure gradient in patients with pulmonary stenosis by quantitative two-dimensional echo Doppler studies. Circulation 1983;67:866–71.

48. Hatle L, Angelsen B. Doppler ultrasound in cardiology. 2nd ed. Philadelphia: Lea & Febiger, 1985:148.

49. Ward JM, Baker DW, Rubenstein SA, Johnson SL. Detection of aortic insufficiency by pulsed Doppler echocardiography. J Clin Ultrasound 1977;5:5–10.

50. Quinones MA, Young JB, Waggoner AD, Ostojic MC, Ribeiro LGT, Miller RR. Assessment of pulsed Doppler echocardiography in detection and quantification of aortic and mitral regurgitation. Br Heart J 1980;44:612–20.

51. Ciobanu M, Abbasi AS, Allen M, Hermer A, Spellberg R. Pulsed Doppler echocardiography in the diagnosis and estimation of severity of aortic insufficiency. Am J Cardiol 1982;49:339–43.

52. Veyrat C, Ameur A, Gourtchiglouian C, Lessana A, Abitbol G, Kalmanson D. Calculation of pulsed Doppler left ventricular outflow tract regurgitant index for grading the severity of aortic regurgitation. Am Heart J 1984;108:507–15.

53. Esper RJ. Detection of mild aortic regurgitation by range-gated pulsed Doppler echocardiography. Am J Cardiol 1982;50:1037–43.

54. Saal AK, Gross BW, Franklin DW, Pearlman AS. Noninvasive detection of aortic insufficiency in patients with mitral stenosis by pulsed Doppler echocardiography. J Am Coll Cardiol 1985;5:176–81.

55. Boughner DR. Assessment of aortic insufficiency by transcutaneous Doppler ultrasound. Circulation 1975;52:874–9.

56. Hatteland K, Semb B. Assessment of aortic regurgitation by means of pulsed Doppler ultrasound. Ultrasound Med Biol 1982;8:1–5.

57. Diebold B, Peronneau P, Blanchard D, et al. Noninvasive quantification of aortic regurgitation by Doppler echocardiography. Br Heart J 1983;49:167–73.

58. Garcia-Dorado Garcia AD, Lopez Bescos L, Almazan Ceballos A, Alvarez Diaz R. Velocimetria Doppler transcutanea de la arteria subclavia en el estudio de la valvulopathia aortica. Rev Esp Cardiol 1980;33:249–57.

59. Stevenson JG, Kawabori I, Guntheroth WG. Differentiation of ventricular septal defects from mitral regurgitation by pulsed Doppler echocardiography. Circulation 1977;56:14–8.

60. Miyatake K, Kinoshita N, Nagata S, et al. Intracardiac flow pattern in mitral regurgitation studied with combined use of the ultrasonic pulsed Doppler technique and cross-sectional echocardiography. Am J Cardiol 1980;45:155–62.

61. Abbasi AS, Allen MW, De Christofaro D, Ungar J. Detection and estimation of the degree of mitral regurgitation by range-gated pulsed Doppler echocardiography. Circulation 1980;61:143–7.

62. Veyrat C, Ameur A, Bas S, Lessana A, Abitbol G, Kalmanson D. Pulsed Doppler echocardiographic indices for assessing mitral regurgitation. Br Heart J 1984;51:130–8.

63. Blanchard D, Diebold B, Peronneau P, et al. Noninvasive diagnosis of mitral regurgitation by Doppler echocardiography. Br Heart J 1981;45:589–93.

64. Patel AK, Rowe GG, Thomsen JH, et al. Detection and estimation of rheumatic mitral regurgitation in the presence of mitral stenosis by pulsed Doppler echocardiography. Am J Cardiol 1983;51:986–91.

65. Hatle L, Angelsen B. Doppler ultrasound in cardiology. 2nd ed. Philadelphia: Lea & Febiger, 1985:39,180.

66. Nichol PM, Boughner DR, Persaud JA. Noninvasive assessment of mitral regurgitation by transcutaneous Doppler ultrasound. Circulation 1976;54:656–61.

67. Stewart WJ, Palacios I, Jiang L, Dinsmore RE, Weyman A. Doppler measurement of regurgitant fraction in patients with mitral regurgitation: a new quantitative technique, abstracted. Circulation 1983;68(suppl III):111.

68. Skjaerpe T, Hatle L. Diagnosis and assessment of tricuspid regurgitation with Doppler ultrasound. In: Rijsterborgh H, ed. Echocardiology. The Hague; the Netherlands: Martinus Nijhoff, 1981:299–304.

69. Waggoner AD, Quinones MA, Young JB, et al. Pulsed Doppler echocardiographic detection of right-sided valve regurgitation. Am J Cardiol 1981;47:279–86.

70. Yock PG, Naasz C, Schnittger I, Popp RL. Doppler tricuspid and

pulmonic regurgitation in normals: is it real? abstracted. Circulation 1984;70(suppl II):40.

71. Skjaerpe T, Hatle L. Noninvasive estimation of pulmonary artery pressure by Doppler ultrasound. In: Spencer M, ed. Cardiac Doppler diagnosis. The Hague, the Netherlands: Martinus Nijhoff, 1983:247–54.

72. Yock PG, Popp RL. Noninvasive estimation of right ventricular systolic pressure by Doppler ultrasound in patients with tricuspid regurgitation. Circulation 1984;70:657–62.

73. Veyrat C, Kalmanson D, Farjou M, Manin JP, Abitbol G. Noninvasive diagnosis and assessment of tricuspid regurgitation and stenosis using one and two dimensional echopulsed Doppler. Br Heart J 1982;47:596–605.

74. Miyatake K, Okamoto M, Kinoshita N, et al. Evaluation of tricuspid regurgitation by pulsed Doppler and two-dimensional echocardiography. Circulation 1982;66:777–84.

75. Benchimol A, Harris CL, Desser KB. Noninvasive diagnosis of tricuspid insufficiency utilizing the external Doppler flowmeter probe. Am J Cardiol 1973;32:868–73.

76. Sivaciyan V, Ranganathan N. Transcutaneous Doppler jugular venous flow velocity recording. Circulation 1978;57:930–9.

77. Garcia-Dorado D, Falzgraf S, Almazan A, Delcan JL, Lopez-Bescos L, Menarguez L. Diagnosis of functional tricuspid insufficiency by pulsed-wave Doppler ultrasound. Circulation 1982;66: 1316–21.

78. Sakai K, Nakamura K, Satomi G, Kondo M, Hirosawa K. Evaluation of tricuspid regurgitation by blood flow pattern in the hepatic vein using pulsed Doppler ultrasound technique. Am Heart J 1984;108:516–23.

79. Pennestri F, Loperfido F, Salvatori MP, et al. Assessment of tricuspid regurgitation by pulsed Doppler ultrasonography of the hepatic veins. Am J Cardiol 1984;54:363–8.

80. Stevenson JG, Kawabori J, Guntheroth W. Detection of pulmonary insufficiency by pulsed Doppler echocardiography: validation, sensitivity, specificity and correlation with M-mode echo, abstracted. Circulation 1980;62(suppl III):251.

81. Takao S, Miyatake K, Dzumi S, Kinoshita N, Sakakibara H, Nimura J. Physiological pulmonary regurgitation detected by the Doppler technique and its differential diagnosis, abstracted. J Am Coll Cardiol 1985;5:499.

82. Hatle L, Angelsen B. Doppler ultrasound in cardiology. 2nd ed. Philadelphia: Lea & Febiger, 1985:188–205.

83. Holen J, Simonsen S, Frøysaker T. An ultrasound Doppler technique for the noninvasive determination of the pressure gradient in the Bjørk-Shiley mitral valve. Circulation 1979;59:436–42.

84. Canale JM, Sahn DJ, Copeland JG, et al. Two-dimensional Doppler echocardiographic/M-mode echocardiographic and phonocardiographic method for study of extracardiac heterograft valved conduits in the right ventricular outflow tract position. Am J Cardiol 1982;49:100–7.

85. Reeder GS, Currie PJ, Fyfe D, Hagler DJ, Seward JB, Tajik AJ. Extracardiac conduit obstruction: initial experience in the use of Doppler echocardiography for noninvasive estimation of pressure gradient. J Am Coll Cardiol 1984;4:1006–11.

86. Hatle L, Angelsen B. Doppler ultrasound in cardiology. 2nd ed. Philadelphia: Lea & Febiger, 1985:205–17.

87. Hoffmann A, Burckhardt D. Evaluation of systolic murmurs by Doppler ultrasonography. Br Heart J 1983;50:337–42.

88. Richards KL, Hockenga DE, Leach JK, Blaustein JC. Doppler cardiographic diagnosis of interventricular septal rupture. Chest 1979;76:101–3.

89. Recusani F, Raisaro A, Sgalambro A, et al. Ventricular septal rupture after myocardial infarction: diagnosis by two-dimensional and pulsed Doppler echocardiography. Am J Cardiol 1984;54:277–81.

90. Kitabatake A, Inoue M, Asao A, et al. Noninvasive estimation of pulmonary hypertension by a pulsed Doppler technique. Circulation 1983;68:302–9.

91. Hatle L, Angelsen B. Doppler ultrasound in cardiology. 2nd ed. Philadelphia: Lea & Febiger, 1985:252–64.

92. Okamoto M, Miyatake K, Kinoshita N, Sakakibara H, Nimura Y. Analysis of blood flow in pulmonary hypertension with a pulsed Doppler flowmeter combined with cross-sectional echocardiography. Br Heart 1984;51:407–415.

5

An Integrated Approach to the Noninvasive Assessment of Left Ventricular Systolic and Diastolic Performance

Kenneth Borow

INTRODUCTION

The integration of M-mode, two-dimensional, and Doppler echocardiographic findings with pulse recordings provides an exceptionally powerful tool for the noninvasive physiologic assessment of left ventricular (LV) performance. Before one can understand the full clinical utility of cardiac ultrasound as a physiologic tool, however, it is necessary to become familiar with the applications and limitations of certain cardiovascular principles. To begin with, it is important to differentiate between overall cardiac performance and myocardial contractility. *Overall cardiac performance* reflects the interaction of the heart, blood vessels, and blood volume. These component parts work together to determine the extent of LV fiber shortening during systole, the magnitude of ventricular wall thickness and mass, and the size of the LV throughout the cardiac cycle. Impaired overall cardiac performance can be due to abnormal LV loading conditions (for example, decreased intravascular blood volume or acute systemic hypertension) as well as structural changes in the heart valves or pericardium. These factors can interfere with cardiac filling or emptying in the presence of normal contractile function, and thus can depress traditional indices of LV function, such as ejection fraction, percent fractional shortening, stroke volume, or cardiac output. In contrast to overall cardiac performance, contractility is an intrinsic property of the ventricular muscle fiber. It reflects the chemical and mechanical processes that lead to force generation and fiber shortening within the LV (1). Depression in LV contractility is most often secondary to myocardial ischemia, viral myocarditis, cardiac toxins, systemic hypertension, or long-standing valvular heart disease.

It is also important to remember that throughout the cardiac cycle, the LV undergoes complex biochemical and conformational changes that result in marked interdependence of systolic and diastolic events. Evaluation of LV physiology throughout the *entire* cardiac cycle is therefore necessary. Under most circumstances, these data should be obtained serially. Exercise and pharmacologic stress testing frequently give important additional information regarding cardiac performance. Finally, the manner in which the heart and its peripheral vascular bed are coupled to supply blood and oxygen to the body must be assessed.

This chapter pursues a physiologically oriented ap-

DETERMINANTS OF LEFT VENTRICULAR SHORTENING

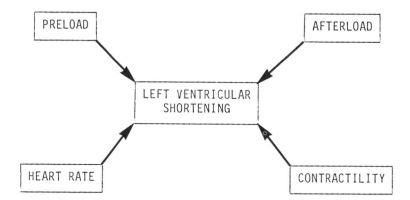

Figure 5.1 The extent and velocity of left ventricular fiber shortening reflects the complex interaction of preload, afterload, heart rate, and contractility.

proach to the noninvasive assessment of both left ventricular and systemic arterial function. The chapter is divided into two sections. The first deals with methods of assessing LV systolic performance. The second section addresses the complexities involved in the evaluation of LV diastolic filling characteristics and chamber compliance. Current approaches and limitations are emphasized. Each section is introduced by a discussion of pertinent cardiac physiology followed by discussions of the use of M-mode, two-dimensional, and Doppler echocardiographic techniques for data acquisition and analysis. Finally, an integrated noninvasive approach to the assessment of LV performance in the clinical setting is presented. It is our hope that the coupling of cardiac physiology with ultrasound imaging will significantly improve the physician's ability to diagnose and understand disease states as well as determine the efficacy of therapy. This is especially important when cost containment issues are superimposed on the need for serial assessment of cardiac performance.

ASSESSMENT OF LEFT VENTRICULAR SYSTOLIC PERFORMANCE

Physiology

Determinants of Overall Cardiac Performance

Overall LV performance reflects the interplay of preload, afterload, heart rate, and contractility (Fig. 5.1) (2). The inability of traditional indices of LV performance to distinguish changes in contractility from alterations in loading conditions or heart rate has been a major problem for the clinician and clinical investigator for years (3–5). Recently, several noninvasively obtained load independent contractility indices have been described. This represents an important advance,

since it is LV contractile state rather than overall ventricular performance that frequently determines long-term prognosis (1, 4, 5). For example, patients with chronic mitral regurgitation exhibit preload augmentation secondary to LV volume overload, as well as afterload reduction due to LV ejection of blood into the low pressure left atrium. This frequently results in maintenance of normal myocardial fiber shortening. It is only with valve replacement and subsequent restoration of more normal LV loading conditions that the underlying contractile abnormality is unmasked. To understand more fully how preload, afterload, contractility, and heart rate affect overall LV systolic performance, each of these factors will be considered separately.

Preload

This is described classically as the force or load acting to stretch the left ventricular fibers at end-diastole (1, 7). As such, it sets the maximal resting length of the sarcomeres. Preload is commonly estimated as the LV end-diastolic pressure or end-diastolic dimension (or volume). More accurately, it is the force on the myocardial fibers per unit cross-sectional area of muscle, and is best expressed as end-diastolic wall stress. It is well known that LV stroke volume and stroke work are dependent on LV end-diastolic fiber load. This relationship is the basis of the Frank-Starling law of the heart (1–9). The level of LV preload reflects many factors, including chamber stiffness, the pumping ability of the heart, the intravascular blood volume and its distribution, the atrial contribution to LV filling, intrapericardial and intrathoracic pressures, as well as the ability of the peripheral circulation to return blood to the heart (1, 8, 10, 11). In addition, the level of end-diastolic wall stress appears to act as the stimulus for LV

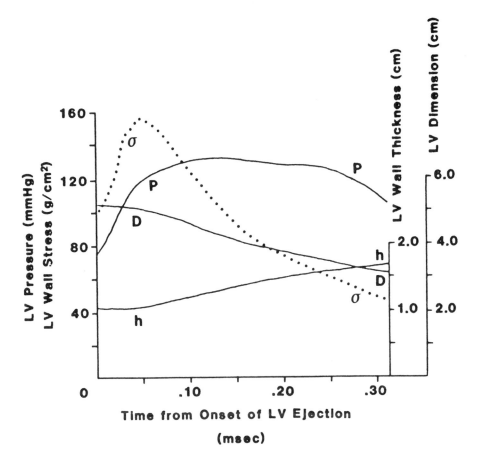

Figure 5.2 Left ventricular afterload [i.e., wall stress (σ)] calculated over the course of ejection from simultaneous measurements of pressure (P), dimension (D), and wall thickness (h) in a normal subject. Systolic wall stress peaks soon after onset of ejection, and then declines throughout the remainder of systole.

hypertrophy in lesions such as chronic aortic regurgitation (12).

Afterload

Left ventricular afterload can be thought of as the force opposing ventricular fiber shortening after the onset of ejection (7, 13). It is not synonymous with peripheral arterial pressure, peripheral vascular tone, or systemic vascular resistance. For example, the calculation of systemic vascular resistance assumes that the LV is a nonpulsatile pump with steady state hemodynamics throughout the cardiac cycle. This is obviously not an accurate description of the pumping nature of the left ventricle. Afterload is much better defined as LV wall stress at the time of ejection. According to the modified LaPlace's law, LV wall stress is directly related to chamber dimension and pressure, and inversely related to wall thickness (1–8, 10, 13–17). During the ejection phase of the cardiac cycle, the LV dimension decreases, while ventricular pressure and wall thickness increase (Fig. 5.2). Thus, LV afterload varies in magnitude throughout ventricular ejection. Normally, LV afterload (wall stress) peaks during the first one-third of ventricular ejection and then declines throughout the remainder of systole. By end-ejection, wall stress in the normal subject is less than 50% of its peak value. Left ventricular wall stress curves throughout systole are

quite different from intraventricular pressure curves. This is illustrated when one compares a dilated thin-walled LV to a ventricle with normal size and wall thickness. Both chambers can generate similar peak systolic pressures, but afterload, as measured by wall stress, is much greater for the dilated heart (Fig. 5.3) (18). In addition, it is thought that increased wall stress in an area of infarcted myocardium is an important contributor to systolic bulging and subsequent aneurysm formation (19).

That afterload varies during the cardiac cycle is important in understanding cardiac physiology. For example, it is the level of *peak* systolic wall stress that is one of the most important stimuli for LV hypertrophy in chronic pressure overload states such as systemic hypertension, valvular aortic stenosis, or coarctation of the aorta (20–24). On the other hand, the integral of LV systolic wall stress, along with heart rate and contractile state, are major determinants of myocardial oxygen requirements (MVO$_2$) (25–27). Finally, the wall stress at end-systole, rather than the wall stress during the course of ventricular ejection, is inversely related to the overall extent and mean velocity of fiber shortening at a given level of contractility (10, 28–34). This important relationship reflects a fundamental property of cardiac muscle. In addition, changes in the pressure-dimension (volume) pathway followed during ejection

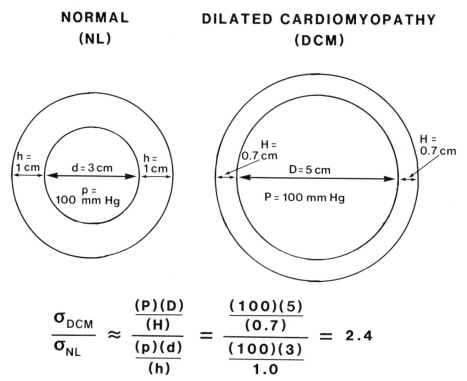

NORMAL (NL) **DILATED CARDIOMYOPATHY (DCM)**

$$\frac{\sigma_{DCM}}{\sigma_{NL}} \approx \frac{\frac{(P)(D)}{(H)}}{\frac{(p)(d)}{(h)}} = \frac{\frac{(100)(5)}{(0.7)}}{\frac{(100)(3)}{1.0}} = 2.4$$

Figure 5.3 Comparison of calculated wall stress values for a normal left ventricle (NL) versus one with dilated cardiomyopathy (DCM). Despite the same intracavitary pressure (i.e., p = P = 100 mm Hg), the dimensions (d, D) and wall thicknesses (h, H) are quite different. This results in a much higher wall stress for the dilated cardiomyopathic ventricle.

do not significantly alter the extent of LV fiber shortening. It is becoming increasingly clear that end-systolic wall stress determines the size of the LV at end-ejection, and in turn becomes a major determinant of LV stroke volume and cardiac output (1, 4, 5, 17, 18, 35, 36).

Heart Rate
In humans, heart rate significantly affects cardiac output. This is true under resting conditions as well as during dynamic exercise (1). With increasing heart rate, the time available for LV filling during diastole is shortened. In normal subjects, this is not a problem because most of LV filling occurs very early in diastole. When mitral valve obstruction or marked abnormalities in LV compliance are present, however, decreased ventricular preload can lead to reduced overall LV performance despite normal LV afterload and contractility. Although increases in heart rate can increase inotropic state in isolated muscle preparations and various animal models, the importance of this force-frequency relationship in humans remains controversial.

Contractile State
As noted earlier, left ventricular contractility reflects the chemical and mechanical processes leading to force generation and fiber shortening within the myocardium (11, 17, 29). Traditionally, a change in contractility in the intact heart can be defined as an alteration in overall cardiac performance that occurs independent of alterations in preload, afterload, or heart rate. Because of the latter confounding variables, it has been

difficult to assess LV contractility in humans (2). Recently, several indices of LV performance that relate physiologic events measured at end-systole have been shown to be independent of ventricular loading conditions, and thus are useful as clinical measures of contractility (8, 30, 31, 34). The most promising of these are the end-systolic pressure-dimension (or volume) relation, end-systolic wall stress-dimension (or volume) relation, and the end-systolic wall stress-rate corrected velocity of fiber shortening relation.

Unlike skeletal muscle, cardiac muscle is not usually fully activated during contraction (11). The capacity of the ventricle to augment contractile state to improve overall performance is an important compensatory mechanism in many disease states. Actual quantitation of LV contractile reserve has become possible using either pharmacologic agents (such as dobutamine or isuprel) or dynamic exercise testing techniques.

Traditional Measures of Left Ventricular Systolic Performance

Frank-Starling Law of the Heart
The classic method used to assess LV systolic performance is to relate ventricular filling pressure, dimension, or volume to the pressure generated, volume displaced (i.e., stroke volume or cardiac output), or work performed (1). This approach utilizes the Frank-Starling relation of the heart. In theory, an increase in end-diastolic pressure, dimension, or volume results in an increase in muscle fiber length. This allows for

augmentation of actin and myosin interaction without changing the LV contractile state (8). However, these changes in diastolic measurements do not bear a predictable relation to diastolic wall stress (i.e., presumed measure of true preload) or to sarcomere length (1). In addition, factors such as pericardial disease, restrictive myocardial disease, cardiac hypertrophy, or abnormalities in LV volume status can alter the Frank-Starling relation in the absence of derangements in LV contractile state (8, 9, 37). In effect, the Frank-Starling relation represents a combination of preload and afterload effects acting in conjunction with a constant or changing contractile state (1, 9, 37).

Isovolumic Indices

The isovolumic indices of left ventricular performance are determined from pressure transients recorded during the pre-ejection period of ventricular systole prior to opening of the aortic valve (1, 7, 17). The simplest and most commonly used of the isovolumic indices is the maximal rate of LV pressure rise (i.e., peak positive dP/dt) (38). The major limitation of peak positive dP/dt as a left ventricular contractility index is its sensitivity to LV preload as well as low aortic diastolic pressures (7, 8, 37, 38). While peak positive dP/dt reflects the maximal rate of LV pressure rise prior to aortic valve opening, it fails to predict the ventricle's ability to undergo fiber shortening when afterload is increased (16, 38). This is particularly true in patients with severe congestive heart failure, where the use of ejection phase indices of LV performance recorded in conjunction with measurements of LV wall stress are more clinically useful than the isovolumic indices (39). Recent animal studies have suggested that the slope of the LV (dP/dt$_{max}$) end-diastolic volume relation may be a sensitive load independent index of LV contractility (40, 41).

Ejection Phase Indices

These are measures of overall LV performance that use data collected during ventricular ejection. In general, they are preload, afterload, heart rate, and contractility-dependent. As such, they are unable to distinguish abnormalities in contractile state from compensatory or detrimental alterations in loading conditions (7–9, 34, 37). They cannot, therefore, be used in isolation as measures of LV contractility. The commonly used ejection phase indices include LV volume or work output, systolic time intervals, ejection fraction (EF), percent fractional shortening (%ΔD), and mean velocity of LV fiber shortening (V_{cf}).

LV VOLUME OR WORK OUTPUT

1. *Stroke volume* is the amount of blood ejected from the ventricle per beat and is a function of the overall extent of LV fiber shortening.

2. *Cardiac output* is stroke volume times heart rate. Through the use of compensatory mechanisms, the dilated, cardiomyopathic LV may still eject a normal or near normal cardiac output, despite significant depression in contractility (1, 8, 9, 18).

3. *Stroke work* is the product of stroke volume and mean systolic pressure. It has been used as an index of LV performance, especially in conjunction with measures of LV preload.

4. *Stroke power* is stroke work per unit time. It reflects the relationship between instantaneous LV pressure and flow. It can be thought of as the rate at which energy is expended in performing LV work. Stroke power during systole has steady state as well as pulsatile components. It can be used as a measure of how efficiently the pumping function of the LV is coupled to its peripheral arterial circulation.

SYSTOLIC TIME INTERVALS. Systolic time intervals (STI) have been used for many years as measures of overall LV performance in patients with suspected or known heart disease. They can be calculated noninvasively using three methods, including 1) simultaneous recording of the electrocardiograms, carotid pulse tracing, and phonocardiogram; 2) simultaneous M-mode echocardiographic and electrocardiographic tracings; and 3) simultaneous Doppler echocardiographic and electrocardiographic recordings (Fig. 5.4). The four measures most commonly used in clinical practice are the *total electromechanical systole*, the *LV ejection time*, the *pre-ejection period*, and the *ratio of pre-ejection period to LV ejection time*.

1. Total electromechanical systole is measured from the onset of the QRS complex to end ejection. It reflects the combination of electromechanical association time, isovolumic contraction time, and LV ejection time.

2. LV ejection time measures the period of blood flow across the aortic valve. It is influenced by heart rate, stroke volume, preload, afterload, and contractile state. Ejection time shortens with mitral regurgitation as well as LV failure. In these cases, it primarily reflects decreased forward stroke volume. LV ejection time increases with compensated aortic stenosis, aortic regurgitation, and high cardiac output states.

3. Pre-ejection period is calculated as total systole minus LV ejection time. It is influenced by heart rate, aortic diastolic pressure, duration of intraventricular conduction, LV end-diastolic pressure, and contractile state. The pre-ejection period lengthens with LV failure primarily due to a reduction in the rate of LV pressure rise during isovolumic systole.

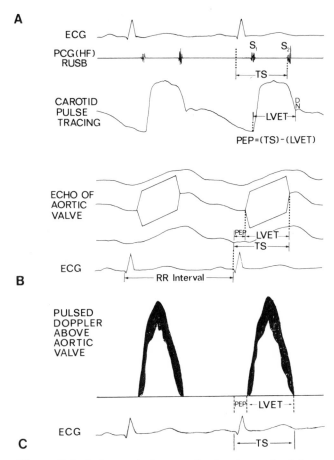

Figure 5.4 Left ventricular systolic time intervals. Schematic drawings indicate the major intervals derived from (*A*) simultaneous phonocardiogram (PCG), indirect carotid pulse tracing, and electrocardiogram (ECG); (*B*) echocardiogram of the aortic valve and ECG; (*C*) pulsed Doppler tracing recorded above the aortic valve and ECG. HF = high frequency; RUSB = right upper sternal border; S_1 = first heart sound; S_2 = second heart sound; DN = dicrotic notch; TS = total electromechanical systole; LVET = left ventricular ejection time; PEP = pre-ejection period; RR = beat cycle length.

4. The ratio of pre-ejection period to LV ejection time is relatively heart rate–independent. However, its clinical utility is markedly limited by its dependence on afterload, preload, and contractility. Increases occur with LV failure, decreased intravascular volume, and mitral regurgitation. Decreases occur with compensated aortic stenosis and/or regurgitation.

EJECTION FRACTION. EF is calculated as LV stroke volume normalized to the initial volume (i.e., end-diastolic volume). Since it is a ratio reflecting the percent of LV end-diastolic volume ejected in a single beat, it is dimensionless. Although this measure of LV systolic performance is adequate for a gross assessment of overall pump function, it is unable to separate

changes in LV contractility from alterations in the other determinants of LV fiber shortening (i.e., preload, afterload, and heart rate). As such, LV ejection fraction reflects a complex interaction between ventricular loading conditions and contractile state (1, 8, 9, 34). For example, in the normal heart, an increase in LV afterload is associated with an increase in end-systolic volume. This leads to an increase in end-diastolic volume with maintenance of stroke volume. If the increase in LV afterload becomes excessive for a given level of contractility, the rise in end-systolic volume may exceed the ventricle's ability to augment end-diastolic volume, resulting in a fall in stroke volume (8, 38). This is known as exhaustion of preload reserve, and reflects a mismatch between afterload, preload, and contractility. The net result is a fall in ventricular ejection fraction, despite stable LV contractility. This is a frequent occurrence in patients with dilated myopathic ventricles. Other examples of conditions in which ejection fraction can give misleading data regarding intrinsic LV contractile properties include aortic stenosis or regurgitation, mitral stenosis or regurgitation, decreased intravascular volume, hypertension or hypotension, and the response to cardioactive pharmacologic agents. It becomes readily apparent that in most pathologic states, LV ejection fraction must be interpreted in conjunction with measures of myocardial loading conditions (3, 7, 9, 34).

Numerous studies of LV function have used the ejection fraction response to dynamic exercise as a measure of contractility and contractile reserve. However, certain acute physiologic adjustments to dynamic exercise result in an increase in ejection fraction, including peripheral vasodilation in exercising muscles, neurally mediated increases in sympathetic tone to the heart and periphery, the release of catecholamines from the adrenal medulla, and changes in venous return and preload. The associated use of preload reserve is highly dependent on LV chamber compliance. Derangement in *any one* of these mechanisms can result in a decrease or failure to increase LV ejection fraction without a concomitant abnormality in LV contractility or contractile reserve. The ejection fraction response to dynamic exercise must be thought of as a nonspecific measure of LV performance that is dependent upon multiple, simultaneously changing variables. Therefore, it is not diagnostic of an alteration in contractile state.

PERCENT FRACTIONAL SHORTENING. This is the echocardiographic equivalent of ejection fraction, in which LV dimensions are substituted for LV volumes. It has all the limitations just discussed for ejection fraction.

MEAN VELOCITY OF LV FIBER SHORTENING. This measures the mean velocity of ventricular fiber shortening at the level of the LV minor axis (7, 38). It is calculated as the percent fractional shortening divided by the LV ejection time. This value is normalized for end-diastolic chamber size, and therefore is useful for comparisons between patients. V_{cf} is relatively preload-independent. However, it is highly afterload-, contractility-, and heart rate–dependent. A heart rate corrected V_{cf} value (Vcf_c) has been clinically useful when plotted against a measure of ventricular afterload (31). Rate corrected V_{cf} is calculated by multiplying V_{cf} by the square root of the preceding RR-interval measured from the electrocardiogram.

M-Mode Echocardiography

Introduction

Traditional M-mode echocardiography employs an independent high-frequency transducer to send sound waves in a narrow beam through the heart. This technique uses 1 microsecond burst of high-frequency sound waves followed by a receiving period of 999 microseconds. Since one complete cycle of sending and receiving an M-mode ultrasound signal requires less than 1 millisecond in humans, a sampling rate in excess of 1000 times per second can be achieved. The net effect is a high time resolution of motion that can be accurately recorded (42–44). Most cardiac ultrasound laboratories now use M-mode tracings derived from targeted two-dimensional images rather than performing independent M-mode transducer studies. Temporal resolution and image quality are less for two-dimensional echocardiography as compared to M-mode techniques, since the video frame rate is only 33 per second. Despite the fact that the frame repetition rate of two-dimensional echocardiography is generally too low to record high frequency vibrations (45), derived and independent M-mode measurements of LV dimensions correlate well (46). The use of two-dimensional targeting for M-mode echocardiographic data acquisition significantly increases inter- and intra-patient reproducibility and allows accurate serial determinations to be performed (44, 47).

Indirect Measures of Left Ventricular Function

Mitral Valve

1. Decreased mitral valve early closing velocity. Decreased mitral valve early closing velocity (i.e., E-F slope) may occur in patients without intrinsic mitral valve disease if low cardiac output or diminished LV compliance are present (44).
2. B bump or AC notch. A prominent B bump or AC notch on the anterior leaflet of the mitral valve suggests that the left atrial component of the LV diastolic pressure is at least 8 mm HG (Fig. 5.5). In many cases, this finding correlates with LV end-diastolic pressures in excess of 20 mm Hg (42, 44, 48–51).
3. Mitral valve E point–septal separation. Mitral valve E point–septal separation in excess of 7 mm has been reported to correlate well with significant depression in overall systolic performance in patients with dilated left ventricles (49, 52–54). This empiric finding reflects a combination of changes characteristic of the dilated LV. As the ventricle enlarges, the left septal surface moves toward the anterior chest wall. This occurs in association with decreased diastolic flow into the LV, resulting in diminished opening excursion (E point) of the mitral valve. Thus, the distance between the septum and anterior leaflet of the mitral valve increases (Fig. 5.5). Increased E point–septal separation has relatively high specificity, but low sensitivity for dilated cardiomyopathy (44, 53, 55). This index is preload- and afterload-dependent. Any intrinsic abnormality within the mitral valve or any process that impedes mitral valve opening (e.g., aortic regurgitation) further compromises the utility of this index.

Aortic Valve

1. Early systolic partial closure. Early systolic partial closure of the aortic valve leaflets has been described in dilated cardiomyopathy as well as other conditions that interrupt normal forward blood flow (e.g., ventricular septal defect, mitral regurgitation, or subaortic obstruction) (Fig. 5.6) (56). Early partial closure generally occurs within the first 20% of mechanical systole and does not correlate well with the severity of LV systolic dysfunction.
2. Systolic time intervals. Systolic time intervals can be measured using a simultaneously recorded electrocardiogram and echocardiogram of the aortic valve. From these tracings, it is possible to determine electromechanical systole, LV ejection time, and LV pre-ejection period (57). The limitations of this technique for assessing LV contractility were discussed previously.

Measures of Left Ventricular Chamber Dimensions and Wall Mass

Chamber Dimension

The LV internal dimension is usually measured at the level of the chordae tendinae or just below the tips of the anterior leaflet of the mitral valve. This provides a measure of the LV size between the left septal surface

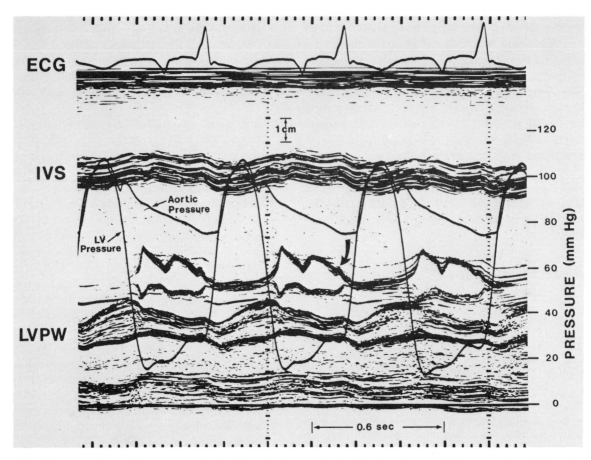

Figure 5.5   M-mode echocardiogram recorded at the mitral valve level with simultaneous left ventricular (LV) and central aortic pressures from a patient with severe dilated cardiomyopathy. There is a prominent B bump (large arrow) associated with large E point–septal separation. Left ventricular end-diastolic pressure was 26 mm Hg. The left atrial contribution of the LV diastolic pressure was 11 mm Hg. ECG = electrocardiogram; IVS = interventricular septum; LVPW = left ventricular posterior wall.

and the endocardial surface of the posterior LV wall. Increased diastolic dimensions correlate well with the existence of ventricular dilatation. The systolic dimension provides a measure of end-systolic size and overall function if the ventricle contracts symmetrically (58–61). The magnitude of posterior wall and septal excursion has been used to assess regional hypokinesis. The maximal rate of change of LV chamber dimension during systole can be determined by digitizing the M-mode tracing using a computer. This value gives a gross measure of overall LV performance (44). Left ventricular end-diastolic dimensions change with the respiratory cycle, becoming smaller with inspiration and larger with expiration (42). Right ventricular dilatation can decrease LV minor axis dimensions disproportionate to other dimensions, thereby making this measure poorly representative of total LV volume. Left ventricular dimensions alone have been used as contractility indices as well as criteria for surgical intervention for LV volume overload lesions (such as aortic regurgitation) (6, 34, 59, 60, 62). Left ventricular dimensions are highly preload-, afterload-, heart rate–, and

contractility-dependent. This limits markedly their clinical utility when used as isolated measurements.

Wall Thickness
Accurate M-mode echocardiographic determinations of LV posterior wall and septal thicknesses depend on the presence of an ultrasound beam that is positioned perpendicular to the region of interest (1, 57). These measurements require careful delineation of the right and left septal surfaces, as well as epicardial and endocardial surfaces of the posterior wall (42). Wall thicknesses can be determined at any time in the cardiac cycle, thus allowing assessment of systolic and diastolic changes. The mechanisms involved in systolic wall thickening include thickening of individual fibers and rearrangement of individual fiber layers to a more radial alignment (37). Systolic thickening of the septal and LV posterior wall can be calculated as

$$\% \text{ thickening} = \left(\frac{h_{es} - h_{ed}}{h_{ed}}\right)(100)$$

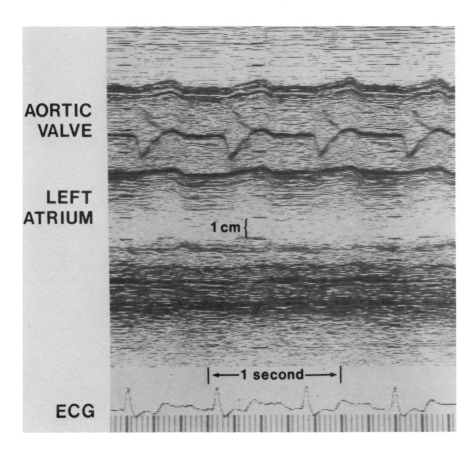

Figure 5.6 M-mode echocardiogram of the aortic valve from a patient with decreased forward cardiac output. There is normal initial leaflet excursion followed by gradual closure over the course of systole. ECG = electrocardiogram.

where h_{es} is end-systolic thickness and h_{ed} is end-diastolic thickness (50, 57). In the patient with a symmetrically contracting LV, the percent change in LV thickening correlates well with overall ventricular performance (47). All measurements of LV wall thickness including percent thickening are load- and contractility-dependent.

Left Ventricular Volume

M-mode echocardiographic estimates of LV volume depend on multiple factors besides accuracy of dimension measurements. Complex geometric modeling of the ventricle is performed from a limited one-dimensional data base. It is necessary to assume that the LV conforms to a prolate ellipse shape with a major and

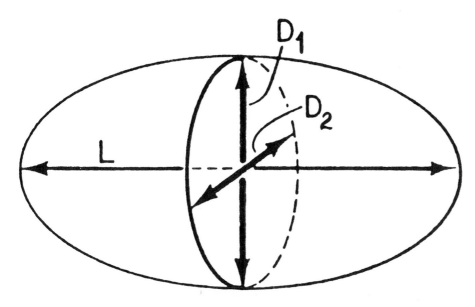

Figure 5.7 Schematic representation of a prolate ellipsoid. D_1 and D_2 are the minor axis dimensions, while L is the long axis length. (Reproduced with permission from Triulzi MO, Wilkins GT, Gillam LD, et al. Normal adult cross-sectional echocardiographic values: Left ventricular volumes. Echocardiography 1985;2:153–169.)

two equal minor axes (Fig. 5.7) (47, 49, 50, 57, 63). As an initial approximation, it is further assumed that the long axis to minor axis ratio is 2:1. The volume of a prolate ellipse is

$$V = \left(\frac{4}{3}\pi\right)\left(\frac{L}{2}\right)\left(\frac{D_1}{2}\right)\left(\frac{D_2}{2}\right)$$

where L = long axis length, and D_1 and D_2 are the minor axis dimensions. However, $D_1 = D_2$ and $L = 2D_1$. Making these substitutions,

$$V = \left(\frac{4}{3}\pi\right)\left(\frac{2D_1}{2}\right)\left(\frac{D_1}{2}\right)\left(\frac{D_1}{3}\right)$$

$$= \frac{\pi}{3}(D_1)^3 \approx (D_1^3)$$

Therefore, in its simplest form, LV volume for a prolate ellipse can be approximated by the cube of the minor axis dimension (47, 50, 57, 63, 64). While this method gives reasonably accurate estimates of LV end-diastolic and end-systolic volumes in normally shaped ventricles, it becomes less accurate when LV shape is abnormal. Typically, the dilated ventricle becomes more spherical. This results from a disproportionate increase in the minor axes relative to the long axis (47, 50, 57). The net result is a decrease in the long axis to minor axis ratio. The cube formula for LV volume therefore grossly overestimates volumes in dilated ventricles (47, 63). Teichholz et al. have derived a formula that attempts to correct for the change in long axis to minor axis ratio occuring with increasing LV volumes.

$$V = \left(\frac{7.0}{2.4 + D}\right)(D)^3$$

where D is the LV minor axis dimensions (47, 50). With this formula, echocardiographic and single-plane angiographic LV volumes correlate well (r = 0.97) in the absence of regional wall motion abnormalities (63). This fact was confirmed by Kronik et al., who found the formula of Teichholz et al. to correlate better than seven other commonly used M-mode echocardiographic methods for determining LV volumes in patients with symmetrically or nearly symmetrically contracting ventricles (65). Using this approach, LV stroke volume can be estimated as the difference between end-diastolic and end-systolic volumes. Cardiac output can then be calculated as LV stroke volume times heart rate. Normalization of cardiac output for body surface area allows more meaningful comparisons between patients.

Left Ventricular Wall Mass
Left ventricular hypertrophy, defined as an increase in wall mass, is a fundamental compensatory response to

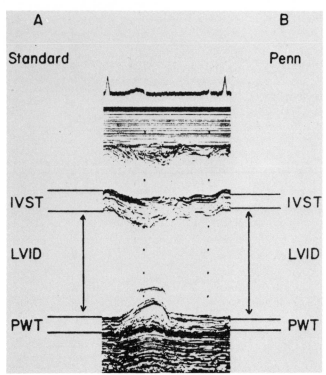

Figure 5.8 Methods for echocardiographic measurement of interventricular septal thickness (IVST), left ventricular internal dimension (LVID), and posterior wall thickness (PWT). Panel A: The standard measurement convention includes the thickness of the right and left septal endocardial echoes in IVST and includes posterior wall endocardial echoes in PWT. Panel B: The Penn Convention excludes right and left septal endocardial echo thickness from IVST and excludes posterial wall endocardial echo thickness from PWT. Left septal endocardial echo thickness and posterial wall endocardial echo thickness are thus included in LVID by this method. (Reproduced by permission of the American Heart Association, Inc. from Devereux RB, Reichek N. Echocardiographic determination of left ventricular mass in man: Anatomic validation of the method. Circulation 1977;55:613–618.)

chronic pressure or volume overload (66). Hypertrophy is one of the ventricle's most effective ways of maintaining systolic performance under circumstances of altered loading conditions (18, 66, 67). By decreasing systolic wall stress, hypertrophy reduces LV afterload and myocardial oxygen requirements.

Ventricular mass reflects both chamber volume and wall thickness. An increased LV wall thickness does not necessarily mean that LV hypertrophy (i.e., increased mass) is present. This is especially true for the small, hypovolemic ventricle. To calculate LV mass using M-mode echocardiography, it is necessary to assume that the volume of the myocardium is equal to the total volume enclosed by the epicardial surfaces of the ventricle minus the chamber volume (44, 50, 68–75). In all cases, the interventricular septum is considered to be part of the left ventricle. The most commonly used M-mode method for measuring LV wall thickness and chamber area is the Penn convention (Fig. 5.8) (66, 75–77). This requires that the thickness of endocardial interfaces is excluded from measurements of septal and posterior wall thickness and included in measurements of LV dimensions. Using this approach, the M-mode echocardiographic formula for LV mass is:

$$LVM = (1.05)[(D + PWT + IVS)^3 - (D)^3] - 14 \text{ g}$$

where D is left ventricular minor axis dimension in cm, PWT is posterior wall thickness in cm, IVS is interventricular septal thickness in cm, 1.05 is the specific gravity of muscle, and 14 g is part of the "regression-corrected cube formula" for LV mass. Using this formula, numerous investigators have shown that M-mode echocadiographic LV mass calculation is superior to echocardiographic LV posterior wall or septal thicknesses as well as ECG criteria for the autopsy diagnosis of LV hypertrophy (70, 71, 74, 76). In addition, a high correlation (r = 0.96) was noted between noninvasively estimated LV mass obtained just before death and actual LV weight measured at autopsy (44, 69, 73, 74). Since LV mass in normal subjects is closely related to lean body mass, indexation by body surface area eliminates intragroup differences in body habitus (75). The 97th percentile of LV mass index reported by Devereux et al. was 136 g/m² for men and 112 g/m² for women (75).

Measures of Overall Left Ventricular Systolic Performance

Percent Fractional Shortening

Percent fractional shortening (%ΔD) measures the extent of minor axis change as a percent of end-diastolic dimension (44, 47, 50, 63, 78). It is a pure number because it is dimensionless, and it is calculated as

$$\%\Delta D = \frac{D_{ed} - D_{es}}{D_{ed}}$$

Percent fractional shortening is predominantly preload-, afterload-, and contractility-dependent. This limits its utility as a contractility index in patients with LV volume overload states (such as mitral or aortic regurgitation), acute alterations in LV afterload, hypovolemia, etc. (44, 47). In patients with regional wall motion abnormalities, %ΔD may not accurately reflect overall ventricular shortening characteristics.

Ejection Fraction

The ejection fraction can be derived from M-mode echocardiographic volumes by dividing stroke volume (SV) by end-diastolic volume (V_{ed}) (42, 44, 47, 49, 50, 63, 79). Similar to %ΔD, it is highly preload-, afterload-, and contractility-dependent. M-mode echocardiographic estimates of LVEF require a symmetrically contracting

ventricle. The above noted limitations to LV volume determinations by M-mode echocardiography also apply to EF calculations.

Velocity of LV Shortening

This value describes the velocity of LV fiber shortening at a specific diameter of the ventricular ellipsoid (37). It does not truly represent the rate of fiber shortening, rather, it is a measure of rate of change of LV size in diameters per second (49). It is calculated as the change in LV internal circumference divided by LV ejection time. The latter can be measured noninvasively from echocardiographic images of the aortic valve or from a carotid pulse tracing, and invasively from a central aortic pressure tracing. Normalization of LV velocity of shortening is performed by dividing by end-diastolic circumference to allow comparisons of LV chambers of differing sizes. Derivation of the commonly used mean velocity of LV shortening is as follows (50):

$$
\begin{aligned}
\text{mean } V_{cf} &= \frac{\text{Change in LV internal circumference}}{(\text{End-diastolic circumference})(\text{LV ejection time})} \\
&= \frac{(\pi D_{ed}) - (\pi D_{es})}{(\pi D_{ed})(LVET)} = \frac{\pi(D_{ed} - D_{es})}{\pi(D_{ed})(LVET)} \\
&= \left(\frac{D_{ed} - D_{es}}{D_{ed}}\right)\left(\frac{1}{LVET}\right) = \frac{\%\Delta D}{LVET}
\end{aligned}
$$

There is a high correlation between mean V_{cf} values calculated using this formula and values obtained at angiography in ventricles without regional wall motion abnormalities (11, 47, 64). Like %ΔD and EF, mean V_{cf} is afterload-, heart rate–, and contractility-dependent. Studies performed in animals as well as humans suggest that mean V_{cf} is relatively preload-independent (31, 80, 81). The effect of heart rate can be eliminated by multiplying the V_{cf} value by the square root of the preceding RR interval as measured from the electrocardiogram (31). This value has been termed the rate corrected mean velocity of shortening (Vcf_c). Thus, Vcf_c is independent of preload and heart rate, while remaining afterload-dependent. When Vcf_c is related to a measure of LV afterload, the resultant index is sensitive to contractile changes, yet independent of rate and loading conditions (31).

Exercise M-Mode Echocardiography

Numerous studies of LV performance and wall motion have been performed using M-mode echocardiography during dynamic exercise (82–86). These studies have been limited by the narrow imaging window available in M-mode echocardiography, changes in heart position in the chest due to body motion, problems in imaging secondary to lung interference, and changes in imaging planes associated with ventricular hyperkinesis and increased heart rate.

Limitations of M-Mode Echocardiography

The major limitation of independently acquired M-mode echocardiographic imaging is the lack of planar or three-dimensional information (9, 44, 45, 50, 57, 87–92). This becomes particularly important in patients with regional wall motion abnormalities, aneurysms, or markedly enlarged chambers. The use of a spatially corrected two-dimensional image to target M-mode data acquisition has greatly enhanced measurement reliability and reproducibility, and thus has increased the quantitative and diagnostic yield of M-mode echocardiography (79).

Two-Dimensional Echocardiography

Introduction

For the assessment of left ventricular function, M-mode and two-dimensional echocardiography assume synergistic rather than merely additive roles. While M-mode echocardiography allows continuous tracings appropriate for quantitation of LV performance in the region visualized within the ultrasound beam, only two-dimensional echocardiography allows acquisition of simultaneous morphologic, anatomic, and functional data. Because two-dimensional echocardiography results in excellent spatial orientation, measurements of chamber and myocardial wall areas can be performed. This makes serial, quantitative, noninvasive assessment of global as well as regional left ventricular performance possible (9, 45, 47, 57, 87–90).

To date, data acquired at the time of cardiac catheterization has been used as the "gold standard" for all noninvasive imaging techniques. It has been assumed that any disparity between the invasive and echocardiographic findings is due to inherent inaccuracies or technical problems with ultrasound imaging. Indeed, there are enough differences between angiographic and cardiac ultrasound methods to raise major questions about the validity of such comparisons (42, 62, 87, 93). These include:

- Much of the data acquired from LV angiograms is semiquantitative with potential reproducibility problems (62).
- Angiographic techniques visualize cavity silhouettes while two-dimensional echocardiography gives detailed data on intracardiac anatomy and wall thicknesses.
- Angiography is limited to several standard views while two-dimensional echocardiography allows

multiple tomographic cuts and visually determined three-dimensional reconstruction.

- Cardiovascular physiology at the time of catheterization may not be representative of the patient's true hemodynamics due to the effects of medications given prior to or during the procedure; increased sympathetic tone secondary to patient anxiety or discomfort; and the effects of iodinated contrast materials on LV contractility, peripheral vascular tone, and intravascular volume status.
- Since angiographic contrast material is usually cleared from the LV within three to five beats, only a limited number of hemodynamically stable beats are available for data analysis. In addition, cardiac rhythm is frequently unstable during ventriculography. With two-dimensional echocardiography, LV performance can be assessed serially in an unlimited number of cardiac cycles without the use of physiologically active contrast agents or exposure to ionizing radiation.

Measures of Left Ventricular Size and Wall Mass

All of the two-dimensional echocardiographic indices of LV systolic performance are directly or indirectly dependent on calculation of ventricular cross-sectional areas in various planes of interest, or on estimations of LV intracavity volumes and myocardial wall thicknesses. A critical appraisal of the methodologic and mathematical problems encountered with this approach to assessing LV function is necessary if these techniques are to be used in the clinical setting.

Left Ventricular Volumes

Reliable determination of LV volumes using two-dimensional echocardiographic techniques depends on numerous factors. These include adequate imaging of the LV endocardial border, reproducible transducer positioning, and proper alignment of imaging planes to obtain true long and short axes tomographic cuts of the ventricle (57, 94–96). The ease and flexibility of acquiring data using two-dimensional echocardiography have resulted in many geometric and mathematical models for calculation of LV volume. The three basic approaches (42, 64, 87, 94, 96) most commonly employed include:

1. use of the volume of a single figure, usually a prolate ellipse, to represent LV volume.
2. the sum of multiple cross-sectional cuts to "reconstruct" the LV (Simpson's rule method).
3. the combination of different geometric shapes to form a new geometric figure. The shapes most commonly used as building blocks are the cylinder, cone, and hemiellipse.

Each of these overall approaches to LV volume determination will be discussed.

PROLATE ELLIPSE METHOD. Two basic approaches to LV volume calculation exist using the prolate ellipse model (Fig. 5.7). In its simplest form (*length-diameter approach*) the minor axes as well as long axis dimensions are measured directly from the two-dimensional image. Using the *area-length approach*, the minor dimension is calculated rather than measured directly. Since the length-diameter approach is highly dependent on assumptions regarding LV base-to-apex shape, it is inherently less accurate than the area-length approach and should not be heavily relied upon for LV volume calculations (42, 96). Therefore, only the area-length approach will be discussed in detail. Data are obtained using the apical or parasternal views of the LV (42). Biplane versions use information from the apical four-chamber and an additional perpendicular view. The latter includes either the short axis parasternal plane at the level of the mitral valve or the apical long-axis view (96). The use of the apical four chamber and long-axis views together results in reliable definition of ventricular base-to-apex shape. The formula using this approach is a modification of the basic prolate ellipsoid formula:

$$V = \left(\frac{4}{3}\pi\right)\left(\frac{L}{2}\right)\left(\frac{D_1}{2}\right)\left(\frac{D_2}{2}\right)$$

where L is the long axis and D_1 and D_2 are the minor axes. For each orthogonal view of the LV, area can be calculated as $(\pi)(D/2)(L/2)$. Rearranging this equation and substituting into the basic prolate ellipsoid formula one obtains:

$$V = \left(\frac{4}{3}\pi\right)\left(\frac{L}{2}\right)\left[\frac{4A_1}{\pi L/2}\right]\left[\frac{4A_2}{\pi L/2}\right]$$

$$V = \frac{8(A_1)(A_2)}{3\pi L}$$

where A_1 is the area obtained using the four chamber view and A_2 is the area obtained using the apical long axis view. When the apical four chamber view and short axis parasternal view at the mitral valve level are used, the resultant prolate ellipsoid formula is:

$$V = \left(\frac{4}{3}\pi\right)\left(\frac{L}{2}\right)\left[\frac{4A_1}{\pi L/2}\right]\left[\frac{4A_3}{\pi D_1/2}\right]$$

$$V = \frac{8(A_1)(A_3)}{3\pi D_1}$$

where A_3 is the area obtained using the short axis parasternal view and D_1 is the anteroposterior short-axis (96). This approach can be further simplified using the short axis area (A_3) and the LV long axis length.

$$A_3 = \pi\left(\frac{D_1}{2}\right)\left(\frac{D_2}{2}\right)$$

Substitution back into the basic prolate ellipsoid formula yields:

$$V = \left(\frac{4}{3}\right)(A_3)\left(\frac{L}{2}\right)$$

$$V = \left(\frac{2}{3}\right)(A_3)(L)$$

The single-plane prolate ellipsoid formula uses only the LV length and area acquired from either apical view. The formulas (96) are:

$$V = \frac{8(A_1)^2}{3\pi L} \qquad \text{apical four-chamber view}$$

$$\text{or}$$

$$V = \frac{8(A_2)^2}{3\pi L} \qquad \text{apical long-axis view}$$

Wyatt et al. have suggested that LV volumes can be calculated from a single plane short axis view of the LV at the high papillary muscle level (A_{pap}). The proposed formula is:

$$V = \frac{5}{6}(A_{pap})(L)$$

where L is the LV length from mitral valve annulus to apical endocardium as measured in the apical four chamber view. Data gathered using the single plane formulas typically do not correlate as well with angiographic volumes as data collected using orthogonal views.

SIMPSON'S RULE METHOD. The prolate ellipse method tends to be unreliable when ventricular geometry deviates from that of a prolate ellipse of revolution. Examples of this include the vigorously contracting normal ventricle at end-systole as well as the LV with significant regional dyskinesis or aneurysmal dilatation (42). An alternative approach uses the angiographically validated method called Simpson's rule. The mathematical basis for Simpson's rule relies on the fact that the volume of any object, regardless of shape, equals the sum of the volumes of multiple individual slices of known thickness that compose the object. The more irregularly shaped the object, the larger the number of individual slices required for accurate volume determination. Each of these slices can be represented by a series of ellipsoid cylinders (Fig. 5.9). Thus, total LV volume can be represented as

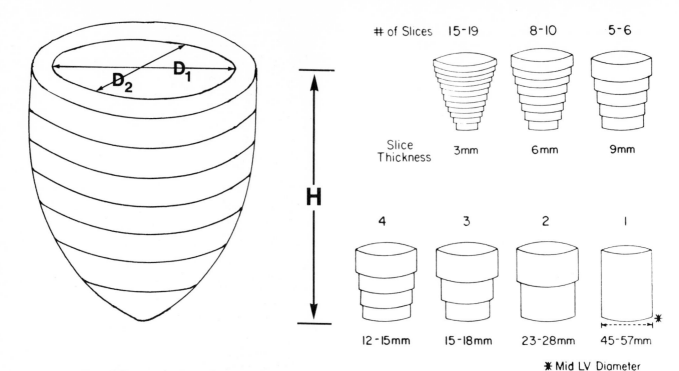

Figure 5.10 Representation of a ventricular (LV) chamber as a series of cross-sectional echocardiographic slices of various thicknesses. (Reproduced by permission of the American Heart Association, Inc. from Weiss JL, Eaton LW, Kallman CH, et al. Accuracy of volume determination by two-dimensional echocardiography. Circulation 1983;67: 889–895).

$$V = \frac{\pi}{4}\left(\frac{H}{n}\right) \sum_{0}^{n} (D_1)(D_2)$$

Figure 5.9 Illustration of the use of Simpson's rule to determine left ventricular volume. The chamber is represented by a series of ellipsoid cylinders. The sum of the volumes of the individual slices gives total chamber volume. V = volume; H = the height of the chamber; n = number of slices; D_1 and D_2 are minor axis dimensions.

$$V = \sum_{0}^{N} (A)(H)$$

$$= \sum_{0}^{N} \left[\pi\left(\frac{D_1}{2}\right)\left(\frac{D_2}{2}\right)\right][H]$$

$$= \frac{\pi}{4}(H) \sum_{0}^{N} (D_1)(D_2)$$

where A = short axis LV area, H = the height of individual slices, D_1 and D_2 are the orthogonal diameters, and N = the number of slices used to construct the ventricle. Using an isolated contracting canine heart preparation, Weiss et al. demonstrated that as the number of slices used to approximate a conical shape decreased, the more the cone resembled a cylinder (Fig. 5.10) (97). The standard error of the estimate (a predictor of accuracy of the test) fell substantially when less than four cross-sectional slices were used. It appears therefore that at least four slices are required to get highly accurate estimates of LV geometry and volume using Simpson's rule, especially if the ventricle is abnormally shaped. Left ventricular volume can also be determined from two cross-sectional views that are orthogonal about the long axis and with the LV divided into even slices along the common axis. The Simpson's rule method is attractive as a means of calculating LV volume because it avoids geometric assumptions and is usable even when ventricular shape has become markedly distorted. The limitations of this method include the need for numerous scan planes as well as the complexity of summing multiple individual volumes. Computer assistance is required since hand calculations are laborious and time-consuming.

COMBINED GEOMETRIC SHAPES. In this approach to ventricular volume determination, short axis planes are used to divide the LV into two or more geometric figures. The shapes most frequently used are the cylinder, cone, truncated cone, and ellipsoid. The three most commonly employed combined geometric figures are the cylinder-cone (Fig. 5.11), cylinder-hemiellipse (also called the bullet) (Fig. 5.12), and the cylinder-truncated cone-cone (Fig. 5.13). To date, the cylinder-hemiellipse model has been used most extensively.

Overall correlations using combined geometric shapes are usually better than those found with the ellipsoid model (96). The Simpson's rule approach is, in general, more reliable than the combined geometric

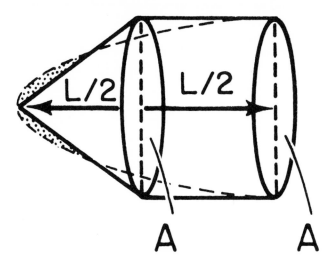

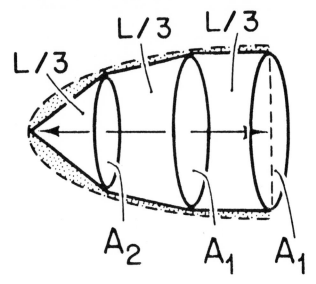

Figure 5.11 Cylinder-cone method of estimating left ventricular volume. L = base to apex length; A = short axis area at the level of the mitral valve. (Reproduced with permission from Triulzi MO, Wilkins GT, Gillam LD, et al. Normal adult cross-sectional echocardiographic values: Left ventricular volumes. Echocardiography 1985;2:153–169.)

Figure 5.13 Cylinder-truncated cone-cone method of estimating left ventricular volume. L = ventricular length measured from an apical view; A_1 and A_2 = areas at the mitral and midpapillary muscle levels, respectively. (Reproduced with permission from Triulzi MO, Wilkins GT, Gillam LD, et al. Normal adult cross-sectional echocardiographic values: Left ventricular volumes. Echocardiography 1985;2:153–169.)

shapes models, especially when LV shape is highly distorted. In most cases in which severe shape distortion is not present, however, volume calculations are easier to perform using the combined geometric shapes or ellipsoidal models than with Simpson's rule (96).

In most studies comparing contrast angiographic and two-dimensionally determined LV volumes, the ultrasound volumes are smaller than those calculated using invasive techniques (87, 94, 96, 98). There are multiple explanations for these results.

1. Two-dimensional echocardiography may give tangential cross-sectional cuts of the LV long axis rather than true measures of the long axis (94). Erbel et al. found this to be the case in 44 of the 46 patients they studied by simultaneous cineangiographic and two-dimensional echocardiographic techniques (94). Whether this represents limitations of a specific laboratory's imaging technique or a generalized imaging problem remains to be determined.

2. The radio-opaque dye used in cineangiography fills in the intertrabecular spaces, making the cardiac silhouette appear larger than it really is. This results in overestimation of true LV size. On the other hand, echocardiography suffers from the inability to image the spaces between trabeculae. This results in incorporation of intertrabecular spaces into the endocardial border, resulting in underestimation of true LV size.

3. "Slice-thickness" artifacts due to transducer mean width may result in deviations from the "thin slice" assumptions used as the basis for all LV volume models.

4. During ventricular systole, the LV moves through multiple imaging planes. Therefore, measurements made during LV systole and diastole may not represent the same region throughout the entire cardiac cycle (98, 99).

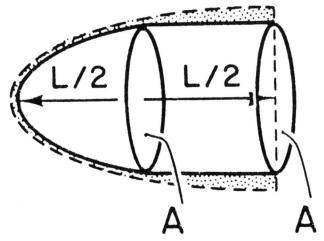

Figure 5.12 Cylinder-hemiellipse method of estimating left ventricular volume. L = ventricular length measured from an apical view; A = area of the short axis plane taken at the midpapillary muscle level. (Reproduced with permission from Triulzi MO, Wilkins GT, Gillam LD, et al. Normal adult cross-sectional echocardiographic values: Left ventricular volumes. Echocardiography 1985;2:153–169.)

Left Ventricular Wall Thickness

Two-dimensional echocardiography has been reported to allow measurement of myocardial wall thickness both in relative and absolute terms (100). This is useful for assessing the extent of global thickening and thinning, as well as identifying hypokinetic, akinetic, and dyskinetic segments. When imaging is performed in the short axis parasternal planes, however, difficulties frequently arise in distinguishing epicardial borders and underestimating the LV cavity area. The net result is overestimation of LV wall thicknesses and myocardial area (53, 64, 77). When imaging is performed with the transducer in the apical position, poor endocardial resolution is a common problem, resulting in underestimation of lateral wall thicknesses. Tangential viewing of the LV apical region is another common problem, leading to spuriously high wall thickness values.

Left Ventricular Wall Mass

As noted earlier in this chapter, LV wall mass can be estimated accurately in the normally shaped, symmetrically contracting ventricle using M-mode echocardiographic techniques. In the abnormally shaped or grossly dilated ventricle, two-dimensional echocardiography is required for LV wall mass determination. As with M-mode echocardiography, two-dimensional techniques require calculation of total volume enclosed within the epicardial borders minus the LV cavity volume (66, 101, 102). In theory, any one of the volume formulas described above can be used (64, 77). In practice, those techniques using short axis images have proved most accurate (77). This is due to better endocardial delineation using short axis rather than apical long axis imaging planes. Simpson's rule approximations seem best suited for this approach. However, multiple short axis images are needed since no long axis data regarding overall LV size and shape are available. Wyatt et al. have tried to overcome this problem by using a single short axis view at the high papillary muscle level in conjunction with an apical LV length (64, 77, 103). Initial data using this approach are encouraging for a more simplified method of LV wall mass calculation. The most promising of the combined geometric shapes model is the cylinder-hemiellipsoid (i.e., bullet) approach. Using this model,

$$V = \frac{5}{6}(A)(L)$$

where A = area measured directly from a short axis view of the LV at the high papillary muscle level, and L = length taken from base to the apical endocardial and epicardial borders, respectively. The formula can be used to calculate the difference between epicardial and endocardial volumes. The resultant wall volume is then multiplied by the density of LV muscle (1.05 g/cm^3) to give LV wall mass. Thus,

$$LVM = (1.05)\left[\left(\frac{5}{6}A_t L_t\right) - \left(\frac{5}{6}A_c L_c\right)\right]$$
$$= (1.05)\left[\left(\frac{5}{6}\right)(A_t L_t - A_c L_c)\right]$$

where $\frac{5}{6}A_t L_t$ is the epicardial volume and $\frac{5}{6}A_c L_c$ is the endocardial volume.

Three-Dimensional Reconstruction of the Left Ventricle

Numerous approaches for three-dimensional assessment of LV volume and wall mass have been proposed (91, 98, 99, 104–107). These include a modified Simpson rule (98, 107), randomly recorded multiple short axis images (105), a pyramid summation algorithm (106), and a method involving transducer rotation over 180 degrees (91). Three-dimensional reconstruction has the potential to allow for the direct calculation of LV volume without need for geometric assumptions. It is yet to be determined if the difficulties associated with two-dimensional echocardiographic imaging of endocardial borders as well as problems associated with rotational, longitudinal, and transverse dynamic motion of the LV can be overcome. High quality, accurate, and reproducible three-dimensional reconstruction using ultrasound imaging is needed if echocardiography is to remain competitive with newer imaging techniques, such as rapid acquisition computerized tomography and cine magnetic resonance imaging.

Measures of Overall Left Ventricular Systolic Performance

Fractional Area Change

This is calculated as the reduction in planimetered LV chamber cross-sectional area from end-diastole to end-systole divided by the end-diastolic cross-sectional area (108). Measurements are usually made at the level of the papillary muscles as seen in the short-axis view. Although this is similar in concept to the M-mode echocardiographic percent fractional shortening, it has the advantage of allowing more accurate assessment of ventricles with regional wall motion abnormalities (109).

Ejection Fraction

Left ventricular ejection fraction has the same physiologic limitations whether determined by M-mode or two-dimensional echocardiography. If ejection fraction is to be determined, however, two-dimensional echocardiography has the obvious advantage of better spatial orientation and geometric modeling. Not surprisingly, LV ejection fraction determinations by two-dimensional echocardiography have less inter-method variability than is found for estimations of either end-systolic or end-diastolic volumes (64, 110). This reflects the canceling out of certain systematic errors inherent in a given geometric or mathematical model of the LV. Despite the limitations involved with two-dimensional echocardiographic determination of ejection fraction, clinical applications have been successfully performed (79, 111).

Left Ventricular Wall Motion
Two-dimensional echocardiographic imaging in conjunction with targeted M-mode recordings allow qualitative as well as quantitative assessment of LV regional wall motion and performance. Analysis of regional wall thickening in conjunction with assessment of regional wall motion give relatively precise information that allows discrimination of viable from nonviable myocardium (112, 113). Correlations with measures of LV preload, afterload, and contractile state should markedly increase our understanding of the physiology of LV wall motion and thickening abnormalities. An extensive discussion addressing quantitative assessment of LV regional wall motion abnormalities in patients with ischemic heart disease is discussed elsewhere (Chapter 10) (114, 115).

Intraoperative Use of Echocardiography
Ultrasound imaging of the LV has been accomplished in the operating room using several techniques (99, 109, 113–121). One approach uses a gas-sterilized hand-held transducer, which is placed directly on the heart to record multiple short axis and long axis views of the LV. The study by Dubroff et al. demonstrates the potential use of this technique (109). The LV in 44 adult patients with acquired heart disease was imaged before and immediately after cardiopulmonary bypass. Percent of short axis area change was calculated at the level of the maximum LV diameter. In addition, multiple short and long axis views of the LV were recorded. Surgical correction of chronic mitral or aortic valvular heart disease produced characteristic changes in overall systolic performance, which were evident immediately after valve replacement. Since no sophisticated measures of ventricular loading conditions were made, interpretation of changes in LV shortening characteristics is difficult. However, it is clear that use of intraoperative echocardiographic imaging can increase our understanding of the changes that occur in myocardial physiology during the immediate pre- and postoperative periods.

Another approach to intraoperative LV imaging uses a miniature two-dimensional transducer attached to a commercially available gastrofiberscope. This is in-serted into the esophagus. Images of the heart can be recorded continuously from the base to the apex as the transducer is withdrawn or advanced in the esophagus (99, 116). In contrast to imaging with the transducer directly on the heart, transesophageal echocardiography allows a stable transducer position with monitoring that can be performed without interfering with the operative procedure. In addition, reproducible images can be obtained before the chest is opened and while it is being closed, without concern about transducer sterility (119). Regional and overall LV performance has been studied using this technique in patients with valvular as well as ischemic heart disease (113, 118–121). Clinically useful information has been obtained regarding the effects of myocardial revascularization on LV wall thickening, the importance of the pericardium in relation to LV diastolic filling and systolic output, and the ventricle's immediate response to valve replacement (113, 119, 121).

Interventional Two-Dimensional Echocardiography

For years it has been known that LV performance under resting conditions may be within the normal range, despite the presence of pre-clinical ventricular dysfunction or underlying coronary artery disease. In part, this represents a problem with the wide range of normal values noted for most ejection phase and isovolumic indices of LV systolic performance. Recently there has been much interest in ways to combine two-dimensional and targeted M-mode echocardiographic imaging with interventions adequate to unmask LV dysfunction or provoke myocardial ischemia. The following approaches have been utilized.

Isometric Exercise
A standard isometric exercise stress consists of 3 to 4 minutes of sustained handgrip (usually at 30% to 50% of maximal voluntary contraction). The hemodynamic response in normal subjects is increased aortic mean pressure and heart rate in association with little or no change in LV end-diastolic dimension, and at most only slight change in end-systolic dimension (1). In contrast, patients with preclinical myopathy may increase heart size, decrease overall performance, and develop regional thickening and wall motion abnormalities (9, 42, 82). However, these findings are relatively nonspecific. Poor patient compliance, lack of reproducibility, and the inability to significantly increase myocardial oxygen demand are major limitations of this technique.

Pharmacologic Interventions
Pharmacologic interventions with methoxamine, phenylephrine, angiotensin, isoproterenol, or dobutamine have been used to assess the LV response to

afterload augmentation and measure LV contractile reserve. These studies have been conducted in normal subjects as well as patients with preclinical or overt cardiac disease (9, 18, 36, 42, 99, 122). These forms of pharmacologic stress testing are ideally suited for assessment of cardiovascular physiology using echocardiographic imaging, since they allow optimal imaging to be performed without lung interference or problems with patient compliance.

Dynamic Exercise

Dynamic exercise in conjunction with electrocardiography or radionuclide angiography has had proven value in the diagnosis and clinical assessment of coronary artery disease (82, 87, 122–125). The normal response to dynamic exercise is an increase in stroke volume (1). This occurs as a result of a significant decrease in LV end-systolic volume, while end-diastolic volume falls slightly or remains unchanged at low to moderate levels of exercise, or increases slightly during more vigorous exercise. This latter change represents use of LV preload reserve (i.e., Frank-Starling law of the heart). In the late 1970s, Wann et al. used two-dimensional echocardiography in conjunction with dynamic exercise to detect regional ischemia (82). This study used ultrasound imaging during exercise, usually using the subcostal transducer position (82). However, deep and rapid breathing frequently prevented adequate visualization of LV myocardium. Recently, "stress-echo" studies have been performed prior to and immediately after exercise using an apical imaging window (48, 99, 122). Apical four chamber or long axis planes were chosen, since there is relatively little lung tissue overlying the LV apex. In these studies, abnormalities in LV regional wall motion and thickening frequently lasted several minutes after cessation of exercise. This was especially true if the patient assumed a recumbent position, in which increased venous return led to augmented LV wall stress and increased myocardial oxygen requirements. The sensitivity of this technique for detection of ischemic heart disease is highest in patients with severe multivessel coronary narrowings. When compared with radionuclide angiographic studies performed during dynamic exercise, "stress-echo" has numerous potential advantages (82, 122–124). These include the ability to assess beat-to-beat performance, as well as more extensively assess regional wall motion and wall thickness changes. In addition, ultrasound imaging can be obtained serially without cumulative radiation risk.

Current problems with "stress-echo" still exist and include (42, 82):

1. Problems with both qualitative and quantitative assessment of wall motion and thickness abnormalities. Exercise induced hyperventilation as well as ventricular hyperkinesis make reproducible assessment of the same regions of the LV difficult under pre- and postexercise conditions. This is compounded by the presence of heterogeneity of wall motion and thickening in normal subjects, especially involving the inferior wall of the LV in the area of the posteromedial papillary muscle.

2. Difficulty with adequate endocardial border delineation when imaging is performed from the apical transducer position. This is further compromised by the tachycardia usually present in the immediate postexercise period.

3. In cases of exercise-induced diffuse hypokinesis (as opposed to akinesis or dyskinesis), it may be difficult to visually determine affected areas of the LV, since no other region of the chamber is sufficiently different to allow adequate comparison.

4. As noted earlier in this chapter, calculation of left ventricular volumes is complicated and somewhat cumbersome, especially in the presence of regional wall motion abnormalities. This problem is further exacerbated by the tendency to foreshorten the LV cavity when imaging is performed from the apical transducer position. Increased chest wall motion and lung expansion during and immediately after exercise further complicate the issue.

5. Finally, it is important to remember that dynamic exercise is associated with simultaneous changes in preload, afterload, peripheral vascular resistance, contractility, and heart rate. These alterations occur at a time when parasympathetic tone is withdrawn, sympathetic tone is increased, and adrenocortical hormones are being released. Changes in left ventricular wall motion, wall thickness, volumes, ejection fraction, etc., reflect the net effect of extremely complicated physiologic alterations, many of which are occurring external to the heart. Thus, specific conclusions regarding the LV contractile response to dynamic exercise are difficult to make and must be accepted with a high degree of caution.

Doppler Echocardiography

Introduction

Assessment of overall left ventricular performance using M-mode and two-dimensional echocardiography is based on geometric assumptions of chamber size and shape. In contrast, Doppler echocardiography provides LV blood flow velocity, acceleration rate, and volume output data without the need for LV geometric assumptions. It measures the net result of the pumping action of the left ventricle using principles that are different from those associated with anatomic imaging. The Doppler derived indices described in this section are influenced by alterations in LV preload, afterload, heart rate, and contractile state (1, 37). As such, they behave like all other ejection phase indices of LV performance and cannot be used as isolated measures of LV contractility. Doppler measurements of LV performance can be divided into 1) blood flow velocity and acceleration rate indices, and 2) blood volume output indices.

Measures of Overall Left Ventricular Systolic Performance

Blood Flow Velocity and Acceleration Rate

Since the mid-1960s, the peak blood flow velocity and maximal acceleration rate of blood in the ascending aorta have been proposed as indices of LV function. Until the advent of Doppler echocardiography, these measures could be determined only by using invasive techniques (126, 127). Recently, Doppler determined blood flow velocity measurements recorded from a suprasternal notch transducer position have been shown to be reproducible to within 13% in animals as well as humans using commercially available equipment (128–131). Gardin et al. reported values for seven easily determined blood flow parameters recorded from the proximal aorta and pulmonary artery in 20 normal adult subjects (130). These included:

1. peak flow velocity in cm/sec
2. average acceleration rate in cm/sec^2
3. acceleration time in msec
4. deceleration time in msec
5. average deceleration rate in cm/sec^2
6. ejection time in msec
7. aortic flow velocity integral in cm

Data indicated that despite a four to five times higher arterial resistance in the systemic circuit compared to pulmonary circuit, blood was accelerated two to three times more rapidly in the ascending aorta than in the pulmonary artery. Also, the peak flow velocity was higher and occurred earlier in the aorta than in the pulmonary artery. These measurements in normal subjects were used to evaluate flow velocity patterns in 12 patients with moderate to severe dilated cardiomyopathy (mean LV percent fractional shortening of 15 ± 4) (132, 133). Peak aortic flow velocity and aortic flow velocity integral were significantly lower for the cardiomyopathy patients compared to normal subjects, with no overlap of data between the groups ($p < 0.001$) (Fig. 5.14). This probably reflected low LV stroke volume in the myopathy patients (132, 133). In contrast, average aortic acceleration rate and aortic ejection time were less useful discriminators (Fig. 5.15). In another study from the same laboratory, 13 patients treated with vasodilator therapy for congestive heart failure were assessed pre- and post-therapy using Doppler aortic blood flow measurements (Fig. 5.16) (134). A poor correlation was found between absolute values for Doppler determined peak aortic flow velocity, ejection time, and flow velocity integral, and systemic vascular resistance (SVR) measured invasively. In contrast, a high correlation was noted between percent changes in aortic peak flow velocity and SVR (r = -0.89) and between percent changes in Doppler aortic flow velocity integral and stroke volume (r = 0.88). In all of these reports, the patients demonstrated clinical symptoms of congestive heart failure. In a study by Kolettis et al., aortic peak flow velocity and maximal acceleration rate failed to distinguish between three groups of patients described as having "good, moderate, or poor LV function" (126). The authors concluded that these indices had limited value in the clinical setting for identification of preclinical as well as mild to moderate LV dysfunction. While it appears that Doppler blood flow indices can identify patients with moderate to severe LV dysfunction, it remains to be proven how well these indices will identify preclinical or mild abnormalities in LV contractility and overall performance.

Blood Volume Output Indices

METHODS. It is well established that in the absence of valvular stenosis, changes in the Doppler flow velocity integral are directly proportional to changes in stroke volume (135–137). Attempts at calculating absolute stroke volume using Doppler echocardiography have been performed using the following formula:

$$SV = (FVI)(CSA)$$

where FVI is the Doppler flow velocity integral in cm, and CSA is the cross-sectional area in cm^2 of the orifice through which blood flows (127, 138–140). Cardiac output in cm^3/min can then be calculated as the stroke volume times heart rate in beats/min. In practical terms, these calculations require accurate measurement of the cross-sectional area of the orifice or vessel, an accurate temporal representation of the blood flow velocity across the area of interest, and knowledge of the angle of incidence of the Doppler ultrasound beam with respect to the mean vector for blood flow velocity. Use of either pulsed or continuous-wave Doppler echocardiography in conjunction with two-dimensional echocardiographic imaging allows these calculations to be performed (137, 138, 141–147). Data have been collected from several sites including:

1. *Ascending aorta.* Continuous-wave Doppler flow from the ascending aorta in conjunction with CSA at the level of the aortic valve annulus appears to be most accurate with the best interobserver and intraobserver reproducibility (Fig. 5.17) (139, 141, 144, 147, 148). This is the most commonly used site

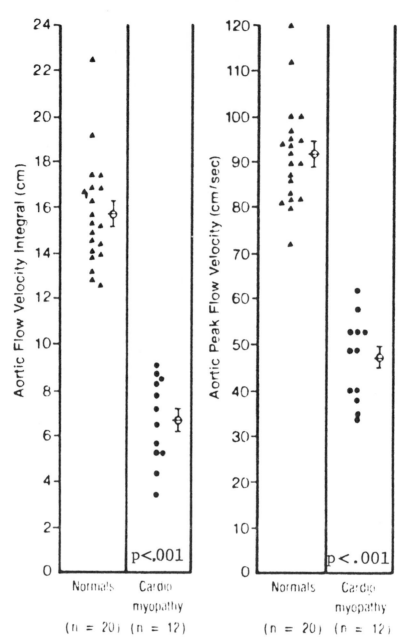

Figure 5.14 Plot of aortic flow velocity integral and peak flow velocity in normal subjects and in patients with cardiomyopathy. Data for both measurements separated normal subjects from patients with cardiomyopathy to a similar degree. (Reproduced with permission from Gardin JM, Tommaso CL, Talano JV, et al. Evaluation of dilated cardiomyopathy by pulsed Doppler echocardiography. Am Heart J 1983;106:1057–1065.)

for stroke volume calculations. Recently, it has been shown that in patients with low flow states, the best correlations are obtained using the separation of the basal aspects of the leaflets to calculate effective cross-sectional area (149).

2. *Pulmonary artery.* Pulmonary flow velocity integral is recorded in conjunction with the pulmonary artery diameter. This latter measurement is frequently difficult to perform accurately, and it is the major source of error in pulmonary artery derived output calculations (148).

3. *LV inflow.* These calculations are based on LV diastolic inflow velocities, and either the maximal mitral orifice as planimetered from the parasternal short axis two-dimensional echocardiographic image or from the mitral annulus diameter (142, 148). Assumptions of an elliptical rather than circular orifice result in closer correlations with invasively determined stroke volume. This approach to stroke volume measurement is frequently difficult to perform in adult patients. Recently, high correlations with measurements of

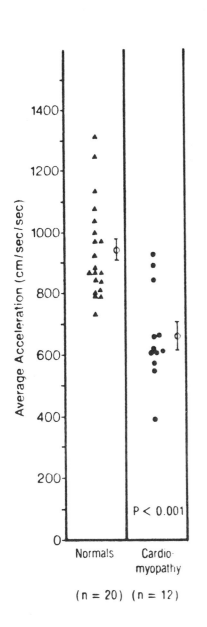

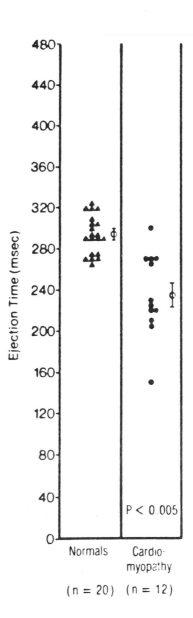

Figure 5.15 Average acceleration and left ventricular ejection time compared in normal subjects and in patients with cardiomyopathy. Note the overlap of data between the groups. (Reproduced with permission from Gardin JM, Tommaso CL, Talano JV, et al. Evaluation of dilated cardiomyopathy by pulsed Doppler echocardiography. Am Heart J 1983;106:1057–1065.)

mitral flow volume have been made using an ellipse shaped inlet and outlet to the valve (150).

4. *RV inflow*. Based on transtricuspid valve Doppler velocity during diastole and tricuspid valve annular size, this approach has resulted in variable results (148).

Regardless of the method used to calculate LV stroke volume or cardiac output, it is essential to remember that these measures of forward blood flow do not define whether the LV has normal contractility or performance. Cardiac output reflects preload, afterload, heart rate, and contractile conditions working together to transfer blood from the ventricle to the periphery. A markedly dilated LV, through an increase in its end-diastolic volume, can frequently maintain a normal or near-normal output, despite decreased overall performance and a markedly depressed contractile

state. In contrast, a left ventricle that is preload-deficient may demonstrate decreased cardiac output and diminished overall performance, yet still have normal contractility. Despite these physiologic limitations in the use of stroke volume and cardiac output measurements, certain clinical applications do exist.

CLINICAL APPLICATIONS OF BLOOD VOLUME OUTPUT INDICES

Effect of Therapeutic Interventions. Cardiac output measurements under baseline conditions, especially when performed in conjunction with other hemodynamic measurements, can be helpful in clinical decision making regarding critically ill patients. Since percent changes in Doppler outputs are more reliable than absolute values, serial measurements can provide useful data (134, 140). This approach has been used to test the

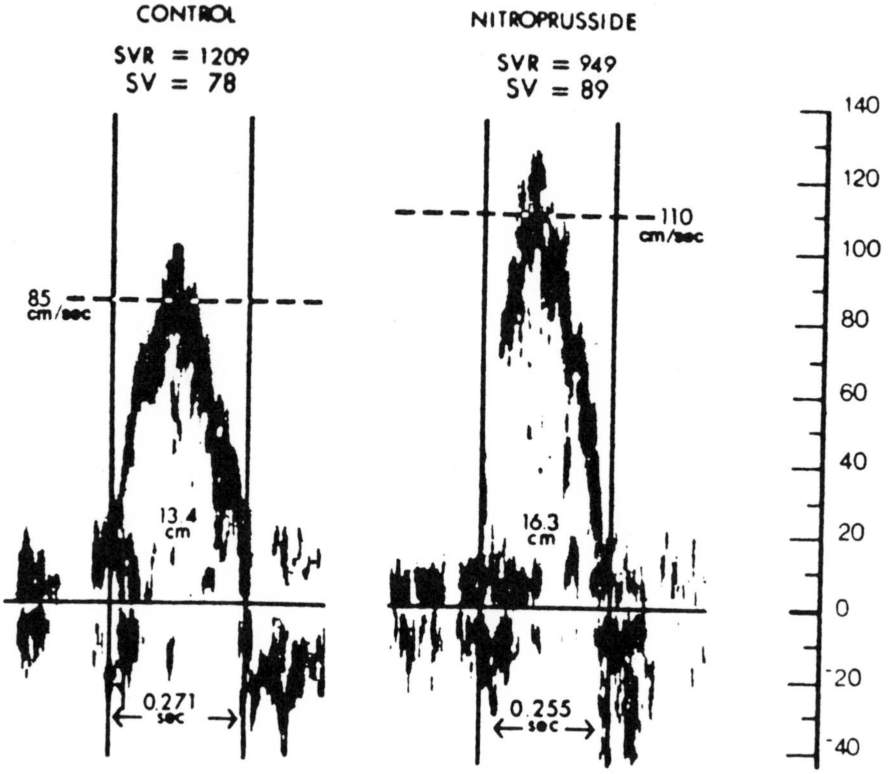

Figure 5.16 Ascending aortic blood flow recordings under control conditions and during nitroprusside infusion in a patient with dilated cardiomyopathy. Left ventricular (LV) stroke volume (SV) increased by 14% in association with a 21% fall in systemic vascular resistance (SVR) and a 6% decrease in LV ejection time. (Reproduced by permission of the American Heart Association, Inc. from Elkayam U, Gardin JM, Berkey R, et al. The use of Doppler flow velocity measurement to assess the hemodynamic response to vasodilators in patients with heart failure. Circulation 1983;67:377–383.)

effectiveness of therapy with positive inotropic agents, vasodilator therapy, diuretics, and chronotropic agents (134, 143, 145, 146).

Evaluation of Pacemaker Hemodynamics. Doppler echocardiography has been useful in assessing the hemodynamics of patients with artificial pacemakers. This has been particularly true in cases of "physiologic" dual chamber devices. Doppler-determined cardiac outputs have been used to determine optimal pacing mode, atrioventricular conduction sequencing, and pacing rate (151–154).

Response to Dynamic Exercise. Doppler echocardiography has been used to demonstrate a fall in stroke volume with dynamic exercise in patients with extensive coronary artery disease as opposed to normal subjects. In addition, this technique has been useful in assessing nearly instantaneous changes in aortic flow velocity and volume during steady state supine and upright exercise (155, 156).

Calculation of Regurgitant Fraction. The regurgitant fraction in patients with isolated aortic regurgitation has been determined by Doppler echocardiography using systolic aortic and pulmonary volume flows (127, 157). By assuming that an excess in aortic volume flow (AF) compared with the pulmonary volume flow (PF) was due to aortic regurgitant flow, the aortic regurgitant fraction (RF%) could be calculated:

$$RF\% = \left(\frac{AF - PF}{AF}\right)(100)$$

Kitabatake et al. reported that RF%, which never exceeded 10% in normal subjects, correlated relatively well (r = 0.80) with semiquantitative cine-aortographic grades of aortic regurgitation (157).

Intra- and Extracardiac Shunt Calculations. Doppler determined volume flow has been used to calculate pulmonary to systemic blood flow ratios (Q_p/Q_s) in neonates, children, and adults (158–162). In general, Doppler Q_p/Q_s estimates have correlated relatively well (r = 0.85) with those derived from cardiac catheterization or radionuclide angiography. The Q_p/Q_s ratio is dependent on multiple factors, including the pulmonary to systemic artery resistance and impedance ratios, the size of the intracardiac communication, and the hemodynamic derangements due to associated lesions. Accordingly, Doppler calculations of Q_p/Q_s are most helpful when done as serial studies and in conjunction with Doppler estimates of right ventricular and pulmonary artery pressures.

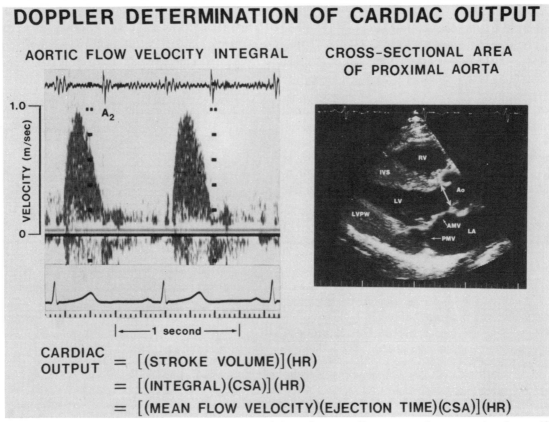

DOPPLER DETERMINATION OF CARDIAC OUTPUT

Figure 5.17 Continuous-wave Doppler flow velocity integral from the ascending aorta and cross-sectional area (CSA) at the level of the aortic valve annulus are used to calculate cardiac output and left ventricular (LV) stroke volume (SV). The phonocardiogram (PCG) recorded from the right upper sternal border defines the end of LV ejection. HR = heart rate; Ao = aorta; LA = left atrium; IVS = septum; RL = Right ventricle; AMV = anterior mitral valve leaflet; PMV = posterior mitral valve leaflet; LVPW = left ventricular posterior wall; A$_2$ = aortic component of the second heart sound.

LIMITATIONS. As noted above, relative changes in Doppler echocardiographically determined LV stroke volume or cardiac output are more reliable than absolute changes. This is a consequence of the multiple simplifying assumptions required to perform these calculations (140, 146, 147, 163). For the purpose of this discussion, only the ascending aorta method of output determination will be addressed.

Cross-Sectional Area (CSA) Measurement. It is assumed that the aorta is perfectly circular in shape without change in CSA throughout the cardiac cycle. In reality, the aorta is not perfectly circular, nor are its systolic and diastolic sizes exactly equal. These problems are minor in comparison to the error introduced by small measurements in measuring the diameter or planimetering the CSA, since the calculated output estimate is proportional to the square of the aortic diameter.

Blood Flow Velocity Distribution. It is assumed that the blood flow velocity profile is flat or blunt over most of the cross-sectional area of the ascending aorta. This

appears to be a reasonable assumption in the absence of LV outflow tract obstruction.

Doppler Angle. It is assumed that the Doppler ultrasound beam is directed parallel to aortic blood flow. Thus, the angle of incidence is small and does not significantly affect volume output calculations. For incident angles less than 20°, the error will be less than 6%.

Integrated Approach to Assessment of Left Ventricular Performance

As noted throughout this chapter, clinicians have been searching for years for an easily obtainable measure of LV contractility that is preload-, afterload-, and heart rate–independent. Such an index, especially if obtained using noninvasive techniques, would be ideal for 1) preclinical detection of cardiomyopathic or cardiotoxic conditions; 2) studies of the effects of therapeutic interventions, such as vasodilator or positive inotropic therapy, in patients with LV systolic dysfunction; and 3) assessment of the progression or recovery of contractile abnormalities in various cardiac disease states. All of the traditional indices described in the first portion of this chapter are highly load-dependent, and thus reflect overall LV performance rather than contractility. However, using various combinations of these measures, it is possible to eliminate loading conditions and heart rate as confounding variables. The net results are highly sensitive load- and rate-independent indices of LV contractile state. The next part of this chapter will describe how the integration of M-mode, two-dimensional, and Doppler echocardiography, in conjunction with noninvasively determined instantaneous LV systolic pressures, can be clinically useful while providing physiologically accurate information. In this manner, measures of LV size, overall pump performance, afterload, preload, myocardial mass, and contractility can be interrelated to provide a noninvasively derived framework for the study of cardiovascular function. Since the problems related to coronary artery disease will be discussed in detail in Chapter 10, only those issues directly applicable to ventricles without significant regional wall motion abnormalities will be addressed in this chapter.

Methods

Noninvasive Determination of Instantaneous LV Systolic Pressure

The shape of the externally recorded carotid pulse and subclavian artery tracings (CPT, SCAT) closely parallels the morphology of the central aortic and LV pressure tracings over the course of ventricular ejection. In addition to this qualitative relationship, these tracings can be used to noninvasively estimate LV systolic pressures in the absence of LV outflow tract obstruction. This was demonstrated in a study of 20 subjects undergoing cardiac catheterization, and in whom pressure tracings in the ascending aorta were simultaneously recorded with externally derived carotid pulse tracings. Peak systolic and diastolic blood pressure determinations were made with a microprocessor-based, noninvasive blood pressure monitor device (Dinamap™, Critikon, Tampa, Florida). This device accurately estimates central aortic pressures over a wide range of systolic and diastolic values independent of the patient's cardiac index, systemic vascular resistance, LV ejection fraction, and body surface area (164, 165). By setting the noninvasively determined aortic peak systolic pressure to the peak of the CPT and the aortic diastolic pressure to the nadir of the CPT, it was possible to use linear interpolation to obtain instantaneous LV pressure values throughout all of ventricular ejection (165). The noninvasive estimation of pressure was excellent, with a maximum difference of 3.4 mm Hg compared with invasively measured

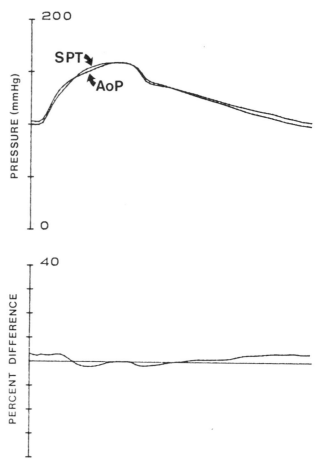

Figure 5.18 Comparison of directly measured high-fidelity central aortic pressure (AoP) and pressure estimated simultaneously by peripheral blood pressure calibration of the subclavian artery pulse tracing (SPT) in a representative subject.

values. This difference occurred within the first third of ejection and was reduced by mid-ejection. At end-ejection, invasively and noninvasively measured pressures were virtually identical. By substituting calibrated subclavian artery pulse tracings for calibrated CPT, this small early systolic difference between invasive and noninvasive pressure measurements can be eliminated (Figs. 5.18 and 5.19). Thus, calibrated indirect carotid and subclavian artery pulse tracings provide an "open window" to the LV pressure tracing over the course of ventricular ejection.

Measures of Ventricular Afterload

The concepts and determinants of LV afterload have been discussed in detail earlier in this chapter. Briefly, afterload is best measured as the force or wall stress developed by the myocardium after the onset of ejection. Its value at any moment during ejection is determined by the instantaneous LV systolic pressure, dimension, and wall thickness. In the normal heart, afterload peaks shortly after aortic valve opening,

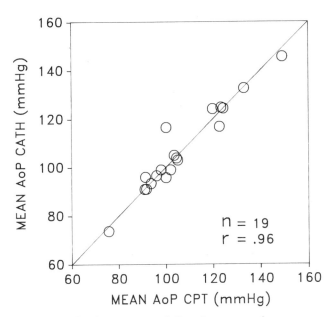

Figure 5.19 Comparison of directly measured mean central pressure values (AoP) with those derived from calibrated carotid pulse tracings (CPT) in 19 adult patients.

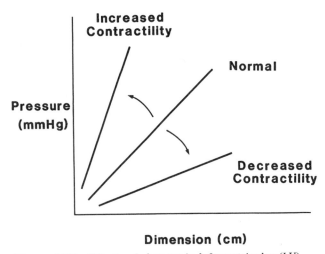

Figure 5.20 Effects of changes in left ventricular (LV) contractility on the LV end-systolic pressure-volume relation. An increase in contractile state shifts the line upward and to the left. A decrease in contractility has the opposite effect.

when wall thickness is still minimal and chamber size is large. It then declines throughout the remainder of ejection. The LV is thus able to partially unload itself. Two different wall stresses can be measured.

MERIDIONAL WALL STRESS. Meridional wall stress (σ_m) measures the forces acting on the LV fibers along the chamber's longitudinal axis (10, 29, 30, 166, 167). The equation for meridional wall stress requires instantaneous chamber pressure (P), wall thickness (h), and minor axis dimension (D). Targeted M-mode echocardiograms of the LV can be recorded with simultaneous calibrated CPT. The calibrated CPT is time corrected for pulse transmission delay by aligning the dicrotic notch of the CPT with the first high-frequency component of the aortic second heart sound recorded by phonocardiogram. Left ventricular meridional wall stress can then be calculated using the angiographically validated formula:

$$\sigma_m = \frac{(P)(D)(1.35)}{(h)(1 + h/D)(4)}$$

where σ is in g/cm^2, P is in mm Hg, D and h are in cm, and 1.35 is the factor to convert pressure from mm Hg to g/cm^2. Peak systolic and end-systolic wall stresses can be determined. Mean ejection wall stress can be calculated as the average of instantaneous wall stress values over ventricular ejection. Left ventricular stress versus time (g-sec/cm^2) and stress versus dimension (g/cm) plots can be constructed. From these curves, the integral of instantaneous stress-time and stress-dimension can be calculated and used as indices of

myocardial oxygen requirement and systolic stroke work, respectively (23, 25, 27, 168, 169). Both indices can be multiplied by heart rate to obtain LV stress-time per minute and LV minute work. Meridional wall stress can also be calculated using two-dimensional echocardiographic short axis imaging of the LV at the high papillary muscle level (166).

CIRCUMFERENTIAL WALL STRESS. Circumferential wall stress (σ_c) measures the forces acting on the LV wall along its minor axis. Absolute values for circumferential wall stress are higher than absolute values for meridional stress because of differences in radii of curvature in circumferential and meridional planes (18). Calculation of circumferential wall stress requires chamber pressure and wall thickness, as well as minor and long axes dimensions. This can be accomplished using time-corrected, calibrated carotid pulse tracings in conjunction with combined M-mode and two-dimensional echocardiography (18), or two-dimensional echocardiography alone.

End-Systolic Indices of LV Performance
These indices relate a measure of LV performance to the physiologic forces acting on the myocardium at end-systole (10, 29–31, 170–172). The fundamental principle on which these indices are based is the fact that for any level of contractility, the end-systolic fiber length is linearly related to the end-systolic forces (i.e., end-systolic wall stress). This means that the LV acts as if fiber shortening continues until the force generated by the myocardium equals the maximal force-generating capacity at that fiber length. At this point, the active state ends and ventricular shortening is terminated.

Figure 5.21 The effect of dobutamine on the echocardiogram of the left ventricle of a single subject. The end-systolic pressure (P_{es}) was the same for both panels. The end-systolic dimension (D_{es}) was significantly smaller during the dobutamine infusion than under control conditions. LVPW = left ventricular posterior wall; D_{ed} = end-systolic dimension; PCG = phonocardiogram; CPT = carotid pulse tracing; S_2 = second heart sound recorded at the right upper sternal border. (Reproduced by permission of the American Heart Association, Inc. from Borow KM, Propper R, Bierman FZ, et al. Sensitivity of end-systolic pressure-dimension and pressure-volume relations to inotropic state in humans. Circulation 1982;65:988–997.)

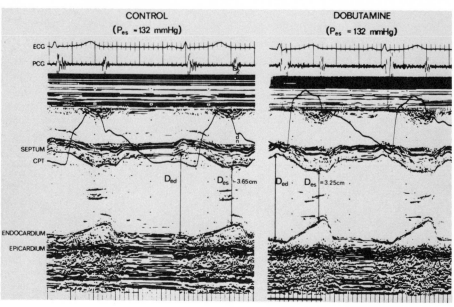

END-SYSTOLIC PRESSURE-DIMENSION (VOLUME) RELATION. The points relating end-systolic pressure and dimension (or volume) form a linear relation that is preload-independent while incorporating afterload (9, 10, 29, 170, 171). Multiple end-systolic pressure-dimension (volume) coordinates can be obtained in the clinical setting by manipulating afterload and preload with drugs (methoxamine or nitroprusside), or with acute changes in LV volume (e.g., IVC balloon occlusion). Changes in end-systolic pressure are directly related to changes in ventricular dimension (or volume). The steepness of the slope of such relations is directly related to LV contractile state (Fig. 5.20) (9, 38). End-systolic pressures can be measured noninvasively using calibrated carotid pulse tracings, while end-systolic dimensions (or volumes) can be measured using targeted M-mode or two-dimensional echocardiographic recordings (Fig. 5.21). Numerous investigators have normalized LV dimension (or volume) for body size in an attempt to compare data from different patients, especially those with chronic heart disease (7, 173). Because of LV shape changes that occur in dilated myopathic ventricles, the LV end-systolic pressure-dimension relation is less sensitive to inotropic state changes in these patients (174).

Attempts to simplify data acquisition by substituting peak systolic pressure for end-systolic pressure, or by using a resting end-systolic pressure to dimension (or volume) ratio are complicated by numerous theoretical as well as physiologic problems (34, 171, 175–177). This is particularly true when the effects of drugs with vasodilator or positive inotropic effects are being evaluated (Fig. 5.22).

END-SYSTOLIC STRESS-DIMENSION (VOLUME) RELATION. Since LV end-systolic pressure is not a complete measure of ventricular afterload, the use of end-systolic wall stress rather than pressure is an attractive alternative (10, 29, 34). This allows incorporation of LV chamber size and wall thickness as well as pressure into the analysis, and thus reduces variability introduced by differing patient body sizes (30, 32, 34, 178). All of the variables required to construct the end-systolic stress-dimension (volume) relation can be acquired using echocardiography and calibrated carotid pulse tracings. Although the LV end-systolic stress-dimension (or volume) relation has been reported to be sensitive to changes in contractility (7, 34, 179), this finding remains controversial (30, 180). Unlike the slope of the end-systolic pressure-dimension (or volume) relation, the slope of the end-systolic stress-dimension (or volume) relation has not been a useful index of contractile state (30, 34). Several investigators have used the ratio of end-systolic stress to volume as a contractility index. However, this measure assumes that the end-systolic stress-volume line goes through the origin (Fig. 5.23). This is usually not the case, and therefore markedly limits the clinical and physiologic utility of this index (34).

END-SYSTOLIC STRESS-PERCENT FRACTIONAL SHORTENING RELATION. Left ventricular percent fractional shortening (%ΔD) is a measure of overall performance, which is afterload-, preload-, and contractility-dependent. By plotting %ΔD against a measure of LV afterload (i.e., end-systolic stress), the afterload dependency of %ΔD can be eliminated. To determine normal values, the σ_{es} versus %ΔD relation was determined using totally noninvasive methods in 26 normal subjects. Afterload

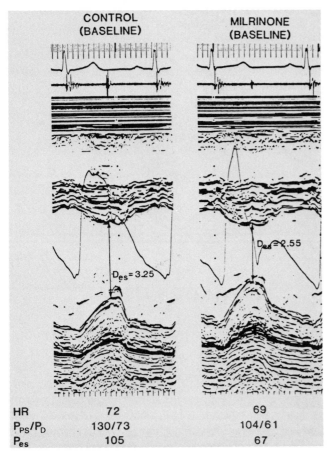

CONTROL (BASELINE)   **MILRINONE (BASELINE)**

$D_{es} = 3.25$ $D_{es} = 2.55$

HR	72	69
P_{PS}/P_D	130/73	104/61
P_{es}	105	67

Figure 5.22 Simultaneous recordings of the left ventricular (LV) echocardiogram, phonocardiogram, carotid pulse tracing, and electrocardiogram under control baseline conditions and during milrinone administration. Milrinone, a peripheral vasodilator and positive inotropic agent, markedly decreased the position of the carotid pulse dicrotic notch and the LV end-systolic pressure (P_{es}). In addition, the LV systolic pressure peaked early in systole followed by a rapid decline, reflecting the significant vasodilator effect of the drug. The fall in LV end-systolic dimension (D_{es}) resulted from the combination of increased contractility and decreased afterload. HR = heart rate; P_{ps} = aortic peak systolic pressure; P_d = aortic diastolic pressure.

was augmented with methoxamine, while contractility was increased with 5 μg/kg/min of dobutamine (30). The relationship between σ_{es} and %ΔD was inversely linear (r = −0.83) for 130 control points. With dobutamine infusion, 43 of 43 σ_{es} versus %ΔD points were greater than 2 standard deviations above the mean for the regression line (Fig. 5.24). In all cases, dobutamine infusion resulted in higher %ΔD for any σ_{es}. From this data, a plot of low, appropriate, and high %ΔD values for any level of LV afterload was constructed. However, the σ_{es} versus %ΔD relation remains preload-dependent (31). In patients with normal intravascular volume, this index has been useful as a clinical measure of LV contractile state (177, 181, 182).

END-SYSTOLIC STRESS-RATE CORRECTED VELOCITY OF FIBER SHORTENING RELATION. As previously stated, the velocity of LV fiber shortening (V_{cf}) is a measure of overall ventricular performance that can be determined accurately by noninvasive methods. Although sensitive to contractile state, its usefulness is limited by dependence on LV loading conditions. Recently, a study was performed investigating the relationship of V_{cf} and LV meridional wall stress in an attempt to develop an index of contractility that is independent of preload and heart rate while incorporating afterload. Calibrated carotid pulse tracings were used to calculate end-systolic pressure and ejection time. V_{cf} was heart rate corrected (Vcf_c) by dividing by the square root of the preceding RR interval. Studies were performed on 68 normal subjects (aged 3 to 70 years) under baseline and afterload augmented conditions (Fig. 5.25). Recordings were also made after increased preload (dextran infusion) and during enhanced LV contractility (dobutamine). The σ_{es} versus Vcf and σ_{es} versus Vcf_c relations were inversely linear with correlation coefficients of −0.72 and −0.84, respectively. For any level of σ_{es}, the 95% confidence intervals for the σ_{es} versus Vcf_c relation were tighter than for the σ_{es} versus V_{cf} relation. The relation between σ_{es} and Vcf_c was not altered by afterload augmentation or combined increase in afterload and preload (Fig. 5.26). During inotropic stimulation, Vcf_c was higher for any given level of σ_{es}, with 93% of σ_{es} versus Vcf_c points above the normal range (Fig. 5.27). Appropriate, high, and low Vcf_c values were determined for a wide range of afterload (σ_{es}) conditions (Fig. 5.28). The σ_{es} versus Vcf_c relation has been useful clinically because it is highly sensitive to LV contractility, incorporates afterload, and is heart rate–independent (23, 168, 169, 183). It should be noted that these studies used meridional wall stress. In cases of dilated, myopathic ventricles, circumferential wall stress as well as meridional wall stress should be calculated.

Left Ventricular-Systemic Arterial Coupling
Overall cardiac performance is determined by the mechanical interaction between the pumping action of the heart and the opposition to blood flow created by the peripheral circulation (170). The traditional measures of this opposing force, mean aortic pressure and systemic vascular resistance (SVR), assume that the heart is a steady state rather than a pulsatile pump. Unlike SVR, aortic impedance incorporates both the steady and pulsatile components of blood pressure and flow waves in the arterial circulation (170, 184–191). Additional information available through impedance calculations includes the magnitude of reflected waves from peripheral reflectance sites, aortic power spectrum, the phase relationship between aortic flow and pressure, and data regarding the intrinsic properties of

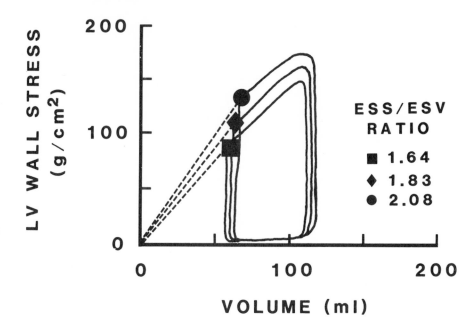

Figure 5.23 Plot of left ventricular (LV) wall stress versus volume for a single subject under control conditions and during nitroprusside infusion. Despite no change in LV contractility, the LV end-systolic stress-volume ratio fell with the nitroprusside infusion. This demonstrates a significant limitation of this ratio as a contractility index.

the aorta (192). The clinical importance of aortic impedance has been demonstrated (192–195). However, the utility of aortic impedance has been limited by the need for cardiac catheterization to measure this important parameter. This is no longer the case. Doppler echocardiography allows noninvasive assessment of LV and aortic blood flow in humans. The combination of simultaneously recorded aortic flow (from suprasternal Doppler) and aortic pressure (from calibrated subclavian artery pulse tracings corrected for pulse transmission time) permits assessment of instantaneous LV and systemic arterial hemodynamics (Fig. 5.29).

Analysis of LV energetics can be performed using this type of approach. Total LV power (TP), which is defined as the energy or work expended by the ventricle per unit time, incorporates instantaneous aortic

pressure and flow, and therefore is an index of performance of the coupled LV-arterial system. Total or generated power is more sensitive to changes in hemodynamic conditions than either pressure or flow considered alone. Total power can be divided into: 1) mean (or delivered) power (MP), which maintains forward blood flow; and 2) oscillatory (or wasted) power (OP), which is energy lost in vascular pulsations of the arterial system. Only mean power results in effective peripheral perfusion. The efficiency of the LV-arterial coupling is inversely proportional to the ratio of oscillatory to total power (OP/TP).

The data generated by these techniques may have particular importance regarding patients with congestive heart failure, systemic hypertension, valvular heart disease, and high cardiac output states such as chronic

Figure 5.24 Plot of the LV end-systolic wall stress (σ_{es})–shortening (%ΔD) relation, showing its sensitivity to inotropic state. All of the σ_{es}-%ΔD points obtained during the dobutamine infusion were greater than two standard deviations above the mean value for the regression line generated from 130 control points. (Reproduced with permission from Borow KM, Green LH, Grossman W, et al. Left ventricular end-systolic stress-shortening and stress-length relations in humans: Normal values and sensitivity to inotropic state. Am J Cardiol 1982;50:1301–1308.)

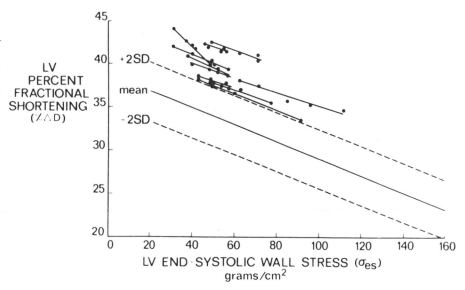

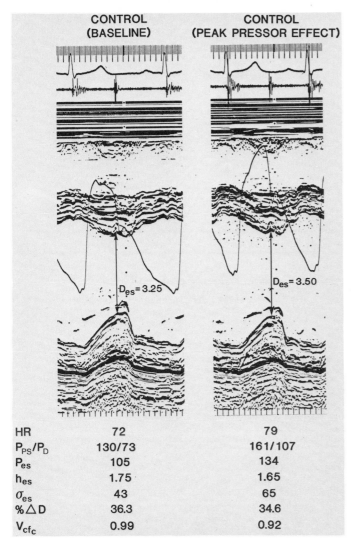

Figure 5.25 Recordings of simultaneously obtained left ventricular (LV) echocardiogram, carotid pulse tracing (CPT), phonocardiogram, and electrocardiogram in a representative subject under control baseline conditions and at peak pressor effect secondary to methoxamine infusion. Note the late peaking of the CPT that occurs with methoxamine. Methoxamine increased end-systolic dimension (D_{es}), aortic peak systolic and diastolic pressures (P_{ps}, P_d), LV end-systolic pressure (P_{es}), and afterload as measured by end-systolic wall stress (σ_{es}). It decreased LV end-systolic wall thickness (h_{es}), percent fractional shortening (%ΔD), and rate corrected velocity of fiber shortening (Vcf_c). Heart rate (HR) did not change significantly.

anemia. In addition, more complete assessment of the effects of cardioactive drugs on the LV-arterial coupling can now be performed.

Clinical Applications

Baseline Contractility and Response to Pharmacologic Interventions

NORMAL SUBJECTS: DOBUTAMINE VERSUS MILRINONE (168, 177). Milrinone and dobutamine are positive inotropic

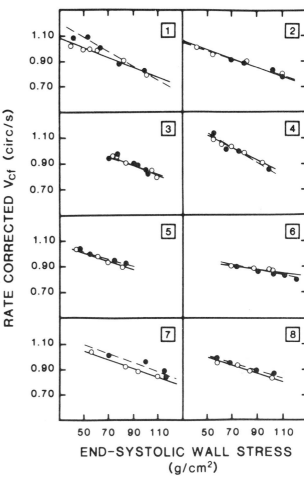

Figure 5.26 Relation of end-systolic wall stress to rate-corrected velocity of fiber shortening (V_{cf}) in eight subjects before (closed circles) and after (open circles) preload augmentation over a wide range of afterload conditions. There was no significant change. Linear regression lines before (solid) and after (dashed) dextran infusion are illustrated. (Reproduced with permission from Colan SD, Borow KM, Neumann A. Left ventricular end-systolic wall stress-velocity of fiber shortening relation: A load-independent index of myocardial contractility. J Am Coll Cardiol 1984;4:715–724.)

agents with complex mechanisms of action. Traditional indices of left ventricular function are unable to determine how much of the improvement in cardiac performance induced by these drugs is due to augmented inotropy and how much is the result of afterload reduction. The end-systolic wall stress (σ_{es}) – rate corrected velocity of fiber shortening relation (Vcf_c), a sensitive measure of contractility that is independent of preload while incorporating afterload, was measured in two groups of normal subjects (n = 8 per group) over a wide range of aortic pressures generated by methoxamine administration prior to and during milrinone or dobutamine infusion. Studies were performed using echocardiographic and calibrated carotid

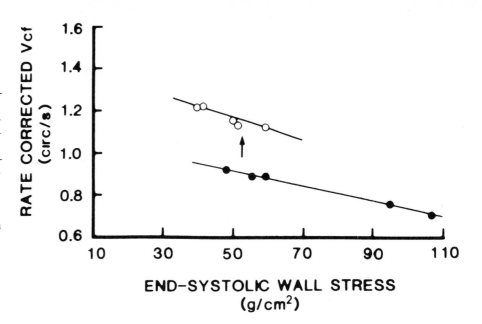

Figure 5.27 Comparison of base-line (closed circles) and increased contractile state (open circles) values of the end-systolic wall stress–rate-corrected velocity of fiber shortening (V_{cf}) relation in a representative subject. During the dobutamine infusion, velocity of fiber shortening was higher for any equivalent end-systolic wall stress. (Reproduced with permission from Colan SD, Borow KM, Neumann A. Left ventricular end-systolic wall-stress velocity of fiber shortening relation: A load-independent index of myocardial contractility. J Am Coll Cardiol 1984;4:715–724.)

pulse tracings. Milrinone and dobutamine produced similar increases in overall LV performance (Fig. 5.30). Milrinone decreased end-systolic dimension (D_{es}) by 15% and end-systolic pressure (P_{es}) by 22%, while increasing end-systolic wall thickness (h_{es}) by 14%. This resulted in a 43% decline in LV afterload as measured by σ_{es}. In contrast, dobutamine decreased D_{es} by 11%, while increasing h_{es} by 14% and P_{es} by 22%. Despite the increase in LV pressure, σ_{es} fell by 20%. Since afterload reduction alone results in increased LV shortening, analysis of LV performance was performed for both drugs at matched levels of σ_{es} under control and positive inotropic conditions. Twenty-nine percent of the improvement in Vcf_c produced by milrinone was due to a decrease in afterload as compared to 18% for dobutamine. Myocardial oxygen requirements (as assessed by the integral of LV systolic wall stress per minute) fell with milrinone but remained unchanged with dobutamine. Thus, milrinone uses advantageous changes in LV afterload conditions and oxygen demands to produce increases in overall LV systolic performance that are comparable to those found with dobutamine. At the doses studied, milrinone was a less potent positive inotropic agent than dobutamine. If only ejection phase indices of LV performance were analyzed, a different conclusion would have been reached.

HYPERTHYROIDISM: RESPONSE TO THERAPY (169). The cardiovascular effects of hyperthyroidism include LV hyperkinesis, a positive chronotropic effect, and reduced systemic vascular resistance (SVR). It is possible that reduced afterload and increased heart rate rather than augmented contractility account for much of the increase in LV performance noted previously in these patients. To investigate this hypothesis, 11 hyperthy-

roid patients were evaluated serially over 4 ± 2 months. With therapy, serum total T4 fell from 21 ± 6 to 5 ± 3 μg/dl (p < 0.001) (normal = 5–12 μg/dl). LV hemodynamics were assessed by two-dimensionally targeted M-mode echocardiograms and calibrated carotid pulse tracings. LV preload was estimated by end-diastolic dimension (D_{ed}), while afterload was

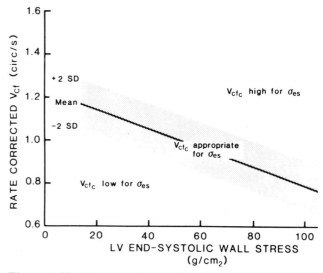

Figure 5.28 Diagram of the end-systolic wall stress (σ_{es})–rate-corrected velocity of fiber shortening (V_{cf}) relation. Depressed contractile state (V_{cf} low for the level of σ_{es}) may be distinguished from situations in which contractility is normal but afterload is increased (V_{cf} appropriate for the level of σ_{es}). A velocity of fiber shortening that is high for the level of end-systolic wall stress is characteristic of increased inotropic state. (Reproduced with permission from Colan SD, Borow KM, Neumann A. Left ventricular end-systolic wall stress-velocity of fiber shortening relation: A load-independent index of myocardial contractility. J Am Coll Cardiol 1984;4:715–724.)

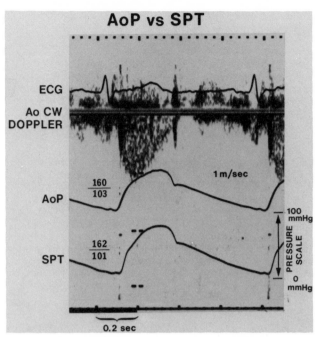

Figure 5.29 Simultaneously recorded aortic blood flow velocity (by continuous-wave Doppler), aortic pressures [from high-fidelity central aortic pressure (AoP) tracing and calibrated subclavian artery pulse tracings (SPT)], and electrocardiogram (ECG) in a representative subject. From this data, the LV and systemic arterial instantaneous blood flow and pressure relationships can be noninvasively determined.

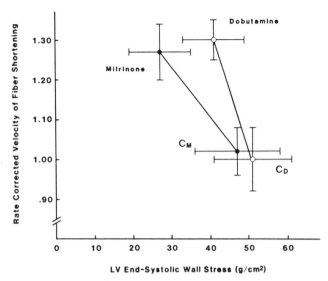

Figure 5.30 The effect of milrinone and dobutamine on the baseline left ventricular (LV) end-systolic wall stress–rate-corrected velocity of fiber shortening relation under control (C_M, C_D) and drug conditions for each study group. Both drugs produced similar increases in overall LV performance (as measured by rate-corrected velocity of fiber shortening). However, milrinone decreased afterload (i.e., end-systolic wall stress) by 43%, while dobutamine decreased afterload by 20%. Thus, milrinone and dobutamine exert very different effects on LV mechanics. (Reproduced by permission of the American Heart Association, Inc. from Borow KM, Neumann A, Lang R. Milrinone versus dobutamine: Contribution of altered myocardial mechanics and augmented inotropic state to improved left ventricular performance. Circulation, in press.)

measured as end-systolic wall stress (σ_{es}). LV contractility was determined using the load-independent relation between σ_{es} and rate corrected velocity of LV fiber shortening (Vcf$_c$). Overall LV performance was quantitated by the extent of shortening (%ΔD) and Vcf$_c$ as well as Doppler echocardiographically derived cardiac output. LV systolic stress-length and stress-time relations were used to assess myocardial work and oxygen consumption, respectively. With therapy, LV performance as well as total minute work declined significantly ($p < 0.001$). These changes occurred in association with a 24% fall in heart rate ($p < 0.001$), a 32% increase in SVR ($p < 0.001$), and no change in LV end-diastolic dimension or end-systolic wall stress. In all cases, the σ_{es} versus Vcf$_c$ relation fell with attainment of normal thyroid status (Fig. 5.31). This is characteristic of a decline in LV contractility. There was a strong positive correlation between LV contractility and serum thyroid hormone level ($r = 0.83$). Thus, the hyperkinesis of hyperthyroidism in human subjects reflects augmented contractility rather than altered loading or chronotropic conditions.

RELATIONSHIP BETWEEN BLOOD IONIZED CALCIUM AND LV CONTRACTILITY. The purpose of this study was to determine the effect of variations in blood ionized calcium

(Ca^{2+}) on myocardial contractility in humans independent of changes in loading conditions and other biochemical variables (36). The study design consisted of hemodialysis performed in a randomized, double-blind manner with dialysates differing only in calcium concentration. Left ventricular contractility was assessed using the load- and heart rate–independent relationship between end-systolic wall stress (σ_{es}) and rate-corrected velocity of fiber shortening (Vcf$_c$). Seven patients with stable, chronic renal failure maintained on regular hemodialysis were studied. Each patient was dialyzed three times within one week, with dialysates differing only in calcium concentration. Ultrafiltration was adjusted to achieve the same postdialysis weight. After dialysis, three statistically distinct levels of Ca^{2+} were achieved. When Ca^{2+} was 1.34 $\pm$ 0.03 m mol/L, Vcf$_c$ [calculated at a common level of afterload (σ_{es} = 50 g/cm^2)] was 1.01 $\pm$ 0.05 circ/sec; at low Ca^{2+} (1.02 $\pm$ 0.02 m mol/L), Vcf$_c$ fell to 0.89 $\pm$ 0.04 circ/sec ($p < 0.001$ compared with medium); at high Ca^{2+} (1.68 $\pm$ 0.07 m mol/L) Vcf$_c$ rose to 1.10 $\pm$ 0.03 circ/sec ($p < 0.001$ compared with medium and low). Thus, this study of a metabolically important ion demonstrated for the first time in humans that variations in plasma

Figure 5.31 Mean (solid line) and ±2 standard deviation confidence limits (dashed lines) for end-systolic stress–rate-corrected velocity of shortening relation determined from a group of normal subjects. Vertical deviation from the mean regression line reflects a change in contractility for a given level of end-systolic wall stress independent of heart rate, preload, and afterload. The end-systolic stress–rate-corrected velocity of shortening relation for the 11 hyperthyroid subjects before (solid squares) and after (open squares) therapy is shown. Prior to treatment, all subjects were above the mean regression line, reflecting increased contractile state; eight of the 11 points were above the ±2 standard deviation confidence limits. Following therapy, all subjects showed a decline in the end-systolic stress–rate-corrected velocity of shortening relation. One subject seen below the −2 standard deviation confidence limit (lower left) was hypothyroid. (Reproduced with permission from Feldman T, Borow KM, Sarne DH, et al. Myocardial mechanics in hyperthyroidism: Importance of left ventricular loading conditions, heart rate and contractile state. J Am Coll Cardiol 1986;7: 967–974.

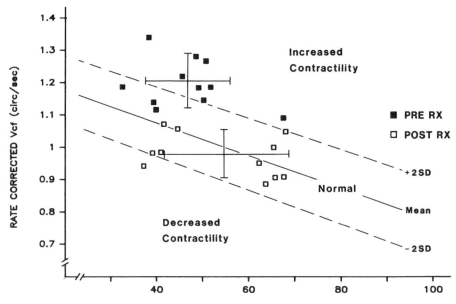

Ca^{2+} are directly correlated with clinically significant changes in myocardial contractility.

DILATED CARDIOMYOPATHY: RESPONSE TO POSITIVE INOTROPIC THERAPY. Clinical trials in patients with dilated cardiomyopathy (DCM) have shown a wide disparity in the hemodynamic responses to positive inotropic therapy. In addition, the response of the failing left ventricle to positive inotropic agents reflects the net interaction of multiple factors, including the magnitude of contractile abnormality and compensatory mechanisms. In this study, left ventricular geometry, loading conditions, and contractile state were assessed in 13 patients with nonischemic DCM using simultaneous high-fidelity pressure measurements and echocardiographic recordings. Comparisons were made with echocardiographic and calibrated carotid pulse data acquired in nine age-matched normal subjects. The patients with DCM were divided according to the left ventricular end-diastolic wall thickness-to-dimension ratio into groups with "appropriate" hypertrophy (i.e., ≤ 2 SDs from mean normal, n = 5: group 1) and "inadequate" hypertrophy (i.e., > 2 SDs from mean normal, n = 8: group 2). Age, New York Heart Association functional class,

	LV SHAPE $(L/D)_{ed}$	ADEQUACY OF LVH $\left(\frac{2h}{D}\right)_{ed}$	BASELINE AFTERLOAD $(\sigma_{es})_c$	BASELINE CONTRACTILITY Vcf_c at $(\sigma_{es})_c$ of 200 g/cm²	CONTRACTILE RESPONSE Vcf_c Shift from NP or Methox Line
NORMAL	D = 1.0 L = 1.7	100%	100%	100%	100%
GROUP 1	D = 1.0 L = 1.5	98%	168%	61%	52%
GROUP 2	D = 1.0 L = 1.2	58%	203%	44%	22%

Figure 5.32 Summary of the major derangements and compensatory mechanisms noted in the described patients with dilated cardiomyopathy. L = LV long axis dimension; D = LV minor axis dimension; h = LV wall thickness; $(\sigma_{es})_c$ = LV circumferential end-systolic wall stress; Vcf_c = rate corrected velocity of fiber shortening; NP = nitroprusside; Methox = methoxamine). (Reproduced by permission of the American Heart Association, Inc. from Borow KM, Lang RM, Neumann A, et al. Physiologic mechanisms governing hemodynamic responses to positive inotropic therapy in patients with dilated cardiomyopathy. Circulation 1988;77:625–637.)

LV wall mass index, and LV end-diastolic pressure and dimension were similar for both DCM groups. Baseline left ventricular afterload (defined as circumferential end-systolic wall stress, σ_{es}) was 168% and 203% greater than normal in groups 1 and 2, respectively. The administration of the β-adrenoceptor agonist dobutamine decreased left ventricular afterload by 12% in the normal subjects and by 10% in group 1 patients, while augmenting afterload by 5% in group 2 patients. The latter response occurred despite a 17% fall in systemic vascular resistance. Overall left ventricular performance, as assessed by the rate-corrected mean velocity of fiber shortening (Vcf_c), was related to left ventricular afterload (i.e., σ_{es}). The resultant σ_{es} versus Vcf_c relationship was determined over a wide range of afterload conditions generated by methoxamine (normal subjects) or nitroprusside (DCM). Baseline left ventricular contractile state was 61% of normal for group 1 and 44% of normal for group 2. The contractile response to dobutamine infusion was 52% of normal for group 1 and only 22% of normal for group 2 (Fig. 5.32). Thus, positive inotropic therapy with dobutamine in patients with DCM was limited by 1) an attenuated contractile response and 2) elevated left ventricular afterload, which may be augmented further during its administration. The ability to separate and quantify abnormalities in left ventricular geometry, loading conditions, and contractile state allowed a more comprehensive interpretation of the hemodynamic responses to a positive inotropic agent. Similar studies have been performed with dopamine (196) and the β-2 adrenoceptor agonist dopexamine (197).

The ability to use ultrasound imaging in conjunction with aortic and LV pressure tracings in patients with dilated cardiomyopathy allowed an accurate assessment of the complex changes in LV afterload and contractility induced by therapeutic agents. This would not have been possible if traditional indices (such as SVR or peak positive dP/dt) had been used alone.

Unmasking Contractile Abnormalities Secondary to Cardiac Toxins

DOXORUBICIN (182). The usual indices of left ventricular systolic performance have been incapable of accurately recognizing early myocardial impairment in many patients treated with doxorubicin, a commonly used antineoplastic agent. In this study, the end-systolic pressure (P_{es}) – dimension (D_{es}) slope value and the σ_{es} – %ΔD relation were used to assess 46 patients receiving low-dose or high-dose doxorubicin. Results were compared with data from 30 healthy subjects. Resting %ΔD failed to accurately recognize left ventricular dysfunction in nine of 17 patients with low normal values. These patients had reduced afterload, as measured by σ_{es}, permitting normal extent of left ventricular fiber shortening despite impaired contractility, as quantified by diminished $P_{es} - D_{es}$ slope values. There was 98% concordance between the relative position of the $\sigma_{es} - \%\Delta D$ relation under resting conditions and the slope value of the $P_{es} - D_{es}$ relation. These indices offered an improved means of recognizing and quantitating preclinical contractility abnormalities in patients treated with doxorubicin.

ALCOHOL (183). Alcohol reduces systemic vascular resistance (SVR), while having variable effects on LV shortening characteristics. It was hypothesized that afterload reduction may mask contractile abnormalities not evident from resting LV shortening characteristics. The $\sigma_{es} - Vcf_c$ relation was determined using echocardiography and calibrated carotid pulse tracings for nine normal nonalcoholic male subjects before and after 1.15 gr/kg body weight of 90% proof whiskey. Mean plasma level 50 minutes post-ingestion was 1.08 $\pm$ 0.25 mg/dl. Under both pre- and postalcohol conditions, afterload was augmented with methoxamine. This allowed comparison of data over comparable ranges of end-systolic wall stress. Cardiac outputs were calculated from suprasternal Doppler tracings of aortic blood flow velocity in conjunction with two-dimensional imaging for aortic annular size. Aortic mean pressure was measured using a microprocessor-based automatic blood pressure monitor device. From this data, total SVR was calculated.

Although baseline end-systolic stress and SVR were significantly lower (p < 0.05) after alcohol ingestion (44 $\pm$ 6 g/cm^2 versus 36 $\pm$ 7 g/cm^2 and 1270 $\pm$ 232 versus 1085 $\pm$ 222 $dyne\text{-}sec\text{-}cm^{-5}$, respectively), no significant associated changes in LV shortening characteristics were noted. However, when rate-corrected velocity of fiber shortening values at the same level of afterload ($\sigma_{es} = 50$ g/cm^2) were compared, a significant decrease in Vcf_c was noted (1.05 $\pm$ 0.05 before alcohol ingestion versus 0.94 $\pm$ 0.03 after alcohol ingestion; p < 0.001). When the relation of σ_{es} and Vcf_c was assessed under control conditions and after alcohol ingestion over a wide range of afterload values, a relatively parallel downward shift of the mean regression line occurred. This is consistent with a significant depression in LV contractile state.

The reason that alcohol's myocardial depressant effect was previously underestimated can be shown graphically using data from a representative subject. In Figure 5.33A, the rate-corrected velocity of fiber shortening is plotted on the y-axis with left ventricular end-systolic wall stress on the x-axis. The triangle labeled C represents the value obtained under control resting conditions. The remaining triangles represent values obtained with the initial methoxamine chal-

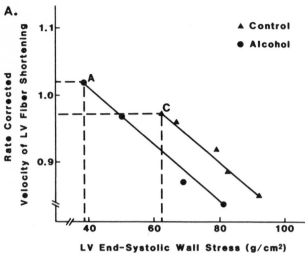

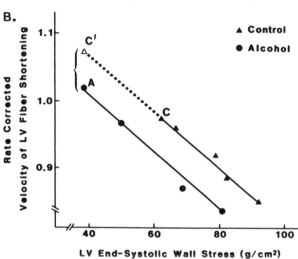

Figure 5.33 Plot of left ventricular end-systolic wall stress–rate-corrected velocity of fiber shortening relations before and after alcohol ingestion for a representative subject. See text for detailed explanation. (Reproduced with permission from Lang RM, Borow KM, Neumann A, et al. Adverse cardiac effects of acute alcohol ingestion in young adults. Ann Int Med 1985;102:742–747.)

lenge. The circle labeled A is the resting value obtained after alcohol ingestion. The remaining circles represent the data points obtained during the second methoxamine challenge. As can be seen, baseline rate-corrected velocity of fiber shortening increased after alcohol ingestion going from point C to point A. Without the aid of load-independent indices of left ventricular contractility, one could conclude that alcohol ingestion resulted in improvement in left ventricular performance. However, when left ventricular afterload (as measured by end-systolic stress) is considered, it becomes apparent that this improvement occurred under different afterload conditions. After alcohol ingestion, baseline end-systolic wall stress fell by 40%, going from 63 to 38 g/cm^2. Because the relationship between rate-cor-

rected velocity of fiber shortening and end-systolic wall stress is linear, it is possible to predict a value for Vcf_c at any level of wall stress over the physiologic range, as demonstrated by the dotted line in Figure 5.33B. Point C′ (open triangle) represents the predicted value for Vcf_c at the same level of wall stress as that measured for baseline after alcohol ingestion (point A). At σ_{es} of 38 g/cm^2, the difference between the predicted (point C′) and actual (point A) values for rate-corrected velocity of fiber shortening defines the true negative inotropic effect of alcohol when afterload is eliminated as a confounding variable. Thus, alcohol decreased left ventricular contractile state despite an increase in baseline Vcf_c. This study demonstrates the utility of noninvasive load-independent indices of LV performance to unmask contractile abnormalities not evident using traditional tests of LV function.

Valvular Heart Disease

VALVULAR AORTIC STENOSIS VERSUS COARCTATION OF THE AORTA (23). Despite similar degrees of left ventricular systolic hypertension, shortening characteristics are usually greater in patients with congenital valvular aortic stenosis (VAS) than in patients with coarctation of the aorta (CoA). It has been hypothesized that these dissimilarities are caused by differences in myocardial mechanics rather than by alterations in contractile state. To test this hypothesis, 11 patients with VAS (ages 6 to 41 years) and 11 with CoA were matched for age, body surface area, and peak systolic ejection gradient. Results were compared with data from 22 normal subjects matched for age and body surface area. Echocardiographic tracings of the left ventricle were recorded in conjunction with left ventricular pressure measurements (VAS) or calibrated carotid pulse tracings (CoA and normal subjects). Peak and end-systolic wall stresses, as well as left ventricular shortening fraction (%ΔD) and rate corrected velocity of fiber shortening (Vcf_c), were calculated. No differences for left ventricular dimensions, heart rate, or peak wall stress were present. Ventricular peak systolic pressures and wall mass were higher for the patients with VAS or CoA than for the normal subjects (p < 0.001). These parameters did not differ between the VAS and CoA groups. The patients with VAS had higher %ΔD and Vcf_c than either the CoA or normal groups (p < 0.01) (Fig. 5.34). Afterload, as quantified by end-systolic stress, was 41% lower than normal for the patients with VAS (p < 0.001) and 13% higher than normal for those with CoA (p < 0.05). Left ventricular contractility as assessed by load-independent indices (i.e., end-systolic stress-%ΔD and end-systolic stress-Vcf_c relations) was depressed in three of 11 patients with CoA. All of these patients were over 20 years of

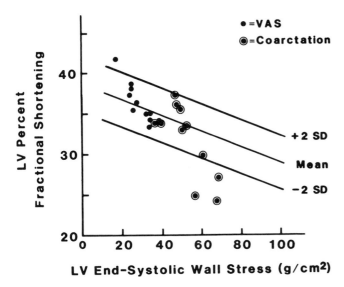

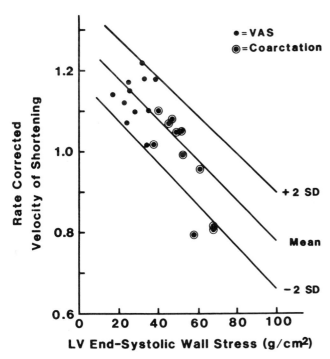

Figure 5.34 Data from valvular aortic stenosis (VAS) and coarctation of the aorta (CoA) groups plotted against normal values for the left ventricular end-systolic stress-shortening (%ΔD) (*top*) and end-systolic stress–rate-corrected velocity of shortening (Vcf$_c$) (*bottom*) relations. All of the patients with VAS and eight of 11 patients with CoA had normal left ventricular contractile state. The three patients with CoA who had depressed left ventricular contractility were all over 20 years of age. (Reproduced by permission of the American Heart Association, Inc. from Borow KM, Colan SD, Neumann A, et al. Altered left ventricular mechanics in patients with valvular aortic stenosis and coarctation of the aorta: Effects on systolic performance and late outcome. Circulation 1985;72:515–522.)

age. In contrast, the increased systolic performance noted in the patients with VAS was caused by reduced afterload at end-systole rather than by altered contractile state. Thus, the extent and velocity of left ventricular shortening is lower in patients with CoA than in those with VAS because of disadvantageous afterload conditions as well as an age-related depression in contractile state.

AORTIC REGURGITATION (108). Wall stress and left ventricular architecture were assessed noninvasively in 15 asymptomatic patients with severe chronic aortic regurgitation, at rest and after load manipulations, with sublingual nitroglycerin. Resting end-systolic meridional and circumferential wall stresses were increased in patients with aortic regurgitation (114 ± 29 and $260 \pm 51 \times 10^3$ dynes/cm^2) compared with those in normal subjects (86 ± 15 and $214 \pm 29 \times 10^3$ dynes/cm^2) (both $p < 0.01$). These wall-stress parameters remained significantly greater than normal after nitroglycerin. Meridional stress values obtained from two-dimensional echocardiographic studies correlated closely ($r = 0.89$) with values calculated from simultaneously recorded M-mode echocardiograms. Ejection fraction in patients with aortic regurgitation and normal subjects were similar at rest ($55 \pm 10\%$ versus $59 \pm 6\%$), and were unchanged by nitroglycerin. In spite of the increased left ventricular mass in patients with aortic regurgitation (227 ± 60 g versus 130 ± 22 g in normal subjects), the mass to volume ratio and the ratio of muscle to cavity area in diastole in patients with aortic regurgitation were significantly lower than normal [0.90 ± 0.23 versus 1.30 ± 0.21 and 0.91 ± 0.23 versus 1.11 ± 0.18 ($p < 0.005$ and $p < 0.02$)]. These differences were exaggerated after nitroglycerin, while concomitant changes in relative wall thickness were almost undetected by M-mode echocardiography. Furthermore, the mean slopes of the circumferential stress-diameter and meridional stress-length lines, which represent load-independent indices of myocardial contractile state, were similar in the group of patients with asymptomatic aortic regurgitation and normal subjects, indicating that overall myocardial contractility was still normal. Thus, this technique can be used for early recognition of afterload excess and changes in left ventricular architecture in patients with aortic regurgitation.

Cardiac Surgery: Orthotopic Heart Transplantation (181, 198)

Limited data are available concerning left ventricular contractility and contractile reserve in the chronically denervated, transplanted human heart. In this study, load-independent end-systolic indices of left ventricular contractility were measured by echocardiography

Table 5.1

	Normals	HTN (NL AC)	HTN (↓ AC)
Age (years)	48 ± 16	47 ± 12	47 ± 20
Mean 24-hour BP	89 ± 10	112 ± 5[a]	116 ± 9[a]
CI (L/m/m²)	2.9 ± 0.4	3.6 ± 0.7[a]	2.8 ± 0.5[b]
SVR (d-s/cm⁵)	1445 ± 281	1316 ± 313	1990 ± 487[ab]
AC (ml/mm Hg)	1.8 ± 0.5	1.8 ± 0.3	1.2 ± 0.3[ab]

[a] $p < 0.01$ versus NL.
[b] $p < 0.01$ versus HTN (NL AC).

Table 5.2

	Invasive	Noninvasive
AOP (mm Hg)	107 ± 17	106 ± 18
SVR (d-s-cm⁻⁵)	1499 ± 130	1510 ± 131
MP (mwatt)	1380 ± 518	1390 ± 540
OP (mwatt)	230 ± 158	215 ± 154
TP (mwatt)	1610 ± 630	1605 ± 670
OP/TP	0.14 ± 0.05	0.13 ± 0.04
Z_c (d-s-cm⁻⁵)	111 ± 25	102 ± 25

and calibrated carotid pulse tracings in ten patients who had undergone orthotopic cardiac transplant (age 48 ± 4 years; interval from operation to study 1.2 ± 0.8 years) and in 10 normal control subjects (age 25 ± 4 years) matched for donor heart age (25 ± 6 years). None of the transplant patients had evidence of rejection as determined by endomyocardial biopsy. Baseline left ventricular contractility was assessed over a wide range of afterload generated by infusion of methoxamine. Contractile reserve was measured as the response to an infusion of dobutamine plus methoxamine. Before afterload augmentation, baseline left ventricular percent fractional shortening was higher for the transplant patients than for the control subjects (36.5 ± 5.7% versus 32.1 ± 2.1%, $p < 0.05$). These differences occurred at a time when end-systolic wall stress (i.e., afterload) was significantly lower for the transplant patients (38 ± 16 versus 50 ± 9 g/cm², $p < 0.05$). When the left ventricular end-systolic pressure-dimension and stress-shortening relationships were determined for the transplant and control subjects, no differences in contractility or contractile reserve were noted. Thus, the chronically denervated, transplanted, non-rejecting human left ventricle demonstrates normal contractile characteristics and reserve, despite elevated LV shortening characteristics under baseline conditions.

Noninvasive Assessment of Systemic Arterial Pressure-Flow Interaction

NONPULSATILE ANALYSIS. Total systemic vascular resistance, a measure of arteriolar tone that assumes non-pulsatile hemodynamics, can be readily calculated using noninvasive measures of mean systemic arterial pressure and cardiac output. Arterial compliance (i.e., the change in aortic volume with incremental changes in aortic pressure) can also be assessed using a totally noninvasive method that we have recently developed. This method, which uses Doppler echocadiography to determine cardiac output and a calibrated subclavian or carotid pulse tracing to determine the rate of aortic pressure decay, is analogous to the invasive method of Yin et al. and employs the Windkessel model of the arterial system (199). In 12 normals and 18 untreated hypertensive patients, continuous-wave Doppler was used to measure instantaneous aortic flow, while simultaneously recorded calibrated carotid pulse tracings were used to determine the rate of aortic pressure decay. From these data, arterial compliance was determined. Sustained hypertension was confirmed by ambulatory 24-hour blood pressure monitoring. The hypertensive patients were divided into those with normal ($n = 9$) versus low ($n = 9$) arterial compliance (AC). (See Table 5.1.) The hypertensive patients with decreased arterial compliance had lower aortic flow and higher SVR than hypertensive patients with normal arterial compliance. This was true despite similar mean 24-hour blood pressures and age. Thus, this easily performed noninvasive method for determining arterial compliance identified differences in LV-peripheral vascular coupling that were not evident from blood pressure measurements alone.

PULSATILE ANALYSIS. Aortic impedance is a physiologic measure of LV-aortic coupling. However, its clinical utility has been limited by the need for cardiac catheterization. To circumvent this problem, we have developed a noninvasive technique for calculating aortic impedance in humans based on our previous work using Doppler instantaneous blood flow and calibrated subclavian artery (SCA) pulse tracings. In ten adult patients, simultaneous microtip central aortic pressure, continuous-wave aortic Doppler, and calibrated subclavian artery tracings were obtained. Fourier analysis was performed on aortic pressure-flow data. Comparisons were made between data acquired using invasive versus noninvasive pressures in conjunction with Doppler instantaneous aortic flow. Heart rate and cardiac output were 69 ± 9 bpm and 5.7 ± 1.3 L/min, respectively. The following were assessed (see Table 5.2):

1. Aortic mean pressure (AP) = steady state pressure component
2. Systemic vascular resistance (SVR) = mean arterial tone
3. Left ventricular mean power (MP) = effective LV work per unit time
4. Left ventricular oscillatory power (OP) = wasted LV work per unit time
5. Total power (TP) = total energy generated per beat
6. OP/TP ratio = measure of LV pump efficiency

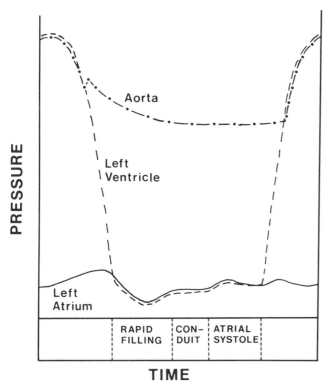

Figure 5.35 Schematic representation of simultaneous left ventricular, left atrial, and aortic pressure tracings demonstrating normal temporal relationships. Diastole is divided into rapid filling, conduit, and atrial systolic phases.

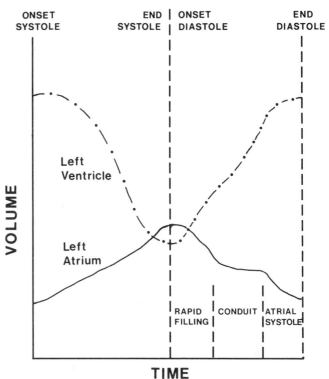

Figure 5.36 Schematic representation of left atrial and left ventricular volume curves from a normal subject during systole and diastole. Note the phases of diastolic filling.

7. Characteristic impedance (Z_c) = index of vascular stiffness

No differences were noted between invasive and noninvasive data. Thus, it is now possible to accurately obtain sophisticated measures of left ventricular–systemic arterial coupling using easily performed, readily available totally noninvasive techniques.

ASSESSMENT OF LEFT VENTRICULAR DIASTOLIC PERFORMANCE

Recently, derangements in the diastolic properties of the left ventricle have been shown to make a major contribution to the clinical manifestations of congestive heart failure. This reflects the interdependence of systole and diastole on overall cardiac performance, as well as the effects of altered diastolic properties on LV filling pressures and subsequent pulmonary venous congestion. Indeed, many forms of heart disease have been associated with early alterations in LV diastolic performance. For example, in such pathophysiologic conditions as LV hypertrophy, diabetes mellitus, anthracycline cardiotoxicity, and myocardial ischemia, disturbances of diastolic function may be detectable before the onset of any impairment in contractile performance (200–204). This section of the chapter

addresses the determinants of the LV diastolic pressure-volume relation; continues with a discussion of traditional measures of diastolic performance; and concludes with the clinical applications of M-mode, two-dimensional, and Doppler echocardiography in the assessment of LV diastolic physiology.

Physiology

Left Atrial–Left Ventricular Interaction

The relationship between left atrial and left ventricular diastolic pressures and volumes reflects multiple factors intrinsic as well as extrinsic to the ventricle. Figure 5.35 shows simultaneous LV, LA, and aortic pressure tracings. These relationships are extremely important because blood flows in the direction of the pressure gradient between chambers. Figure 5.36 illustrates the resultant LA and LV volume curves throughout the cardiac cycle. During isovolumic relaxation (i.e., period from aortic valve closure to mitral valve opening), LV pressure decreases without a change in ventricular volume. Throughout this portion of the cardiac cycle, the left atrium is serving as a reservoir for blood returning to the heart via the pulmonary veins. With continued LV relaxation, the pressure in the ventricle falls below LA pressure, resulting in mitral valve opening. Flow of blood across the mitral valve

Figure 5.37 Left ventricular diastolic pressure-volume relations (*left*) and chamber stiffness–pressure relations (*right*). Operating chamber stiffness (dP/dV) may increase by virtue of an increase in volume (preload-dependent change in stiffness); alternatively, a leftward shift of the pressure-volume relation may cause an increase in dP/dV. If the diastolic pressure-volume relation is exponential, the relation between dP/dV and pressure is linear; the slope of this line is the chamber stiffness constant (k_c). (Reproduced with permission from Hoshino PK, et al. Diastolic dysfunction in left ventricular hypertrophy. Heart Failure 1985;1: 220–230.)

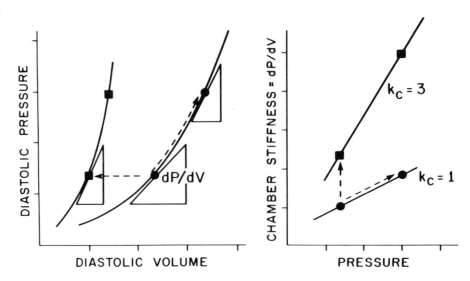

commences and left ventricular volume starts to increase. Initial filling is rapid because the atrioventricular pressure gradient is relatively high. As the LV fills, chamber stiffness properties act to oppose continued rapid filling. This results in a decrease in the rate of LV filling. At this point, the mitral valve is passively held open, and blood flows from the pulmonary veins, through the left atrium, and into the left ventricle. Thus, the volume of LV filling prior to left atrial contraction reflects the combined effects of LA emptying (reservoir volume) and blood flowing from the pulmonary veins to the LV (conduit volume). In the normal subject, left atrial contraction occurs immediately prior to LV systole. This results in augmentation of ventricular preload at the time that the Frank-Starling relationship is most important relative to overall LV systolic performance. Thus, atrial systole allows the LV to maximize myocardial fiber stretch at end-diastole (i.e., preload) without having to maintain high LV pressures throughout the entire diastolic phase of the cardiac cycle.

Determinants of the Left Ventricular Diastolic Pressure-Volume Relation

Factors Intrinsic to the Left Ventricle

CHAMBER PROPERTIES (OPERATING CHAMBER STIFFNESS). The left ventricle can be considered a blood-filled chamber enclosed by a wall of muscle. Increases in LV volume result in distension of the chamber. Since there is conservation of muscle mass throughout diastole, the increase in LV size must result in stretching and thinning of the chamber wall. Because of the viscoelastic material properties of the muscle, chamber enlargement results in elevations of chamber pressure. This increase in chamber pressure, in conjunction with the simultaneously occurring changes in volume (i.e.,

the pressure-volume relation), reflects the distending force required to stretch the chamber wall (205). As with the LV ejection phase indices of systolic performance, the diastolic pressure-volume relation reflects overall LV chamber properties in a multifactorial manner. This includes the interaction of factors intrinsic (e.g., material properties, wall thickness, active relaxation, etc.) as well as extrinsic (e.g., pericardium, RV-LV interaction, etc.) to the ventricle (7, 205).

In a broad sense, overall diastolic function of the LV can be described as chamber (or volume) stiffness (7, 47). This is defined as the increment in LV pressure (dP) required to produce a given change in ventricular volume (dV). While chamber stiffness can be thought of as dP/dV, chamber compliance is the reciprocal of this ratio (i.e., dV/dP). Both of these indices refer to the net effects of multiple factors on the behavior of the entire chamber and not the specific properties of individual LV muscle units (47, 206). Conceptually, LV chamber stiffness is a measure of the resistance met by blood entering the LV chamber at any instant in time during diastole. This pressure-volume relation is curvilinear. This means that in the normal heart at low LV diastolic pressures, large changes in volume are accompanied by small changes in pressure (dP). In contrast, at high diastolic pressures, a comparable change in LV volume results in a much larger change in chamber pressure (dP) (Fig. 5.37, *left*). Thus, as the LV operates further out on its diastolic pressure-volume curve, dP/dV increases despite the absence of changes in myocardial fiber structure. The slope of a tangent to this curvilinear diastolic pressure-volume relation defines the *operating chamber stiffness* (dP/dV) at each level of filling pressure (7). The relation between dP/dV and diastolic pressure is linear; the slope of this line is the chamber stiffness constant (K_C) (Fig. 5.37, *right*) (7).

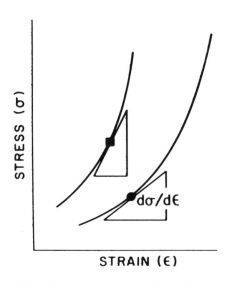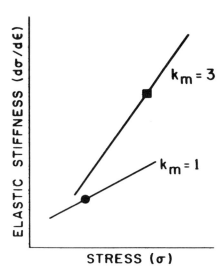

Figure 5.38 Myocardial stress-strain relations (*left*) and elastic stiffness–stress relations (*right*). Similar to the pressure-volume analysis, myocardial elastic stiffness (d_σ/d_ϵ) will increase as strain increases; alternatively, a leftward shift of the stress-strain relation results in high d_σ/d_ϵ. The relation between elastic stiffness (d_σ/d_ϵ) and stress is linear, and the slope of this line is the myocardial stiffness constant (k_m). (Reproduced with permission from Hoshino PK, et al. Diastolic dysfunction in left ventricular hypertrophy. Heart Failure 1985;1:220–230.)

Therefore, neither end-diastolic pressure nor end-diastolic volume alone are measures of diastolic stiffness (47). It must be noted that operating chamber stiffness (dP/dV) is preload-dependent, and can therefore change by virtue of changes in LV volume without alteration in intrinsic muscle fiber properties (7). For example, the value for dP/dV will differ for the same heart when assessed at small as compared to large LV diastolic volumes, even though material properties of the muscle have not changed. If a comparison between hearts of differing mass and volume is to be made, the analysis must be performed at equal levels of diastolic pressure and should include normalization for chamber volume.

MUSCLE PROPERTIES (STRESS-STRAIN RELATIONS). Myocardial stiffness refers to the intrinsic material properties of

the muscle rather than to the pressure-volume relation of the entire chamber (7, 38, 207, 208). It reflects the stiffness properties of each unit of muscle and can be expressed in a manner similar to that used for operating chamber stiffness. In this case, however, the equation describes the LV diastolic stress-strain relation at various levels of wall stress (Fig. 5.38) (7, 209). To perform this analysis, *wall stress* (i.e., force per unit cross-sectional area) is calculated from simultaneously measured LV pressure, diameter, and wall thickness. Simultaneous assessment of *wall strain* (i.e., the resultant effect of an application of stress measured as the fractional change in dimension or size from a reference or unstressed dimension) is determined from measurements of chamber geometry (207, 209). This diastolic stress-strain relation is curvilinear. Elastic stiffness is the slope of a tangent at any point on the

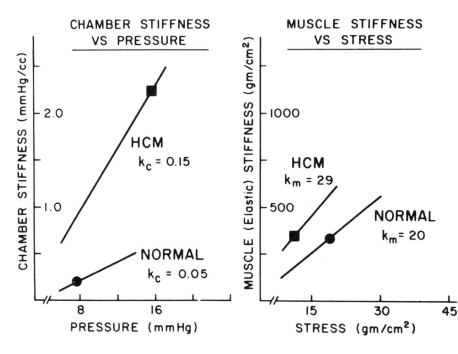

Figure 5.39 Data from representative patients. Left ventricular chamber stiffness is plotted against pressure on the *left*, and myocardial stiffness is plotted against stress on the *right*. The modulus of chamber stiffness (k_c) in the patient with hypertrophic cardiomyopathy (HCM) is three times the k_c in a person without HCM, but the modulus of muscle stiffness is only 50% greater than normal. In this example, the abnormal chamber stiffness is due to a combination of increased myocardial mass and increased intrinsic myocardial stiffness. (Reproduced with permission from Hoshino PK, et al. Diastolic dysfunction in left ventricular hypertrophy. Heart Failure 1985;1:220–230).

stress-strain curve (7). As such, it can be considered as the change in stress per increment of strain (208). The myocardial stiffness constant (K_m) is the slope of the linear relation between muscle elastic stiffness and LV diastolic wall stress (Fig. 5.38). When values for operating chamber stiffness and muscle stiffness constants are compared, it is common to find differences, especially in the presence of LV hypertrophy and cardiomyopathy (Fig. 5.39) (210). This suggests that overall operating chamber stiffness and intrinsic muscle properties are not necessarily synonymous. Thus, complete analysis of diastolic properties should include both pressure-dimension and stress-strain calculations performed over a wide range of filling pressures and chamber volumes.

RELAXATION. Relaxation is the process of restoring the left ventricle from its end-systolic configuration to its end-diastolic size and wall stress (211). Its early period is active (i.e., energy consuming) and leads to the disappearance of force generating sites (i.e., actin-myosin cross bridges). This is followed by a passive filling period (212). The timing and magnitude of overlap of these two periods depend on the uniformity and completeness of the active relaxation process (212, 213). In the presence of LV pressure overload, ischemia, and hypertrophic cardiomyopathy, abnormalities of the active phase of myocardial relaxation may occur with prolongation and slowing of diastolic relaxation (20, 214). This slow and possibly incomplete relaxation may be due to cellular calcium overload, as well as improper energy utilization or production (214). This results in slowly falling LV pressure, with delayed mitral valve opening and increased LV diastolic pressures. The situation may be further complicated by asynchronous wall relaxation, as has been described with myocardial ischemia and hypertrophic cardiomyopathy (207, 213).

FIBER RESTORING FORCES. Several investigators have postulated that internal restoring forces within the cardiac fibers, and external restoring forces resulting from deformation of the LV wall during contraction contribute to ventricular filling in early diastole (213). This concept of active "suction" of blood from the left atrium to the left ventricle has been supported by a direct correlation between early diastolic peak velocity of fiber lengthening and the extent of systolic shortening (215–217). The significance of internal and external restoring forces during early diastole, however, remains controversial (213).

Factors Extrinsic to the Left Ventricle

PERICARDIUM. In normal subjects, the intrapericardial pressure is approximately 0 mm Hg. As a result, the pericardium does not typically exert a significant effect on the left ventricle's pressure-volume relations. However, in pathologic conditions such as constrictive pericarditis or acute cardiac tamponade, decreased forward cardiac output in association with elevated LV filling pressures can occur, despite normal myocardial stiffness and normal LV contractile state (9, 218–221). In these cases, the entire LV diastolic pressure-volume relation is shifted upward due, at least in part, to changes in intrapericardial pressure. In a similar manner, the structurally normal pericardium can adversely affect LV hemodynamics during acute changes in LV loading conditions, or in the patient with a dilated cardiomyopathy (219–222). This is due to limitation of pericardial expansion, and is characterized by an upward shift of the diastolic pressure-volume relation.

Therapy with nitroprusside can decrease heart size and thus decrease total intrapericardial volume, resulting in restoration of a more normal diastolic pressure-volume relation (9, 219, 222).

RIGHT VENTRICULAR–LEFT VENTRICULAR INTERACTION. In situations of significant right ventricular pressure or volume overload, LV chamber stiffness can increase due to a shift of the interventricular septum in a right-to-left direction (17, 205, 219, 220). With each increment in RV filling volume or pressure, the LV becomes functionally less distensible, leading to an upward and leftward shift of the diastolic pressure-volume relation. The presence of an intact pericardium can augment the degree of RV-LV interaction, and thus further elevate LV operating chamber stiffness and filling pressures. An extreme example of this occurs with pulsus paradox in the setting of cardiac tamponade. The effects of the RV on LV diastolic filling is also commonly seen with acute right ventricular infarction and chamber dilatation. The RV-LV interaction becomes less hemodynamically significant in the presence of an open pericardium.

CORONARY ARTERY PERFUSION. The sudden onset of a pressure gradient between the central aorta and the LV wall during diastole results in abrupt filling of the coronary arterial vessels, capillaries, and venules. This engorgement of the coronary reservoir can act as an intramural compressive force on the relaxing myocardial fibers, thus altering the diastolic pressure-volume relation in the absence of intrinsic abnormalities in the muscle fibers themselves (213).

TRANSTHORACIC PRESSURE. Left ventricular diastolic pressures are usually measured with reference only to the position of the heart in the chest cavity. Increases in intrathoracic pressure will be transmitted to the LV, resulting in an upward shift of the diastolic pressure-volume relation. Correction for transthoracic pressure has been performed by subtracting esophageal pressure from LV diastolic pressure. In this manner, ventricular pressure readings reflect more accurately intrachamber pressures alone, having eliminated intrathoracic pressure as a confounding variable.

EXTRINSIC COMPRESSION OF THE HEART. This is most often secondary to infiltrating tumor involving structures adjacent to the heart (e.g., lung, breast, mediastinal lymph nodes). Left ventricular diastolic pressures may be elevated with either right or left ventricular compression.

Traditional Indices of LV Diastolic Relaxation

Pressure-Derived Indices

PEAK NEGATIVE DP/DT. Measurements of the maximal rate of LV pressure decay (peak negative dP/dt) are performed during the isovolumic relaxation phase of the cardiac cycle (213). This index requires use of a high-fidelity manometer in the LV during cardiac catheterization. It is dependent on active LV relaxation as well as ventricular loading conditions. Peak negative dP/dt is a measurement of the rate of pressure change at a single instant in time. It does not consider the effects of chamber size, mass, or systolic performance.

TIME CONSTANT OF ISOVOLUMIC PRESSURE DECLINE. The time constant (τ) is determined from the plot of the natural logarithm (ln) of LV isovolumic pressure versus time beginning at aortic valve closure and ending at mitral valve opening (213). Since LV pressure decline is exponential, the plot of ln P versus time is a straight line. The time constant (τ) is calculated as (-1/slope). This index has been used extensively to assess the effects of myocardial ischemia on altered LV relaxation (223, 224). For a more complete discussion of the time constant of isovolumic pressure decline, see Carroll et al. (223, 224). The usefulness of pressure-derived indices is limited by their dependence on ventricular loading conditions, inotropic state, pericardial factors, and the neurohumoral milieu (38, 213).

Volume-, Dimension-, or Wall Thickness–Derived Indices

These are most commonly measured as rapid filling period indices of overall LV relaxation. They can be divided into two subgroups.

INDICES OF DIMENSION OR WALL THICKNESS CHANGE

1. LV dimension change during diastolic filling
2. LV posterior wall excursion during the rapid filling period
3. Percent of LV diastolic dimension change during the rapid filling period

4. LV posterior wall diastolic thickness change
5. Fractional wall thinning

INDICES OF RATE OF LV VOLUME, DIMENSION, OR WALL THICKNESS CHANGE

1. Peak LV filling rate often measured as the peak rate of dimension enlargement during early diastole
2. Peak LV posterior wall thinning rate

These indices can be obtained using M-mode and two-dimensional echocardiography. However, they are load- as well as contractility-dependent.

Interval-Derived Indices

1. Isovolumic relaxation period (IRP) indices. The IRP indices usually measure the time from aortic valve closure or minimum LV dimension to mitral valve opening (A_2-MVO). They have been used extensively in studies of LV relaxation in patients with hypertrophic cardiomyopathy. The major failing of this method is the omission of a measure of the LA-LV pressure gradient as a factor influencing mitral valve opening.
2. Time to peak LV filling rate. This is measured as the time to peak rate of LV dimension increase.
3. Time to peak LV posterior wall thinning rate.

These load-dependent indices are also influenced by the magnitude of wall thickening and extent of chamber shortening during systole.

M-Mode Echocardiographic Indices of Diastolic Function

Indices Using the Mitral Valve

Normal Diastolic Motion Pattern

In the absence of intrinsic mitral valve pathology, the motion pattern of the leaflets is determined by the combined effects of blood flow characteristics through the valve and the motion of the heart within the chest relative to the fixed precordial transducer position. The normal mitral valve opens rapidly in early diastole (D to E points). This motion corresponds to the period of rapid transmitral flow and rapid filling of the left ventricle. This is followed by early diastolic partial closure (E to F points), which occurs as the rapid filling period ends and the slow filling or conduit phase begins. There is frequently partial reopening of the mitral valve leaflets during this portion of diastole, especially if the heart rate is less than 80 beats per minute. With atrial systole, the valve reopens and reaches a peak (A point) just prior to LV systole. With onset of ventricular contraction, LV pressure exceeds LA pressure and the mitral valve closes (C point). The transition from the A to C point is normally smooth and rapid without interruption (i.e., absent B notch).

Abnormal Diastolic Motion Pattern

DECREASED LEAFLET EXCURSION. This is a nonspecific finding which occurs with a nonpliable valve in mitral stenosis, in decreased cardiac output states associated with low pulmonary venous flow through the LA and mitral valve, and in conditions of decreased LV compliance (Fig. 5.5).

DECREASED D TO E SLOPE. This reflects decreased initial diastolic flow between the left atrium and left ventricle (225, 226). It can be caused by elevated initial LV diastolic pressures with decreased LA-LV pressure gradient, decreased left atrial reservoir function during systole secondary to low cardiac output, and by a jet of aortic regurgitation impeding early diastolic opening of the mitral valve into the region of the LV outflow tract.

DECREASED E TO F SLOPE. A decreased E to F slope of the anterior leaflet of the mitral valve occurs in mitral stenosis, and in any condition associated with decreased LV compliance. It reflects increased resistance either at the valvular or ventricular level to early diastolic flow from LA to LV (225, 227). In general, an abnormal EF slope is not a sensitive index of abnormalities in LV end-diastolic pressure or compliance.

PROMINENT A WAVE. Exaggerated reopening of the mitral valve with atrial systole is demonstrated on the M-mode echocardiogram as a prominent A point, usually higher than the accompanying E point. This is due to increased LA to LV flow late in diastole in association with decreased transmitral flow during the rapid filling and conduit periods of ventricular filling. Thus, when LV stroke volume is relatively normal, a prominent A wave is due to a redistribution of much of transmitral flow from early to late diastole. A prominent A wave is often evident when LV hypertrophy and diminished compliance are present.

A-C NOTCH (B NOTCH). This abnormality in late mitral valve closure has been associated with an elevated left atrial contribution to LV end-diastolic pressure (Fig. 5.5). In most cases, LV end-diastolic pressure is in excess of 20 mm Hg. It is a relatively insensitive index of abnormal LV compliance (228, 229).

Indices Using the Left Atrium

Left Atrial Size

This is a nonspecific index of pathologic changes in LV compliance. Left atrial enlargement can occur in many conditions, including mitral stenosis and/or regurgitation, ventricular septal defect, and presbycardia.

Left Atrial Emptying Index

The LA emptying index (LAEI) has been used in patients with systemic hypertension (230) and congestive heart failure as an indirect measure of LV compliance. It is calculated from the motion pattern of the posterior wall of the aorta, which reflects changes in LA volume. The LAEI represents the fraction of atrial emptying that occurs in the first third of diastole. It assumes that the aorta is of normal size and shape, and that the left atrium is not grossly distorted in morphology.

Indices Using the Left Ventricle

End-Diastolic Dimension

The LV end-diastolic dimension (Fig. 5.40) has been used by numerous investigators as a measure of ventricular preload. Similar to LV end-diastolic volume, LV end-diastolic dimension fails to measure the forces acting on myocardial fibers at end-diastole (i.e., true preload). It cannot be used as a measure of diastolic function since it is altered by many factors intrinsic and extrinsic to the ventricle. Among these are age, body size, intravascular volume status, LV pressure and wall mass, RV-LV interaction, status of the pericardium, etc.

Peak Rate of Change of Dimension and Wall Thickness

These indices measure the peak rate at which the end-diastolic muscle length and thickness are being

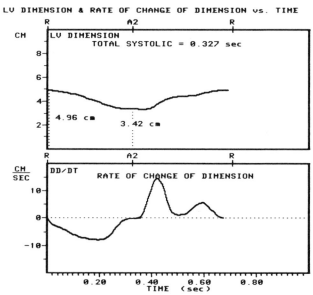

Figure 5.40 Plot of left ventricular dimension and rate of change of dimension (dD/dt) versus time for a normal subject. Note that the derivative of the dimension curve during diastole resembles a Doppler determined velocity profile. The maximal value for dD/dt is the peak filling rate. R = timing of peak QRS complex; A₂ = aortic valve closure sound.

re-established after completion of ventricular systole. The peak rate of LV dimension enlargement [dD/dt)$_{max}$] is calculated as the maximum value of the first derivative of LV dimension during early diastole (Fig. 5.40) (212, 213, 217, 231). Similarly, the peak posterior wall thinning rate [(−dh/dt)$_{max}$] is calculated as the greatest negative value of the first derivative of LV wall thinning during early diastole (Fig. 5.41) (212, 217, 231, 232). These indices have been used to assess ventricular diastolic performance in humans with valvular regurgitation (232), cardiac amyloidosis (233), physiologic cardiac hypertrophy (212), and ischemic heart disease (234). Although correlations between abnormalities of diastolic function and these indices have been reported, both (dD/dt)$_{max}$ and (−dh/dt)$_{max}$ are dependent on ventricular loading conditions, heart rate, contractility, and systolic performance (217, 231). The best method for adjusting these indices for ventricular size and systolic function remains controversial. A commonly used approach relates (dD/dt)$_{max}$ to absolute or percent change in thickening during systole (212, 217, 235). While these normalization factors improve the clinical utility of (dD/dt)$_{max}$ and (−dh/dt)$_{max}$, they fail to overcome the interactive nature of multiple variables and complex physiology during early diastole.

Interval-Derived Indices

ISOVOLUMIC RELAXATION PERIOD (IRP). This index of early diastolic relaxation has been determined noninvasively in several ways. The most commonly used approaches measure the time from aortic valve closure to mitral

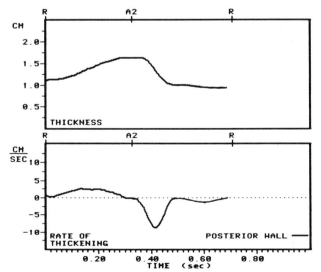

THICKNESS & RATE OF THICKENING vs. TIME

Figure 5.41 Plot of left ventricular posterior wall thickness (h) and a rate of change (dh/dt) versus time. The maximal negative value for dh/dt during diastole is −8.1 cm/sec. Abbreviations as in Figure 5.40.

valve opening (236, 237) and the time from minimum LV dimension to mitral valve opening (Figs. 5.35 and 5.36) (238). The value for the IRP is dependent on many factors, including the rate of active LV diastolic relaxation, the aortic end-systolic pressure, the left atrial–left ventricular interaction, and intrinsic myocardial factors. Despite these limitations, the IRP indices have been used to assess LV diastolic performance in patients with systemic hypertension as well as hypertrophic cardiomyopathy (237–243).

TIME TO PEAK FILLING RATE AND PEAK WALL THINNING RATE. The combination of a digitized M-mode echocardiogram and the aortic valve closure sound (A$_2$) on phonocardiogram is used to determine these indices. The specific measurements are the time between A$_2$ and the peak rate of LV dimension enlargement [dD/dt)$_{max}$] and the time between A$_2$ and the peak rate of LV posterior wall thinning [(−dh/dt)$_{max}$] (Figs. 5.40 and 5.41). Both of these indices of diastolic function are afterload- and contractile state–dependent (217). In addition, they are unable to distinguish between abnormalities in myocardial stiffness and abnormalities in active LV relaxation.

Combined Hemodynamic-Echocardiographic Studies

COMPARISON WITH HEMODYNAMIC-ANGIOGRAPHIC STUDIES. As noted earlier, because of the complexity of LV diastolic function, a quantitative approach using ventricular pressure, volume (or dimension), and wall thickness has the most promise as a means of distinguishing abnormalities in overall chamber characteristics from derangements in LV muscle physiology. Traditionally, these studies have been performed in the cardiac catheterization laboratory using combined hemodynamic and angiographic methods. However, several practical as well as methodologic problems exist with this approach.

1. Left ventricular cineangiography for volume determination requires injection of 30 to 50 cc of viscous contrast media (e.g., renografin-76) into the ventricular cavity. This can alter LV shape, volume, and wall stress while depressing contractile state. Thus, measurements made using this technique may not be representative of steady state myocardial mechanics.
2. Angiographic measurements are limited to a few cardiac cycles, may be complicated by ventricular ectopic beats, and cannot safely be repeated more than two or three times due to the toxicity of intravascular accumulation of contrast material.
3. Determination of LV volume, dimension, and mass requires laborious frame-by-frame analysis of the cineangiogram.

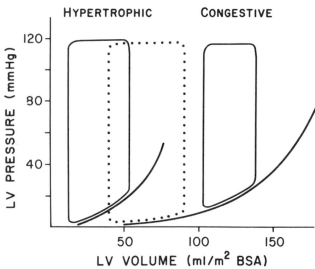

Figure 5.42 Schematic diagram of left ventricular (LV) pressure-volume loops in hypertrophic and idiopathic dilated congestive cardiomyopathy. The dotted line represents a normal ventricle. In congestive cardiomyopathy, the chamber is dilated and shortening is decreased; as a consequence of increased chamber volume, the end diastolic pressure is increased. In hypertrophic cardiomyopathy, the chamber volume is normal or small, the ejection fraction is supernormal, and increased chamber stiffness results in elevated and diastolic pressure. (Reproduced with permission from Gaasch WH, Zile MR. Evaluation of myocardial function in cardiomyopathic states. Prog CV Dis 1984;27: 115–132.)

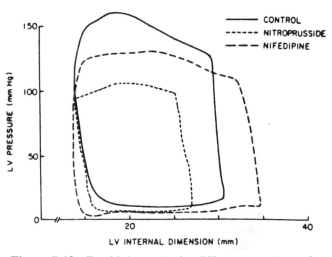

Figure 5.43 Total left ventricular (LV) pressure–internal dimension relations obtained from a single patient with hypertrophic cardiomyopathy. Individual loops were generated under control conditions as well as during nitroprusside and nifedipine administration. (Reproduced with permission from Paulus WJ, Lorell BH, Craig WE, et al. Comparison of the effects of nitroprusside and nifedipine on diastolic properties in patients with hypertrophic cardiomyopathy: Altered left ventricular loading conditions or improved muscle inactivation. J Am Coll Cardiol 1983;2: 879–886.)

Many of these problems can be overcome using two-dimensionally targeted M-mode echocardiograms recorded simultaneously with high-fidelity LV pressure tracings in the cardiac catheterization laboratory. This allows excellent time resolution for data acquisition without alteration of myocardial mechanics. In addition, data can be acquired continuously and serially during acute interventions with pharmacologic agents, pacing stress testing, etc.

CLINICAL APPLICATIONS

Valvular Heart Disease. Data have been acquired using combined hemodynamic-echocardiographic techniques in patients with LV pressure overload or volume overload due to valvular heart disease. Several of these studies have used the ratio between the increment of LV pressure to the increment in LV dimension associated with left atrial contraction as an index of LV chamber stiffness (12, 206, 244, 245). The resultant slope was found to be steep in patients with LV pressure or volume overload (9.0 ± 1.8 mm Hg/mm for pressure overload, 5.6 ± 0.9 mm Hg/mm for volume overload) compared with a control group (2.2 ± 0.2 mm Hg/mm). When this slope was normalized for

operating diastolic pressure (i.e., the mean LV pressure during atrial systole), chamber stiffness remained high in the pressure-overloaded ventricles but only slightly increased in the volume-overloaded ventricles. Thus, chronic pressure overload, but not chronic volume overload, resulted in significantly increased normalized LV diastolic chamber stiffness despite increased LV wall mass for both groups. It should be noted that this approach for quantitation of LV diastolic stiffness involves several simplistic assumptions. The most important of these is the fact that LV diastolic performance during atrial systole is assumed to be representative of ventricular diastolic characteristics for all phases of LV filling. This approach is therefore not ideal for assessment of muscle stiffness. Similar approaches could be applied to other portions of the diastolic pressure-volume relation to determine LV diastolic stress-strain relations.

Hypertrophic Cardiomyopathy (HCM). Left ventricular diastolic performance is abnormal in many patients with hypertrophic cardiomyopathy (Fig. 5.42). Administration of a calcium channel blocking agent has been reported to improve diastolic performance in many of these patients (237, 240–242, 245). However, the mechanism of action of these drugs is complex. Accordingly, a study using combined hemodynamic-echocardiographic methods was performed to determine whether the diastolic effects of these drugs reflected improvement in myocardial inactivation or merely systemic vasodilation and LV unloading. Ten patients with nonobstructive HCM were studied prior to and during administration of the calcium channel blocking agent nifedipine and the vasodilator nitroprusside. Left ventricular peak systolic pressure was comparable during nitroprusside infusion (132 ± 38 mm Hg) and after nifedipine (132 ± 32 mm Hg). During nitroprusside infusion, a decrease in left ventricular end-diastolic pressure (22 ± 11 to 17 ± 11 mm Hg, p < 0.05) was associated with a decrease in left ventricular end-diastolic dimension (Fig. 5.43). In contrast, the decrease in left ventricular end-diastolic pressure after nifedipine (22 ± 11 to 18 ± 10 mm Hg, p < 0.05) was associated with no reduction of left ventricular end-diastolic dimension, suggesting an increase in left ventricular distensibility. Compared with nitroprusside, nifedipine was associated with less prolongation of the left ventricular isovolumic relaxation time and less depression of the peak LV posterior wall thinning rate [$(-dh/dt)_{max}$] and peak filling rate [$(dD/dt)_{max}$]. These data suggest that the effects of nifedipine on diastolic mechanics in hypertrophic cardiomyopathy result not only from systemic vasodilation but also from improved cardiac muscle inactivation. Findings such as these are particularly important to the clinician who has to manage patients with severe LV diastolic dysfunction. A study of this type was feasible only because of the availability of combined invasive and noninvasive techniques to maximize data collection. Repeated LV angiographic assessment of chamber volume and function would have jeopardized patient safety due to the adverse hemodynamic and renal effects of angiographic contrast agents.

Congestive Cardiomyopathy. Symptoms of congestive heart failure frequently reflect abnormalities of both systolic and diastolic performance. While much work has been reported on the mechanisms by which positive inotropic and vasodilator therapy affect systolic performance, little is known about their effect on diastolic function. Twelve patients with diffuse dilated cardiomyopathies were studied using micromanometer left ventricular and aortic pressure measurements recorded simultaneously with two-dimensional targeted M-mode echocardiograms and thermodilution determined cardiac output (222). Each patient received dopamine (2, 4, and 6 μg/kg/min) and dobutamine (2, 6, and 10 μg/kg/min).

Baseline hemodynamics were characterized by low cardiac index (2.1 ± 0.7 L/min/M², mean ± S.D.), high LV end-diastolic pressure (24 ± 10 mm Hg), and increased end-diastolic (6.8 ± 1.0 cm) and end-systolic dimensions (6.0 ± 1.0 cm). All patients had abnormal

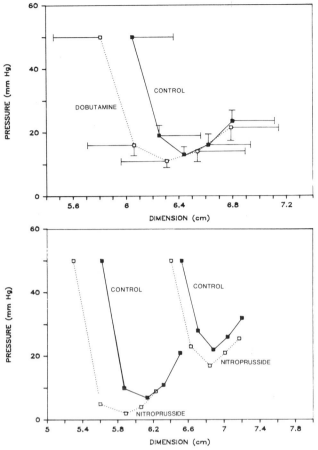

Figure 5.44 *Top*: Diastolic pressure-dimension relations constructed for each patient are shown under control conditions and at maximum dobutamine dose. In early diastole, dobutamine caused a leftward shift due to the reduced end-systolic chamber size and reduced pressures relative to chamber diameter. After the diastolic pressure nadir, the diastolic pressure-dimension relation for dobutamine was superimposable on the control state relation. Dobutamine also increased peak filling rate from 6.4 ± 3.2 to 9.4 ± 2.6 cm/s (p < 0.01). *Bottom*: The average diastolic pressure-dimension relations are shown before and after nitroprusside for two groups of patients separated by right atrial pressure values. Those on the left had normal right atrial pressures and responded to nitroprusside with a reduction in pressure and chamber size. Those on the right had elevated right atrial pressures and responded to nitroprusside with a reduction in intracavitary pressure out of proportion to any change in chamber size, suggesting that pericardial restraint and/or ventricular interaction was operative. (Reproduced by permission of the American Heart Association, Inc. from Carroll JD, Lang R, Neumann A, et al. Differential effects of positive inotropic and vasodilator therapy on diastolic properties in dilated cardiomyopathy. Circulation 1985;72:III–368.)

LV pressure decay with a prolonged time constant (67 ± 20 ms) and reduced peak filling rates (6.4 ± 3.2 cm/s). Dopamine and dobutamine decreased the time constant of relaxation and increased the peak filling rate. Dobutamine also reduced the minimum diastolic

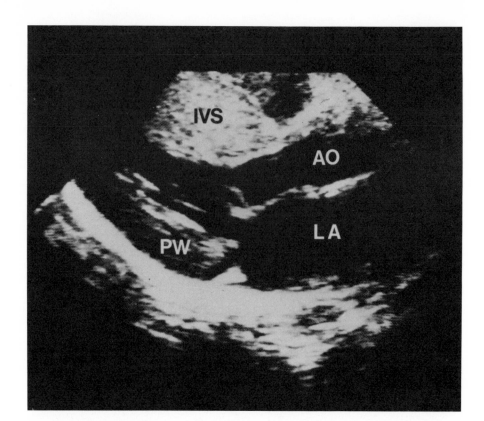

Figure 5.45 Two-dimensional echocardiographic image recorded from a long axis parasternal transducer position in a 22-year-old patient with hypertrophic cardiomyopathy. The septum is disproportionately thickened. There is also hypertrophy of the LV posterior wall, as well as left atrial enlargement.

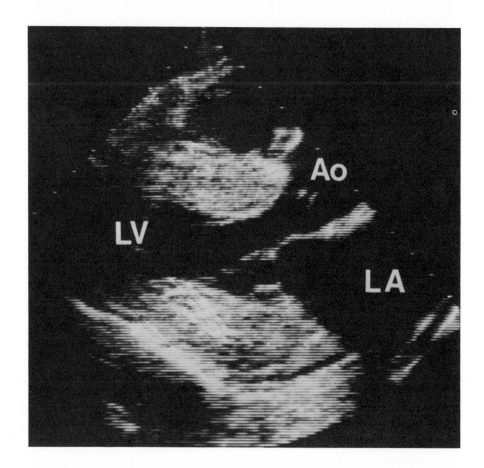

Figure 5.46 Two-dimensional long axis parasternal image from a 47-year-old patient with cardiac amyloidosis. The ventricular walls are thickened and demonstrate a diffuse speckled appearance. This patient's apical four chamber view showed a thickened interatrial septum with decreased left atrial systolic performance.

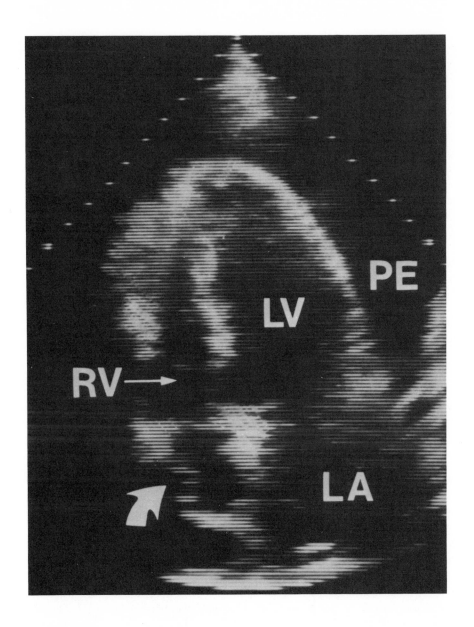

Figure 5.47 Apical four chamber echocardiographic image from a 44-year-old patient with cardiac tamponade. There is a large pericardial effusion (PE), as well as marked right atrial early diastolic collapse (*curved white arrow*).

pressure from 14 ± 7 to 10 ± 9 mm Hg (p < 0.01); neither drug reduced end-diastolic pressure. Diastolic pressure-dimension relations after dopamine and dobutamine showed a leftward shift with a reduced end-systolic chamber size, but otherwise no significant alterations (Fig. 5.44, *top*).

Nitroprusside decreased LV minimum diastolic pressure by 4 mm Hg and end-diastolic pressure by 7 ± 4 mm Hg (p < 0.01). It did not accelerate ventricular pressure decay. The decreased end-diastolic pressure with nitroprusside was due to a reduced end-diastolic dimension in five patients (Fig. 5.44, *bottom left*). In the other patients diastolic pressure-dimension relations showed a parallel downward shift after nitroprusside (Fig. 5.44, *bottom right*). All five of these patients had elevated right atrial pressures. This response is strongly suggestive of relief of pericardial restraining forces as a partial cause for the elevated pressure-dimension curves.

Thus, positive inotropic therapy with β-1 adrenoceptor agonists enhances early diastolic distensibility by accelerating relaxation, augmenting filling, and reducing end-systolic chamber size. Vasodilator therapy is much more effective in lowering diastolic pressures. In some patients this is due to a reduction in extrinsic restraint of the pericardium and/or right ventricular interaction, while in others it simply reflects a decrease in chamber size.

Two-Dimensional Echocardiographic Assessment of LV Diastolic Function

Two-dimensional echocardiography allows excellent spatial orientation in conjunction with high-quality

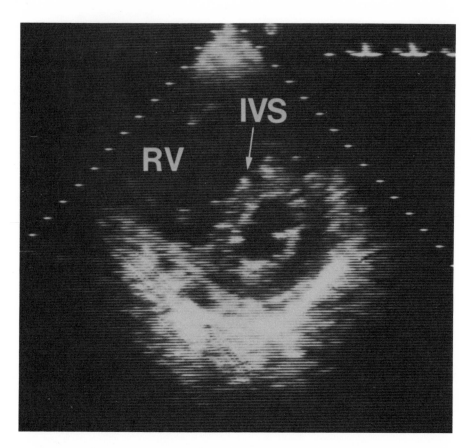

Figure 5.48 Short axis parasternal view demonstrating a grossly enlarged right ventricle (RV) in a 44-year-old patient with severe pulmonary artery hypertension. The interventricular septum (IVS) is flattened, reflecting marked right ventricular diastolic pressure and volume overload. There is extrinsic compression of the LV chamber with elevated LV pressures throughout diastole.

anatomic detail. However, it does not have the temporal resolution of M-mode imaging, Doppler echocardiography, or physiologic pulse recordings. This is due to the relatively slow sampling rate for two-dimensional imaging (i.e., 33 msec/frame), as compared with that of the other imaging techniques (i.e., approximately 1–5 msec). It is therefore not surprising that two-dimensional echo with its video-format images is limited in its ability to assess rapidly occurring, physiologically complex motion patterns during diastole. In some circumstances, however, one can be alerted by two-dimensional images to the probability of existing diastolic abnormalities and proceed to more appropriate quantitate techniques for further assessment. In particular, real-time two-dimensional images are useful in determining whether abnormalities in LV diastolic function are due to factors intrinsic or extrinsic to the left ventricle.

Intrinsic Factors (Diseases of the
Left Ventricular Myocardium)

Ventricular Hypertrophy
Two-dimensional echocardiography is an excellent tool for diagnosing concentric as well as asymmetric types of LV hypertrophy (Fig. 5.45). This is important information in the evaluation of ventricular diastolic

function since LVH is frequently associated with an upward and leftward shift of the ventricular pressure-volume relation. This results in increased operating chamber stiffness (Figs. 5.37 and 5.42). The most common etiologies for LVH (measured as increased wall mass by two-dimensional echocardiographic imaging) include chronic systemic hypertension, idiopathic hypertrophic cardiomyopathy, and valvular aortic stenosis. Ventricular hypertrophy by two-dimensional echo usually is accompanied by LVH on the scalar electrocardiogram.

Infiltrative Disease
These conditions are characterized by markedly increased LV wall thickness, usually without LVH on electrocardiogram. In these patients, the acoustic signature of the myocardium is typically altered to produce a speckled or ground-glass appearance. The classic example of this type of process is cardiac amyloidosis (Fig. 5.46). Infiltration of cardiac valves as well as the interatrial septum (especially in amyloidosis) are common associated abnormalities. Other infiltrative diseases include hemochromatosis, glycogen storage disease, and neoplastic invasion (Chapter 11). Left ventricular distensibility is decreased by all of the infiltrative diseases involving the myocardium. At the present time, attempts at tissue characterization of

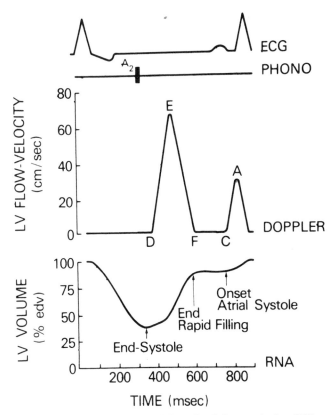

Figure 5.49 Superimposed Doppler left ventricular (LV) diastolic flow velocity waveform (*middle*) and radionuclide angiographic (RNA) time-activity curve (*bottom*) obtained in a normal subject. Cycle length (878 ms) was identical in the two studies. Changes in flow velocity appear to occur at the same time as changes in relative volume. The early diastolic flow velocity peak occurs during the period of left ventricular (LV) rapid filling. At the end of rapid filling, flow velocity begins to decrease and reaches zero baseline at the beginning of diastasis. At the end of diastasis and after atrial systole (A), both flow velocity and filling rate increase again. A_2 = aortic component of the second heart sound in the phonocardiogram (PHONO); ECG = electrocardiogram; edv = end-diastolic volume. (Reproduced with permission from Spirito P, Maron BJ, Bonow RO, et al. Noninvasive assessment of left ventricular diastolic function: Comparative analysis of Doppler echocardiographic and radionuclide angiographic techniques. J Am Coll Cardiol 1986;7:518–526.)

two-dimensional images are progressing slowly due to technical difficulties in data acquisition and analysis.

Dilated Congestive Cardiomyopathy

Since there is an intricate interaction between LV systolic and diastolic performance (e.g., systolic loading conditions, elastic recoil, extent of LV fiber shortening), it is not surprising that left ventricular filling characteristics are abnormal in congestive cardiomyopathy. This is illustrated in Figure 5.42, where it is seen that the LV in idiopathic congestive cardiomyopathy operates on a higher portion of the normal diastolic

pressure-volume curve. This results in elevated LV filling pressures and increased operating chamber stiffness. Two-dimensional imaging is useful for assessing 1) the extent of chamber dilatation and wall thinning, 2) the presence of regional wall motion abnormalities, and 3) the severity of LV systolic dysfunction (Chapter 11).

Ischemic Cardiomyopathy

Real-time imaging allows assessment of left ventricular wall motion, wall thickening and thinning, and overall as well as regional chamber morphology. Both upward and leftward shifts in the position of the LV diastolic pressure-volume relation occur in patients with coronary artery disease and active ischemia. In more chronically ischemic or infarcted myocardium, ventricular walls are often fibrotic, thin, and highly ultrasound reflective (Chapter 10).

Extrinsic Factors

Abnormalities Involving the Pericardium

1. Cardiac tamponade. Cardiac tamponade is characterized by an impairment of ventricular filling secondary to an accumulation of pericardial fluid and subsequent rise in intrapericardial pressure. This results in hemodynamic compromise, systemic and venous vascular congestion, and decreased cardiac output. On two-dimensional echocardiographic imaging, the most specific and sensitive mechanical correlate of cardiac tamponade is the degree and duration of right ventricular and/or right atrial inversion (Fig. 5.47). This marker may not be very reliable, however, in the presence of significant right ventricular hypertrophy.
2. Constrictive pericarditis. There are no specific or objective markers for the diagnosis of constrictive pericarditis using two-dimensional echocardiographic imaging. However, in severe forms it may be possible to appreciate abrupt cessation of early diastolic filling. When this is observed in conjunction with a thickened, adherent, or calcified pericardium, the possibility of constriction should be considered. These features are subjective and require considerable interpretive experience, and they are especially difficult when the rapid heart rate that most often accompanies this disorder is present.

RV-LV Interaction

As discussed in an earlier section of this chapter, clinical situations resulting in significant right ventricular volume or pressure overload may alter left ventricular filling properties secondary to a diastolic shift of the interventricular septum in a right to left

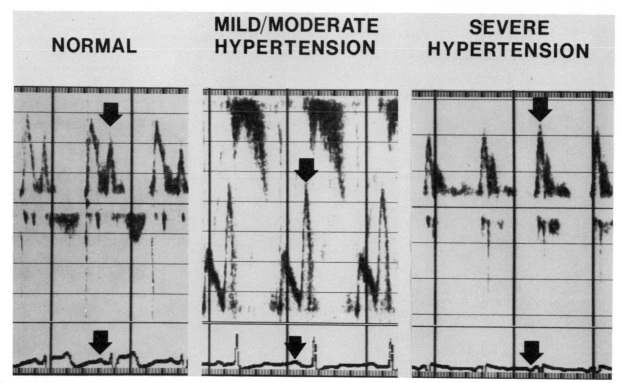

Figure 5.50 Simultaneously recorded pulsed Doppler echocardiogram and surface electrocardiogram (EKG). Doppler data were acquired with the sample site in the LV inflow area. The arrows indicate the A wave on the Doppler tracing and the P wave on the EKG. In the normal subject, peak early diastolic velocity exceeds late diastolic velocity (A/E < 1). In the patient with mild to moderate systemic hypertension, the timing and pattern of predominant transmitral diastolic flow has shifted into late diastole (A/E > 1). In the case of a patient with severe hypertension and marked LVH on EKG, nearly all transmitral flow occurs in late diastole, with negligible left atrial to left ventricular flow during early and mid-diastole.

direction (Fig. 5.48). The two-dimensional morphologic expression of this phenomenon is recognized by a D-shaped (as opposed to the normal circular-shaped) left ventricle on two-dimensional parasternal short axis views. Real-time imaging is also helpful in diagnosing RV infarction as the cause of LV hemodynamic derangements.

Doppler Echocardiographic Indices of Diastolic Function

The commonly used Doppler echocardiographic indices of LV diastolic function are acquired in the pulsed mode with the sample site just distal to the mitral annulus in the LV inflow area. To assess the rate of blood flow (cm³/sec) into the LV during diastole, both the velocity profile across the mitral orifice and the instantaneous mitral valve area need to be considered. In most cases, however, it appears that the transmitral blood flow velocity pattern is similar to the rate of LV volume change during diastole (246, 247). This was recently confirmed in a comparison study of LV filling characteristics performed with pulsed Doppler echo-

cardiography and LV cineangiography (247). Despite this fact, there is a poor correlation between mitral valve diastolic motion by M-mode echocardiography and transmitral valve flow velocity by Doppler (248). All of the Doppler changes noted with ventricular hypertrophy, cardiomyopathy, myocardial ischemia, etc., reflect changes in the physiologic relationship between the LA and LV during rapid filling, conduit, and atrial systolic periods of ventricular filling (Fig. 5.36). As such, the Doppler indices of diastolic function demonstrate the same basic physiologic limitations noted previously for M-mode echocardiography (202, 204). These include dependence on completeness of LV active relaxation, myocardial tissue characteristics, ventricular dimensions, and LV loading conditions (249–251). In addition, age-related differences have been reported in normal subjects for many of these indices (252–254). This raises the issue of whether the patient's age and heart rate need to be eliminated as confounding variables when using Doppler echocardiography to compare diastolic performance in normal and diseased hearts.

Specific Doppler Indices

Early Diastolic Flow (Rapid Filling)

PEAK EARLY DIASTOLIC FLOW VELOCITY. This is measured directly from the Doppler echocardiographic tracing as the peak early diastolic flow velocity during the LV rapid filling period (Fig. 5.49). It has been reported to be reduced in the presence of systemic hypertension, hypertrophic cardiomyopathy, and myocardial ischemia or infarction (246, 255, 256). Other studies have suggested that there is no change from normal for this index in patients with valvular aortic stenosis or congestive cardiomyopathy (257).

INTERVAL FROM AORTIC VALVE CLOSURE TO ONSET OF DIASTOLIC FLOW. This index measures the LV isovolumic relaxation period. It is measured as the time interval from the aortic closing component of the second heart sound by phonocardiogram to onset of the diastolic flow velocity waveform by Doppler (Fig. 5.49) (258). This index has been shown to correlate well with negative $(dp/dt)_{max}$ (259).

DURATION OF EARLY DIASTOLIC FLOW. It is controversial how to best measure this index. In some studies, it is defined as the time interval from the onset of diastolic flow velocity to the time when the waveform returns to baseline (258). Other authors measure it as the width of the rapid inflow wave at the level of one-half of the peak velocity (252).

DECELERATION RATE. This is usually determined as the slope of a straight line drawn between the peak of early diastolic inflow and a point at half peak velocity on the down-side of the velocity envelope (246, 258). It is reduced in patients with systemic hypertension, hypertrophic cardiomyopathy, and old myocardial infarction (246).

Late Diastolic Flow (Atrial Contraction)

PEAK LATE DIASTOLIC FLOW VELOCITY. This is measured as the height of the late diastolic peak of the Doppler waveform (Fig. 5.50). It correlates with transmitral flow associated with atrial systole (260). Increases occur in patients with systemic hypertension, valvular aortic stenosis, and ischemic heart disease (246, 256, 257) but not necessarily with congestive cardiomyopathy (257).

LATE DIASTOLIC FLOW VELOCITY INTEGRAL. The late diastolic flow velocity integral measures the area under the late diastolic flow velocity waveform (256, 261). When multiplied by the mitral valve cross-sectional area during atrial systole, it gives an approximation of transmitral blood flow volume associated with LA contraction.

Ratio of Peak Late Diastolic to Peak Early Diastolic Flow Velocities

This index has been shown to be highly age-dependent in a study of 69 normal subjects aged 21 to 70 years (252). It is increased in systemic hypertension, hypertrophic cardiomyopathy, and myocardial ischemia/infarction (246, 252, 255, 262). In LV infiltrative processes such as cardiac amyloidosis, this ratio may be markedly diminished, despite significantly increased ventricular wall thicknesses. This apparent incongruity probably reflects diminished LA contractile function, thereby rendering this index unhelpful as a measure of LV diastolic filling properties.

Left Atrial Systolic Time Intervals

These measurements are obtained from LV inflow Doppler tracings. In a recent study of 47 patients with systemic hypertension, left atrial systolic time intervals (STIs) correlated well with the presence of a fourth heart sound and with LV wall thickness (263).

Limitations of Doppler Indices of LV Diastolic Function

All of the Doppler echocardiographic indices of LV diastolic performance are highly load- and heart rate–dependent. They reflect physiologic changes in the timing and magnitude of transmitral velocity and flow. However, they also reflect complex interactions between the left atrium and left ventricle, as well as structures extrinsic to the heart itself. As such, they do not assess ventricular operating chamber stiffness since the relationship between LV pressure and volume is not evaluated. In addition, the issue of myocardial stiffness (i.e., properties of the myocardial fibers themselves) is totally ignored. While trends have been described using Doppler diastolic indices, their application for assessing true myocardial diastolic properties is unproven.

REFERENCES

1. Braunwald E, Ross J Jr. Control of cardiac performance. In: Handbook of physiology: The cardiovascular system. Vol. 1. Baltimore: Williams and Wilkins Co, 1979, pp. 533–580.
2. Borow KM. Clinical assessment of contractility in the symmetrically contracting left ventricle. Mod Concepts Cardiovasc Dis, 1988;57:29–34.
3. Marantz PR, Tobin JN, Wassertheil-Smoller S, et al. The relationship between left ventricular systolic function and congestive heart failure diagnosed by clinical criteria. Circulation 1988;77:607–612.
4. Wisenbaugh T. Does normal pump function belie muscle dysfunction in patients with chronic severe mitral regurgitation? Circulation 1988;77:515–525.
5. Carabello BA, Usher BW, Hendrix GH, Assey ME, Crawford FA, Leman RB. Predictors of outcome for aortic valve replacement

in patients with aortic regurgitation and left ventricular dysfunction: A change in the measuring stick. J Am Coll Cardiol 1987;10:991–997.

6. Borow KM. Surgical outcome in chronic aortic regurgitation: A physiologic framework for assessing preoperative predictors. J Am Coll Cardiol 1987;10:1165–1170.

7. Gaasch W, Zile MR. Evaluation of myocardial function in cardiomyopathic states. Prog CV Dis 1984;27:115–132.

8. Ross J Jr. The failing heart and the circulation. Hosp Practice 1983;151–169.

9. Hurst JW. The heart. 5th ed. New York: McGraw-Hill Book Co., 1982.

10. Weber KT, Janicki JS. Afterload and the failing heart. Practical Cardiology 1980;6:35–45.

11. Braunwald E. Determinants and assessment of cardiac function. N Eng J Med 1977;296:86–89.

12. Grossman W, Barry WH. Diastolic pressure-volume relations in the diseased heart. Federation Proc 1980;39:148–155.

13. Tarazi RC, Levy MN. Cardiac responses to increased afterload. Hypertension 1982;4:II8–II11.

14. Quinones MA. Concepts of ventricular contractility in pressure and volume overload. Texas Heart Inst J 1982;9:463–465.

15. Pouleur H, Covell JW, Ross J Jr. Effects of alterations in aortic input impedance on the force-velocity-length relationship in the intact canine heart. Circ Res 1979;45:126–135.

16. Weber KT, Janicki JS, Shroff SG, Laskey W. The mechanics of ventricular function. Hosp Practice 1983;113–125.

17. Weber KT, Janicki JS, Hunter WC, Shroff S, Pearlman ES, Fishman AP. The contractile behavior of the heart and its functional coupling to the circulation. Progr in Cardiovasc Dis 1982;24:375–400.

18. Borow KM, Lang RM, Neumann A, Carroll JD, Rajfer SI. Physiologic mechanisms governing hemodynamic responses to positive inotropic therapy in patients with dilated cardiomyopathy. Circulation 1988;77:625–637.

19. Noma S, Askenase AD, Agarwal JB, Helfant RH. The effect of changes in afterload on systolic bulging. Circulation 1988;77:221–226.

20. Grossman W, Carabello BA, Gunther S, Fifer MA. Ventricular wall stress and the development of cardiac hypertrophy and failure. In: Albert NR, ed. Perspectives in cardiovascular research: Myocardial hypertrophy and failure. Vol. 7. New York: Raven Press, 1983, pp. 1–18.

21. Grossman W, Jones D, McLaurin LP. Wall stress and patterns of hypertrophy in human left ventricle. J Clin Invest 1975;56:56–64.

22. Dodge HT, Stewart DK, Frimer M. Implications of shape, stress, and wall dynamics in clinical heart disease. In: Fishman AP, ed. Heart failure. Washington, DC: Hemisphere Publ Corp, 1978, pp. 43–54.

23. Borow KM, Colan SD, Neumann A. Altered LV mechanics in patients with valvular aortic stenosis and coarctation of the aorta: Effects on systolic performance and late outcome. Circulation 1985;72:515–522.

24. Gould KL, Lipscomb K, Hamilton GW, Kennedy JW. Relation of left ventricular shape, function, and wall stress in man. Am J Cardiol 1974;34:627–634.

25. Weber KT, Janicki JS. Myocardial oxygen consumption—The role of wall force and shortening. Am J Physiol 1977;233:H421.

26. Strauer BE. Myocardial oxygen consumption in chronic heart disease: Role of wall stress, hypertrophy, and coronary reserve. Am J Cardiol 1979;44:730–740.

27. Lang RM, Borow KM, Neumann A, Marcus R, Sareli P. Analysis of the variable effects of positive inotropic therapy on determinants of myocardial oxygen consumption in dilated cardiomyopathy (abstr.). Circulation 1988;in press.

28. Ross J Jr. Applications and limitations of end-systolic measures of ventricular performance. Fed Proc 1984;43:2418–2422.

29. Weber KT, Janicki JS. The dynamics of ventricular contraction: Force, length and shortening. Fed Proc 1980;39:188–195.

30. Borow KM, Green LH, Grossman W, Braunwald E. Left ventricular end-systolic stress-shortening and stress-length relationships in humans: Normal values and sensitivity to inotropic states. Am J Cardiol 1982;50:1301–1308.

31. Colan SD, Borow KM, Neumann A. The left ventricular end-systolic wall stress-velocity of fiber shortening relation: A load independent index of myocardial contractility. J Am Coll Cardiol 1984;4:715–724.

32. Reichek N, Wilson J, St John Sutton M, Plappert TA, Goldberg S, Hirshfeld JW. Noninvasive determination of left ventricular end-systolic stress: Validation of the method and initial application. Circulation 1982;65:99–108.

33. Zile MR, Gaasch WH, Levine HJ. Left ventricular stress-dimension-shortening relations before and after correction of chronic aortic and mitral regurgitation. Am J Cardiol 1985;56:99–105.

34. Carabello BA, Spann JF. The uses and limitations of end-systolic indexes of LV function. Circulation 1984;69:1058–1064.

35. Weber KT, Likoff MJ, Janicki JS, Andrews V. Advances in the evaluation and management of chronic cardiac failure. Chest 1984;85:253–259.

36. Lang RM, Fellner SK, Neumann A, Bushinsky DA, Borow KM. Left ventricular contractility varies directly with blood ionized calcium. Ann Intern Med 1988;108:524–529.

37. Krayenbuehl HP, Hess OM, Turina J. Assessment of left ventricular function. Cardiovasc Med 1978;3:883–908.

38. Grossman W. Evaluation of systolic and diastolic function of the myocardium. In: Grossman W, ed. Cardiac catheterization and angiography. 3rd ed. Philadelphia: Lea and Febiger, 1986, pp. 301–319.

39. Borow KM, Neumann A, Lang RM, Sareli P, Marcus R, Rajfer SI. Assessment of left ventricular contractility in dilated cardiomyopathy: Comparison of non-ejection phase indices (abstr.). J Am Coll Cardiol 1988;11:142A.

40. Little WC. The left ventricular dP/dt$_{max}$-end diastolic volume relation in closed chest dogs. Circ Res 1985;56:808–815.

41. Little WC, Park RC, Freeman GL. Effects of regional ischemia and ventricular pacing on LV dP/dt$_{max}$-end diastolic volume relation. Am J Physiol 1987;252 (Heart Circ Physiol 21):H933–H940.

42. Feigenbaum H. Echocardiography. 3rd ed. Philadelphia: Lea and Febiger, 1981.

43. Parisi A. Echocardiography as an index of cardiac performance. Hosp Practice 1978;101–111.

44. Popp RL. M-mode echocardiographic assessment of LV function. Am J Cardiol 1982;49:1312–1318.

45. Hurst JW. The heart. New York: McGraw-Hill, 1982, pp. 1790–1793.

46. Panidis IP, Ross J, Ren JF, Kotler MN, Mintz GS. Comparison of independent and derived M-mode echocardiographic measurements. Amer J Cardiol 1984;54:694–696.

47. Mason SJ, Fortuin NJ. The use of echocardiography for quantitative evaluation of LV function. Prog CV Dis 1978;21:119–132.

48. Braunwald E, ed. Heart disease: A textbook of cardiovascular medicine. 2nd ed. Philadelphia: Saunders, 1984.

49. Shine KI, Perloff JK, Child JS, Marshall RC, Schelbert H. Noninvasive assessment of myocardial function. Annals Int Med 1980;92:78–90.

50. Nanda NC, Gramiak R. Clinical echocardiography. St. Louis: CV Mosby Co, 1978.

51. Jugdutt MB, Lee SJK, McFarlane D. Noninvasive assessment of left ventricular function from mitral valve echogram: Relation of final anterior mitral leaflet closing velocity to peak dp/dt and aortic velocity. Circulation 1978;58:861–871.

52. Lehman KC, Johnson AD, Goldberger AL. Mitral valve E point–septal separation as an index of LV function with valvular heart disease. Chest 1983;83:102–108.

53. Lew W, Henning H, Schelbert H, Karliner JS. Assessment of mitral valve E point–separation as an index of LV performance in patients with acute and previous myocardial infarction. Am J Cardiol 1978;41:836–845.

54. Ahmadpour H, Shah AA, Allen JW, Edmiston WA, Kim SJ, Haywood LJ. Mitral E point–septal separation: A reliable index of LV performance in coronary artery disease. Am J Heart 1983;106:21–28.

55. Matzer L, Cortada X, Ferrer P, DeArmendi F, Kinney EL. Widened E point–septal separation in a normal pediatric population. Chest 1985;87:73–77.

56. Gardin JM, Tommaso CL, Talano JV. Echographic early systolic partial closure (notching) of the aortic valve in congestive cardiomyopathy. Am Heart J 1984;107:135–142.

57. Ratshin RA, Rackley CE, Russell RO. Determination of left ventricular preload and afterload by quantitative echocardiography in man. Circ Res 1974;34:711–718.

58. Packer M, Meller J, Medina N, Sorlin R, Herman MV. Importance of left ventricular chamber size in determining the response to hydralazine in severe chronic heart failure. N Eng J Med 1980; 303:250–255.

59. Henry WL, Bonow RO, Rosing DR, Epstein SE. Observations on the optimum time for operative intervention for aortic regurgitation: II. Serial echocardiographic evaluation of asymptomatic patients. Circulation 1980;61:484–492.

60. Henry WL, Bonow RO, Borer JS, et al. Observations on the optimum time for operative intervention for aortic regurgitation: I. Evaluation of the results of aortic valve replacement in symptomatic patients. Circulation 1980;61:471–483.

61. Henry WL, Ware J, Gardin JM, Hepner S, McKay J, Weiner M. Echocardiographic measurements in normal subjects: Growth-related changes that occur between infancy and early adulthood. Circulation 1978;57:278–288.

62. Gibson D. Echocardiography and valve replacement. Echocardiography 1984;1:397–402.

63. Parisi AF, Tow DE, eds: Noninvasive approaches to CV diagnosis. New York: Appleton-Century-Crofts, 1979.

64. Reichek N. Echocardiographic assessment of LV structure and function in hypertension. Am J Med 1983;73:19–25.

65. Kronik G, Slany J, Mösslacher H. Comparative value of eight M-mode echocardiographic formulas for determining left ventricular stroke volume: A correlative study with thermodilution and LV single-plane cineangiography. Circulation 1979;60:1308–1316.

66. Panidis IP, Kotler MN, Ren JF, Mintz GS, Ross J, Kalman P. Development and regression of LV hypertrophy. J Am Coll Cardiol 1984;3:1309–1320.

67. Tarazi RC. The progression from hypertrophy to heart failure. Hosp Practice 1983;101–122.

68. Troy BL, Pombo J, Rackley CE. Measurement of LV wall thickness and mass of echocardiography. Circulation 1972;45:602–610.

69. Devereux RB, Reichek N. Echocardiographic determination of LV mass in man: Anatomic validation of the method. Circulation 1977;55:613–618.

70. McFarland TM, Alam M, Goldstein S, Pickard SD, Stein PD. Echocardiographic diagnosis of LV hypertrophy. Circulation 1978;57:1140–1144.

71. Reichek N, Devereux RB. LV hypertrophy: Relationship to anatomic, echocardiographic and electrocardiographic findings. Circulation 1981;63:1391–1398.

72. Abi-Samra F, Fouad FM, Tarazi RC. Determinants of LV hypertrophy and function in hypertensive patients—An echocardiographic study. Am J Med 1983;73:26–33.

73. Dreslinksi GR. Identification of LV hypertrophy: Chest roentgenography, echocardiography, and electrocardiography. Am J Med 1983;73:47–50.

74. Woythaler JN, Singer SL, Kwan OL, et al. Accuracy of echocardiography versus electrocardiography in detecting LV hypertrophy: Comparison with postmortem mass measurements. J Am Coll Cardiol 1983;2:305–311.

75. Devereux RB, Lutas EM, Casale PN, et al. Standardization of M-mode echocardiographic LV anatomic measurements. J Am Coll Cardiol 1984;4:1222–1230.

76. Ditchey RV, Schuler G, Peterson KL. Reliability of echocardiographic and electrocardiographic parameters in assessing serial changes in LV mass. Am J Med 1981;70:1042–1050.

77. Reichek N, Helak J, Plappert T, St John Sutton MS, Weber KT. Anatomic validation of LV mass estimates from clinical two-dimensional echocardiography: Initial results. Circulation 1983; 67:348–352.

78. Bonow RO, Rosing DR, Mason BJ, et al. Reversal of LV dysfunction after aortic valve replacement for chronic aortic regurgitation: Influence of duration of preoperative LV dysfunction. Circulation 1984;70:570–579.

79. Van der Bossche JL, Kramer BL, Massie BM, Morris DL, Karliner JS. Two-dimensional echocardiographic evaluation of the size, function and shape of the left ventricle in chronic aortic regurgitation: Comparison with radionuclide angiography. J Am Coll Cardiol 1984;4:1195–1206.

80. Mahler F, Ross J Jr, O'Rourke RA, Covell JW. Effects of changes in preload, afterload, and inotropic state on ejection and iso-volumic phase measures of contractility in the conscious dog. Am J Cardiol 1975;35:626–634.

81. Nixon JV, Murray RG, Leonard PD, Mitchell JH, Blomquist CG. Effect of large variations in preload on left ventricular performance characteristics in normal subjects. Circulation 1982;65:698–703.

82. Quinones MA. Exercise two-dimensional echocardiography. Echocardiography. 1984;1:151–163.

83. Dancy M, Leech G, Leatham A. Changes in echocardiographic left ventricular minor axis dimensions during exercise in patients with aortic stenosis. Br Heart J 1984;52:446–450.

84. Lowe DK, Rothbaum DA, McHenry PL, Corya BC, Knoebel SB. Myocardial blood flow response to isometric handgrip and treadmill exercise in coronary artery disease. Circulation 1975;51:126–131.

85. Redwood DR, Henry WL, Goldstein S, Smith ER. Design and function of a mechanical assembly for recording echocardiograms during upright exercise. Cardiovasc Res 1975;9:145–149.

86. Mason SJ, Weiss JL, Weisfeldt ML, Garrison JB, Fortiun NJ. Exercise echocardiography: Detection of wall motion abnormalities during ischemia. Circulation 1979;59:50–59.

87. Henry WL. Evaluation of ventricular function using two-dimensional echocardiography. Am J Cardiol 1982;49:1319–1323.

88. McGillem MJ, Mancini GBJ, DeBoe SF, Buda AJ. Modification of the centerline method for assessment of echocardiographic wall thickening and motion: A comparison with areas of risk. J Am Coll Cardiol 1988;11:861–866.

89. Zoghbi WA, Charlat ML, Bolli R, Zhu WX, Hartley CJ, Quinones MA. Quantitative assessment of left ventricular wall motion by two-dimensional echocardiography: Validation during reversible ischemia in the conscious dog. J Am Coll Cardiol 1988;11:851–860.

90. Mehta PM, Alker KJ, Kloner RA. Functional infarct expansion, left ventricular dilation and isovolumic relaxation time after coronary occlusion: A two-dimensional echocardiographic study. J Am Coll Cardiol 1988;11:630–636.

91. Joynt L, Popp RL. The concept of three-dimensional resolution in echocardiographic imaging. Ultrasound in Med and Biol 1982;8:237–247.

92. Miller JL, Nanda NC. Echocardiography in the MI workup. Diagnosis 1984;75–90.

93. Cohn PF, ed: Diagnosis and therapy of CAD. Boston: Little Brown and Co, 1979.

94. Erbel R, Schweizer P, Lambertz H, et al. Echoventriculography—A simultaneous analysis of two-dimensional echocardiography and cineventriculography. Circulation 1983;67:205–215.

95. Kornfeld J. Artful echo learns to quantify. Cardio 1984;22–29.

96. Triulzi MO, Wilkins GT, Gillam LD, Gentile F, Weyman AE. Normal adult cross-sectional echocardiographic values: LV volumes. Echocardiography 1985;2:153–170.

97. Weiss JL, Eaton LW, Kallman CH, Maughan WL. Accuracy of volume determination by two-dimensional echocardiography: Defining requirements under controlled conditions in the ejecting canine left ventricle. Circulation 1983;67:889–895.

98. Nixon JV, Saffer SI, Lipscomb K, Blomqvist CG. Three-dimensional echoventriculography. Am Heart J 1983;435–443.

99. Feigenbaum H. Future applications for the evaluation of ventricular function using echocardiography. Am J Cardiol 1982;49:1330–1336.

100. Feneley MP, Hickie JB. Validity of echocardiographic determination of left ventricular systolic wall thickening. Circulation 1984;70:226–232.

101. Helak JW, Reichek N. Quantitation of human left ventricular

mass and volume by two-dimensional echocardiography: In vitro anatomic validation. Circulation 1981;63:1398–1407.

102. Schiller NB, Skioldebrand CG, Schiller EJ, et al. Canine LV mass estimation by two-dimensional echocardiography. Circulation 1983;68:210–216.

103. Wyatt HL, Heng MK, Meerbaum S. Cross-sectional echocardiography. I. Analysis of mathematic models for quantifying mass of the left ventricle in dogs. Circulation 1979;60:1104–1113.

104. Ghosh A, Nanda NC, Maurer G. Three-dimensional reconstruction of echocardiographic images using the rotation method. Ultrasound in Med and Biol 1982;8:655–661.

105. Sawada H, Fujii J, Kato K, Onoe M, Kuno Y. Three-dimensional reconstruction of the LV from multiple cross-sectional echocardiograms: Value for measuring LV volume. Br Heart J 1983;50: 438–442.

106. Ariet M, Geiser EA, Lupkiewicz SM, Conetta DA, Conti CR. Evaluation of a three-dimensional reconstruction to compute left ventricular volume and mass. Am J Cardiol 1984;54:415–420.

107. Stickels KR, Wann LS. An analysis of three-dimensional reconstructive echocardiography. Ultrasound in Med and Biol 1984; 10:575–580.

108. St John Sutton MG, Pappert TA, Hirshfeld JW, Reichek N. Assessment of left ventricular mechanics in patients with asymptomatic aortic regurgitation: A two-dimensional echocardiographic study. Circulation 1984;69:259–268.

109. Dubroff JM, Clark MB, Wong CYH, Spotnitz AJ, Collins RH, Spotnitz HM. Left ventricular ejection fraction during cardiac surgery: A two-dimensional echocardiographic study. Circulation 1983;68:95–103.

110. Schiller N. A review of the echo literature for 1983. Echocardiography 1985;2:171–190.

111. Jardin F, Gueret P, Prost JF, Farcot JC, Ozier LY, Bowrdarias JP. Two-dimensional echocardiographic assessment of left ventricular function in chronic obstructive pulmonary disease. Am Rev Respir Dis 1984;129:135–142.

112. Lieberman AN, Weiss JL, Jugdutt BI, et al. Two-dimensional echocardiography and infarct size: Relationship of regional wall motion and thickening to the extent of myocardial infarction in the dog. Circulation 1981;63:739–746.

113. Topol EJ, Weiss JL, Guzman PA, et al. Immediate improvement of dysfunctional myocardial segments after coronary revascularization: Detection by intraoperative transesophageal echocardiography. J Am Coll Cardiol 1984;6:1123–1134.

114. Lang RM, Briller R, Neumann A, Borow KM. Assessment of global and regional left ventricular mechanics: Applications to myocardial ischemia. In: Kerber RE, ed. Echocardiography in coronary artery disease. Mt. Kisco, New York: Futura Publishing Co, 1988, pp. 221–257.

115. Borow KM. Clinical assessment of contractility in the ischemic left ventricle. In: Modern concepts in cardiovascular disease (in press).

116. Hisanaga K, Hisanaga A, Nagata K, Ichie Y. Transesophageal cross-sectional echocardiography. Am Heart J 1980;100:605–609.

117. Histand MB, Wells MK, Reeves JT, Sodal IE, Adamson HP, Willson JT. Ultrasonic pulsed Doppler transesophageal measurement of aortic hemodynamics in humans. Ultrasonics 1979;17:215–218.

118. Shively B, Watters T, Benefiel D, Cahalan M, Botvinick EH, Schiller NB. The intraoperative detection of myocardial infarction by transesophageal echocardiography. J Am Coll Cardiol 1986;7:2A.

119. Konstadt S, Thys D, Mindich BP, Kaplan J, Goldman ME. Validation of quantitative intraoperative transesophageal echocardiography. Anesthesiology 1986;65:418–421.

120. Goldman ME, Mindich BP, Nanda NC. Intraoperative echocardiography: Who monitors the flood once the flood gates are opened? J Am Coll Cardiol 1988;6:1362–1364.

121. Smith JS, Calahan MK, Benefiel DJ. Intraoperative detection of myocardial ischemia in high risk patients: Electrocardiography versus two-dimensional transesophageal echocardiography. Circulation 1985;75:1015–1021.

122. Child JS. Stress echocardiography: A technique whose time has come. Echocardiography 1984;1:107–110.

123. Ryan T, Vasey CG, Presti CF, O'Donnell JA, Feigenbaum H, Armstrong WF. Exercise echocardiography: Detection of coronary artery disease in patients with normal left ventricular wall motion at rest. J Am Coll Cardiol 1988;11:993–999.

124. Armstrong WF. Exercise echocardiography: Ready, willing and able. J Am Coll Cardiol 1988;11:1359–1361.

125. Bairey CN, Rozanski A, Berman DS. Exercise echocardiography: Ready or not? J Am Coll Cardiol 1988;11:1355–1358.

126. Kolettis M, Jenkins BS, Webb-Peploe MM. Assessment of left ventricular function by indices derived from aortic flow velocity. Br Heart J 1976;38:18–31.

127. Pearlman AS. Evaluation of ventricular function using Doppler echocardiography. Am J Cardiol 1982;49:1324–1330.

128. Gisvold SE, Brubakk AO. Measurement of instantaneous blood-flow velocity in the human aorta using pulsed Doppler ultrasound. Cardiovasc Res 1982;16:26–33.

129. Gardin JM, Cabestani A, Matin K, Allfie A, Russell D, Henry WL. Reproducibility of Doppler aortic blood flow measurements: Studies on intraobserver, interobserver and day-to-day variability in normal subjects. Am J Cardiol 1984;54:1092–1098.

130. Gardin JM, Burn CS, Childs WJ, Henry WL. Evaluation of blood flow velocity in the ascending aorta and main pulmonary artery of normal subjects by Doppler echocardiography. Am Heart J 1984;107:310–318.

131. Wilson N, Goldberg SJ, Dickinson DF, Scott O. Normal intracardiac and great artery blood velocity measurements by pulsed Doppler echocardiography. Br Heart J 1985;53:451–458.

132. Gardin JM, Iseri LT, Elkayam U, et al. Evaluation of dilated cardiomyopathy by pulsed Doppler echocardiography. Am Heart J 1983;106:1057–1065.

133. Colocousis JS, Huntsman LL, Curreri PW. Estimation of stroke volume changes by ultrasound Doppler. Circulation 1977;56: 914–917.

134. Elkayam U, Gardin JM, Berkey R, Hughes CA, Henry WL. The use of Doppler flow velocity measurement to assess the hemodynamic response to vasodilators in patients with heart failure. Circulation 1983;67:377–383.

135. Light LH. Non-injurious ultrasonic techniques for observing flow in the human aorta. Nature 1969;224:1119–1121.

136. Light LH. Initial evaluation of transcutaneous aortovelography —A new non-invasive technique for hemodynamic measurements in the major thoracic vessels. In: Reneman RS, ed. Cardiovascular applications of ultrasound. New York: Elsevier, 1974, pp. 325–360.

137. Colocousis JS, Huntsman LL, Curreri PW. Estimation of stroke volume changes by ultrasonic Doppler. Circulation 1977;56:914–917.

138. Magnin PA, Stewart JA, Myers S, von Romm O, Kisslo JA. Combined Doppler and phased-array echocardiographic estimation of cardiac output. Circulation 1981;63:388–392.

139. Voyles WF, Miranda IP, Greene ER, Reilly PA, Caprihan A. Observer variability in serial noninvasive measurements of stroke index using pulsed Doppler flowmetry. Biomed Sci Instrumentation 1982;18:67–75.

140. Schuster AH, Nanda NC. Doppler echocardiography—Doppler cardiac output measurements. Echocardiography 1984;1:45–54.

141. Huntsman LL, Stewart DK, Barnes SR, Franklin SB, Colocousis JS, Hessel EA. Noninvasive Doppler determination of cardiac output in man—Clinical validation. Circulation 1983;67:595–602.

142. Fisher DC, Sahn DJ, Friedman MJ, et al. The mitral valve orifice method for noninvasive two-dimensional echo Doppler determinations of cardiac output. Circulation 1983;67:872–877.

143. Rose JS, Nanna M, Rahimtoola SH, Elkayam U, McKay C, Chandraratna PAN. Accuracy of determination of cardiac output by transcutaneous continuous-wave Doppler computer. Am J Cardiol 1984;54:1099–1101.

144. Loeppky JA, Hockenga DE, Greene ER, Luft UC. Comparison of noninvasive pulsed Doppler and Fick measurements of stroke volume in cardiac patients. Am Heart J 1984;107:339–346.

145. Ihlen H, Amlie JP, Dale J, et al. Determination of cardiac output by Doppler echocardiography. Br Heart J 1984;51:54–60.

146. Nusgunyra RA, Callahan MJ, Schaff HV, Ilstrup DM, Miller FA, Tajik AJ. Noninvasive measurement of cardiac output by continuous-wave Doppler echocardiography—Initial experience and review of the literature. Mayo Clin Proc 1984;59:484–489.

147. Chandraratna PA, Nanna M, McKay C, et al. Determination of cardiac output by transcutaneous continuous-wave ultrasonic Doppler computer. Am J Cardiol 1984;53:234–237.

148. Loeber CP, Goldberg SJ, Allen HD. Doppler echocardiographic comparison of flows distal to the four cardiac valves. J Am Coll Cardiol 1984;4:268–272.

149. Neumann A, Spencer KT, Lang RM, et al. Is it possible to obtain an accurate Doppler estimate of stroke volume in patients with decreased forward flow? (abstr.). J Am Coll Cardiol 1988;11: 121A.

150. deZuttere D, Touche T, Saumon G, Nitenberg A, Prasquier R. Doppler echocardiographic measurement of mitral flow volume: Validation of a new method in adult patients. J Am Coil Cardiol 1988;11:343–350.

151. Schuster AH, Nanda NC. Doppler echocardiography and cardiac pacing. Pace 1982;5:607–612.

152. Labovitz AJ, Williams GA, Redd RM, Kennedy HL. Noninvasive assessment of pacemaker hemodynamics by Doppler echocardiography—Importance of left atrial size. J Am Coll Cardiol 1985;6:196–200.

153. Iliceto S, Amico A, Marangelli V, D'Ambrosio G, Rizzon P. Doppler echocardiographic evaluation of the effect of atrial pacing-induced ischemia on left ventricular filling in patients with coronary artery disease. J Am Coll Cardiol 1988;11:953–961.

154. Buckingham TA, Woodruff RC, Pennington DG, et al. Effect of ventricular function on the exercise hemodynamics of variable rate pacing. J Am Coll Cardiol 1988;11:1269–1277.

155. Loeppky JA, Greene ER, Hoekenga DE, Caprihan A, Luft UC. Beat-by-beat stroke volume assessment by pulsed Doppler in upright and supine exercise. J Appl Physiol 1981;50:1173–1182.

156. Harrison MR, Smith MD, Nissen SE, Grayburn PA, DeMaria AN. Use of exercise Doppler echocardiography to evaluate cardiac drugs: Effects of propranolol and verapamil on aortic blood flow velocity and acceleration. J Am Coll Cardiol 1988;11:1002–1009.

157. Kitabatake A, Ito H, Inoue M, et al. A new approach to noninvasive evaluation of aortic regurgitant fraction by two-dimensional Doppler echocardiography. Circulation 1985;72: 523–529.

158. Sanders SP, Yeager S, Williams RG. Measurement of systemic and pulmonary blood flow and Qp/Qs using Doppler and two-dimensional echocardiography. Am J Cardiol 1983;51:952–956.

159. Vargas Barron J, Sahn DJ, Valdes-Cruz LM, Lima CO, Goldberg SJ, Grenadier E. Clinical utility of two-dimensional Doppler echocardiographic techniques for estimating pulmonary to systemic blood flow ratios in children with left-to-right shunting atrial septal defect, ventricular septal defect or patent ductus arteriosus. J Am Coll Cardiol 1984;3:169–178.

160. Valdes-Cruz LM, Horowitz S, Mesel E, Sahn DJ, Fisher DC, Larson D. A pulsed Doppler echocardiographic method for calculating pulmonary and systemic blood flow in atrial level shunts: Validation in animals and initial human experience. Circulation 1984;69:80–86.

161. Kitabatake A, Inouie M, Asao M, et al. Noninvasive evaluation of the ratio of pulmonary to systemic flow in atrial septal defect by duplex Doppler echocardiography. Circulation 1984;69:73–79.

162. Dittmann H, Jacksch R, Voelker W, Karsch KR, Seipel L. Accuracy of Doppler echocardiography in quantification of left to right shunts in adult patients with atrial septal defect. J Am Coll Cardiol 1988;11:338–342.

163. Schuster AH, Nanda NC. Doppler echocardiographic measurement of cardiac output: Comparison with a non-golden standard. Am J Cardiol 1984;53:257–259.

164. Borow KM, Newburger JW. Noninvasive estimation of central aortic pressure using the oscillometric method for analyzing systemic artery pulsatile blood flow: Comparative study of indirect systolic, diastolic, and mean brachial artery pressure with simultaneous direct ascending aortic pressure measurements. Am Heart J 1982;103:879–886.

165. Colan SD, Borow KM, Neumann A. Use of the calibrated carotid pulse tracing for calculation of left ventricular pressure and wall stress throughout ejection. Am Heart J 1985;109:1306–1310.

166. Mirsky I. Review of various theories for evaluation of left ventricular wall stresses. In: Mirsky I, Chiston DN, Sandler H, eds. Cardiac mechanics: Physiological, chemical, and mathematical considerations. New York: John Wiley and Sons, Inc, 1974.

167. Yin FCP. Ventricular wall stress. Circ Res 1981;49:829–842.

168. Borow KM, Neumann A, Lang R. Milrinone versus dobutamine: Contribution of altered myocardial mechanics and augmented inotropic state to improved left ventricular performance. Circulation 1986;73:III153–III161.

169. Feldman T, Borow KM, Sarne DH, Neumann A, Lang RM. Myocardial mechanics in hyperthyroidism: Importance of left ventricular loading conditions, heart rate, and contractile state. J Am Coll Cardiol (in press).

170. Grossman W, Braunwald E, Mann T, et al. Contractile state of the left ventricle in man as evaluated from end-systolic pressure-volume relations. Circulation 1977;56:845–852.

171. Borow KM, Neumann A, Wynne J. Sensitivity of end-systolic pressure-dimension and pressure-volume relations to inotropic state in humans. Circulation 1982;65:988–997.

172. Kass DA, Maughan WL. From "E_{max}" to pressure-volume relations: A broader view. Circulation 1988;77:1203–1212.

173. Borow KM, Propper R, Bierman FZ, Grady S, Inati A. The left ventricular end-systolic pressure-dimension relation in patients with thalassemia major: A new noninvasive method for assessing contractile state. Circulation 1982;66:980–985.

174. Borow KM, Neumann A, Lang RM. The end-systolic pressure-dimension relation: A reliable measure of left ventricular contractility in myopathic ventricles? (abstr.). J Am Coll Cardiol 1988;11:244A.

175. Maughan WL, Sunagawa K. Factors affecting the end-systolic pressure-volume relationship. Fed Proc 1984;43:2408–2410.

176. Kono A, Maugham WL, Sunagawa K, Hamilton K, Sagawa K, Weisfeldt ML. The use of LV end-ejection pressure and peak pressure in the estimation of the end-systolic pressure-volume relationship. Circulation 1984;70:1057–1065.

177. Borow KM, Come PC, Neumann A, Baim DS, Braunwald E, Grossman W. Physiologic assessment of the inotropic, vasodilator and afterload reducing effects of milrinone in subjects without cardiac disease. Am J Cardiol 1985;55:1204–1209.

178. Takahashi M, Sasayama S, Kawai C, Kotoura H. Contractile performance of the hypertrophied ventricle in patients with systemic hypertension. Circulation 1980;62:116–126.

179. Smucker ML, Sanford CF, Lipscomb KM. Effects of hydralazine on pressure-volume and stress-volume relations in congestive heart failure secondary to idiopathic dilated cardiomyopathy. Am J Cardiol 1985;56:690–695.

180. Colan SD, Borow KM, Gamble WJ, Sanders SP. Effects of enhanced afterload (methoxamine) and contractile state (dobutamine) on the LV late systolic wall stress-dimension relation. Am J Cardiol 1985;52:1304–1309.

181. Borow KM, Neumann A, Arensman FW, Yacoub MH. LV contractility and contractile reserve in humans after cardiac transplantation. Circulation 1985;71:866–872.

182. Borow KM, Henderson IC, Neumann A, et al. Assessment of left ventricular contractility in patients receiving doxorubicin. Ann Int Med 1983;99:750–756.

183. Lang RM, Borow KM, Neumann A, Feldman T. Adverse cardiac effects of acute alcohol ingestion in young adults. Ann Int Med 1985;102:742–747.

184. O'Rourke ME. Steady and pulsatile energy losses in the systemic circulation under normal conditions and in simulated arterial disease. Cardiovasc Res 1967;1:313–326.

185. O'Rourke, MF. The arterial pulse in health and disease. Am Heart J 1971;82:687–702.

186. McDonald DA. Blood flow in arteries. 2nd ed. Baltimore: The Williams and Wilkins Co, 1974.

187. Milnor WR. Arterial impedance as ventricular afterload. Circ Res 1975;36:565–570.
188. Nichols WW, Conti CR, Walker WE, Milnor WR. Input impedance of the systemic circulation in man. Circ Res 1977;40:451–458.
189. O'Rourke MF. Vascular impedance in studies of arterial and cardiac function. Physiological Reviews 1982;62:570–623.
190. Nichols WW, Pepine CJ. Left ventricular afterload and aortic input impedance: Implications of pulsatile blood flow. Progr Cardiovasc Dis 1982;24:293–306.
191. O'Rourke M, Yaginuma T. Wave reflections and the arterial pulse. Arch Intern Med 1984;144:366–371.
192. Laskey WK, Kussmaul WG, Martin JL, Kleaveland JP, Hirshfeld JW, Shroff S. Characteristics of vascular hydraulic load in patients with heart failure. Circulation 1985;72:61–71.
193. O'Rourke M. Arterial hemodynamics in hypertension. Circ Res 1970;16/17:II123–II133.
194. Pepine CJ, Nichols WW, Conti CR. Aortic input impedance in heart failure. Circulation 1978;58:460–465.
195. Pepine CJ, Nichols WW, Curry RC, Conti CR. Aortic input impedance during nitroprusside infusion. J Clin Invest 1979;64:643–654.
196. Rajfer SI, Borow KM, Lang RM, Neumann A, Carroll JD. Effects of dopamine on left ventricular afterload and contractile state: Relationship to the activation of beta$_1$-adrenoceptors and dopamine receptors. J Am Coll Cardiol 1988;12:498–506.
197. Lang RM, Borow KM, Neumann A, et al. Role of the beta-2 adrenoceptors in mediating positive inotropic activity in the failing heart and its relationship to the hemodynamic actions of dopexamine. Am J Cardiol 1988;62:46c–52c.
198. Borow KM, Neumann A, Arensman F, Yacoub M. Clinical evidence for differential sensitivity of alpha and beta adrenergic receptors after cardiac transplantation. Circulation 1985;72:III-29.
199. Yin CPF. Aging and vascular impedance. In: Yin CPF, ed. Ventricular/vascular coupling. Springer-Verlag, 1987, pp. 115–139.
200. Bonow RO, Rosing DR, Bacharach SL, et al. Effects of verapamil on left ventricular systolic function and diastolic filling in patients with hypertrophic cardiomyopathy. Circulation 1981;64:787–796.
201. Fouad FM, Slominski JM, Tarazi RC. Left ventricular diastolic function in hypertension: Relation to LV mass and systolic function. J Am Coll Cardiol 1984;3:1500–1506.
202. Topol EJ, Traill TA, Fortuin NJ. Hypertensive hypertrophic cardiomyopathy of the elderly. N Engl J Med 1985;312:277–283.
203. Maron BJ, Spirito P, Green KJ, Wesley YE, Bonow RO, Arce J. Noninvasive assessment of left ventricular diastolic function by pulsed Doppler echocardiography in patients with hypertrophic cardiomyopathy. J Am Coll Cardiol 1987;10:733–742.
204. Spirito P, Maron BJ. Doppler echocardiography for assessing left ventricular diastolic function. Ann Int Med 1988;109:122–126.
205. Janicki JS, Weber KT. Factors influencing the diastolic pressure-volume relation of the cardiac ventricles. Federation Proc 1980;39:133–140.
206. Grossman W, McLaurin LP, Stefadouros MA. Left ventricular stiffness associated with chronic pressure and volume overloads in man. Circ Res 1974;35:793–800.
207. Rankin JS, Arentzen CE, Ring WS, Edwards CH, McHale PA, Anderson RW. The diastolic mechanical properties of the intact left ventricle. Federation Proc 1980;39:141–147.
208. Yoshii K, Iwao H, Fukuda S, Mizoguchi LY, Sunagawa H, Honda S. Left ventricular diastolic pressure-volume and stress-strain relationship in children. Japanese Circulation Journal 1985;49:385–394.
209. Yang SS, Bentivoglio LG, Maranhao V, Goldberg H. From cardiac catheterization data to hemodynamic parameters. 2nd ed. Philadelphia: FA Davis Co, 1978, pp. 327–335.
210. Peterson KL, Tsuji J, Johnson A, DiDonna J, LeWinter M. Diastolic left ventricular pressure-volume and stress-strain relations in patients with valvular aortic stenosis and LV hypertrophy. Circulation 1978;58:77–89.
211. Shimizu G, Zile MR, Blaustein AS, Gaasch WH. Left ventricular chamber filling and midwall fiber lengthening in patients with LV hypertrophy: Overestimation of fiber velocities by conventional midwall measurements. Circulation 1985;71:266–272.
212. Colan SD, Sanders SP, MacPherson D, Borow KM. Left ventricular diastolic function in elite athletes with physiologic hypertrophy. J Am Coll Cardiol 1985;6:545–549.
213. Brutsaert DL, Rademakers FE, Sys SU, Gillebert TC, Housmans PR. Analysis of relaxation in the evaluation of ventricular function of the heart. Prog CV Dis 1985;28:143–163.
214. Borow KM, Grossman W. Clinical use of pressure-dimension and stress-shortening relations in systole and diastole. Fed Proc 1984;43:2414–2417.
215. Sabbah HN, Stein PD. Pressure-diameter relations during early diastole in dogs. Incompatibility with the concept of passive left ventricular filling. Circ Res 1981;45:357–365.
216. Caillet D, Crozatier B. Role of myocardial restoring forces in the determination of early diastolic peak velocity of fiber lengthening in the conscious dog. Cardiovasc Res 1982;16:107–112.
217. Colan SD, Borow KM, Neumann A. Effects of loading conditions and contractile state (methoxamine and dobutamine) on LV early diastolic function in normal subjects. Am J Cardiol 1985;55:790–796.
218. Shirato K, Shabetai R, Bargava V. Alterations of left ventricular diastolic pressure-segment length relation produced by the pericardium: Effects of cardiac distension and afterload reduction in conscious dogs. Circulation 1978;57:1191–1198.
219. Ross J Jr. Acute displacement of the diastolic pressure-volume curve of the left ventricle: Role of the pericardium and right ventricle. Circulation 1979;59:32–37.
220. Janicki JS, Weber KT. The pericardium and ventricular interaction, distensibility and function. Am J Physiol 1980;238:H494–H503.
221. Shabetai R. Pericardial and cardiac pressure. Circulation 1988;77:1–5.
222. Carroll JD, Lang R, Neumann A, Borow KM, Rajfer S. Differential effects of positive inotropic and vasodilator therapy on diastolic properties in dilated cardiomyopathy. Circulation 1985;72:III368.
223. Carroll JD, Hess OM, Hirzel HO, Krayenbuehl HP. Exercise-induced ischemia: The influence of altered relaxation on early diastolic pressures. Circulation 1983;67:521–528.
224. Carroll JD, Hess OM, Hirzel HO, Krayenbuehl HP. Dynamics of left ventricular filling at rest and during exercise. Circulation 1983;68:59–67.
225. Quinones MA, Gaasch WH, Waisser E, Alexander JK. Reduction in the rate of diastolic descent of the mitral valve echogram in patients with altered LV diastolic pressure-volume relations. Circulation 1974;49:246–254.
226. Rubenstein JJ, Pohost GM, Dinsmore RE, Harthorne JW. The echocardiographic determination of mitral valve opening and closure: Correlation with hemodynamic studies in man. Circulation 1975;51:98–104.
227. Lancado S, Yellin E, Kother M, Levy L, Stadler J, Terdiman R. A study of the dynamic relations between the mitral valve echogram and phasic mitral flow. Circulation 1975;51:104–110.
228. Koecke LL, Feigenbaum H, Chang S, Corya BC, Fischer JC. Abnormal mitral valve motion in patients with elevated left ventricular diastolic pressures. Circulation 1973;47:989–994.
229. Ambrose JA, Teichholz LE, Meller J, Weintraub W, Pichard AD. The influence of left ventricular late diastolic filling on the A wave of the left ventricular pressure tracing. Circulation 1979;60:510–515.
230. Dreslinski GR, Frohlich ED, Dunn FG, Messerli FH, Suarez DH, Rersin E. Echocardiographic diastolic ventricular abnormality in hypertensive heart disease: Atrial emptying index. Am J Cardiol 1981;47:1087–1090.
231. Bahler RC, Vrobel TR, Martin P. The relation of heart rate and shortening fraction to echocardiographic indexes of left ventricular relaxation in normal subjects. J Am Coll Cardiol 1983;2:926–933.
232. Gibson DG, Brown D. Measurement of instantaneous left ven-

tricular dimension and filling rate in man using echocardiography. Br Heart J 1973;35:1141–1149.

233. St John Sutton MS, Reichek N, Kastor JA, Giuliani ER. Computerized M-mode echocardiographic analysis of LV dysfunction in cardiac amyloid. Circulation 1982;66:790–799.

234. DeCoodt P, Mathey D, Swan HJC. Assessment of left ventricular filling by echocardiography in normal subjects and in subjects with coronary artery disease and with asymmetric septal hypertrophy. Acta Cardiologica 1979;34:11–33.

235. Fifer MA, Borow KM, Colan SD, Lorell BH. Early diastolic left ventricular function in children and adults with aortic stenosis. J Am Coll Cardiol 1985;5:1147–1154.

236. Sanderson JE, Traill TA, St John Sutton MS, Brown DJ, Gibson DG, Goodwin JF. LV relaxation and filling in cardiomyopathy — An echocardiographic study. Br Heart J 1978;40:595–601.

237. Suwa M, Hirota Y, Kawamura K. Improvement in LV diastolic function during intravenous and oral diltiazem therapy in patients with hypertrophic cardiomyopathy: An echocardiographic study. Am J Cardiol 1984;54:1047–1053.

238. Hanrath P, Mathey DG, Siegert R, Bleifeld W. Left ventricular relaxation and filling pattern in different forms of left ventricular hypertrophy: An echocardiographic study. Am J Cardiol 1980;45:15–23.

239. Gamble WH, Shaver JA, Alvares RF, Salerni R, Reddy PS. A critical appraisal of diastolic time intervals as a measure of relaxation in left ventricular hypertrophy. Circulation 1983;68: 76–87.

240. Lorell BH, Paulus WJ, Grossman W, Wynne J, Cohn PF. Modification of abnormal left ventricular diastolic properties by nifedipine in patients with hypertrophic cardiomyopathy. Circulation 1982;65:499–507.

241. Paulus WJ, Lorell BH, Craig WE, Wynne J, Murgo JP, Grossman W. Comparison of the effects of nitroprusside and nifedipine on diastolic properties in patients with hypertrophic cardiomyopathy: Altered left ventricular loading or improved muscle inactivation? J Am Coll Cardiol 1983;2:879–886.

242. Hanrath P, Mathey DG, Kremer P, Sonntag F, Bleifeld W. Effects of verapamil on left ventricular isovolumic relaxation time and regional left ventricular filling in hypertrophic cardiomyopathy. Am J Cardiol 1980;45:1258–1264.

243. Inouye I, Massie B, Loge D. Abnormal left ventricular filling: An early finding in mild to moderate systemic hypertension. Am J Cardiol 1984;53:120–126.

244. Grossman W, McLaurin LP, Moos SP, Stefadouros M, Young DT. Wall thickness and diastolic properties of the left ventricle. Circulation 1974;49:129–135.

245. Lorell BH, Paulus WJ, Grossman W, Wynne J, Cohn PF, Braunwald E. Improved diastolic function and systolic performance in hypertrophic cardiomyopathy after nifedipine. N Engl J Med 1980;303:801–803.

246. Kitabatake A, Inoue M, Asao M, et al. Transmitral blood flow reflecting diastolic behavior of the left ventricle in health and disease—A study by pulsed Doppler technique. Jap Circulation J 1982;46:92–102.

247. Rokey R, Kuo LC, Zoghbi WA, Limacher MC, Quinones MA. Determination of parameters of left ventricular diastolic filling with pulsed Doppler echocardiography: Comparison with cineangiography. Circulation 1985;71:543–550.

248. Douglas PS, Berko BA, Ioli A, Reichek N. Variable relationships of mitral valve motion and flow. J Am Coll Cardiol 1986;7:244A.

249. Choong CY, Herrmann HC, Weyman AE, Fifer MA. Preload dependence of Doppler-derived indexes of left ventricular diastolic function in humans. J Am Coll Cardiol 1987;10:800–808.

250. David D, Lang RM, Neumann A, et al. Reliability of Doppler derived indices of left ventricular diastolic function in patients with dilated cardiomyopathy: Comparison with simultaneously obtained left atrial and ventricular micromanometer pressures. (abstr.). J Am Coll Cardiol 1988;11:119A.

251. Leeman DE, Levine MJ, Come PC. Doppler echocardiography in cardiac tamponade: Exaggerated respiratory variation in transvalvular blood flow velocity integrals. J Am Coll Cardiol 1988;11: 572–578.

252. Miyatake K, Okamoto M, Kinoshita N, et al. Augmentation of atrial contribution of left ventricular flow with aging as assessed by intracardiac Doppler flowmetry. Am J Cardiol 1984;53:586–589.

253. Kuo LC, Quinones MA, Rokey R, Sartori M, Abinader EG, Zoghbi WA. Quantification of atrial contribution to left ventricular filling by pulsed Doppler echocardiography and the effect of age in normal and diseased hearts. Am J Cardiol 1987;59:1174–1178.

254. Sartori MP, Quinones MA, Kuo LC. Relation of Doppler-derived left ventricular filling parameters to age and radius/thickness ratio in normal and pathologic states. Am J Cardiol 1987;59: 1179–1182.

255. Rosoff M, Funai J, Wang SS, Pandian N. Left ventricular diastolic filling dynamics in acute myocardial infarction: Immediate effects of ischemia, time course in first 6 hours and relation to infarct size. J Am Coll Cardiol 1986;7:227A.

256. Wind BE, Dilworth LR, Buda AJ, Snider AR. Doppler evaluation of left ventricular diastolic filling in ischemic heart disease. Circulation 1985;72:III-59.

257. St John Sutton MS, Plappert T. Relation between instantaneous Doppler velocity across the mitral valve and changes in left ventricular volume in normal, dilated and hypertrophied hearts. J Am Coll Cardiol 1986;7:227A.

258. Spirito P, Maron BJ, Bonow RO. Noninvasive assessment of left ventricular diastolic function: Comparative analysis of Doppler echocardiographic and radionuclide angiographic techniques. J Am Coll Cardiol 1986;7:518–526.

259. Drinkovic N, Wisenbaugh T, Kwan OL, Elion J, Smith M, DeMaria AN. Assessment of diastolic left ventricular function by Doppler: Comparison with catheterization measurements. J Am Coll Cardiol 1986;7:227A.

260. Ryan T, Armstrong WF, Feigenbaum H. Doppler assessment of left ventricular filling during experimental myocardial ischemia. Circulation 1985;72:III-59.

261. Freidman B, Drinkovic N, Miles H, Stipp V, Mazzoleni A. DeMaria AN. Assessment of left ventricular diastolic function: Comparison of Doppler and blood pool scintigraphy. Circulation 1985;72:III-429.

262. Visser CA, de Koning H, Delmarre B, Koolen JJ, Dunning AJ. Pulsed Doppler-derived mitral inflow velocity in acute myocardial infarction: An early prognostic indicator. J Am Coll Cardiol 1986;7:136A.

263. Abe H, Yokouchi M, Deguchi F, et al. Measurement of left atrial systolic time intervals in hypertensive patients using Doppler echocardiography: Relation to fourth heart sound and left ventricular wall thickness. J Am Coll Cardiol 1988;11:800–805.

6
Assessment of Right Ventricular Function

Gary Mintz
Ioannis Panidis

To understand the echocardiographic approach to the analysis of right ventricular function, it is first necessary to review those factors that affect right ventricular function during normal and pathophysiologic states.

VENTRICULAR INDEPENDENCE AND INTERDEPENDENCE

The right and left ventricles are not independent in function. The preload and afterload of one chamber affects the other; this interdependence is mediated via the septum and pericardium (1).

Preload

Enlargement of either ventricle alters the geometry and compliance of the opposite ventricle (2–8). As right ventricular volume increases, the left ventricular pressure-volume curve shifts to the left and becomes steeper. As the right ventricle gets larger, changes in right ventricular volume have greater effects than usual on left ventricular geometry and compliance. Furthermore, the secondary effects on the left ventricle are approximately proportional to the primary changes in the right ventricle (4, 7). In a similar manner, changes in left ventricular preload affect right ventricular geometry and compliance (9). The mechanism for this interaction appears to be a diastolic alteration in ventricular configuration caused by contralateral ventricular volume changes mediated by the interventricular septum. Increasing right ventricular volume shifts the septum toward the left ventricle during diastole, causing a decrease in septal to posterior (or lateral)

wall dimension. These changes occur in the presence or absence of the pericardium (5–7). Thus, right ventricular volume overload from an atrial septal defect or tricuspid or pulmonic insufficiency causes increased right ventricular end-systolic and end-diastolic volumes while maintaining a normal right ventricular ejection fraction (10, 11). Because of the diastolic shifts of the septum into the left ventricle, left ventricular geometry is altered and left ventricular preload is reduced. During systole, the left ventricle resumes a normal or nearly normal shape. The decreased left ventricular end-diastolic volume, the limit to which left ventricular end-systolic volume can be decreased to match the decreased end-diastolic volume, and the necessary resumption of normal shape to maximize ejection efficiency, probably account for the reduced left ventricular ejection fraction commonly observed in right ventricular volume overload states (12, 13), even though left ventricular muscle function is normal (9, 14). The systolic shift of the septum into the right ventricle may account for normal right ventricular ejection fraction even though right ventricular muscle function may be abnormal.

Normal right ventricular function is associated with inspiratory augmentation in venous return and an inspiratory augmentation in right ventricular preload with a concomitant decrease in left ventricular preload. This can be observed by viewing the inferior vena cava. The venae cavae are the reservoir vessels from which this increased return comes. This respiratory variation is blunted or absent in hemodynamically significant pericardial disease or severe right ventricular dysfunction in which there is a shift in the compliance or pressure–volume curve (15). The right ventricle is more compliant than the left ventricle; thus, it is better able to handle a volume load than a pressure load. Unless pulmonary hypertension occurs to superimpose a pressure load on the volume load, a pure volume-loaded right ventricle has moderately increased contractile function, develops only mild to moderate hypertrophy, and is subject to a slow rate of wear; there is a long period of time before functional reserves are exhausted.

Afterload

In a similar manner, right ventricular pressure overload distorts left ventricular end-diastolic volume and geometry. However, in a pure pressure-overloaded state, the left ventricle does not return to its normal geometry during systole (16, 17). The right ventricle is more compliant and is better able to handle a volume load than a pressure load. In contrast, the left ventricle is more able to handle a pressure load than a volume load. Small acute increases in pulmonary artery pressure cause sharp decreases in right ventricular stroke volume. In response to chronic pressure loads, significant changes develop in the geometric configuration, mass, and functional characteristics of the right ventricle, although the rate at which these changes occur is unknown. However, in contrast to volume loading, pressure loading results in marked right ventricular hypertrophy and a relatively fast rate of wear. Initially, mass increases to normalize wall stress. When the increased muscle mass is no longer an adequate compensatory mechanism, right ventricular muscle function deteriorates and an increase in right ventricular preload (volume) comes into play as a secondary compensatory mechanism.

Contraction

When the right ventricle is severely damaged, particularly if damage is limited to the free wall, right ventricular systolic function may be maintained by left ventricular assistance (1, 18, 19). Again, the septum mediates ventricular interdependence (20). However, if the right ventricle is adequately stressed by a concomitant pressure or volume overload and the interventricular septum is damaged, or if there is concomitant left ventricular dysfunction, then left ventricular assistance may be either inadequate or absent and right ventricular dysfunction will be manifested (9, 19).

The Pericardium

Although diastolic interdependence between the two ventricles can be shown with the pericardium removed, it is considerably stronger with the pericardium intact. Because altered diastolic properties influence systolic function of each ventricle, the intact pericardium (and pericardial diseases) can affect right and left ventricular contraction and their interdependence. However, the effects on systolic function are considerably less than the effects on diastolic function (21).

RIGHT VENTRICULAR PATHOPHYSIOLOGY

Most causes of right ventricular dysfunction do not cause primary right ventricular contraction abnormalities but alter right or left ventricular preload and afterload and secondarily affect right ventricular contraction. Long-standing alterations in right or left ventricular preload and afterload may lead to permanent changes in right ventricular systolic function.

Chronic Obstructive Pulmonary Disease

Right ventricular ejection fraction is depressed in most patients with decompensated cor pulmonale and in approximately 15 percent of patients without cor pulmonale (22–24). More severe compromise of pulmonary function is associated with a greater depression of right ventricular function. Even in patients with normal resting right ventricular function, stress such as exercise may cause an abnormal response (1, 25). Increases in right ventricular afterload from hypoxemia and severe airway obstruction appear to be important mechanisms both at rest and with stress. Similar observations have been made in patients with other lung diseases such as cystic fibrosis (26–29). The hemodynamic changes observed during positive end-expiratory pressure ventilation have been attributed to right ventricular pressure overload with displacement of the interventricular septum into the left ventricle and its resultant impairment of left ventricular systolic performance (30, 31).

Valvular Heart Disease

Right ventricular function in valvular heart disease is affected by the degree of pulmonary hypertension, compensatory hypertrophy (which tends to normalize wall stress), intrinsic changes in contractility, changes in preload from primary or secondary tricuspid insufficiency, and the duration of the disease (32–36). Of the left-sided valvular lesions, mitral stenosis causes right ventricular dysfunction more often than mitral insufficiency. Aortic valve disease rarely causes right ventricular dysfunction (1, 36).

Right Ventricular Blood Flow

The right coronary artery is the main source of blood supply to the right ventricular free wall; both the right coronary artery and the left anterior descending coronary artery perfuse the interventricular septum (37). Right ventricular coronary blood flow is less than left ventricular coronary blood flow; the right ventricle extracts less oxygen than does the left ventricle; and unlike left coronary artery blood flow, which is mainly diastolic, right coronary artery blood flow is biphasic and similar in systole and diastole. Right coronary blood flow increases linearly in pressure overload, but not in volume overload states. The increased flow is mainly diastolic; and the increased flow is to both the free wall and the right side of the interventricular septum (38–41). Thus, disease of the right coronary artery limits the ability of the right ventricle to adapt to pressure overload, perhaps even more so than to volume overload.

Chronic Coronary Artery Disease

Resting right ventricular function is normal in the vast majority of patients with chronic coronary artery disease. Abnormal resting right ventricular function is usually only seen in patients with three-vessel disease or multiple infarcts, and stress may unmask right ventricular dysfunction in these patients as it does in those with chronic lung disease. The pathophysiologic and anatomic explanations for stress-induced right ventricular dysfunction include right coronary artery disease, resting or exercise-induced left ventricular dysfunction, and stress-induced pulmonary hypertension and right ventricular pressure overload (1, 42–50).

Acute Myocardial Infarction

Some patients with acute myocardial infarction but *no* right ventricular infarction have right ventricular dysfunction. The etiologies of this dysfunction include the degree of left ventricular dysfunction and the development of pulmonary hypertension, but septal involvement does not appear to be important (1, 9, 51, 52).

Right Ventricular Infarction

Right ventricular infarction is more common than is clinically apparent and certainly more frequent than right ventricular infarction associated with hemodynamic compromise. Pathologically, right ventricular infarction is seen in approximately 25 percent of patients with an inferior or posterior infarction. It is less common in the absence of a transmural infarction and more common in the presence of a transmural infarction that involves the interventricular septum (53). Right ventricular infarction occurs exclusively in the setting of an inferior or posterior left ventricular infarction; isolated right ventricular infarction is rare

(54). Hemodynamically, right ventricular infarction in which right atrial pressure is equal to or greater than left atrial pressure and right ventricular end-diastolic pressure is equal to or greater than left ventricular end-diastolic pressure is much less common, occurring in perhaps 5 percent of patients with inferior or posterior infarction (55–57). The important pathophysiologic factors that make a right ventricular infarction hemodynamically significant include the size of the right ventricular infarction, the size of the left ventricular infarction, the development of pulmonary hypertension secondary to left ventricular failure, and involvement of the interventricular septum limiting left ventricular assistance to right ventricular function (1, 9, 45, 58–60).

Cardiomyopathies

The right ventricle may be involved primary or secondary to pulmonary hypertension in congestive, restrictive, infiltrative, or hypertrophic myopathy. An unusual form of cardiomyopathy, arrhythmogenic right ventricular dysplasia, primarily affects the right ventricle and frequently presents with ventricular arrhythmias. The right ventricle may be more susceptible to radiation injury in patients receiving mediastinal irradiation because of its anterior location in the chest (61).

CARDIAC ULTRASOUND

Cardiac ultrasound analysis of right ventricular diastolic and systolic function is complicated by the difficulties in selecting a satisfactory hemodynamic model for its geometry (Fig. 6.1). Paradoxically, the ability of cardiac ultrasound to analyze the interventricular septum has provided important physiologic information on the interdependence of the left and right ventricles.

Ultrasound Anatomy

Unlike the left ventricle, the right ventricle is a geometrically complex structure. When viewed from the side, it appears triangular. In cross section, it is crescent shaped: The interventricular septum forms the medial wall, and the right ventricular free wall forms the lateral wall. Numerous two-dimensional echocardiographic planes can be used to visualize the right ventricle: the parasternal long- and short-axis views, the parasternal right ventricular inflow tract view, the apical four-chamber and the apical two-chamber (right ventricle–right atrial) views, and the subcostal four-chamber and short-axis views (62). From a practical standpoint, the apical four- and two-chamber views and the subcostal four-chamber view have provided the most information concerning right ventricular size and function. The parasternal short-axis view has

Figure 6.1. The volume of the right ventricle can be assessed with the use of one area and one length from each of two intersecting views. When A_1 is the area in one view and L_2 is the long axis of the intersecting view, right ventricular volume is $2(A_1)(L_2)/3$. (*A*) through (*G*) show geometric models that can be described by $V = 2AL/3$. (*A*) A prolate ellipsoid constructed by moving the right ventricular outflow tract from the center of the long axis to approximate a triangular pyramid. (*B*) A half-cylindric, half-conical structure. Models (*C*) through (*E*) are tapering structures with rectangular (*C*), trapezoidal (*D*), and triangular (*E*) bases. Model (*F*) is the most flexible (and complex) one. (*G*) is similar to *F* without the flanking structure that tapers. A = area; a_1, a_2, a_3 = fractions of area A_1 contributed by different portions of the model; b_1, b_2 = fractions of lengths L_1, L_2 contributed by the rectangular portion of the model; d = fraction of the width D contributed by the rectangular portion; PV = pulmonic valve; TV = tricuspid valve. (Reproduced by permission of The American Heart Association from Levine RA, et al. Echocardiographic measurement of right ventricular volume. Circulation 1984;69:497–505.)

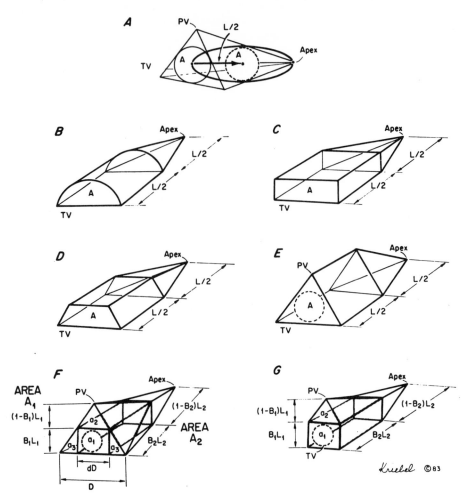

provided the most information concerning the interventricular septum.

Right Ventricular Volume

Measurement of right ventricular volume must take into account not only the complex geometry of the normal-sized right ventricle, but also the equally complex way in which this geometry changes as the right ventricle enlarges to become more spheric and less triangular and crescent shaped. In addition, there are difficulties in 1) defining the right ventricular endocardium because of its near-field location and heavy trabeculation, 2) standardizing views to visualize the complete right ventricular circumference, and 3) obtaining two perpendicular views that enable calculation of right ventricular volume from right ventricular angiograms. The most useful paired angiographic views are the anteroposterior and lateral views and the 30-degree right and 60-degree left anterior oblique views (63). Equivalent views are difficult to obtain using two-dimensional echocardiography.

Ultimately, a flexible three-dimensional reconstructive model using multiple views should allow measure-

ment of right ventricular volume (63). As of 1986, paired- or single-plane models have yielded only moderate success compared to in vivo angiographic or in vitro casted right ventricular volumes (64–70). At this time, right ventricular volume cannot be measured accurately in vivo by ultrasound.

Volume Overload

Although the measurement of right ventricular volume is difficult, the detection of a right ventricular volume overload state is important. Volume overload alters both right ventricle size and shape. In the parasternal long-axis view, the right ventricle is larger than normal in both its anteroposterior and superoinferior axes; the right ventricular apex may be distal to the left ventricular apex (Fig. 6.2). In the apical and subcostal four-chamber views, the right ventricle becomes less triangular and more elliptic (Fig. 6.3). In the parasternal short-axis view, the right ventricle is no longer crescent shaped but is more spherical; conversely, the left ventricle becomes less spherical and more crescent-shaped. During diastole, the septum is displaced into the left ventricle. During systole, the septum moves

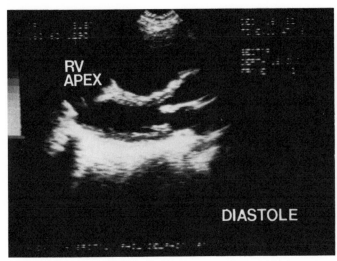

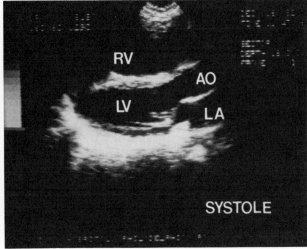

Figure 6.2. Diastolic and systolic frames of parasternal long-axis view of an example of right ventricular volume overload. In particular, note that the right ventricular (RV) apex is distal to the left ventricular (LV) apex. AO = aorta; LA = left atrium.

paradoxically toward the right ventricular free wall, and the left ventricle becomes more spherical (Fig. 6.4) (71). Paradoxic septal motion can be seen in other views as well. Causes of right ventricular volume overload include atrial septal defect, partial or total anomalous pulmonary venous return, tricuspid insufficiency, pulmonic insufficiency, left ventricular–right atrial shunting, and rupture of an aortic sinus into the right atrium.

Pressure Overload

Cardiac ultrasound can determine a right ventricular pressure overload state and, consequently, right ventricular hypertrophy. Two approaches have been used to estimate right ventricular systolic pressure: an ana-

tomic two-dimensional echocardiographic method and a Doppler ultrasound method. The right ventricle alters its geometry in pressure overload states less than in volume overload states. Normal right ventricular geometry is unsuited for ejecting blood against resistance. However, in a pressure overload state, the interventricular septum shifts somewhat toward the left ventricle, and the right ventricle becomes more spherical (16, 17). This spherical shape is adaptive; it is more efficient for ejecting against resistance (9). The degree of septal displacement is an approximate index of the severity of the pressure overload (72). Assuming the absence of tricuspid stenosis, ventricular systolic pressure can be estimated more accurately with Doppler ultrasound by 1) detecting tricuspid insufficiency, 2) measuring the

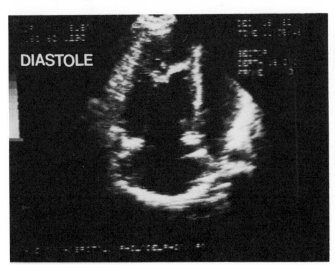

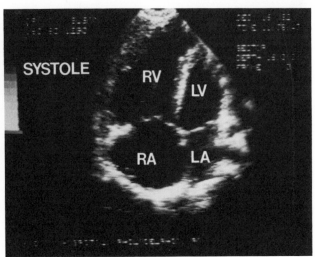

Figure 6.3. Diastolic and systolic frames of apical four-chamber view of an example of right ventricular (RV) volume overload. In diastole, the left ventricle (LV) is "compressed" by the displaced interventricular septum; in systole, septal motion is paradoxic (toward the RV). As is typical of a dilated RV, the RV is more elliptic and less triangular. LA = left atrium; RA = right atrium.

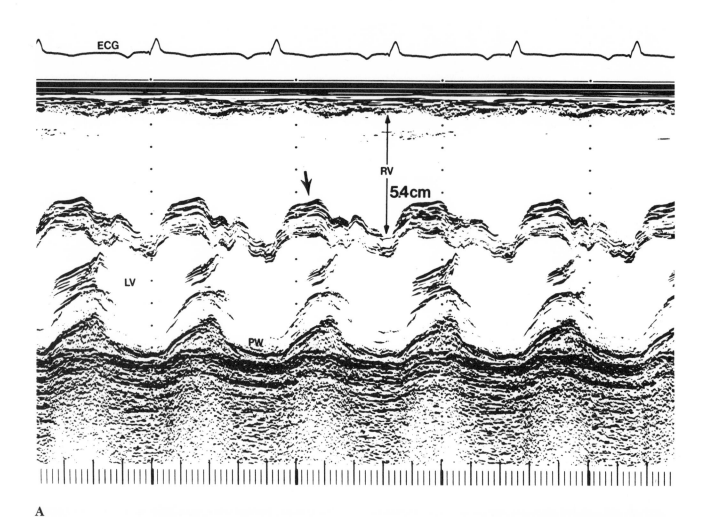

A

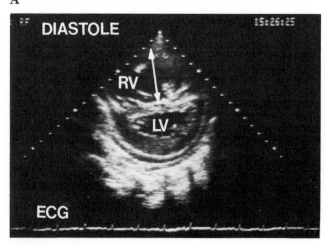

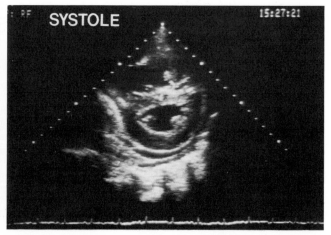

B

Figure 6.4. (*A*) An M-mode echocardiogram showing right ventricular (RV) enlargement measuring 5.4 centimeters and paradoxic septal motion (*dark arrow*). Note that septal thickening is normal. The mechanism of paradoxic septal motion is seen in (*B*), a parasternal short-axis view of an example of RV volume overload. In diastole, the septum is displaced into the left ventricle (LV), causing it to be less spherical and more crescent shaped. In systole, the contracting LV attempts to become more spherical (a more efficient shape for ejecting blood against a resistance). To do so, the septum must be displaced toward the LV. Paradoxic septal motion is seen in other conditions where there is no RV volume overload (e.g., following pericardiectomy, when septal thickening is normal, and in conduction disturbances, when septal thickening is abnormal). ECG = electrocardiogram; PW = posterior wall.

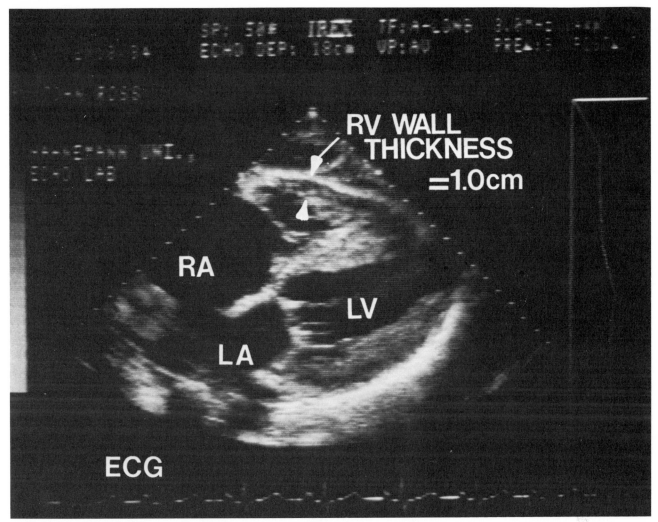

**RV WALL
THICKNESS
=1.0cm**

RA

LV

LA

ECG

Figure 6.5.   This subcostal four-chamber view shows right ventricular (RV) hypertrophy: an RV wall thickness of 1.0 cm. ECG = electrocardiogram; LA = left atrium; LV = left ventricle; RA = right atrium.

velocity of the tricuspid insufficiency jet, 3) calculating the right ventricular–right atrial pressure difference (4 × (tricuspid insufficiency peak velocity)^2), and 4) adding the right atrial pressure estimated from the jugular venous pressure (73). In the absence of right ventricular outflow tract obstruction, right ventricular systolic pressure equals pulmonary artery systolic pressure. This technique is applicable to 87 percent of patients with right ventricular pressure overload who have tricuspid insufficiency.

Any right ventricular pressure overload state can cause right ventricular hypertrophy. Initially, right ventricular hypertrophy is adaptive in normalizing right ventricular wall stress and in improving the ability of the right ventricle to eject against resistance. However, chronic right ventricular pressure overload ultimately has a deleterious effect on right ventricular function. Right ventricular hypertrophy is diagnosed by a right ventricular free wall thickness of greater than 5 millimeters. M-mode and two-dimensional echocardiog-

raphy from either the parasternal or subcostal window is useful (Fig. 6.5) (74). This criterion has a sensitivity of at least 70 percent and a specificity approaching 100 percent (75, 76). It is far more accurate than electrocardiography (77). Right ventricular pressure overload states include pulmonary hypertension and any form of anatomic right ventricular outflow tract obstruction. An increased right ventricular free wall thickness also occurs in infiltrative cardiomyopathy and is indistinguishable from true right ventricular hypertrophy.

Some causes of right ventricular volume overload such as atrial septal defect can lead to right ventricular pressure overload through development of pulmonary hypertension; right ventricular pressure overload can lead to right ventricular volume overload because of the development of tricuspid insufficiency. As the right ventricle becomes more dilated, the septum is further displaced into the left ventricle during diastole; and as the abnormal load increases, the left ventricle becomes less able to assume spherical geometry during systole and may maintain a crescent shape throughout the cardiac cycle (78). It is important to distinguish between volume overload causing pressure overload and pressure overload causing volume overload. The former may be surgically correctable, but the latter is not. This distinction can sometimes be made by two-dimensional echocardiography alone, is facilitated by Doppler ultrasound study, but may require invasive study.

Right Ventricular Function and Dysfunction

Despite the geometric difficulties that hinder accurate measurement of right ventricular volume, the complex geometry of the right ventricle causes a constant and systematic difficulty in both systole and diastole. Thus, it is possible to calculate right ventricular ejection fraction by two-dimensional echocardiography. Both biplane and single-plane techniques have been proposed. Biplane techniques use either paired apical four-chamber and subcostal four-chamber views (79, 80), paired apical four-chamber and two-chamber views (68, 79), paired subcostal views (66, 81), or paired apical four-chamber and parasternal short-axis views (67, 82) employing either the area-length method or Simpson's rule (Fig. 6.6). Paired planes can be obtained in 65 percent to 90 percent of patients (81,

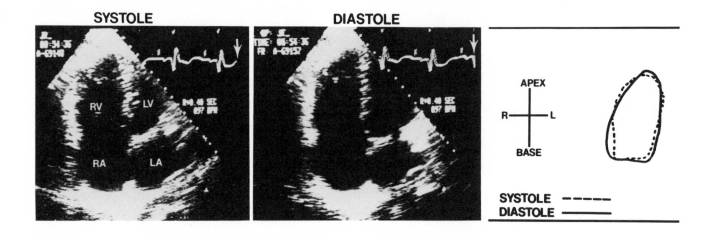

A

B

Figure 6.6.   Paired apical four-chamber (*A*) and two-chamber (*B*) views of the right ventricle (RV) at end systole and end diastole are used to calculate RV ejection fraction. The end diastole (solid line) and end systole (dotted line) are shown to the right. Usng these views to compare the two-dimensional echocardiographic RV ejection fraction to the first-pass radionuclide RV ejection fraction, and using either the area-length method or Simpson's rule, we found regression equations of $y = 1.4 \times -12$, $R = 0.76$ (area-length), or $y = 1.3 \times -5$, $R = 0.78$ (Simpson's). In addition, note that in the apical two-chamber view, the RV becomes more elliptic (less trapezoidal) as it enlarges and the RV outflow tract is no longer seen. L = left; LA = left atrium; LV = left ventricle; R = right; RA = right atrium. (Reproduced by permission from Panidis IP, Kotler MN, Mintz GS, et al. Right ventricular function in coronary artery disease as assessed by two-dimensional echocardiography. Am Heart J 1984;107:1187–94.)

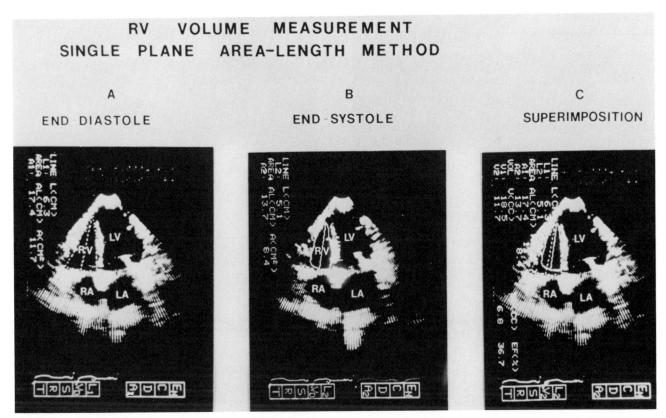

Figure 6.7. Using only the apical four-chamber view, it is possible to estimate right ventricular (RV) ejection fraction by generating equivalent frontal and lateral view dimensions (via correlation with RV angiograms). The formula is V = (C)(A$_1$)(A$_2$)/L$_{common}$. Also note that the normal-sized RV is triangular in the apical four-chamber view. As the RV enlarges, it becomes more elliptic. (*A*) End diastole with RV endocardium as a dotted line. (*B*) End systole with RV endocardium as a solid line. (*C*) The superimposition of the two. LA = left atrium; LV = left ventricle; RA = right atrium.

83). Single-plane techiques generally use the apical four-chamber view (Fig. 6.7) (65, 68). Both yield statistically acceptable results. Right ventricular ejection fraction calculated from single or paired echocardiographic planes and right ventricular ejection fraction calculated from biplane angiography or radionuclide angiography have a correlation coefficient of approximately 0.80 in most studies. Identification of the right ventricular endocardium can be improved by peripheral contrast injection that "outlines" the right ventricular cavity (Fig. 6.8) (84). In addition, in severe right ventricular dysfunction, inspiratory augmentation of venous return is reduced, and the inferior vena cava remains dilated with reduction or absence of the normal inspiratory reduction in caliber (Fig. 6.9) (15). Echocardiographic detection of right ventricular dysfunction is limited, however, by the technical difficulty of studying right ventricular function during stress. Many disease states are associated with normal resting ejection fraction, but stress may result in decreased right ventricular ejection fraction.

Coronary Artery Disease

Segmental right ventricular wall motion abnormalities (akinesia or dyskinesia) are almost always present in patients with clinical and hemodynamic criteria diagnostic of right ventricular infarction (Fig. 6.8) (85–88). The right ventricle is enlarged, and there may be displacement of the interventricular septum into the left ventricle during diastole, with paradoxic motion of the septum during systole (85, 86). These wall motion abnormalities can be detected in approximately 25 percent of patients with an inferior or posterior infarction who do not have clinical or hemodynamic criteria of a right ventricular infarction (83, 88, 89). Thus, two-dimensional echocardiography is more sensitive than hemodynamic monitoring in detecting right ventricular infarction. The prevalence approximates that found during pathologic examination (53). However, the right ventricular dysfunction and infarction may not be clinically significant. Complications of right ventricular infarction are hypotension, atrioventricular block, sinus node dysfunction, atrial and ventricular

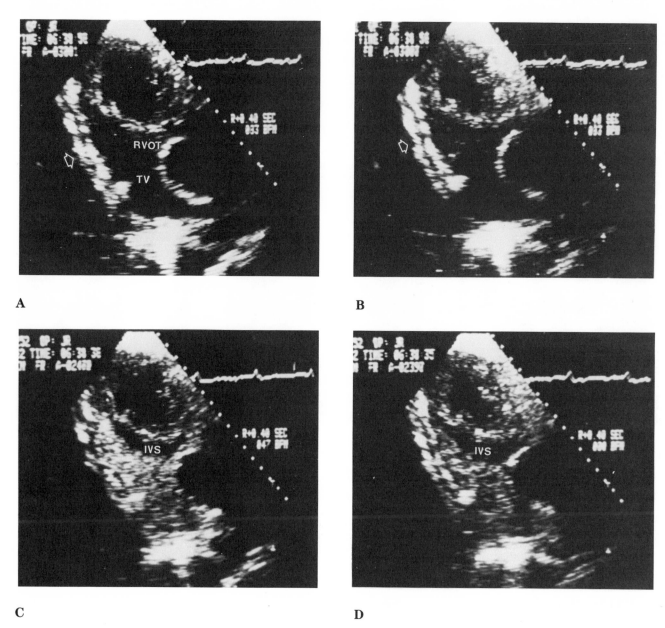

A   **B**

C   **D**

Figure 6.8. Identification of the right ventricular endocardium can be improved by peripheral contrast injection. (*A*) End diastole without contrast. (*B*) End systole without contrast. Although the inferior wall (*open white arrow*) is obviously akinetic and "scarred," the septum and its contraction are not well defined. (*C*) End diastole after contrast injection. (*D*) End systole after contrast injection. The interventricular septum (IVS), its thickness, and its systolic thickening are well defined. In this apical two-chamber view of a normal-sized right ventricle, the right ventricle is roughly trapezoidal in shape; the sides of the trapezoid are the inferior wall, the IVS, the right ventricular outflow tract (RVOT), and the plane of the tricuspid valve (TV). In this view, as the right ventricle enlarges, it becomes more elliptic (see Fig. 6.6). In this patient with an inferior wall infarction, the right ventricular ejection fraction measured 27 percent.

arrhythmias, ventricular fibrillation during temporary pacing, right-to-left shunting through a patent foramen ovale, cardiogenic shock, and tricuspid insufficiency. Because the most common presentation is hypotension, other causes must be excluded. Two-dimensional echocardiography is useful in detecting hemodynamically significant pericardial disease such as constriction, tamponade, and hypovolemia (in which the infe-

rior vena cava appears smaller than normal, indicating volume depletion) that may be mistaken for right ventricular infarction.

Generalized right ventricular dysfunction without segmental wall motion abnormalities can be seen in some patients with extensive left ventricular infarction, with multiple infarctions, or with severe three-vessel coronary artery disease (1, 83).

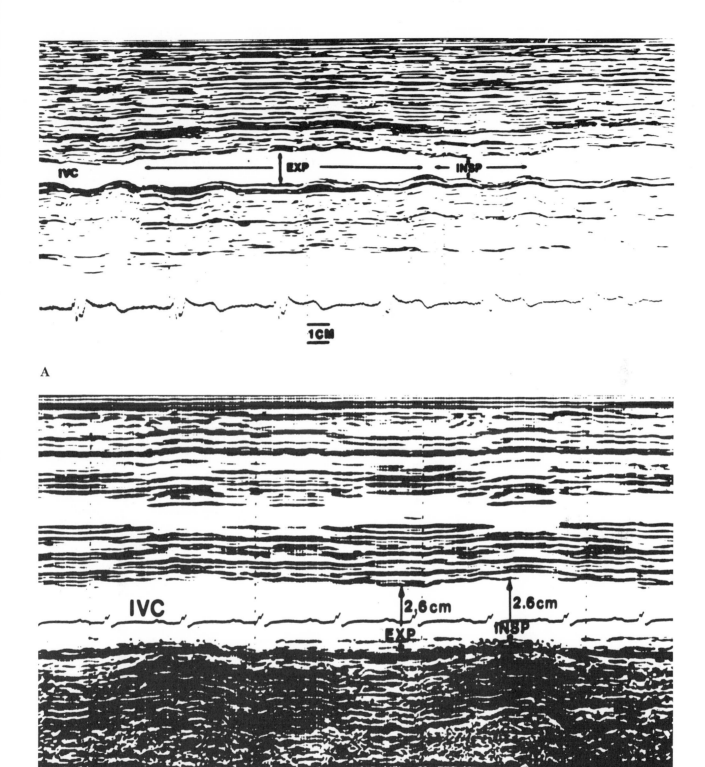

A

B

Figure 6.9. (*A*) A normal inferior vena caval (IVC) echogram showing an inspiratory (INSP) decrease in caliber compared to expiration (EXP). (*B*) An abnormal IVC echogram from a patient with a cardiomyopathy. The IVC is dilated (indicating a high central venous pressure); there is no inspiratory decrease in caliber. This pattern is seen in severe right ventricular dysfunction or hemodynamically significant pericardial disease.

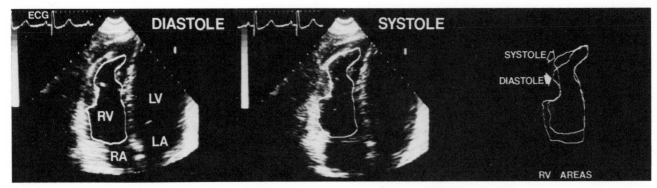

Figure 6.10.   These diastolic and systolic apical four-chamber views show arrhythmogenic right ventricular (RV) dysplasia. End-diastolic and end-systolic RV endocardial tracings are superimposed at the right (RV areas). Note the areas of akinesis and dyskinesis. ECG = electrocardiogram; LA = left atrium; LV = left ventricle; RA = right atrium.

Arrhythmogenic Right Ventricular Dysplasia

Arrhythmogenic dysplasia primarily or exclusively affects the right ventricle and has characteristic two-dimensional echocardiographic features (Fig. 6.10). Left ventricular function is normal. The right ventricle is enlarged, and the free wall is thin and typically distorted in shape. There is generalized hypokinesis and frequent segmental wall motion abnormalities usually involving the free wall (90, 91). Although these patients have normal exercise tolerance and no evidence of right heart failure—possibly because of ventricular interdependence with left ventricular assistance of right ventricular output—they are prone to serious arrhythmias.

REFERENCES

1. Manno BV, Iskandrian AS, Hakki AH. Right ventricular function: methodologic and clinical considerations in non-invasive scintigraphic assessment. J Am Coll Cardiol 1984;3:1072–81.
2. Bemis CE, Serus JR, Borkenhagen D, et al. Influence of right ventricular filling pressure on left ventricular pressure and dimension. Circ Res 1974;34:498–504.
3. Elzinga G, van Grandelle R, Westerhof N, et al. Ventricular interference. Am J Physiol 1974;226:941–47.
4. Santamore WP, Lynch PR, Meier GM, et al. Myocardial interaction between the ventricles. J Appl Physiol 1976;41:362–68.
5. Janicki JS, Weber KT. Ventricular action pre and post pericardiectomy. Fed Proc 1978;37:776.
6. Rabson J, Permut S. The role of the pericardium in diastolic interdependence of the right and left ventricles. Fed Proc 1978;37:778.
7. Glantz SA, Misbach GA, Moores WY, et al. The pericardium substantially affects the left ventricular diastolic pressure volume relationship in the dog. Circ Res 1978;42:433–41.
8. Ludbrook PA, Byrne JD, McKnight RC. Influence of right ventricular hemodynamics on left ventricular pressure volume relations in man. Circulation 1979;59:21–31.
9. Bove AA, Santamore WP. Ventricular interdependence. Prog Cardiovasc Dis 1981;23:365–88.
10. Flamm MD, Cohn KE, Hancock EW. Ventricular function in atrial septal defect. Am J Med 1970;48:286–94.
11. Mathew R, Thilenius OG, Arcilla RA. Comparative response of right and left ventricles to volume overload. Am J Cardiol 1976;38:209–17.
12. Levin AR, Liebson PR, Ehlers KH, et al. Assessment of left ventricular function in secundum atrial septal defect. Pediatr Res 1975;9:894–9.
13. Popio KA, Gorlin R, Teichholtz LE, et al. Abnormalities of left ventricular function and geometry in adults with an atrial septal defect. Am J Cardiol 1975;36:302–8.
14. St. John Sutton MG, Tajik AJ, Mercier LA, et al. Assessment of left ventricular function in secundum atrial septal defect by computer analysis of the M-mode echocardiogram. Circulation 1979;60:1082–90.
15. Mintz GS, Kotler MN, Parry WR, Iskandrian AS, Kane SA. Real-time inferior vena caval ultrasonography: normal and abnormal findings and its use in assessing right-heart function. Circulation 1981;64:1018–25.
16. Stool EW, Mallins CB, Leshin SJ, et al. Dimensional changes of the left ventricle during acute pulmonary arterial hypertension in dogs. Am J Cardiol 1974;33:868–75.
17. Machida K, Rapaport E. Left ventricular function in experimental pulmonary embolism. Jpn Heart J 1971;12:221–32.
18. Seki S, Ohba O, Tanizaki M, et al. Construction of a new right ventricle on the epicardium. J Thorac Cardiovasc Surg 1975;70:330–7.
19. Seki S, Ona K, Tanizaki M, et al. Role of contraction and size of right ventricular free wall performance of the heart. Jpn J Thorac Surg 1977;29:731–40.
20. Sawatani S, Mandell C, Kusaba E, et al. Ventricular performance following ablation and prosthetic replacement of right ventricular myocardium. Trans Am Soc Artif Intern Organs 1974;20:629–36.
21. Shabetai R, Mangiardi L, Bargava V, et al. The pericardium and cardiac function. Prog Cardiovasc Dis 1979;22:107–34.
22. Berger HJ, Matthay RA, Loke J, et al. Assessment of cardiac performance with quantitative radionuclide angiography: right ventricular ejection fraction with reference to findings in chronic obstructive pulmonary disease. Am J Cardiol 1978;41:897–905.
23. Ellis JH, Kirk D, Steele PP. Right ventricular ejection fraction in severe chronic airway obstruction. Chest 1977;71:281–2.
24. Slutsky RA, Ackerman W, Karliner JS, et al. Right and left ventricular dysfunction in patients with chronic obstructive lung disease. Am J Med 1978;68:197–205.
25. Matthay RA, Berger HJ, Davies R, et al. Right and left ventricular exercise performance in chronic pulmonary disease. Ann Intern Med 1980;93:234–9.
26. Matthay RA, Berger HJ, Loke J, et al. Right and left ventricular performance in ambulatory young adults with cystic fibrosis. Br Heart J 1980;43:474–80.
27. Chipps BE, Anderson PO, Roland JMA, et al. Non-invasive evaluation of ventricular function in cystic fibrosis. J Pediatr 1979;95:373–84.
28. Jacobstein MD, Hirschfeld SS, Winnie G, et al. Ventricular interdependence in severe cystic fibrosis. A two-dimensional echocardiographic study. Chest 1981;80:399–404.
29. Panidis IP, Ren JF, Holsclaw DS, Mintz GS, Kotler MN, Ross J.

Cardiac function in patients with cystic fibrosis: evaluation by two-dimensional and Doppler echocardiography. J Am Coll Cardiol 1985;6:701–6.

30. Jardin F, Farot JC, Boisante L, et al. Influence of positive end-expiratory pressure on left ventricular performance. N Engl J Med 1981;364:387–92.

31. Jardin F, Farcot JC, Gueret P, et al. Echocardiographic evaluation of ventricles during continuous positive airway pressure breathing. J Appl Physiol 1984;56:619–27.

32. Berger HJ, Matthay RA. Radionuclide right ventricular ejection fraction. Applications in valvular heart disease. Chest 1981;79:497–8.

33. Winzelberg GG, Boucher CA, Pohost GA, et al. Right ventricular function in mitral and aortic valve disease: relation of gated first-pass radionuclide angiography to clinical and hemodynamic findings. Chest 1981;79:520–8.

34. Korr RS, Gandsman EJ, Winkler ML, et al. Hemodynamic correlates of right ventricular ejection fraction measured with gated radionuclide angiography. Am J Cardiol 1982;49:71–7.

35. Iskandrian AS, Hakki AH, Ren JF, et al. Correlation among right ventricular preload, afterload, and ejection fraction in mitral valve disease. J Am Coll Cardiol 1984;3:1403–11.

36. Henze E, Schelbert HR, Wisenberg G, et al. Assessment of regurgitant fraction and right and left ventricular function at rest and during exercise. Am Heart J 1981;104:953–62.

37. James TN. The arteries of the free ventricular walls in man. Anat Rec 1960;136:371–9.

38. Braunwald E, Sobel BE. Coronary blood flow and myocardial ischemia. In: Braunwald E, ed. Heart disease: a textbook of cardiovascular medicine. Philadelphia: WB Saunders, 1980:1279–1308.

39. Monroe GA, Knapp RS, Fixler DE, et al. Effect of acute pulmonary arterial obstruction on right ventricular volume and coronary blood flow in closed chest anesthetized dogs, abstracted. Circulation 1973;48:IV-97.

40. Lowensohn HS, Khouri EM, Crigg DE, et al. Phasic right coronary artery blood flow in conscious dogs with normal and elevated right ventricular pressures. Circulation 1976;39:760–6.

41. Manohan M, Biscard GE, Bullard V, et al. Regional myocardial blood flow and myocardial function during acute right ventricular pressure overload in calves. Circ Res 1979;44:531–9.

42. Steele P, Kirch D, LeFree M, Battock D. Measurement of right and left ventricular ejection fractions by radionuclide angiography in coronary artery disease. Chest 1976;70:51–6.

43. Ferlinz J, Gorlin R, Cohn PF, et al. Right ventricular performance in patients with coronary artery disease. Circulation 1975;52:608–15.

44. Ferlinz J, Delvicario M, Gorlin R. Incidence of right ventricular asynergy with coronary artery disease. Am J Cardiol 1976;38:557–63.

45. Blesa ES, Boak JG, Bove AA, et al. Right ventricular function in coronary artery disease. Circulation 1975;52:II-162.

46. Maddahi J, Berman DS, Matsuoka DT, et al. A new technique for assessing right ventricular ejection fraction using rapid multiple-gated equilibrium cardiac blood scintigraphy. Circulation 1979;60:581–9.

47. Berger HJ, Johnstone DE, Sands JM, et al. Response of right ventricular ejection fraction to upright bicycle exercise in coronary artery disease. Circulation 1979;60:1292–1300.

48. Johnson LL, McCarthy DM, Sciacca RR, et al. Right ventricular ejection fraction during exercise in patients with coronary artery disease. Circulation 1979;60:1284–91.

49. Maddahi J, Berman DS, Matsuoka DT, et al. Right ventricular ejection fraction during exercise in normal subjects and in coronary artery disease patients. Circulation 1980;62:133–40.

50. Slutsky R, Hooper W, Gerberk K, et al. Assessment of right ventricular function at rest and during exercise in patients with coronary heart disease. Am J Cardiol 1980;45:63–71.

51. Marmar A, Geltman EM, Biello DR, et al. Functional response of the right ventricle to myocardial infarction. Circulation 1981;64:1005–11.

52. Reduto LA, Berger AJ, Cohen LS, et al. Sequential radionuclide assessment of left and right ventricular performance after acute myocardial infarction. Ann Intern Med 1978;89:441–7.

53. Isner JM, Roberts WC. Right ventricular infarction complicating left ventricular infarction secondary to coronary heart disease. Am J Cardiol 1978;42:885–94.

54. Rackley CE, Russel RO Jr, Mantle JA, et al. Right ventricular infarction and function. Am Heart J 1981;101:215–8.

55. Cohn JN. Right ventricular infarction revisited. Am J Cardiol 1979;43:666–8.

56. Lorell B, Leinbach RC, Pohost GM, et al. Right ventricular infarction. Am J Cardiol 1979;43:465–71.

57. Lopez-Sendon J, Coma-Canella I, Gamallo C. Sensitivity and specificity of hemodynamic criteria in the diagnosis of acute right ventricular infarction. Circulation 1981;64:515–25.

58. Russel R, Dowling JT, Burdeshaw J, et al. Comparison of right and left ventricular function in acute myocardial infarction. Cathet Cardiovasc Diagn 1976;2:253–67.

59. Rackley CE, Russell RO. Right ventricular function in acute myocardial infarction. Am J Cardiol 1974;33:927–9.

60. Raabe DS, Chester AC. Right ventricular infarction. Chest 1978;73:96–9.

61. Burns RJ, Bar-Shlomo B, Druck MN, et al. Detection of radiation cardiomyopathy by gated radionuclide angiography. Am J Med 1983;74:297–302.

62. Tajik AJ, Seward JB, Hagler DJ, et al. Two-dimensional real-time ultrasonic imaging of the heart and great vessels. Mayo Clin Proc 1978;53:271–303.

63. Linker DT, Pearlman AS, Moritz WE, Huntsman LH. A new method for right ventricular volume calculation from a three-dimensional echocardiographic reconstruction. Circulation 1982;66:II-338.

64. Lange PE, Onnasch D, Farr FL, Heintzen PH. Angiographic right ventricular volume determination. Eur Heart J 1978;8:477.

65. Bommer W, Weinert L, Neumann A, et al. Determination of right atrial and right ventricular size by two-dimensional echocardiography. Circulation 1979;60:91–100.

66. Saito A, Ueda K, Nakano H. Right ventricular volume determination by two-dimensional echocardiography. J Cardiogr 1981;11:1159–68.

67. Ninomiya K, Duncan WJ, Cook DH, et al. Right ventricular ejection fraction and volumes after Mustard report. Correlation of two-dimensional echocardiograms and cineangiograms. Am J Cardiol 1981;48:317–24.

68. Watanabe R, Katsume H, Matsukobo H, et al. Estimation of right ventricular volume with two-dimensional echocardiography. Am J Cardiol 1982;49:1946–53.

69. Hiraishi S, DiSessa TG, Jarmakani JM, et al. Two-dimensional echocardiographic assessment of right ventricular volume in children with congenital heart disease. Am J Cardiol 1982;50:1368–75.

70. Levine RE, Gibson TC, Aretz T, et al. Echocardiographic measurement of right ventricular volume. Circulation 1984;69:497–505.

71. Weyman AE, Wann S, Feigenbaum H, et al. Mechanism of abnormal septal motion in patients with right ventricular volume overload. Circulation 1976;54:179–86.

72. Watanabe K. Evaluation of right ventricular pressure by two-dimensional echocardiography. Jpn Heart J 1984;25:523–31.

73. Yock PG, Popp RL. Non-invasive estimation of right ventricular systolic pressure by Doppler ultrasound in patients with tricuspid regurgitation. Circulation 1984;70:657–62.

74. Cooper MJ, Teitel DF, Silverman NH, Enderlein M. Comparison of M-mode echocardiographic measurement of right ventricular wall thickness obtained by the subcostal and parasternal approach in children. Am J Cardiol 1984;54:835–8.

75. Baker BJ, Scovil JA, Kane JJ, Murphy ML. Echocardiographic detection of right ventricular hypertrophy. Am Heart J 1983;105:611–4.

76. Cacho A, Prakash R, Sarma R, Kaushik VS. Usefulness of two-dimensional echocardiography in diagnosing right ventricular hypertrophy. Chest 1983;84:154–7.

77. Prakash R. Echocardiographic diagnosis of right ventricular hypertrophy. Cathet Cardiovasc Diagn 1981;7:179–84.

78. Shimada R, Takeshita A, Nakamura M. Non-invasive assessment of right ventricular systolic pressure in atrial septal defect. Am J Cardiol 1984;53:117–23.

79. Panidis IP, Ren JF, Kotler MN, et al. Two-dimensional echocardiographic estimation of right ventricular ejection fraction in patients with coronary artery disease. J Am Coll Cardiol 1983;2: 911–8.

80. Kaul S, Tei C, Hopkins JM, Shah PM. Assessment of right ventricular function using two-dimensional echocardiography. Am Heart J 1984;107:526–31.

81. Starling MR, Crawford MH, Sorenson SG, O'Rourke RA. A new two-dimensional echocardiographic technique for evaluating right ventricular size and performance in patients with obstructive lung disease. Circulation 1982;66:612–20.

82. Silverman NH, Hudson S. Evaluation of right ventricular volume and ejection fraction in children by two-dimensional echocardiography. Pediatr Cardiol 1983;4:197–203.

83. Panidis IP, Kotler MN, Mintz GS, et al. Right ventricular function in coronary artery disease as assessed by two-dimensional echocardiography. Am Heart J 1984;107:1187–94.

84. Lange PE, Seiffert PA, Preis F, et al. Value of image enhancement and injection of contrast medium for right ventricular volume determination by two-dimensional echocardiography in congenital heart disease. Am J Cardiol 1985;55:152–7.

85. D'Arcy B, Nanda NC. Two-dimensional echocardiographic features of right ventricular infarction. Circulation 1982;65:167–73.

86. Lopez-Sendon J, Garcia-Fernandez MA, Coma-Canella I, et al. Segmental right ventricular function after acute myocardial infarction. Am J Cardiol 1983;51:390–6.

87. Jugdutt BI, Sussex BA, Sivaram CA, Rossall RE. Right ventricular infarction. Two-dimensional echocardiographic evaluation. Am Heart J 1984;107:505–18.

88. Vannucci A, Cecchi F, Zuppiroli A, et al. Right ventricular infarction. Clinical, hemodynamic, mono and two-dimensional echocardiographic features. Eur Heart J 1983;4:854–64.

89. Cecchi F, Zuppiroli A, Favilli S, et al. Echocardiographic features of right ventricular infarction. Clin Cardiol 1984;7:405–12.

90. Marcus FI, Fontaine GH, Guirandon G, et al. Right ventricular dysplasia. Circulation 1982;65:384–98.

91. Rowland E, McKenna WJ, Sugrue D, et al. Ventricular tachycardia of left bundle branch block configuration in patients with isolated right ventricular dilatation. Br Heart J 1984;51:15–24.

7

Acquired Mitral and Tricuspid Valve Disease

Charles Pollick
Martin St. John Sutton

Three decades have elapsed since the first M-mode echocardiographic study of the mitral valve was obtained. During this time, there have been many technologic advances in instrumentation; the development of two-dimensional echocardiography; and pulsed, continuous, and color-flow Doppler. Current Doppler echocardiographic techniques allow accurate assessment of the anatomy of the mitral valve leaflets, subvalve tensor apparatus and annulus, characterization of the leaflet texture and mobility, assessment of the hemodynamics in terms of transvalve gradients and valve orifice areas, and evaluation of the effects of mitral stenosis and regurgitation on left ventricular filling and pump function.

MITRAL STENOSIS

The M-mode echocardiogram of the normal mitral valve demonstrates abrupt anterior motion of the anterior leaflet and posterior motion of the posterior leaflet (D to E points) as the valve opens; partial closure in early diastole (E to F points), followed by reopening of the leaflets (F to A point) by atrial systole, and finally coaption of the cusps (A to C points) at end diastole (Fig. 7.1). The mitral leaflet motion pattern in mitral stenosis is remarkably different, and the first clinical application of M-mode echocardiography was in the noninvasive diagnosis and evaluation of rheumatic mitral stenosis (1, 2). M-mode echocardiographic findings are still of diagnostic value in mitral stenosis, and demonstrate 1) thickening and often calcification of the anterior and posterior mitral valve leaflets, 2)

characteristic diastolic motion with reduced excursion and decreased diastolic closing velocity (EF slope) of the anterior leaflet, 3) anterior motion of the posterior mitral valve leaflet, 4) slow and prolonged increase in left ventricular dimension during diastolic filling, and 5) enlargement of the left atrium (1–8) (Fig. 7.2). The pathognomonic echocardiographic abnormality of mitral stenosis is the anterior motion of the posterior leaflet (8). This is due to commissural fusion, and it is the hallmark of rheumatic mitral valve disease. The diastolic closing velocity of the anterior mitral valve leaflet (EF slope) has been used as an index of the severity of mitral stenosis (1–3, 5, 6) (Fig. 7.3). The flatter the EF slope, the more hemodynamically important the mitral stenosis. Patients with closing velocities of less than 36 mm/sec were regarded as having clinically significant mitral stenosis (2, 3). The EF slope varies with cardiac cycle length however, and this poses problems in accurately assessing the severity of mitral stenosis because the natural history of the disease is the development of atrial fibrillation (3) (Fig. 7.4). Furthermore, the EF slope does not correlate with mitral valve area calculated at cardiac catheterization (3, 9, 10), and provides no information regarding coexistent mitral regurgitation, even when this is the dominant lesion.

An alternative method of estimating the severity of mitral stenosis, which has had limited use, is continuous digitization of the endocardial surface of the left side of the interventricular septum and the endocardium of the posterior left ventricular wall (11, 12) (Fig.

169

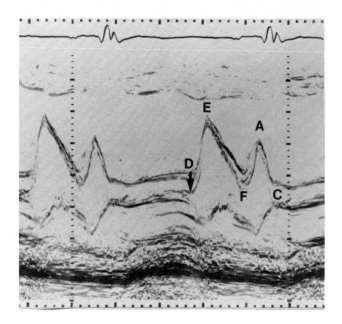
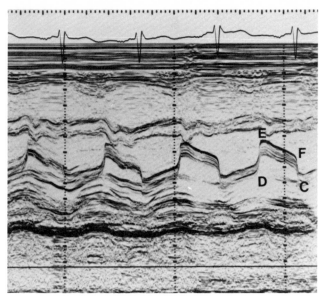

A   **B**

Figure 7.1.   M-mode echocardiogram (*A*) of the left ventricle showing the anterior and posterior leaflets of a normal mitral valve. The mitral valve (MV) leaflets open at the onset of diastole from the coaption point (D point, *black arrow*). The anterior leaflet moves anteriorly to its maximum amplitude (E point), while the posterior leaflet moves posteriorly. In early diastole, the anterior leaflet drifts posteriorly toward the closed position (F point), and is reopened by atrial contraction and moves anteriorly again (A point), and finally closes by moving posteriorly to coapt with the posterior cusp (C point). In systole the two leaflets move slightly anteriorly before reopening with the onset of the next diastole. By contrast, the mitral valve in rheumatic mitral stenosis appears thickened and less mobile than normal (*B*). The anterior leaflet moves anteriorly (D point to E point) with the onset of diastole, and instead of the posterior leaflet moving posteriorly, it too moves anteriorly. Anterior motion of the posterior mitral valve leaflet indicates commissural fusion and is pathognomic of rheumatic mitral stenosis. The EF slope or early diastolic closing velocity of the anterior leaflet is slower than normal. The increased thickness of the leaflets can be seen in diastole as an increased number of echoes emanating from the cusps. At end-diastole, the mitral valve leaflet moves posteriorly (C point).

7.5). This assumes that the left ventricle contracts concentrically and that the area of the left ventricle sampled by the M-mode echo beam is representative of the ventricle as a whole. Digitization of the left ventricular boundaries enables quantitation of both the peak diastolic left ventricular filling rate and the duration of the rapid filling period. In severe mitral stenosis, the peak rate of increase in left ventricular diameter is reduced, and the discrete rapid filling phase and the normal period of diastasis are lost because filling continues slowly throughout diastole (Fig. 7.5) (11–13).

Other M-mode echocardiographic findings in patients with severe mitral stenosis include left atrial enlargement, dilatation of the right ventricular outflow tract, and diminished or reversed septal motion. Reversed septal motion is due to different diastolic filling rates of the two ventricles, and is similar to that occurring in pulmonary hypertension and with right ventricular volume overload from tricuspid regurgitation.

Two-dimensional echocardiographic imaging of the mitral valve in orthogonal long and short axis views from the left parasternal region and in the apical two and four chamber views enables detailed description of all the component parts of the mitral valve unit—the leaflets, chordae, papillary muscles, and the valve ring. In mitral stenosis, the valve leaflets are thickened due to fibrosis, often with additional calcification, and their surface areas are reduced due to cicatrization, which contributes to their limited mobility. In the two-dimensional echocardiographic parasternal short axis view at the base of the left ventricle, the mitral commissures are thickened and fused, especially at the outer margins, and the extent of commissural adhesion determines the severity of the mitral stenosis (Fig. 7.6). The line of the commissures is often distorted due to scarring of the mitral valve, so that the orifice area, in addition to being narrowed, may no longer be in the center of the valve but displaced toward the septal or free wall commissure. Fusion of the commissures results in the mitral valve having an abrupt opening movement.

The anterior cusp takes origin from approximately 45%, and the posterior leaflet takes origin from approximately 55% of the mitral valve ring circumference, but their respective surface areas are similar. When the commissures are partially fused due to rheumatic

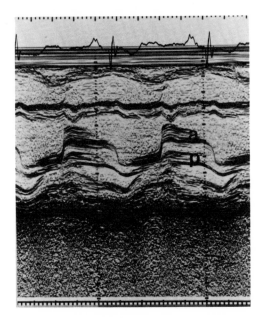

A

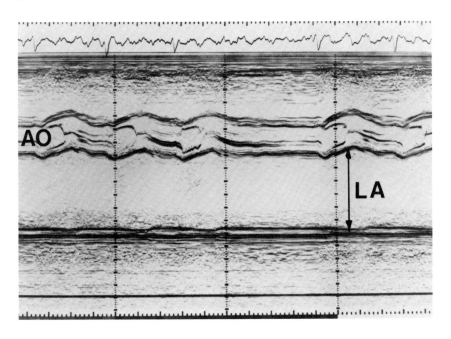

B

Figure 7.2. M-mode echocardiogram of a patient with rheumatic mitral stenosis. The anterior (a) and posterior (p) mitral valve leaflets are calcified (*A*) and both move anteriorly when the valve opens. The slow EF slope indicates moderately severe mitral stenosis. M-mode echocardiogram of the right ventricular outflow tract, aorta, and left atrium from a patient with rheumatic mitral stenosis (*B*) shows an enlarged left atrium of 6.4 cm in diameter (normal = less than 4.0 cm) and minor rheumatic thickening of the aortic valve leaflets, which open fully.

mitral stenosis, the two leaflets move in the same direction when the valve opens. The mitral valve orifice has a fishmouth appearance with thickening of the free edges of the cusps. The valve orifice is clearly visualized in the short axis view of the left ventricle obtained from the left parasternal position (Fig. 7.6), and the mitral valve orifice area can be measured by planimetry in approximately 80% to 90% of cases. When the mitral valve area is planimetered, care must be taken to image the valve at the level of the tips of the mitral valve leaflets, not at the base of the mitral valve funnel

because this will result in a falsely large orifice area. The latter can be avoided by determining the maximal vertical diastolic separation of the leaflet tips from the parasternal long axis view and rotating the transducer 90° to the short axis. From the short axis view, the transducer is angled and a sweep is performed along the long axis of the left ventricle toward the papillary muscles, and then angled slowly cephalad to the point at which the mitral leaflet tips first reappear (14, 15). The inside edge of the valve is planimetered, regardless of how thick and immobile the leaflets appear, and the

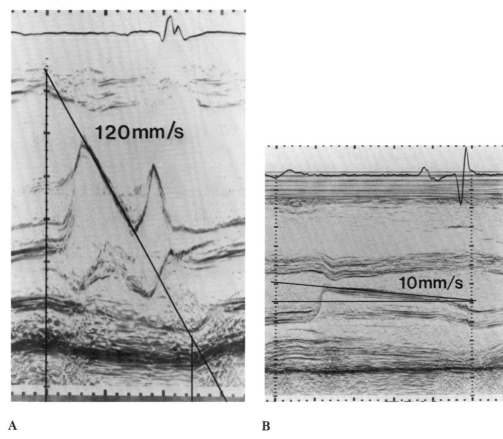

A   B

Figure 7.3. M-mode echocardiogram of a normal mitral valve showing partial closure of the anterior leaflet in early diastole (EF slope). A tangent to the anterior leaflet enables calculation of the peak diastolic closing velocity, which in this normal subject is 120 mm/sec (*A*). By contrast, a tangent to the anterior mitral valve leaflet in a patient with rheumatic mitral stenosis (*B*) demonstrates an EF slope or peak diastolic closing velocity of 10 mm/sec (moderately severe mitral stenosis was described initially as a closing velocity less than 36 mm/sec).

gain settings adjusted to obtain clear images without "blooming," since too much gain will result in underestimation of the mitral orifice area (Fig. 7.7). Mitral valve orifice areas measured by planimetry from two-dimensional echocardiograms have correlated closely with those calculated using the Gorlin hydraulic formula at cardiac catheterization (14–17) (Fig. 7.8). In 5% to 10% of patients, the images of the mitral valve leaflets are unsatisfactory because the orifice is eccentric and the opening cannot be completely visualized in

Figure 7.4. M-mode echocardiogram from a patient with severe calcific rheumatic mitral stenosis with atrial fibrillation, showing variation in the EF slope with cycle length. There is also calcification of the mitral subvalve apparatus.

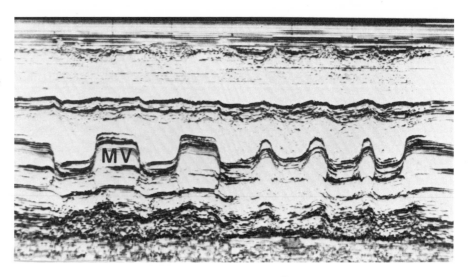

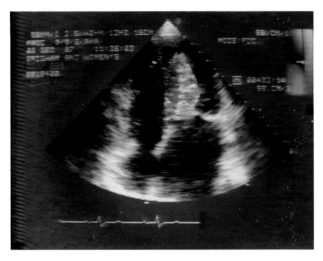

A

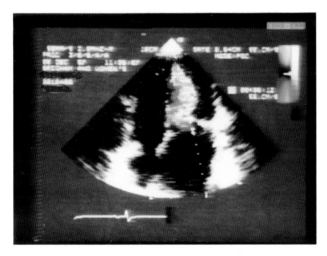

B

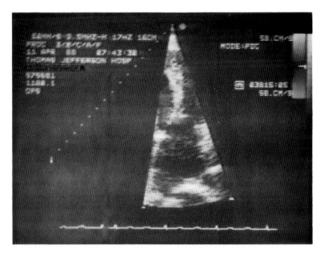

C

Figure 7.18. Two-dimensional echocardiogram of the apical four chamber view with color-flow Doppler in mitral stenosis. The flame shaped high-velocity signal extends almost to the left ventricular apex. The mosaic colored signal represents aliasing of the high velocity turbulent transmitral blood flow. All panels show similar signals to identify the area of the jet, which is used to position the pulsed-wave sample volume and to demonstrate the direction of the jet for subsequent nonimaging continuous-wave Doppler recordings.

Plate IV

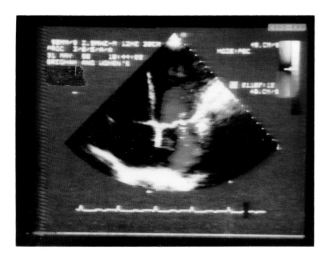

A

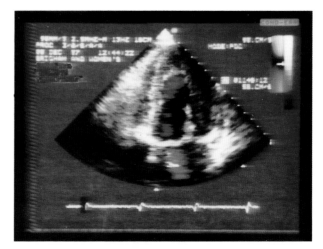

B

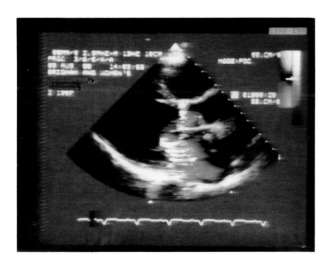

C

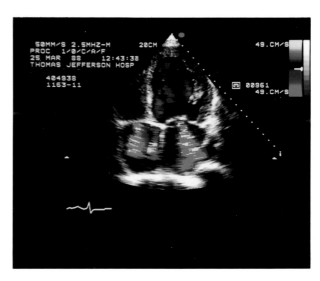

D

Figure 7.40. Color-flow Doppler demonstrating the regurgitant blood flow of mitral regurgitation as a blue signal in systole (blood flow away from the transducer encoded in blue) in the apical four chamber view (*A*) and apical two chamber view (*B*). The width and area of the regurgitant jet is also visible in the parasternal long axis view (*C*). Color-flow map in the apical four chamber view in a patient with co-existent mitral regurgitation and tricuspid regurgitation (*D*). The mitral regurgitant jet has a narrow initial width, but extends to the roof of the left atrium and into the left inferior pulmonary vein.

Plate V

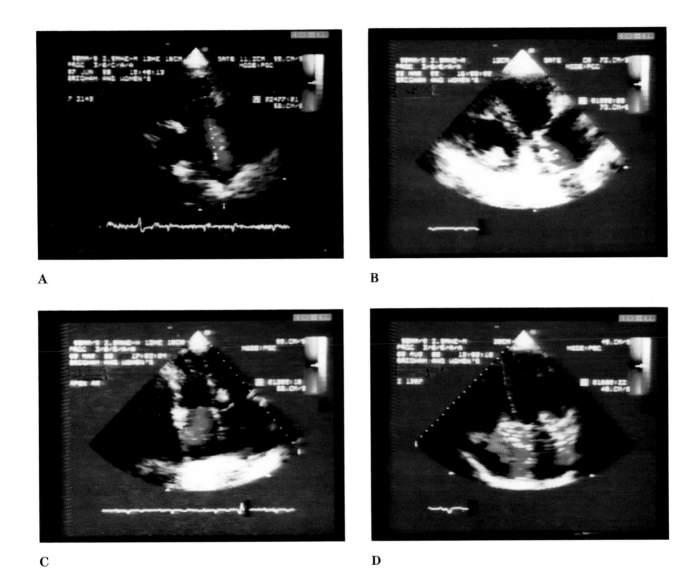

A

B

C

D

Figure 7.81. Color-flow Doppler velocity maps showing tricuspid regurgitation as a blue mosaic colored jet from the right ventricular inflow view (*A* and *B*) and from the apical four chamber view (*C*). There is coexistent mitral regurgitation (*D*).

Plate VI

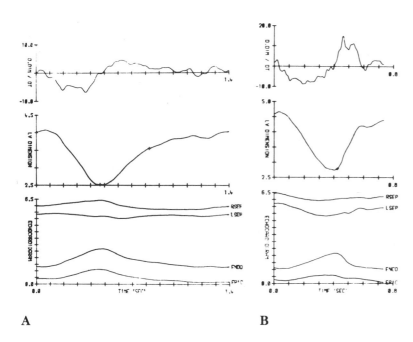

A   B

Figure 7.5. Computer output of a digitized M-mode echocardiogram from a patient with mitral stenosis (*A*, bottom graph), showing the *xy* coordinates of the right side of the septum and the posterior wall endo- and epicardium. In the second graph is continuous left ventricular dimension with time, showing no discrete rapid filling phase. Left ventricular dimension increases steadily and slowly throughout diastole. The peak rate of increase in left ventricular dimension in the top graph is 5 cm/sec (normal 14 ± 3 cm/sec). A computer output of a digitized M-mode echocardiogram from a normal subject shows the *xy* coordinates of the echocardiogram (*B*, bottom graph). In the second graph is continuous left ventricular dimension, which shows a discrete rapid filling phase followed by a slow filling phase. In the top graph is the peak rate of change of left ventricular dimension, which is 14 cm/sec.

a single plane. This occurs more often following mitral valvotomy, when attempts to measure valve area may be unrewarding (18).

In the parasternal long axis view of the left ventricle, mitral valve leaflet motion can be visualized in profile (Fig. 7.9). Fusion of the commissures, and thickening and shortening of the chordae tendineae result in sudden diastolic arrest of the tip of the anterior leaflet, so that the body of the leaflet has a characteristic "bent-knee" deformity in mild to moderate stenosis. As the leaflets increase in thickness and become heavily calcified, there is further restriction of movement due to chordal shortening and cicatrization, and the bent-knee deformity is lost (Fig. 7.10). The leaflets then exhibit either minimal excursion or appear immobile from diastole to systole, often with development of concomitant mitral regurgitation.

The rheumatic process involves the whole of the mitral valve unit (19), so that the mitral valve leaflets, subvalve apparatus, chordal length, and the degree of thickness of the mitral valve annulus should all be carefully assessed by two-dimensional echo. This is particularly important in two circumstances: first, in the preoperative selection of patients for mitral valve reconstruction surgery, which should be contemplated in all patients because primary bioprosthetic failure occurs in 25% of patients at 10 years and because of the risks of hemorrhagic complications from long-term anticoagulation with mechanical prostheses (20, 21); and second, in selecting patients for mitral balloon valvuloplasty and predicting the success of this new

form of therapy. The chordae tendineae in severe calcific rheumatic mitral valve disease may be very thick, shortened, and fused, causing retraction and eversion of the cusps, with heavy calcification extending from the leaflets to the tips of the hypertrophied papillary muscles (19) (Fig. 7.10). Furthermore, calcification may spread circumferentially around the mitral valve annulus, and on occasion result in mitral inflow obstruction below the level of the valve leaflets (22).

In pure rheumatic mitral stenosis, left ventricular dimensions and wall thickness and function are normal, although septal motion may be abnormal when pulmonary hypertension or severe tricuspid regurgitation supervene (23). The left atrium is invariably enlarged and may be aneurysmal, with thrombus formation occurring most commonly in the appendage. Whenever left atrial thrombus is suspected, it should be diagnosed only if it is visualized as a filling defect in at least two orthogonal echocardiographic views (Fig. 7.11).

In isolated mild rheumatic mitral stenosis, the right ventricular and right atrial chamber sizes are usually normal (Fig. 7.12). With increasing severity of mitral stenosis, there is progressive left atrial hypertension and dilatation of the right heart chambers (Fig. 7.13) due to increased pulmonary artery pressure with subsequent development of tricuspid regurgitation. The thickened mitral leaflets and their restricted excursion, as well as the sizes of the right heart chambers, should be inspected from the apical two as well as the four chamber and apical left ventricular long axis views

A

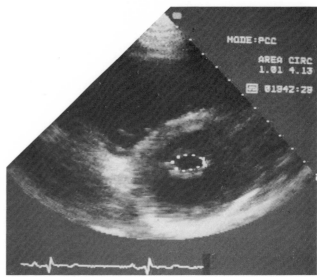

B

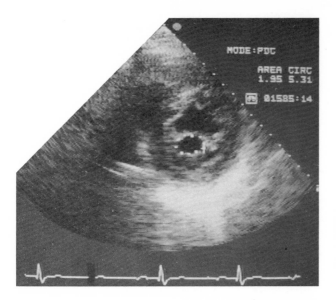

C

Figure 7.6. Two-dimensional echocardiogram of the LV short axis at mitral valve level, showing the mitral valve leaflets with thickened and calcified septal and lateral commissures and a reduced mitral valve orifice, in three patients with rheumatic mitral stenosis with increasing severity from A–C. Mitral valve area is 1.9 cm^2 in A, and 1.0 cm^2 in B. The patient in B also has a large right ventricle and flat interventricular septum. The patient shown in C has a mitral valve orifice area of 0.8 cm^2, abnormal septal motion, and an enlarged right ventricle.

(Figs. 7.14, 7.15). Approximately 85% of patients with pulmonary artery systolic pressures of >40 mmHg have tricuspid regurgitation (24). Tricuspid regurgitation is associated with further right ventricular dilatation and alteration of chamber architecture with disruption of the normal tricuspid valve unit and increased tricuspid ring circumference, which results in more severe tricuspid incompetence and reversed interventricular septal motion. In rheumatic mitral valve disease, the tricuspid valve may itself be involved in varying degrees in the rheumatic process, with fibrous thickening and retraction of the leaflets, and restricted leaflet motion with resultant stenosis and/or regurgitation (25–27) (Fig. 7.16).

Because the tricuspid and aortic valves are also frequently involved in rheumatic heart disease, they should be carefully examined with two-dimensional echo and with pulsed, continuous-wave, and color-flow Doppler mapping. The presence and severity of pulmonary hypertension should be estimated with continuous-wave Doppler from the peak velocity of the tricuspid regurgitant jet (vide infra) because pulmonary hypertension is a major determinant of prognosis following mitral valve surgery.

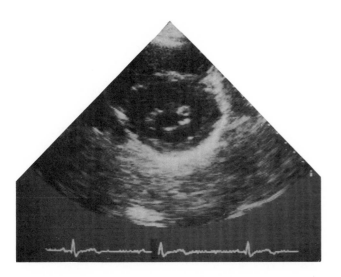

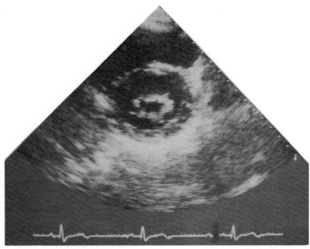

A   **B**

Figure 7.7. Two-dimensional echocardiogram of the short axis of the left ventricle at mitral valve level (*A*). The same patient is shown with the gain setting increased (*B*) so more echoes emanate from the mitral valve leaflets, resulting in a calculated mitral valve orifice area that is spuriously low.

DOPPLER

Doppler has added a hemodynamic limb to the two-dimensional echocardiographic assessment of mitral stenosis (28–33). The instantaneous pressure gradient across the mitral valve can be calculated from the transmitral blood flow velocity using the Bernoulli equation, which relates the pressure difference across the stenosis to the flow velocity distal to the stenosis, flow acceleration, and viscous frictional resistance:

$$P_1 - P_2 = \underbrace{\tfrac{1}{2}\rho\,(V_2^{\,2} - V_1^{\,2})}_{\substack{\text{convective}\\\text{acceleration}}} + \underbrace{\rho \int_1^2 \frac{dv}{dt}\,ds}_{\substack{\text{flow}\\\text{acceleration}}} + \underbrace{R(v)}_{\substack{\text{viscous}\\\text{friction}}}$$

The viscous friction component in the human heart is small because the cross-sectional area of the flow stream is large relative to its perimeter, so that the proportion of blood in contact with the vessel wall is relatively small. For all practical purposes the viscous friction component can be omitted. The flow acceleration term is only relevant over the short period during which the valve opens and closes. In addition, the flow velocity proximal to the stenosis is usually less than 1.0 m/sec, so that when squared, it becomes inconsequentially small. The Bernoulli equation can therefore be greatly simplified to

$$P_1 - P_2 = 4(V_{max})^2.$$

Thus, in mitral stenosis, the pressure difference across the valve and the velocity downstream are quadratically related. The peak, mean, and end-diastolic mitral valve gradients calculated from the Doppler signals are of clinical importance as noninvasive indices of the severity of mitral stenosis. The Doppler pulsed-wave sample volume is positioned immediately downstream

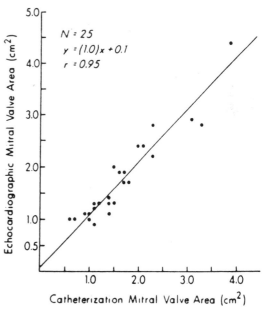

Figure 7.8. Comparison between mitral valve orifice area calculated by planimetry from stop action frames from two-dimensional echocardiograms and mitral valve orifice area calculated from the hemodynamics obtained at cardiac catheterization employing the Gorlin formula show close correlation between the two techniques. (Reproduced with permission of the American Heart Association, Inc. from Nichol PM, Gilbert BW, Kisslo JA. Two dimensional echocardiographic assessment of mitral stenosis. Circulation 1977;55:124.)

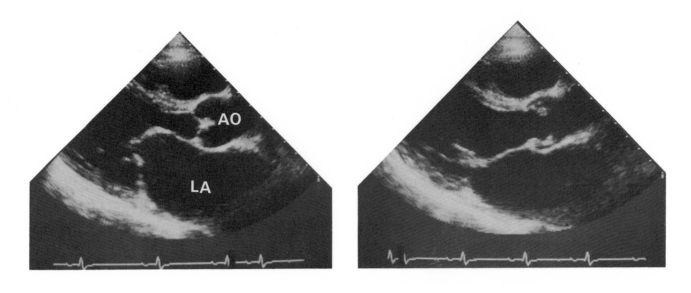

A   **B**

Figure 7.9.   Two-dimensional echocardiogram of the long axis view of the left ventricle in rheumatic mitral stenosis shows the characteristic bent-knee deformity of the anterior leaflet in diastole (*A*) due to the chordal shortening of the thickened mitral valve leaflets. The left atrium is enlarged and the aortic valve commissures are thickened, indicating a rheumatic valve etiology. In systole (*B*), the thickened aortic valve leaflets can be better visualized.

from the stenotic mitral valve with simultaneous two-dimensional echo imaging, and it is moved with the guidance of the audio signal until it is located in the high-velocity jet coming through the mitral orifice. The Doppler sample volume is then repositioned until the velocity spectral envelope with the maximum amplitude is obtained (Fig. 7.17). Location of the high-velocity antegrade jet can be facilitated with color-flow

Doppler from the apical four chamber view (Fig. 7.18, Plate IV). The high-velocity jet can be recognized as a flame shaped, multicolored area of red and blue in the center, with a mosaic of yellow-green around it, which may extend from the mitral valve leaflets for a variable distance toward the left ventricular apex (34). The yellow-green mosaic appearance represents turbulence, while in the central area the red surrounded by

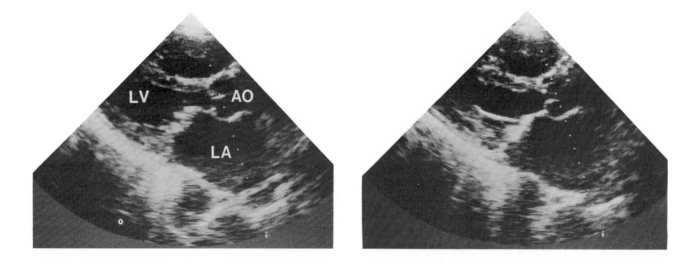

A   **B**

Figure 7.10.   Two-dimensional echocardiogram of the LV long axis showing heavily calcified mitral valve leaflets with severely restricted motion in diastole (*A*) and in systole (*B*). There is no bent-knee deformity consistent with severe calcific rheumatic mitral stenosis (*A*). Calcification extends into the subvalve structures, resulting in markedly thickened and shortened chordae. Aortic valve leaflets are also thickened and their motion restricted due to commissural adhesions. The left atrium is markedly enlarged.

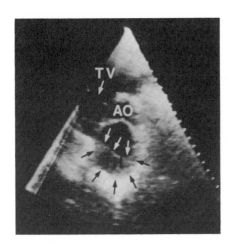

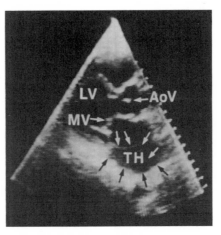

A   **B**

Figure 7.11. Two-dimensional echocardiogram of the left ventricle in short axis from a patient with rheumatic mitral stenosis, demonstrating an enlarged left atrium with thrombus on the posterior left atrial wall (*A*), which is seen in the orthogonal view of the short axis of the aorta and left atrium (*B*).

blue, often in several alternating layers, represents aliasing because the peak velocity exceeds the Nyquist limit of the color flow system (see Chapter 2). In severe mitral stenosis, the peak velocity may exceed 2 m/sec, and depending upon the depth of the sample volume and the transducer frequency, may result in aliasing of the velocity signal if pulsed-wave Doppler is used. Antegrade mitral valve flow velocity should always be recorded with continuous-wave Doppler (Fig. 7.19), even when the velocity signal does not alias with pulsed-wave, so that the maximum velocity spectrum is obtained, from which hemodynamic calculations are made.

The characteristic Doppler features of mitral steno-sis are increased peak velocity, reduced rate of decrease in velocity with time, and augmentation of the velocity signal due to atrial contraction in those patients in sinus rhythm (Fig. 7.20). The increased transmitral blood flow velocity profile and its slow decline indicate a pressure gradient across the valve continuing throughout diastole. The pressure gradients across the mitral valve at any point in time are estimated employing the modified Bernoulli equation ($P_1 - P_2 = 4V^2$) and these values correlate closely with those calculated at cardiac catheterization from the Gorlin equation (Fig. 7.21).

In addition to calculation of the pressure gradients across the valve, the mitral valve orifice area can be

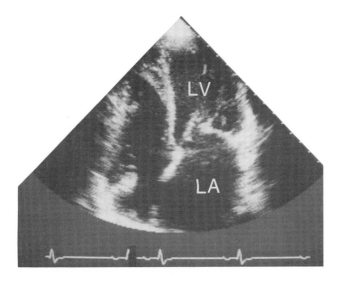

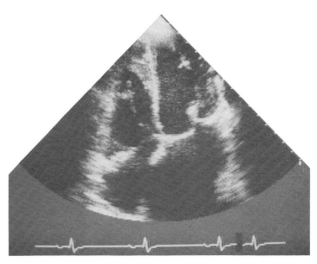

A   **B**

Figure 7.12. Two-dimensional echocardiogram of the apical four chamber view in rheumatic mitral stenosis. The restricted excursion of the anterior leaflet and fixed posterior leaflet allows only minimal separation of the cusps of the leaflets in diastole (*A*). The left ventricle is of normal size, and the calcification involves the valve leaflets and extends into the subvalve apparatus (*A* and *B*). The left atrium is markedly enlarged with the interatrial septum bulging toward the right atrium.

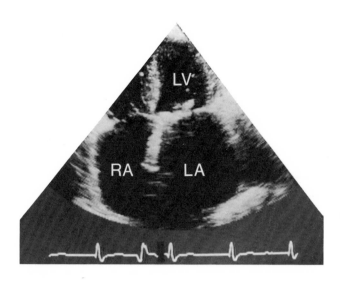

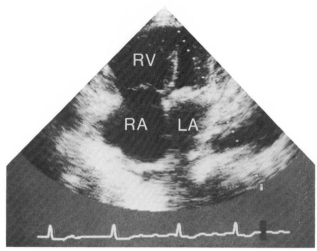

A

B

Figure 7.13.   Two-dimensional echocardiogram of the apical four chamber view from two patients with severe calcific rheumatic mitral stenosis. The left atrium and right atrium are considerably enlarged (*A*) due to pulmonary venous hypertension and tricuspid regurgitation, while the left ventricular size remains normal. There is severe pulmonary hypertension with massive dilatation of the right ventricle and right atrium, compared to the left ventricle, due to associated functional tricuspid regurgitation secondary to untreated chronic severe rheumatic mitral stenosis (*B*).

determined by estimating the transmitral diastolic pressure half-time (35, 36). The mitral pressure half-time can be calculated from the velocity signal as the time interval over which the velocity falls from its maximum value to its maximum value divided by the square root of 2 (Fig. 7.22). Since the transmitral pressure gradient and blood flow velocity is related by a square power function, mitral valve orifice area is obtained from the following relationship:

$$MVA = 220/t_{1/2},$$

where 220 is a constant, and $t_{1/2}$ is the pressure half-time (35, 36).

The normal pressure half-time is less than 100 msec; in mild mitral stenosis, it is approximately 160 msec, and in severe MS is 220 msec, consistent with a mitral valve orifice area of 1.0 cm^2. Transmitral Doppler flow velocity signals can be obtained in virtually every patient, even when two-dimensional echocardiographic imaging of the valve itself is technically unsatisfactory. This is especially true in patients post–mitral

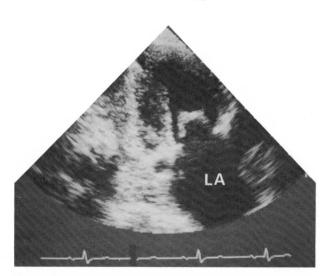

Figure 7.14.   Two-dimensional echocardiogram of the apical two chamber view, showing a thickened calcified mitral valve in a patient with rheumatic mitral stenosis and marked left atrial dilatation.

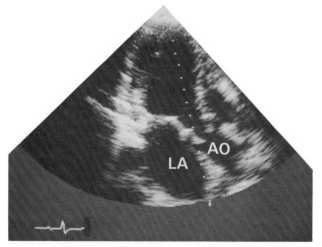

Figure 7.15.   Two-dimensional echocardiogram of the apical LV long axis in the same patient as Fig. 7.14, showing the calcification involving the mitral valve leaflets, and rheumatic thickening and reduced excursion of the aortic valve leaflets.

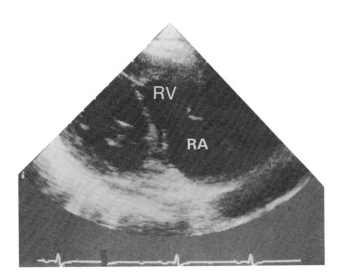

A

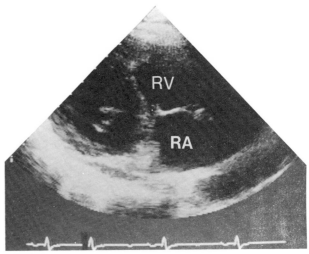

B

Figure 7.16.   Two-dimensional echocardiogram of the right ventricular inflow tract, showing restricted diastolic motion (*A*) and nodular thickening of the septal and anterior tricuspid valve leaflets in systole (*B*).

valvotomy, when the mitral valve orifice usually cannot be imaged in a single plane (18). The mitral valve orifice areas calculated from pressure half-times measured from transmitral flow velocity recordings have in general corresponded closely with nonsimultaneous estimates of valve area obtained at cardiac catheterization using the Gorlin formula (Fig. 7.23) (37).

Mitral valve area can also be calculated using the continuity principle (37), which states that volume flow per unit time through a stenosis is equal to the volume flow either proximal and/or distal to the stenosis, provided cardiac output does not change between the recordings. Volume flow is assessed as the product of the flow velocity integral (FVI) and the cross-sectional area of the flow stream (Fig. 7.24). Applying the continuity equation,

volume flow in the nonstenotic zone = volume flow at stenosis

$$FVI_1 \times CSA_1 = FVI_2 \times CSA_2$$

Mitral valve orifice area in mitral stenosis is therefore determined by solving the continuity equation for the one unknown, that is, CSA of the mitral orifice. The aortic or the pulmonary artery cross-sectional areas are calculated from measurements of vessel diameter because they can be regarded as circular in cross-section. The blood flow velocity spectra are recorded either in the proximal aorta or the proximal pulmonary artery, where the vessel diameters are measured. The blood flow velocity spectrum across the stenosed mitral valve orifice is obtained either with pulsed- or continuous-wave Doppler. The mitral valve area is then computed as the product of the aortic or pulmonary artery cross-sectional area and the ratio of the flow

velocity integral of the aortic or pulmonary artery to that of the mitral stenotic jet (37):

$$CSA_2 = \frac{FVI_1}{FVI_2} \times CSA_1$$

The mitral valve areas calculated from Doppler recordings employing the continuity equation correlate closely with the mitral valve areas calculated at cardiac

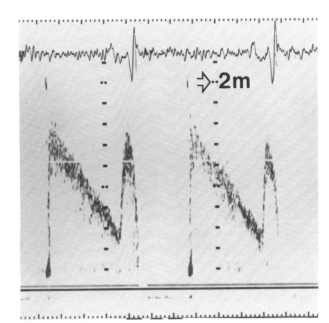

Figure 7.17.   Pulsed-wave Doppler blood flow velocity signal across the mitral valve in mild mitral stenosis. Peak velocity is increased above normal with a maximum velocity of 1.4 m/sec, followed by slow deceleration and further increase in velocity during atriosystolic contraction.

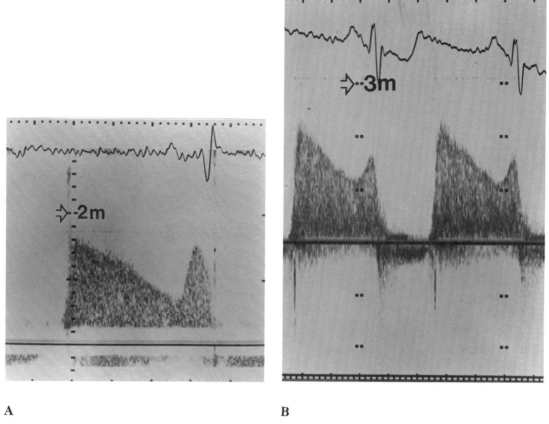

A   B

Figure 7.19. Continuous-wave Doppler flow velocity signals from two patients with rheumatic mitral stenosis in sinus rhythm. Peak velocity approaches 1.6 m/sec in a patient with mild mitral stenosis, with a peak gradient of 10 mmHg (*A*). It exceeds 2 m/sec in a patient with severe mitral stenosis and a peak gradient of 18 mmHg (*B*). High-quality velocity signals are of paramount importance if transmitral valve gradients or pressure half times are to be estimated.

Figure 7.20. Continuous-wave Doppler signal from a patient with rheumatic mitral stenosis in atrial fibrillation. The peak velocity varies little (1.8 to 2.0 m/sec), consistent with a gradient of approximately 13 to 16 mmHg in early diastole. The velocity decays to zero by end diastole with long cycle lengths, so that there is equilibration of the pressures across the mitral valve at end diastole. Consecutive velocity signals in atrial fibrillation show zero gradient after long cardiac cycles, but 4 to 5 mmHg gradients with short cycle lengths.

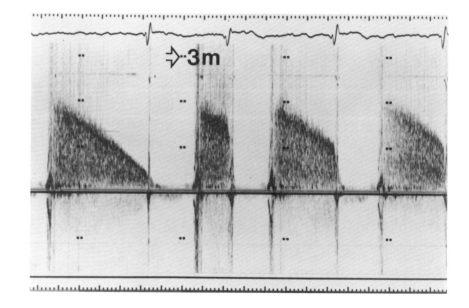

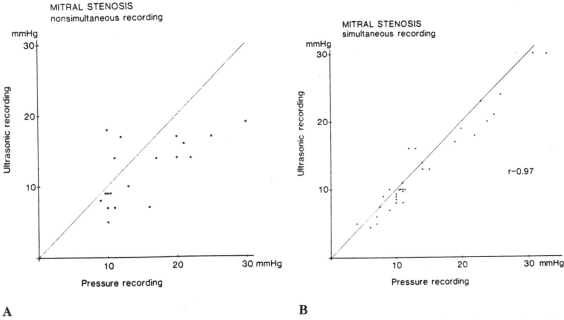

Figure 7.21.   Comparison of transmitral valve gradients estimated by Doppler and by cardiac catheterization when the studies were performed simultaneously (*A*) show a closer correlation than when the studies were not performed simultaneously (*B*). (Reproduced with permission from Hatle L, Angelson B. Doppler ultrasound in cardiology. 2 ed. Lea & Febiger, 1985, p. 117.)

catheterization (37) (Fig. 7.25), and with Doppler calculations of mitral valve area using the pressure half-time methods in those patients with pure mitral stenosis. In patients with mitral stenosis and concomitant aortic regurgitation, the pressure half-time methods for calculating mitral valve area result in significant overestimation of the true mitral valve area (37) (Figs. 7.23, 7.26). By contrast, mitral valve area calculated from Doppler recordings using the continuity equation correlate well with measurements made at cardiac catheterization, regardless of the presence of aortic regurgitation (37) (Fig. 7.25). Thus, in patients with mitral stenosis and co-existent aortic regurgitation, the continuity equation should be used to quantify mitral valve area noninvasively.

MITRAL REGURGITATION

Mitral regurgitation can result from primary disease in any one of the component parts of the mitral valve—in the valve leaflets (from rheumatic mitral valve disease and endocarditis), the chordal structures (from elongation or rupture, as may occur in mitral valve prolapse), the papillary muscles (when they become dysfunctional from myocardial infarction), and the annulus (when it dilates secondary to left ventricular chamber enlargement). Mitral regurgitation may also result from changes in left ventricular cavity architecture, as in dilated cardiomyopathy in which the left ventricle becomes more spherical than ellipsoidal. Left

ventricular dilatation results in displacement of the papillary muscles laterally with respect to the long axis of the left ventricle so that they are further apart than normal. Since there is no change in the length of the chordae, the leaflets are unable to coapt normally.

In a series of 97 consecutive patients undergoing mitral valve surgery for chronic severe isolated mitral regurgitation, 60 had mitral valve prolapse, and 13 of those had ruptured chordae tendinae, 20 had papillary muscle dysfunction, 6 had infective endocarditis, and 2 had rheumatic involvement (38).

The echocardiographic appearance of the mitral valve leaflets in mitral regurgitation may be completely normal, but often their appearance provides insight into the patho-etiology of the regurgitation. The secondary effects of the volume overload on left atrial and left ventricular sizes, left ventricular remodeling, and residual left ventricular contractile function vary with the severity and the time course of mitral regurgitation. In chronic severe mitral regurgitation, the left ventricle and the left atrium are enlarged, and ventricular function ranges from supranormal to severely subnormal. By contrast, in acute severe mitral regurgitation, the left atrium and ventricle may be normal size, but the left ventricle is usually hyperdynamic.

The diagnosis of mitral regurgitation by M-mode echocardiography is made indirectly from the combination of an enlarged volume-overloaded left ventricle with vigorous endocardial motion, the abnormal appearance of the mitral valve leaflets (Fig. 7.27), a

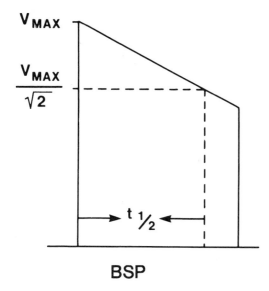

A

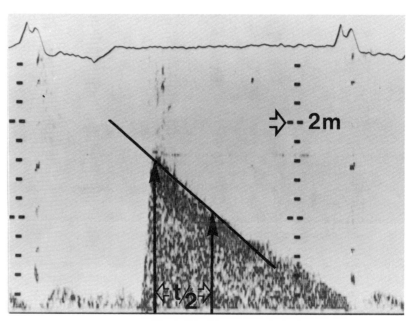

B

Figure 7.22. Schematic showing how to calculate the pressure half-time from a Doppler velocity signal. Since the transmitral pressure gradient is related to the blood flow velocity immediately distal to the stenotic valve by a square power function, the pressure half-time ($t_{1/2}$) can be calculated as the time during which the maximum velocity (V_{max}) decays to $V_{max}/\sqrt{2}$. The mitral valve area can be calculated from the $t_{1/2}$ as: MVA = $220/t_{1/2}$ (*A*). Doppler transmitral flow velocity signal is shown in *B*, where the $t_{1/2}$ has been calculated to be approximately 200 msec, which corresponds to mitral valve orifice area of 1.1 cm^2.

dilated left atrium, and sometimes early closure of the aortic valve as left ventricular ejection continues into the low resistance left atrium (39–45) (Fig. 7.28). The mitral leaflets often demonstrate the patho-etiology of the regurgitation, such as leaflet prolapse (Fig. 7.29), flail leaflets, vegetations (Fig. 7.30), rheumatic commissural thickening (Fig. 7.31), etc. (39–43). The M-mode echocardiographic findings of severe chronic mitral regurgitation include markedly increased left ventricular end-diastolic dimension, usually with equivalent increase in septal and posterior left ventricular wall endocardial excursion (Fig. 7.27). The increased endocardial motion in diastole is due to the rapid inflow of blood from the left atrium, and in systole because a

proportion of the stroke volume is ejected into the left atrium against minimal resistance. Left ventricular fractional shortening may be normal, increased, or decreased. Exaggerated wall motion is not specific for mitral regurgitation and may occur in any condition that results in volume overload of the left ventricle, for example, profound anemia, aortic regurgitation, and extreme bradycardia. The left ventricular rapid early diastolic filling is highly suggestive of mitral regurgitation, however, and computer analysis of the digitized M-mode echocardiogram demonstrates markedly elevated peak rates of increase in left ventricular dimension (peak filling rates) (11, 12) (Fig. 7.32) and acquisition of maximum left ventricular dimension early in

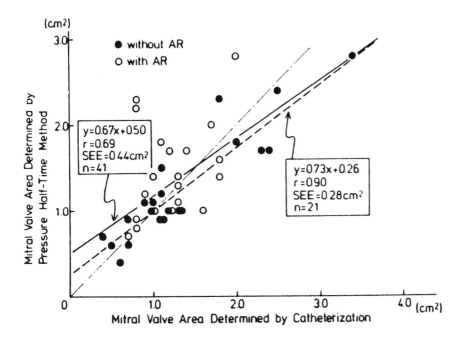

Figure 7.23. Comparison of mitral valve area estimated by Doppler and by cardiac catheterization demonstrates a closer correlation in patients with mitral stenosis and no aortic regurgitation (N = 21, r = 0.90), than in patients with mitral stenosis and concomitant aortic regurgitation (N = 41, r = 0.69.) (Reproduced by permission of the American Heart Association, Inc., from Nakatani S, Masuyama T, Kodama K, et al. Value and limitations of Doppler echocardiography in the quantification of stenotic mitral valve area: comparison of the pressure half-time and the continuity equation methods. Circulation; 1988:7:81.)

diastole. When mitral regurgitation occurs in dilated cardiomyopathy, or following myocardial infarction involving the papillary muscles, the left ventricle is dilated, but wall motion is decreased, mitral valve closure is incomplete (46), and systolic expansion of the left atrium is not apparent because of the impaired left ventricular pump function and diminished stroke volume.

The left atrium is usually dilated in mitral regurgitation and measurements of the rate of left atrial emptying are increased (47–49). However, left atrial emptying rate has not proved useful clinically because of overlap between mild and severe mitral regurgitation (48). The posterior aortic root motion is exaggerated in mitral regurgitation compared to normal, but this varies greatly with different transducer placement and angulation and also with left ventricular contractile function (48).

Two-dimensional echocardiography enables characterization and quantitation of the changes in left ventricular architecture and function that occur as the left ventricle remodels in response to the chronic volume overload of mitral regurgitation. The left ventricular cavity is not only dilated (Figs. 7.33, 7.34), but becomes more globular than ellipsoid in shape, with increase in the radius of curvature of the left side of the septum (Fig. 7.35). The alteration in ventricular shape occurs because, as the volume overload increases in severity, the left ventricle dilates by increasing its short axis to a greater extent than its long axis. The short/long axis ratio approaches unity, thereby achieving the largest possible chamber volume per unit perimeter. In chronic severe mitral regurgitation, left ventricular wall and septal motion are characteristically equally

increased, and this can be visualized in real time in the conventional left ventricular short axis images obtained from the left parasternal region. Furthermore, maximum left ventricular volume occurs very early in diastole. In the apical four chamber view, the enlarged left atrium may expand in systole (Fig. 7.36). In severe mitral regurgitation, the size of the right heart chambers may be normal initially, but when the mitral regurgitation is not corrected, myocardial contractile dysfunction develops due to cavity dilatation with concomitant increased wall stress. This leads to left ventricular failure (50) and, in time, dilatation of the right heart chambers due to secondary pulmonary hypertension and consequent tricuspid regurgitation.

When mitral regurgitation develops due to papillary muscle dysfunction in coronary artery disease or from left ventricular dilatation in dilated cardiomyopathy, segmental wall motion abnormalities, the size of the left ventricle, and the severe global dysfunction, respectively, are the stigmata that indicate the likely etiology (Fig. 7.37).

Although the diagnosis of mitral regurgitation can be made only inferentially by echocardiographic imaging, it can be established unequivocally by Doppler (29, 51–57). Mitral regurgitation can be detected with pulsed-wave Doppler when the sample volume is positioned in the left atrium immediately proximal to the mitral valve in the apical four, apical two chamber or apical long axis views, and the presence of high velocity turbulent retrograde systolic flow demonstrated (Fig. 7.38). Mitral regurgitation should be not just diagnosed, but its severity at least semiquantitated by flow mapping of the left atrium (52). Left atrial flow mapping entails placing the Doppler sample volume at increasing dis-

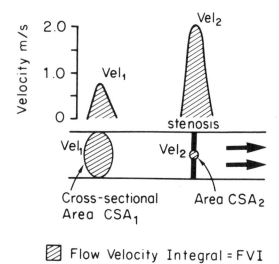

Continuity Equation:

$$FVI_1 \times CSA_1 = FVI_2 \times CSA_2$$

$$CSA_2 = \frac{FVI_1}{FVI_2} \times CSA_1$$

Figure 7.24. Schematic showing the continuity principle, which states that flow proximal to the stenosis is equal to flow through the stenosis. Flow is calculated as the product of the flow velocity integral, which is the area under the velocity signal, and the cross-sectional area of the flow stream. The flow velocity integral (FVI) proximal and distal to the stenosis and the area proximal to the stenosis can be calculated by Doppler echocardiography. The unknown stenotic valve orifice area can be calculated by solving the continuity equation for the stenotic valve area, which equals the ratio of FVI proximal and FVI distal multiplied by the cross-sectional area proximal to the stenosis.

tances from the mitral valve annulus, and progressively sampling for the presence of the regurgitant jet by moving the sample volume laterally from the interatrial septum to the free left atrial wall (52) (Fig. 7.39). Mild or 1+ mitral regurgitation is diagnosed when systolic retrograde flow is detected within a 1 cm radius of the mitral valve plane, and severe or 4+ mitral regurgitation is diagnosed when systolic regurgitant high-velocity flow is detectable throughout the left atrium (52). Problems in grading the severity of mitral regurgitation by flow mapping arise when the regurgitant jet is narrow, but reaches the roof of the left atrium and still is not detectable throughout the left atrium. These problems can be minimized if the jet area is expressed as a ratio of the total left atrial area. Care must be taken not to position the sample volume in the mitral valve

orifice because a systolic signal will be obtained, suggesting mitral regurgitation, as the leaflets normally bulge backward toward the left atrium during systole. The timing of the peak velocity in relation to the onset of systole has been suggested to indicate the severity of regurgitation. Thus, in severe mitral regurgitation, the peak velocity occurs early in systole, while in mild to moderate mitral regurgitation, the peak velocity occurs in mid- to late systole.

Color-flow Doppler is invaluable in establishing the diagnosis of mitral regurgitation (58–60), especially when it is mild or has unusual jet directions, as often occurs with mitral valve prolapse (Fig. 7.40, Plate V). Measurements of mitral regurgitant jet length, width, height, and area appear promising in semiquantitating mitral regurgitation (58–60) by color flow mapping.

The severity of mitral regurgitation has also been assessed by determining the regurgitant fraction (61, 62). Regurgitant fraction is obtained by estimating volume flow through the mitral valve orifice as the product of mitral annular cross-sectional area (which is assumed to be circular and constant throughout diastole) and the area under the transmitral blood flow velocity integral, and subtracting from it the volume flow through the aortic valve, which is estimated as the product of the cross-sectional area of the aorta and the aortic flow velocity integral. The difference between mitral and aortic volume flow expressed as a percentage of total transmitral volume flow is the regurgitant fraction. Doppler estimates of mitral regurgitant fraction have compared favorably with regurgitant fraction assessed at cardiac catheterization (60, 61) (Fig. 7.41).

MITRAL VALVE LEAFLET PROLAPSE

The first clinical description of mitral valve prolapse was in the early 1960s (65, 66) with subsequent angiographic demonstration in the mid-1960s (65, 66), and echocardiographic characterization in the early 1970s (67, 68). M-mode echocardiography reveals two characteristic patterns, namely, mid- to late systolic buckling and pan-systolic bowing of the mitral leaflets toward the posterior left atrial wall (Figs. 7.42, 7.43). Many attempts have been made to examine the sensitivity of echocardiography in the diagnosis of mitral valve prolapse, but a major confounding problem is that there is no gold standard for its diagnosis. It has been suggested that the auscultatory findings of a mid-systolic click or late systolic murmur should be the diagnostic criteria for mitral valve prolapse, and many echocardiographic studies have been based on this assumption (69).

In an M-mode echocardiographic study of 100 consecutive healthy young females, mid- or pan-systolic posterior motion of the mitral leaflets more than 2 mm

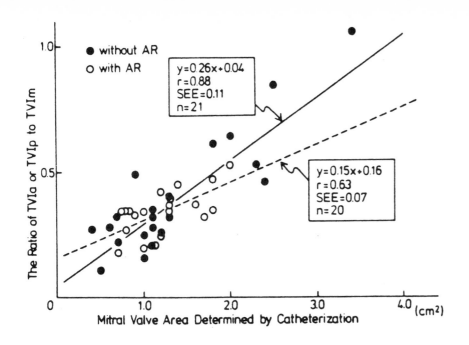

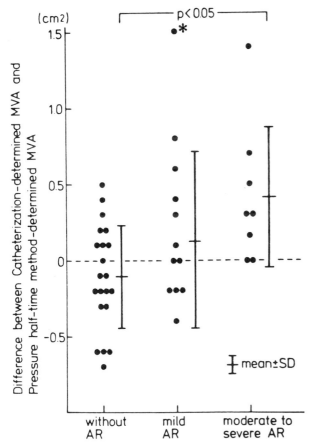

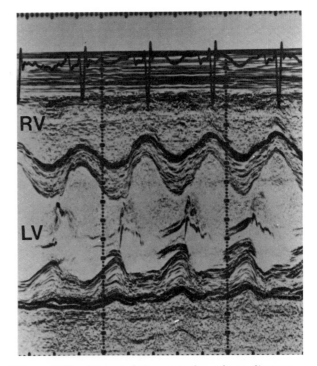

Figure 7.25. Comparison of mitral valve orifice areas calculated from Doppler velocity signals employing the continuity equation, and mitral valve areas calculated at cardiac catheterization. The closed symbols represent patients with mitral stenosis and no aortic regurgitation, and the open symbols represent patients with mitral stenosis and co-existent aortic regurgitation. The correlation was closer between the two techniques for patients with mitral stenosis and no aortic regurgitation (r = 0.88) than for patients with mitral stenosis and aortic regurgitation (r = 0.63). TVI_m is the time velocity integral of the stenotic mitral valve jet, and TVI_a and TVI_p are the time velocity integrals of the flow at aortic and pulmonic valve annuli, respectively. (Reproduced by permission of the American Heart Association, Inc., from Nakatani S, Masuyama T, Kodama K, et al. Value and limitations of Doppler echocardiography in the quantification of stenotic mitral valve area. Circulation; 1988;7:81.)

Figure 7.26. The discrepancy between the mitral valve area determined at cardiac catheterization, and the mitral valve area determined by pressure half-time using the Doppler velocity in rheumatic mitral stenosis increases progressively with increasing severity of concomitant aortic regurgitation. (Reproduced by permission of the American Heart Association, Inc. from Nakatani S, Masuyama T, Kodama K, et al. Value and limitations of Doppler echocardiography in the quantification of stenotic mitral valve area: comparison of the pressure half-time and the continuity equation methods. Circulation; 1988:7:82.)

Figure 7.27. M-mode left ventricular echocardiogram from a patient with chronic severe mitral regurgitation, showing a dilated left ventricular cavity, a vigorous contraction pattern due to volume overload, and increased excursion of the septum and posterior left ventricular wall. The anterior mitral valve leaflet is thickened in this patient because of mitral valve vegetative endocarditis.

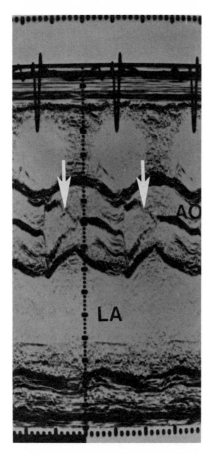

Figure 7.28. M-mode echocardiogram of the aorta, aortic valve, and left atrium from a patient with severe mitral regurgitation showing early aortic valve closure (*arrows*), which occurs before end ejection. Blood is ejected preferentially into the enlarged left atrium against low resistance.

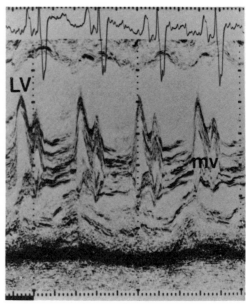

Figure 7.30. M-mode echocardiogram showing a mildly dilated left ventricle with an increased number of echoes emanating from the mitral valve leaflets because of mitral valve vegetative endocarditis.

below the CD line had a sensitivity of 59% and a specificity of 87% for auscultatory mitral valve prolapse (70). By contrast, the same echocardiographic signs of mid- and pan-systolic posterior movement in 100 patients with auscultatory evidence of mitral valve prolapse and 100 normal subjects were 85% sensitive and 99% specific for auscultatory mitral valve prolapse (71). The sensitivity and specificity of several other M-mode signs have been described in mitral valve prolapse. The following four M-mode echocardiographic signs were

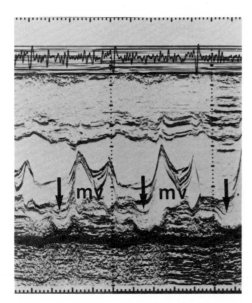

Figure 7.29. M-mode echocardiogram from a patient with mild mitral regurgitation due to late systolic mitral valve prolapse (*arrows*).

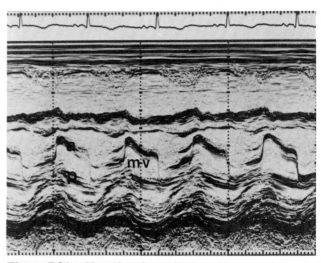

Figure 7.31. M-mode echocardiogram from a patient with moderate rheumatic mitral stenosis, showing the characteristic leaflet thickening, restricted excursion of the leaflets, and anterior motion of the posterior cusp. Left ventricular size and wall thickness are normal.

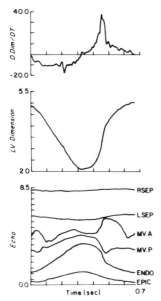

Figure 7.32. Computer output of the digitized M-mode echocardiogram from a patient with mitral regurgitation. The *XY* coordinates of the septum and posterior left ventricular wall are shown in the bottom graph. Above that is the continuous left ventricular dimension, which shows a brisk rapid filling phase. The top graph shows the increased peak rate of left ventricular filling (40 cm/sec; normal = 14.0 ± 2.0 cm/sec). Mitral regurgitation is characterized by rapid left ventricular filling and early acquisition of the maximum left ventricular dimension.

100% specific for mitral valve prolapse but had low sensitivity.

1. Anterior motion of the leaflets in early systole, followed by notching in mid-systole and late systolic posterior motion (10% sensitivity).

2. Systolic echoes in the mid left atrium (8% sensitivity).
3. Early diastolic (paradoxical) anterior motion of the posterior mitral leaflet (5% sensitivity).
4. Shaggy or multiple cascading echoes posterior to the mitral valve in diastole (3% sensitivity).

Three other echocardiographic signs, including multiple parallel systolic mitral valve echoes, increased early diastolic excursion of the anterior mitral leaflet (more than or equal to 25 mm), and abutment of the anterior mitral leaflet against the septum in early diastole, are also frequent findings in mitral valve prolapse.

When the diagnosis of mitral valve prolapse is anticipated, it is important to align the transducer perpendicular to the valve because incorrect angulation may produce both false negative and false positive results (72). Prolapse should not be diagnosed in patients with pericardial effusions because excessive cardiac motion within the pericardium may lead to "pseudo prolapse" (73).

Two-dimensional echocardiography has provided further insight into the pathophysiology of mitral valve prolapse (74). (Figs. 7.44–7.46). Several authors have suggested that the demonstration of one or both leaflets or the coaptation point superior to the plane of the mitral annulus in systole in either the parasternal or apical four chamber views should be considered as diagnostic of mitral leaflet prolapse (75, 76) (Figs. 7.44, 7.45). In a study of 70 patients with auscultatory mitral valve prolapse and 100 normal controls, these criteria provided 84% sensitivity and 97% specificity for mitral

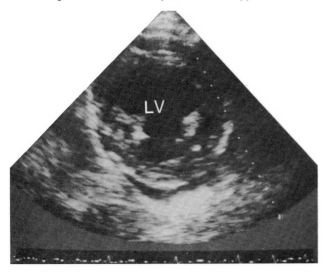

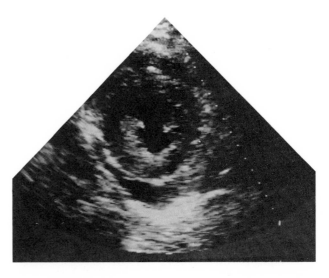

A   **B**

Figure 7.33. Two-dimensional echocardiogram of the left ventricular short axis from a patient with severe mitral regurgitation. The left ventricle is enlarged with an end-diastolic diameter of 7.2 cm (*A*) and an end-systolic diameter of 4.7 cm (*B*). There is mild left ventricular hypertrophy and good systolic contractile function. A small posterior pericardial effusion is also present.

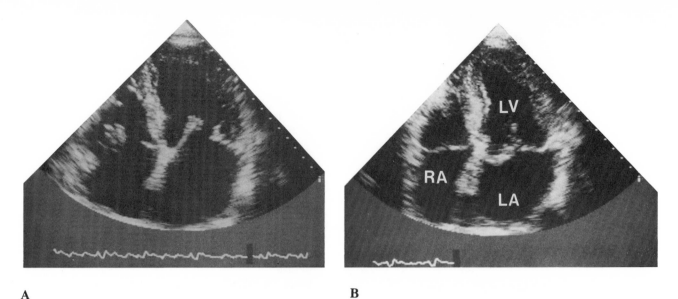

A   **B**

Figure 7.34. Two-dimensional echocardiogram of the apical four chamber view from a patient with severe mitral regurgitation, showing a dilated left ventricle and left atrium. The interatrial septum bulges toward the right atrium, and a myxomatous tricuspid valve leaflet is visualized in diastole (*A*). The mitral valve leaflets, which are thickened due to myxomatous changes in the cusps, prolapse into the left atrium in systole (*B*).

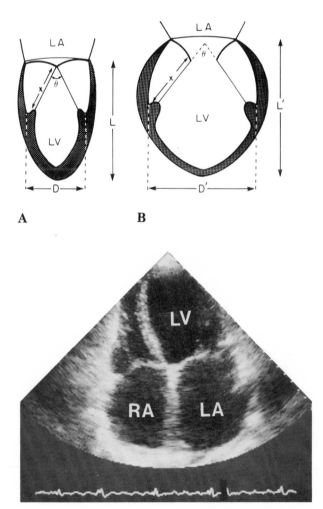

Figure 7.35. Schematic demonstrating the possible mechanism of mitral regurgitation. Left ventricular dilatation due to volume overload results in the left ventricle becoming more spherical (*A*, *B*). The mitral valve ring circumference increases. The angle subtended by the papillary muscles to the mitral annulus increases, but there is no elongation of the mitral valve leaflets or chordae, which results in incomplete cusp coaption and mitral regurgitation. Two-dimensional echocardiogram of the apical four chamber view showing a dilated left ventricle with increased radius of curvature of the interventricular septum as the left ventricle becomes more globular in shape (*C*). The left atrium is markedly dilated. The LV cavity has become more globular than spherical in shape, so the maximum left ventricular minor diameter is no longer at the base of the ventricle, but more toward the middle of the left ventricular long axis.

188

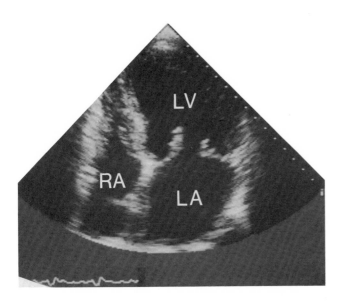

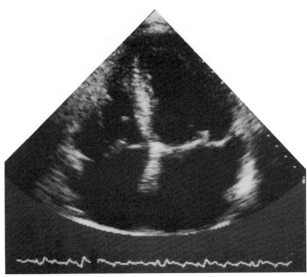

A

B

Figure 7.36. Two-dimensional echocardiogram of the apical four chamber view from a patient with severe mitral regurgitation, demonstrating increase in left atrial size from diastole (*A*) to systole (*B*) due to systolic expansion by the regurgitant blood flow.

prolapse (76). There were few false positives: the anterior leaflet bowed superior to the mitral annulus in three normal controls, two of whom also had bowing of the posterior leaflet. Other signs, such as excessive motion of the posterior mitral ring and whiplike motion of the mitral leaflets, were not significantly associated with the mitral prolapse, and had low sensitivities, 38% and 23%, respectively, with specificities of 88% and 87%, respectively. Similar findings were recorded by Spaccavento et al. (77), who reported 89% sensitivity and 93% specificity for these criteria, with false positives due to superior motion of either leaflet in only two of

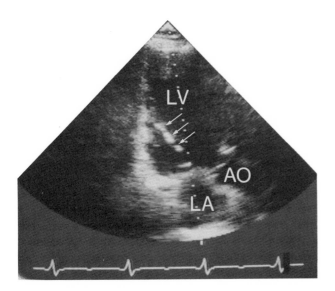

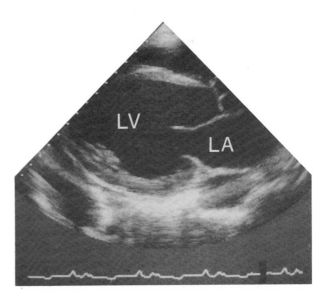

A

B

Figure 7.37. Two-dimensional echocardiogram of the apical LV long axis from a patient with mitral regurgitation due to posteroinferior myocardial infarction. There is scarring and fibrosis of the papillary muscle, which appears brighter than the adjacent myocardium (*A*). Two-dimensional echocardiogram of the LV long axis from the parasternal view route showing an enlarged globular left ventricle due to dilated cardiomyopathy, with mitral regurgitation resulting from left ventricular remodeling (*B*). The mitral valve ring is dilated, and the papillary muscles subtend a larger-than-normal angle to the mitral valve annulus; although the leaflets and chordae are intrinsically normal, they cannot coapt normally.

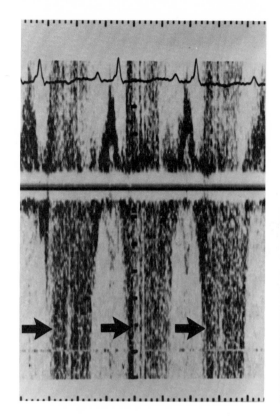

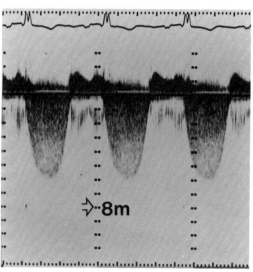

A   B

Figure 7.38.   Doppler velocity signal recorded with the sample volume in the left atrium in a patient with mitral regurgitation. The high velocity of the regurgitant blood flow into the left atrium in systole exceeds the Nyquist limit, resulting in aliasing (*A*). The velocity signal thus also appears on the upper register. The velocity signal recorded with continuous-wave Doppler from the apex in a patient with severe mitral regurgitation (*B*) shows mid-systolic peaking with a maximum velocity approaching 6 m/sec. Note that the duration of the velocity signal is holosystolic.

27 normals. False positive echocardiographic findings of mitral valve prolapse are reported more frequently (up to 23%) from the apical four chamber view due to superior displacement of one or both leaflets or the coaptation point, and can be provoked in approximately 50% of normal subjects with amyl nitrate inhalation (78).

One hundred presumed normal healthy subjects were evaluated in our laboratory (79) by auscultation and by combined M-mode and two-dimensional echocardiography. Five subjects had auscultatory evidence of prolapse, and three had M-mode evidence of prolapse (mid- or pan-systolic motion more than 2 mm below the CD line). By two-dimensional echocardiography, four had superior displacement in the parasternal long axis view. However, all five had superior displacement in the apical four chamber view. Of the 95 remaining subjects without auscultatory evidence of prolapse, three had M-mode evidence of mitral valve prolapse, two had superior displacement of only the posterior leaflet in the parasternal long axis view, and 23 had superior displacement of the anterior leaflet in the apical four chamber view. The discrepancies be-

tween findings of leaflet displacement or prolapse in the apical four chamber and long axis views of the left ventricle most probably result from the fact that the human mitral annulus, which is used as a reference, is saddle-shaped and nonplanar (80). Therefore careful consideration should be given to the relationship between mitral annular shape and leaflet motion during systole (80).

On the basis of a combination of our own study, previous reports, and in particular that of Devereux et al. (81–83), we suggest that the echocardiographic diagnosis of mitral valve prolapse be made when there is either M-mode evidence of mitral prolapse, or superior displacement of one or more of the valve leaflets or the coaptation point more than 2 mm behind the mitral annulus from the parasternal long axis view on two-dimensional echocardiograms (81–83). In addition to the characteristic pattern of motion described above, the mitral valve leaflets in mitral valve prolapse often appear thickened (Figs. 7.47, 7.48). In contrast to rheumatic mitral stenosis, however, they exhibit no commissural fusion and the leaflet mobility is excessive and not restricted. The apparent thickening is due

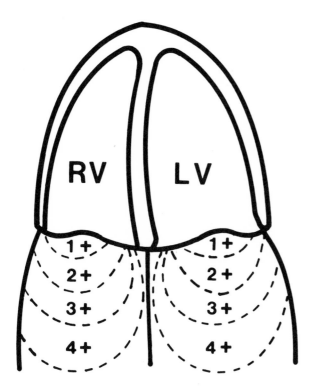

Figure 7.39. Schematic showing how the severity of mitral regurgitation and tricuspid regurgitation are semiquantitated by pulsed-wave Doppler flow mapping. The atria are each divided into four regions. When the pulsed-wave sample volume detects only high velocity systolic flow close to the mitral valve, mitral regurgitation is designated 1+ or mild. When the signal is detected throughout the left atrium, mitral regurgitation is severe or 4+.

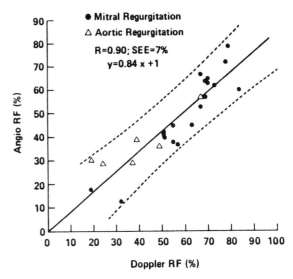

Figure 7.41. Comparison of the estimates of regurgitant fraction in mitral regurgitation (and aortic regurgitation) by angiography and Doppler shows close correlation between the techniques (r = 0.90). (Reproduced with permission from Rokey R, Sterling LL, Zoghi WA et al. Determination of regurgitant fraction in isolated mitral or aortic regurgitation by pulsed Doppler two-dimensional echocardiography. J Am Coll Cardiol 1986;7:1273–1278.)

to bending and scalloping of the free edges of the cusps, and also to myxomatous change and thickening of the leaflets themselves. Their increased motion may also come from minor third generation chordal rupture, which can be visualized in the apical two and four chamber views. The tensor apparatus and, in particular, the chordae tendineae to the two leaflets are elongated, resulting in overlap of the cusps during coaptation with increased vibratory motion of the chordae and papillary muscles.

The long-term prognosis of mitral valve prolapse documented echocardiographically has been examined in three studies, which have reported markedly different incidences of complications (84–86). Nishimura et al. (84) suggested in their six-year follow-up of 237 patients that survival was not different from age-matched normals, but a left ventricular end-diastolic dimension greater than 60 mm was the best predictor of the subsequent need for mitral valve replacement. Patients with redundant mitral leaflets have an increased risk (10.3%) of sudden death, infective endocarditis, and cerebral embolism, and these patients were identifiable by echocardiography (84). McMahon et al. (85) found that endocarditis in mitral valve

prolapse predominated in males over 45 years old who had systolic murmurs on auscultation (85). In the only prospective study of patients followed long-term with echocardiographic mitral valve prolapse, serious complications including sudden death, ventricular tachycardia, severe mitral regurgitation, cerebrovascular accidents, and infective endocarditis occurred in one-third (33%) of the total population over a six-year follow-up (86). The differences between these two large series are most probably explained by differences in inclusion criteria in the two studies.

CHORDAL RUPTURE

Mitral leaflet prolapse may be complicated by rupture of the chordae tendinae, which may be visualized on M-mode echocardiograms as a flail or excessively mobile mitral leaflet. The M-mode appearances vary and include fine systolic valve flutter (87), coarse diastolic anterior mitral leaflet flutter (88), and chaotic or paradoxical diastolic posterior leaflet motion (89). By two-dimensional echocardiography, the affected leaflet tip does not coapt with the other leaflet tip, and moves from the point of coaptation back into the left atrium during systole (90, 91) (Fig. 7.49). The leaflets may also prolapse in late diastole, even before the QRS complex (92). In some patients it is not possible to distinguish between severe prolapse and a true flail leaflet.

Mintz et al. (93) reported on the sensitivity and specificity of M-mode and two-dimensional echocardiographic signs of flail mitral leaflets in 45 patients

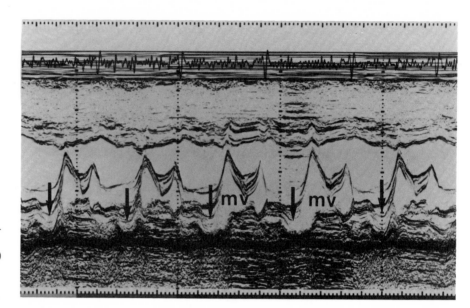

Figure 7.42. M-mode echocardiogram showing mid-systolic bowing of the mitral valve leaflets (*arrows*) due to mid-systolic mitral valve prolapse, which was confirmed by two-dimensional echocardiography.

who underwent surgery for pure mitral regurgitation. Twenty-six patients had ruptured chordae tendinae and 19 patients had intact chordae tendinae. M-mode echocardiographic findings had low sensitivity (60%), low specificity (53%), and a predictive accuracy of only 63%. The two-dimensional echocardiographic diagnosis of a flail mitral leaflet had a sensitivity of 96%, specificity of 84%, and a predictive accuracy of 89%. While the appearance of a flail mitral leaflet is often dramatic, its presence does not necessarily indicate that the patient requires corrective surgery. De Pace et al. (94) reported a group of 11 of 91 patients with a diagnosis of flail mitral leaflet who were treated successfully med-

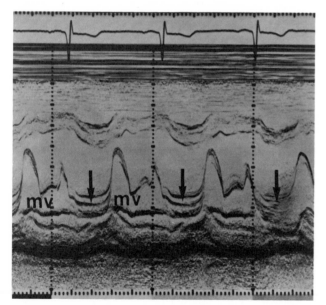

Figure 7.43. M-mode echocardiogram showing holosystolic bowing or hammocking of the mitral valve leaflets (*arrows*). Two-dimensional echocardiography demonstrated holosystolic mitral valve prolapse.

ically and remained hemodynamically stable without surgery at followup.

MITRAL ANNULAR CALCIFICATION

Mitral annular calcification is demonstrated by M-mode echocardiography as a dense band posterior to the mitral leaflets (Fig. 7.50), and by two-dimensional echocardiography as a dense mass posterior to the posterior mitral leaflet at the atrioventricular junction (Fig. 7.51). It may completely encircle the mitral valve annulus and extend into the aortic root (Fig. 7.52).

Calcification of the mitral annulus is one of the most common cardiac abnormalities seen at autopsy, occurring in 10% of autopsies in patients over 50 years of age (95), and with increased frequency with increasing age (96, 97). The incidence of mitral annular calcification assessed by M-mode echocardiography in 5694 subjects under the age of 59 in the Framingham study was less than 1% for both men and women, but it was 3% for both men and women aged 60–69. In women in the 70–79 age group and in the over 80 age group, the incidence was 12% and 22%, compared to 6% and 6% for men, respectively. However, a recent study has reported equal frequency in men and women (96).

The patho-etiology of mitral annular calcification is not known, but its incidence is increased in systemic hypertension and left ventricular outflow tract obstruction (98–100). This has led to the suggestion that elevated left ventricular pressure may in some way be a causative factor (98–101). However, Pomerance (95) and Nair (102) did not find a significant difference in the incidence of hypertension between age- and sex-matched groups with and without annular calcification.

Abnormalities of the mitral valve have also been associated with mitral annular calcification. Mitral

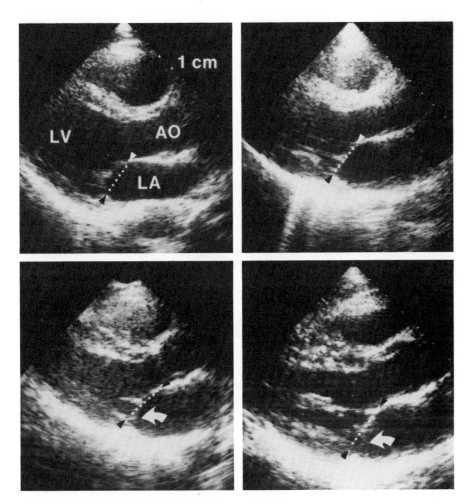

Figure 7.44.   Two-dimensional echocardiogram of the left ventricular long axis showing the plane of the mitral valve annulus, designated by a line joined by arrows. The leaflets of the mitral valve prolapse onto the left atrial side of that plane in systole, indicating the presence of mitral valve prolapse.

valve prolapse has been reported in 3% and 14% of two separate series of patients with annular calcification (65). An association has been proposed between mitral annular calcification and Marfan's syndrome (103, 104). Mitral annular calcification is also more frequent in a number of metabolic disorders such as Hurler's syndrome (105), Paget's disease (106), and the bone dystrophy of chronic renal failure (107).

On M-mode echocardiography (Fig. 7.50), the band of annular calcification may involve the posterior mitral valve leaflet, but is usually visualized between this leaflet and the left ventricular endocardium. The band can be distinguished from the posterior left ventricular wall by its increased echogenicity and relatively little movement. The severity of mitral annular calcification on M-mode echocardiography has been correlated with its complications. Mellino et al. (108) reported that when the width of the band exceeded 5 mm, there was a significant increase in the incidence of conduction defects, atrial fibrillation, and heart failure compared to those patients with a band less than 5 mm. Extensive mitral annular calcification is also associated with a greater incidence both of cerebral and retinal embolism (109, 110).

Mitral annular calcification in its mildest form appears as a small dense mass adjacent to the posterior mitral leaflet at the atrioventricular junction in the parasternal long axis and apical four chamber two-dimensional echocardiographic views. In the short axis view of the left ventricle from the left parasternal region, there is a semicircular linear band beneath the posterior leaflet at the base of the mitral valve (Fig. 7.51). The absence of a true anatomic anterior mitral annulus may explain why mitral annular calcification does not often occur anteriorly (111).

Detection of mitral annular calcification by two-dimensional echocardiography and fluoroscopy has been compared. The presence of annular calcification was diagnosed when the echo density at the annulus was 1.5 mm or more in diameter, and persisted after the suppression of aortic root echoes when transducer transmission was gradually reduced (112). Two-dimensional echocardiography detected 13 of 17 patients with fluoroscopically detectable mitral annulus calcification (sensitivity 76%), and echocardiography suggested mitral annular calcification in six of 96 patients without fluoroscopically detectable mitral annulus calcification (specificity 94%). Mitral annular calcification

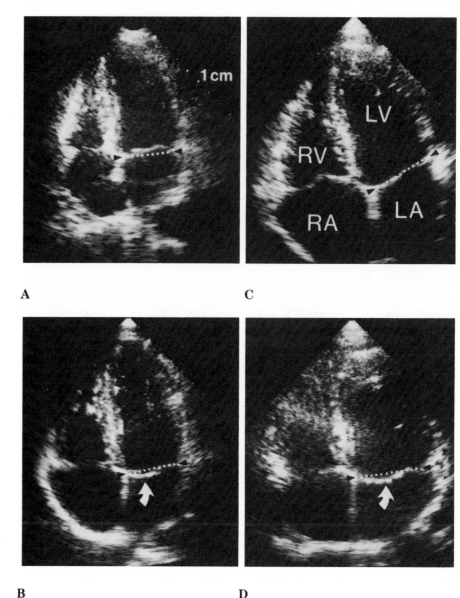

Figure 7.45. Two-dimensional echocardiograms of the apical four chamber view demonstrating the plane of the mitral valve annulus by a line joining two arrows (*A* and *C*). The mitral valve leaflets prolapse beyond this plane in systole, indicating the presence of mitral leaflet prolapse (*B* and *D*).

can be overlooked by two-dimensional echocardiography when the amount of calcification is small. Conversely, echocardiography may suggest calcification when thickening of the annulus is due to fibrosis alone.

Mitral annular calcification may extend into the posterior leaflet and render the leaflet immobile (Fig. 7.52). Associated calcification may involve the body and tip of the anterior leaflet and chordae tendinae, leading to left ventricular inflow tract obstruction simulating rheumatic mitral stenosis. Massive mitral annular calcification may occasionally protrude into the left ventricle or left atrium and mimic a cardiac tumor (113). However, the characteristic relation to the posterior leaflet at the atrioventricular junction in the parasternal long axis view should differentiate these conditions. Calcification of the mitral annulus may also originate from calcification outside the annulus but

project into it. What is commonly referred to as mitral annular calcification consists of calcific deposits situated in the angle between the posterior mitral leaflet and the subjacent left ventricular posterior wall—the posterior submitral angle—and should in reality be termed "submitral calcification" (114).

INFECTIVE ENDOCARDITIS

Echocardiography is the most sensitive method for detecting valvular vegetations in patients with endocarditis. The M-mode diagnosis of a vegetation on the mitral valve is based on shaggy thickening of the valve leaflets and abnormal diastolic motion of the mitral leaflets (Fig. 7.53), which may vary from cycle to cycle (115–117). Similar appearances may occur in patients with nonspecific mitral valve leaflet thickening or

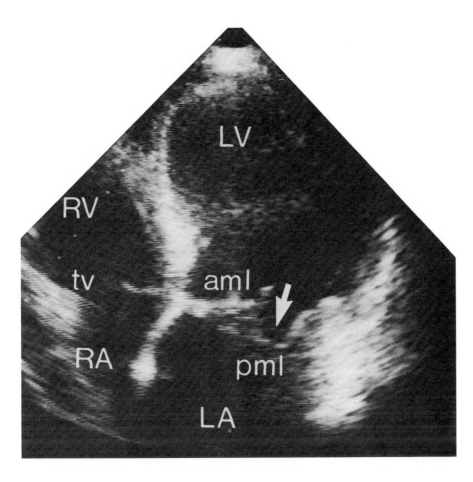

Figure 7.46. Two-dimensional echocardiogram of the apical four chamber view showing dramatic prolapse of the posterior mitral valve leaflet (pml) into the left atrium in systole, while the motion of the anterior leaflet (aml) is normal.

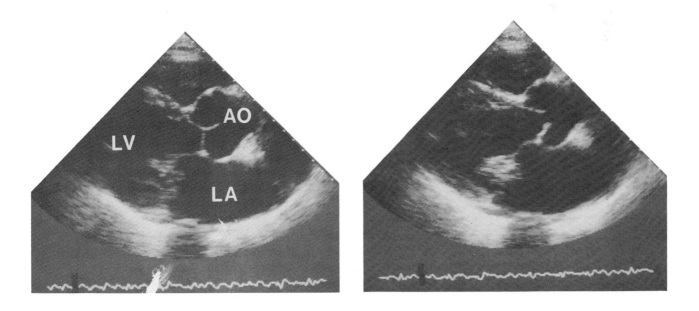

A

B

Figure 7.47. Two-dimensional echocardiograms from a patient with thickened but excessively mobile mitral valve leaflets, suggesting myxomatous degeneration of the leaflets. The long axis view of the left ventricle demonstrates the increased mitral valve leaflet thickness (*A*) and the systolic prolapse (*B*).

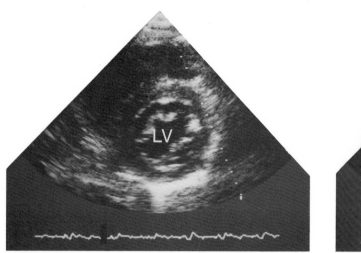

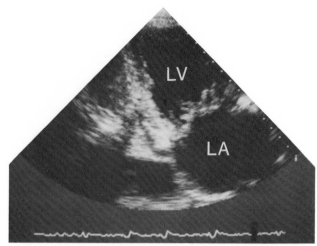

A   B

Figure 7.48.   Two-dimensional echocardiogram of the short axis (*A*) and apical long axis of the left ventricle (*B*), showing the increased thickness of the voluminous mitral valve leaflets in a patient with myxomatous changes in the cusps.

myxomatous degeneration of the cusps, with or without prolapse, because the leaflets are often excessively mobile and that makes differentiation from vegetative endocarditis difficult by M-mode echocardiography alone (118) (Fig. 7.54).

Mitral valve vegetations appear on two-dimensional echocardiography as irregular echogenic masses attached to one or both of the valve leaflets (119–123) (Figs. 7.55, 7.56). Valvular vegetations as small as 2 mm in diameter are detectable. They are usually visualized best in the parasternal long and short axis views, but are usually also clearly visible in the apical two and four chamber views (Figs. 7.57, 7.58). Vegetations may be sessile or pedunculated, and have been reported as large as 40 mm in diameter. They may occasionally obstruct the mitral orifice (124). Vegetations move in concert with the leaflet when firmly adherent to it, or almost independently of valve leaflet motion when pedunculated. Mitral vegetations may also be erroneously diagnosed by two-dimensional echocardiograms in patients with mitral valve prolapse and thickened myxomatous valves (125, 126) (Fig. 7.59).

The differential diagnosis of echocardiographic masses involving the mitral valve should include mitral valve tumors, such as myxoma, fibroma (127), and lipoma (128). These masses have different morphologies. Fibromas and lipomas are usually round and discrete, while myxomas are friable and cystic compared to the fluffy homogeneous appearance of acute valvular vegetations (Figs. 7.55–7.58).

In infective endocarditis, the presence of vegetations was believed initially to be associated with an increased risk of systemic embolization, heart failure, need for surgery, and death, compared to patients with

endocarditis but without echocardiographically demonstrable vegetations (129–132). A recent prospective two-dimensional echocardiographic study of patients with infective endocarditis with and without vegetations demonstrated that thromboembolism, heart failure, and the need for surgery were similar in the two groups. Furthermore, there was no association between either the size of the vegetation or the causative micro-organism and any systemic complication (133). The majority (70%) of vegetations remain unchanged in size after initial detection following the clinical presentation with endocarditis (132). On rare occasions vegetations may enlarge significantly (134), but more commonly, the vegetations decrease and disappear with or without clinical evidence of systemic embolization, if their size changes at all.

The diagnosis of infective endocarditis is primarily clinical and should not rest on the echocardiographic detection of vegetations, since pathologic studies indicate that up to 50% of patients dying of acute endocarditis do not have vegetations (135). In a review of the literature, mitral valve vegetations were detected by M-mode echocardiography in 14% to 65% (mean 52%), and by two-dimensional echocardiography in 43% to 100% (mean 80%) of patients with clinical evidence of infective endocarditis (129). Thus, even when the mitral valve appears entirely normal, infective endocarditis cannot be excluded (135). Mitral valve prolapse (136), rheumatic valvulitis, papillary muscle dysfunction with secondary mitral regurgitation, and mitral annular calcification (137) account for the majority of valvular abnormalities that predispose to endocarditis.

The echocardiographic detection of mitral valve vegetations in the absence of clinical infective endo-

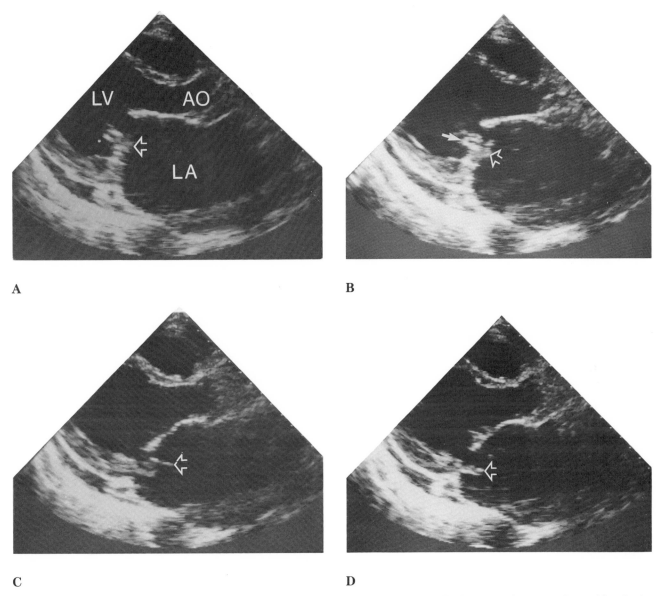

A   B

C   D

Figure 7.49. Serial two-dimensional echocardiographic frames of the left ventricular long axis from a patient with mitral regurgitation due to rupture of the chordae to the posterior mitral valve cusp, which resulted in a flail leaflet. The thickened posterior cusp begins to fold upon itself (*A*) and continues to move posteriorly (*B, open arrow*), with a ruptured chordae appearing as a sigmoidal structure (*closed arrow*) attached to the ventricular surface of the leaflet. The posterior cusp then moves progressively further back into the left atrium (*C, D, open arrow*).

carditis may represent healed or indolent endocarditis (138). Such vegetations may appear more echo dense than "active" vegetations (139), but chronic vegetations usually cannot be distinguished from acute or new vegetations. There is no data to indicate that surgical removal of the vegetations, however large or mobile echocardiographically, is beneficial in the absence of emboli, hemodynamic compromise, or heart failure from valve perforation or chordal rupture.

The echocardiographic manifestations of mitral valve endocarditis are not limited to the detection of vegetations. Infective endocarditis of the mitral valve may also lead to perforation (140) or aneurysm of the valve leaflets (141), development of paravalvular abscesses, ruptured chordae tendinae, and flail leaflets with varying degrees of mitral regurgitation. All the potential complications of endocarditis should be looked for with meticulous two-dimensional echocardiographic imaging, and the competence of the mitral valve assessed by pulsed, continuous-wave, and color-flow Doppler. Furthermore, the size of the mitral valve vegetations, the intracardiac hemodynamics, and left ventricular function should be assessed serially in patients with infective endocarditis.

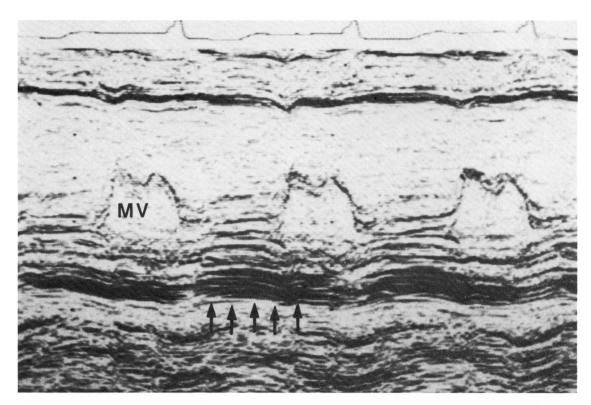

Figure 7.50. M-mode echocardiogram of the left ventricle demonstrating mitral valve annular calcification as a heavy echo reflection posterior to the posterior mitral valve leaflet (*arrows*).

MITRAL VALVE ABNORMALITIES AND OTHER CONDITIONS

Aortic Regurgitation

In aortic regurgitation, the regurgitant jet of blood may impinge on the mitral leaflets and subvalve apparatus, on the interventricular septum, or less frequently on the posterior left ventricular wall, producing high-frequency vibrations of these structures in early diastole (142–148) (Fig. 7.60). The frequency of oscillation of these structures is in the range of 30–40 Hz, and is therefore detected better by M-mode than two-dimensional echocardiography because of its higher sampling frequency (1000 vs. 30 Hz).

Skorton et al. (146) examined the sensitivity and specificity of diastolic flutter in aortic regurgitation and found an overall sensitivity of 66% and specificity of 83%. With severe aortic regurgitation, however, the sensitivity approaches 100%. The overall sensitivity of interventricular septal diastolic flutter was 36%, but its specificity was 98%. Diastolic anterior mitral leaflet flutter has also been reported in tetralogy of Fallot (145), mitral regurgitation (147), and repaired D-transposition (148).

There are three other echocardiographic findings in aortic regurgitation that relate to the mitral valve: 1) reversed doming of the anterior mitral leaflet (149,

150), 2) increased E point septal separation, and 3) presystolic closure of the mitral valve when aortic regurgitation is acute and severe (151, 152), so that the mitral valve closes before the QRS complex on the simultaneously recorded electrocardiogram (Fig. 7.61). Premature mitral valve closure occurs when the left ventricular diastolic pressure exceeds left atrial pressure, which it does early in diastole when there is a free communication between the aorta and left ventricle (152). Premature mitral valve closure also occurs in patients with first-degree atrioventricular block.

Systolic Anterior Motion

Angiographic demonstration of abnormal systolic motion of the mitral valve in hypertrophic cardiomyopathy was first reported in 1961 (153), and subsequently confirmed by others (154, 155). The same finding was described by M-mode echocardiography and termed systolic anterior motion (SAM) of the mitral valve (156, 157) (Fig. 7.62). (See Chapter 11.)

Gilbert et al. (158) studied 70 patients with hypertrophic cardiomyopathy and found that severe SAM (i.e., prolonged mitral-septal contact for 30% or more of systole) was present in all patients with resting gradients across the left ventricular outflow tract. In patients with no left ventricular outflow tract gradient at

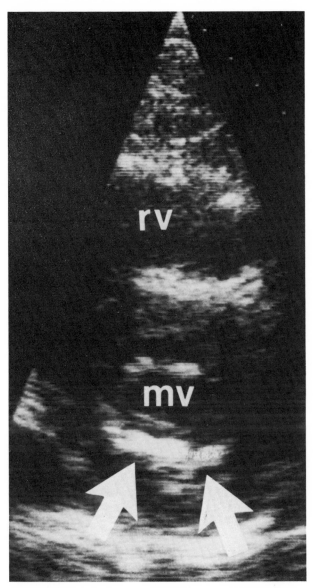

Figure 7.51. Two-dimensional echocardiogram of the left ventricle in short axis, showing heavy calcification of the mitral annulus (*arrows*), which is posterior to the posterior mitral valve leaflet but anterior to the endocardium of the inferoposterior LV wall.

rest, but who developed pressure gradients on provocation, SAM was mild, with a minimal mitral-septal distance of more than 10 mm.

A close temporal relation has been demonstrated between the onset of mitral-septal contact and the onset of the subaortic pressure gradient, suggesting that systolic anterior motion is the cause of the pressure gradient (159) (Fig. 7.62). Furthermore, a quantitative relationship has been demonstrated between the duration of mitral-septal contact and the pressure gradient across the left ventricular outflow tract (160,

161) (Fig. 7.63). An index based on these observations—the "time-period" index—has been derived as follows: (duration of septal contact divided by the time from the onset of SAM to the onset of septal contact) × 25 + 26 (mmHg) (Figs. 7.64, 7.65). This "time-period" index correlates well with hemodynamically derived pressure gradients (r = 0.90, p = 0.001, SE ± 15 mmHg [Fig. 7.65]). Moreover, SAM without septal contact was not associated with significant pressure gradients.

SAM occurs in conditions other than hypertrophic cardiomyopathy. Mild degrees of SAM may be seen in normal, usually young subjects in hypovolemic states, during inotropic stimulation (162), and in hypercontractile states (163). SAM may also occur in hypertensive patients (164), in amyloid heart disease (165), Pompes disease (166), Friedrich's ataxia (167), and in the infants of diabetic mothers (168). In these conditions, SAM is usually mild or moderate.

Two-dimensional echocardiography has provided further insight into the etiology of SAM (169, 170). Mild to moderate SAM usually originates from chordal anterior motion, whereas severe SAM involves the body of the anterior mitral leaflet (170). Spirito and Maron (171) reported on a variety of patterns of SAM using two-dimensional echocardiography in 62 patients with hypertrophic cardiomyopathy. In 36 patients, both anterior and posterior leaflets contributed to SAM, although mitral septal contact, when it occurred, originated from the anterior leaflet. In 19 patients, SAM was produced selectively by the posterior mitral leaflet. In only 16 patients was the anterior leaflet alone responsible for SAM, and in one patient the chordae tendinae appeared to be primarily responsible for SAM (171). SAM was severe in four of the 19 (21%) patients with posterior leaflet SAM versus 26 of the 43 (60%) patients with other patterns of SAM involving the anterior leaflet (171).

THE MITRAL VALVE AS A MIRROR OF CARDIAC FUNCTION

Left Ventricular Diastolic Function

Several abnormalities of mitral valve motion have been described in patients with decreased left ventricular compliance and/or elevated left ventricular end-diastolic pressure. Zaky et al. (172) reported "incomplete closure of the mitral valve in pre-systole," demonstrated by prolongation of the AC interval on M-mode echocardiograms in patients with elevated mean left atrial and left ventricular end-diastolic pressures (Fig. 7.66). Since the duration of the AC interval depends on atrioventricular conduction, measurements of the electrocardiographic PR interval minus the echocardiographic AC interval have been used to correct for atrioventricular conduction time. Konecke et al. (173)

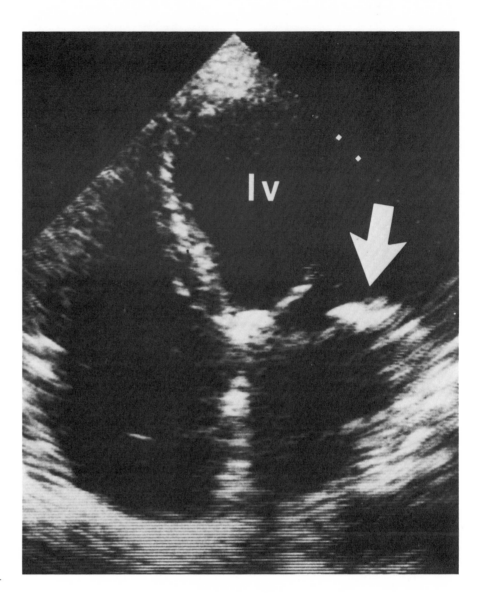

Figure 7.52. Two-dimensional echocardiogram of the apical four chamber view (*A*), showing the mitral valve annular calcification (*arrow*).

A

evaluated 14 patients with left ventricular end-diastolic pressures greater than 20 mmHg and atrial components of LV diastolic pressure greater than 8 mmHg. These patients all had a PR-AC interval less than 60 msec, and 11 of the patients had a prolonged AC segment or plateau at the B point (Fig. 7.66). Wilson et al. (174) reported a significant correlation between PR-AC interval and left ventricular ejection fraction.

Initial M-mode studies of the mitral valve indicated that the EF slope may reflect the rate of left ventricular filling (172, 175, 176). DeMaria et al. (177) correlated the EF slope with left ventricular inflow in the first third of diastole (r = 0.87, p < 0.001), but found no direct relationship between EF slope and indices of left ventricular diastolic compliance. Wilson et al. (174) found no correlation between the EF slope and mean pulmonary wedge pressure.

Transmitral blood flow velocity profiles have also been used to describe left ventricular diastolic function (178–180). In the normal heart, there is a rapid increase in the velocity of blood flow into the left ventricle immediately following mitral valve opening (E wave). The peak velocity of the E wave varies from 0.4 to 1.0 m/sec during the rapid left ventricular diastolic filling period (178–180) (Fig. 7.67). The velocity declines in early to mid-diastole, and increases again as left atrial systole propels blood into the left ventricle (A wave). The peak velocity of the A wave in normal subjects is less than the peak velocity during rapid filling (E wave) (Fig. 7.67). The ratio of E wave to A wave velocity (E/A) is greater than unity during early life, but decreases toward unity with increasing age. Some authors have expressed this inversely as the ratio of atrial to rapid filling velocities (designated A/R ratio) and demon-

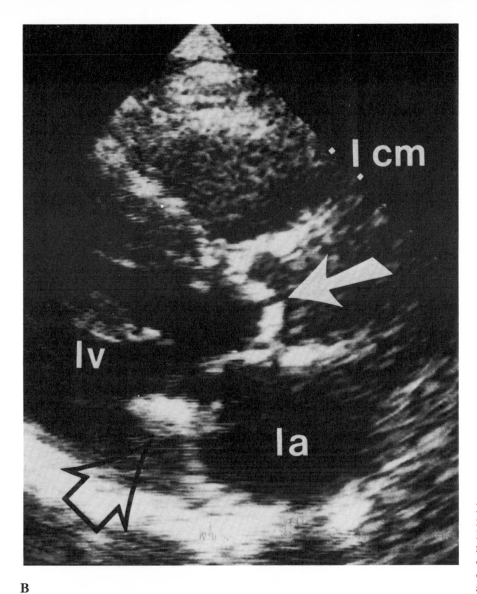

1 cm

lv

la

B

Figure 7.52 (cont'd.). Two-dimensional echocardiogram of the LV long axis from left parasternal region (B) in a patient with severe calcific aortic stenosis with calcification involving the mitral valve annulus (*black arrow*).

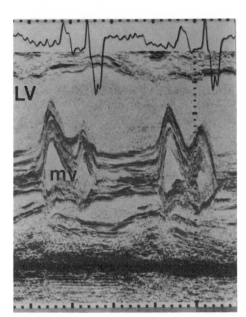

LV

mv

Figure 7.53. M-mode echocardiogram showing an increased number of echos emanating from both mitral valve leaflets, due to adherent vegetations, in a patient with vegetative endocarditis involving the mitral leaflets.

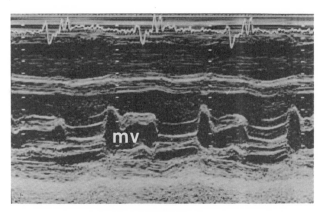

mv

Figure 7.54. M-mode echocardiogram showing increased echos from both mitral valve leaflets in a patient with thickened but excessively mobile myxomatous mitral valve leaflets and systolic leaflet prolapse by two-dimensional echo (which is not apparent on the M-mode recording). The patient had associated mitral regurgitation.

201

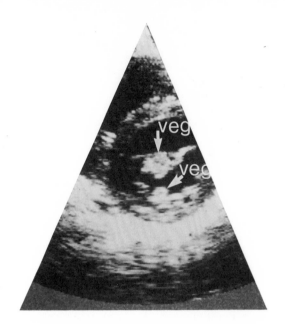

A

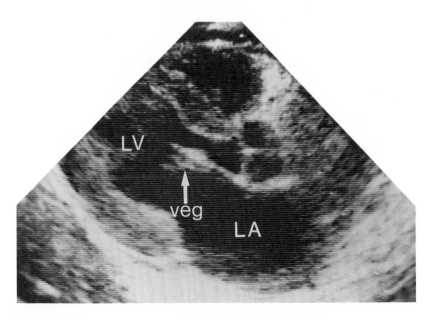

Figure 7.55. Two-dimensional echocardiogram of the left ventricle in short axis (*A*), showing thickening of both anterior and posterior mitral valve leaflets due to vegetations (*arrows*). Two-dimensional echocardiogram of the left ventricular long axis, showing a florid vegetation on the anterior mitral valve cusp (*B, arrow*).

B

strated that it increases with age (181) (Fig. 7.68). In patients with decreased left ventricular compliance due to severe left ventricular hypertrophy, myocardial infarction, and primary muscle disease, the E wave tends to be smaller and its duration prolonged, suggesting increased resistance to left ventricular filling, while the peak A wave velocity increases so that the E/A ratio is less than unity (182–184) (Fig. 7.69). This E/A ratio has been advocated as an indicator of impaired diastolic left ventricular function. However, no predictable correlation between the E/A ratio and left ventricular compliance, or absolute left ventricular mass or vol-

ume has been demonstrated, although the E/A ratio does correlate with left ventricular architecture when expressed as the ratio of left ventricular mass/volume (185). The initial ethusiasm for using the E/A velocity ratio as an index of diastolic function has declined because it varies markedly with age, heart rate, and left ventricular loading conditions.

Left Ventricular Systolic Function

Rasmussen et al. (186) demonstrated a significant correlation between the maximal separation of the

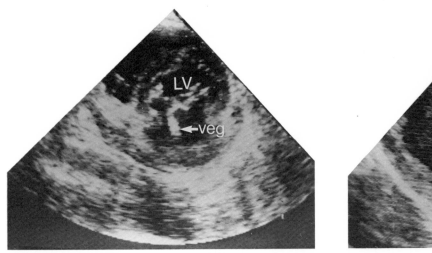 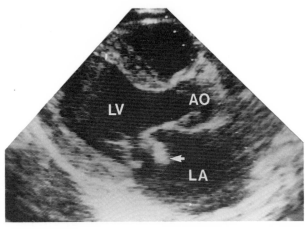

A   **B**

Figure 7.56. Two-dimensional echocardiogram of the left ventricular short axis (*A*) and long axis (*B*), showing a very mobile mitral valve vegetation on the anterior leaflet, which prolapses into the left atrium in systole (*arrow*).

anterior and posterior cusps at the E point, and between the DE slope and cardiac output, in patients without mitral regurgitation. They derived an index based on the EE separation and the DE slope to calculate stroke volume and cardiac output. However, subsequent examination of the same index revealed a poor correlation with stroke volume measured by either thermodilution or angiography (187).

Reduced EE separation commonly occurs in low cardiac output states in M-mode echocardiograms (Fig. 7.70), and a reduced mitral orifice is seen on two-dimensional echocardiography (Fig. 7.71). However,

the valve is intrinsically normal and does not exhibit doming or thickening as in rheumatic mitral stenosis (188). Massie et al. (189) found a strong negative correlation between the distance between the E point of the anterior mitral valve leaflet and the left side of the interventricular septal surface and left ventricular ejection fraction. Thus, reduced excursion of the anterior leaflet resulting in mitral E point septal separation of more than 8 mm, in the absence of mitral stenosis, aortic regurgitation, and proximal septal dyskinesis or paradoxical motion, is an indicator of reduced left ventricular function, assessed either by fractional

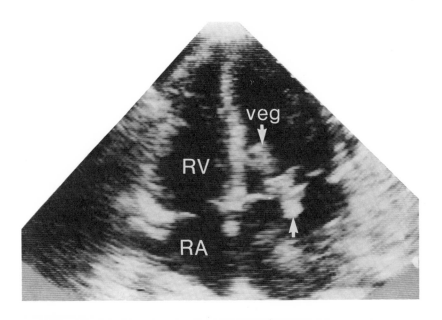

Figure 7.57. Two-dimensional echocardiogram of the apical four chamber view, showing an extensive vegetation attached to the anterior mitral valve leaflet, which is visible in the left ventricular body and the left atrium (*arrows*).

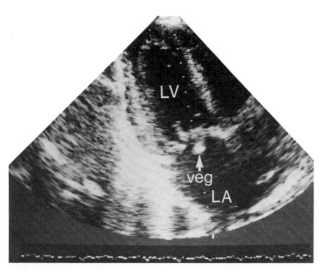

Figure 7.58. Two-dimensional echocardiogram of the LV apical long axis showing mitral valve vegetations (*arrow*).

shortening or by ejection fraction (Fig. 7.72). This relationship is independent of left ventricular size (190).

TRICUSPID VALVE

Tricuspid Stenosis

Occasionally tricuspid stenosis develops secondary to carcinoid, in which deposits of fibrous tissue and

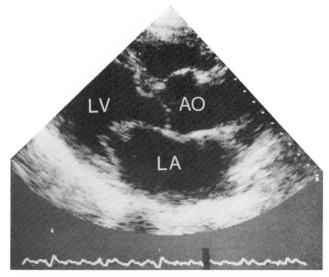

Figure 7.59. Two-dimensional echocardiogram of the LV long axis demonstrating thickened mitral valve leaflets due to myxomatous changes in the leaflets, which may resemble mitral valve vegetations.

mucopolysaccharide material are laid down on the tricuspid leaflets and on the atrial endocardium (191). Tricuspid leaflet motion is severely reduced (Fig. 7.73), often with the leaflets becoming fixed in the partially open position so that there is concomitant tricuspid regurgitation. However, tricuspid stenosis almost al-

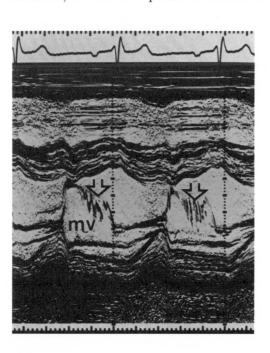

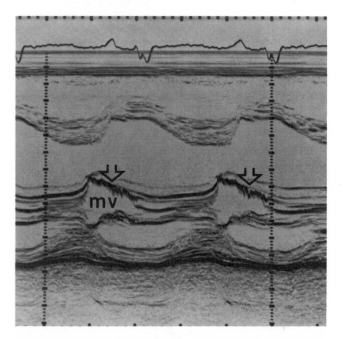

A

B

Figure 7.60. M-mode echocardiogram showing high-frequency diastolic flutter of the anterior mitral valve leaflet due to aortic regurgitation in two patients (*arrows*). One patient had moderately severe aortic stenosis with mild aortic regurgitation (*A*). One had chronic severe aortic regurgitation (*B*). Diastolic flutter of the mitral valve does not correlate with the severity of aortic regurgitation.

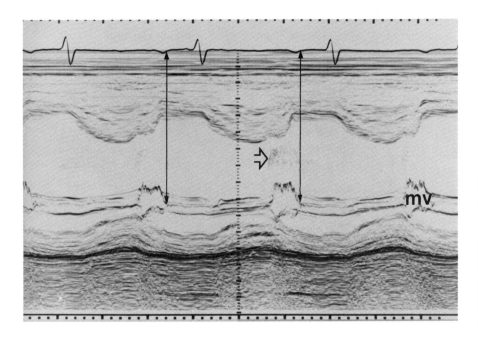

Figure 7.61. M-mode echocardiogram showing premature closure of the mitral valve approximately 100 msec before the onset of the QRS complex (*vertical arrows*) in a patient with sudden worsening in the severity of chronic severe aortic regurgitation due to an aortic vegetation (*horizontal arrow*), which prolapses into the left ventricular outflow tract. Note also the diastolic flutter on the anterior and posterior mitral valve leaflets.

ways results from rheumatic heart disease and is invariably associated with mitral stenosis (192). The M-mode echocardiographic findings of the rheumatically stenosed tricuspid valve are similar to those in mitral stenosis. The leaflets are thickened, their motion is restricted, the diastolic EF slope of the anterior and

posterior leaflet are reduced (193) (Fig. 7.74), and the right atrium is enlarged.

The typical two-dimensional echocardiographic findings in tricuspid stenosis include leaflet thickening and restricted motion, often with diastolic doming of the anterior leaflet due to fibrosis and shortening of

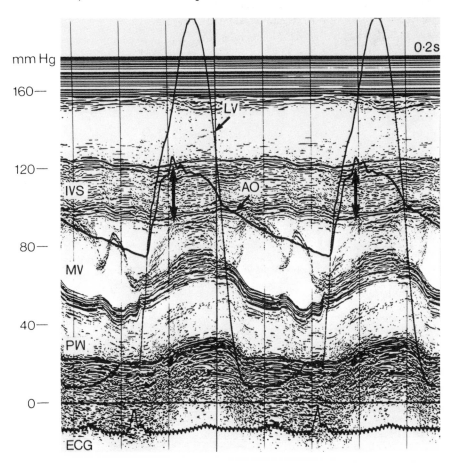

Figure 7.62. M-mode echocardiogram from a patient with hypertrophic cardiomyopathy HCM, showing a small left ventricular cavity with SAM, whose onset (*black vertical arrow*) coincides with the beginning of the pressure gradient between the aorta and left ventricle. Pressure equilibration between the aorta and left ventricle coincides with the offset of SAM, indicating a cause-and-effect relationship between SAM and the LV outflow tract gradient.

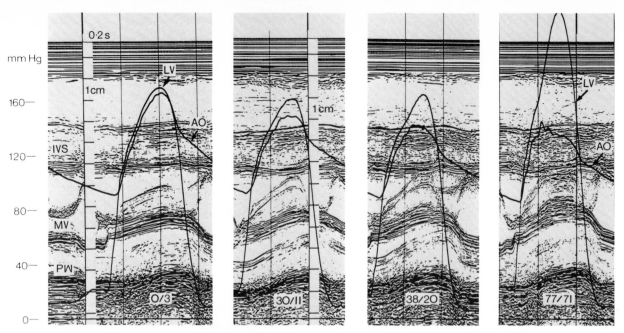

Figure 7.63. Serial M-mode echocardiograms from a patient with HCM, and simultaneous aortic and left ventricular pressures, showing increasing duration of SAM from left to right, resulting in increasing magnitude of the pressure difference between the left ventricle and aorta. (Reproduced by permission of the American Heart Association, Inc. from Pollick C, Rakowski H, Wigle ED. Muscular subaortic stenosis: the quantitative relationship between systolic anterior motion and the pressive gradient. Circulation; 1984:69:46.)

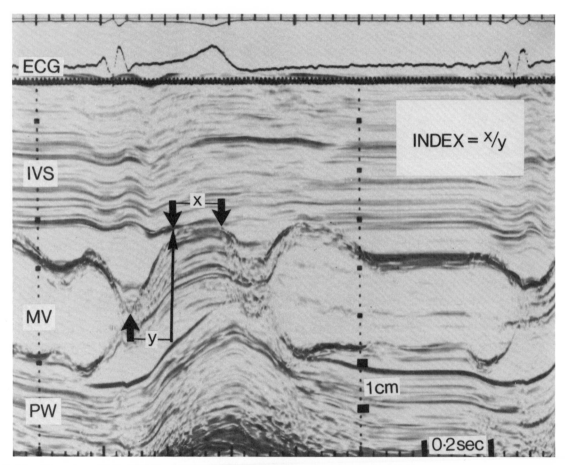

Figure 7.64. M-mode echocardiogram from a patient with HCM with SAM and ASH, showing derivation of the time period index, which is the duration of mitral-septal contact (x) divided by the time from the onset of SAM to the onset of septal contact (y) (index = x/y). (Reproduced by permission of the American Heart Association, Inc. from Pollick C, Rakowski H, Wigle ED. Muscular subaortic stenosis: the quantitative relationship between systolic anterior motion and the pressure gradient. Circulation; 1984:69:46.)

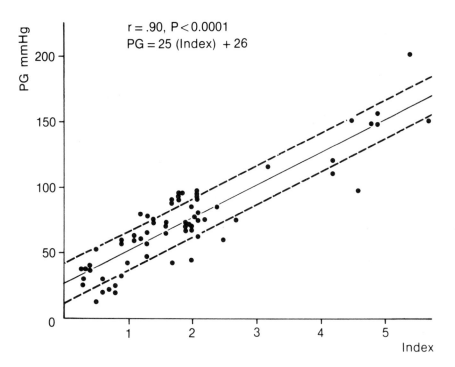

r = .90, P < 0.0001
PG = 25 (Index) + 26

Figure 7.65. Comparison of the time period index and the left ventricular outflow pressure gradient at cardiac catheterization shows close correlation between the two techniques (r = 0.90). (Reproduced by permission of the American Heart Association. Inc. from Pollick C, Rakowski H, Wigle ED. Muscular subaortic stenosis: the quantitative relationship between systolic anterior motion and the pressure gradient. Circulation; 1984:69:47.)

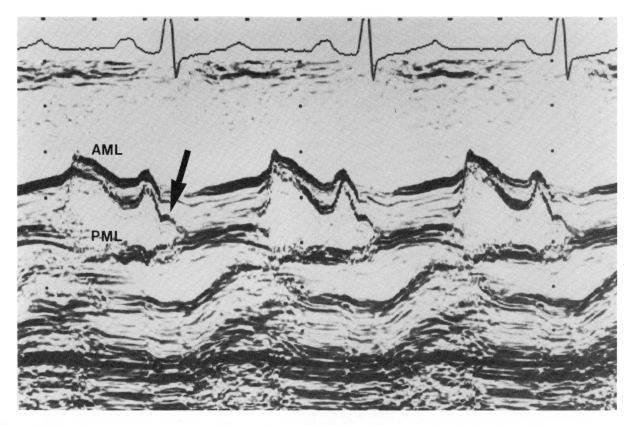

Figure 7.66. M-mode echocardiogram of the mitral valve showing an inflection on the closing slope of the anterior and posterior leaflets (beta bump), with prolongation of the interval between the A wave and the closing point C (AC segment), suggesting elevation of left ventricular end-diastolic pressure.

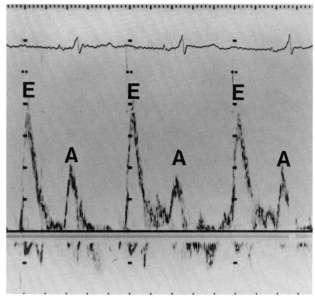

Figure 7.67. Pulsed-wave Doppler flow velocity signal across the mitral valve recorded from the apical four chamber view. There is an increase in blood flow velocity (E wave) with a peak of 0.8 m/sec during rapid diastolic left ventricular filling, which decays quickly and is followed by a second smaller peak (A wave) of 0.3 to 0.4 m/sec during atriosystolic filling.

the chordal structures, and decreased separation of the leaflet tips (194–197). These changes in the valve leaflets and subvalve apparatus should be carefully assessed in multiple views, including the right ventricular inflow tract from the left parasternal position, and the apical and subcostal four chamber views.

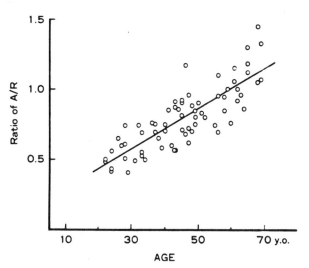

Figure 7.68. The ratio of the velocities during atriosystolic contraction and during the rapid diastolic filling period increases linearly with age in normal subjects. (Reproduced with permission from Miyatake K, Okamoto M, Kinoshita N, et al. Augmentation of atrial contribution of left ventricular inflow with aging as assessed by intracardiac Doppler flowmetry. Am J. Cardiol 1984; 53:589.)

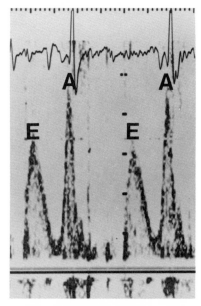

Figure 7.69. Pulsed-wave Doppler flow velocity signal from a patient with severe left ventricular dysfunction secondary to cardiomyopathy shows the peak E wave velocity of 0.62 m/sec during the rapid filling phase and the large A wave during atriosystolic contraction with a velocity of .95 m/sec, suggesting "decreased compliance."

Guyer et al. (195) found a tricuspid valve gradient at cardiac catheterization in 13 patients, nine of whom had echocardiographic evidence of tricuspid stenosis. Only one of the 10 patients with echocardiographic

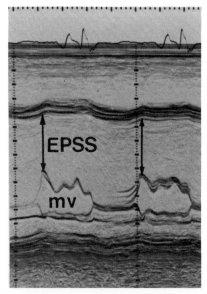

Figure 7.70. M-mode echocardiogram from a patient with severe left ventricular dilatation and poor contractile function, showing an increased E point–septal separation (*arrow*), that is, an increased distance between the maximum excursion of the mitral valve (E point) and the left side of the interventricular septum. There is also a prolonged AC segment.

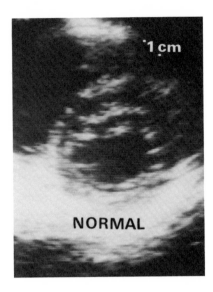
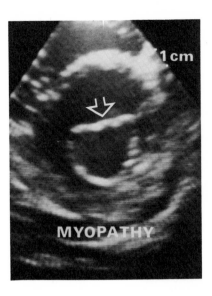

Figure 7.71. Two-dimensional echocardiogram of the left ventricle in short axis at the base, showing the distance between anterior mitral valve leaflet and the left side of the interventricular septum at the timing of the E point in a normal subject (less than 0.8 cm) and the increased distance (E point–septal separation) in a patient with dilated cardiomyopathy (*arrow*).

evidence of tricuspid stenosis had no tricuspid gradient. Thus, echocardiographically detectable tricuspid stenosis was 90% predictive of a tricuspid gradient. However, Daniels et al. (196) detected a tricuspid valve gradient in only four of 19 patients, with echocardio-

graphic evidence of tricuspid stenosis giving a predictive accuracy of 21%.

Doppler echocardiography is of diagnostic value in tricuspid stenosis (198–200). When the sample volume is placed in the right ventricle immediately down-

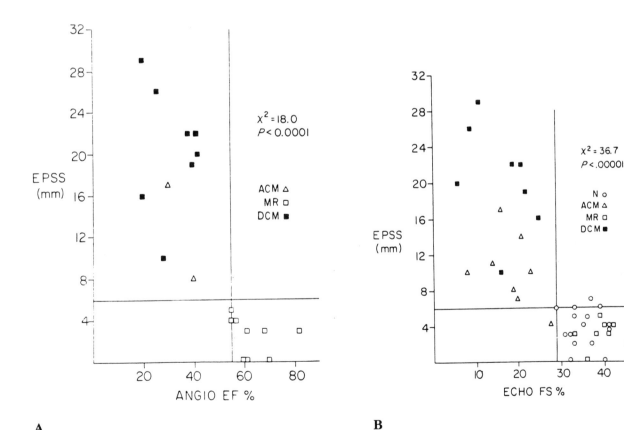

A   **B**

Figure 7.72. There is an inverse relationship between E point–septal separation (EPSS) and fractional left ventricular shortening by echo (*A*) and ejection fraction by angiography (*B*). (Reproduced with permission from Child JS, Krivokapich J, Perloff JK. Effect of left ventricular size on mitral E point to ventricular septal separation in assessment of cardiac performance. Am Heart Journal; 1981:101:798,800.)

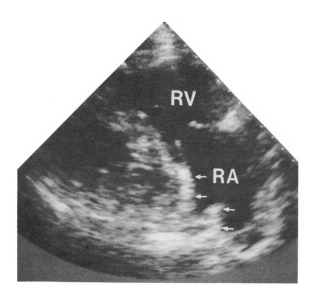

Figure 7.73.   Two-dimensional echocardiogram of the right ventricular inflow tract from a patient with carcinoid. The opening of the tricuspid valve is restricted, and the leaflets are thickened with plaques of carcinoid, which extend onto the right side of the interatrial septum and coronary sinus, resulting in increased echo reflectance (*arrows*).

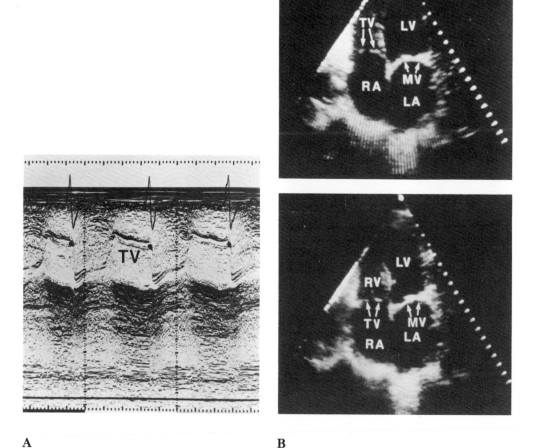

A   B

Figure 7.74.   M-mode echocardiogram shows thickened tricuspid valve leaflets, restricted motion, and a flat EF slope (*A*). Two-dimensional echocardiogram of the apical four chamber view from a patient with rheumatic mitral stenosis and tricuspid stenosis in diastole (*B*) and systole (*C*) demonstrates thickened mitral and tricuspid leaflets with restricted leaflet motion and biatrial enlargement.

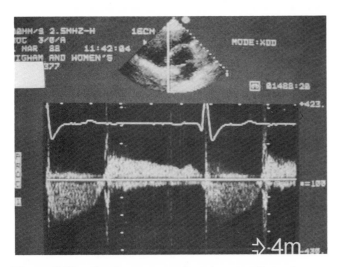

Figure 7.75. Continuous-wave Doppler recordings obtained with simultaneous two-dimensional echocardiographic imaging from a patient with rheumatic tricuspid stenosis and regurgitation, demonstrating a markedly increased peak antegrade transtricuspid valve velocity of 1.3 m/sec, and tricuspid regurgitation with a peak velocity of 2.1 m/sec.

stream of the tricuspid valve, a high-velocity jet is recorded with a spectral envelope similar to that in mitral stenosis, but with a lower peak velocity. Particular attention should be paid to aligning the ultrasound beam parallel to the direction of blood flow, and only well-defined velocity spectra should be analyzed (Fig. 7.75) because transvalve gradients in tricuspid stenosis are small and the potential for error is therefore comparatively large. The elevated transvalve flow velocity in tricuspid stenosis and its slow rate of decline in diastole theoretically allows derivation of the pressure half-time and calculation of the tricuspid valve orifice area, although how useful this will be has yet to be determined (199).

Tricuspid Regurgitation

Tricuspid regurgitation may be due to primary disease of the valve leaflets and subvalvar apparatus as in rheumatic heart disease, carcinoid, leaflet prolapse, chordal rupture, bacterial endocarditis, and papillary muscle dysfunction, or it may develop secondary to changes in right ventricular configuration (201–215). The most frequent change in right ventricular architecture is dilatation due to chronic elevation of left heart filling pressures and subsequent development of pulmonary hypertension. Tricuspid regurgitation may also result from changes in RV configuration due to increased pulmonary blood flow as occurs in the intracardiac shunts, especially at atrial level. When pulmonary artery systolic pressure exceeds 40 mmHg, the incidence of tricuspid regurgitation approaches 90%,

and in severe pulmonary hypertension, the incidence of tricuspid regurgitation is close to 100% (24).

The echocardiographic diagnosis of tricuspid regurgitation is made indirectly from a combination of findings, which include abnormalities of tricuspid leaflets and subvalve apparatus, increased right ventricular size with a vigorous volume overload contraction pattern, increased right atrial size with systolic expansion, and a dilated inferior vena cava that expands in systole. In the apical four chamber view, the right ventricle is dilated. With severe tricuspid regurgitation, septal motion is flattened or reversed, and the right ventricle becomes globular and forms the apex of the heart (Figs. 7.76–7.78). Tricuspid regurgitation also occurs secondarily when the right ventricle dilates, as in primary myocardial failure due to concomitant increase in the tricuspid valve ring circumference.

Contrast injection into a peripheral vein may be helpful in establishing the diagnosis of tricuspid regurgitation and in semiquantifying its severity (216–218). Tricuspid regurgitation, however, can be diagnosed directly and unequivocally and its severity assessed with Doppler echocardiography (24, 198, 219–224). Tricuspid regurgitation is detected with pulsed-wave and/or color-flow Doppler (58, 221, 225). The Doppler sample volume is positioned in the right atrium immediately proximal to the tricuspid valve in the apical four chamber view, and tricuspid regurgitation is diagnosed when high velocity turbulent retrograde systolic flow is recorded (Fig. 7.79). The right atrium is subdivided into four regions and flow mapping performed to semiquantitate the severity of tricuspid regurgitation. Detection of retrograde systolic flow only within 1 cm of the tricuspid valve is designated mild or 1+ tricuspid regurgitation. Detection of the jet throughout the right atrium represents severe or 4+ tricuspid regurgitation (Fig. 7.39). Right atrial flow mapping for tricuspid regurgitation can also be performed from the parasternal right ventricular inflow view. Pulsed-wave Doppler may also be used to examine the superior and inferior vena cavae and the middle hepatic vein for the presence of tricuspid regurgitation, which is detected as high-velocity systolic retrograde blood flow away from the heart (Fig. 7.80). Color-flow Doppler is also useful in diagnosing tricuspid regurgitation in the apical four chamber and RV inflow views (Fig. 7.81, Plate VI). The regurgitant jet is represented as a blue, flame-shaped signal in the right atrium whose length, width, and area can be measured, which provides a semiquantitative estimate of the severity of tricuspid regurgitation. Color-flow Doppler is especially useful in detecting the presence of mild tricuspid regurgitation, which is auscultatorily silent, and also in locating regurgitant jets, which may not be diagnosed even after meticulous flow mapping with pulsed-wave Doppler. The severity

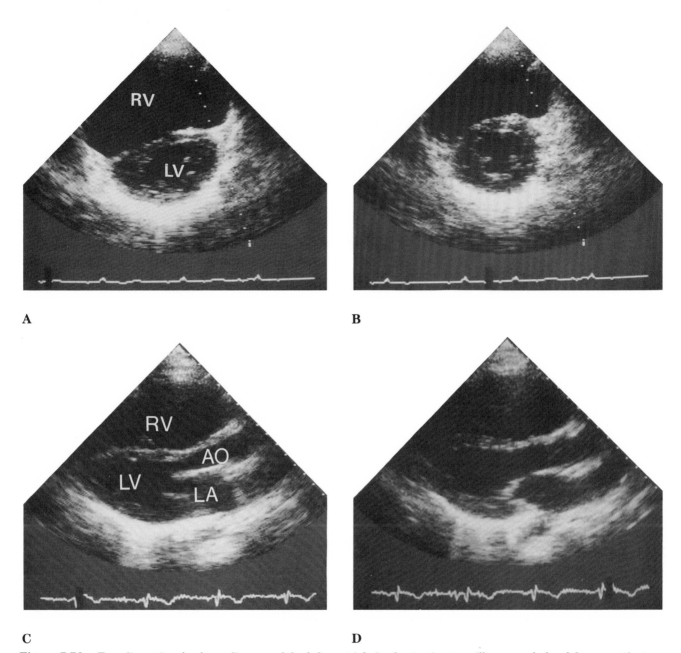

A

B

C

D

Figure 7.76. Two-dimensional echocardiogram of the left ventricle in short axis at papillary muscle level from a patient with severe tricuspid regurgitation, showing a flattened interventricular septum in diastole (*A*) and almost normal septal configuration in systole (*B*). The right ventricle, which is anterior to the interventricular septum, is greatly enlarged. The left ventricle in long axis is shown in diastole (*C*) with septal flattening and a very large right ventricle anteriorly, with restoration of the normal septal curvature in systole (*D*). The dilated right ventricle and abnormal septal motion are due to tricuspid regurgitation.

of tricuspid regurgitation can theoretically be quantitated by estimating the regurgitant fraction, which is the difference between volume across the tricuspid and pulmonary valves. Each is calculated as the product of their respective flow velocity integrals and cross-sectional areas of the flow streams expressed as a percentage of the total flow across the tricuspid valve.

Continuous-wave Doppler recordings of the tricus-

pid jet should be used routinely to confirm the presence of tricuspid regurgitation (Fig. 7.82) and to calculate the right atrial–right ventricular systolic pressure difference from the modified Bernoulli equation ($\Delta p = 4V^2$), using the peak velocity of the regurgitant signal (24, 233, 224). Pulmonary artery systolic pressure can be obtained by the addition of the clinical estimate of the height of the jugular venous pressure (24), or

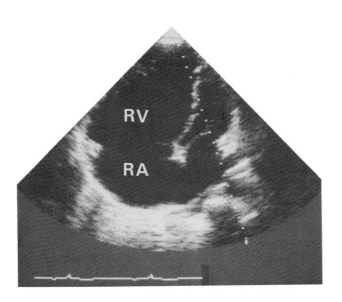

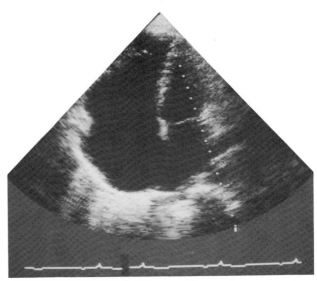

A   **B**

Figure 7.77.   Two-dimensional echocardiogram of the apical four chamber view shows a greatly dilated right ventricle and right atrium due to tricuspid regurgitation, with abnormal septal position in diastole, and a small left ventricle and left atrium with clearly visible pulmonary veins (*A*). Septal position is near normal in systole (*B*).

adding 14 mmHg, which was derived from a regression equation in which simultaneous Doppler recordings and direct measurements of pulmonary artery pressure were compared (223, 224) (Fig. 7.83).

Acute tricuspid regurgitation develops when pulmo-

nary arterial pressure increases abruptly following pulmonary embolism. In patients with major pulmonary embolism, calculation of pulmonary systolic pressure by continuous-wave Doppler echocardiography and measurement of right ventricular dimensions seri-

Figure 7.78.   M-mode echocardiogram from a patient with severe (4+) tricuspid regurgitation, showing a normal size left ventricle at high papillary muscle level, with abnormal septal motion (*A*), and at mitral valve level (*B*).

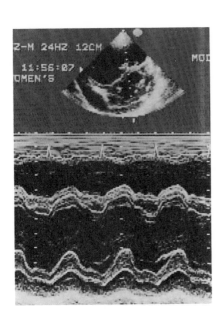

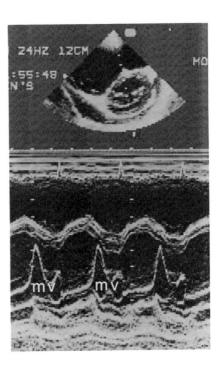

A   **B**

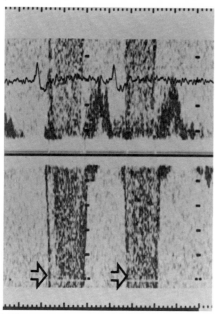

Figure 7.79. Pulsed-wave Doppler velocity signal obtained from the apex with the sample volume positioned in the right atrium. The velocity exceeds the Nyquist limit (*arrows*), resulting in aliasing and appearance of the velocity signal on the upper register. One-cm calibration marks represent 20 cm/sec.

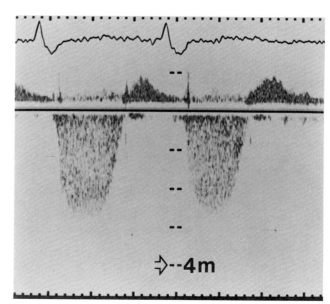

Figure 7.82. Continuous-wave Doppler velocity signals from a patient with tricuspid regurgitation obtained from the apex. Note the high holosystolic timing of the signal, the mid-systolic peaking, and the maximum velocity of 2.6 m/sec. The right atrial–right ventricular gradient can be calculated from the peak velocity of the tricuspid regurgitant jet using the Bernoulli equation ($\Delta P = 4V^2$, which equals 27 mmHg).

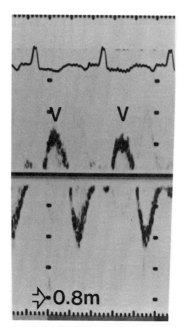

Figure 7.80. Pulsed-wave Doppler velocity signal recorded from the inferior vena cava, showing a systolic wave (V) in the upper register with a peak velocity of 0.25 m/sec, indicating the presence of tricuspid regurgitation.

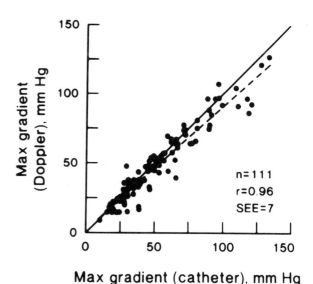

Figure 7.83. Comparison between the maximum right atrial–right ventricular gradient calculated from Doppler, and the maximum gradient measured at cardiac catheterization, in patients with pulmonary hypertension shows excellent correlation between the two techniques. (Reproduced with permission from Currie PJ, Seward JB, Chan K-L et al. Continuous wave Doppler determination of right ventricular pressure. A simultaneous Doppler-catheterization study in 127 patients. J Am Coll Cardiol 1985;6:750–756.)

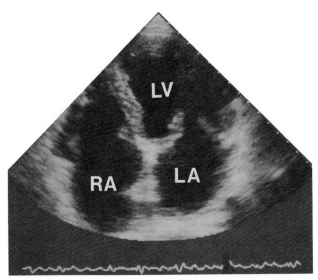

Figure 7.84. Two-dimensional echocardiogram of the apical four chamber view from a patient with thickened and myxomatous mitral and tricuspid valve leaflets.

ally after treatment with thrombolytic therapy provide important noninvasive information regarding hemodynamics and right heart function (226).

Ruptured Chordae Tendinae

Ruptured chordae tendinae of the tricuspid valve have been described on M-mode and two-dimensional echocardiographic studies (203–206). Irregular low-frequency diastolic fluttering, wide excursion of the anterior leaflet, and chaotic paradoxical motion of the posterior leaflet have all been reported on M-mode echocardiography. Ruptured chordae appear on two-

dimensional echocardiography as marked prolapse of the tricuspid valve into the right atrium beyond the valve annulus with loss of the normal leaflet coaptation. Tricuspid regurgitation invariably results from ruptured chordae with right ventricular dilatation; vigorous contractile function; and a dilated, pulsatile right atrium on two-dimensional echo with incomplete closure of the tricuspid valve leaflets. Incomplete closure is defined as failure of the tricuspid leaflet tips to reach within 1 cm of the plane of the tricuspid valve annulus in systole (201). This is best visualized in the apical four chamber view.

Tricuspid Valve Prolapse

The true incidence of tricuspid valve prolapse is unknown, and there are no generally accepted criteria for its diagnosis, but it has been reported in association with mitral valve prolapse more frequently than as an isolated finding. The reported incidence of tricuspid valve prolapse has emanated from autopsy studies, but these studies have varied markedly. In a series of 3083 autopsies (207), myxomatous degeneration of the mitral valve occurred in 30 (1%); in nine of these the tricuspid valve leaflets were myxomatous and voluminous, consistent with prolapse (0.3%) (Fig. 7.84). Davies et al. (208) detected mitral valve prolapse in 102 of 1376 (7.4%) autopsies, of which 41 also had tricuspid valve prolapse (3.0%). M-mode echocardiographic tricuspid valve motion patterns in tricuspid prolapse demonstrate mid- and pan-systolic buckling resembling mitral valve prolapse (210). On two-dimensional echocardiography, prolapse of the septal, anterior, and posterior leaflets, individually or together, superior to

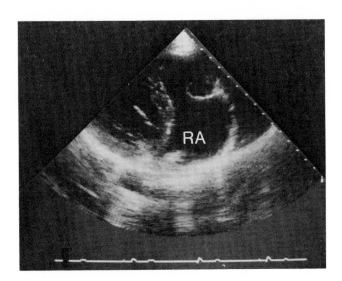

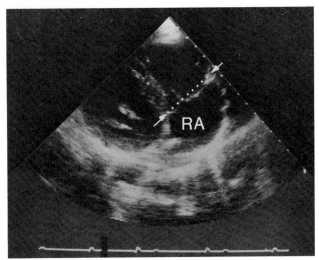

A   **B**

Figure 7.85. Two-dimensional echocardiogram of the right ventricular inflow tract from a patient with mild tricuspid regurgitation and tricuspid valve prolapse in diastole (*A*) and in systole (*B*). The plane in the tricuspid valve is shown by the line joining the arrows. The septal and anterior leaflets prolapsed beyond this plane into the right atrium in systole (*B*).

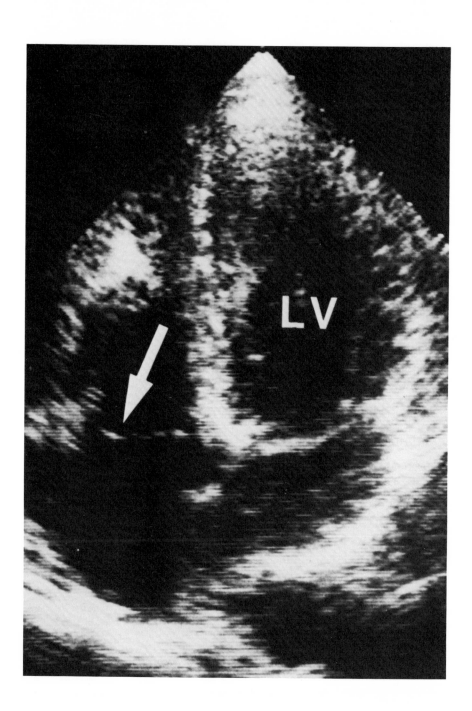

Figure 7.86. Two-dimensional echocardiogram of the apical four chamber view, showing the systolic bowing of the tricuspid valve (*arrow*).

the tricuspid annulus have been described in 19 to 50% of patients with mitral valve prolapse (211, 212) (Figs. 7.85, 7.86).

Tricuspid Annular Calcification

Calcification of the tricuspid annulus is much more rare than calcification of the mitral annulus, but it also occurs more often in the elderly. Mattelman et al. (227) studied 80 patients retrospectively with a two-dimensional echocardiographic diagnosis of mitral annular calcification, and detected only one patient with tricuspid annular calcification. By M-mode echocardiography, calcification of the tricuspid valve annulus appears as a uniform dense band beneath the tricuspid valve and it parallels the motion of the right ventricular endocardium. Two-dimensional echocardiography demonstrates increased reflectiveness of the posterior tricuspid annulus in the apical four chamber view and in the right ventricular two chamber view. Tricuspid annular calcification is associated with longstanding pressure or volume overload of the right ventricle from pulmonic stenosis, atrial septal defect, or cor pulmo-

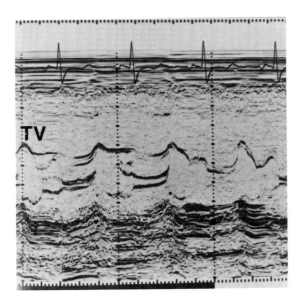

A

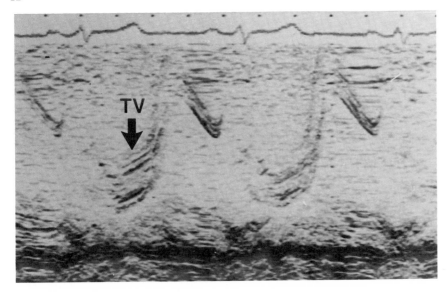

B

Figure 7.87. M-mode echocardiogram of a normal tricuspid valve (A), and of tricuspid valve vegetations, which present as thickened leaflets with increased echos emanating from them (B).

nale (228, 229). Thus, the difference in incidence of calcification of the right and left atrioventricular valve annuli is believed to be related to the difference in right and left heart pressures.

Infective Endocarditis

Right-side infective endocarditis occurs less commonly than left-side endocarditis. Of 137 hearts with infective endocarditis, Arnett (230) reported 23 (17%) with right-side vegetations, and in 13 only the tricuspid valve was involved. Although intravenous drug abuse is the most common cause of right-side infective vegetative endo-

carditis, noninfective vegetations consisting of thrombotic material may occur rarely in patients with disseminated intravascular coagulation or in patients with mucus secreting neoplasms involving the gastrointestinal or the genitourinary tract (213–215, 231–233).

Vegetations associated with tricuspid valve endocarditis vary greatly in size, but are usually larger than aortic or mitral valve vegetations and frequently occur on previously normal valve leaflets. They appear on M-mode (213, 232) as thickened leaflets (Fig. 7.87), and on two-dimensional echocardiography (215, 231, 232) as sessile or pedunculated irregular masses attached to one or more leaflets (Figs. 7.88–7.90). It is therefore

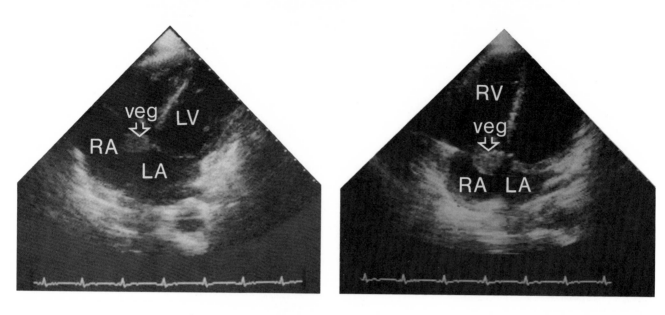

A   **B**

Figure 7.88. Two-dimensional echocardiogram of the four chamber view showing a large vegetation attached to the septal leaflet of the tricuspid valve (*A* and *B, arrow*).

crucially important to examine the tricuspid valve carefully with two-dimensional echocardiography in multiple orthogonal views, including the parasternal right ventricular inflow view, in all patients referred with suspected infective endocarditis (Figs. 7.89, 7.90). Ginzton et al. (215) followed eight patients with tricuspid valve vegetations for a mean of 11 months. In four the vegetation disappeared, in three it was smaller, and in one it remained the same size. The presence of a vegetation at followup study and rate of regression does not correlate with clinical outcome during the acute illness or with functional class at late followup.

Tricuspid Valve in Pulmonary Regurgitation

The jet of pulmonary regurgitation may impinge on the tricuspid valve leaflets, producing high-frequency diastolic flutter of one or more leaflets. This is uncommon in mild pulmonary regurgitation because the tricuspid valve is not situated directly below the pulmonary valve, but it often occurs in severe pulmonary regurgitation because right ventricular dilatation results in the tricuspid valve being more in the direct line of the regurgitant jet (234, 235).

TRICUSPID VALVE AS A MIRROR OF RIGHT VENTRICULAR FUNCTION

Right ventricular dysfunction may produce changes in tricuspid valve motion analogous to those of mitral valve motion in the presence of left ventricular dys-

function. Starling et al. (236) studied nine patients with right heart failure and 10 normal subjects. In all nine patients, the AC interval was prolonged beyond the normal range of 84 to 124 msec (Fig. 7.91), and the PR-AC interval was less than the normal range of 46 to 130 msec in all but one patient. However, there was only a mild correlation between right ventricular end-diastolic pressure and AC (r = 0.42), and PR-AC intervals (r = 0.52). A plateau at the B point was present in all nine patients in whom right ventricular end-diastolic pressure was elevated from 9 to 19 mmHg, but not in those in whom it was normal. In two patients, right ventricular end-diastolic pressure decreased from 14 to 6 mmHg, and 10 to 4 mmHg following treatment for heart failure, and the B notch disappeared in both patients. These results parallel the effects of left ventricular dysfunction on mitral valve motion, indicating that the tricuspid valve provides some insight into right ventricular dysfunction.

Iwasaki et al. (237) described a "monophasic triangular wave" in the M-mode appearance of the tricuspid valve in diastole in five patients with pulmonary embolism. The pattern resembles the fusion of EA points, which occurs in normal patients with tachycardia, or the extremely slow DE slope on the mitral valve, which is associated with left ventricular dysfunction.

A diminished EF slope may also be visualized in situations when right ventricular diastolic pressure is elevated. Nanda et al. (194) detected a reduced EF slope in seven patients with pulmonary hypertension, in the absence of tricuspid stenosis.

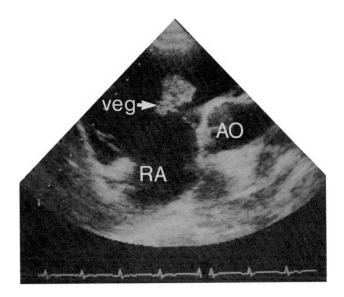

A

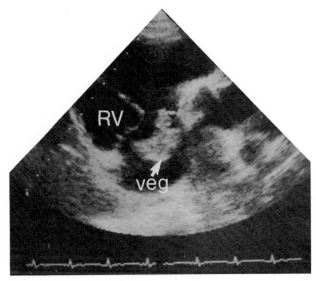

B

C

Figure 7.89.   Serial two-dimensional echocardiogram showing a large tricuspid valve vegetation in diastole (*A*), in systole (*B*), and in the short axis view of the aorta in systole (*C*).

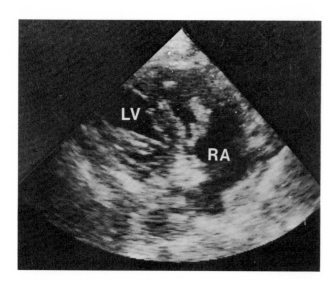

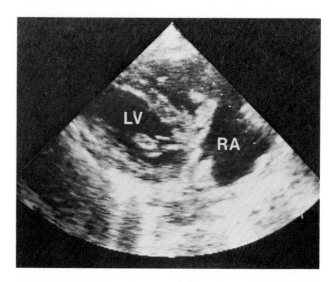

A   B

Figure 7.90.   Two-dimensional echocardiogram of the right ventricular inflow tract demonstrating an extensive vegetation on the septal leaflet of the tricuspid valve. (*A* and *B*).

Figure 7.91.   M-mode echocardiogram of the tricuspid valve from a patient with severe pulmonic hypertension, demonstrating prolongation of the AC segment (*arrows*).

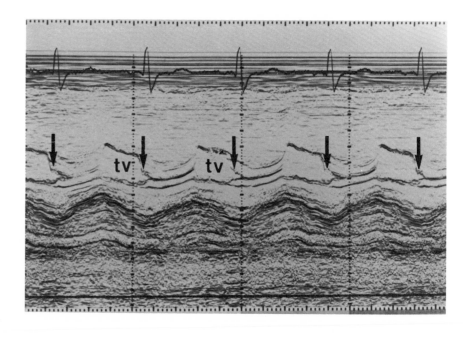

REFERENCES

1. Edler I. Ultrasound cardiogram in mitral valve disease. Acta Chir Scand 1956;3:230.
2. Edler I, Gustafson A. Ultrasonic cardiogram in mitral stenosis. Acta Med Scand 1957;159:85.
3. Edler I. Ultrasoundcardiography in mitral valve stenosis. Am J Cardiol 1967;19:18–31.
4. Segal BI, Likoff W, Kingsley B. Echocardiography: Clinical application in mitral stenosis. JAMA 1966;195:161–166.
5. Gustafson A. Correlation between ultrasound cardiography, hemodynamics and surgical findings in mitral stenosis. Am J Cardiol 1967;19:32–41.
6. Effert S. Pre- and postoperative evaluation of mitral stenosis by ultrasound. Am J Cardiol 1967;19:59–64.
7. Zaky A, Nasser WE, Feigenbaum H. Study of mitral valve action recorded by reflected ultrasound and its application in the diagnosis of mitral stenosis. Circulation 1968;37:789.
8. Duchak JM, Chang S, Feigenbaum H. The posterior mitral valve echo and the echocardiographic diagnosis of mitral stenosis. Am J Cardiol 1972;29:628–632.
9. Cope GD, Kisslo JA, Johnson ML, Behar VS. Reassessment of the echocardiogram in mitral stenosis. Circulation 1975;52:664–670.
10. Hall R, Austin A, Hunter S. M-mode echogram as a means of distinguishing between mild and severe mitral stenosis. Br Heart J 1981;46:486–491.
11. Gibson DG, Brown D. Measurement of instantaneous left ventricular dimension and filling rate in man, using echocardiography. Br Heart J 1973;35:1141–1149.
12. Upton MT, Gibson DG. The study of left ventricular function from digitized echocardiograms. Prog Cardiovasc Dis 1978;20:359–384.
13. St. John Sutton MG, Traill TA, Ghafour AS, Brown DJ, Gibson DG. Echocardiographic assessment of left ventricular filling after mitral valve surgery. Br Heart J 1977;39:1283.
14. Henry WL, Griffith JM, Michaelis LL, McIntosh CL, Morrow AG, Epstein SE. Measurement of mitral orifice area in patients with mitral valve disease by real time, two-dimensional echocardiography. Circulation 1975;51:827–831.
15. Wann LS, Weyman AE, Feigenbaum H, Dillon JC, Johnston KW, Eggleton RC. Determination of mitral valve area by cross-sectional echocardiography. Ann Int Med 1978;88:337–341.
16. Nichol PM, Gilbert BW, Kisslo JA. Two-dimensional echocardiographic assessment of mitral stenosis. Circulation 1977;55:120–133.
17. Martin RP, Rakowski H, Kleiman JH, Beaver W, London E, Popp RL. Reliability and reproducibility of two-dimensional echocardiographic measurement of the stenotic mitral valve orifice area. Am J Cardiol 1979;43:560–568.
18. Smith MD, Handshoe R, Handshoe S, Dwan OL, DeMaria AN. Comparative accuracy of two-dimensional echocardiography and Doppler pressure half-time methods in assessing the severity of mitral stenosis in patients with and without prior commissurotomy. Circulation 1986;73:100–107.
19. Come PC, Riley MF. M-mode and cross-sectional echocardiographic recognition of fibrosis and calcification of the mitral valve chordae and left ventricular papillary muscles. Am J Cardiol 1982;49:461.
20. Cohn LH, Alfred EN, Cohn LA, et al. Early and late risk of mitral valve replacement—A 12-year concomitant comparison of the porcine bioprosthetic and prosthetic disc mitral valves. J Thorac Cardiovasc Surg 1985;90:872.
21. Edmunds LH. Thromboembolic complications of current cardiac valvular prostheses. Ann Thor Surg 1982;34:96–106.
22. Ramirez J, Flowers NC. Severe mitral stenosis secondary to massive calcification of the mitral annulus with unusual echocardiographic manifestations. Clin Cardiol 1980;3:284.
23. Weyman AE, Heger JJ, Kronik G, Wann LS, Dillon JC, Feigenbaum H. Mechanism of paradoxical early diastolic septal motion in patients with mitral stenosis: Cross-sectional echocardiographic study. Am J Cardiol 1977;40:691.
24. Yock PB, Popp RL. Non-invasive estimation of right ventricular systolic pressure by Doppler ultrasound in patients with tricuspid regurgitation. Circulation 1984;70:657–662.
25. Joyner CR, Hey EB, Johnson J, Reid JM. Reflected ultrasound in the diagnosis of tricuspid stenosis. Am J Cardiol 1967;19:66–73.
26. Daniels SJ, Mintz GS, Kotler MN. Rheumatic tricuspid valve disease. Two-dimensional echocardiography, hemodynamic and angiographic correlations. Am J Cardiol 1983;51:491–496.
27. Veyrat C, Kalmanson D, Farjon M, Manin J, Abitbolg P. Non-invasive diagnosis and assessment of tricuspid regurgitation and stenosis using one- and two-dimensional echo-pulsed Doppler. Br Heart J 1982;47:596–605.
28. Kalmanson D, Veyrat C, Bouchareine F, Degroote A. Non-invasive recording of mitral valve flow velocity patterns using pulsed Doppler echocardiography: Application to diagnosis and evaluation of mitral valve disease. Br Heart J 1977;39:517–528.
29. Hatle L, Brubakk A, Tromsdal A, Angelsen B. Noninvasive assessment of pressure drop in mitral stenosis by Doppler ultrasound. Br Heart J 1978;40:131.
30. Holen J, Simonsen S. Determination of pressure gradient in mitral stenosis with Doppler echocardiography. Br Heart J 1979;41:529.
31. Diebold B, Theroux P, Bourassa MG, et al. Non-invasive pulsed Doppler study of mitral stenosis and mitral regurgitation: Preliminary study. Br Heart J 1979;42:168.
32. Thuillez C, Theroux P, Bourassa MG, et al. Pulsed Doppler echocardiographic study of mitral stenosis. Circulation 1980;61:381.
33. Stamm RB, Martin RP. Quantification of pressure gradients across stenotic valves by Doppler ultrasound. J Am Coll Cardiol 1983;2:707.
34. Kandheria BK, Tajik AJ, Reeder GS, et al. Doppler color flow imaging: A new technique for visualization and characterization of the blood flow jet in mitral stenosis. Mayo Clinic Proc 1986;61:623–630.
35. Hatle L, Angelsen B, Tromsdal B. Non-invasive assessment of pressure half-time by Doppler ultrasound. Circulation 1980;60:1096.
36. Hatle L, Angelson B. Doppler ultrasound in cardiology. 2nd ed. Philadelphia: Lea and Febiger, 1985.
37. Nakatani S, Masuyama T, Kodama K, Kitabatake A, Fujii K, Kamada T. Value and limitations of Doppler echocardiography in the quantification of stenotic mitral valve area: Comparison of the pressure half-time and the continuity equation methods. Circulation 1988;77:78–85.
38. Waller BF, Morrow AG, Maron BJ. Etiology of clinically severe, isolated chronic mitral regurgitation: Analysis of 97 patients over 30 years of age having mitral valve replacement. Am Heart J 1982;104:276–288.
39. Segal BL, Likoff W, Kingsley B. Echocardiography: Clinical application in mitral regurgitation. Am J Cardiol 1967;19:50–58.
40. Winters WL, Hafter J, Soloff LA. Abnormal mitral valve motion as demonstrated by the ultrasound technique in apparent pure mitral insufficiency. Am Heart J 1969;77:196.
41. Millward DK, Mclaurin PL, Craige E. Echocardiographic studies of the mitral valve in patients with congestive cardiomyopathy and mitral regurgitation. Am Heart J 1973;85:413.
42. Burgess J, Clark R, Kamingaki M, Cohn K. Echocardiographic findings in different types of mitral regurgitation. Circulation 1973;48:97.
43. Wann LS, Feigenbaum H, Weyman AE, Dillon JC. Cross-sectional echocardiographic detection of rheumatic mitral regurgitation. Am J Cardiol 1978;41:1258.
44. Patton R, Dragatakis L, Marpole D, Sniderman A. The posterior left atrial echocardiogram of mitral regurgitation. Circulation 1978;57:1134–1139.
45. Tei C, Tanaka H, Nakao S, et al. Motion of the interatrial septum in acute mitral regurgitation. Circulation 1980;62:1080–1088.
46. Godley RW, Wann LS, Rogers EW, Feigenbaum H, Weyman AE. Incomplete late mitral leaflet closure in patients with papillary muscle dysfunction. Circulation 1981;63:565–571.
47. Lewis BS, Hasin Y, Pasternak R, Gotsman S. Echocardiographic aortic root motion in ventricular volume overload and the effect of mitral incompetence. Eur J Cardiol 1979;10:375.

48. Hall RJC, Clark SE, Brown D. Evaluation of posterior aortic wall echogram in the diagnosis of mitral valve disease. Br Heart J 1979;41:522–528.

49. Ren J-F, Kotler MN, DePace NL, et al. Two-dimensional echocardiographic determination of left atrial emptying volume. A non-invasive index in quantifying the degree of non-rheumatic mitral regurgitation. J Am Coll Cardiol 1983;2:729.

50. Zile MR, Gaasch WH, Levine HJ. Left ventricular stress-dimensional-shortening before and after correction of chronic aortic and mitral regurgitation. Am J Cardiol 1985;56:99.

51. Nichol PM, Boughner DR, Persaud JA. Noninvasive assessment of mitral insufficiency by transcutaneous Doppler ultrasound. Circulation 1976;54:656.

52. Abbasi AS, Allen MW, DeCristofaro D, Ungar I. Detection and estimation of the degree of mitral regurgitation by range-gated pulsed Doppler echocardiography. Circulation 1980;61:143–147.

53. Areias JC, Goldberg SJ, Villeneuve VH. Use and limitations of the time interval histogram output from echo Doppler to detect mitral regurgitation. Am Heart J 1981;101:805.

54. Miyatake K, Kinoshita N, Nagata S, et al. Intracardiac flow pattern in mitral regurgitation studied with combined use of the ultrasonic pulsed Doppler technique and cross-sectional echocardiography. Am J Cardiol 1980;45:155.

55. Quinones MA, Young JB, Waggoner AD, Ostojic MC, Ribeiro LE, Miller RR. Assessment of pulsed Doppler echocardiography and detection and quantitation of aortic and mitral regurgitation. Br Heart J 1980;44:612–620.

56. Blanchard D, Diebold B, Perroneau P, et al. Non-invasive diagnosis of mitral regurgitation by Doppler echocardiography. Br Heart J 1981;45:589.

57. Veyrat C, Ameur A, Bas S, Lessana A, Abitbol G, Kalmanson D. Pulsed Doppler echocardiographic indices for assessing mitral regurgitation. Br Heart J 1984;51:130.

58. Omoto R, Yokotey Takamoto S, Kyo S, et al. The development of real-time two-dimensional Doppler echocardiography and its clinical significance in acquired valvular diseases. With special reference to the evaluation of valvular regurgitation. Jpn Heart J 1984;25:325.

59. Helmcke F, Nanda NC, Hsiung MC, et al. Color Doppler assessment of mitral regurgitation in orthogonal planes. Circulation 1987;75:175–183.

60. Miyatake K, Izumi S, Okamoto M, et al. Semiquantitative grading of severity of mitral regurgitation by real-time two-dimensional Doppler flow imaging technique. J Am Coll Cardiol 1986;7:82–88.

61. Rokey R, Sterling LL, Zoghbi WA, et al. Determination of regurgitation fraction in isolated mitral or aortic regurgitation by pulsed Doppler two-dimensional echocardiography. J Am Coll Cardiol 1986;7:1273–1278.

62. Blumlein S, Bouchard A, Schiller NB, et al. Quantitation of mitral regurgitation by Doppler echocardiography. Circulation 1986;74:306–314.

63. Barlow JB, Pocock WA, Marchand P, Denny M. The significance of late systolic murmurs. Am Heart J 1963;28:443–452.

64. Hancock EW, Cohn K. The syndrome associated with mid systolic click and late systolic murmur. Am J Med 1966;41:183–196.

65. Criley JM, Lewis KB, Humphries JO, Ross RS. Prolapse of the mitral valve: Clinical and cineangiographic findings. Br Heart J 1966;488–496.

66. Linhart JW, Taylor JW. The late apical systolic murmur: Clinical, hemodynamic and angiographic observations. Am J Cardiol 1966;18:164–168.

67. Kerber RE, Isaeff DM, Hancock EW. Echocardiographic patterns in patients with the syndrome of systolic click and late systolic murmur. N Engl J Med 1971;284:691-693.

68. Dillon JC, Haisse CL, Chang S, Feigenbaum H. Use of echocardiography in patients with prolapsed mitral valve. Circulation 1971;43:503.

69. Barlow JB, Pocock WA. The mitral valve prolapse enigma—Two decades later. Med Con Card Dis 1984;53:13–17.

70. Markiewicz W, Stoner J, London E, Hunt SA, Popp RL. Mitral valve prolapse in 100 presumably healthy young females. Circulation 1976;53:464–473.

71. Haikal M, Alpert MA, Whiting RB, Ahmed M, Kelly D. Sensitivity and specificity of M-mode echocardiographic signs of mitral valve prolapse. Am J Cardiol 1982;50:185–190.

72. Markiewicz W, London E, Popp RL. Effect of transducer placement on echocardiographic mitral valve motion. Am Heart J 1978;96:595–556.

73. Levisman JA, Abbasi AA. Abnormal motion of the mitral valve with pericardial effusion: Pseudo-prolapse of the mitral valve. Am Heart J 1976;91:18–20.

74. Gilbert BW, Schatz RA, Von Ramm OT, Behar VS, Kisslo JA. Mitral valve prolapse. Two-dimensional echocardiographic and angiographic correlation. Circulation 1976;54:716–723.

75. Morganroth J, Mardelli TJ, Naito M, Chen CC. Apical cross-sectional echocardiography, standard for the diagnosis of idiopathic mitral valve prolapse syndrome. Chest 1981;79:23–38.

76. Alpert MA, Carney RJ, Flaker GC, Sanfelippo JF, Webel RR, Kelly DL. Sensitivity and specificity of two-dimensional echocardiographic signs of mitral valve prolapse. Am J Cardiol 1984;54:792–796.

77. Spaccavento LJ, Hopkins DG, Popp RL. The sensitivity and specificity of two-dimensional echocardiography in mitral valve prolapse (abstr). Circulation 1983;68:III–366.

78. Gavin WA, Pearlman AS, Saal AK. Abnormal mitral leaflet coaptation: A non-specific two-dimensional echo finding (abstr). Circulation 1983;68:III–365.

79. Pollick C, Wilansky S, Parker S. Mitral valve prolapse; clinical and echocardiographic perspectives. Can Med A J 1986;135:277–280.

80. Levine RA, Triulzi MO, Harrigan P, Weyman AE. The relationship of mitral annular shape to the diagnosis of mitral valve prolapse. Circulation 1987;75:756–767.

81. Pollick C, Wilansky S. Echocardiography reports and data-base by microcomputer. Echocardiography 1985;2:393–400.

82. Devereux RB, Kramer-Fox R, Shear MK, Kligfield P, Pini R, Savage D. Diagnosis and classification of severity of mitral valve: Methodologic, biologic and prognostic considerations. Am Heart J 1987;113:1265–1280.

83. Krivokapich J, Child JS, Dadourian BJ, Perloff JK. Reassessment of echocardiographic criteria for diagnosis of mitral valve prolapse. Am J Cardiol 1988;61:131–135.

84. McMahon SW, Roberts JK, Kramer-Fox R, Zucker DM, Roberts RB, Devereux RB. Mitral valve prolapse and infective endocarditis. Am Heart J 1987;113:1291–1298.

85. Nishimura RA, McGoon MD, Shub C, Miller FA, Ilstrup DM, Tajik AJ. Echocardiographically documented mitral valve prolapse: Long-term follow-up of 232 patients. N Engl J Med 1985;313:1305–1309.

86. Duren DR, Becker AE, Dunning AJ. Long-term follow-up of idiopathic mitral valve prolapse in 300 patients: A prospective study. J Am Coll Cardiol 1988;2:42–47.

87. Meyer JF, Frank MJ, Goldberg S, Chen TO. Systolic mitral valve flutter, an echocardiographic clue to the diagnosis of ruptured chordae tendinae. Am Heart J 1977;93:308.

88. Duchak JM, Change S, Feigenbaum H. Echocardiographic features of torn chordae tendinae (abstr). Am J Cardiol 1972;29:260.

89. Burgess J, Clark R, Kamagaki M, Cohn K. Echocardiographic findings in different types of mitral regurgitation. Circulation 1973;48:97–106.

90. Humphries WC, Hammer WJ, McDonough MT. Echocardiographic equivalent of a flail mitral leaflet. Am J Cardiol 1977;40:802–807.

91. Mintz GS, Kotler MN, Segal BS, Parry WR. Two-dimensional echocardiographic recognition of ruptured chordae tendinae. Circulation 1978;57:244–250.

92. Cherian GC, Tei C, Shah PM, Wong M. Diastolic prolapse in the flail mitral valve syndrome: A new observation providing differentiation from the mitral valve prolapse syndrome. Am Heart J 1982;103:1074–1075.

93. Mintz GS, Kotler MN, Parry WR, Segal BL. Statistical comparison of M-mode and two-dimensional echocardiographic diagnosis of flail mitral leaflets. Am J Cardiol 1980;45:253–259.

94. DePace NL, Mintz GS, Ren J-F, et al. Natural history of the flail

mitral leaflet syndrome: A serial two-dimensional echocardiographic study. Am J Cardiol 1983;52:789–795.

95. Pomerance A. Pathological and clinical study of calcification of the mitral valve ring. J Clin Path 1970;23:354–360.

96. Roberts WC. Morphological features of the normal and abnormal mitral valve ring. Am J Cardiol 1983;51:1005–1028.

97. Pomerance A, Davies MJ. The pathology of the heart. Oxford: Blackwell Scientific Publications, 1975.

98. Savage DD, Garrison RJ, Castelli WP, et al. Prevalence of sub mitral (annular) calcium and its correlates in a general population based sample (Framingham Study). Am J Cardiol 1983;51: 1375–1378.

99. Tajik AJ, Giuliani ER, Frye RL, Davies GD, McGoon DC, Brandenberg RO. Mitral valve and/or annulus calcification associated with IHSS. Circulation 1972;46:III 228.

100. Kronzon I, Glassman E. Mitral ring calcification in IHSS. Am J Cardiol 1978;42:60–66.

101. Roberts WC, Perloff JK, Kostantino T. Severe valvular aortic stenosis in patients over 65 years of age. Am J Cardiol 1971;27: 497–506.

102. Nair CK, Aronow WS, Sketch MH, et al. Clinical and echocardiographic characteristics of patients with mitral annular calcification. Am J Cardiol 1983;51:992–995.

103. Goodman HB, Dorney ER. Marfan's syndrome with massive calcification of the mitral annulus at age 26. Am J Cardiol 1969; 24:426–431.

104. Grossman M, Knott AP, Jacoby WJ. Calcified annulus fibrosus with mitral insufficiency in the Marfan's syndrome. Arch Intern Med 1968;121:561–566.

105. Schieken RM, Kerber RE, Ionasescu W, Zellweger H. Cardiac manifestations of the mucopolysaccharidoses. Circulation 1975; 52:700–705.

106. Harrison CV, Lennox B. Heart block in osteitis deformans. Br Heart J 1948;10:167–173.

107. Nestico PF, DePace NL, Kotler MN, et al. Calcium phosphorus metabolism in dialysis patients with and without mitral annular calcium. Am J Cardiol 1983;51:497–500.

108. Mellino M, Salcedo EE, Lever HM, Vasudeven G, Kramer J. Echographic quantified severity of mitral annulus calcification. Am Heart J 1982;103:222–225.

109. DeBono DP, Warlow CP. Mitral annulus calcification and cerebral or retinal ischemia. Lancet 1979;2:383–385.

110. Meltzer RS, Martin RP, Robbins BS, Popp RL. Mitral annular calcification: Clinical and echocardiographic features. Acta Cardiologica 1980;35:189–202.

111. Chiechi MA, Lees WM, Thompson R. Functional anatomy of the normal mitral valve. J Thorac Surg 1956;32:378–398.

112. Wong M, Tei C, Shah PM. Sensitivity and specificity of two-dimensional echocardiography in the detection of valvular calcification. Chest 1983;84:423–427.

113. Korn D, DeSanctis RW, Sell S. Massive calcification of the mitral annulus. N Engl J Med 1962;267:900–909.

114. D'Cruz I, Panetta F, Cohen H, Glick G. Sub mitral calcification or sclerosis in elderly patients. Am J Cardiol 1979;44:31–38.

115. Dillon JC, Feigenbaum H, Konecke LL, Davis RH, Chang S. Echocardiographic manifestations of valvular vegetations. Am Heart J 1973;86:698–704.

116. Roy P, Tajik AJ, Giuliani ER, Schattenberg TT, Gau GT, Frye RL. Spectrum of echocardiographic findings in bacteria endocarditis. Circulation 1976;53:474–482.

117. Wann LS, Dillon JC, Weyman AE, Feigenbaum H. Echocardiography in bacterial endocarditis. N Engl J Med 1976;295:135.

118. Chandraratna PAN, Langevin E. Limitations of echocardiograms in diagnosing valvular vegetations in patients with mitral valve prolapse. Circulation 1977;56:436–438.

119. Gilbert BW, Haney RS, Crawford F, et al. Two-dimensional echocardiographic assessment of vegetative endocarditis. Circulation 1977;55:346–353.

120. Mintz GS, Kotler MN, Segal BL, Parry WR. Comparison of two-dimensional and M-mode echocardiography in the evaluation of patients with endocarditis. Am J Cardiol 1979;43:738–744.

121. Martin RP, Meltzer RS, Chia BL. Clinical utility of two-dimensional echocardiography in infective endocarditis. Am J Cardiol 1980;46:379.

122. Wann LS, Hallan CC, Dillon JC, Weyman AE, Feigenbaum H. Comparison of M-mode and cross-sectional echocardiography in infective endocarditis. Circulation 1979;60:728.

123. Mintz GS, Kotler MN. Clinical value and limitations of echocardiography. Arch Intern Med 1980;140:122.

124. Grenadier E, Schuger C, Palant A, Ben Ari J. Echocardiographic diagnosis of mitral obstruction in bacterial endocarditis. Am Heart J 1983;106:591–593.

125. Chun PKC, Sheehan MW. Myxomatous degeneration of the mitral valve. M-mode and two-dimensional echocardiographic findings. Br Heart J 1982;47:404–408.

126. Hickey AJ, Wolfers J. False positive diagnosis of vegetations on a myxomatous mitral valve using two-dimensional echocardiography. Aus NZ J Med 1982;12:540–542.

127. Fowles RE, Miller DC, Egbert BM, Fitzgerald JW, Popp RL. Systemic embolization from a mitral valve papillary endocardial fibroma detected by two-dimensional echocardiography. Am Heart J 1981;102:128–130.

128. Behnam R, Williams G, Gerlis L, Walker D, Scott O. Lipoma of the mitral valve and papillary muscle. Am J Cardiol 1983;51: 1459–1460.

129. O'Brien JT, Geiser EA. Infective endocarditis and echocardiography. Am Heart J 1984;108:386–394.

130. Mills J, Utley J, Abbott J. Heart failure in infective endocarditis: Predisposing factors, course and treatment. Chest 1974;66:151–157.

131. Pratt C, Whitcomb C, Neuman A, Mason DT, Amsterdam EA, DeMaria AN. Relationship of vegetations on echocardiogram to the clinical course and systemic emboli in bacterial endocarditis. Am J Cardiol 1978;41:384.

132. Stewart JA, Silimperi D, Horace P, Wise NK, Fraber TD, Kisslo JA. Echocardiographic documentation of vegetative lesions in infective endocarditis: Clinical implications. Circulation 1980; 61:374–399.

133. Lutas EM, Roberts RB, Devereux RB, Prieto LM. Relations between the presence of echocardiographic vegetations and the complication rate in infective endocarditis. Am Heart J 1986; 112:107–113.

134. Buda AJ, MacDonald IL, David TE, Kerwin AJ. Rapidly progressive vegetative endocarditis. Acta Cardiol (Brux) 1982;37:85–92.

135. Buchbinder NA, Roberts WC. Left sided valvular active infective endocarditis: A study of 45 necropsy patients. Am J Med 1972; 53:20–34.

136. Corrigall D, Bolen J, Hancock EW, Popp RL. Mitral valve prolapse and infective endocarditis. Am J Med 1977;63:215–222.

137. D'Cruz IA, Collison HK, Gerardo L, Hensel P. Two-dimensional echocardiographic detection of staphylococcal vegetation attached to calcified mitral annulus. Am Heart J 1982;103:295–298.

138. Rubenson DS, Tucker CR, Stinson EB, et al. The use of echocardiography in diagnosing culture-negative endocarditis. Circulation 1981;64:641–646.

139. Stafford A, Wann LS, Dillon JC, Weyman AE, Feigenbaum H. Serial echocardiographic appearance of healing bacterial vegetations. Am J Cardiol 1979;44:754–760.

140. Matsumoto M, Strom J, Hirose H, Abe H. Preoperative echocardiographic diagnosis of anterior mitral valve leaflet fenestration associated with infective endocarditis. Br Heart J 1982;48:538–540.

141. Enia F, Celona G, Filippone V. Echocardiographic detection of mitral valve aneurysm in patient with infective endocarditis. Br Heart J 1983;49:98–100.

142. Dillon J, Haine CL, Chang S, Feigenbaum H. Significance of mitral fluttering in patients with aortic insufficiency (abstr). Clin Res 1970;18:304.

143. Winsberg F, Gabor GE, Hernberg JG, Weiss B. Fluttering of the mitral valve in aortic insufficiency. Circulation 1970;41:225–229.

144. Cope GD, Kisslo JA, Johnson ML, Myers S. Diastolic vibration of the interventricular septum in aortic insufficiency. Circulation 1975;51:589–593.

145. D'Cruz I, Cohen HC, Prabhu R, Ayabe T, Glick G. Flutter of left ventricular structures in patients with aortic regurgitation, with

special reference to patients with associated mitral stenosis. Am Heart J 1976;92:684–691.

146. Skorton DJ, Child JS, Perloff JK. Accuracy of the echocardiographic diagnosis of aortic regurgitation. Am J Med 1980;69:377–382.

147. Meyer R, Bloon K, Schwartz D, Kaplan S. Mitral flutter without aortic incompetence (abstr). Circulation 1973;48:IV 81.

148. Hagler DJ, Tajik AJ, Ritter DG. Fluttering of atrio-ventricular valves in patients with D-transposition of the great arteries after Mustard operation. Mayo Clin Proc 1975;50:69–75.

149. Rowe DW, Pechacek LW, DeCastro CM, Garcia E, Hall RJ. Initial diastolic indentation of the mitral valve in aortic insufficiency. J Clin Ultrasound 1980;8:53–57.

150. Robertson WS, Stewart J, Armstrong WF, Dillo JC, Feigenbaum H. Reverse doming of the anterior mitral leaflet with severe aortic regurgitation. JACC 1984;3:431–436.

151. Pridie RB, Benham R, Oakley CM. Echocardiography of the mitral valve in aortic valve disease. Br Heart J 1971;33:296–304.

152. Botvinick EH, Schiller NB, Wickramasekaran R, Klausner SC, Gertz E. Echocardiographic demonstration of early mitral valve closure in severe aortic insufficiency—Its clinical implications. Circulation 1975;51:836–847.

153. Bjork VO, Hultquist G, Lodin H. Subaortic stenosis produced by an abnormally placed anterior mitral leaflet. J Thorac Cardiovasc Surg 1961;41:659–669.

154. Dinsmore RE, Sanders CA, Harthorne JW. Mitral valve regurgitation in idiopathic hypertrophic subaortic stenosis. N Engl J Med 1976;275:1225–1230.

155. Simon AI, Ross J Jr, Gault JH. Angiographic anatomy of the left ventricle and mitral valve in idiopathic hypertrophic subaortic stenosis. Circulation 1967;36:852–890.

156. Shah PM, Gramiak R, Kramer DH. Ultrasound localization of left ventricular outflow obstruction in hypertrophic obstructive cardiomyopathy. Circulation 1969;40:3–11.

157. Popp RL, Harrison DC. Ultrasound in the diagnosis and evaluation of therapy of idiopathic hypertrophic subaortic stenosis. Circulation 1969;40:905–914.

158. Gilbert BW, Pollick C, Adelman AG, Wigle ED. Hypertrophic cardiomyopathy: Subclassification by M-mode echocardiography. Am J Cardiol 1980;45:861–872.

159. Pollick C, Morgan CD, Gilbert BW, Rakowski H, Wigle ED. Muscular subaortic stenosis: The temporal relationship between systolic anterior motion and the anterior mitral leaflet and the pressure gradient. Circulation 1982;66:1087–1094.

160. Pollick C, Rakowski H, Wigle ED. Muscular subaortic stenosis: The quantitative relationship between systolic anterior motion and the pressure gradient. Circulation 1984;69:43–49.

161. Pollick C. Unlocking the mystery of systolic anterior motion: The key is timing. Can J Cardiol 1985;1:33–34.

162. Bulkley BH, Fortuin NJ. Systolic anterior motion of the mitral valve without asymmetric septal hypertrophy. Chest 1976;69:694–696.

163. Come PC, Bulkley BH, Goodman ZD, Hutchins GM, Pitt B, Fortuin NJ. Hypercontractile cardiac states simulating hypertrophic cardiomyopathy. Circulation 1977;55:901–908.

164. Wilansky S, Marquez-Julio A, Ogilvie RI, Cardella C, Leenan FH, Pollick C. Are hypertensive patients predisposed to hypertrophic obstructive cardiomyopathy? (abstr) Circulation 1985; Suppl III 131.

165. Sedlis SO, Saffitz JE, Schwob VS, Jaffe AS. Cardiac amyloidosis simulating hypertrophy cardiomyopathy. Am J Cardiol 1984;53:969–970.

166. Rees A, Elbl F, Minhas K, Solinger R. Echocardiographic evidence of outflow tract obstruction in Pompe's disease (glycogen storage disease of the heart). Am J Cardiol 1976;37:1103–1106.

167. Gattiker HF, Davignon A, Bozio A, et al. Echocardiographic findings in Friedreich's ataxia. Can J Neurol Sci 1976;3:321–332.

168. Way GL, Ruttenberg HD, Eshaghpour E, Nora JJ, Wolfe RR. Hypertrophic obstructive cardiomyopathy in infants of diabetic mothers (abstr). Circulation 1976;54:II 105.

169. Henry WL, Clark CE, Griffith JM, Epstein SE. Mechanism of left ventricular outflow obstruction in patients with obstructive asymmetric septal hypertrophy (idiopathic hypertrophic subaortic stenosis). Am J Cardiol 1975;35:337–345.

170. Martin RP, Rakowski H, French J, Popp RL. Idiopathic hypertrophic subaortic stenosis viewed by wide-angle, phased array echocardiography. Circulation 1979;59:1206–1217.

171. Spirito J, Maron BJ. Patterns of systolic anterior motion of the mitral valve in hypertrophic cardiomyopathy: Assessment by two-dimensional echocardiography. Am J Cardiol 1984;54:1039–1046.

172. Zaky A, Steinmetz E, Feigenbaum H. Role of atrium in closure of mitral valve in man. Am J Physiol 1969;217:1652–1659.

173. Konecke LL, Feigenbaum H, Chang S, Corya BC, Fischer JC. Abnormal mitral valve motion in patients with elevated left ventricular diastolic pressures. Circulation 1973;47:989–996.

174. Wilson JR, Robertson JF, Holford F, Reichek N. Evaluation of M-mode echographic estimates of left ventricular function: Relationship of selective ultrasonic and hemodynamic perimeters. Am Heart J 1981;101:249–254.

175. McLaurin LP, Gibson TC, Waider W, Grossman W, Craige E. An appraisal of mitral valve echocardiograms mimicking mitral stenosis in conditions with right ventricular pressure overload. Circulation 1973;48:801–809.

176. Laniado S, Yellin E, Kotler MN, Levy L, Stadler J, Turdiman R. A study of the dynamic relations between the mitral valve echogram and phasic mitral flow. Circulation 1975;51:104–113.

177. DeMaria AN, Miller RR, Amsterdam EA, Markson W, Mason DT. Mitral valve early diastolic closing velocity in the echocardiogram: Relation to sequential diastolic flow and ventricular compliance. Am J Cardiol 1976;37:693–700.

178. Rokey R, Kuo LC, Zoghbi WA, Limacher MC, Quinones MA. Determination of parameters of left ventricular diastolic filling with pulsed Doppler echocardiography: Comparison with cineangiography. Circulation 1985;71:543–550.

179. Kitabatake A, Inove M, Asao M, et al. Transmitral blood flow reflecting diastolic behaviour of the left ventricle in health and disease—A study by pulsed Doppler technique. Japan Circ J 1986;46:92–102.

180. Spirito P, Maron BJ, Bonow RO. Noninvasive assessment of left ventricular diastolic function: Comparative analysis of Doppler echocardiographic and radionuclide angiographic techniques. J Am Coll Cardiol 1986;7:518–526.

181. Miyatake K, Okamoto M, Kinoshita N, et al. Augmentation of atrial contribution of left ventricular inflow with aging as assessed by intracardiac Doppler flowmetry. Am J Cardiol 1984; 53:586–589.

182. Snider AR, Giddings SS, Rochini AP, et al. Doppler evaluation of left ventricular filling in children with systemic hypertension. Am J Cardiol 1985;56:921–926.

183. Takenaka K, Dabestani A, Gardon JM, et al. Pulsed Doppler echocardiographic study of left ventricular filling in dilated cardiomyopathy. Am J Cardiol 1986;58:143–147.

184. Fujii J, Yazaki Y, Sawada H, Aizawa T, Watanabe H, Kato K. Noninvasive assessment of left and right ventricular filling in myocardial infarction with a two-dimensional Doppler echocardiographic method. J Am Coll Cardiol 1985;5:1155–1160.

185. Kenny J, Plappert T, St. John Sutton M. Relationship between instantaneous Doppler velocity across the mitral valve and instantaneous left ventricular volume in normal and hypertrophied hearts. Br Heart J, in press.

186. Rasmussen S, Corya BC, Feigenbaum H, et al. Stroke volume calculated from the mitral valve echogram in patients with and without ventricular dyssynergy. Circulation 1978;58:125–133.

187. Kronik G, Slany J, Mosslacher H. Comparative value of eight M-mode echocardiographic formulas for determining left ventricular stroke volume. Circulation 1975;60:1308–1316.

188. Pollick C, Pittman M, Filly K, Fitzgerald PJ, Popp RL. Mitral and aortic valve orifice area in normal subjects and in patients with congestive cardiomyopathy: Determination by two-dimensional echocardiography. Am J Cardiol 1982;49:1191–1196.

189. Massie BM, Schiller MB, Ratshin RA, Parmley WW. Mitral-septal separation: New echocardiographic index of left ventricular function. Am J Cardiol 1977;39:1008–1016.

190. Child JS, Krivokapich J, Perloff JK. Effect of left ventricular size

on the mitral E point to ventricular septal separation in assessment of cardiac performance. Am Heart J 1981;101:797–802.

191. Ross EM, Roberts WC. The carcinoid syndrome: Comparison of 21 necropsy subjects with carcinoid heart disease to 15 necropsy subjects without carcinoid heart disease. Am J Med 1985;79:339–354.

192. Waller BF. Morphological aspects of valvular heart disease: Part II. Curr Prob Card 1984;9:40.

193. Joyner CR, Hey BE Jr, Johnson J, Reid JM. Reflected ultrasound in the diagnosis of tricuspid stenosis. Am J Cardiol 1967;19:66–73.

194. Nanna M, Chandraratna PA, Reid C, Nimalasuriya A, Rahimtoola SH. Value of two-dimensional echocardiography in detecting tricuspid stenosis. Circulation 1983;67:221–224.

195. Guyer DE, Gillam LD, Foale RA, et al. Comparison of echocardiographic and hemodynamic diagnosis of rheumatic tricuspid stenosis. J Am Coll Cardiol 1984;3:1135–1144.

196. Daniels SJ, Mintz GS, Kotler MN. Rheumatic tricuspid valve disease: Two-dimensional echocardiographic, hemodynamic, and angiographic correlations. Am J Cardiol 1983;51:492–496.

197. Shimada R, Takeshita A, Nakamura M, Tokunaga K, Hirata T. Diagnosis of tricuspid stenosis by M-mode and two-dimensional echocardiography. Am J Cardiol 1984;53:164.

198. Veyrat C, Kalmanson D, Farjon M, Mann J, Abitbolg P. Noninvasive diagnosis and assessment of tricuspid regurgitation and stenosis using one and two dimensional echo pulsed Doppler. Br Heart J 1982;47:596–605.

199. Dennig GK, Henneke KH, Rudolph W. Assessment of tricuspid stenosis by Doppler echocardiography. J Am Coll Cardiol 1987; 9:237A.

200. Parris TM, Panidis IP, Ross J, Mintz GS. Doppler echocardiographic findings in rheumatic tricuspid stenosis. Am J Cardiol 1987;60:1414–1416.

201. Gibson TC, Foale RA, Guyer DE, Weyman AE. Clinical significance of incomplete tricuspid valve closure seen on two-dimensional echocardiography. JACC 1984;4:1052–1057.

202. Howard RJ, Drobac M, Rider WD, et al. Carcinoid heart disease: Diagnosis by two-dimensional echocardiography. Circulation 1982;66:1059–1065.

203. Watanabe T, Katsume H, Matsukubo H, Furukawa K, Ijichi H. Ruptured chordae tendinae of the tricuspid valve due to nonpenetrating trauma. Chest 1981;80:751–753.

204. Donaldson RM, Ballester M, Rickards AF. Rupture of a papillary muscle of the tricuspid valve. Br Heart J 1982;48:291–293.

205. Oliver J, Benito F, Gallego FG, Sotillo J. Echocardiographic findings in ruptured chordae tendinae of the tricuspid valve. Am Heart J 1983;105:1033–1035.

206. Bates ER, Sorkin RP. Echocardiographic diagnosis of flail anterior leaflet in tricuspid endocarditis. Am Heart J 1983;106:161–163.

207. Pomerance A. Ballooning deformity of atrioventricular valves. Br Heart J 1969;31:343.

208. Davies MJ, Moore BP, Brainbridge MV. The floppy mitral valve: Study of incidence, pathology and complication in surgical, necropsy and forensic material. Br Heart J 1978;40:468.

209. Rippe JM, Angoff G, Sloss LJ, Wynne J, Alpert JS. Multiple floppy valves: An echocardiographic syndrome. Am J Med 1979;66:817.

210. Chandraratna PSN, Lopez JM, Fernandez JJ, Cohen LS. Echocardiographic detection of tricuspid valve prolapse. Circulation 1975;51:823–826.

211. Schlamowitz RA, Gross S, Keating E, Pitt W, Mazur J. Tricuspid valve prolapse: A common occurrence in the click murmur syndrome. J Clin Ultrasound 1982;10:435–439.

212. Brown GK, Anderson V. Two-dimensional echocardiography and the tricuspid valve. Br Heart J 1983;49:495–500.

213. Lee CC, Ganguly SN, Magnisalis K, Robin E. Illustrative echocardiogram: Detection of tricuspid valve vegetations by echocardiography. Chest 1974;66:432–433.

214. Crawford FA Jr, Wechsler AS, Kisslo JA. Tricuspid endocarditis in a drug addict: Detection of tricuspid vegetations by two-dimensional echocardiography. Chest 1978;74:473–475.

215. Ginzton LE, Siegel RJ, Criley JM. Natural history of tricuspid

valve endocarditis: A two-dimensional echocardiographic study. Am J Cardiol 1982;49:1853–1859.

216. Lieppe W, Behar VS, Scallion R, Kisslo JA. Detection of tricuspid regurgitation with two-dimensional echocardiography and peripheral vein injections. Circulation 1978;57:128.

217. Meltzer RS, Vered Z, Benjamin P, Hegesh J, Visser CA, Neufeld HN. Diagnosing tricuspid regurgitation by direct imaging of the regurgitant flow in the right atrium using contrast echocardiography. Am J Cardiol 1983;52:1050.

218. Wise NK, Myers S, Fraker TD, Stewart JA, Kisslo JA. Contrast M-mode ultrasonography of the inferior vena cava. Circulation 1981;63:1100.

219. Miyatake K, Okamoto M, Kinoshita N, et al. Evaluation of tricuspid regurgitation by pulsed Doppler and two-dimensional echocardiography. Circulation 1982;66:777.

220. Skjaerpe T, Hatle L. Diagnosis of tricuspid regurgitation sensitivity of Doppler ultrasound compared with contrast echocardiography. Eur Heart J 1985;6:429–436.

221. Suzuki Y, Kambara H, Kadota K, et al. Detection and evaluation of tricuspid regurgitation using a real time, two-dimensional, color-encoded, Doppler flow imaging system: Comparison with contrast two-dimensional echocardiography and right ventriculography. Am J Cardiol 1986;57:811–815.

222. Sakai K, Nakamura K, Satomi G, Kondo M, Kirosawa K. Hepatic vein blood flow pattern measured by Doppler echocardiography as an evaluation of tricuspid valve insufficiency. J Cardiogr 1983;13:33.

223. Currie PJ, Seward JB, Chan K-L, et al. Continuous wave Doppler determination of right ventricular pressure: A simultaneous Doppler-catheterization study in 127 patients. J Am Coll Cardiol 1985;6:750–756.

224. Chan K-L, Currie PJ, Seward JB, Hagler DJ, Mair DD, Tajik AJ. Comparison of three Doppler ultrasound methods in the prediction of pulmonary artery pressure. J Am Coll Cardiol 1987;9:549–554.

225. Nishimura RA, Miller FA Jr, Callahan MJ, Benassi RC, Seward JB, Tajik AJ. Doppler echocardiography: Instrumentation, technique and application. Mayo Clin Proc 1985;60:321–343.

226. Come PC, Kim D, Parker JA, et al. Early reversal of right ventricular dysfunction in patients with acute pulmonary embolism after treatment with intravenous tissue plasminogen activator. J Am Coll Cardiol 1987;10:971–978.

227. Mattleman S, Panidis I, Kotler MN, et al. Calcification of the tricuspid annulus diagnosed by two-dimensional echocardiography. Am Heart J 1984;107:986–988.

228. Rogers JV Jr, Chandler NW, Franch RH. Calcification of the tricuspid annulus. Am J Radiol 1969;106:550.

229. Bonchek LI. Calcification of the annulus of the tricuspid valve. Chest 1972;61:307.

230. Arnett EN, Roberts WC. Active infective endocarditis: A clinical pathological analysis of 137 necropsy patients. Curr Prob Cardiol 1976;1:1.

231. Panidis IP, Kotler MN, Mintz GS, Segal BL, Ross JJ. Right heart endocarditis. A two-dimensional echocardiographic study. Am Heart J 1984;107:759.

232. Kisslo JA, Von Ramm OT, Harvey R, Jones R, Juk SS, Behar VS. Echocardiographic evaluation of tricuspid valve endocarditis. An M-mode and two-dimensional study. Am J Cardiol 1976;38:302.

233. St. John Sutton M, Lie JT. Clinical importance and recognition of nonbacterial thrombotic endocarditis. Practical Cardiology 1985;2:45–57.

234. Gramiak R, Shah PM. Cardiac ultrasonography: A review of current applications. Radiol Clin North Am 1971;9:469.

235. Nanda NC. The tricuspid valve. In: Kraus, ed. The practice of echocardiography. New York: John Wiley, 1985.

236. Starling MR, Crawford MH, Walsh RA, O'Rourke RA. Value of the tricuspid valve echogram for estimating right ventricular end diastolic pressure during vasodilator therapy. Am J Cardiol 1980;45:966–972.

237. Iwasaki T, Tanimoto M, Yamamoto T, Makihata S, Kayai Y, Yorifugi S. Echocardiographic abnormalities of tricuspid valve motion in pulmonary embolism. Br Heart J 1982;47:454–460.

8
Acquired Aortic and Pulmonary Valve Disease

Martin St. John Sutton
John Kenny
Ted Plappert
Paul Oldershaw

Clinical evaluation of aortic valve disease is often difficult, but the combination of M-mode and two-dimensional Doppler echocardiography enables the correct diagnosis to be established and the severity of the disease to be quantified accurately in the majority of patients.

NORMAL AORTIC VALVE

Two-dimensional echocardiographic imaging of the aortic valve from the left parasternal long axis view visualizes the right cusp anteriorly and the noncoronary cusp posteriorly (Fig. 8.1). In diastole a thin linear echo is visible in the center of the aorta parallel to the long axis of the aorta (Fig. 8.1); this image is produced by the line of coaption of the free edges of the two aortic cusps. The bodies of the leaflets are parallel to the ultrasonic beam in this view and are usually not well visualized. The leaflets move apart in systole and lie parallel to the walls of the aortic root (Fig. 8.1), where they may be difficult to distinguish from the images produced by the anterior and posterior aortic walls. The normal M-mode echocardiographic recording illustrates the normal pattern of motion of the aortic valve leaflets (Fig. 8.2). In systole the leaflets open widely and coapt briskly following left ventricular ejection, forming a box-shaped structure. During dias-

tole, there is a discrete closure line, which is usually centrally placed in the aorta when the aortic valve is tricuspid (Fig. 8.2). Occasionally, the left coronary aortic leaflet can be seen in the normal M-mode recording in systole as a linear echo in the center of the box-shaped structure. Excursion of the aortic valve leaflets is dependent, not only on valve mobility, but also on volume flow through the valve. Reduced blood flow results in decreased rate, amplitude, and duration of leaflet opening (Fig. 8.3). Fine systolic fluttering of the aortic leaflets is seen occasionally by M-mode echocardiography and is normal, indicating that the leaflet tissue is sufficiently pliable to vibrate at high frequency (Fig. 8.4). The positions of the commissures and the three cusps of the aortic valve are demonstrated in two-dimensional echocardiographic short axis views of the aorta, obtained from the left parasternal region (Fig. 8.5). The leaflets move apart in systole and come to rest in their respective sinuses, forming a triangular-shaped orifice with curved edges (Fig. 8.5). The aortic valve can also be imaged throughout the cardiac cycle from the apical five chamber view (Fig. 8.6), but it may be difficult to assess accurately movement of the individual cusps from this position. The apical long axis view of the left ventricle also demonstrates the aortic valve (Fig. 8.7), and is similar to that obtained from the parasternal long axis view. Short

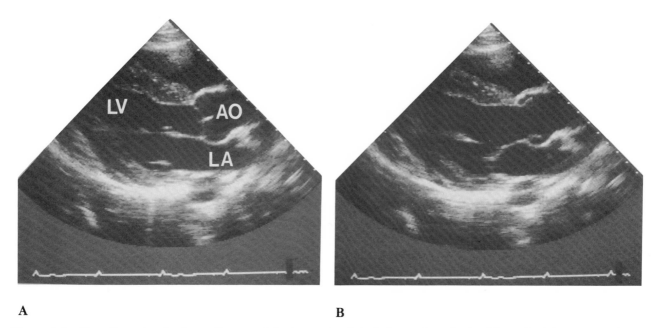

A   B

Figure 8.1. Two-dimensional echocardiogram of the long axis of the left ventricle obtained from the left parasternal region, showing the aortic valve leaflets in apposition during diastole. The right coronary leaflet is superior and the noncoronary leaflet is inferior (*A*). The leaflets open in systole and can be seen in their respective coronary sinuses (*B*).

axis images of the aortic valve can be obtained from the subcostal route, and this may be invaluable when the aortic leaflets cannot be visualized from the left parasternal and/or apical routes (Fig. 8.8).

Blood flow velocity spectra in the left ventricular outflow tract can be recorded from the apical five chamber or from the apical long axis view using pulsed wave Doppler echocardiography to position the sample volume immediately proximal to the aortic valve. The normal peak velocity (Fig. 8.9) ranges from 0.7 to 1.5 m/s and tends to increase as recordings are made

closer to the valve. Flow velocity increases further when the blood flow velocity is recorded distal to the valve in the proximal ascending aorta. Although the contour of the blood flow velocity spectral envelopes obtained proximal and distal to the aortic valve are similar, the peak velocity distal to the valve is frequently higher and may reach 1.5 m/s. When blood flow velocity is recorded from the ascending aorta, there is often a short negative velocity signal indicating reversed flow associated with aortic valve closure. The maximum blood flow velocity is usually recorded ei-

Figure 8.2. M-mode echocardiogram showing the aorta with the left atrium posterior to it. The aortic leaflets open briskly in systole and remain widely open as the aortic root moves anteriorly during left ventricular ejection. The leaflets close rapidly at end ejection with a centrally placed closure line between the anterior and posterior aortic root.

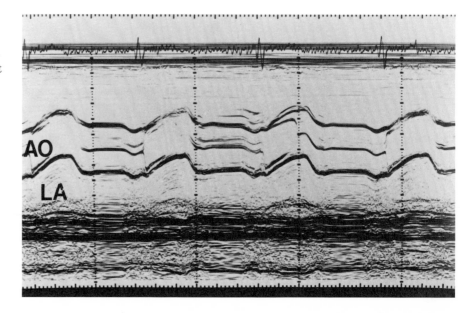

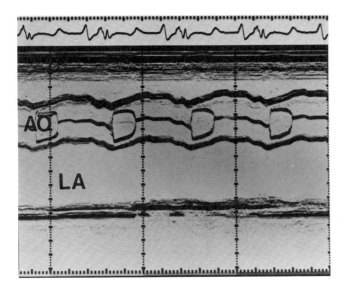

Figure 8.3. M-mode echocardiogram from a patient with severe primary left ventricular dysfunction. The left atrium is enlarged, and the aortic valve leaflets drift open rather than open briskly and they do not approximate the aortic walls. Having opened, they drift slowly into closed position.

ther at valve level or within the first 2 cm of the ascending aorta. When blood flow velocity profiles are recorded from the ascending aorta, it should be appreciated that the velocity spectra may vary depending on the precise location of the sample volume. Velocity spectra obtained close to the inferior wall on the lesser curvature of the aortic arch may have lower velocities than those obtained close to the superior wall on the greater curvature of the aortic arch. Sometimes an abnormal blood flow velocity spectrum showing an

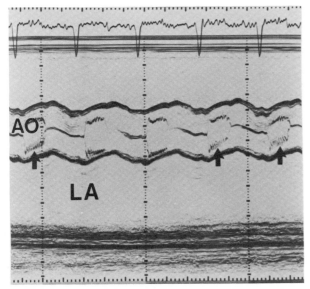

Figure 8.4. M-mode echocardiogram showing high frequency vibrations on the right and noncoronary leaflets (*arrow*)—a normal finding indicating that the leaflets are texturally normal and able to resonate at high frequency.

early peak with a reduced late flow is obtained close to the inferior wall, similar to that recorded from patients with hypertrophic cardiomyopathy. Normal blood flow velocity spectra can be obtained when the transducer is repositioned in the center of the aorta. Continuous-wave Doppler flow velocity profile amplitudes are similar to those obtained with pulsed-wave Doppler and can be recorded with the transducer at the apex, the right parasternal, and the suprasternal positions.

BICUSPID AORTIC VALVE

Approximately 1% of the population have bicuspid aortic valves (1). Bicuspid valves often produce a clicking sound or ejection click as the cusps evert upon opening. The ejection click is usually followed by an ejection systolic murmur generated by turbulent blood flow through the valve orifice. M-mode echocardiography demonstrates that the leaflets open widely in systole, but the diastolic closure line is usually, although not always, eccentrically placed (Fig. 8.10). An eccentricity index has been derived from M-mode echo recordings of bicuspid valve (2):

Eccentricity index (mm) =

$$\frac{\frac{1}{2} \times \text{width of aortic lumen at beginning of diastole}}{\text{maximum distance of diastolic cusp echo from nearest aortic margin}}$$

This index is usually in excess of 1.5 in bicuspid aortic valves, but it may also exceed 1.5 in patients with congenitally stenosed trileaflet aortic valves. This eccentricity index has been of limited value in detecting bicuspid aortic valves in children (3).

Two-dimensional echocardiograms of bicuspid aortic valves in short axis obtained from the left parasternal region have shown that the two leaflets are usually equal in size, with the commissure running obliquely from left to right (Fig. 8.11). However, there are many variations in the anatomy of the cusps and commissures, with raphe's or incomplete commissures being common (Fig. 8.11). In childhood and early adult life, the bicuspid valve is usually not stenotic, but has a propensity to calcify early and may become stenotic by the fifth to sixth decade.

AORTIC STENOSIS

Left ventricular outflow obstruction occurs most commonly at aortic valve level, but may occur above the valve (congenital supravalvar stenosis) or below the valve (congenital subvalvar stenosis). Aortic valve stenosis may be congenital or acquired. Congenitally

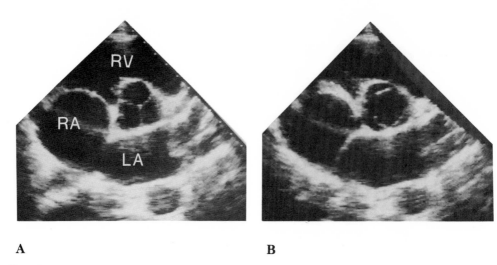

A   **B**

Figure 8.5. Two-dimensional echocardiogram obtained from the left parasternal region showing the aorta and aortic valve in short axis with the leaflets closed in diastole (*A*) and open in systole (*B*). The commissures between the three leaflets are clearly visualized with the superior right coronary cusp; the noncoronary cusp, positioned inferiorly and to the left; and the left coronary cusp, inferiorly and to the right. The tricuspid valve is visualized to the left of the aortic root, the right ventricular outflow tract wraps around the aorta superiorly, and the left atrium is posterior to the aorta.

abnormal stenotic valves may be unicuspid, bicuspid, or tricuspid, or may be due to a dome-shaped diaphragm. Unicuspid valves usually produce severe aortic stenosis in infancy, while bicuspid and tricuspid valves rarely cause stenosis before adult life. The abnormal architecture of congenitally abnormal bicuspid and tricuspid valves results in turbulent flow across the valve. This turbulent flow is believed to be an important etiological factor in the progressive damage to the leaflets culminating in fibrosis, calcification, and stenosis. Acquired aortic stenosis may be rheumatic or due to degenerative senile calcification. In rheumatic aortic stenosis, the pathologic hallmark is commissural fusion with cuspal thickening, which is almost always

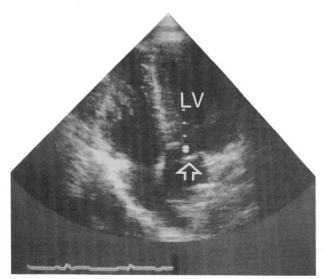

Figure 8.6. Two-dimensional echocardiogram of the apical five chamber view in diastole, showing the aortic leaflets (*arrow*).

associated with similar commissural thickening and fusion of the mitral valve leaflets. By contrast, in degenerative or senile calcific aortic stenosis, the calcific changes occur in the leaflets themselves, with no commissural fusion. The accumulation of calcium begins at the bases of the leaflets and slowly involves the bodies of the valve leaflets, rendering them rigid and immobile with progressive reduction in the aortic valve orifice area. Degenerative calcific aortic stenosis is a disease occurring late in life (in the seventh and eighth decades) and has a predilection for bicuspid valves a decade earlier than tricuspid valves. Degenerative calcific aortic stenosis is often accompanied by calcification of the mitral annulus and subvalve apparatus, occasionally also involving the mitral valve leaflets themselves.

The characteristic M-mode echocardiographic findings in aortic stenosis are marked thickening of the leaflets and reduced leaflet separation in systole (Fig. 8.12). It is important to realize, however, that thickening and/or calcification of the leaflets alone does not necessarily indicate hemodynamically important aortic stenosis. Measurements of aortic leaflet separation by M-mode echocardiography have correlated poorly with the clinical severity of aortic stenosis and with aortic valve gradients and valve orifice areas measured at cardiac catheterization (4–6).

The poor correlations between M-mode echocardiography and hemodynamics in aortic stenosis is due to a combination of factors. The M-mode echo beam only transects the right and noncoronary aortic leaflets, both of which may be fixed, while the left coronary leaflet may be normally mobile. The aortic valve may be extensively calcified so that the aortic root is filled

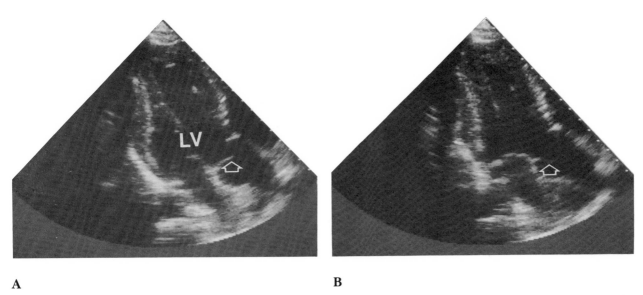

A   **B**

Figure 8.7. Two-dimensional echocardiogram showing the left ventricular long axis from the apex. The anterior mitral valve leaflet is contiguous with the aortic root. The aortic leaflets coapt in diastole (*arrow*, *A*) and open in systole (*arrow*, *B*) while the mitral leaflets are visualized in the closed position.

with echoes throughout systole and diastole (Fig. 8.12), and leaflet separation may be impossible to visualize. Aortic valve leaflet separation may vary depending upon where the beam passes through the valve orifice. For example, if the ultrasound beam passes through the partially fused commissures, the valve may appear more stenotic than if it passes through the central orifice. This is particularly important in congenital aortic stenosis, in which the valve domes in systole. The M-mode beam may pass through the base of the pliable leaflets and show normal cusp opening, whereas in reality there is severe aortic stenosis with a pinhole orifice at the top of the doming leaflets. Thus, the true aortic valve orifice may be very small, while leaflet separation recorded at the base of the valve appears normal. Attention should not be confined to the echocardiographic appearances of valve leaflets in aortic stenosis. Aortic stenosis is an obstruction to left ventricular ejection, which is associated with development of left ventricular hypertrophy to overcome the increased work of ejection. In significant aortic stenosis, left ventricular wall thickness is increased, while

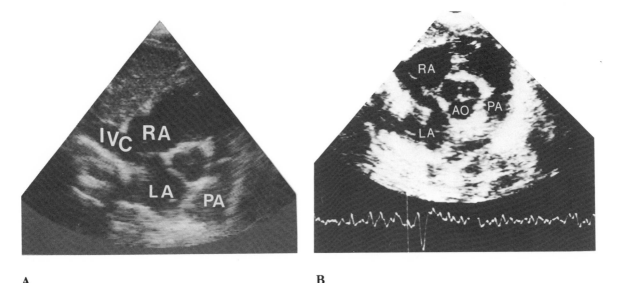

A   **B**

Figure 8.8. Two-dimensional echocardiogram of the aorta and aortic valve in cross-section, obtained from the subcostal. The tricuspid valve is superior to the aorta; the right atrium is to the left with the interatrium septum running horizontally and leftward toward the inferior vena cava. The pulmonary valve is to the right of the aorta and the right ventricular outflow tract and main pulmonary artery run vertically from top to bottom, to the right of the aorta (*A*). The aortic valve commissures are better visualized in (*B*).

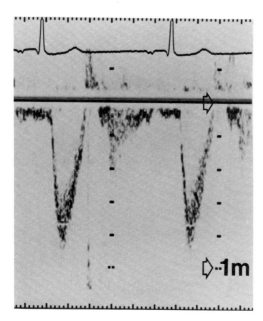

Figure 8.9.   Pulsed-wave Doppler velocity profile, obtained from the LV outflow tract, showing rapid acquisition of the peak velocity (0.8 m/sec), and a slower deceleration toward the end of left ventricular ejection. The velocity spectral envelope is narrow, indicating laminar blood flow.

the cavity dimension initially remains normal (Fig. 8.13). When the capacity to develop left ventricular hypertrophy has been exhausted, however, the left ventricle dilates, end-systolic wall stress increases as predicted by Laplace's Law, and contractile function decreases. Thus, left ventricular cavity dimension and wall thickness should be measured in aortic stenosis; if these are both normal, the aortic stenosis is trivial, regardless of the appearance of the valve leaflets themselves.

Two-Dimensional Echocardiography

Two-dimensional echocardiography overcomes some of the problems encountered with M-mode echocardiography (6, 7). The combination of high quality left parasternal long and short axis views and apical long axis left ventricular views enables accurate assessment of the aortic valve by two-dimensional echocardiography (Figs. 8.14, 8.15). As aortic stenosis develops, the valve leaflets initially appear thickened, resulting in an increased number of echoes. As the disease process progresses, the valve becomes fibrosed and calcified, with progressive decrease in both leaflet separation and valve orifice area. In some individuals the valve becomes so heavily calcified that it is impossible to discern any cusp motion or any aortic valve orifice. In congenital aortic stenosis, the characteristic systolic doming of the valve leaflets is visualized best in the left parasternal long axis view, in which the echoes from the leaflet edges curve inward toward the center of the aortic root in systole, and do not run parallel to the wall of the aorta. In rheumatic aortic stenosis, the thickened valve commissures are well demonstrated in the para-

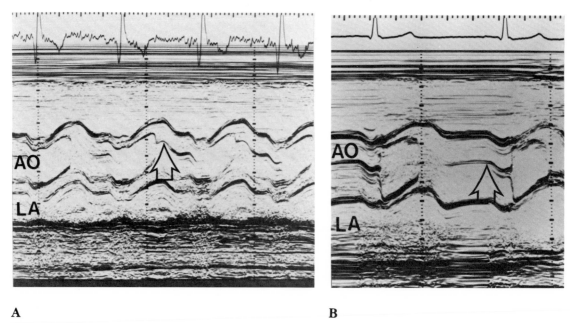

A   B

Figure 8.10.   M-mode echocardiogram of the aortic valve, aorta, and left atrium from two patients with bicuspid aortic valves by two-dimensional echocardiography. The aortic leaflets open fully in systole in both patients, but the closure line in diastole is eccentric in one (*A*), and almost central in the other (*B*). Although eccentricity of the aortic valve closure line (*arrows*) is common in bicuspid valves, the commissural and leaflet anatomy can usually be determined only by two-dimensional echocardiography.

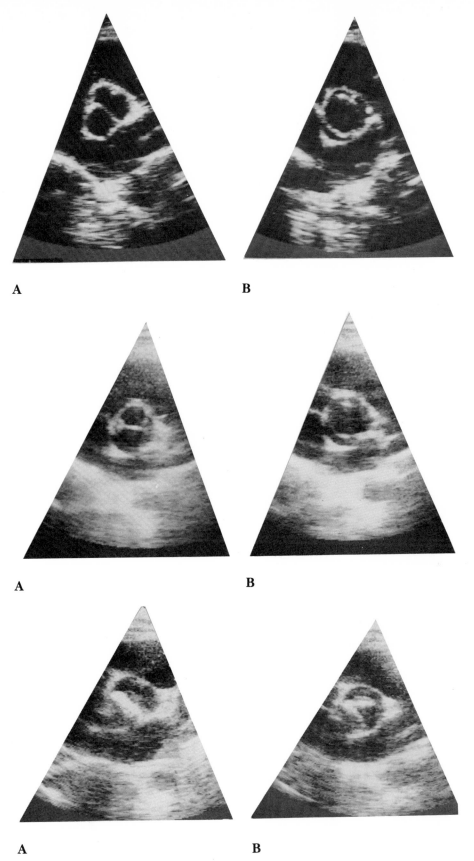

A   B

A   B

A   B

Figure 8.11. Two-dimensional echocardiograms of the short axis view of the aorta and aortic valves from three patients with bicuspid aortic valves. The commissural anatomy is seen easily in diastole when the leaflets are in apposition (*A*). The aortic leaflets are shown open in systole (*B*). The valves in the two upper panels open fully, while the valve in the bottom panel is calcified, and leaflet opening is reduced, consistent with moderate aortic stenosis.

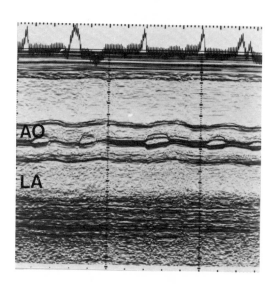

A

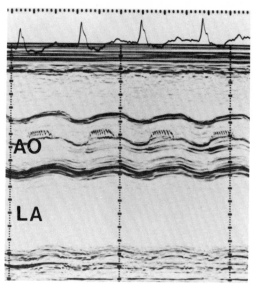

B

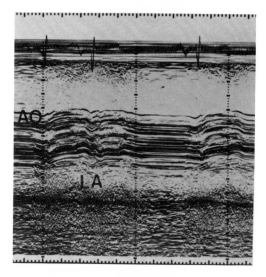

C

Figure 8.12.   M-mode echocardiograms from three patients with aortic valve stenosis of varying severity. The leaflets are thickened but there is observable leaflet separation (*A*). The right coronary leaflet (*B*) vibrates at high frequency, but the noncoronary leaflet is thickened and immobile. There is extreme calcification of the aortic valve leaflets with linear echos filling the aortic root (*C*) and no clearly defined leaflet separation.

sternal short axis view (Fig. 8.16). In systole the triangular orifice of the stenotic aortic valve becomes increasingly smaller and ultimately slitlike (Fig. 8.16). In the degenerative type of aortic stenosis, the deposits of calcium can be seen well in the left parasternal short axis view of the aorta in the body, base, and free edges of the valve leaflets, but there is no fusion of the commissures (Fig. 8.14).

Although M-mode and two-dimensional echocardiography have been useful in the detection of aortic stenosis, attempts to assess its severity by visualization of the valve leaflet motion have been less reliable. The aortic valve orifice has been measured from two-dimensional long axis (7–9) and short axis (10) views,

and results compared with hemodynamic measurements obtained at cardiac catheterization. An early study reported an excellent correlation between maximum cusp separation and aortic valve area assessed at cardiac catheterization when cusp separation was expressed as a percentage of aortic root diameter to compensate for patient size (7). An average maximum value for aortic leaflet separation in normal subjects was 73%, compared to a mean of 53% in patients with mild aortic stenosis and 30% in patients with moderate to severe stenosis. Subsequent studies have indicated that aortic stenosis is likely to be severe if leaflet separation is less than 8 mm (8, 9). Although calculation of group mean values for cusp separation is

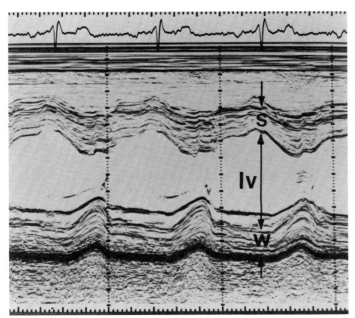

Figure 8.13.   M-mode echocardiogram of the left ventricle, at the level of the tips of the mitral valve leaflets, from a patient with moderately severe aortic valve stenosis. The LV cavity is of normal size, and endocardial motion of the septum and posterior left LV wall are normal and equal. The septum (S) and left ventricular posterior wall thicknesses (W) are equivalently increased, indicating moderate concentric LV hypertrophy.

helpful in separating populations of patients with mild aortic stenosis from those with severe obstruction, there is considerable overlap between mild and moderate and between moderate and severe obstruction. These measurements are of limited clinical value in the

management of individual patients (Fig. 8.17). Attempts to measure aortic valve area from short axis views (10) have been less successful because the orifice is irregularly shaped, and it is technically difficult to planimeter the orifice area in the majority of patients. A qualitative estimate of the severity of aortic stenosis can be made by examining the mobility of individual leaflets in long and short axis (9) and assessing left ventricular chamber size, the degree of hypertrophy, and pump function. Aortic stenosis is characterized by slow but progressive development of concentric hypertrophy and reduction in left ventricular cavity volume, so that end-systolic wall stress is normal and systolic contractile function preserved. Parasternal short and long axis and apical four chamber two-dimensional echocardiographic sections through the left ventricle clearly demonstrate the characteristic alterations in left ventricle architecture of chronic severe pressure overload (Figs. 8.18, 8.19, 8.20).

Indirect methods of assessing the severity of aortic stenosis by estimation of left ventricular peak pressure have been described noninvasively in adults and in children (11, 12). They involve M-mode echocardiographic measurements of end-systolic wall thickness and end-systolic left ventricular cavity radius (10–14). This end-systolic relationship between cavity dimension and wall thickness correlates with peak left ventricular pressure measured at cardiac catheterization better in children than in adults (12) (Fig. 8.21). The reliability in predicting the severity of aortic stenosis by this method is based on the concept of normalized end-systolic wall stress (15, 16). This determination makes the assumption that, in patients with compen-

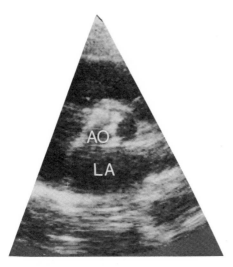

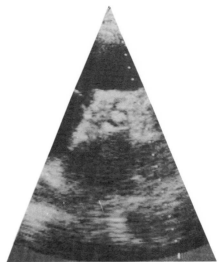

A   B

Figure 8.14.   Two-dimensional echocardiogram of the short axis of a heavily calcified trileaflet aortic valve in a patient with severe aortic stenosis. The calcified leaflets in diastole (*A*) and in systole (*B*) demonstrate severely reduced leaflet excursion, consistent with hemodynamically important aortic stenosis.

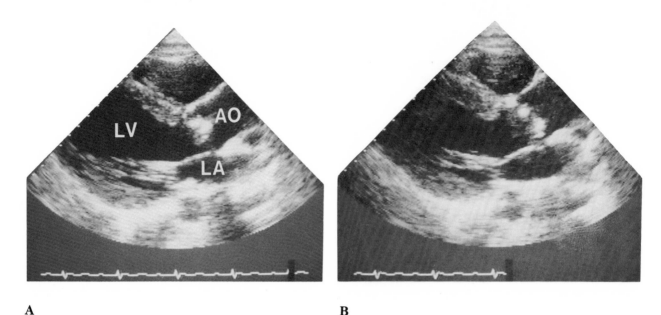

A   **B**

Figure 8.15.   Two-dimensional echocardiogram of the LV long axis in aortic stenosis, showing heavily calcified aortic valve leaflets in diastole (*A*) and restricted opening in systole (*B*). Note the normal LV cavity dimensions, and hypertrophied septum and posterior wall.

sated aortic stenosis, left ventricular hypertrophy develops in response to chronic pressure overload to normalize end-systolic wall stress (afterload), which is the force that the myocardium must overcome to eject a normal stroke volume (15). If the left ventricular cavity is not dilated, left ventricular wall stress is relatively constant and the estimated left ventricular peak systolic pressure (LVPSP) is described by the equation

$$LVPSP = 225 \times PWS/LVESD,$$

where 225 is a constant value of wall stress, PWS is peak wall thickness at end systole, and LVESD is left ventricular end-systolic chamber dimension. If cuff systolic blood pressure and the left ventricular echocardiogram are recorded simultaneously, left ventricular pressure and the peak systolic gradient across the aortic valve can be calculated (16) (Fig. 8.22). The reliability of such quantitative methods depends upon obtaining high quality left ventricular echocar-

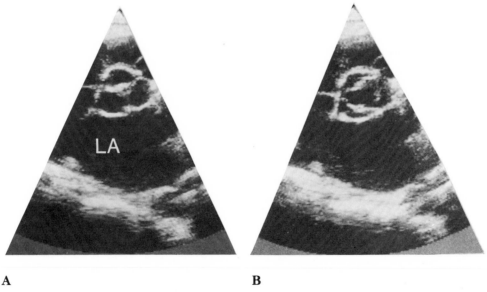

A   **B**

Figure 8.16.   Two-dimensional echocardiogram of the aorta in short axis from a patient with mild rheumatic aortic stenosis. The commissural thickening, which is pathognomonic of rheumatic valve disease, is seen easily in diastole (*A*), while the adhesions between the leaflets, which are mild in this patient, are best appreciated in systole (*B*).

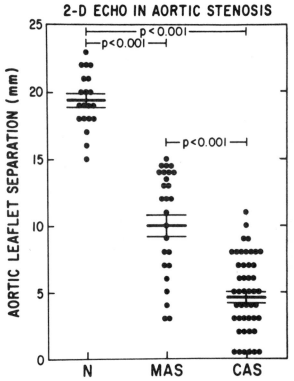

2-D ECHO IN AORTIC STENOSIS

Figure 8.17.   Measurement of the aortic leaflet separation by two-dimensional echocardiography does enable separation of patients with mild aortic valve stenosis from those with critical aortic valve stenosis, in terms of population means. However, the considerable overlap in leaflet separation between these hemodynamically different groups does not enable assessment of the severity of aortic stenosis in individual patients. (Reproduced by permission of the American Heart Association, Inc. from DeMaria A, Bommer W, Joye J. Value and limitations of cross-sectional echocardiography of the aortic valve in the diagnosis and quantification of valvular aortic stenosis. Circulation; 1980:62:309.)

diograms; for this, and a variety of unrelated reasons, this quantitative method has proved disappointing in the clinical assessment of patients with aortic stenosis.

Doppler Assessment

The introduction of Doppler echocardiography has greatly improved the detection and quantification of aortic stenosis. When blood passes through a narrowed aortic valve, as in aortic stenosis, the flow velocity increases and flow becomes turbulent. The increase in blood flow velocity distal to the stenosis is quadratically related to the pressure gradient across the stenosis, as shown by the Bernoulli equation:

$$P_1 - P_2 = \frac{1}{2}\rho\,(V_2^2 - V_1^2) + \rho\int_1^2 \frac{dv}{dt}ds + R(v)$$

convective acceleration   flow acceleration   viscous friction

Early studies attempted to quantify the severity of aortic stenosis by analyzing the amount of turbulent flow detected by pulsed-wave Doppler, but such methods were unsatisfactory for routine clinical use (17). In subsequent studies, continuous-wave Doppler has been used to measure the peak blood flow velocity distal to the valve and the aortic gradient calculated from a modification of the Bernoulli equation (18). The Bernoulli equation relates the pressure drop across a stenosis, not only to the velocity of blood flow proximal and distal to the stenosis, but also to the viscous friction and convective acceleration of flow. Viscous friction is small in large vessels with laminar flow, however, and the convective acceleration term can be ignored when flow velocity is unchanging. Thus, for practical purposes the Bernoulli equation can be simplified to

$$P_1 - P_2 = 4V_2^2,$$

where $P_1 - P_2$ represents the pressure gradient across the valve, and V_2 represents the peak velocity distal to the valve. This modified equation can ignore the blood flow velocity proximal to the valve, since blood flow in the left ventricular outflow tract is usually approximately 1.0 m/s; it must be taken into account if it is much above unity as occurs with increased volume flow, such as in aortic regurgitation (vide infra). An example of the high velocity jet recorded with continuous-wave Doppler in a patient with aortic stenosis obtained with the transducer at the apex is shown in Figure 8.23. A number of investigators have used the modified Bernoulli equation to calculate transaortic gradients from Doppler velocity recordings, and these have correlated closely with aortic valve gradients measured at cardiac catheterization (19–26). The correlations between Doppler and hemodynamic assessment of aortic valve gradients are better when the studies are performed simultaneously (23–26) (Fig. 8.24) than when Doppler and catheter studies are performed at different times (18–22). These discrepancies are probably due to variations in resting cardiac outputs between the two studies. Some workers have suggested that high pulse repetition frequency pulsed-wave Doppler can be used to make similar measurements of transaortic pressure gradients (16), but there is evidence to suggest that this technology may underestimate the true pressure gradient (27).

When the severity of aortic stenosis is assessed using Doppler derived transaortic pressure gradients, there are a number of theoretical and practical considerations that warrant careful consideration.

1. It is important that the ultrasound beam is aligned parallel to the high velocity jet for accurate measurement because the velocity varies inversely with the cosine of the angle between

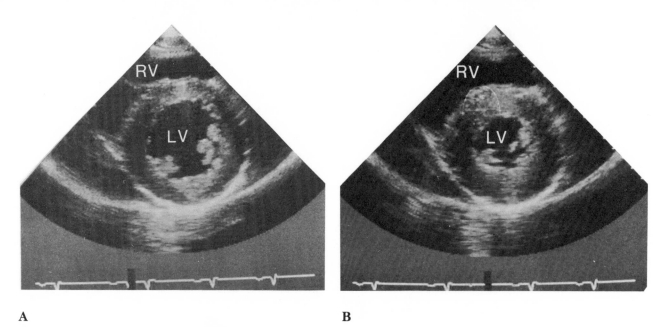

A   **B**

Figure 8.18.   Two-dimensional echocardiogram of the short axis of the LV at high papillary muscle level, from a patient with severe aortic stenosis, obtained from the left parasternal region in diastole (*A*) and systole (*B*). The LV size is normal, but there is severe concentric LV hypertrophy.

the Doppler beam and the direction of blood flow ($v = f_d \cdot c/2f_t \cdot \cos \theta$). This can be achieved by positioning the transducer at the apex, at the right upper sternal border, or in the suprasternal notch. All three acoustic windows should be used (Fig. 8.25). Failure to align the Doppler beam parallel to the direction of blood flow results in a predictable underestimation of the true transaortic pressure gradient. This may partly explain the differences in estimates of transaortic gradients

by catheter and Doppler when the studies are not performed simultaneously (18, 19, 21). Aortic stenosis is a disease with its maximum incidence in the seventh to eighth decade, and in such individuals the aorta is often unfolded and therefore more horizontal than normal. This potential for misalignment of the Doppler beam must be taken into account when assessing the severity of aortic stenosis, since most ultrasound systems have "nonimaging" continuous-wave Doppler transduc-

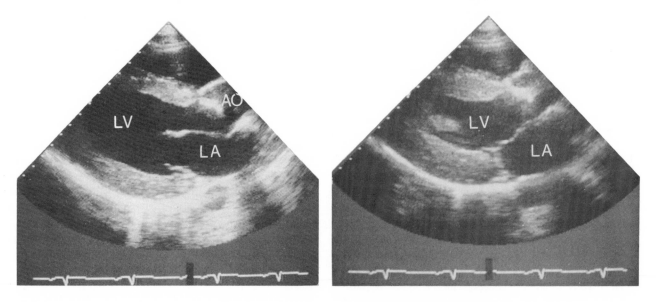

A   **B**

Figure 8.19.   Two-dimensional echocardiogram of the long axis of the LV in the same patient with severe AS in diastole (*A*) and in systole (*B*), showing the calcified immobile aortic valve, normal cavity size, and severe concentric hypertrophy.

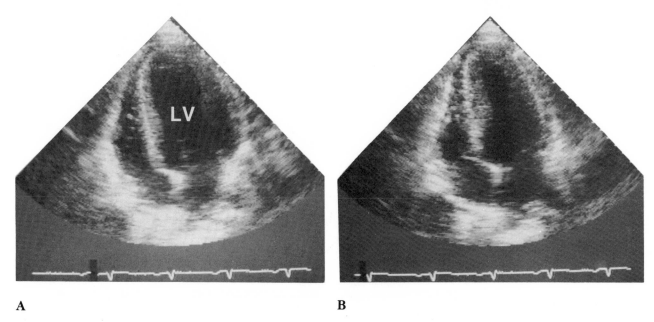

A   **B**

Figure 8.20.   Two-dimensional echocardiogram of the apical four chamber in stenosis, showing the extent of the concentric hypertrophy in diastole (*A*) and almost complete cavity obliteration in systole (*B*).

ers. The echocardiographer therefore relies on the acoustic signal to identify the peak transaortic velocity, which may not be appreciated by the inexperienced technologist. Thus, there are several potential sources of error in beam alignment, which will result in underestimation of the true transaortic gradient.

2. The aortic gradient calculated from the peak blood flow velocity obtained by Doppler represents the peak instantaneous gradient and not the peak-to-peak gradient measured at cardiac catheterization (Fig. 8.26) (23). This difference can be

overcome for practical purposes if the mean gradients derived from the Doppler velocity integral are compared with mean catheter gradients (Fig. 8.27).

3. Recent studies have indicated that Doppler estimation of the aortic valve gradient may be greater than the pressure gradient measured at cardiac catheterization in patients with concomitant aortic regurgitation (28–30) (Fig. 8.28). The increased blood flow velocity in the left ventricular outflow tract (V_1) is due to the augmented volume flow in this condition. This discrepancy

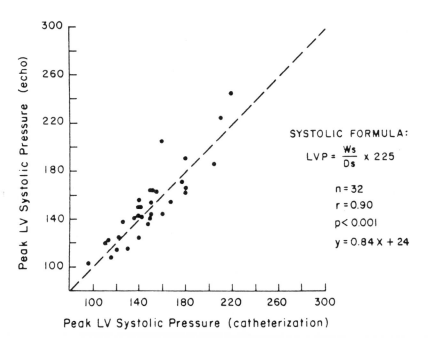

SYSTOLIC FORMULA:

$$LVP = \frac{Ws}{Ds} \times 225$$

n = 32
r = 0.90
p < 0.001
y = 0.84 X + 24

Figure 8.21.   The relationship between the peak LV systolic pressure determined by echocardiography from the ratio of LV wall thickness and LV cavity diameter in systole, and peak LV systolic pressure measured at cardiac catheterization in children with aortic stenosis. The close correlation between echocardiographic and hemodynamic measurements enables assessment of the severity of aortic stenosis in children. (Reproduced with permission from Gewitz HM, Werner JC, Kleinman CS, et al. Role of echocardiography in aortic stenosis: pre- and postoperative studies. Am J Cardiol; 1979:43:68.)

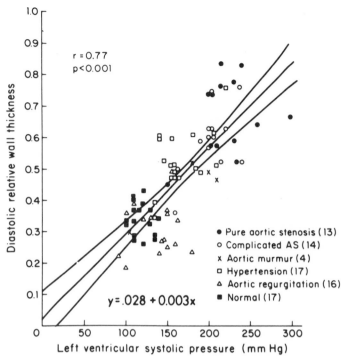

Figure 8.22. The relationship between diastolic relative LV wall thickness and LV systolic pressure in adults with mixed aortic valve disease. The correlation is not as close as that in children. (Reproduced with permission from Reichek N, Devereux RB. Reliable estimation of the peak left ventricular systolic pressure by M mode echocardiography of severe valvular aortic stenosis in adult patients. Am Heart J; 1982:103:203.)

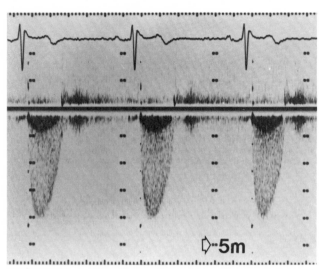

Figure 8.23. Velocity tracing obtained from the apex of the heart with continuous-wave Doppler from a patient with aortic valve stenosis. There is acquisition of a maximum velocity early in systole. The peak velocity is 4.0 m/sec (normal range 0.7 to 1.5 m/sec), which is equivalent to a peak transaortic valve gradient of 64 mmHg, using the modified Bernoulli equation ($p = 4V^2$).

between Doppler and catheter gradients can be accounted for by including the increased velocity proximal to the valve (V_1) in the modified Bernoulli equation:

$$P_1 - P_2 = 4(V_2^2 - V_1^2)^2$$

4. Operator experience may also account for discrepancies in estimates of aortic valve gradients between Doppler and cardiac catheterization (23, 29). Operator inexperience may be manifested 1) by failure to obtain the maximal velocity by not recording velocities from all the potential recording sites (the apex, suprasternal notch, and the second right intercostal space), and 2) failure to obtain technically adequate signals. Whenever aortic valve gradients are calculated from Doppler recordings, the velocity signals must have well-defined spectral envelopes throughout ejection (Fig. 8.29) with no early systolic spiking. Only the maximum or mean velocities are utilized to calculate transaortic gradients.

5. Transaortic pressure gradients determined by cardiac catheterization and by Doppler are dependent not only on valve area but also on cardiac output. Thus, the severity of aortic stenosis may be underestimated in a patient with poor left ventricular function and reduced cardiac output if the gradient alone is relied upon.

The single most important piece of information in the assessment of aortic stenosis is the aortic valve

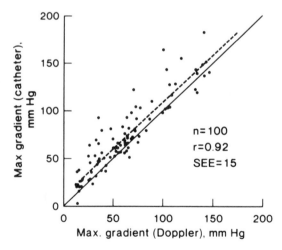

Figure 8.24. Comparison of the maximum gradient measured at cardiac catheterization and the maximum gradient estimated by Doppler in 100 consecutive patients with the diagnosis of aortic valve stenosis. (Reproduced by permission of the American Heart Association, Inc. from Currie PJ, Seward JB, Reeder GS, et al. Continuous wave Doppler echocardiographic assessment of severity of calcific aortic stenosis: a simultaneous Doppler-catheter correlative study in 100 patients. Circulation; 1985:71:1164.)

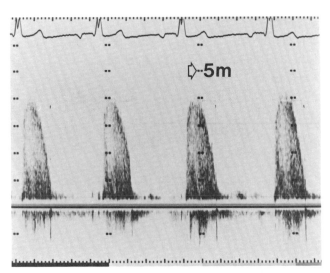

Figure 8.25. Velocity recordings obtained from the right parasternal region by continuous-wave Doppler in a patient with moderate aortic stenosis (peak velocity 4.0 with a peak gradient of 64 mmHg). The maximum velocity signal was obtained only from this transducer position. No technically satisfactory velocity signals were obtained from the apex and the suprasternal notch.

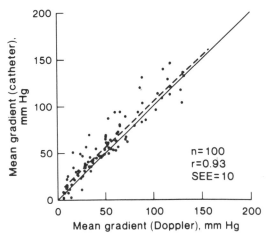

Figure 8.26. Comparison of the mean aortic valve gradient measured at cardiac catheterization and the mean Doppler gradient in 100 consecutive patients with aortic stenosis demonstrated a closer correlation between the mean gradients than the maximum gradients. (Reproduced by permission of the American Heart Association, Inc. from Currie PJ, Seward JB, Reeder GS, et al. Continuous wave Doppler echocardiographic assessment of severity of calcific aortic stenosis: a simultaneous Doppler-Catheter correlative study in 100 patients. Circulation; 1985:71:1164.)

area because, unlike transvalve gradients, it is independent of left ventricular performance and concomitant aortic regurgitation. Several methods have been described to assess aortic valve area. Some have required assessment of cardiac output or stroke volume, and have used this in combination with the transaortic pressure gradient to calculate the valve area. Cardiac output has usually been measured by thermodilutation or carbon dioxide rebreathing techniques (31, 32). Recently, however, noninvasive methods using Doppler echocardiography have been derived employing the concept of a continuity equation (22, 33–36). Most methods apply the direct continuity equation across the aortic valve to blood flow velocities recorded from the left ventricular outflow tract and in the proximal aorta (33–36), although some investigators have recommended using the ratio of antegrade blood flow velocities through the mitral and aortic valves (33, 35). The theoretical basis for the continuity equation is that when volume flow is maintained constant across a partial obstruction in a flow channel, the volume flow per unit time in the partially obstructed region and in the nonobstructed parts of the flow channel are equal. Thus, the product of the flow velocity integral and cross-sectional area is equal in the partially obstructed and the nonobstructed regions (Fig. 8.30). The aortic valve area can be calculated using the continuity equation because the cross-sectional area of the left ventricular outflow tract, the flow velocity integral in the left ventricular outflow tract (that is, the area under

the instantaneous velocity envelope), and the flow velocity integral distal to the aortic valve can all be measured, leaving the aortic valve area as the only unknown:

$$A_A \times FVI_A = A_{OT} \times FVI_{OT},$$

where A_A is the stenotic aortic valve area, A_{OT} is the cross-sectional area of the left ventricular outflow tract calculated from two-dimensional echo measurements of outflow tract diameter (Fig. 8.31), and V_A and V_{OT} are the velocities in the aorta and left ventricular outflow tract, respectively. The equation can be rearranged to solve for the unknown aortic valve area (A_A):

$$A_A = \frac{A_{OT} \times FVI_{OT}}{FVI_A}$$

Peak velocities can be substituted for flow velocity integrals in the continuity equation, but either velocities or velocity integrals must be used throughout. For routine purposes, peak velocities are easier to measure than the flow velocity integrals and give similar results (33) (Fig. 8.32). The diameter of the left ventricular outflow tract is measured immediately below the aortic valve, and the cross-sectional area is calculated assuming that the left ventricular outflow tract is circular (33). The diameter should be measured close to the valve to avoid septal and anterior mitral valve motion (Fig. 8.31). The trailing edge to leading edge diameter, the leading edge to leading edge diameter, or the

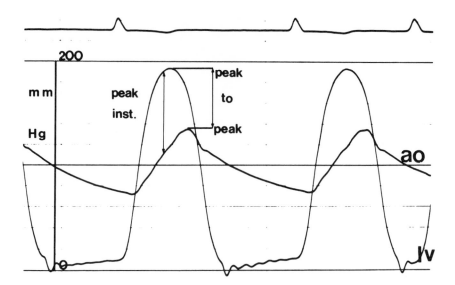

Figure 8.27. Strip chart recording of simultaneous LV and ascending aortic pressures. Peak pressure gradients determined by Doppler estimate the peak instantaneous transaortic gradients, while peak gradients measured by cardiac catheterization estimate peak-to-peak gradients.

average of the two diameters may be used to calculate cross-sectional area (30, 33). Blood flow velocity may be difficult to measure in the left ventricular outflow tract with pulsed Doppler, as it may suddenly increase and alias close to the valve orifice. Velocity is best measured where it is stable in the left ventricular outflow tract, 1–2 cm proximal to the valve. The velocity distal to the aortic valve is recorded using

continuous-wave Doppler in the conventional manner to obtain the maximum velocity with the minimum angle between the ultrasound beam and direction of blood flow. Aortic valve areas calculated from Doppler velocities using these methods correlate closely with aortic valve areas calculated at cardiac catheterization using the Gorlin hydraulic formula, in patients with or without significant aortic regurgitation (30, 33) (Fig. 8.32).

SUPRAVALVULAR AORTIC STENOSIS

Supravalvular aortic stenosis is a congenital anomaly of the ascending aorta that takes the form of a localized or diffuse narrowing of the aorta, usually beginning immediately distal to the origin of the coronary arteries. In most cases supravalvar stenosis occurs in association with abnormal, "elfin-like" facies and mental retardation. The most common M-mode abnormality in supravalvar stenosis is a reduction of the anteroposterior diameter of the aorta above the level of the aortic valve when the transducer scans cephalad through the center of the aorta beginning at the aortic valve (37–41). The location, extent, and severity of the narrowing can be visualized directly using two-dimensional echocardiography from the parasternal long axis and suprasternal views (42). Quantification of the narrowing by two-dimensional echocardiography is based on comparison between the diameter of the aorta measured at the site of the obstruction and the diameter of the aorta measured at the aortic annulus. The proximal aorta is mapped from the aortic valve ring using pulsed-wave Doppler, by moving the sample volume progressively along the aorta and noting the location at which the blood flow velocity profile increases and flow becomes turbulent. The trans-stenotic pressure

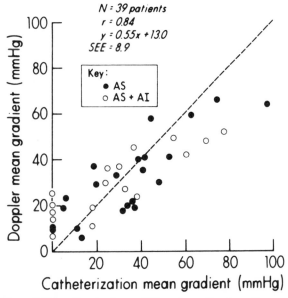

Figure 8.28. Comparison of Doppler estimates of mean transaortic valve gradients and mean gradients at cardiac catheterization show that Doppler may both under- and overestimate transaortic valve gradients in aortic stenosis, especially when there is concomitant aortic regurgitation. (Reproduced with permission from Krafchek J, Roberts JH, Radford M, et al. A reconsideration of Doppler assessed gradients in suspected aortic stenosis. Am Heart J; 1985: 110:771.)

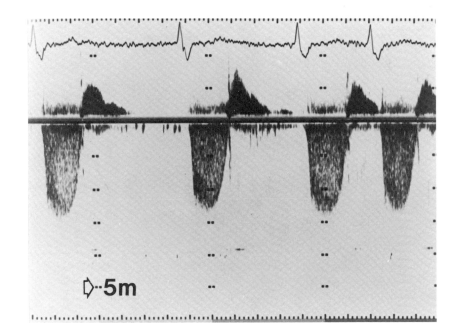

Figure 8.29.   Continuous-wave Doppler velocity signals from a patient with aortic stenosis and atrial fibrillation, showing clearly defined spectral envelopes that enable accurate assessment of transvalve gradients from a series of different cardiac cycle lengths.

gradient, which is usually only mild to moderate, can be quantified using continuous-wave Doppler and the modified Bernoulli equation.

SUBVALVULAR AORTIC STENOSIS

Subaortic stenosis may be dynamic, as in hypertrophic obstructive cardiomyopathy, or fixed as a discrete crescent-shaped shelf or collar encircling the left ventricular outflow tract close to the aortic valve. Dynamic subaortic stenosis due to hypertrophic obstructive cardiomyopathy is described in Chapter 11. The discrete form of subaortic stenosis, whether a shelf, membranous diaphragm, or fibrous collar, is situated most commonly 1 to 2 mm proximal to the aortic valve, and usually results in the development of symptoms of left ventricular outflow tract obstruction in the first three decades of life. Associated cardiac anomalies, such as defects in the atrial septum primum, stenoses on the left side of the heart at supra-mitral valve and supra-aortic levels, and coarctation of the aorta at the level of the ligamentum arteriosum, should be excluded by two-dimensional echocardiography. The M-mode features of this condition have been described (43–48). Although it is often difficult to directly visualize the subaortic membrane per se as a discrete echo in the left ventricular outflow tract with M-mode echocardiography, its presence may be suggested by the combination of early systolic closure of the aortic valve, left ventricular hypertrophy, and high frequency diastolic flutter of the mitral valve leaflets due to associated aortic regurgitation. Aortic regurgitation occurs because the subaortic shelf is in close apposition to the

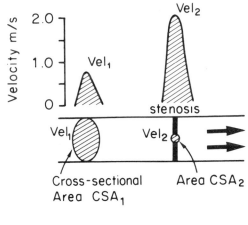

Continuity Equation :

$$FVI_1 \times CSA_1 = FVI_2 \times CSA_2$$

$$CSA_2 = \frac{FVI_1}{FVI_2} \times CSA_1$$

Figure 8.30.   Blood volume flow can be estimated as the product of the flow velocity integral and the cross-sectional area of the flow stream. The continuity equation states that in a closed system, such as the cardiovascular system, volume flow proximal to and through a stenosis are equal. Thus, the area of the stenosis can be determined as the product of the ratio of the flow velocity integrals proximal to and at the stenosis, and the cross-section area of the flow stream proximal to the stenosis.

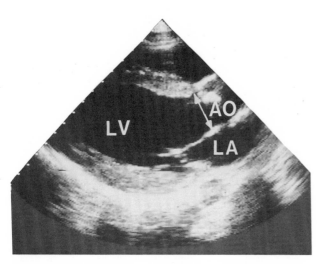

Figure 8.31. Two-dimensional echocardiogram of the left ventricular long axis in a patient with aortic stenosis demonstrating where the LV outflow tract diameter is measured.

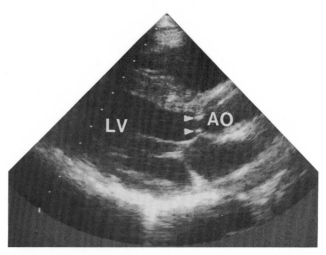

Figure 8.33. Two-dimensional echocardiogram of the LV long axis from a patient with discrete subaortic stenosis. The LV is normal size with marked concentric LVH. There is a discrete collar (*white arrows*) encircling the left ventricular outflow tract immediately proximal to the aortic valve, seen on the left side of the septum and on the ventricular surface of the mitral valve, resulting in obstruction to left ventricular ejection.

Figure 8.32. Correlation between Doppler echocardiographic estimates of aortic valve area from the flow velocity integrals, and aortic valve area estimated at cardiac catheterization, in patients with aortic stenosis and no or only mild aortic regurgitation (*A*, left), and in patients with aortic stenosis with coexistent aortic regurgitation (*A*, right). Comparison between Doppler echocardiographic estimates of aortic valve area based on peak velocity measurements and aortic valve areas determined at cardiac catheterization in patients with little or no aortic regurgitation (*B*, left) and those with co-existent aortic regurgitation (*B*, right). (Reproduced by permission of the American Heart Association, Inc. from Skjaerpe T, Hegrenaes L, Hatle L. Non-invasive estimation of valve area in patients with aortic stenosis by Doppler ultrasound and 2 dimensional echocardiography. Circulation; 1985:72:815.)

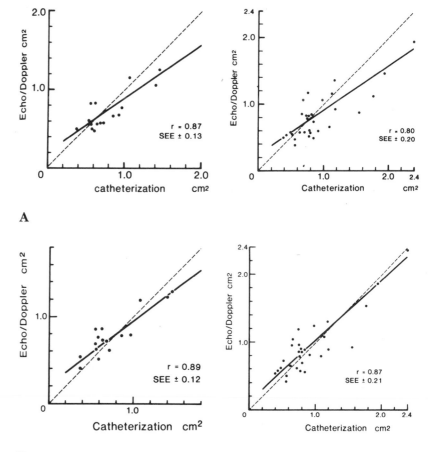

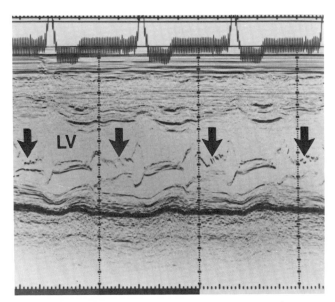

Figure 8.34.   M-mode echocardiogram from a patient with aortic regurgitation, showing high-frequency diastolic flutter of the anterior mitral valve leaflet (*black arrows*).

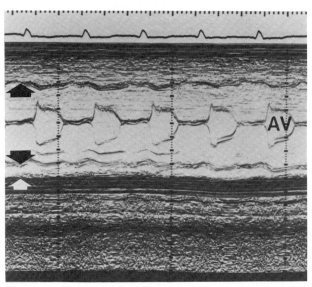

Figure 8.36.   M-mode echocardiogram from a patient with severe dilatation of the aortic root and ascending aorta. The aorta is 5.8 cm in diameter (*black arrows*), while the posterior left atrium appears small (1 cm). The presence of a small left atrium should suggest aortic dilatation.

aortic valve and interferes with leaflet function. Two-dimensional echocardiographic examination from the left parasternal long axis or apical long axis view of the left ventricle allows accurate localization of stenosis below the aortic valve. The shelf or collar often appears as a bright echo protruding from the proximal septum below the aortic valve, and often extends around the left ventricular outflow tract onto the ventricular surface of the anterior mitral valve leaflet

(Fig. 8.33). Rarely, subaortic narrowing is due to subvalvar fibromuscular hyperplasia (47, 48), which presents in early childhood and is also readily demonstrated using two-dimensional echocardiography.

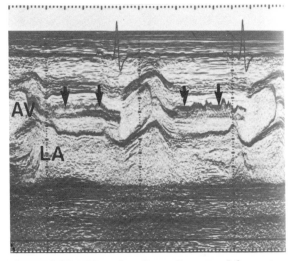

Figure 8.35.   M-mode echocardiogram of the aorta, aortic valve, and left atrium from a patient with aortic regurgitation due to fenestration of one of the aortic valve leaflets, which has resulted in high-frequency flutter of the aortic leaflets in diastole (*arrows*).

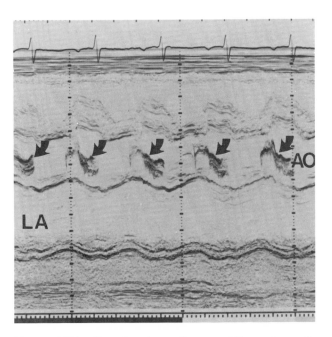

Figure 8.37.   M-mode echocardiogram of the aorta, aortic valve, and left atrium from a patient with severe aortic regurgitation due to vegetative endocarditis involving the aortic valve leaflets. The vegetations appear as increased echo densities attached to the aortic leaflets, best visualized in diastole (*black arrows*).

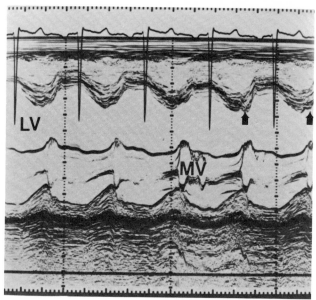

LV

MV

Figure 8.38. M-mode echocardiogram of the left ventricle at mitral valve level from a patient with chronic severe aortic regurgitation, demonstrating marked left ventricular dilatation (left ventricular end-diastolic dimension of 7.4 and end-systolic dimension of 5.2 cm). There is a characteristic bump or posterior excursion of ventricular septum in early diastole (*arrow*), which occurs commonly in aortic regurgitation.

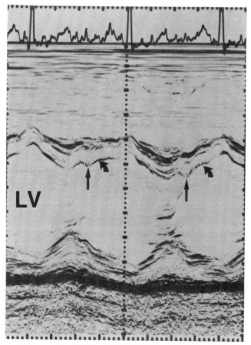

LV

Figure 8.39. M-mode echocardiogram of the left ventricle in a patient with mild aortic regurgitation, in whom there is the commonly occurring posterior motion of the septum in early diastole (*straight arrow*), and also high frequency flutter of the left side of the ventricular septum (*curved arrow*), indicating the presence of aortic regurgitation.

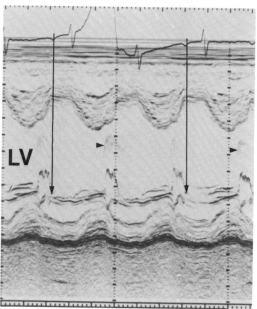

LV

Figure 8.40. M-mode echocardiogram of the left ventricle from a patient with severe acute on chronic aortic regurgitation. The left ventricle is greatly enlarged, with a vigorously contracting volume-overloaded cavity and an aortic vegetation prolapsing into the LV outflow tract (*horizontal arrow*). The mitral valve closes early (*vertical black arrow*), well before the onset of a QRS complex on EKG, indicating marked elevation in left ventricle diastolic pressure, which quickly exceeds left atrial pressure and closes the mitral valve prematurely.

Some investigators have found echocardiography superior to angiography in detecting and localizing discrete as well as dynamic subaortic stenosis (47).

Although two-dimensional echocardiography enables localization of the subaortic stenosis, it provides only indirect information about the severity by the presence and degree of left ventricular hypertrophy. Pulsed-wave Doppler can accurately localize the site of stenosis, but usually the peak velocity exceeds the Nyquist limit of the pulsed-wave systems, resulting in aliasing and inability to measure the peak velocity. Thus continuous-wave Doppler is necessary to quantify the trans-stenotic pressure gradient (49–51). The trans-aortic pressure gradients in both discrete and dynamic subaortic stenosis determined by continuous-wave Doppler using the modified Bernoulli equation have correlated closely with those obtained at cardiac catheterization. Mild regurgitation is often present in discrete subaortic stenosis and should be assessed by pulsed-wave Doppler flow mapping of the left atrium.

AORTIC REGURGITATION

Although there are many individual etiologies of aortic regurgitation, it results either from diseases involving

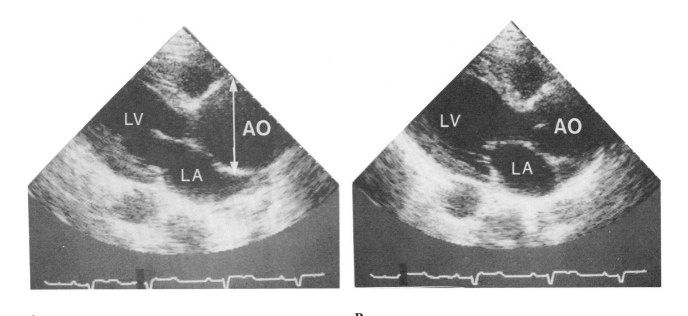

A   **B**

Figure 8.41.   Two-dimensional echocardiogram of the left ventricle in long axis from the left parasternal region in systole (*A*), and diastole (*B*) from a patient with chronic aortic regurgitation due to gross dilatation of the ascending aorta. The aortic diameter is 7.5 cm.

the aortic valve leaflets themselves or from diseases involving the aortic wall. Diseases of the aorta are discussed elsewhere (Chapter 14). M-mode, two-dimensional echocardiography, and Doppler echocardiography are extremely useful in detecting aortic regurgitation and establishing its etiology, but have proved less helpful in assessing the severity of aortic regurgitation and in determining its management, particularly in deciding the optimal timing of aortic valve replacement.

M-Mode Assessment

The M-mode echocardiographic abnormality that is pathognomonic of aortic regurgitation is high-frequency diastolic fluttering of the mitral valve leaflets (52–54) (Fig. 8.34). Similar diastolic fluttering may occur on the left side of the interventricular septum and the mitral chordae tendinae, and this may be a useful finding (53, 55, 56) when the regurgitant jet occurs predominantly through the posterior or noncoronary cusp (57). In patients with coexistent severe calcific mitral stenosis, diastolic fluttering may not be present since the leaflets are thickened and are thus not able to resonate at high frequency. Prosthetic mitral valves also do not exhibit fluttering, even if aortic regurgitation is present. In these two circumstances, diastolic fluttering of the septum should be looked for as an indicator of aortic regurgitation. Although these high-frequency oscillations of the mitral valve are a sensitive marker of the presence of

aortic regurgitation, they are not useful in estimating either its severity or etiology.

There are no specific M-mode echocardiographic features of aortic regurgitation apparent from examining the aortic leaflets per se, although clues as to the etiology may be identified. Low-frequency fluttering of the aortic valve closure line during diastole is pathognomonic of cusp rupture or fenestration (Fig. 8.35) (58–60). Rupture of aortic valve leaflets is usually due to bacterial endocarditis but may also result from myxomatous degeneration (61, 62). Other etiologies recognizable by M-mode recordings include an eccentric closure line, which is suggestive but not diagnostic of a bicuspid aortic valve (Fig. 8.11); dilatation of the aortic root, with or without aortic dissection (Fig. 8.36); and direct visualization of vegetations (Fig. 8.37) or myxomatous valve leaflets.

The characteristic M-mode echocardiographic findings in patients with aortic regurgitation include progressive left ventricular dilatation and exaggerated motion of the septum and posterior wall (58–62) (Fig. 8.38). These findings reflect volume overload of the left ventricle, and similar abnormalities are seen in significant mitral regurgitation. Patients with aortic regurgitation often demonstrate a characteristic abnormality of septal motion, which consists of an exaggerated early diastolic dip (Fig. 8.39) not encountered in other conditions that produce left ventricular volume overload. The mechanism of this septal movement is unexplained. Acute severe aortic regurgitation can be recognized by M-mode echocardiography by premature

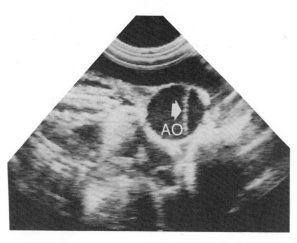

A

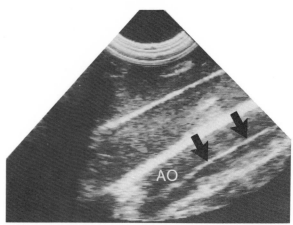

B

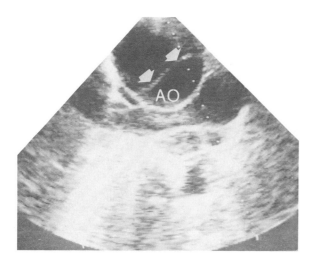

C

Figure 8.42.   Two-dimensional echocardiogram, obtained intraoperatively, of an aortic dissection showing the descending thoracic aortic lumen with an intimal flap in cross-section (*A, arrow*), and in long axis (*B, arrows*). A two-dimensional echocardiogram in another patient (*C*), in whom there was dilatation of the aorta due to dissection with an intimal flap visualized in cross-section (*white arrow*).

diastolic mitral valve closure (52, 54, 61–70) (Fig. 8.40). The mitral valve closes before the onset of the QRS complex on the simultaneously recorded electrocardiogram, and does not reopen with atrial systole. This premature mitral valve closure occurs because, in acute severe aortic regurgitation, the left ventricle and aorta communicate freely, and left ventricular diastolic and aortic diastolic pressures are similar. Thus, the greatly increased left ventricular diastolic pressure quickly exceeds left atrial pressure, resulting in premature closure of the mitral valve. Premature mitral valve closure also occurs in first degree atrioventricular block and when this coexists with aortic regurgitation, premature mitral closure must be interpreted with caution. Another useful diagnostic M-mode echo sign in chronic severe aortic regurgitation occurs when the left ventricular diastolic pressure is so elevated that it exceeds aortic diastolic pressure (which is usually

lower than normal) and opens the aortic valve prematurely (71, 72).

Two-Dimensional Assessment

Two-dimensional echocardiography provides additional information in elucidating the etiology of aortic regurgitation. Direct examination of the aortic root, from the right and left parasternal and suprasternal views, may demonstrate aneurysmal dilatation (Fig. 8.41) (73–75) or proximal (type A) dissection when a mobile intimal flap can often be visualized in orthogonal scan planes (Fig. 8.42) (76–78). Other etiologies of aortic regurgitation determined by two-dimensional echocardiography include bicuspid aortic valve (Fig. 8.11), idiopathic senile calcific degeneration (Fig. 8.14), rheumatic commissural fusion with leaflet deformation (Fig. 8.16), and aortic valve prolapse (Fig. 8.43) (79–81).

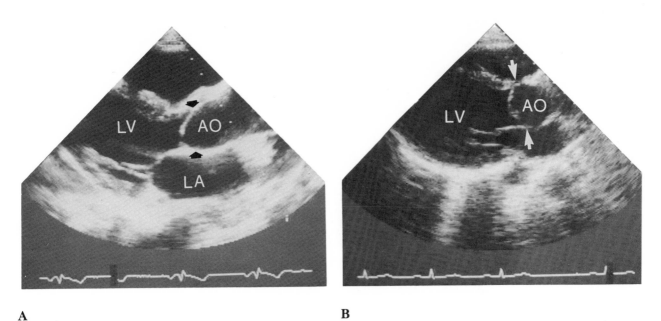

A   **B**

Figure 8.43.   Two-dimensional echocardiogram of the left ventricle in long axis from two patients with a bicuspid aortic valve (*A* and *B*) in whom the aortic valve ring is indicated by arrows, demonstrating prolapse of two aortic valve leaflets into the left ventricular outflow tract in diastole.

The mitral valve leaflet motion may also be abnormal in aortic regurgitation by two-dimensional echocardiography. The anterior mitral leaflet often becomes distorted with indentation in the short axis view (82) and reversed doming, with the leaflet curved so that the convexity is toward the mitral orifice in both the long axis and the apical four chamber views (83), a finding that usually indicates the presence of severe aortic regurgitation (83) (Fig. 8.44).

The LV cavity is dilated and there is concentric hypertrophy in chronic severe aortic regurgitation (Fig.

8.45); the more severe the regurgitation, the larger the left ventricular cavity. The left ventricle becomes more globular in shape as it dilates (Fig. 8.46). Initially, contractile function is preserved. But as the cavity continues to dilate, wall stress increases and finally, the increase in muscle mass is no longer able to parallel the changes in cavity volume, and end-systolic wall stress is not normalized and becomes elevated. Thus, in severe progressive aortic regurgitation, a state of inadequate hypertrophy results, with further increase in end-systolic stress and concomitant decrease in myocardial contractile function.

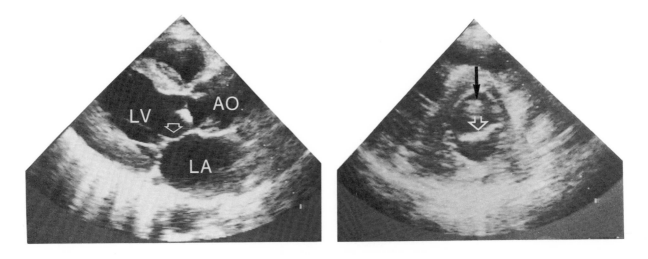

A   **B**

Figure 8.44.   Two-dimensional echocardiogram of the left ventricle from a patient with severe aortic regurgitation due to vegetative endocarditis with reversed doming of the anterior mitral valve leaflet in long axis (*A, white arrow*) and in short axis (*B, white arrow*). The prolapsing vegetation is seen in the left ventricular outflow tract in both long and short axis (*black arrows*).

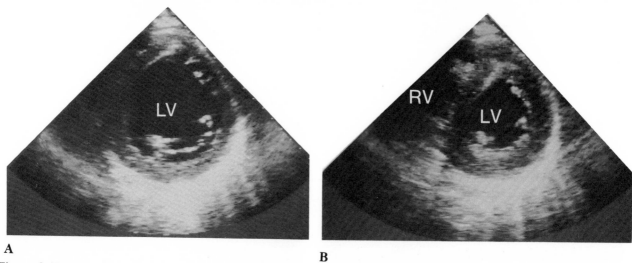

Figure 8.45. Two-dimensional echocardiogram of the short axis of the left ventricle from a patient with chronic severe aortic regurgitation in diastole (*A*) and in systole (*B*), demonstrating marked left ventricular chamber dilatation and severe, concentric left ventricular hypertrophy.

Many attempts have been made using echocardiography to identify 1) the optimal timing of aortic valve replacement in aortic regurgitation, and 2) preoperative factors that might predict prognosis and postoperative left ventricular function at long-term followup (65–67). Left ventricular cavity size, end-diastolic pressure, pressure/volume relationships, afterload, varying indices of contractility, and ejection phase indices have all been advocated, respectively (65–67, 84–94). End-systolic dimension of greater than 55 mm and/or a percentage fractional shortening of less than 25% assessed by M-mode echocardiography have been suggested as indications for valve replacement in asymptomatic as well as symptomatic patients with chronic aortic regurgitation (66, 67). There is considerable

variability, however, in repetitive M-mode echocardiographic measurements of left ventricular cavity size at end-systole and at end-diastole by the same or different observers at any one point in time (95, 96). This variability results either because, in large hearts with volume overload, the ultrasound beam transects a chord and not the diameter of the left ventricle (96), or because the ultrasound beam does not pass through the major "minor" axis. The latter occurs because the left ventricle becomes more spherical in aortic regurgitation, as the increasing volume is accommodated with minimal change in chamber perimeter, and the maximum short axis diameter (the major "minor" axis) moves more toward the apex of the left ventricle and away from the tips of the mitral valve leaflets (Fig.

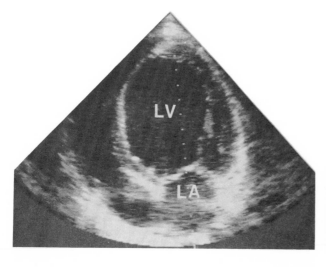

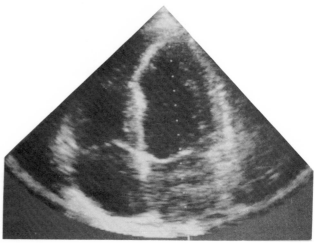

Figure 8.46. Two-dimensional echocardiogram of the apical four chamber view in chronic severe aortic regurgitation in diastole (*A*) and systole (*B*), showing a very dilated globular-shaped left ventricle with concentric hypertrophy.

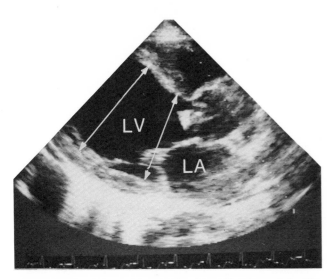

Figure 8.47. Two-dimensional echocardiogram of the LV long axis from a patient with severe aortic regurgitation due to vegetative endocarditis. Note that the left ventricle is more spherical than normal, and the left ventricular architecture has remodeled consequent to the chronic volume overload. The major "minor" axis of the left ventricle is no longer at the base of the LV at mitral valve level, but occurs at midcavity level, that is, further toward the apex than normal.

8.47). Furthermore, left ventricular end-systolic diameter varies widely in the same subject over short periods of time because it is exquisitely sensitive to even minor alterations in left ventricular afterload (97) (Fig. 8.48).

Ejection phase indices in aortic regurgitation are also load-dependent and tend to overestimate left ventricular function, so that incipient and irreversible myocardial contractile dysfunction may be overlooked (93, 94). In an attempt to overcome these difficulties, attention has focused upon developing two-dimensional-echocardiographic, load-independent indices of left ventricular performance, most of which require calculation of end-systolic or peak stress from the combined use of cuff systolic blood pressure and two-dimensional imaging. When these calculations are made at rest and following minor perturbations in afterload, induced either pharmacologically or by isometric exercise (such as handgrip), load-independent indices of myocardial contractility can be obtained from the slopes of the end-systolic stress versus LV systolic diameter and end-systolic stress versus LV systolic volume relationships (94, 97) (Fig. 8.49). The slopes of these lines can be recalculated during serial followup, and progressive decline in the slope over serial studies, at least theoretically, indicates progressive reduction in myocardial contractility. These and similar echo techniques have been used intraoperatively pre- and post-bypass in an attempt to identify preoperative measurements of afterload or chamber architecture that may

predict prognosis and left ventricular pump function at long-term followup (98).

Diastolic dimensions, wall thickness, and left ventricular stress/strain relationships have also been used as prognostic indicators (84–87), but there is considerable doubt about how effective these preoperative indices of left ventricular function are in predicting prognosis following valve replacement (88–91). Part of the difficulty in assessing stress/strain relationships with M-mode echocardiography is because M-mode dimensions in patients with volume overloaded left ventricles do not correlate well with ventricular volumes calculated angiographically (96). To overcome such difficulties, more sophisticated determinations of the end-systolic stress/dimension relationship using two-dimensional echocardiography have been proposed to identify those patients with irreversible impaired left ventricular function (93, 94, 97). Further work is required to determine their clinical usefulness.

Doppler Assessment

Doppler echocardiography is a sensitive (99) and widely used noninvasive tool for quantifying the severity of aortic regurgitation. Aortic regurgitation is best detected with the Doppler pulsed-wave sample volume positioned in the left ventricular outflow tract, immediately proximal to the aortic valve from the apical five chamber view. Aortic regurgitation may also be detected from the left and right parasternal long axis views, and from the suprasternal notch as reversed flow in the ascending or descending aorta. A Doppler blood flow velocity profile recorded from the left ventricular outflow tract in a patient with aortic regurgitation obtained from the apical five chamber view shows a turbulent high velocity flow signal during diastole (Fig. 8.50). Aortic regurgitation may occasionally be difficult to detect clinically in patients with concomitant severe mitral stenosis. Pulsed Doppler is extremely useful in this situation, however, and by careful flow mapping of the left ventricular outflow tract in both the apical five chamber and the apical long axis views, the presence of co-existing aortic regurgitation can be confirmed unequivocally (100). On rare occasions, the Doppler velocity signal of mitral stenosis may be difficult to differentiate from that of aortic regurgitation when the blood flow through the deformed mitral orifice is deflected into the left ventricular outflow tract. If the diastolic flow commences before mitral valve opening, however, the signal is due to aortic regurgitation. Continuous-wave Doppler in aortic regurgitation, in contrast to mitral stenosis, will demonstrate a holodiastolic velocity signal in excess of 2 m/sec (Fig. 8.51).

Doppler echocardiography can also provide important information regarding the severity of aortic regur-

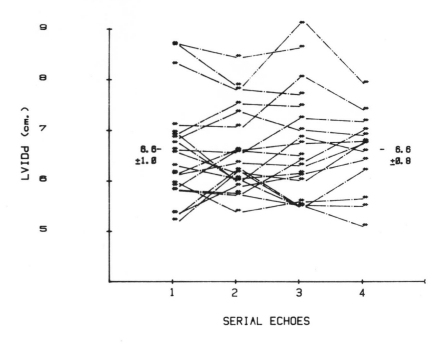

A

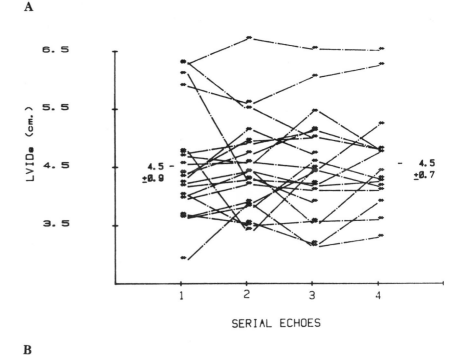

Figure 8.48. Serial, two-dimensionally directed, M-mode echocardiographic measurements of left ventricular dimension in diastole (*A*) and in systole (*B*) from 19 patients with chronic aortic regurgitation. They were followed at 6-month intervals for an eighteenmonth period. The mean LV dimensions in diastole and systole for the whole population were unchanged over the duration, but there were major alterations in left ventricular size in some individuals, due to the extreme sensitivity to changes in afterload in the volume-overloaded ventricles of aortic regurgitation.

B

gitation. The simplest semiquantitative technique involves flow mapping of the left ventricle. The turbulent diastolic flow is mapped by moving the sample volume throughout the left ventricle from the apical LV long axis or parasternal long axis view. The severity of aortic regurgitation is graded from I+ to IV+, in increasing order of severity, based on the location of the turbulent diastolic blood flow velocity signal: Grade 1+ (mild)—aortic regurgitation is present when the turbulent diastolic flow is detected only immediately subjacent to the aortic valve (Fig. 8.52); grade 2+—when the signal is detectable in the left ventricular outflow tract; grade 3+—when the regurgitant signal is detectable as far as the papillary muscles; grade 4, that is, severe aortic regurgitation, is diagnosed when the high velocity diastolic signal is detectable throughout the LV, even at the apex (Fig. 8.52). This grading of aortic regurgitation by pulsed-wave Doppler correlates well with the semiquantitative assessment of the severity of aortic regurgitation by contrast aortography (101,

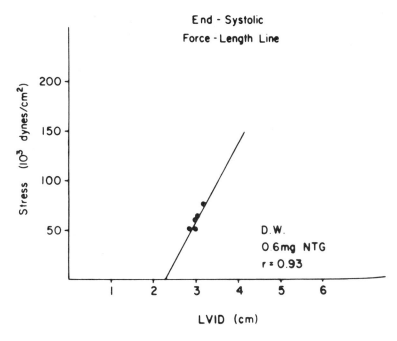

End - Systolic
Force - Length Line

Figure 8.49. The slope of the relationship between the peak or end-systolic stress and left ventricular dimensions, in a patient in whom afterload was perturbed by nitroglycerin, may be utilized as a load-independent index of left ventricular contractility. (Reproduced by permission of the American Heart Association, Inc. from Reichek N, Wilson J, St. John Sutton M, et al. Non-invasive determination of left ventricular end-systolic stress validation of a method and initial application. Circulation; 1982: 65:106.)

102). Flow mapping of the aortic orifice in diastole has also been used to determine the severity of aortic regurgitation (103). The introduction of color-flow Doppler has considerably facilitated the recognition and semiquantitation of aortic regurgitation by flow mapping (Fig. 8.53, Plate VII). This technique enables the area of the regurgitant diastolic jet of high velocity turbulent flow to be directly visualized and quantitated

in the left ventricle from the apical five chamber and the apical LV long axis view as a mosaic of colors (104) (Fig. 8.53).

Alternative Doppler methods of quantitating the severity of aortic regurgitation involve the determination of regurgitant fraction (105–107). This requires Doppler calculations of volume flow through the pulmonary or mitral valve and through the aortic valve. Volume flow through these valves is obtained as the product of the cross-sectional area of the valve orifice and the respec-

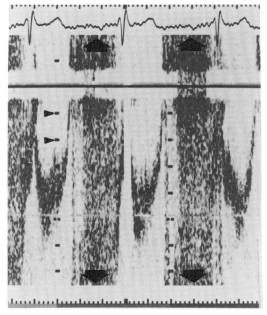

Figure 8.50. Pulsed-wave Doppler velocity signal obtained in the left ventricular outflow tract from the apical five chamber view. The aliased high-velocity signal in diastole (*black vertical arrows*) indicates regurgitant blood flow of aortic regurgitation. The small horizontal arrows identify the calibration markers of 20 cm/sec.

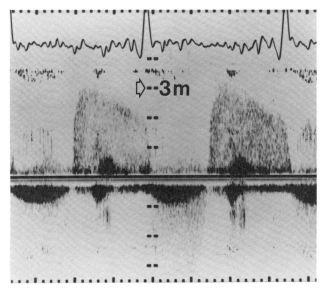

Figure 8.51. Continuous-wave Doppler velocity signals in a patient with aortic regurgitation. The velocity signals are holodiastolic with a peak of approximately 3 m/sec and a slow decay, suggesting mild to moderate aortic regurgitation.

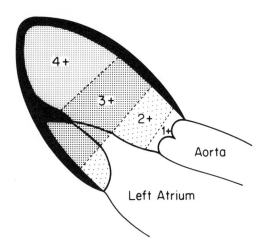

APICAL L.V. LONG AXIS VIEW

Figure 8.52. Diagram of the left ventricular long axis from the apex, showing the left ventricle divided into regions for assessing the extent of the regurgitant jet in aortic regurgitation. Mild aortic regurgitation, designated 1+, is when the signal is detected immediately under the aortic valve within the first cm of the left ventricular outflow tract. Grade 2+ is designated when it is detectable up to the tips of the mitral valve leaflets, grade 3+ when the signal is detectable as far as the papillary muscle, and grade 4+ when the velocity signal is obtainable throughout the left ventricle.

tive flow velocity integral. Regurgitant fractions are obtained by expressing the difference between pulmonary (or mitral) volume flow and aortic volume flow as a percentage of aortic flow:

$$\frac{FVI_{A_o} \times CSA_{A_o} - FVI_{PA} \times CSA_{PA}}{FVI_{A_o} \times CSA_{A_o}} \times 100\%$$

These measurements correspond closely to regurgitant fraction assessed at cardiac catheterization (Fig. 8.54). When pulmonary flow is used, aortic regurgitant fractions are relatively accurate, even in the presence of associated mitral disease (105).

The Doppler flow velocity spectra recorded by continuous-wave Doppler in aortic regurgitation are characterized by increased early peak velocity with a variable rate of deceleration (108). The severity of aortic regurgitation can be estimated by measuring the rate of velocity decline, which is greater in severe aortic regurgitation (Fig. 8.55).

Aortic regurgitation, similar to mitral stenosis, results in left ventricular filling as the diastolic pressure across the valve decreases (109). The severity of aortic regurgitation can be quantitated using continuous-wave Doppler by measuring the time taken for the aortic peak diastolic velocity to decay by 29%, which corresponds to the time at which the diastolic transaortic pressure decays by 50% (since pressure and velocity are quadratically related). This time interval

is called the "velocity half time." This correlates closely with the pressure half time and varies inversely both with regurgitant fraction (Fig. 8.56) and contrast angiographic grading of the severity of aortic regurgitation (Fig. 8.57).

Aortic regurgitation can also be assessed by pulsed-wave and continuous-wave Doppler studies of blood flow velocity profiles in the aorta. Regurgitation is indicated by reversed flow in the aorta in diastole (Fig. 8.58). However, a small degree of reversed flow can occur in early diastole in normal subjects immediately following aortic valve closure, and reversed flow also occurs with patent ductus arteriosus. The degree of aortic regurgitation can be assessed by quantifying the ratio of the flow velocity integrals of the forward and reversed flow signals (110–113). The regurgitant fraction can also be assessed by pulsed-wave Doppler technique as the ratio of diastolic to systolic blood flow in the aortic arch (114) (Fig. 8.59).

INFECTIVE ENDOCARDITIS OF THE AORTIC VALVE

The diagnosis of infective endocarditis of the aortic valve is usually made clinically and confirmed when the etiologic organism is isolated from blood cultures and identified by standard microbiologic techniques. Echocardiography provides confirmation of the diagnosis when valvular vegetations and their associated hemodynamic abnormalities produced by valvular dysfunction are demonstrated.

Aortic valve vegetations are detected echocardiographically by the combination of increased echoes emanating from or associated with the valve leaflets, and abnormal motion of the valve leaflets themselves (115–118). Vegetations often appear as shaggy thickening of the valve leaflets by M-mode echocardiography and are visualized better in diastole (Figs. 8.37, 8.40). Differentiation from fibrotic thickening of the leaflets is usually possible because valve motion is exaggerated by adherent vegetations. Leaflet motion is restricted when the leaflets are thickened and fibrotic. It may be difficult to diagnose vegetations in the presence of co-existing rheumatic aortic valve fibrosis or calcification by M-mode echocardiography alone.

Detection of vegetations by two-dimensional echocardiography is considerably easier than with M-mode (119–121). Vegetations appear as very mobile, globular, polypoid masses adherent to the valve leaflets, often prolapsing into the left ventricle during diastole, or the leaflets appear thickened but unusually mobile when the vegetations are small and sessile (Figs. 8.60, 8.61) (121–123). When aortic vegetative endocarditis is suspected, the aortic valve should be meticulously exam-

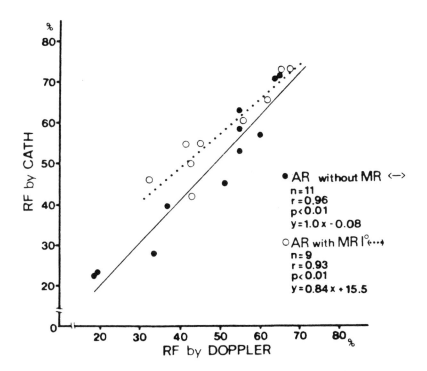

Figure 8.54. Comparison of estimates of regurgitant fraction (RF) by Doppler and cardiac catheterization in patients with aortic regurgitation, with and without mitral regurgitation, shows high correlation between the two techniques. (Reproduced by permission of the American Heart Association, Inc. from Kitabatake A, Ito H, Inove M, et al. A new approach to non-invasive evaluation of aortic regurgitant fraction by 2 dimensional Doppler echocardiography. Circulation; 1985:72:527.)

ined both in short and long axis, and individual leaflet motion inspected with the images magnified using the zoom feature option when available. Vegetations on the aortic valve are usually attached to the ventricular surface of the leaflets. Vegetations of 1 mm or less are sufficiently small, however, as not to interfere with aortic valve leaflet motion patterns, and thus may not be detected by two-dimensional echocardiography, since the axial resolution of the most commonly used 2.2 MHz transducers is 1 mm, with lateral resolution close to 2 mm. Serial echocardiographic studies may be required in patients with acute bacterial endocarditis to detect the vegetations as they increase in size.

The frequency with which patients with proven bacterial endocarditis show vegetations on echocardiographic examination varies greatly. In a recent review, vegetations were detected by M-mode echocardiography in 52% of cases and by two-dimensional echocardiography in 80% of cases (121). It is important to realize that the absence of vegetations on echocardiographic study does not exclude the diagnosis of bacterial endocarditis. Moreover, two-dimensional echocardiography cannot reliably distinguish between active and old vegetations (123), although serial examinations may show a progressive reduction in vegetation size and increasing echo density during the healing process (124, 125). In addition to the vegetations themselves, the complications of endocarditis should be assessed with great care, since these can change dramatically over short periods of time. These include leaflet fenestration, aortic ring abscesses (Fig. 8.62), septal tracks (suggested by prolongation of the PR interval on electrocardiogram), and satellite lesions in the septum and on the mitral valve. Other valve involvement with vegetations should be looked for carefully echocardiographically. The presence of hemodynamic alterations and, particularly, deterioration in cardiac output consequent to increasing severity of aortic regurgitation can be identified by the development of early mitral valve closure and by changes in the Doppler blood flow velocities profiles in diastole, such as shortening of the diastolic pressure half-time.

Despite enthusiastic initial reports regarding the role of two-dimensional echocardiography in the management of patients with vegetative endocarditis, measurements of vegetation size, mobility, and location have not proved useful clinically. Recent prospective studies have demonstrated that the presence or absence of vegetations in endocarditis does not correlate with the incidence of thromboembolic phenomena, valve rupture, or the need for urgent surgery (126). By contrast a number of retrospective studies have shown that patients with vegetations are at risk of developing peripheral emboli and heart failure, and have an increased likelihood of proceeding to valvular surgery (122, 123). However, early recognition of the complications of aortic valve endocarditis, including acute severe aortic regurgitation due to a flail leaflet, early mitral valve closure, aortic root or ring abscesses (127–129) (Fig. 8.62), and satellite lesions on the septum and anterior mitral valve (130), is of paramount importance. Echocardiography may have prognostic importance in detecting early mitral valve closure in aortic regurgitation, which, similar to ruptured chordae

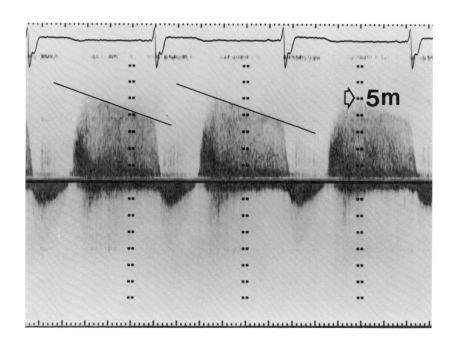

A

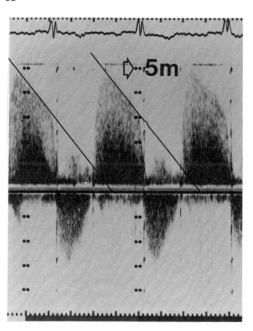

Figure 8.55. Continuous-wave Doppler velocity tracings from two patients with aortic regurgitation (AR), in whom the peak velocity is approximately 5 m/sec. The deceleration rate (indicated by the slope) is markedly slower in *A*—the pressure half time ($t_{1/2}$) of 520 m/sec indicates mild AR. In *B*, the deceleration rate is rapid, with a $t_{1/2}$ of 200 m/sec, indicating that the aortic regurgitation is vere.

B

in mitral regurgitation, is associated with an increased likelihood of valve replacement (126).

AORTIC VALVE PROLAPSE

Aortic valve prolapse is an uncommon condition of the aortic valve that is recognized with increasing frequency by two-dimensional echocardiography (79, 81, 131). It is best appreciated in the parasternal long axis view (Figs. 8.43, 8.63), and is recognized by downward displacement of one or more cusps of the aortic valve below a line joining the points of attachment of the aortic valve leaflets. The valve leaflets often have a fluffy appearance, indicating increased thickness, but paradoxically have increased rather than decreased mobility suggestive of myxomatous change (81). Aortic valve prolapse is most commonly reported in association with bicuspid aortic valve or with mitral valve prolapse (131). Other causes include aortic root dilatation, endocarditis, and severe mitral regurgitation. Aor-

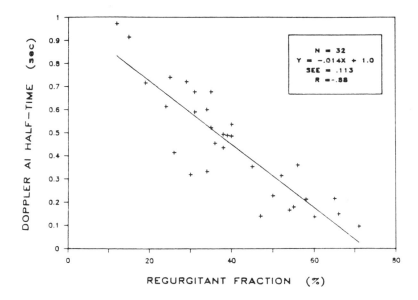

Figure 8.56. Doppler estimation of the pressure half time correlates inversely with regurgitant fraction in patients with aortic regurgitation. (Reproduced with permission from Teague SM, Heinsimer JA, Anderson JL et al. Quantitation of aortic regurgiation utilizing continuous wave Doppler ultrasound. J Am Coll Cardiol 1986;8:592–599.).

tic valve prolapse may result in hemodynamically important aortic regurgitation (132), although how frequently this occurs is unknown (131).

THE PULMONARY VALVE

The pulmonary valve may be more difficult to image echocardiographically in the adult than the aortic or the atrioventricular valves, but it is relatively easy to image in infants and children. With careful attention to recording technique, however, it is possible to obtain images of the pulmonary valve in the majority of patients. They provide important diagnostic information in patients with right-side heart disease, and pulmonary parenchymal and pulmonary vascular disease. Even when the pulmonary valve leaflets are difficult to image, blood flow velocity spectra can

usually be recorded with Doppler echocardiography from the right ventricular outflow tract and from the proximal main pulmonary artery.

Imaging Planes

Two-dimensional images of the pulmonary valve are obtained from the left parasternal region in either the third or fourth intercostal space with the transducer angled superiorly toward the left shoulder, so that the scan plane passes through the short axis of the aorta at the level of the aortic valve. In this view, the tricuspid valve is to the left and the right ventricle wraps around the aorta, with the pulmonary valve and main pulmonary artery to the right (Fig. 8.64). Minor angulation of the transducer to the left brings the ultrasound beam parallel to the long axis of the pulmonary trunk, which

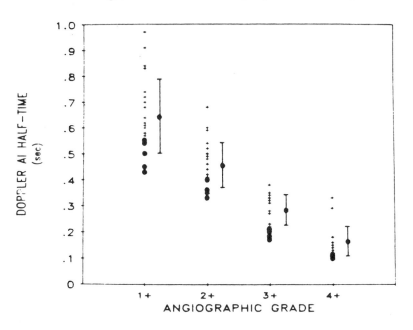

Figure 8.57. There is a close inverse correlation, in patients with aortic regurgitation, between Doppler estimates of pressure half time and contrast angiographic grading of severity of aortic regurgitation. (Reproduced with permission from Teague SM, Heinsimer JA, Anderson JL et al. Quantitation of aortic regurgiation utilizing continuous wave Doppler ultrasound. J Am Coll Cardiol 1986;8:592–599.)

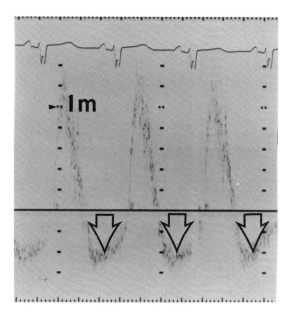

Figure 8.58. Pulsed-wave Doppler velocity signals obtained from the ascending aorta in a patient with aortic regurgitation, showing the positive antegrade signal followed by the negative or reversed flow signal (*arrows*). The ratio of systolic to diastolic flow velocity integrals has been used as an index of the severity of aortic regurgitation.

runs vertically such that the bifurcation into right and left pulmonary arteries can be visualized with the right pulmonary artery passing behind the left atrium. Accurate Doppler blood flow velocity profiles can be recorded from the pulmonary artery and the right ventricular outflow tract from this scan plane as the ultrasound beam is parallel to the direction of blood flow. To record blood flow velocities from the main

pulmonary artery, the pulsed-wave Doppler sample volume is positioned in the middle of the pulmonary artery immediately distal to the valve. Blood flow velocities from the right ventricular outflow tract are obtained by positioning the Doppler sample volume immediately proximal to the pulmonary valve, which enables detection of any retrograde diastolic flow from pulmonary regurgitation.

The long axis view of the right ventricular outflow tract can also be recorded from the subcostal short axis view. With the transducer in the subxiphoid region in the subcostal four chamber orientation, the scan plane is rotated 90° counterclockwise and angled cephalad, until the tricuspid valve, the aortic valve in short axis, the pulmonary artery annulus, and the pulmonary artery bifurcation are all in the same plane (Fig. 8.65). Doppler recordings of blood flow velocity across the pulmonary valve can be obtained from this scan plane. An elongated right oblique view, which is a modification of the subcostal view, may be superior in imaging the right ventricular outflow tract anatomy in children since it allows localization and assessment of the severity of associated infundibular narrowing and/or obstruction (133).

The pulmonary artery and its main branches can also be imaged with the transducer in the suprasternal region (134). In the suprasternal long axis view of the aortic arch, the aorta is superior and curves around the right pulmonary artery, which is imaged in cross-section (Fig. 8.66). Rotation of the transducer 90° from this scan plane brings into view the aorta in cross-section and the right pulmonary artery in long axis. Usually, the first few centimeters of the left pulmonary artery can be visualized from the suprasternal view parallel to the aorta.

The right ventricular outflow tract can occasionally

Figure 8.59. Pulsed-wave Doppler velocity signal recorded from the descending thoracic aorta (*top*) and the change in aortic diameter from systole to diastole (*bottom*). These measurements may be utilized to calculate regurgitant fraction. (Reproduced by permission of the American Heart Association Inc. from Touche T, Prasquier R, Nitenberg A, et al. Assessment and follow-up of patients with aortic regurgitation by an updated Doppler echocardiographic measurements of the regurgitant fraction in the aortic arch. Circulation; 1985: 72:821.)

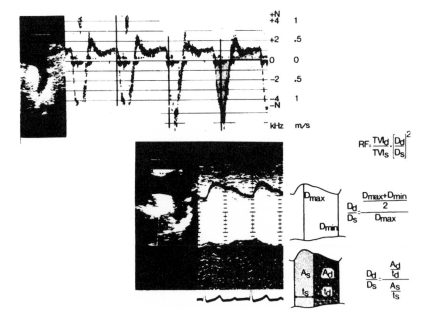

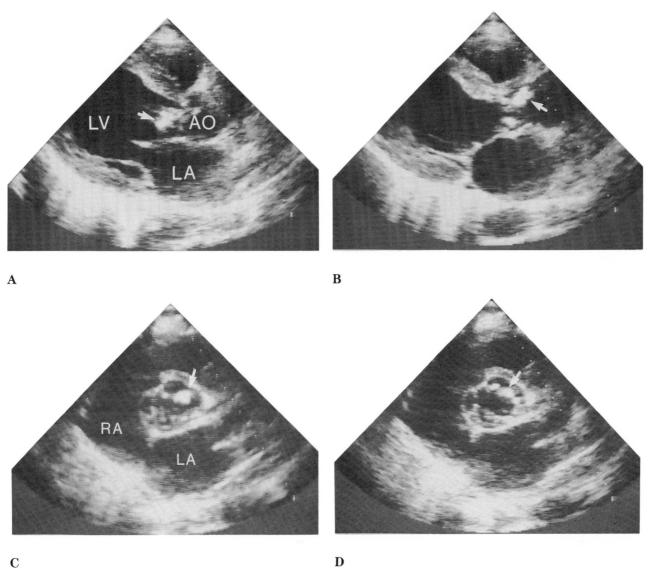

Figure 8.60.   Two-dimensional echocardiogram of the parasternal long axis from a patient with aortic valve endocarditis. Vegetations are visualized prolapsing into the left ventricle during diastole (*A*) and involving both the aortic valve leaflets (*B*). The short axis view shows that the aortic valve is bicuspid, with vegetations attached to both leaflets in diastole (*C*) and in systole (*D*).

be seen from the apex. From the four chamber apical view, superior angulation of the transducer allows imaging of the left ventricular outflow tract. Continued superior angulation demonstrates the right ventricular outflow tract, the pulmonic valve, and the proximal pulmonic artery. Short axis views of the pulmonary valve are difficult to obtain in patients with normally related great vessels.

The Normal Pulmonary Valve

The pulmonary valve leaflets are in apposition in diastole along the line of the annulus. Normal valve leaflets are thin, and often the only structure that can be identified is the area of leaflet coaption represented

by a thin linear structure in the long axis of the pulmonary artery (Fig. 8.64). The valve leaflets open through a 90°-angle in systole and lie parallel to the walls of the pulmonary artery, and are often obscured by echoes from the vessel wall.

The optimal M-mode images of the pulmonary valve are obtained by locating the pulmonary valve using two-dimensional echocardiographic images from the left parasternal short axis view of the aorta. M-mode echocardiographic images of the posterior leaflet of the pulmonary valve are usually obtained only in diastole and early systole (135–137). Occasionally M-mode images of the anterior and posterior cusps of the pulmonary valve can be obtained throughout the cardiac cycle, but this is possible only when the pulmonary

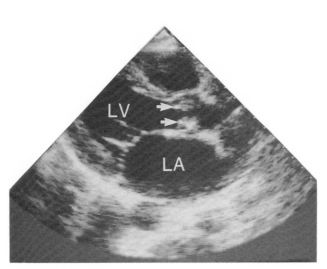

A

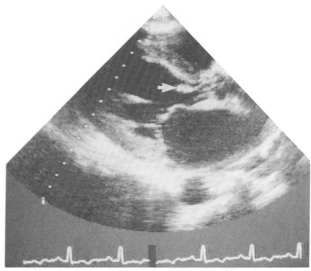

B

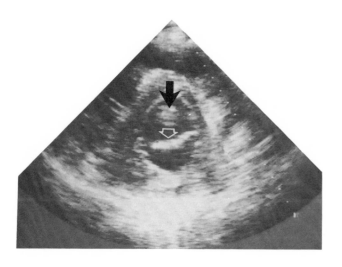

C

Figure 8.61. Two-dimensional echocardiogram of the LV long axis demonstrating vegetations attached to the right and noncoronary aortic valve leaflets (*A*). Pedunculated vegetations are visualized prolapsing into the left ventricular outflow tract in long (*B*) and in short axis (*C, black arrow*). There is reversed doming of the anterior mitral valve leaflets in long and short axis (*B* and *C, white arrow*), indicating severe aortic regurgitation.

artery is dilated (Fig. 8.67). The normal pattern of pulmonary valve motion recorded by M-mode echocardiography is illustrated in Figure 8.67. In early diastole the pulmonary valve moves posteriorly, away from the chest wall, and this is reflected as a gradual downward motion of the M-mode echo. In patients in sinus rhythm, there is abrupt downward motion of the valve leaflet following atrial systole, this is the "a" dip. This "a" dip varies markedly with respiration and is caused by doming of the valve leaflets into the pulmonary artery, which is a result of the rise in right ventricular end-diastolic pressure following atrial systole (138). It has also been suggested that this movement is a reflection of posterior displacement of the entire base of the heart and that variations in "a" wave amplitude result partly from the effects of altered ventricular

geometry and compliance. Other portions of the M-mode echocardiogram of the pulmonary valve have also been labelled (Fig. 8.67). The "b" point represents the onset of ventricular systole, and the maximum excursion of the leaflet during systole is represented by the "c" point. During systole the leaflet moves forward to the "d" point, at which time closure begins. Complete closure of the valve is represented by the "e" point, and the point in diastole immediately prior to the "a" dip is called the "f" point. Usually only the "e" to "f" interval, the "a" dip, and "b" to "c" opening can be identified by M-mode echocardiography.

Blood flow velocity profiles recorded proximal and distal to the pulmonary valve are similar to those obtained from the aortic valve, although peak velocity amplitudes are smaller (Fig. 8.68). Blood flow velocity

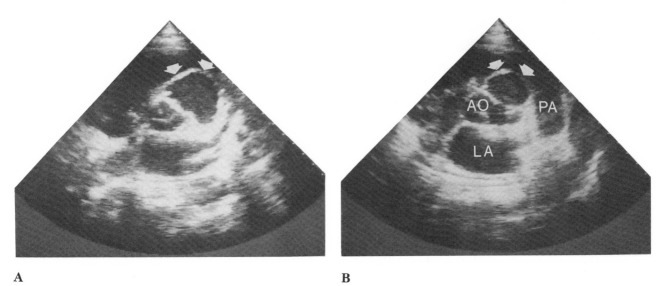

A   **B**

Figure 8.62.   Two-dimensional echocardiogram of the short axis of the aorta, showing a trileaflet aortic valve with a large expansile abscess cavity (*white arrows*) in a patient with vegetative endocarditis involving the aortic valve.

profiles recorded from the right ventricular outflow tract may sometimes show flow away from the transducer in diastole with atrial systole. The blood flow velocity in the pulmonary artery may be higher than in the right ventricular outflow tract, similar to that occurring in the left ventricular outflow tract and aorta. In adults, the peak velocity in the pulmonary artery is approximately 0.75 m/s (139). In children, peak velocity in the pulmonary artery increases from 0.67 m/s in the neonatal period to 0.79 m/s in early childhood (140).

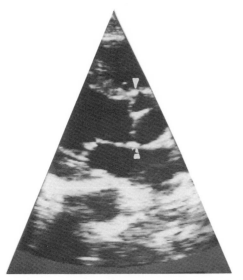

Figure 8.63.   Two-dimensional echocardiogram of the long axis of the left ventricular outflow tract and proximal aorta demonstrating diastolic prolapse of the aortic valve leaflets in a patient with a bicuspid aortic valve. The white arrows point to the aortic valve ring; the leaflets prolapse beyond this into the LV outflow tract.

Pulmonary Stenosis

Obstructions to right ventricular ejection are conventionally classified by their location—valvular, subvalvular, and supravalvular. The most common type of right ventricular outflow obstruction occurs at valve level; however, pulmonary valvular obstruction is often associated with secondary subvalvular obstruction. The presence of combined valve and subvalvular stenosis can be identified with two-dimensional echocardiographic imaging, and by the combination of pulsed- and continuous-wave Doppler.

Valvular Pulmonary Stenosis

Stenosis of the pulmonary valve is almost always congenital in origin. It can be acquired as a result of rheumatic or carcinoid heart disease, although this is rare. Congenital pulmonary stenosis consists of fusion of the cusps at the leaflet edges, which leaves a central perforation. The pliable leaflets of the valve dome during systole because of their restricted opening. Later in life the leaflets become thickened, fibrosed, and may occasionally calcify, which further restricts their movement. Congenital pulmonary valvular stenosis is usually associated with poststenotic dilatation of the main and often the secondary branches of the pulmonary artery. Less frequently congenital pulmonary valve stenosis may be caused by dysplasia of the valve leaflets, which are thickened and fibrotic, and obstruct the right ventricular outflow tract (141). When the valve is dysplastic, it is often associated with marked hypoplasia of the pulmonary valve annulus. Congenital pulmonary stenosis with dysplastic cusps is

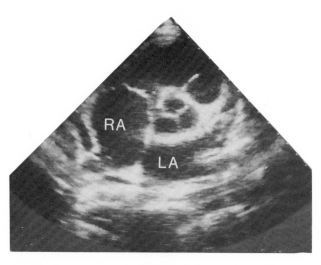

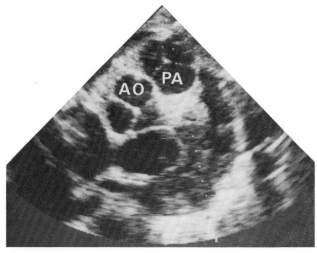

A

B

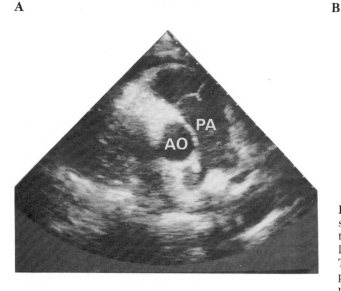

C

Figure 8.64. Two-dimensional echocardiogram of the short axis of the aorta at aortic valve level obtained from the left parasternal region, showing the pulmonary artery in long axis with pulmonary valve leaflets in diastole (*A*). Two-dimensional echocardiogram showing the trileaflet pulmonary valve in cross-section obtained from the left parasternal region (*B*), and the pulmonary artery in its long axis (*C*).

often severe and presents with right ventricular failure in the neonatal period.

The typical two-dimensional echocardiographic appearance of valvular pulmonary stenosis is the restricted motion and doming of the thickened valve leaflets during systole (142). In diastole the leaflets may appear almost normal and only minimally thickened. Valve motion is arrested in systole so that the leaflets lie in the center of the pulmonary artery, and not parallel to the walls of the pulmonary artery as occurs when the valve leaflets are normally mobile (Fig. 8.69). This characteristic domed appearance occurs because the bodies of the leaflets are pliable and the tips are fused. When the valve is dysplastic or becomes heavily fibrosed and calcified, it may not exhibit the characteristic systolic doming in systole. Congenital pulmonary stenosis is suggested by the presence of poststenotic

dilatation of the proximal pulmonary artery, which does not occur in acquired pulmonary stenosis.

The characteristic M-mode echocardiographic pattern in moderate to severe pulmonary stenosis is a large "a" wave (137), which is produced by diastolic movement of the pulmonary valve into the pulmonary artery. In severe pulmonary stenosis, right atrial pressure exceeds pulmonary artery diastolic pressure and the pressure generated by right atrial contraction results in an exaggerated "a" wave on the pulmonary valve and premature pulmonary valve opening. In mild pulmonary stenosis (gradient < 50 mmHg), the "a" wave is usually of normal amplitude. Although it was initially suggested that the maximum depth of the "a" wave reflected the severity of pulmonary stenosis, this has not been substantiated, and the depth of the "a" wave is neither specific nor sensitive for the

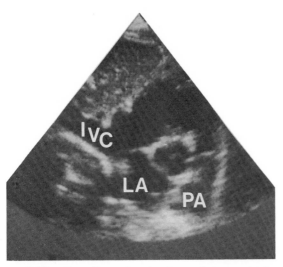

Figure 8.65. Two-dimensional echocardiogram obtained from the subcostal route showing the right atrium, right ventricle, right ventricular outflow tract, and pulmonary artery in long axis. The pulmonary valve is visible in diastole, during which the tricuspid valve is open and the aortic valve closed.

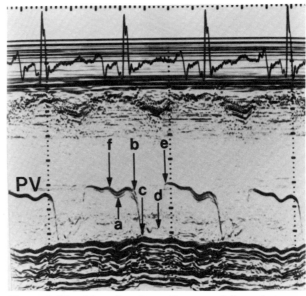

Figure 8.67. M-mode echocardiogram of the pulmonary valve showing the f point immediately prior to the a wave, and the b point, which indicates the onset of ventricular systole. The c point represents the maximum excursion of the leaflet, the d point is when the leaflets begin to move anteriorly, and the e point is the time of complete leaflet closure.

presence or severity of valvular stenosis (142). Although M-mode and two-dimensional echocardiography provide important anatomical information in pulmonary stenosis, the severity of the stenosis can be assessed only indirectly by the presence of right ventricular hypertrophy; right ventricular dilatation; and abnormal septal thickness, position, and motion (143).

The severity of pulmonary valve stenosis can be accurately quantitated by Doppler echocardiography. The high velocity systolic jet is located in the pulmonary artery immediately distal to the valve from the parasternal and subcostal scan planes (Fig. 8.70). The maximum velocity of blood flow distal to the pulmo-

nary valve should be recorded and the peak instantaneous pressure gradient in mmHg calculated using the modified Bernoulli equation [transvalvular gradient = 4 × (peak velocity)^2] (144, 145). Pulsed-wave Doppler echocardiography should be used initially to identify the location of obstruction in the right ventricular outflow tract and pulmonary artery. Mild pulmonary stenosis can be quantitated with pulsed-wave Doppler, but severe stenosis results in aliasing of the velocity

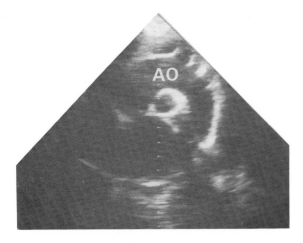

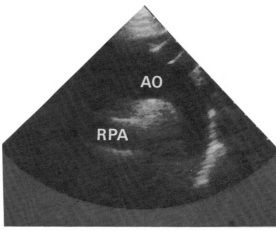

A   **B**

Figure 8.66. Two-dimensional echocardiogram of the aortic arch showing the origins of the brachiocephalic vessels. The right pulmonary artery is seen in cross-section passing under the aortic arch (*A*). The right pulmonary artery can be examined in its long axis if the scan plane is rotated 90° (*B*).

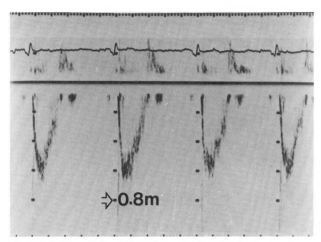

Figure 8.68. Pulsed Doppler velocity signal obtained from the right ventricular outflow tract, showing a peak velocity of 0.6 m/sec, and early to midsystolic peaking.

signal so that the peak amplitude cannot be determined, and therefore high-pulse repetition or continuous-wave Doppler must be used (144, 146). A close correlation has been demonstrated between transvalvular pressure gradients derived from Doppler blood flow velocities in the pulmonary artery and those obtained at cardiac catheterization, although Doppler slightly underestimates the gradient when the obstruction is severe (144, 145) (Fig. 8.71). The pressure gradient across a stenotic valve is dependent not only on the valve area but also on flow through the valve. Thus the severity of right outflow obstruction may be underestimated by a low transvalvular pressure gradient in the presence of right ventricular dysfunction and reduced right ventricular stroke volume. These potential difficulties may be overcome by using a noninvasive method of calculating pulmonary valve area. Pulmonary valve area has been estimated using the formula:

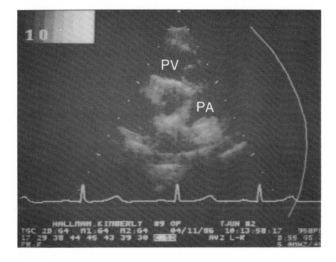

A

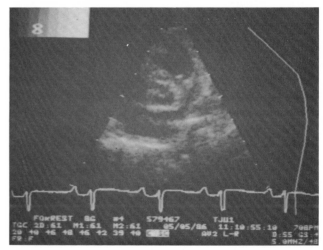

B

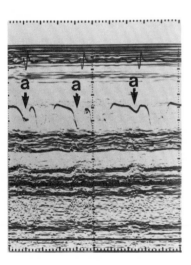

C

Figure 8.69. Two-dimensional echocardiogram of the short axis of the aorta in a newborn, demonstrating the right ventricular outflow tract and pulmonary artery in long axis, and thickened pulmonary leaflets with reduced excursion consistent with moderately severe congenital pulmonary valve stenosis. The leaflets are considerably thickened and dome during systole, with little change in cusp separation from diastole (A) to systole (B). M-mode echocardiogram from a patient with pulmonary valve stenosis showing a deep a wave (C).

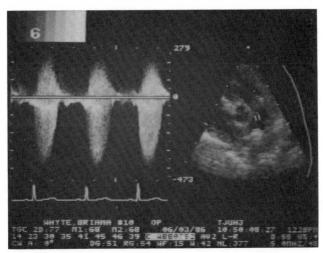

Figure 8.70. Two-dimensional Doppler echocardiogram of the right ventricular outflow tract, pulmonary artery, and pulmonary valve in a patient with pulmonary valve stenosis, showing the thickened leaflets and a Doppler peak velocity of 3.8 m/sec. This is consistent with a peak pressure gradient of between 55 and 60 mmHg, indicating moderate to severe pulmonary valve stenosis.

$$\text{valve area} = \text{SV}(0.88) \times V_2 \times \text{VET},$$

where SV is the stroke volume derived noninvasively by Doppler, V_2 is the maximal velocity distal to stenosis, and VET is ventricular ejection time (22). Valve areas derived by this method correspond closely with those obtained at cardiac catheterization (Fig. 8.72).

Subvalvular Pulmonary Stenosis

Subvalvular or infundibular pulmonary stenosis may occur in association with valvular pulmonary stenosis, ventricular septal defects, transposition of the great vessels, and tetralogy of Fallot. It may also occur as a result of hypertrophic cardiomyopathy or as a result of tumor infiltration. Two-dimensional echocardiography is invaluable in visualizing subvalvular pulmonary stenosis. The characteristic feature is a band of muscle, from the anterior and posterior walls of the infundibulum, that narrows the right ventricular outflow tract, increasing in severity during systole (147). In contrast to valvular stenosis, there is usually no poststenotic dilatation of the pulmonary artery. Subvalvular pulmonary stenosis results in coarse systolic fluttering of the pulmonary valve on M-mode echocardiography (Fig. 8.73) (148, 149), similar to the fluttering of the aortic valve in subaortic stenosis. Fluttering of the pulmonary valve leaflets is caused by turbulent blood flow distal to the stenosis, but it may not be present when there is coexistent valvular stenosis because the valve thickening does not allow the leaflets to resonate at high frequency. This turbulent systolic flow can be identified by Doppler echocardiography as a high velocity jet in the right ventricular outflow tract and main pulmonary trunk, and the site of obstruction can be determined. Similar to pulmonary valve stenosis, the pressure gradient across the subpulmonary or infundibular stenoses can be quantified using continuous-wave Doppler. Thus, with the combination of pulsed-wave and continuous-wave Doppler, the location and severity of stenoses can be accurately determined.

Supravalvular Pulmonary Stenosis

Congenital stenoses of the main or peripheral pulmonary arteries vary greatly in location and severity. The stenoses may be single or multiple, and the morphology of the stenosis may vary from discrete band lesions

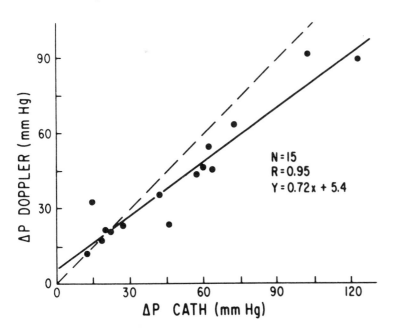

Figure 8.71. Comparison between the transvalve pressure gradients derived from Doppler flow velocities and those obtained at cardiac catheterization in patients with pulmonary valve stenosis show a close correlation, although Doppler slightly underestimates the gradient when the stenoses are severe. (Reproduced with permission from Johnson GL, Kwan OL, Handshoe S, Noonan JA, DeMaria AN. Accuracy of combined two-dimensional echocardiography and continuous wave Doppler recordings in the estimation of pressure gradient in right ventricular outlet obstruction. J Am Coll Cardiol 1984;3:1013.)

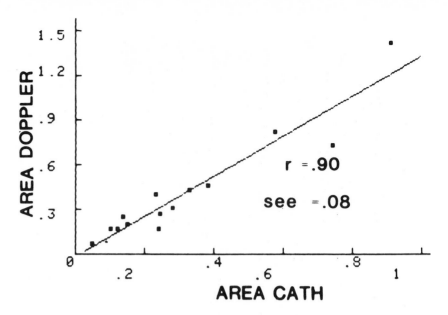

Figure 8.72. Estimates of pulmonary valve orifice area derived noninvasively by Doppler echocardiography correspond closely with those calculated at cardiac catheterization. (Reproduced with permission from Kosturakis D, Allen HD, Goldberg SJ, Sahn D, Valdes-Cruz LM. Non-invasive quantification of stenotic semi-lunar valve areas by Doppler echocardiography. J Am Coll Cardiol 1984;5: 1256–1262.)

to long tubular stenoses. Supravalvular pulmonary stenosis may also result from surgical banding of the main pulmonary artery as a palliative measure to reduce pulmonary blood flow in congenital heart diseases with large intracardiac left to right shunts.

Stenoses in the main pulmonary artery and proximal portions of the right and left pulmonary artery can usually be visualized with two-dimensional echocardiography (150). Similarly the adequacy of banding procedures in reducing the luminal diameter of the pulmonary artery can be assessed by cross-sectional echocardiography (151). Pulmonary bands usually appear as two dense parallel lines, which are often due to surrounding scar tissue, producing marked narrowing of the pulmonary artery beyond the valve. Two-dimensional echocardiography is also useful in detecting the complications of pulmonary banding procedures, in-

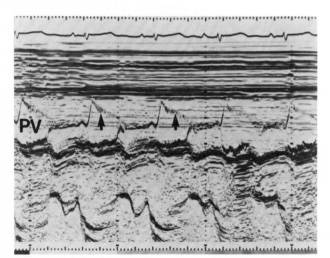

Figure 8.73. M-mode echocardiogram from a patient with subpulmonic stenosis, demonstrating systolic fluttering of the pulmonary valve leaflets.

cluding migration of the band and pseudoaneurysm formation (152). Doppler echocardiography provides important quantitative information regarding pulmonary artery banding procedures and their adequacy, because the pressure gradient across the band can be calculated from blood flow velocity measurements (146, 153).

Pulmonary Regurgitation

Pulmonary regurgitation may result from primary disorder of the valve cusps, or develop secondarily to dilatation of the pulmonary artery. Since the introduction of Doppler echocardiography, mild, hemodynamically unimportant pulmonary regurgitation has been recognized frequently in patients without any clinical evidence of structural heart disease (154). Primary valve disorders include myxomatous degeneration, often as part of the multiple floppy valve syndrome; infective endocarditis; congenital pulmonary stenosis; and congenital absence of the pulmonary cusps. Pulmonary regurgitation occurs secondarily to pulmonary artery dilatation, infective endocarditis involving the pulmonary valve, and following pulmonary valvotomy. Moderate to severe pulmonary regurgitation, resulting from pulmonary artery dilatation due to pulmonary hypertension, may be suspected on the basis of echocardiographic evidence of right ventricular dilatation and diastolic fluttering of the tricuspid valve. Contrast echocardiography has been used in detecting pulmonary regurgitation (155).

Pulmonary regurgitation can be detected accurately using pulsed-wave Doppler echocardiography (154, 156) when the transducer is in the left parasternal position and the sample volume positioned in the right ventricular outflow tract immediately below the pulmonary valve. The regurgitant flow is toward the transducer in diastole, and therefore the velocity spectra are

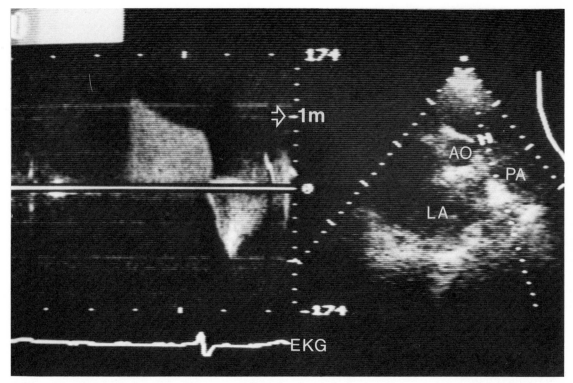

Figure 8.74.   Two-dimensional echocardiogram and Doppler flow velocity signal from a baby with mild pulmonary valve stenosis and regurgitation, showing a holodiastolic velocity signal with a peak of 1.2 m/sec and a slow deceleration rate consistent with pulmonary regurgitation. The systolic signal has a peak velocity of 1.0 m/sec occurring in mid-systole.

displayed in the upper register (Fig. 8.74). The severity of pulmonary regurgitation may be assessed by mapping the area in the right ventricle where the regurgitant jet is detected, but color-flow Doppler is now the technique of choice (Fig. 8.75, Plate VIII). Doppler echocardiography is highly sensitive and specific for pulmonary regurgitation.

The presence of pulmonary regurgitation is a frequent marker of pulmonary hypertension (154). In pulmonary hypertension, the instantaneous flow velocity is sustained at the same signal amplitude throughout diastole. By contrast, when the pulmonary artery pressure is normal, the velocity decreases gradually from early diastole to end diastole (156). The intensity of the regurgitant signal may vary with respiration. In severe pulmonary regurgitation, the velocity may decline to zero before end diastole, indicating diastolic equalization of pressures. The peak velocity recorded at end diastole may be used to calculate pulmonary artery end-diastolic pressure using the modified Bernoulli equation.

Dilatation of the Pulmonary Artery

Dilatation of the main pulmonary artery may be idiopathic, and may occur in pulmonary valve stenosis, Marfan's syndrome, right ventricular volume overload secondary to atrial septal defect or anomalous pulmonary venous drainage, and in severe pulmonary hypertension due either to pulmonary vascular disease or to recurrent thromboembolism. Measurements of the main pulmonary artery diameter can be made from the scan plane which passes through the long axis of the pulmonary artery and short axis of the aortic valve obtained from the left parasternal position (Fig. 8.76). Accurate measurements of pulmonary artery diameter may be difficult in adults because of inadequate definition of the pulmonary artery walls. Two-dimensional echocardiographic measurements of the main pulmonary artery and aortic diameters, and calculation of the ratio of their diameters are useful in estimating the magnitude of left to right shunts at atrial level (157). Measurements of the right pulmonary artery size from two-dimensional echocardiographic images from the suprasternal region may facilitate both the selection and timing of corrective surgery in patients with tetralogy of Fallot (158).

Two-dimensional echocardiography is useful in detecting aneurysms of the pulmonary artery (159), which may be saccular or fusiform, and usually occur in association with congenital heart disease. Dissecting aneurysms of the pulmonary artery may also be identified using cross-sectional echocardiography (160) (Fig. 8.77).

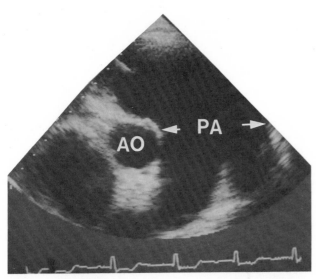

Figure 8.76.   Two-dimensional echocardiogram showing the aorta in cross-section, and the right ventricular outflow tract, pulmonary valve, and main pulmonary artery (PA) in long axis from a patient with severe dilatation of the pulmonary artery secondary to pulmonary hypertension. The pulmonary artery diameter is approximately 6 cm.

Pulmonary Hypertension

The presence of primary and secondary pulmonary hypertension can only be inferred by M-mode and two-dimensional echocardiography. Doppler echocardiography allows calculation of pulmonary artery systolic pressure and therefore assessment of the severity of pulmonary hypertension.

The diagnosis of pulmonary hypertension is suggested by the presence of a dilated pulmonary artery and right ventricular pressure overload in the absence of pulmonary valve disease (Figs. 8.78, 8.79). Abnormalities of septal motion may indicate that the pulmonary artery systolic pressure is elevated (143), and the size of the right pulmonary artery has been used as a measure of the severity of acute pulmonary hypertension following pulmonary embolism (161). There are several M-mode echocardiographic features that suggest the presence of pulmonary hypertension (136). The most frequently utilized signs are an absent or diminished "a" wave (4) and decreased respiratory variation in "a" wave amplitude, which is due to elevated right ventricular end-diastolic pressure (Fig. 8.80). However, the "a" wave may be normal in right heart failure and elevated right ventricular end-diastolic pressure. Although the absence or reduced "a" dip is specific, it does not correlate with the severity of pulmonary hypertension (162). Mid-systolic notching of the pulmonary valve on M-mode echo is another indicator of pulmonary hypertension (136, 162, 163) (Fig. 8.81), but it may also occur in idiopathic dilatation of the pulmonary artery in the absence of pulmonary hypertension (164). Dilatation of the right ventricle and abnormal septal motion also suggest pulmonary hypertension (Fig. 8.82). Systolic flutter of the pulmonary valve, which may resemble mid-systolic notching, also occurs in pulmonary hypertension.

Right ventricular isovolumic relaxation time, which is the time period from pulmonary valve closure to tricuspid valve opening, can be determined by Doppler.

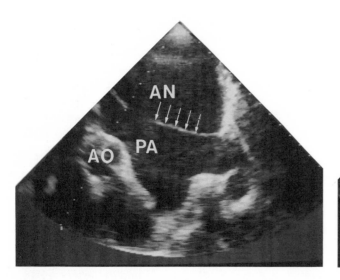

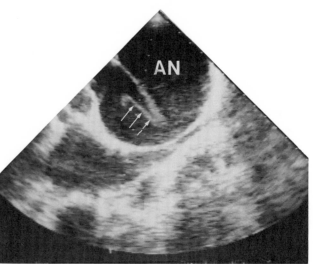

A   **B**

Figure 8.77.   Two-dimensional echocardiogram (*A*) showing the short axis of the aorta (AO) at aortic valve level with the main pulmonary artery (PA) in long axis down to its bifurcation. The main pulmonary artery is massively dilated due to a dissecting aneurysm (AN) with an intimal flap indicated by white arrows. Two-dimensional echocardiogram showing the very dilated pulmonary artery aneurysm with mobile intimal flaps (*B, white arrows*).

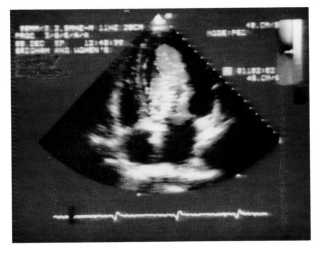

A

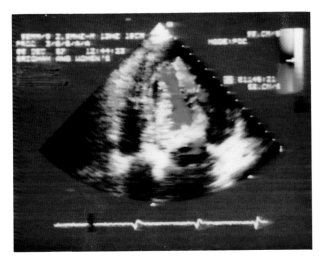

B

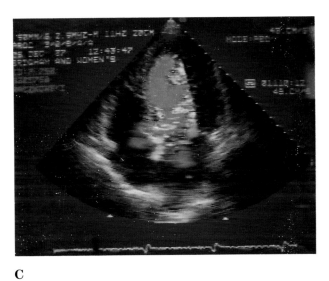

C

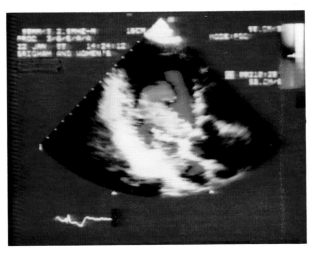

D

E

Figure 8.53. Doppler color-flow maps of aortic regurgitation. The apical four chamber view showing a regurgitant jet of blood in the left ventricle in diastole as a red, yellow, and green aliased high velocity signal (*A*). An apical four chamber view shows two aortic regurgitant jets, one running toward the apex along the interventricular septum, and the other running across the left ventricular inflow tract to the lateral wall (*B*). A wide-based regurgitant aortic jet is shown extending from the aortic valve papillary muscles, indicating 3+ AR (*C*). The width of the jet of the aortic valve occupies between one-third and one-half width of the left ventricular outflow tract (*C*). The jet in (*D*) is narrow compared to the width of the left ventricular outflow tract, but the jet extends almost to the apex of the left ventricle.

Plate VII

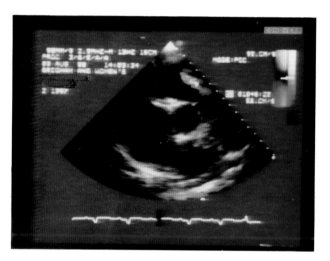 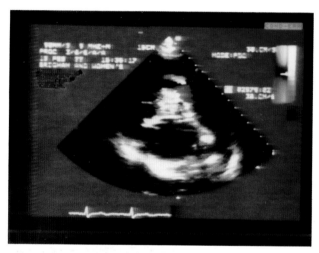

A   **B**

Figure 8.75. Color-flow Doppler velocity flow maps obtained in the short axis view of the aorta, showing the right ventricular outflow tract and the pulmonary artery from the left parasternal region, from two patients with mild pulmonary regurgitation (*A* and *B*). Diastolic retrograde flow is demonstrated as a red, flame-shaped signal in the right ventricular outflow tract immediately proximal to the pulmonary valve (*A* and *B*).

Plate VIII

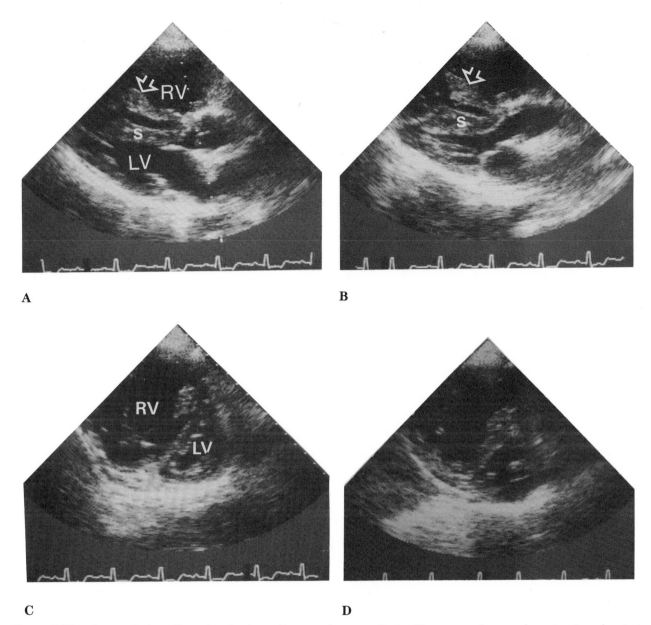

A

B

C

D

Figure 8.78. Composite two-dimensional echocardiograms from a patient with severe pulmonary hypertension, showing the left ventricle in long axis in diastole (*A*) and in systole (*B*). The right ventricle is dilated with a very hypertrophic papillary muscle (*arrow*) crossing the cavity, interventricular septal (s) motion is reversed, and the left ventricle appears small. Short axis views of the left ventricle below the mitral valve level show the enlarged right ventricle, abnormal diastolic septal motion, the large hypertrophic papillary muscle, and the more normal septal configuration during systole (*C*, *D*).

It provides an accurate estimate of pulmonary artery pressure in patients with pulmonary hypertension (165), which correlates closely with pulmonary artery pressure measured at cardiac catheterization. Right ventricular isovolumic relaxation is estimated by measuring the time from the Q wave to the end of the tricuspid regurgitation velocity signal, and subtracting from it the time interval from the Q wave on the electrocardiogram to the termination of the pulmonary artery blood flow velocity signal, and using the predicted pulmonary artery pressure nomogram of Burstin (166). However, the isovolumic RV relaxation period is

heart rate–dependent. Acceleration time (Fy) can be corrected for differing heart rates by dividing it by the electrocardiographic RR interval as a measure of the cardiac cycle length (167). In contrast to the normal pulmonary arterial blood flow velocity signal, the blood flow velocity in pulmonary hypertension increases rapidly and peaks early in systole. In addition, there is a second slow rise in flow velocity during deceleration, resulting in midsystolic notching. A close correlation has been demonstrated between the ratio of the time to peak flow, right ventricular ejection time, and mean pulmonary artery pressure.

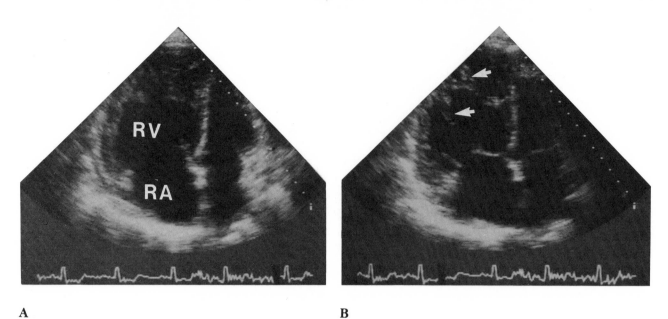

A

B

Figure 8.79. Two-dimensional echocardiogram of the apical four chamber view in a patient with severe pulmonary hypertension, showing the massively dilated right ventricle and right atrium in diastole (*A*) and in systole (*B*). There is marked right ventricular hypertrophy with increased free wall thickness and hypertrophic right ventricular papillary muscles (*B*, *arrows*). Note the abnormal diastolic septal configuration.

Tricuspid regurgitation occurs in the majority of patients with pulmonary hypertension when pulmonary artery systolic pressure exceeds 40 mmHg. This enables quantitation of pulmonary artery systolic pressure with continuous-wave Doppler (168–170) (see Chapter 7). This methodology assumes that the pressure gradient across the tricuspid valve, calculated from the peak velocity of the jet of tricuspid regurgitation using the modified Bernoulli equation, represents the difference in right atrial–right ventricular

systolic pressure. In the absence of pulmonary valve disease, addition of right atrial pressure to the right atrial–right ventricular pressure difference should be equivalent to pulmonary artery systolic pressure. There is controversy about whether it is necessary to add the right atrial pressure, determined by visual inspection of the jugular venous pulse, to the transtricuspid gradient to obtain an accurate measure of pulmonary artery systolic pressure. Some investigators have

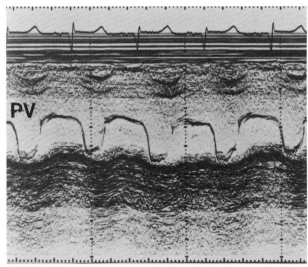

Figure 8.80. M-mode echocardiogram of the pulmonary valve from a patient with severe pulmonary hypertension, showing no a wave on the pulmonary valve during atrial systolic contraction.

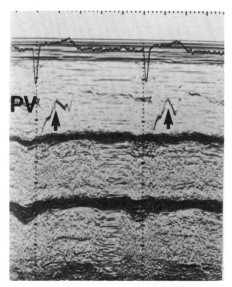

Figure 8.81. M-mode echocardiogram from a patient with pulmonary hypertension showing mid-systolic closure of the pulmonary valve (*arrows*).

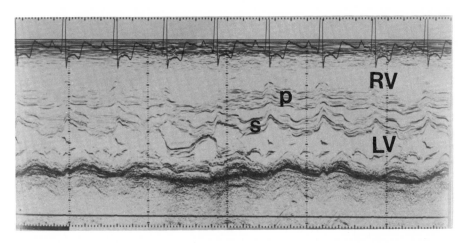

Figure 8.82. M-mode echocardiogram of the left ventricle in a patient with severe pulmonary hypertension, showing the mitral valve, a very enlarged right ventricle with a hypertrophic papillary (p) muscle anterior to the interventricular septum (s), and abnormal septal motion. The left ventricle appears small, but its function is normal. The hypertrophic right ventricular papillary muscle is best identified anterior to the septum when a sweep is performed from the mid- to the basal levels of the ventricular cavity.

added the constant 10 to the gradient or else used a regression equation to obtain a more accurate estimate of pulmonary artery systolic pressure (170). Both methods for calculating pulmonary artery pressure have been shown to correlate well with pulmonary artery systolic pressure measured at cardiac catheterization (171).

Infective Endocarditis

Thrombotic non-infective and infective vegetative endocarditis involving the pulmonary valve is rare. The pulmonary valve is less frequently involved with infective and non-infective endocarditis than the other three cardiac valves. When infective vegetative endocarditis does involve the pulmonary valve, it is usually either in association with congenital heart disease or with intravenous drug abuse. Pulmonary valve endocarditis is usually associated with vegetations on the other valves, but it may be an isolated finding (172, 173). The two-dimensional echocardiographic appearance of pulmonary valve vegetations is of abnormal, shaggy, irregular echoes attached to the valve cusps, causing exaggerated motion of the cusps (Fig. 8.83). Vegetations can be detected by M-mode echocardiography, but their morphologic appearances are better assessed by cross-sectional echocardiography. Differentiation of vegetations from fibrosis, myxomatous degeneration, and primary tumors of the valve cusps may sometimes be difficult to discern echocardiographically. Two-dimensional echocardiography cannot determine whether pulmonary vegetations are active or healed. The ma-

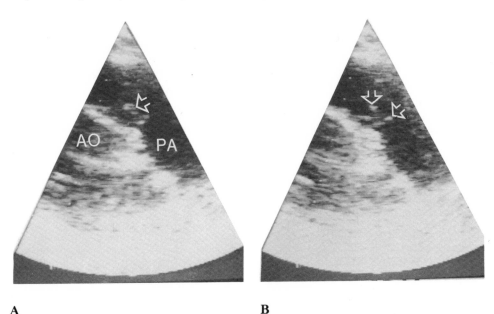

A   **B**

Figure 8.83. Two-dimensional echocardiogram from a patient with pulmonary valve vegetative endocarditis. Mobile vegetation is present (*arrows*), attached to the pulmonary valve leaflets (*A* and *B*). These are visualized best from the left parasternal region.

jority of patients with pulmonary endocarditis have evidence of pulmonary regurgitation by pulsed-wave or color-flow Doppler echocardiography (173).

Miscellaneous Conditions

Congenital absence of the pulmonary valve is a rare congenital anomaly associated with tetralogy of Fallot (174, 175). Two-dimensional echocardiography may show a thick, immobile ridge at valve level extending into the pulmonary artery.

Mid-diastolic opening of the pulmonary valve before or with atrial systole may be observed in conditions such as Uhl's anomaly, extensive right ventricular infarction, constrictive pericarditis, Loeffler's endocarditis, Ebstein's anomaly, pulmonary regurgitation, tricuspid valvulectomy, and rupture of the sinus of Valsalva into the right atrium (176, 177).

Cardiac Output Determinations

Cardiac output may be determined at the pulmonary valve level using Doppler echocardiography (178–180). Cardiac output is derived from the product of the flow velocity integral in the pulmonary artery and the cross-sectional area of the pulmonary artery. This area can be obtained by measuring the internal diameter at valve level from cross-sectional echocardiographic images assuming a circular cross-section. When systemic flow is also measured at the aortic valve using Doppler echocardiography, this technique can accurately estimate pulmonary to systemic flow ratios in patients with cardiac shunts. Because it is often difficult to obtain clearly defined images of the pulmonary artery, cardiac output at this site may not be as accurate as that measured at other sites (181).

REFERENCES

1. Roberts WC. The congenitally bicuspid aortic valve. A study of 85 autopsy cases. Am J Cardiol 1970;26:72–83.
2. Nanda NC, Gramiak R, Manning J, Mahoney EB, Lipchick ED, DeWeese JA. Echocardiographic recognition of the congenital bicuspid aortic valve. Circ 1974;49:870–875.
3. Kececioglu-Drailos Z, Goldberg SJ. Role of M-mode echocardiography in congenital aortic stenosis. Am J Cardiol 1981;47:1267–1272.
4. Chang S, Clements S, Chang J. Aortic stenosis: Echocardiographic cusp separation and surgical description of aortic valve in 22 patients. Am J Cardiol 1977;39:499.
5. Lesbre JP, Scheuble C, Kalisa A, Lalau JD, Andrejak MT. Echocardiography in the diagnosis of severe aortic valve stenosis in adults. Arch Mal Mol Coeur 1983;76:1.
6. Williams DE, Sahn DJ, Friedman WF. Cross-sectional echocardiographic localization of sites of left ventricular outflow tract obstruction. Am J Cardiol 1976;37:250.
7. Weyman AE, Feigenbaum H, Hurwitz RA, Girod DA, Dillon JC. Cross-sectional echocardiographic assessment of the severity of aortic stenosis in children. Circulation 1977;55:773.
8. De Maria AN, Joyce JA, Bommer W, et al. Sensitivity and specificity of cross-sectional echocardiography in the diagnosis and quantification of valvular aortic stenosis. Circulation, Suppl II, 1978;58:232.
9. Godley RW, Green D, Dillon JC, Rogers EW, Feigenbaum H, Weyman AE. Reliability of two-dimensional echocardiography in assessing the severity of valvular aortic stenosis. Chest 1981;79:657.
10. Le LR, Barrett MJ, Leddy CL, Wolf NM, Frankl WS. Determination of aortic valve area by cross-sectional echocardiography. Circulation Suppl II 1979;60:203.
11. Bennett DH, Evans DW, Raj MVJ. Echocardiographic left ventricular dimensions in pressure and volume—Their use in assessing aortic stenosis. Br Heart J 1975;39:971.
12. Gewitz HM, Werner JC, Kleinman CS, Hellenbrandle WE, Talner NS. Role of echocardiography in aortic stenosis: Pre- and postoperative studies. Am J Cardiol 1979;43:67–73.
13. Blackwood RA, Bloom KR, William CM. Aortic stenosis in children. Experience with echocardiographic prediction of severity. Circulation 1978;57:263.
14. Schwartz A, Vignola PA, Walker HJ, King ME, Goldblatt A. Echocardiographic estimation of aortic valve gradient in aortic stenosis. Ann Intern Med 1978;89:329.
15. Grossman W, Jones D, McLaurin LP. Wall stress and patterns of hypertrophy in the human left ventricle. J Clin Invest 1976;56:56.
16. Reichek N, Devereux RB. Reliable estimation of the peak left ventricular systolic pressure by M-mode echocardiography of severe valvular aortic stenosis in adult patients. Am Heart J 1982;103:202.
17. Young JB, Quinones MA, Waggoner AD, Miller RR. Diagnosis and quantification of aortic stenosis with pulsed Doppler echocardiography. Am J Cardiol 1980;45:987.
18. Hatle L, Angelson B, Tromsdal A. Non-invasive assessment of aortic stenosis by Doppler ultrasound. Br Heart J 1980;43:284.
19. Hatle L, Angelson B. Doppler ultrasound in cardiology. 2nd ed. Philadelphia: Lea & Febiger, 1985.
20. Lima CD, Sahn DJ, Valdes-Cruz LM, et al. Prediction of the severity of left ventricular outflow tract obstruction by quantitative two-dimensional echocardiographic Doppler studies. Circulation 1983;68:348.
21. Berger M, Berdoff RL, Gallerstein PE, Goldberg E. Evaluation of aortic stenosis by continuous wave Doppler ultrasound. J Am Coll Cardiol 1984;3:150.
22. Kosturakis D, Allen HD, Goldberg SJ, Sahn DJ, Valdes-Cruz LM. Noninvasive quantification of stenotic semilunar valve areas by Doppler echocardiography. J Am Coll Cardiol 1984;33:1256.
23. Currie PJ, Seward JB, Reeder GS, et al. Continuous wave Doppler echocardiographic assessment of severity of calcific aortic stenosis: A simultaneous Doppler-catheter correlative study in 100 adult patients. Circulation 1985;71:1162.
24. Simpson JA, Houston AB, Sheldon CD, Hutton I, Lawrie TDV. Clinical value of Doppler echocardiography in the assessment of adults with aortic stenosis. Br Heart J 1985;53:636.
25. Smith MD, Dawson PL, Elion JL, et al. Systematic correlation of continuous wave Doppler and haemodynamic measurements in patients with aortic stenosis. Am Heart J 1986;111:245.
26. Otto CM, Jarko C, Prestley R, Seal AK, Pearlman AS. Measurements of peak flow velocity in adults with valvular aortic stenosis using high pulse repetition frequency duplex pulsed Doppler echocardiography (abstr). J Am Coll Cardiol 1984;3:494.
27. Stewart WJ, Galvin KA, Gillam LD, Guyer DE, Weyman AE. Comparison of high pulse repetition frequency and continuous wave Doppler echocardiography in the assessment of high flow velocity in patients with valvular stenosis and regurgitation. J Am Coll Cardiol 1985;6:565.
28. Krafchek J, Roberts JH, Radford M, Adams D, Kisslo J. A reconsideration of Doppler assessed gradients in suspected aortic stenosis. Am Heart J 1985;110:765.
29. Panidis IP, Mintz GS, Ross J. Value and limitations of Doppler ultrasound in the evaluation of aortic stenosis: A statistical analysis of 70 consecutive patients. Am Heart J 1986;112:150.
30. Dawley D, Lilly L, Plappert T, St. John Sutton MG. Prospective Doppler quantitation of aortic stenosis (AS): Overestimation in

concomitant aortic insufficiency (AI) (abstr). Circulation Suppl. III 1985;72:373.

31. Warth DC, Stewart WJ, Block PC, Weyman AE. A new method to calculate aortic valve area without left heart catheterization. Circulation 1984;70:978–983.

32. Ohlsson J, Wranne B. Noninvasive assessment of valve area in patients with aortic stenosis. J Am Coll Cardiol 1986;7:501–508.

33. Skjaerpe T, Hegrenaes L, Hatle L. Noninvasive estimation of valve area in patients with aortic stenosis by Doppler ultrasound and two-dimensional echocardiography. Circulation 1985;72:810–818.

34. Otto CM, Pearlman AS, Comess KA, Reamer RP, Janko CL, Huntsman LL. Determination of the stenotic aortic valve area in adults using Doppler echocardiography. J Am Coll Cardiol 1986;7:509–517.

35. Richards KL, Cannon SR, Miller JF, Crawford MH. Calculation of aortic valve area by Doppler echocardiography: A direct application of the continuity equation. Circulation 1986;73:764–769.

36. Zoghbi WA, Framer KL, Soto JG, Nelson JG, Quinones MA. Accurate noninvasive quantification of stenotic aortic valve area by Doppler echocardiography. Circulation 1986;73:452–459.

37. Usher BW, Goulder D, Murgo JP. Echocardiographic detection of supraventricular aortic stenosis. Circulation 1974;49:1257.

38. Bolen JL, Popp RL, French JW. Echocardiographic features of supravalvular aortic stenosis. Circulation 1975;52:817.

39. Nasrallah AT, Nihill M. Supravalvular aortic stenosis echocardiographic features. Br Heart J 1975;37:662.

40. Ali N, Sheikh M, Mehrotra P, Barker T. Echocardiographic diagnosis of supraventricular aortic stenosis. South Med J 1977;70:759.

41. Mori Y, Nakano H, Kamiya T, Mori C. Echocardiographic and angiographic features of supravalvular aortic stenosis. J Cardiogr 1979;7:339.

42. Weyman AE, Caldwell RL, Hurwitz RA, et al. Cross-sectional echocardiographic characterisation of aortic obstruction. I. Supravalvular aortic stenosis and aortic hypoplasia. Circulation 1978;57:491.

43. David RH, Feigenbaum H, Chang G, Konecke LL, Dillon JC. Echocardiographic manifestations of discrete subaortic stenosis. Am J Cardiol 1974;33:277.

44. Weyman AE, Feigenbaum H, Hurwitz RA, Girod DA, Dillon JC, Chang S. Localisation of left ventricular outflow tract obstruction by cross-sectional echocardiography. Am J Med 1976;60:33.

45. Berry TE, Aziz KU, Paul MH. Echocardiographic assessment of discrete subaortic stenosis in childhood. Am J Cardiol 1979;43:957.

46. Krueger SK, French JW, Forker AD, Caudill CC, Popp RL. Echocardiography in discrete subaortic stenosis. Circulation 1979;59:506.

47. Wilcox WD, Seward JB, Hagler DJ, Mair DD, Tajik AJ. Discrete subaortic stenosis. Two-dimensional echocardiographic features with angiographic and surgical correlation. Mayo Clin Proc 1980;55:425.

48. DiSessa TG, Hagan AD, Isabel-Jones JB, Ti CC, Mercier JC, Friedman WF. Two-dimensional echocardiographic evaluation of discrete subaortic stenosis from an apical long axis view. Am Heart J 1981;101:774.

49. Hatle L. Noninvasive assessment and differentiation of left ventricular outflow obstruction with Doppler obstruction. Circulation 1981;64:381.

50. Valdes-Cruz LM, Jones M, Scagnelli S, Sahn DJ, Tomizuka FM, Pierce JE. Prediction of gradients in fibrous subaortic stenosis by continuous wave two-dimensional Doppler echocardiography: Animal studies. J Am Coll Cardiol 1985;5:1363.

51. Kinney EL, Machado H, Cortada X, Galbot DL. Diagnoses of discrete subaortic stenosis by pulsed and continuous wave Doppler. Am Heart J 1985;110:1069.

52. Pridie RB, Benham R, Oakley CM. Echocardiography of the mitral valve in aortic valve disease. Br Heart J 1971;33:296.

53. D'Cruz I, Cohen HC, Prabhu R, Ayabe T, Glick G. Flutter of left ventricular structure in patients with aortic regurgitation with special reference to patients with associated mitral stenosis. Am Heart J 1976;9:684.

54. Henzi M, Burckhardt D, Raider EA, Folleth F. Echocardiography as a method for the determination of the severity of aortic insufficiency. Schweiz Med Wochenschr 1976;106:1557.

55. Johnson AD, Gosink BB. Oscillation of left ventricular structures in aortic regurgitation. J Clin Ultrasound 1977;5:21.

56. Fujioka T, Beda K, Ohdawa S, et al. A clinicopathological study of aortic regurgitation with septal flutter on echocardiogram. J Cardio 1978;8:697.

57. Nakao S, Tanaka M, Yoshimura K, Sakurai S, Tei C, Kashima T. A regurgitant jet and echocardiographic abnormalities in aortic regurgitation. An experimental study. Circulation 1983;67:860.

58. Estevez CN, Dillon JC, Walker PD, Feigenbaum H, Chang S. Echocardiographic manifestations of aortic cusp rupture in a case of myxomatous degeneration of the aortic valve. Chest 1976;69:544.

59. Rolson WA, Hirshfield DS, Emilson BB, Cheitlin MD. Echocardiographic appearance of ruptured aortic cusp. Am J Med 1977;62:133.

60. Ramirez J, Guardiole J, Flowers NC. Echocardiographic diagnosis of ruptured aortic valve leaflet in bacterial endocarditis. Circulation 1978;57:634.

61. Whipple RL III, Morris DC, Feher JM, Merrill AJ Jr, Miller JI. Echocardiographic manifestations of flail aortic valve leaflets. J Clin Ultrasound 1977;5:417.

62. Chandraratna PAN, Robinson MJ, Byrd C, Pitha JV. Significance of abnormal echoes in left ventricular outflow tract. Br Heart J 1977;39:381.

63. Johnson AD, Alpert JS, Francis GS, Yieweg VR, Ockene I, Hagan AD. Assessment of left ventricular function in severe aortic regurgitation. Circulation 1976;54:975.

64. McDonald IG. Echocardiographic assessment of left ventricular function in aortic valve disease. Circulation 1976;53:860.

65. Cunha CLP, Guiliani ER, Fuster V, Seward JB, Brandenbrug RD. Surgery for aortic insufficiency: Value of M-mode echocardiography as a prognostic indicator: Am J Cardiol 1979;43:406.

66. Henry WL, Bonow RO, Borer JS, et al. Observations on the optimum time for operative interests for aortic regurgitation. I. Evaluation of the results of aortic valve replacement in symptomatic patients. Circulation 1980;61:471.

67. Henry WL, Bonow RO, Rosing DR, Epstein SE. Observations on the optimum time for operative interventions for aortic regurgitation. II. Serial echocardiographic evaluation of asymptomatic patients. Circulation 1980;61:484.

68. Mann T, McLaurin L, Grossman W, Grange E. Assessing the haemodynamic severity of acute aortic regurgitation due to infective endocarditis. N Engl J Med 1975;293:108.

69. Oki T, Matsukisa M, Tsuyuguchi N, et al. Echo patterns of the anterior leaflet of the mitral valve in patients with aortic insufficiency. J Cardiol 1976;6:307.

70. Ambrose JA, Meller J, Teicholz LE, Herman MV. Premature closure of the mitral valve: Echocardiographic clue for the diagnosis of aortic dissection. Chest 1978;73:121.

71. Weaver WF, Wilson CS, Rourke T, Caudrill CC. Mid-diastolic aortic valve opening in severe acute aortic regurgitation. Circulation 1977;55:145.

72. Pietro DA, Parisi AF, Harrington JJ, Askenazi J. Premature opening of the aortic valve: An index of highly advanced aortic regurgitation. J Clin Ultrasound 1978;6:170.

73. D'Cruz TA, Jain DP, Hirsch L, Levinsky R, Cohen HC, Glick G. Echocardiographic diagnosis of dilatation of the ascending aorta using right parasternal scanning. Radiology 1978;129:465.

74. DeMaria AN, Bommer W, Neumann A, Weinart L, Bogren H, Mann DT. Identification and localisation of aneurysms of the ascending aorta by cross-sectional echocardiography. Circulation 1979;59:755.

75. Mintz GS, Kotler MN, Segal BL, Parry WR. Two-dimensional echocardiographic recognition of the descending thoracic aorta. Am J Cardiol 1979;44:232.

76. Brown DR, Popp RL, Kloster FE. Echocardiographic criteria for aortic root dissection. Am J Cardiol 1975;36:17.

77. Krueger SK, Starke H, Forker AD, Eliot RS. Echocardiographic mimics of aortic root dissection. Chest 1975;67:441.

78. Kasper W, Meinertz T, Kerstig F, Lange K, Just H. Diagnosis of dissecting aortic aneurysm with suprasternal echocardiography. Am J Cardiol 1978;42:291.

79. El-Shahawy M, Graybeal R, Pepini CJ, Conte CR. Diagnosis of aortic valvular prolapse by echocardiography. Chest 1976;69:411.

80. Mardelli TJ, Morganroth J, Naito M, Chen CC, Messcell L, Parrotto C. Cross-sectional echocardiographic identification of aortic valve prolapse. Circulation Suppl II 1979;60:797.

81. Shiu MF, Coltart DJ, Braimbridge MV. Echocardiographic findings in prolapsed aortic cusps with vegetations. Br Heart J 1979;41:118.

82. Rowe DE, Pechachek LW, De Castro CM, Carcia E, Hall RJ. Initial diastolic indentation of the mitral valve in aortic insufficiency. J Clin Ultrasound 1982;10:53.

83. Robertson WS, Stewart J, Armstrong WF, Dillon JC, Feigenbaum H. Reversed doming of the anterior mitral leaflet with severe aortic regurgitation. J Am Coll Cardiol 1984;3:431.

84. Schuler G, Peterson KL, Johnson AD, et al. Serial non-invasive assessment of left ventricular hypertrophy and function after surgical correction of aortic regurgitation. Am J Cardiol 1979;44:585.

85. Al-Nouri M, Hellman C, Schmidt DH. Echocardiographic indices predictive of early left ventricular dysfunction in patients with aortic regurgitation. Circulation Suppl II 1979;60:137.

86. Scognamiglio R, Rochardt J, Fasoli G, Marchese D, Prandi A, Stritoni P. Relation between myocardial contractility, hypertrophy and performance in patients with chronic aortic regurgitation. Int J Cardiol 1984;6:473–484.

87. Gaasch WH, Carroll JD, Levine HJ, Criscitiello MG. Chronic aortic regurgitation: Prognostic value of left ventricular end-systolic dimensions and end-diastolic radius/thickness ratio. J Am Coll Cardiol 1983;3:775.

88. Fioretti P, Roelandt J, Bos RJ, et al. Echocardiography in chronic aortic insufficiency. Circulation 1983;67:216.

89. Stone PH, Clark RD, Goldschlager N, Selzer A, Cohn K. Determinants of prognosis of patients with aortic regurgitation who undergo aortic valve replacement. J Am Coll Cardiol 1984;3:1118.

90. Fioretti P, Roelandt J, Sclavo M, et al. Postoperative regression of left ventricular dimensions in aortic insufficiency. A long term echocardiographic study. J Am Coll Cardiol 1985;5:856.

91. Daniel WG, Hood WP, Siart A, et al. Chronic aortic regurgitation: Reassessment of the prognostic value of preoperative left ventricular end-systolic dimension and fractional shortening. Circulation 1985;71:669.

92. Hirshfeld JW Jr, Epstein SE, Roberts AJ, Glancy DL, Morrow AG. Indices predicting long-term survival after valve replacement in patients with aortic regurgitation and patients with aortic stenosis. Circulation 50:1190–1194.

93. Borow KM, Green LH, Mann T, et al. End-systolic volume as a predictor of postoperative left ventricular function in volume overload from valvular regurgitation. Am J Med 1980;68:655.

94. Carabello GA, Spann JF. The uses and limitations of end-systolic indices of left ventricular function. Circulation 1984;69:1058.

95. Crawford MH, Grant D, O'Rourke RA, Starling MR, Groves BM. Accuracy and reproducibility of new M-mode recommendations for measuring left ventricular dimensions. Circulation 1980;66:137.

96. Abdulla AM, Frank MJ, Canedo MI, Stafadouros MA. Limitations of echocardiography in the assessment of left ventricular size and function in aortic regurgitation. Circulation 1980;61:148.

97. St. John Sutton MG, Plappert T, Hirshfeld JW, Reichek N. Assessment of left ventricular mechanics in patients with asymptomatic aortic regurgitation. A two-dimensional echocardiographic study. Circulation 1984;69:259–268.

98. St. John Sutton MG, Plappert T, Spiegel A, et al. Early postoperative changes in left ventricular chamber size, architecture and function in aortic stenosis and in aortic regurgitation and their relation to intraoperative changes in afterload: A prospective 2D echocardiographic study. Circulation 1987;76:77–89.

99. Grayburn PA, Smith MD, Handshoe R, Friedman BJ, De Maria AN. Detection of aortic insufficiency by standard echocardiography, pulsed Doppler echocardiography, and auscultation. Ann Intern Med 1986;104:599.

100. Saal AK, Gross BW, Franklin DW, Pearlman AS. Noninvasive detection of aortic insufficiency in patients with stenosis by pulsed Doppler echocardiography. J Am Coll Cardiol 1985;5:176.

101. Esper RJ. Detection of mild aortic regurgitation by range-gated pulsed Doppler echocardiography. Am J Cardiol 1982;50:1037.

102. Ciobanu M, Abbasi AS, Allen M, Hermer A, Spellberg R. Pulsed Doppler echocardiography in the diagnosis and estimation of severity of aortic insufficiency. Am J Cardiol 1982;49:339.

103. Veyrat C, Lessana A, Abitbol G, Ameur A, Benaim R, Kalmonson D. New indices for assessing aortic regurgitation with two-dimensional Doppler echocardiographic assessment of the regurgitant aortic valvular area. Circulation 1983;68:998.

104. Byard CE, Perry GJ, Roitman DI, Nanda NC. Quantitative assessment of aortic regurgitation by colour Doppler. Circulation Suppl III (abstr) 1985;72:146.

105. Kitabatake A, Ito H, Inoue M, et al. A new approach to noninvasive evaluation of aortic regurgitant fraction by two-dimensional Doppler echocardiography. Circulation 1985;72:523.

106. Rokey R, Sterling L, Zoghbi WA, et al. Determination of regurgitant fraction in isolated mitral or aortic regurgitation by pulsed Doppler two-dimensional echocardiography. J Am Coll Cardiol 1986;7:1273.

107. Zhang Y, Nitter-Hauge S, Ihlen H, Rootwelt K, Myhre E. Measurement of aortic regurgitation by Doppler echocardiography. Br Heart J 1986;55:32.

108. Masuyama T, Kodama K, Kitabatake A, et al. Noninvasive evaluation of aortic regurgitation by continuous wave Doppler echocardiography. Circulation 1986;73:460.

109. Teague SM, Heinsimer JA, Anderson JL, et al. Quantification of aortic regurgitation utilizing continuous wave Doppler ultrasound. J Am Coll Cardiol 1986;8:592–599.

110. Hoffman A, Pfisterer M, Stulz P, Schmitt HE, Burkart F, Burckhardt D. Non-invasive grading of aortic regurgitation by Doppler ultrasonography. Br Heart J 1986;55:283.

111. Sellier P, Maurice P. Non-invasive quantification of aortic regurgitation by Doppler echocardiography. Br Heart J 1983;49:167.

112. Imaizumi T, Orita Y, Kiowaya Y, Hirata T, Nakamura M. Utility of two-dimensional echocardiography in the differential diagnosis of the aetiology of aortic regurgitation. Am Heart J 1982;103:887.

113. Quinones MA, Young JB, Waggoner AD, Ostojic MC, Ribeiro LGT, Miller RR. Assessment of pulsed Doppler echocardiography in detection and quantification of aortic and mitral regurgitation. Br Heart J 1980;44:612.

114. Touche T, Prasquier R, Nitenberg A, DeZuttere D, Gourgon R. Assessment and followup of patients with aortic regurgitation by an updated Doppler echocardiographic measurement of the regurgitant fraction in the aortic arch. Circulation 1985;72:819.

115. Dillon JC, Feigenbaum H, Konecke LL, Davis RH, Chang S. Echocardiographic manifestations of valvular vegetations. Am Heart J 1972;86:698.

116. Martinez EC, Birch BE, Giles TD. Echocardiographic diagnosis of vegetative aortic bacterial endocarditis. Am J Cardiol 1974;34:385.

117. De Maria AN, King JF, Salel AF, Caudill CC, Miller RR, Mason DT. Echography and phonography of acute aortic regurgitation in bacterial endocarditis. Ann Intern Med 1975;82:329.

118. Hirshfield DS, Schiller N. Localisation of aortic valve vegetations by echocardiography. Circulation 1976;53:280.

119. Busch UW, Garcia E, Pechachek LW, De Castro CMJ, Hall RJ. Cross-sectional echocardiographic findings in vegetative aortic valve endocarditis. Cardiovasc Dis 1978;5:328.

120. O'Brien JT, Geiser EA. Infective endocarditis and echocardiography. Am Heart J 1984;108:386.

121. Wann LS, Hallan CC, Dillon JC, Weyman AE, Feigenbaum H. Comparison of M-mode and cross-sectional echocardiography in infective endocarditis. Circulation 1979;60:728.

122. Berger M, Gallerstein PE, Benhuri P, Balla R, Goldberg E. Evaluation of aortic valve endocarditis by two-dimensional echocardiography. Chest 1981;80:61.

123. Steward JA, Silimperi D, Harris P, Wise NK, Fraker TD, Kisslo JA. Echocardiographic documentation of vegetative lesions in infective endocarditis: Clinical implications. Circulation 1980; 61:374.

124. Stafford A, Wann LS, Dillon JC, Weyman AE, Feigenbaum H. Serial echocardiographic appearance of healing bacterial vegetations. Am J Cardiol 1979;44:754.

125. Stafford WJ, Petch J, Radford DJ. Vegetations in infective endocarditis. Clinical relevance and diagnosis by cross-sectional echocardiography. Br Heart J 1985;53:310.

126. Lutas EM, Roberts RB, Deverus RB, Prieto LM. Relation between the presence of echocardiographic vegetations and the complication rate in infective endocarditis. Am Heart J 1986;112:107–113.

127. Wong AM, Oldershaw PJ, Gibson DG. Echocardiographic demonstration of aortic root abscess after infective endocarditis. Br Heart J 1981;46:584.

128. Scanlan JG, Seward JB, Tajik AJ. Valve ring abscess in infective endocarditis. Visualization with wide angle two-dimensional echocardiography. Am J Cardiol 1982;49:1794.

129. Griffiths BE, Petch MC, English TAH. Echocardiographic detection of subvalvular aortic root aneurysm extending to mitral valve annulus as complication of aortic valve endocarditis. Br Heart J 1982;47:392.

130. Nguyen NX, Kessler KM, Bilsker MS, Myerburg RJ. Echocardiographic demonstration of satellite lesions in aortic valve endocarditis. Am J Cardiol 1985;55:1433.

131. Shapiro LM, Thwaites B, Westgate C, Donaldson R. Prevalence and clinical significance of aortic valve prolapse. Br Heart J 1985;54:179.

132. Woldow AB, Parmaeswaran R, Hartman J, Kotler M. Aortic regurgitation due to aortic valve prolapse. Am J Cardiol 1985;55: 1435.

133. Isaaz K, Cloez JL, Danchin N, Marcon F, Worms AM, Pernot C. Assessment of right ventricular outflow tract in children by two-dimensional echocardiography using a new subcostal view. Am J Cardiol 1985;56:539–545.

134. Snider AR, Silverman HN. Suprasternal notch echocardiography: A two-dimensional technique for evaluating congenital heart disease. Circulation 1982;66:652.

135. Gramiak R, Nanda NC, Shah PM. Echocardiographic detection of the pulmonary valve. Radiology 1972;102:152.

136. Weyman AE, Dillon JC, Feigenbaum H, Chang S. Echocardiographic patterns of pulmonary valve motion with pulmonary hypertension. Circulation 1974;50:905.

137. Weyman AE, Dillon JC, Feigenbaum H, Chang S. Echocardiographic patterns of pulmonic valve motion in valvular pulmonary stenosis. Am J Cardiol 1974;34:644.

138. Green SE, Popp RL. The relationship of pulmonary valve motion to the motion of surrounding cardiac structures: A two-dimensional and dual M-mode echocardiographic study. Circulation 1981;64:107.

139. Griffith JM, Henry WL. An ultrasound system for combined cardiac imaging and Doppler blood flow measurements in man. Circulation 1978;57:925.

140. Grenadier E, Lima CO, Allen HD, et al. Normal intracardiac and great vessel Doppler flow velocities in infants and children. J Am Coll Cardiol 1984;4:343.

141. Weyman AE, Murwitz RA, Girod DA, Dillon JC, Feigenbaum H, Green D. Cross-sectional echocardiographic visualization of the stenotic pulmonary valve. Circulation 1977;56:769.

142. LeBlanc MJ, Paquet M. Echocardiographic assessment of valvular pulmonary stenosis in children. Br Heart J 1981;46:363–368.

143. King ME, Braun H, Goldblatt A, Liberthson R, Weyman AE. Interventricular septal configuration as a prediction of right ventricular systolic hypertension in children: A cross-sectional echocardiographic study. Circulation 1983;68:68.

144. Lima CO, Sahn DJ, Valdes-Cruz LM, et al. Noninvasive prediction of transvalvar pressure gradients in patients with pulmo-

nary stenosis by quantitative two-dimensional echocardiographic Doppler studies. Circulation 1983;67:866.

145. Johnson GL, Kwan OL, Handshoe S, Noonan JA, DeMaria AN. Accuracy of combined two-dimensional echocardiography and continuous wave Doppler recordings in the estimation of pressure gradient in right ventricular outlet obstruction. J Am Coll Cardiol 1984;3:1013.

146. Stevenson JG, Kawabori I. Noninvasive determination of pressure gradients in children: Two methods employing pulsed Doppler echocardiography. J Am Coll Cardiol 1984;3:179.

147. Caldwell RL, Weyman AE, Hurwitz RA, Girod DA, Feigenbaum H. Right ventricular outflow tract assessment by cross-sectional echocardiography in tetralogy of Fallot. Circulation 1979;59:395.

148. Weyman AE, Dillon JC, Feigenbaum H, Chang S. Echocardiographic differentiation of infundibular from valvular pulmonary stenosis. Am J Cardiol 1975;36:21.

149. Mills P, Wolfe C, Redwood D, Leech G, Craige E, Leatham A. Non-invasive diagnosis of subpulmonary outflow tract obstruction. Br Heart J 1980;43:276.

150. Tinker DD, Nanda NC, Harris JP, Manning JA. Two-dimensional echocardiographic identification of pulmonary artery branch stenosis. Am J Cardiol 1982;50:814.

151. Ormsond GS, Jaffe RB, Newren L, Ruttenberg HD. Two-dimensional echocardiographic assessment of pulmonary artery band (abstr). Am J Cardiol 1982;49:1027.

152. Foale RA, King ME, Gordon D, Marshall JE, Weyman AE. Pseudoaneurysm of the pulmonary artery after the banding procedure: Two-dimensional echocardiographic description. J Am Coll Cardiol 1984;3:371.

153. Valdes-Cruz LM, Horowitz S, Sahn DJ, Larson D, Lima CO, Mesel E. Validation of a Doppler echocardiographic method for calculating severity of discrete stenotic obstructions in a canine preparation with a pulmonary arterial band. Circulation 1984;69: 1177.

154. Waggoner AD, Quinones MA, Young JB, et al. Pulsed Doppler echocardiographic detection of right-sided valve regurgitation. Experimental results and clinical significance. Am J Cardiol 1981;47:279.

155. Meltzer RS, Vered Z, Hegesh T, et al. Diagnosis of pulmonic regurgitation by contrast echocardiography. Am Heart J 1984;107:102.

156. Miyatake K, Okamoto M, Kinoshita N, et al. Pulmonary regurgitation studied with ultrasonic pulsed Doppler technique. Circulation 1982;65:969.

157. Denef B, Dumoulin M, Van Der Hauwaert LG. Usefulness of echocardiographic assessment of right ventricular and pulmonary trunk-size for estimating magnitude of left-to-right shunt in children with atrial septal defect. Am J Cardiol 1985;55:1571.

158. Lappen RS, Riggs TW, Lapin GD, Paul MH, Muster AJ. Two-dimensional echocardiographic measurement of right pulmonary artery diameter in infants and children. J Am Coll Cardiol 1983;2:121.

159. Bhandari AK, Nanda NC. Pulmonary artery aneurysms: Echocardiographic features in 5 patients. Am J Cardiol 1984;53:1438.

160. Rosenson R, St. John Sutton MG. Dissecting aneurysm of the pulmonary artery diagnosed by Doppler echocardiography. Am J Cardiol 1986;58:1140.

161. Kasper W, Meinertz T, Kersting F, Lollgen H, Limbourg P, Just H. Echocardiography in assessing acute pulmonary hypertension due to pulmonary embolism. Am J Cardiol 1980;45:567.

162. Acquatella H, Schiller NB, Sharpe DN, Chatterjee K. Lack of correlation between echocardiographic pulmonary valve morphology and simultaneous pulmonary arterial pressure. Am J Cardiol 1979;43:946.

163. Tahara M, Tanaka H, Nakao S, et al. Hemodynamic determinants of pulmonary valve motion during systole in experimental pulmonary hypertension. Circulation 1981;64:1249.

164. Bauman W, Wann LS, Childress R, Weyman AE, Feigenbaum H, Dillon J. Mid-systolic notching of the pulmonary valve in the absence of pulmonary hypertension. Am J Cardiol 1979;43:1049.

165. Hatle L, Angelsen B, Tromsdal A. Noninvasive estimation of pulmonary artery systolic pressure with Doppler ultrasound. Br Heart J 1981;45:157.

166. Burstin L. Determination of pressure in the pulmonary artery by external graphic recordings. Br Heart J 1967;29:396–404.

167. Kitabatake A, Inove M, Asao M, et al. Noninvasive evaluation of pulmonary hypertension by a pulsed Doppler technique. Circulation 1983;68:302.

168. Yock PG, Popp RL. Noninvasive estimation of right ventricular systolic pressure by Doppler ultrasound in patients with tricuspid incompetence. Circulation 1984;70:657–662.

169. Berger M, Haimowitz A, Van Tosh A, Berdoff RL, Goldberg E. Quantitative assessment of pulmonary hypertension in patients with tricuspid regurgitation using continuous wave Doppler ultrasound. J Am Coll Cardiol 1985;6:359.

170. Currie DJ, Seward JB, Chan K, et al. Continuous wave Doppler determination of right ventricular pressure: A simultaneous Doppler-catheterization study in 127 patients . J Am Coll Cardiol 1985;6:750.

171. Chan K-L, Currie PJ, Seward JB, Hagler DJ, Mair DD, Tajik AJ. Comparison of three Doppler ultrasound methods in the prediction of pulmonary artery pressure. J Am Coll Cardiol 1987;9:549–554.

172. Nakamura K, Satomi G, Sakai T, et al. Clinical and echocardiographic features of pulmonary valve endocarditis. Circulation 1983;67:198.

173. Cremieux A, Witchitz S, Malergue MC, et al. Clinical and echocardiographic observations in pulmonary valve endocarditis. Am J Cardiol 1985;56:610.

174. Buendia A, Attie F, Ovseyevitz J, et al. Congenital absence of pulmonary valve leaflets. Br Heart J 1983;50:31.

175. Segni ED, Einzig S, Bass JL, Edwards JE. Congenital absence of pulmonary valve associated with Tetralogy of Fallot: Diagnosis by 2-dimensional echocardiography. Am J Cardiol 1983;51:1798.

176. Wann LS, Weyman AE, Dillon JC, Feigenbaum H. Premature pulmonary valve opening. Circulation 1977;55:128.

177. Doyle T, Troup PJ, Wann LS. Mid-diastolic opening of the pulmonary valve after right ventricular infarction. J Am Coll Cardiol 1985;5:366.

178. Barron JV, Sahn DJ, Valdes-Cruz LM, et al. Clinical utility of two-dimensional Doppler echocardiographic techniques for estimating pulmonary to systemic blood flow ratios in children with left to right shunting, atrial septal defect, ventricular septal defect or patent ductus arteriosus. J Am Coll Cardiol 1984;3:169.

179. Sanders SP, Yeager S, Williams RG. Measurement of systemic and pulmonary blood flow and QP/QS ratio using Doppler and two-dimensional echocardiography. Am J Cardiol 1983;51:952.

180. Kenny JF, Plappert T, Doubilet P, et al. Changes in intracardiac blood flow velocities and right and left ventricular stroke volumes in the normal human fetus with gestational age: A prospective Doppler echocardiographic study. Circulation 1986;74:1208.

181. Sahn DJ. Determination of cardiac output by echocardiographic Doppler methods: Relative accuracy of various sites for measurement. J Am Coll Cardiol 1985;6:663.

9
Prosthetic Valves and Malfunction: Noninvasive Evaluation

Morris Kotler
Anthony Goldman
Wayne Parry

INTRODUCTION

The ideal prosthetic valve should consist of lasting geometric features capable of permanent fixation in a normal anatomic site (1). The prosthetic valve should be chemically inert and nonthrombogenic, should not interfere with blood elements, and should open and close promptly during phases of the cardiac cycle. It should offer as little resistance to blood flow as possible in both the resting and exercise states. Most important, it should be possible to evaluate accurately the functioning of the prosthetic valve by noninvasive techniques (2).

Evaluation of a patient with suspected prosthetic heart valve malfunction should begin with a careful history, physical examination, electrocardiogram (ECG), and chest x-ray. The cardiologist should be aware of the exact type of prosthetic heart valve, including the model number and size of each individual valve (3). The commonly used prosthetic valves are listed in Table 9.1. (For the purposes of this chapter, the basic prototype prosthetic valves to be discussed are in italic type.)

The clinician should be aware of the normal auscultatory findings in patients with prosthetic heart valves because auscultatory findings may vary depending on the type and location of the prosthesis. The intensity of the opening and closing clicks and the character of associated murmurs depend on the type of prosthetic

valve, heart rate, rhythm, and the underlying hemodynamic status (4).

NONINVASIVE EVALUATION OF PROSTHETIC VALVE FUNCTION

Listed in Table 9.2 are the various noninvasive parameters that can be employed in evaluating patients with suspected prosthetic valve malfunction.

Phonocardiography

Central Occluder Ball Valves

With regard to the ball valves, the typical Starr-Edwards valve has clearly audible opening and closing sounds. The normal amplitude ratio of the aortic opening to closing sound by phonocardiography is usually greater than 0.5 (Table 9.3) (5). A reduction in this ratio may suggest prosthetic valve malfunction. Low cardiac output and premature ventricular contractions may result in decreased intensity of the aortic prosthetic clicks. A grade II/VI early crescendo-decrescendo systolic murmur that radiates into the carotid vessels is usually present as a result of turbulence, minimal transvalvular gradient, or both. In the aortic position, multiple systolic clicks have been recorded in association with a bouncing poppet (6). An early diastolic murmur is generally regarded as abnormal

Table 9.1. Commonly Used Prosthetic Valves

Mechanical valves
    Central ball occluder
        Starr-Edwards
        Smeloff-Cutter
        Braunwald-Cutter
        Magovern-Cromie
        Harken
        DeBakey-Surgitool
        Hufnagel
    Central disc occluder
        Beall-Surgitool
        Cooley-Cutter
        Kay-Shiley
        Kay-Suzuki
        Cross-Jones
    Eccentric monocuspid disc
        Bjork-Shiley
        Lillehei-Kaster
        Medtronic-Hall
        Wada-Cutter
    Bileaflet prosthesis
        St. Jude
Tissue valves or bioprosthesis
    Hancock
    Carpentier-Edwards
    Ionescu-Shiley

Reprinted with permission from Kotler MN, Mintz GS, Panidis I, et al. Non-invasive evaluation of normal and abnormal prosthetic valve function. J Am Coll Cardiol 1983;2:151–73.

and may be indicative of paravalvular leak or abnormal seating of the ball. In the mitral position, both the opening and closing clicks are well recorded. A prominent opening click usually follows the aortic component of the second heart sound (A_2) by 0.6 to 1.3 seconds (Fig. 9.1).

Disc Valves

Disc valves can be generally classified into the central occluder type, of which the Beall-Surgitool is a prototype, or the eccentric monocuspid valve, of which the Bjork-Shiley is the most commonly implanted valve. The central occluder valves produce loud opening and closing clicks in the mitral position; a prominent closing sound is best heard at the apex (Fig. 9.2). Occasionally, a systolic ejection murmur may be audible as a result of turbulence around the prosthetic valve, which in turn is a result of projection into the outflow tract. In most instances, a diastolic murmur is not recorded. However, when there is tissue valve mismatch or when a larger prosthesis for the mitral annular size is implanted, a diastolic murmur may occur. Central oc-

Table 9.2. Noninvasive Evaluation of Prosthetic Valve Function

Phonocardiography
Spectral analysis
M-mode echocardiography
Two-dimensional echocardiography
Doppler ultrasound
Cinefluoroscopy

Table 9.3. Phonocardiographic Time Intervals

Measurement	Normal Range (s)	Clinical Implications
A_2–MVO	0.06–0.12	Shortened A_2 to MVO indicates mitral obstruction, severe mitral regurgitation, and rarely LV dysfunction. Prolonged A_2 to MVO may indicate sticking valve as with tissue ingrowth or LV dysfunction
A_2–TVO	0.08–0.13	Same as for MV
Q–MI*	0.055–0.09	Markedly prolonged interval indicates high LA pressure and obstruction
S_1–AVO*	0.07–0.09	Markedly prolonged interval indicates *obstruction*
Ratio of AO/AC (Starr-Edwards valve only)	>0.50	<0.50 indicates variance

*Usually of minimal value.
AC = aortic closure click; AO = aortic opening click; AVO = aortic valve opening; A_2 = aortic component of the second heart sound; MVO = mitral valve opening; M_1 = mitral component of the first heart sound; Q = Q wave on ECG; S_1 = first heart sound; TVO = tricuspid valve opening.
Reprinted with permission from Kotler MN, Mintz GS, Panidis I, et al. Non-invasive evaluation of normal and abnormal prosthetic valve function. J Am Coll Cardiol 1983;2:151–73.

cluder discs are not generally inserted in the aortic position.

With regard to the eccentric monocuspid disc valves in the aortic position, a distinct closing sound is produced, and a soft ejection-type systolic murmur is audible. The murmur occurs as a result of turbulence of flow across the unequal orifices. A faint diastolic murmur suggesting minimal aortic regurgitation may be audible in some patients with Bjork-Shiley valves. A mild degree of aortic regurgitation has been documented at the time of cardiac catheterization in patients with aortic Bjork-Shiley valves (7). In the mitral position, a faint opening sound may be produced but generally is not audible; however, a loud closing sound is produced (Fig. 9.3).

The Medtronic-Hall (previously known as the Hall-Kaster) valve is a rod-guided tilting disc valve prosthesis with favorable hemodynamic properties and a low incidence of thrombosis and embolism (8). It has gained popularity in the United States (9, 10) since its introduction in clinical practice in the late 1970s in Norway.

Both opening and closing clicks of the valve can be recorded in the aortic and mitral positions. More than one (generally two to three) opening clicks and two closing clicks are recorded, the latter occurring simultaneously with the onset and completion of valve closure. In the aortic position, an early systolic murmur

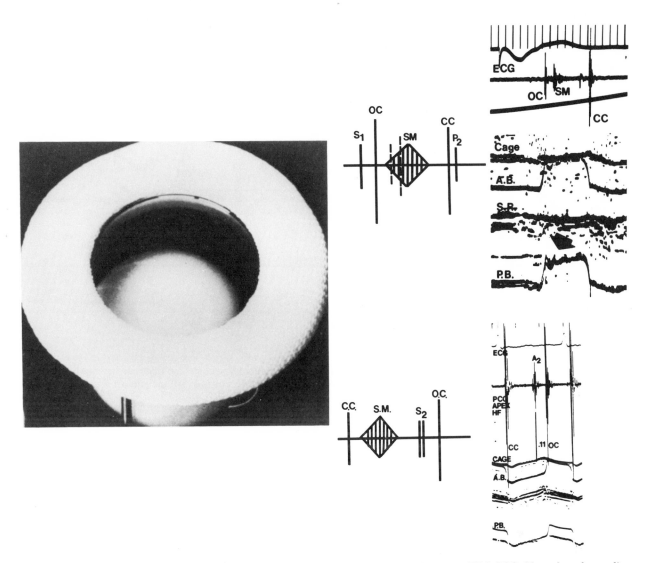

Figure 9.1. Model 6120 Starr-Edwards MV. Phonocardiograms (PCG) and simultaneous ECG PCG. M-mode echocardiograms of the aortic prosthesis (above), and the mitral prosthesis (below). Schematic diagrams of the PCGs. A loud opening click (OC) is produced when the aortic prosthesis poppet moves anteriorly and makes contact with the cage. During systole, bouncing motion of the poppet occurs with opening and reclosing motion. This is especially apparent in the posterior poppet (wide arrow in upper echocardiogram). With closure of the aortic valve, a closure sound (CC) is produced. A short ejection systolic murmur (SM) is recorded. In the mitral position (below), the A_2 to MV opening interval measures 0.11 second. A crisp OC occurs with opening of the poppet against the cage and similarly a CC with closure of the poppet. Because of the apparent discrepancy between the transmission of sound through Silastic, the posterior surface of the ball is recorded posterior to the suture ring. A.B. = anterior ball of poppet; HF = high frequency; P_2 = pulmonary component of the second heart sound; P.B. = posterior ball of poppet; S_1 = first heart sound; S_2 = second heart sound; S.R. = suture ring. (Reproduced by permission from Kotler MN, Mintz GS, Panidis I, et al. Non-invasive evaluation of normal and abnormal prosthetic valve function. J Am Coll Cardiol 1983;2:151–73.)

is audible, and in rare instances, a faint diastolic murmur may be audible (11). In the mitral position, both opening and closing clicks are recorded but the closure sound is generally louder. Rarely is a diastolic murmur recorded.

The Bileaflet St. Jude Cardiac Valve Prosthesis

The auscultatory findings of the bileaflet St. Jude prosthesis are similar to those produced by the monocuspid

valve (12, 13). In the aortic position, an opening sound is not generally audible, although occasionally a soft click can be recorded. A prominent high-pitched metallic sound is audible and coincides with valve closure (Fig. 9.4). A short midsystolic crescendo-decrescendo grade II/VI systolic murmur is often audible at the right second intercostal space. The murmur radiates into the neck and results from turbulence of flow across the valve. An aortic diastolic murmur is distinctly abnormal even though a minimal, clinically insignificant

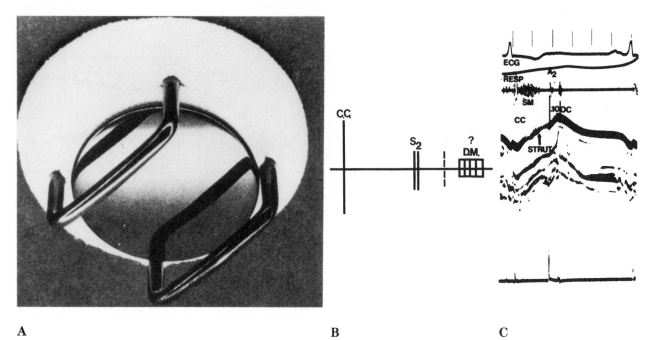

A   **B**   **C**

Figure 9.2. (*A*) Beall-Surgitool 106 pyrolite disc valve with pyrolite struts. (*B*) Schematic diagram of phonocardiogram. (*C*) Combined echophonocardiogram. A distinct opening click sound (OC) is recorded 0.10 second after the aortic component (A$_2$) of the second heart sound (S$_2$). As the pyrolite disc opens, it produces a loud opening sound as the disc abuts the struts. During diastole, the leaflet is in close proximity to the anterior stent. With the onset of systole, a loud closure sound (CC) is produced. A diastolic murmur (D.M.) may be recorded, but it usually represents valve mismatch or tissue ingrowth. The crescendo-decrescendo systolic murmur (SM) recorded in this patient was related to thickening of the aortic valve. RESP = respirations. (Reproduced by permission from Kotler MN, Mintz GS, Panidis I, et al. Non-invasive evaluation of normal and abnormal prosthetic valve function. J Am Coll Cardiol 1983;2:151–73.)

amount of aortic regurgitation can occur as a result of incomplete valve seating (14, 15). In patients with a mitral St. Jude cardiac valve prosthesis, a middiastolic rumble has been recorded and may represent turbulence of flow due to three separate orifices in diastole (12). An opening click is not usually audible although it may be occasionally recorded by phonocardiography.

Bioprosthetic Valves

Bioprosthetic valves usually have auscultatory sounds that are indistinguishable from those of normal valves (Fig. 9.5). In the aortic position, the closure sound is clearly heard in the second right and left intercostal spaces although an opening sound is not audible. A high-frequency grade II/VI early to midsystolic murmur is located in the left sternal border. A diastolic murmur is not heard and, if present, should be considered abnormal in the aortic position. In the mitral position, an opening snap may be detected by auscultation (4). In approximately one-half of patients, a sound occurs 0.07 to 0.11 second after the second heart sound and is usually best auscultated at the apex. In one-half to two-thirds of patients, an apical diastolic murmur has been recorded (16, 17). The diastolic murmur may be

related to turbulence of flow or to a valve gradient caused by small orifice, protruding stents, or a flexible resonating stent. An apical or left sternal midsystolic murmur grade II/VI has been recorded in one-half to two-thirds of patients (18). A systolic murmur will increase following the administration of amyl nitrite, suggesting that the murmur is related to turbulence as a result of the stents projecting into the left ventricular (LV) outflow tract. The mitral closing sound may be indistinguishable from the normal component of the first heart sound.

Spectral Analysis

Spectral analysis evaluates sound emission by monitoring sound frequency and intensity (19). The function of prosthetic valves can be evaluated by determining the frequency profile of the opening and closing clicks for each type of prosthetic valve. A normally functioning prosthesis will produce opening and closing sounds at specific frequencies (the cut-off frequencies) depending on the individual characteristics of that particular valve. Prosthetic valve dysfunction due to thrombus formation or tissue ingrowth will be manifested by a

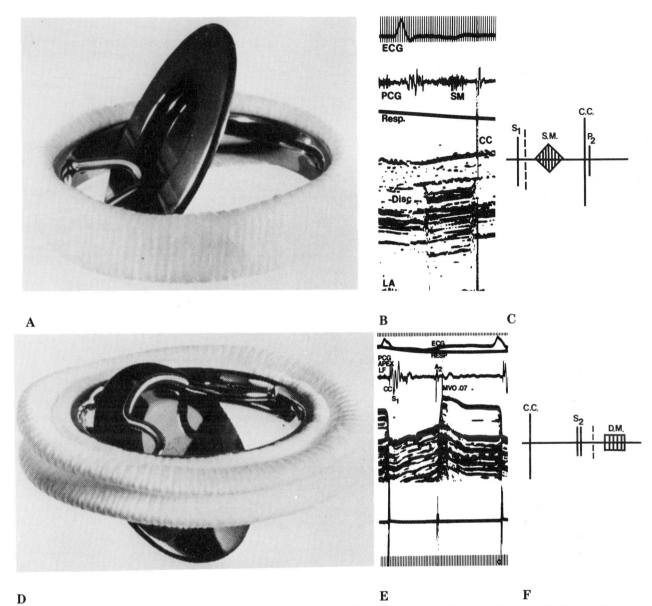

A **B** **C**

D **E** **F**

Figure 9.3. (*A*) Bjork-Shiley aortic valve in the open position. (*B*) Combined echophonocardiogram. (*C*) Schematic representation of the phonocardiographic (PCG) findings. In the aortic position, the disc opens to about 60 degrees from the horizontal plane of the valve, with a minor orifice to the left and a major orifice to the right. A crescendo-decrescendo systolic murmur (SM) is generally recorded as a result of turbulence of flow, and a loud closure sound (CC) is produced as the valve seats itself. Usually, no opening click is recorded in the aortic position. Multiple echoes emanate from the disc and reverberate behind the aortic root into the LA. (*D*) A Bjork-Shiley MV in the open position. (*E*) Combined echophonocardiogram. (*F*) Schematic diagram of low-frequency (LF) PCG. In the mitral position, the valve opens to approximately 50 degrees from the horizontal plane of the valve, and an opening sound is not produced. Therefore, the A_2 to MV opening (MVO) interval has to be measured by simultaneous echophonocardiogram. In this example, the A_2 to MVO interval measures 0.07 second. With the onset of diastole, there is a brisk opening movement, a sharp E point and then a prolonged EF slope. With the onset of systole, the valve closes abruptly and produces a loud CC. A diastolic murmur (D.M.) may be recorded as a result of valve mismatch or obstruction due to tissue ingrowth or clot. P_2 = pulmonary component of second heart sound; Resp. = respiration; S_1 = first heart sound; S_2 = second heart sound. (Reproduced by permission from Kotler MN, Mintz GS, Panidis I, et al. Non-invasive evaluation of normal and abnormal prosthetic valve function. J Am Coll Cardiol 1983;2:151–73.)

lower cut-off frequency than expected for that particular valve. The instrumentation consists of a combination of a filter system and a system for indicating the relative energy that passes through the filter system.

Frequency profiles have been established for normally functioning Starr-Edwards valves and Bjork-Shiley valves. For example, in the aortic Starr-Edwards prosthetic valve, the cut-off frequency is greater than 2000

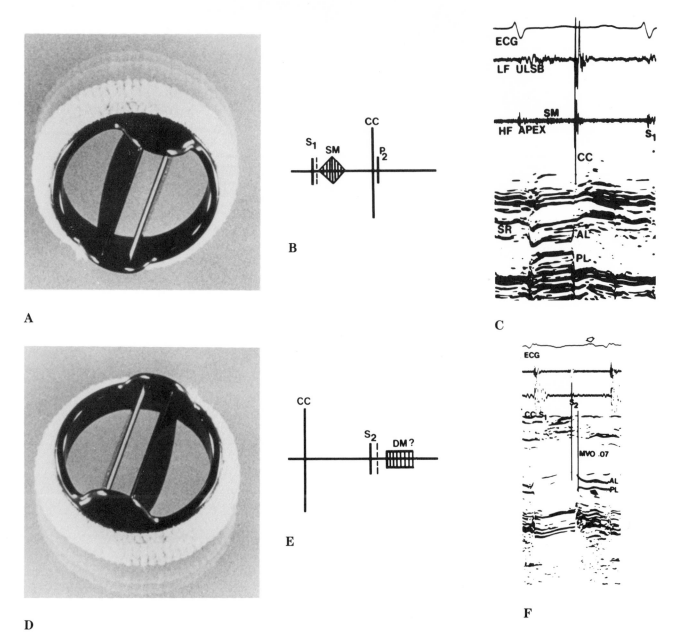

Figure 9.4. (*A*) A St. Jude aortic valve in the open position. (*B*) Schematic phonocardiogram. (*C*) Combined echophono-cardiogram. In the aortic position, a soft crescendo-decrescendo systolic murmur (SM) is recorded. Generally, an opening click is not recorded, and a loud closing click (CC) is recorded coinciding with closure movement of the valve. When the valve is fully closed, the leaflets abut against the suture ring. When they are open, the anterior leaflet (AL) moves posteri-orly and the posterior leaflet (PL) moves anteriorly with some separation between the two leaflets. (*D*) A St. Jude MV in the open position. (*E*) Schematic phonocardiogram. (*F*) Combined echophonocardiogram. In the mitral position, an opening click is not produced, and a diastolic murmur (DM) may be audible as a result of flow through three orifices or valve tissue mismatch. Because the opening click is not always recorded, the A$_2$ to MV opening (MVO) interval has to be measured with simultaneous echophonocardiography. The valve moves from a closed position during systole to an open position with the AL moving posteriorly and the PL moving anteriorly (*small arrow*) separated by a space. A CC is generally recorded as the valve closes in late systole. HF = high frequency; LF = low frequency; P$_2$ = pulmonary component of the second heart sound; S$_1$ = first heart sound; S$_2$ = second heart sound; SR = suture ring; ULSB = upper left sternal border. (Reproduced by permission from Kotler MN, Mintz GS, Panidis I, et al. Non-invasive evaluation of normal and abnormal prosthetic valve function. J Am Coll Cardiol 1983; 2:151–73.)

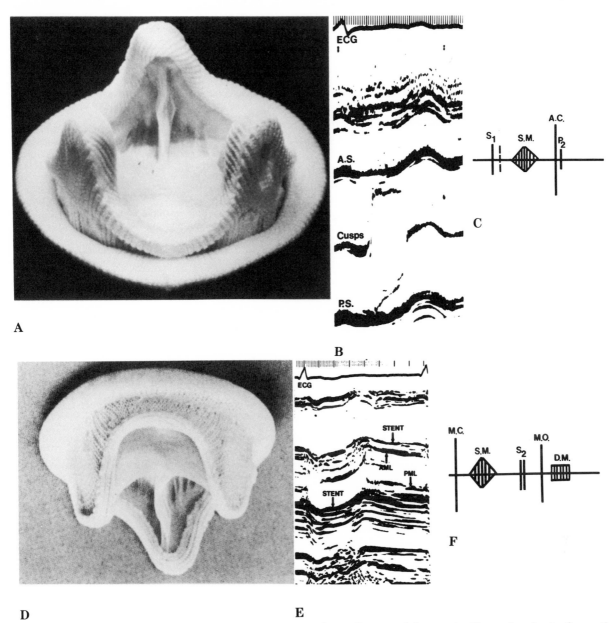

Figure 9.5.   (*A*) Aortic porcine Hancock valve. (*B*) M-mode echocardiogram of the porcine Hancock valve in the aortic position. (*C*) Schematic phonocardiogram of the aortic porcine bioprosthesis. M-mode echocardiogram (*B*) shows the leaflets open in a box-like structure during systole. The anterior and posterior stents (A.S. and P.S.) are clearly recorded. With aortic valve closure, a loud aortic closure sound (A.C.) is produced that is indistinguishable from a normally occurring aortic sound. A systolic murmur (S.M.) is generally recorded, which represents turbulence of flow due to the resting pressure gradient or results from turbulence due to the stents protruding into the aorta (*C*). (*D*) Mitral porcine Hancock valve. In the mitral position, a mitral opening snap (M.O.) occurs coinciding with maximal motion of the leaflets during diastole (*F*). M-mode echocardiogram demonstrates the leaflets remaining in an open position throughout diastole and oppose each other during systole (*E*). Systolic and diastolic (D.M.) murmurs can be recorded (*F*). AML = anterior mitral leaflet; M.C. = mitral closure; P_2 = pulmonary component of the second heart sound; PML = posterior mitral leaflet; S_1 = first heart sound; S_2 = second heart sound.

hertz for the opening and closing clicks, and a cut-off frequency less than 500 Hz is considered abnormal. However, it should be noted that there is a large gray area in which cut-off frequencies between 500 and 2000 Hz are borderline and may sometimes be considered normal and at other times abnormal. Newer techniques

such as the Fourier transform method of spectral analysis and the maximal entropy method, which employ expensive, complex instrumentation, are now available (20–22). Both systems consist of a combination of a filter and a recorder for indicating the relative energy that has passed through the filter system. A transducer preamplifier, octave band analyzer with output in decibels, oscilloscope, and ECG constitute the system. With regard to porcine valves, several investigators have shown that high-resolution spectral analysis of aortic porcine closing sounds will facilitate the diagnosis of intrinsic valve dysfunction caused by leaflet degeneration or infection (21, 22). The Fourier transform method of spectral analysis may be less accurate than the maximal entropy method. In the former system, the frequency resolution is directly proportional to the duration of the signal; but the technique may be limited because aortic porcine valve closing sounds are only 15 to 25 milliseconds in duration. The maximal entropy method is not limited in resolution and therefore may be more accurate for analysis of signals of short duration such as aortic heterograft closure sounds (22). Because of the availability of more accurate and less expensive techniques such as Doppler echocardiography, it is doubtful that these complex methods of sound analysis will become viable or commonly used.

Echocardiography

Several reviews (2, 3) have addressed the question of technique in performing M-mode and two-dimensional echocardiography in patients with prosthetic valves; this is not reviewed in this discussion. When using echocardiography to evaluate patients for suspected

Table 9.4. Echocardiographic Evaluation of Mechanical Valve Prostheses

Initial two-dimensional echocardiographic evaluation
  Overall usefulness in evaluation of LV, LA, right atrial, and right ventricular chamber size
  Determination of LV and right ventricular function
  Exclusion of *large* LA thrombi, large clots, or vegetations attached to prosthetic poppet or disc
  Determination of the precise alignment of the prosthetic valve
    Optimal M-mode cursor evaluation of individual disc or poppet excursion can be accomplished by directing the beam as nearly perpendicular as possible to the plane of motion of the disc or ball
  Evaluation of other valvular abnormalities and exclusion of pericardial effusion
M-mode evaluation of mechanical valve prosthesis
  Prosthetic valve description
    Poppet or disc excursion
    Poppet or disc opening and closing velocities
    Appearance and motion of struts, suture ring, and poppet or disc
  Cardiac chamber evaluation
    LV
      Cavity dimension
      % Fractional shortening
    Ventricular septum
      Paradoxic
      Normal or hyperdynamic
      Diastolic fluttering of IVS
    Outflow tract
      Size
      Presence of extraneous prosthetic echoes
    LA
      Cavity size
      Presence of extraneous prosthetic echoes
      Emptying index
  MV motion and appearance
    Diastolic fluttering
    Premature closure

Table 9.5. Echophonocardiographic Findings of Normal Prosthetic Valves

| Type of Valve | Position | Phonocardiography | | | | Echocardiography |
		OC	CC	SM	DM	
Central ball occluder: Starr-Edwards	Aortic	+	+	+	−	Anterior-posterior poppet with suture ring between (Silastic poppet)
	Mitral	+	+	+	−	
	Tricuspid	+	+	±	−	
Central disc occluder: Beall-Surgitool	Mitral	+	+	−	− or ±	Disc excursion with rapid opening and closing motion. Anterior cage and suture ring recorded
	Tricuspid	+	+	−	− or ±	
Eccentric monocuspid disc: Bjork-Shiley	Aortic	±	+	+	+	Multiple echoes in aortic root and LA
	Mitral	±	+	−	±	Brisk opening and closure motion. Initial sharp E point
Bileaflet prosthesis: St Jude	Aortic	±	+	+	−	Two leafletws separated by a space during opening motion
	Mitral	±	+	−	±	Same as aortic
	Tricuspid	±	+	−	±	Same as aortic
Bioprosthesis (or tissue valve): Hancock	Aortic	±	+	+	−	Leaflets open during systole as boxlike tissue
	Pulmonary	±	+	+	−	
	Mitral	+	+	+	+	Leaflets open as boxlike structure in diastole. Anterior and posterior stents recorded
	Tricuspid	?	+	?	?	

CC = closure click; DM = diastolic murmur; OC = opening click or sound; SM = systolic murmur; + = usually present; ± = may be present; − = absent; ? = unknown.
Reprinted with permission from Kotler MN, Mintz GS, Panidis I, et al. Non-invasive evaluation of normal and abnormal prosthetic valve function. J Am Coll Cardiol 1983;2:151–73.

prosthetic valve malfunction, an initial two-dimensional echocardiographic study should be performed to assess the overall chamber size and LV function (Table 9.4). In addition, determination of precise alignment of the prosthetic valve can be accomplished by directing the M-mode cursor as perpendicularly as possible to the plane of motion of the disc or ball. By combining phonocardiography with M-mode echocardiography, valve motion and its relation to opening and closing sounds can be recorded (Table 9.5). A very valuable interval is the A_2 to mitral valve (MV) opening interval. This interval can be recorded in patients where the opening click is not heard well and the interval from the aortic valve closure sound to maximal opening of the mitral prosthesis recorded by echocardiography can be measured. Dual, simultaneous echocardiography of the aortic valves and MVs can also be used to evaluate this interval. This is particularly relevant with the eccentric monocuspid valves and the St. Jude bileaflet prosthesis. The normal A_2 to MV opening interval measures between 0.06 to 0.12 second (23). A shortened A_2 to MV opening interval indicates mitral obstruction or severe regurgitation; it may also occur in the presence of LV dysfunction. A prolonged A_2 to MV opening interval may indicate a sticking valve as a result of tissue ingrowth or LV dysfunction.

The echocardiographic features of the Starr-Edwards valve consist of motion of the anterior and posterior surface of the poppet or ball as well as motion of the suture ring (Fig. 9.1). Because of the discrepancy between the transmission of sound

through Silastic and soft tissue, the posterior surface of the ball is recorded posterior to the suture ring (24).

With the central occluder disc valve, the Beall-Surgitool mitral prosthetic disc opens briskly in diastole, making contact with the struts, and closes promptly at the start of systole (Fig. 9.2). Two series of Beall-Surgitool valves have been commonly used: models 103 and 104, which have Teflon discs, and models 105 and 106, which have pyrolite carbon discs. The sewing ring and band are covered with a Dacron velour fabric. The approximation of the disc to the cage can also be recognized by echocardiography.

The motion of the Bjork-Shiley disc can be recorded by M-mode echocardiography (25). In patients with a Bjork-Shiley MV, the A_2 to MV opening interval can be measured with a simultaneous phonocardiogram and echocardiogram or with dual simultaneous echocardiograms. In the mitral position, the valve opens to approximately 50 degrees from the horizontal plane of the valve (Fig. 9.3). An opening sound is generally not produced. The A_2 to MV opening is generally shorter than with other prosthetic valves, measuring 0.05 to 0.09 second, and is similar to intervals recorded with other eccentric monocuspid valves (26). With the onset of diastole, there is a brisk opening movement and a sharp E point followed by prolonged EF slope (Fig. 9.3). With the onset of systole, the disc will close abruptly and produce a loud closure sound. A diastolic murmur may be recorded as a result of valve mismatch (4) or obstruction due to tissue ingrowth or clot. The

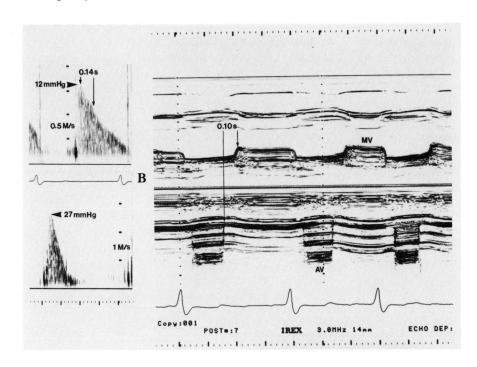

A   **C**

Figure 9.6. (*A*) Dual, simultaneous echocardiographic recording in the mitral Medtronic-Hall valve (top) and aortic Medtronic-Hall valve (bottom). The aortic valve (AV) closure–MV opening interval is normal and measures 0.10 second. Normal MV flow pattern is recorded by Doppler echocardiography (*B*) and normal AV flow pattern (*C*) is demonstrated. The peak gradient across the MV is 12 mm Hg, and the peak gradient across the AV is 27 mm Hg; both values are in the normal range for the Medtronic-Hall valve.

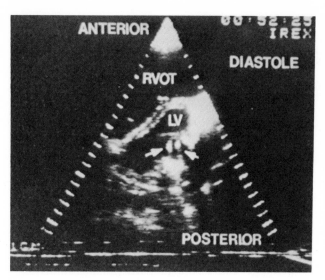

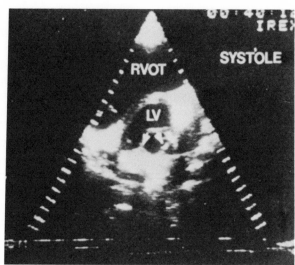

A   **B**

Figure 9.7. Two-dimensional echocardiograms of a patient with a normally functioning St. Jude MV prosthesis. Parasternal short-axis views obtained during diastole (*A*) and systole (*B*). In the open position during diastole, the two leaflets parallel each other (*white arrows*); during systole, the two leaflets are in a closed position producing a V-shaped configuration (*white arrows*). RVOT = right ventricular outflow tract.

motion of the Medtronic-Hall valve is similar to that of the Bjork-Shiley valve (Fig. 9.6).

In patients with St. Jude aortic prostheses, leaflet motion may be recorded by M-mode echocardiography (12, 27, 28). The motion of the leaflets is exactly opposite to the motion of other prosthetic valves (29). In the aortic position, two leaflets may be visualized within the aortic root. During systole, a separation of the anterior and posterior leaflets is present (Fig. 9.4). In the mitral position, the valve opens in diastole with clear separation of the anterior and posterior leaflets (Fig. 9.4) (12). During systole, the valve seats itself against the suture ring, and the leaflets are difficult to separate from the suture ring. The motion of the leaflets during the opening of the valve with the two leaflets opposing each other and an echo-free space separating them was seen in 85 percent of patients with a St. Jude valve in the mitral position and in only 24 percent in the aortic position (Fig. 9.4) (27). Because of reverberation artifacts, the echoes frequently appear within the left atrium (LA). These reverberating echoes also occur in patients with other eccentric aortic monocuspid valves. In a study of 126 patients with St. Jude valve prostheses studied by echophonocardiography, the aortic closure (A_2) to St. Jude MV opening interval measured 0.08 ± 0.02 second in patients with normal St. Jude MVs (27). Other investigators have reported slightly longer (0.10 ± 0.02 second) intervals (29). The tissue annulus diameter is smaller with the St. Jude MV prosthesis than with any other prosthetic valve of similar size.

Two-dimensional echocardiography can sometimes provide direct visualization of the leaflet motion, espe-

cially if the leaflets open in a direction that is perpendicular to the echocardiographic plane of the long axis of the LV (Fig. 9.7) (29, 30). On occasion, there is asynchronous early diastolic closure of the posterior leaflet, which has been observed in patients with atrial fibrillation and long cycle lengths (12, 29).

Echocardiography of the bioprosthetic valves generally demonstrates two strong, distinct parallel bands of echoes from the far and near portions of the circular stent. Within these bands of echoes, individual motion of the aortic leaflets or mitral leaflets can be observed (Fig. 9.5) (31). The outer surface of the anterior band of echoes to the outer surface of the posterior band of echoes corresponds to the actual diameter of the stent. The stent moves anteriorly during systole and posteriorly during diastole. In the aortic position, the leaflet motion occurs during systole, with merging of the leaflets during diastole. In the mitral position, the opening motion of the leaflets occurs during diastole, with merging of the leaflets together at the onset of systole. Individual leaflet motion and valve alignment may be better recognized with two-dimensional echocardiography (32, 33). Several investigators have been able to differentiate valvular problems from LV dysfunction (Fig. 9.8) (34–36). Other parameters of bioprosthetic valve function that can be assessed by echocardiography are outlined in Table 9.6.

Cinefluoroscopy

Two excellent reviews (37, 38) have addressed the question of radiographic identification of prosthetic

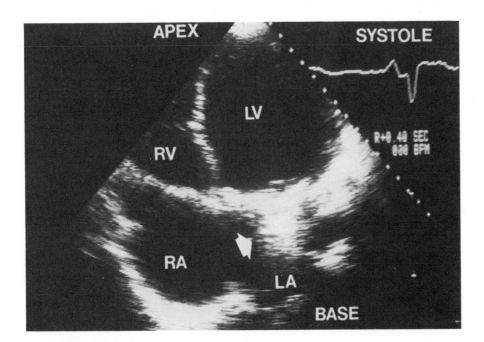

A

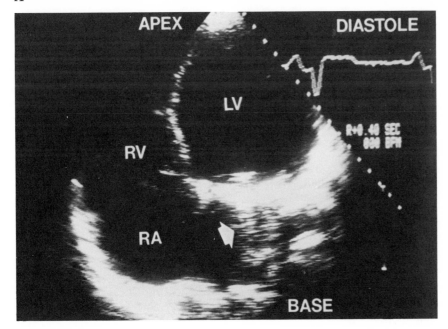

B

Figure 9.8. Apical four-chamber two-dimensional echocardiograms during systole and diastole in a patient with metallic valve prosthesis and severe LV dysfunction. Side-lobe echoes extend from the base of the suture ring laterally and medially. In addition, dense reverberating echoes (*arrows*) from the disc itself are seen in the LA, obscuring the clearly defined motion of the disc and causing confusion with intraatrial masses. The LV is dilated and globular with little reduction in LV cavity size from diastole to systole. RA = right atrium, RV = right ventricle.

heart valves, but the subject is beyond the scope of this chapter. We have found cinefluoroscopy to be particularly useful in evaluating metallic valves, especially the central occluder disc valves. The cinefluoroscopic findings of normally functioning prosthetic valves are shown in Fig. 9.9. The findings, with the degree of normal tilting angle, are listed in Table 9.7 (39–41). Cinefluoroscopy is extremely valuable in diagnosing suspected prosthetic valve dysfunction (42). Bioprosthetic valves that have limited radiopacity are difficult to visualize by cinefluoroscopy. In the case of the St.

Table 9.6. Echocardiography in Evaluation of Bioprosthetic Valves

1. Valve alignment and ring and individual leaflet motion best accomplished by two-dimensional echocardiography
2. Differentiation of valvular from ventricular dysfunction
3. Detection of dehiscence or paravalvular leak
4. Detection of degeneration and calcification
5. Detection of vegetations
6. Detection of thrombotic occlusion
7. Detection of encroachment of LV outflow tract by insertion of too large a prosthesis

Modified from Usher BW. Echocardiographic assessment of patients with bioprosthetic valves. Echocardiography 1984;1:311–32.

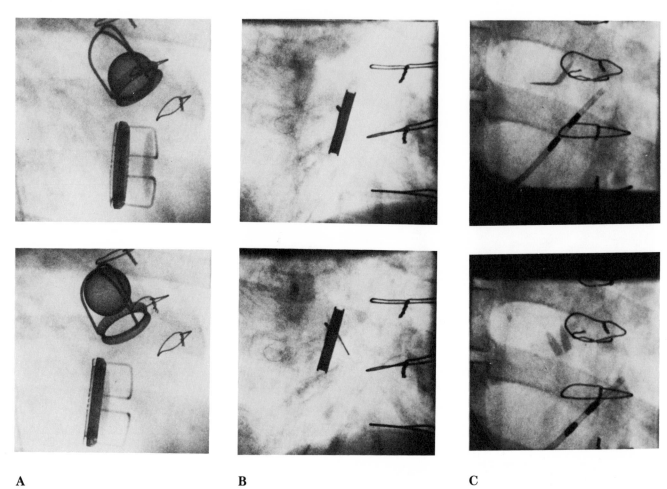

A   **B**   **C**

Figure 9.9. Cinefluoroscopic findings with some of the more commonly used prosthetic valves. (*A*) Upper part shows a Starr-Edwards aortic valve in the closed position during diastole, with a Beall MV in the open position. Lower part shows the aortic Starr-Edwards poppet in the open position during systole and the disc of the Beall valve in the closed position. (*B*) Upper part shows a Bjork-Shiley valve in the mitral position during systole with no apparent disc seen. Lower part shows the disc opening to about 50 degrees from the horizontal baseline during diastole. (*C*) A St. Jude valve in the aortic position. Upper part is during diastole with the leaflets closed (V-shaped configuration), and lower part is with the two leaflets in the opened position during systole.

Jude cardiac valve prostheses, each leaflet is impregnated with tungsten (43). However, cinefluoroscopy cannot always detect individual leaflet motion throughout the phase of the cardiac cycle. A great degree of variability in the motion of the individual leaflets makes alignment of both leaflets tangential to the x-ray beam difficult. Mitral valve motion is moredifficult to evaluate by cinefluoroscopy than is aortic valve motion.

Doppler Echocardiography

Doppler echocardiography measures the direction and velocity of blood flow. Since Doppler techniques are highly reliable in assessing native valve regurgitation (44), the use of Doppler echocardiography to detect

Table 9.7. Cinefluoroscopy

Prosthesis Type	Position	Normal Tilting Angle (degrees)
Starr-Edwards	Mitral	12
Starr-Edwards	Aortic	6
Bjork-Shiley	Mitral	9
Bjork-Shiley	Aortic	10
St. Jude*	Mitral	Normal opening and closing angle of leaflets Opening motion of leaflets 85 Closing angle of leaflets 30–35
St. Jude*	Aortic	Opening motion of leaflets 85 Closing angle of leaflets 30–35
Bjork-Shiley	Mitral	Opening angle of 50 Closing angle of 0
Bjork-Shiley	Aortic	Opening angle of 60 Closing angle of 0

*Great variability in the position of the prosthetic valve in the heart makes alignment of both leaflets tangential to the x-ray beam difficult. Motion of the MV is more difficult to demonstrate by cinefluoroscopy than is aortic valve motion.

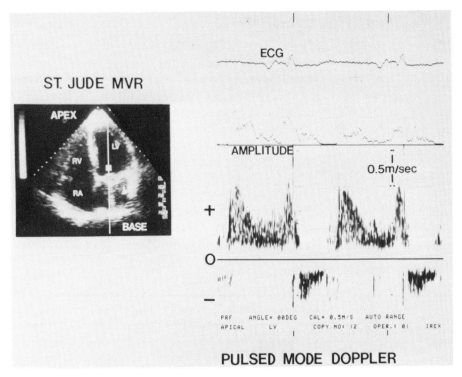

Figure 9.10. Two-dimensional four-chamber view echocardiogram obtained from the apical position and pulsed mode Doppler in a patient with a normally functioning No. 31 St. Jude MV. The sample volume is inferior to the mitral prosthesis (*white box*). The representative Doppler spectra of transmitral flow of the St. Jude prosthesis resemble normal biphasic flow pattern of a native MV. The peak velocity measures 1 m per second with a calculated peak gradient of 4 mm Hg. MVR = mitral valve replacement; RA = right atrium; RV = right ventricle.

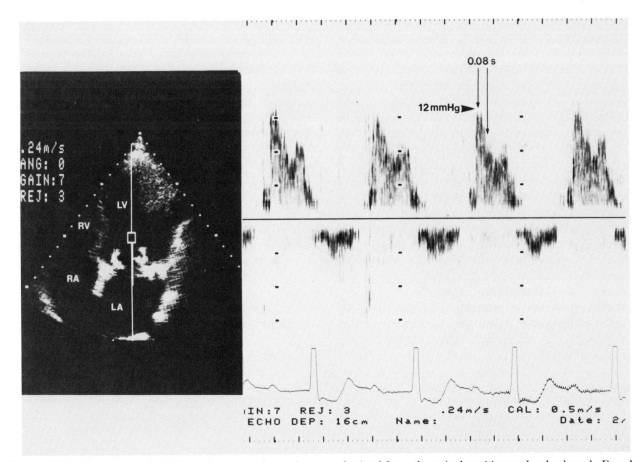

Figure 9.11. Two-dimensional four-chamber echocardiogram obtained from the apical position and pulsed mode Doppler in a patient with a normally functioning Ionescu-Shiley MV. The sample volume is just distal or inferior to the stents. Biphasic mitral flow is evident with a maximal diastolic gradient of 12 mm Hg recorded. The pressure half-time is normal and measures 0.08 second. Calculated MV orifice is 2.8 cm². RA = right atrium; RV = right ventricle.

Table 9.8. Doppler Echocardiography in the Evaluation of Prosthetic Valve Function

1. Provides hemodynamic information with regard to direction and velocity of blood flow through prosthetic valves. Note: Direction of interrogating beam should be as parallel as possible to direction of flow
2. Differentiates laminar from disturbed flow
3. Is useful for calculating pressure gradients across obstructed prosthetic valves
4. Detects regurgitation through or around prosthetic valves

Table 9.9. Limitations of Doppler Echocardiography in the Evaluation of Suspected Prosthetic Valve Malfunction

1. Most reported studies have included a relatively small number of patients
2. In assessing blood flow velocity in prosthetic valves, one should take into account the direction of blood flow since it may vary from valve to valve and may be quite complex
3. Velocity of blood flow through a prosthetic valve is influenced by the kind of prosthesis, its size, the position of implantation and the transvalvular volume flow. "Increased velocities" are not uncommon in "normal" prosthetic valves
4. Regurgitation may occur normally in some prosthetic valves

normal and abnormal prosthetic valve function has generated considerable interest. Several investigators have found Doppler echocardiography to be extremely useful in evaluating patients with suspected prosthetic valve malfunction (45–51). Most Doppler systems employ either pulsed or continuous wave (CW) modes, and newer systems offer both modes of operation. Doppler modular operations are integrated with two-dimensional scanning functions by means of time-sharing, with the Doppler sample indicated by a cursor on the two-dimensional image display (Figs. 9.10 and 9.11). Although the pulsed mode is accurate in defining the exact site of the sample volume, pressure gradients cannot be calculated when the peak velocity exceeds 2 m per second because of aliasing (45). In order to measure significant obstructive gradients, CW Doppler must be utilized, which allows maximal velocities in excess of 10 m per second to be measured. Doppler echocardiography (Table 9.8) provides hemodynamic information about the direction and velocity of blood flow and differentiates laminar from disturbed flow. It is useful in calculating pressure gradients across obstructed valves and particularly in detecting regurgitation through or around prosthetic valves. The Doppler ultrasound beam has to be as parallel as possible to the

direction of blood flow, in contrast to M-mode and two-dimensional echocardiography, which align the transducer in a direction that is perpendicular to leaflet motion to detect maximum valve opening excursions. Continuous wave Doppler has a greater application in measuring transvalvular gradients in central flow metallic prostheses and bioprosthetic valves than in the central occluder caged-ball prostheses.

In examination of the MV, transmitral velocity profiles can be examined by placing the transducer in the apical position (Figs. 9.10 and 9.11). Initial positioning of the sample volume can be obtained with a two-dimensional image. After the data are obtained by pulsed wave mode, one can switch to CW Doppler to measure the maximum velocity. After evaluation of LV inflow is completed, the LA can be examined to determine if there are any paravalvular leaks. With metallic prostheses, the closed disc or poppet will reflect back most or all of the sound when examined from the apex, and the left parasternal position provides a portal for interrogation of the LA. To examine the aortic valve by Doppler, the transducer is generally placed at the apical, left parasternal, suprasternal, or second right intercostal parasternal position. However, the apical and right parasternal positions may be the most useful. It is possible to track the sample volume through the LV outflow tract, the aortic valve, and the ascending aorta using the apical position. Once the LV outflow tract and aortic valve have been identified by pulsed techniques, CW Doppler can be then employed to obtain maximum transvalvular velocity. After aortic outflow is examined, the subvalvular region can be scrutinized for transvalvular and paravalvular leaks. Pulsed wave Doppler appears to be more useful in evaluating aortic prosthetic regurgitation than mitral prosthetic regurgitation. This is probably due to the fact that paravalvular regurgitation produces a localized regurgitant jet that is more widely dispersed in the LA than it is in the LV outflow tract.

Despite the initial enthusiastic reception of Doppler echocardiography, certain pitfalls and limitations can occur when assessing patients with suspected prosthetic valve malfunction (Table 9.9). Doppler velocity measurements may be particularly difficult with certain kinds of prostheses: Blood flow through various types

Table 9.10. Comparison of Velocities for St. Jude Valves and Native Valves

	Aortic				Mitral			
	No.	Maximal Velocity (m/s)	Mean Velocity (m/s)	TTP	No.	Maximal Velocity (m/s)	Mean Velocity (m/s)	TP 1/2 (m/s)
St. Jude valves	7	1.97 ± 0.52	1.23 ± 0.25	82.7 ± 16.5	13	1.38 ± 0.33	0.73 ± 0.16	61.2 ± 16.9
p value		0.001	0.1	0.02		0.001	0.001	NS
Native valves	10	1.22 ± 0.19	0.89 ± 0.14	63.2 ± 14.0	10	0.78 ± 0.20	0.35 ± 0.06	57.2 ± 13.2

TTP = time-to-peak velocity; TP 1/2 = pressure half-time; NS = not significant.
Reprinted with permission from Weinstein IR, Marbarger JP, Perez JE. Ultrasonic assessment of the St. Jude prosthetic valve, M-mode, two-dimensional and Doppler echocardiography. Circulation 1983;68:897–905.

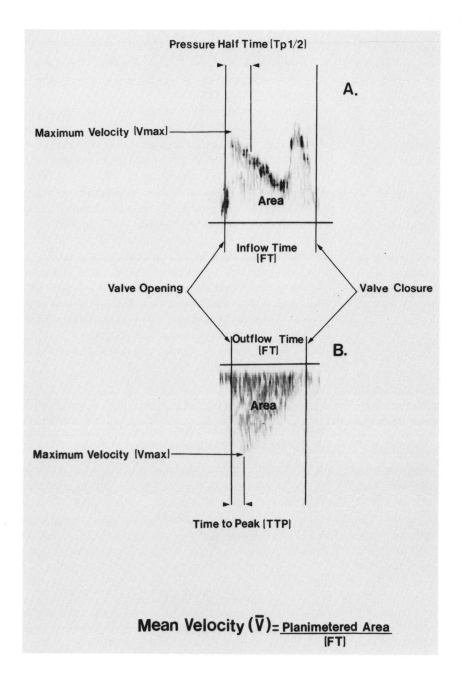

Mean Velocity (V̄)= Planimetered Area
$$\overline{}$$
(FT)

Figure 9.12. Typical Doppler flow velocity spectra of mitral valves (*A*) and aortic valves (*B*) showing the calculated and estimated parameters of flow. Mean velocity is calculated by planimetering the area of the velocity spectrum divided by either inflow or outflow time (FT). (Modified from Weinstein IR, Marbarger JP. Ultrasonic assessment of the St. Jude prosthetic valve: M-mode, two-dimensional and Doppler echocardiography. Circulation 1983;68:897–905.)

of prostheses is complex and multidirectional, and the actual direction of blood flow cannot be imaged in three-dimensional space so that Doppler intercept angles may be difficult to determine. The profile of flow velocities through a prosthesis is complex and varies with the size, position, and volume flow across the prosthesis (51). Thus, nonlaminar flow is frequently seen in patients with ball valve prostheses, where flow occurs at the sides of the cage in the open position, when the ball is at the apex of the cage. In addition, in patients with eccentric monocuspid valves, flow occurs through two orifices, namely, a major and a minor orifice. Flow velocity through the minor orifice may be greater than through the major orifice. Thus, abnormal velocity profiles can be obtained depending on the area

of sampling or interrogation. Increased velocities are not uncommon in prosthetic valves and depend on the position of implant, the transvalvular flow and gradient, and the size of the prosthesis. Therefore, patients with smaller prostheses may have increased velocities that may be normal for that particular valve.

PRESSURE GRADIENTS IN NORMAL PROSTHETIC VALVES

Doppler measurements of pressure gradients across native and prosthetic valves have been correlated with cardiac catheterization measurements (46, 52). Using the simplified Bernoulli equation, the pressure gradient across a valvular obstruction can be calculated by

Doppler echocardiography (45): pressure gradient = 4 × (maximum velocity)^2. In the mitral position, the St. Jude valve has relatively low peak and mean transvalvular velocities (1.38 ± 0.3 m/s and 0.73 ± 0.14 m/s) (47) compared to other prosthetic valves and is slightly higher than native valves (0.78 ± 0.1 m/s and 0.35 ± 0.06 m/s) (Table 9.10).

Mitral valve orifice for a prosthetic valve can be calculated by the pressure half-time technique (P$_{1/2}$) using the equation MV orifice (squared centimeters) = 220 ÷ P$_{1/2}$ (m/s) (Fig. 9.12) (45).

In the mitral position, all valves have similar peak velocities and pressure gradients, but the St. Jude valve has a significantly larger calculated orifice than other prosthetic valves. Holen et al. (46) studied 19 patients with Bjork-Shiley, Hancock, and Lillehei-Kaster mitral prostheses in the immediate postoperative period and found significant obstruction in some, with mean valve gradients ranging from 2 to 12.5 millimeters of mercury. Hatle and Angelsen found mean diastolic gradients generally ranging between 2 and 5 mm Hg with tilting disc valves (45). There is no apparent correlation between valve size and the Doppler-derived gradient (45). In a study of 106 aortic prostheses, Ramirez et al. (53) found a significant negative correlation between valve size and transvalvular flow velocity in several types of mechanical and bioprosthetic valves. These Doppler findings confirm the hemodynamic studies that have demonstrated lower transvalvular gradients and larger effective valve areas, especially in valves with larger annular sizes (54).

Aortic peak and mean Doppler flow velocities were slightly higher in St. Jude valves (1.97 ± 0.52 and 1.23 ± 0.25 m/s) than in the native valves (1.22 ± 0.19 and 0.89 ± 0.14 m/s) (Table 9.10) (47).

DIFFERENTIATION OF "PHYSIOLOGIC" AND PATHOLOGIC REGURGITATION

In the majority of normally functioning aortic and mitral St. Jude or Bjork-Shiley prosthetic valves, mild reflux of contrast medium subvalvularly has been demonstrated by aortography and left ventriculography (55–57). Regurgitation tends to be slightly more in patients with larger valves and tends to be transvalvular rather than paravalvular.

Aortic regurgitation can be detected in 15 percent of patients by auscultation and in 22 percent of patients with normally functioning aortic St. Jude valves by echocardiography (27).

Insignificant aortic regurgitation (detection of a regurgitant jet 2 cm or less into the LV outflow tract) has been reported in 62 percent of patients with metallic disc valves (45). Detection of a regurgitant jet greater than 2 cm into the LV cavity or the LA with maximal recorded velocities of 2 m per second or greater generally indicates significant aortic or mitral regurgitation respectively (45).

"Physiologic" regurgitation has been reported to be less common with Starr-Edwards and tissue prosthetic valves (58). However, regurgitation was reported in 43 percent of patients with bioprosthetic valves (59).

Like M-mode and two-dimensional echocardiography, Doppler techniques are dependent on ultrasound penetration. Thus, recordings of adequate Doppler signals are not always possible. In addition, most prosthetic valves lie at a considerable depth from the transducer and may reflect a substantial amount of sound energy from the proximal surfaces. Because Doppler measurements of flow velocity remain constant and have an excellent reproducibility (60), and because "physiologic" aortic or mitral regurgitation is frequently encountered, initial postoperative baseline Doppler studies are mandatory for serial evaluation of the individual patient.

EFFECT OF CARDIAC ARRHYTHMIAS AND CONDUCTION DISTURBANCES IN PROSTHETIC VALVE MOTION

Various rhythm and conduction disturbances can alter the characteristic echocardiographic motion of valves (Table 9.11) (61). The altered motion patterns may mimic some of the echocardiographic signs of malfunction in prosthetic valves. For example, first-degree atrioventricular (AV) block may produce premature

Table 9.11. Effect of Abnormal Heart Rhythm and Conduction on the Normal Echocardiographic Pattern of Prosthetic Mitral Valves

Normal sinus rhythm
  Late diastolic "bump"
First-degree AV block
  Premature diastolic closure
Atrial fibrillation
  Premature diastolic closure
  Intermittent closure and opening corresponding to coarse fibrillation waves
  Increased separation between ball and anterior cage
Atrial flutter, atrial tachycardia
  Diastolic closure induced by flutter or P waves
Complete heart block
  Diastolic closure and reopening induced by the atrial contraction (corresponding with the P waves)
Pacemakers
  Ventricular pacing: diastolic closure and reopening in the presence of underlying complete heart block
  Atrial or AV sequential pacing: premature diastolic closure in the presence of prolonged AV interval

Reprinted with permission from Kotler MN, Mintz GS, Panidis I, et al. Non-invasive evaluation of normal and abnormal prosthetic valve function. J Am Coll Cardiol 1983;2:151–73.

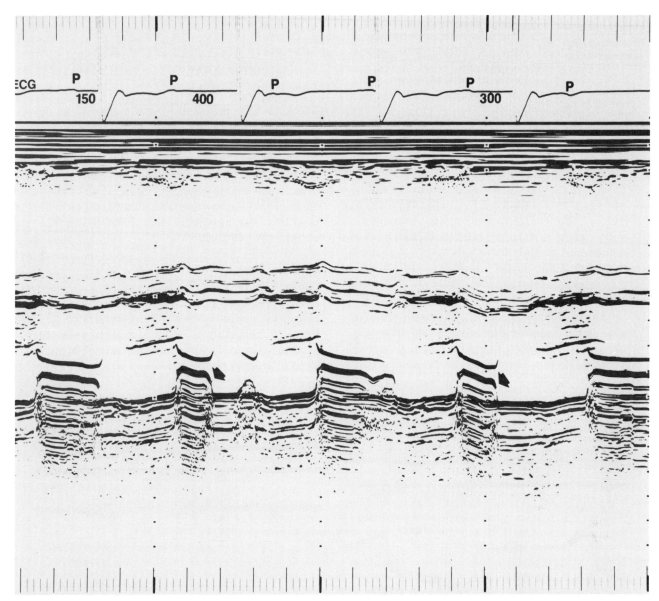

Figure 9.13. M-mode echocardiogram showing motion of a St. Jude MV in a patient with a ventricular pacemaker and AV dissociation. Middiastolic closure of both leaflets (*left wide arrow*) is seen with a PR interval of 400 ms. The valve re-opens slightly in late diastole just before ventricular contraction. With a PR interval of 300 ms, premature late diastolic closure of the valve is noted (*right wide arrow*). When the PR interval is normal (150 ms), no premature closure of the valve is seen. (Reproduced by permission from Kotler MN, Mintz GS, Panidis I, et al. Non-invasive evaluation of normal and abnormal prosthetic valve function. J Am Coll Cardiol 1983;2:151–73.)

Table 9.12. Causes of Malfunctioning Prosthetic Valves

Clot formation and fibrous tissue ingrowth
Paravalvular regurgitation
Variance
Dehiscence
Bacterial endocarditis
Mechanical malfunction
Primary valve failure (bioprosthetic valves)

Reprinted with permission from Kotler MN, Mintz GS, Panidis I, et al. Non-invasive evaluation of normal and abnormal prosthetic valve function. J Am Coll Cardiol 1983;2:151–73.

diastolic closure of the mitral valve due to the ventriculoatrial pressure gradient (62, 63). This should not be confused with significant aortic regurgitation, which produces elevation of end-diastolic pressure and resultant premature MV closure (64, 65). In addition, in patients with atrial fibrillation, complete heart block, or VVI pacemakers (Fig. 9.13), premature diastolic closure may also be present. In addition, reopening motion can occur following atrial contraction. The mechanism of

Table 9.13. Noninvasive Features of Malfunctioning Prosthetic Valves: Clot or Fibrin Tissue Formation

Echocardiography
   Echo-producing mass in the vicinity of the prosthetic valve with
      total absence of disc or ball motion
      False positive responses: reverberations, beam-width artifacts
      Alterations in motion: intermittent, incomplete, or delayed
         opening of the valve
      Short A_2–MVO interval (due to obstruction of flow)
      Early diastolic "bump" (rounding of the initial diastolic
         motion)
Cinefluoroscopy
   Impaired or decreased excursion of poppet or disc
Doppler echocardiography
   Increased maximal velocity of flow and significant valvular
      gradient, especially if changed from initial baseline study

this early closure is unknown but may be related to the development of a critical LV volume or pressure during the prolonged filling period, resulting in closure of the valve before the ventricular contraction (66). Other investigators have demonstrated the influence of gravity on the premature closure of prosthetic MVs (67). Because of premature closure of the MV in patients with atrial fibrillation and long cycle length, the closing click may be absent. The absent or intermittent clicks

should not be confused with prosthetic valve malfunction.

NONINVASIVE EVALUATION OF PROSTHETIC VALVE MALFUNCTION

The causes of prosthetic valve malfunction are presented in Table 9.12. In a patient with a prosthetic valve who presents with signs of thromboembolism, fibrous tissue ingrowth, bacterial endocarditis, and noncardiac causes could account for the event. Symptoms of left- or right-sided congestive heart failure can occur on the basis of prosthetic valve obstruction and paravalvular leak. However, in such individuals, LV dysfunction and constrictive pericarditis must be excluded. Hemolysis, jaundice, and anemia frequently occur as a result of a paravalvular leak. In that setting, with documented noninvasive findings of a paravalvular leak, especially if confirmed by Doppler echocardiography, appropriate measures should be instituted to correct the problem. Fever is frequently a manifestation of endocarditis. Although patients with metallic prosthetic heart valves have a 1 percent to 3 percent yearly incidence of

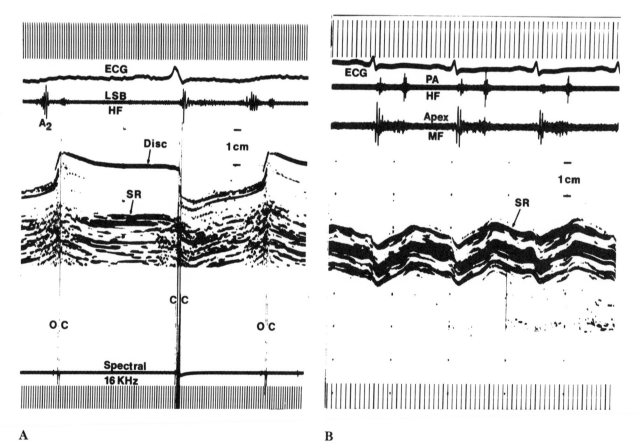

A   **B**

Figure 9.14. (*A*) Combined echophonocardiogram in a patient with a normal Bjork-Shiley MV prosthesis. Brisk opening and closing motion, sharp E point, and prolonged EF slope of the disc are apparent. (*B*) Combined echophonocardiogram in same patient now demonstrates abnormal Bjork-Shiley disc motion, with motion of the disc not going beyond the confines of the suture ring (SR). A systolic murmur is present indicative of mitral insufficiency. CC = closing click; HF = high frequency; LSB = left sternal border; MF = midfrequency; OC = opening click; PA = pulmonary artery.

endocarditis, detection by echocardiography is extremely difficult. However, in bioprosthetic valves, the incidence of detecting distinct vegetations may be similar to that seen in native valves. It is extremely difficult to detect vegetations in metallic prosthetic valves because of reverberation artifacts and side-lobe echoes arising from the suture ring. Frequently, the clinician must rely on the clinical as well as the laboratory documentation of positive blood cultures. However, in the presence of endocarditis, new documentation of paravalvular murmur or confirmation of paravalvular leak by Doppler should immediately arouse suspicion of root abscess and paravalvular leak. The complications of endocarditis such as an aortic root abscess and myocardial abscess can be occasionally detected by two-dimensional echocardiography (68, 69). In patients who present with decreased cardiac output in the immediate postoperative period,

differentiation of LV dysfunction, tamponade due to either pericardial bleeding or a localized hematoma, and prosthetic valve malfunction can readily be accomplished by two-dimensional echocardiography. In our experience, two-dimensional echocardiography has been extremely useful in the surgical intensive care unit regarding decision making in patients with suspected complications following prosthetic valve insertion.

Thrombus Formation: Noninvasive Features of Malfunctioning Prosthetic Valves Secondary to Clot or Fibrin Tissue Formation

Starr-Edwards Valve

The deposition of fibrin and thrombotic material may occur on any part of the prosthetic valve (Table 9.13). Thrombosis of the valve ring or cage strut can prevent complete opening or closing of the poppet, producing

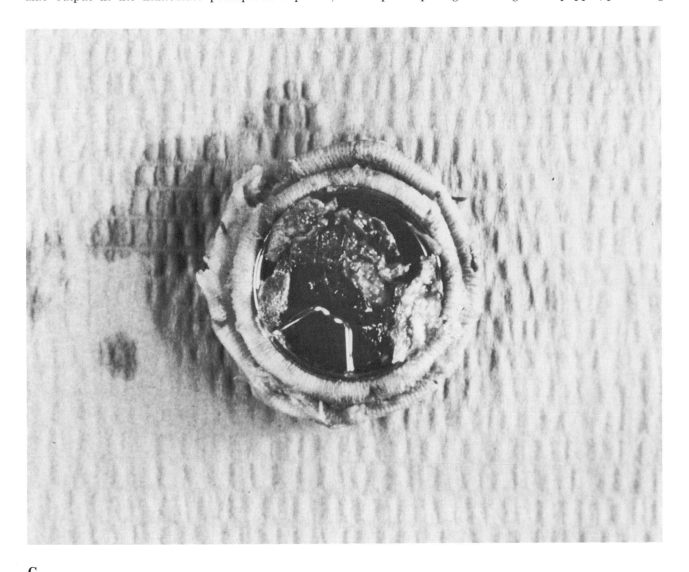

C

Figure 9.14. (*C*). At surgery, a thrombosed disc was found. (Reproduced by permission from Mintz GS, Carlson EB, Kotler MN. Non-invasive evaluation of prosthetic valves. Am J Cardiol 1982;49:39–44.)

obstruction to flow or regurgitation. Thrombosis on the prosthetic valve is often associated with a large mass of echoes that totally obscures the motion of the poppet. Poppet immobilization and thrombosed mitral Starr-Edwards valve can be recognized by the absence of demonstrable independent anterior and posterior poppet motion despite the presence of normal cage and suture rings (70). In addition, thrombus or tissue ingrowth may prevent full excursion of the ball or poppet, especially if reduced intensity of the opening and closing clicks is recorded. Patients with sticking poppets exhibit marked prolongation of the A_2 to MV opening interval generally beyond 0.17 second (71). A thrombus within the valve can be identified by the apparent lack of contact of the anterior ball and cage echoes and by lack of full excursion of the poppet. In the aortic position, the inability to demonstrate multiple clicks associated with a bouncing motion of the poppet may suggest a thrombosed aortic poppet (6). With cinefluoroscopy, restriction of motion of the poppet has been reported (42). In addition, lack of complete seating of the ball within the valve orifice would suggest the presence of thrombus formation, tissue ingrowth, or a combination of the two.

Beall-Surgitool Valve

Delayed opening has been reported in patients with thrombosed Beall-Surgitool valves (72, 73). In one such patient, initial opening occurred at 0.07 second after the second heart sound, but it was delayed to 0.2 second until full opening occurred (2). The delayed, rapid opening may be explained by the development of high LA pressure due to thrombus or tissue ingrowth on the struts to the point of opening the valve in late diastole. On occasion, the valve may only open after atrial contraction. It should be noted that delayed opening can also occur in the absence of a malfunctioning valve as a result of LV dysfunction.

Bjork-Shiley Valve

The mitral Bjork-Shiley prosthesis is more susceptible to thrombus formation than the aortic Bjork-Shiley valve (41). The rounding of the E point may indicate thrombus or obstruction (Fig. 9.14) (75). If there has been significant reduction in excursion in association with marked rounding of the initial motion of the Bjork-Shiley mitral prosthesis as compared to the baseline postoperative study, thrombosis of the valve should be strongly suspected. The thrombosed Bjork-Shiley prosthesis can be recognized echocardiographically by reduced or zero amplitude of valve excursion

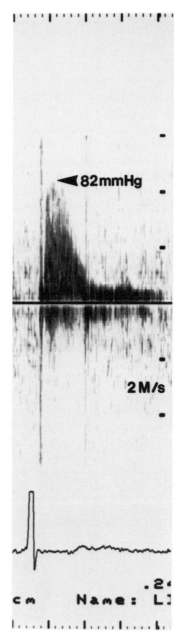

Figure 9.15. Continuous wave Doppler recording in a patient with obstructed aortic Ionescu-Shiley valve demonstrating a maximal gradient of 82 mm Hg across the valve. Recording was obtained from the second right intercostal space.

in association with dense echoes in the region of the suture ring (76). The finding is especially significant in the absence of a demonstrable closing click. On occasion, two-dimensional echocardiography may detect a large thrombus attached to the disc. Patients with extensive clot formation in and around the Bjork-Shiley aortic valve may have a complete absence of disc motion and associated dense echoes in the aortic root (77). Cinefluoroscopy is extremely useful and may demonstrate impaired excursion of the metallic disc,

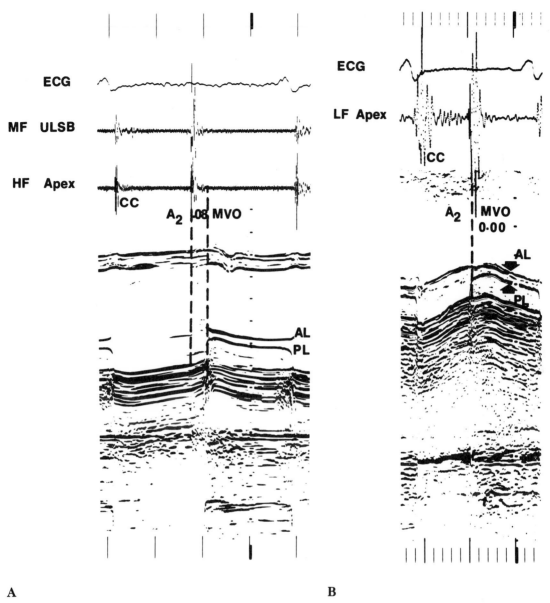

A   **B**

Figure 9.16. (*A*) Simultaneous ECG phonocardiogram and M-mode echocardiogram recorded in a patient with mitral St. Jude cardiac valve. Clear anterior leaflet (AL) and posterior leaflet (PL) motion is seen. The A_2 to MV opening (MVO) interval is normal and measures 0.08 second. (*B*) Simultaneous ECG, phonocardiogram, and M-mode echocardiogram in the same patient 1 month later. The A_2 to MVO interval has considerably shortened, indicative of a high LA pressure. Also, PL motion has a prolonged, rounded appearance in diastole (*dark arrows*) compared with the baseline study in *A*. CC = closure click; HF = high frequency; MF = medium frequency; ULSB = upper left sternal border. (Reproduced by permission from DePace N, Lichtenberg R, Kotler MN, et al. Echocardiographic and phonocardiographic assessment of the St. Jude cardiac valve prosthesis. Chest 1980;80:272–7.)

which is especially well seen if the disc is radiopaque (42). Occasional instances of significant prosthetic stenosis due to thrombosis or tissue valve degeneration have been identified by the findings of very high velocities measured by Doppler echocardiography (Fig. 9.15) (50, 51). The increased peak velocity due to obstruction has to be differentiated from that occurring as a result of paravalvular regurgitation, and careful mapping in the LV outflow tract or LA must be

undertaken to distinguish between these two conditions.

St. Jude Cardiac Valve

In patients with a clotted St. Jude MV prosthesis, the A_2 to MV opening interval may be considerably shortened (Fig. 9.16) (12, 78). In addition, abnormal rounding of the opening motion as compared to a baseline study has been reported (Fig. 9.16).

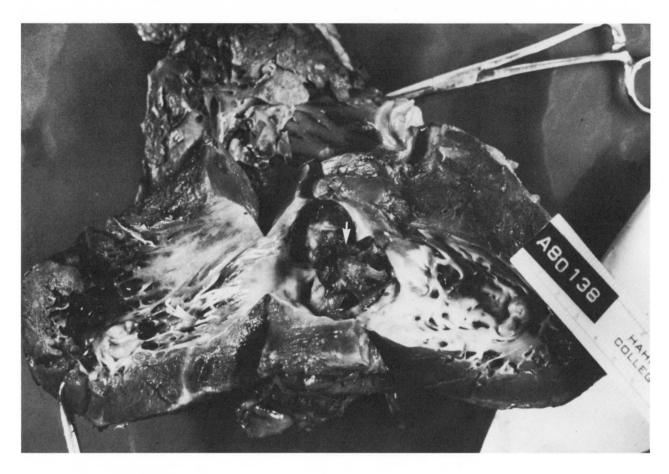

C

Figure 9.16. (*C*) Autopsy heart specimen viewed from the ventricular side showing thrombotic occlusion of the St. Jude MV prosthesis (*arrow*). (Reproduced by permission from DeBakey ME, ed. Advances in cardiac valves. Clinical perspectives. New York: Yorke Medical Books, 1983.)

PARAVALVULAR REGURGITATION

In patients with paravalvular regurgitation, murmurs are generally heard. However, in approximately 20 percent of patients with significant paravalvular regurgitation, no murmurs may be audible. Shown in Table 9.14 are the noninvasive features of malfunctioning prosthetic valves. One group of investigators has shown a high sensitivity and specificity of Doppler echocardiography in demonstrating paraprosthetic regurgitation even in the absence of a clinically suspected murmur (79). In a series of 50 patients with prosthetic valves who underwent angiography, auscultation demonstrated a sensitivity of 71 percent in patients with mitral regurgitation as compared to 86 percent sensitivity by Doppler echocardiography (79). In patients with aortic prosthetic valves and aortic regurgitation, the sensitivity by auscultation was 73 percent, in contrast to Doppler echocardiography, which demonstrated a 91 percent sensitivity. Thus, in patients with suspected prosthetic paravalvular leak,

Doppler echocardiography is the noninvasive technique of choice in its detection (79). In a series reported by Hatle (45), 12 patients with paravalvular mitral leaks had mean diastolic gradients in the 4 to 8

Table 9.14. Noninvasive Features of Malfunctioning Prosthetic Valves: Paravalvular Regurgitation

Doppler echocardiography
  High sensitivity and specificity in demonstrating prosthetic or paraprosthetic regurgitation even in absence of a clinically suspected murmur
Cinefluoroscopy
  Excessive rocking of suture rings
Echophonocardiographic findings
  Short A_2–MVO interval (due to elevated LA pressure)
  False-positive response: LV dysfunction
  Increasing LA and LV dimensions (volume overload)
  Normalization of abnormal septal motion or hyperdynamic septal motion
  Fluttering of MV or IV (in aortic prosthetic valve paravalvular leak)
  Early diastolic "bump"
  Premature MV closure (in acute severe paravalvular regurgitation of aortic prosthetic valve)

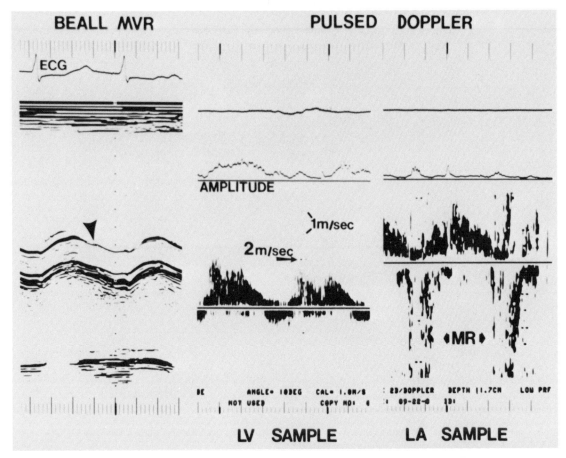

Figure 9.17. M-mode echocardiogram and a representative Doppler spectral. No evidence of disc motion is observed during diastole; however, the suture ring and the struts are seen. The dark arrow in the echocardiogram demonstrates where the normal diastolic position of MV disc should be in relation to its position against the struts. Significant mitral regurgitation (MR) during systole was detected by Doppler. At surgery, the patient had embolized the entire disc. MVR = mitral valve replacement.

mm Hg range. In a study reported by Williams and Labovitz (80), a significant number of patients had moderate to severe valvular regurgitation. Mild aortic regurgitation was seen in 42 percent of Bjork-Shiley valves, 26 percent of porcine valves and two of six Starr-Edwards valves. Mitral regurgitation was found in 11 percent of Bjork-Shiley valves, 19 percent of porcine valves and 30 percent of Starr-Edwards valves (80).

Color flow mapping Doppler can provide important spatial orientation of stenotic and regurgitant flow across prosthetic valves and allow rational correction of Doppler velocities for pressure gradient calculations (81). In patients with known regurgitation, color flow Doppler mapping is useful in localizing regurgitant jets and in distinguishing central valve leaks from paravalvular leaks. In a series reported by Hoit and associates (81), color flow imaging detected regurgitation in eight of nine patients with clinically known regurgitation.

Figures 9.17 and 9.18 show examples of significant paravalvular leaks detected by Doppler echocardiog-

raphy. However, there are limitations when trying to estimate the severity of para- or intraprosthetic valvular regurgitation by Doppler echocardiography (Table 9.15). Care must be taken not to confuse normal MV flow from aortic regurgitation when evaluating a patient with an aortic prosthetic valve (Fig. 9.19). In patients with paravalvular mitral regurgitation, a shortened A_2 to MV opening interval has been demonstrated irrespective of the type of valve prosthesis. However, a shortened A_2 to MV opening interval can occur in patients with LV dysfunction. An early diastolic bump of the Bjork-Shiley mitral prosthetic valve has also been reported in patients with paravalvular leaks (75). In patients with significant mitral paravalvular leak, septal motion is normalized or even hyperdynamic (Fig. 9.18), whereas septal motion is frequently abnormal or paradoxic following cardiac surgery (82). Significant mitral regurgitation secondary to a paravalvular leak is unlikely in patients with hypokinetic or paradoxic septal motion. In addition, the LA is en-

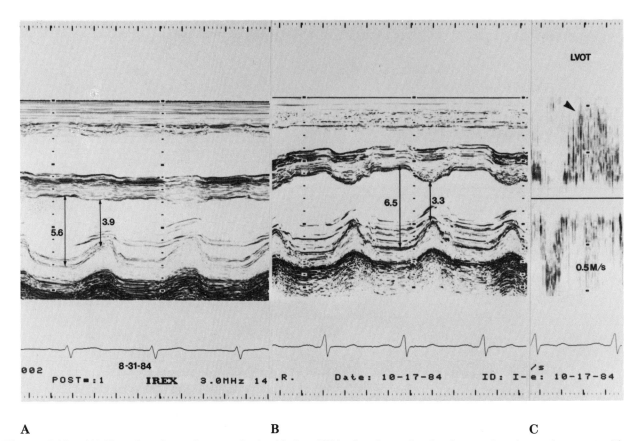

A   **B**   **C**

Figure 9.18. (*A*) M-mode echocardiogram obtained below MV leaflets immediately after aortic valve replacement with an Ionescu-Shiley valve. (*B*) M-mode echocardiogram obtained below MV leaflets 6 weeks after surgery. Note LV internal dimension in diastole has increased from 5.6 to 6.5 cm and systolic dimension has decreased from 3.9 to 3.3 cm. Septal motion has changed from hypokinetic to flat to hyperdynamic consistent with volume overload. (*C*) Pulsed mode Doppler recording obtained from apical five-chamber view in the left ventricular outflow tract (LVOT). Significant diastolic flow (*black arrow*) was obtained consistent with paravalvular aortic regurgitation.

larged. Patients who present with an aortic paravalvular leak may have reversed flow patterns detected in the LV outflow tract by Doppler echocardiography. In addition, fine fluttering of the MV or interventricular septum (IVS) or both may be demonstrated. Premature closure of the native MV in the absence of a prolonged PR interval or atrial fibrillation with long RR interval suggests severe, acute aortic regurgitation (64, 65). If there is greater than 9 to 12 degrees rocking of the suture ring by cinefluoroscopy, mitral paravalvular leaks should be suspected (39). Greater than 6 to 10 degrees rocking motion of the aortic valve is suggestive of a paravalvular leak.

BALL OR DISC VARIANCE

Listed in Table 9.16 are the features of prosthetic valve variance. The old Starr-Edwards aortic valve and Beall-Surgitool 103 and 104 MVs were prone to develop variance. The process of curing the silicone rubber ball

was changed in 1965, and ball variance is not seen with the newest Starr-Edwards aortic prosthesis. With the Beall-Surgitool 103 and 104 mitral disc valves, abnormal systolic seating of the valves as a sign of disc variance has been reported (2). In addition, a shortened A_2 to MV opening interval and a loud systolic murmur are characteristic of variance. Cinefluoroscopy may be particularly useful in documenting systolic sticking or "cocking" (33). In addition, abnormal motion suggestive of trapping of the disc within the valve orifice can occur (41). The disc generally develops erosion and notching, and complete extrusion or disc entrapment

Table 9.15. Limitations of Estimating Severity of Mitral Regurgitation by Doppler Echocardiography

Low cardiac output of large LA may underestimate severity of mitral regurgitation (MR)

Extension of regurgitant jet out of the examining plane may lead to underestimation of severity of MR

Overestimation of regurgitation when a high-velocity jet reaches deep into the LA especially when the jet is narrow and limited to a small area

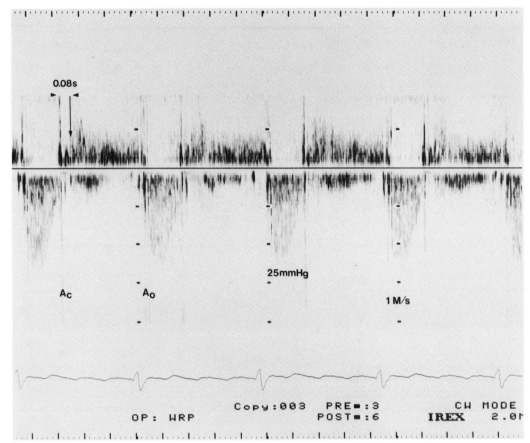

Figure 9.19. Continuous wave Doppler recording from the apical position in a patient with Bjork-Shiley mitral and aortic prostheses. During systole, the aortic valve opening (A_o) and closing (A_c) clicks are well recorded. A peak systolic velocity of 2.5 m per second in the ascending aorta indicates a peak instantaneous aortic valve gradient of 25 mm Hg. During diastole, flow toward the transducer suggests prosthetic aortic valve regurgitation. On close examination of the first beat, an 0.08 second hiatus is noted separating the onset of diastolic flow from aortic valve closure, indicating that this is normal flow through the prosthetic MV and not aortic regurgitation.

can occur. Varying intensity of the systolic murmur and variable A_2 to MV opening intervals may occur in patients with mitral Beall-Surgitool valve variance (Fig. 9.20). In such patients, mitral regurgitation is frequently

Table 9.16. Noninvasive Features of Malfunctioning Prosthetic Valves: Valve Variance

Echophonocardiography
  Reduced motion of the valve increased distance of ball from the cage
  Early diastolic notch (Beall, Starr-Edwards valves)
  Premature diastolic closure (due to notching or scalloping of a Beall valve)
  Short A_2–MVO interval (Beall mitral valve)
  Abnormal seating during systole (Beall mitral valve)
Cinefluoroscopy
  Mitral disc valves
    Absent or sticking motion suggestive of entrapment of the disc within the valve orifice
    In advanced situations, complete extrusion or disc entrapment can occur
  Starr-Edwards aortic valve
    Includes restriction of motion or extrusion of the poppet or excessive mobility of cage or both
Doppler Echocardiography
  Demonstration of prosthetic valvular regurgitation

present by Doppler echocardiography. Shown in Figure 9.17 is the value of Doppler echocardiography in detecting severe mitral regurgitation in a patient who had disc embolization with a Beall-Surgitool 103 valve. In this particular instance, the disc itself was not visualized either by cinefluoroscopy or echocardiography.

Valve Dehiscence

Valve dehiscence is generally caused by disruption of suture lines securing the prosthesis to the sewing bed or by loosening, breaking, or avulsion of the sutures from the supporting tissues (42). Dehiscence results in severe valve regurgitation or heart failure or both. M-mode and two-dimensional echocardiographic features include detection of motion of the valve within the LA and abnormal excursion with an echo-free space between the suture lines and the mitral annulus. Excessive abnormal excursion can occur in the aortic position (Fig. 9.21). Cinefluoroscopy is particularly helpful in diagnosing dehiscence and is characterized

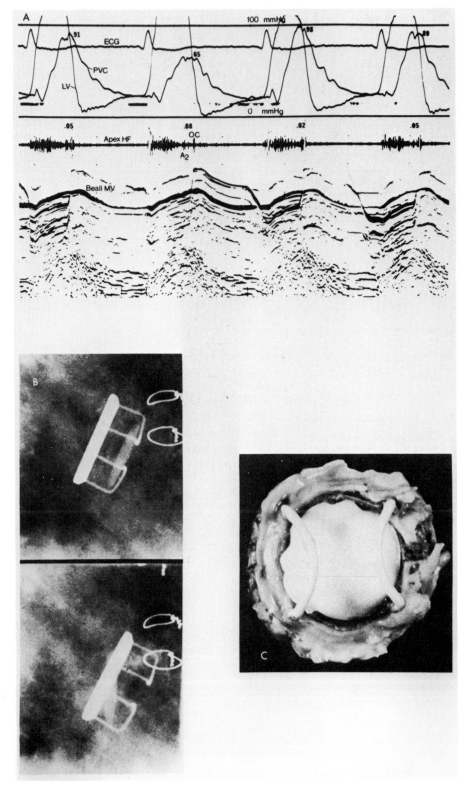

Figure 9.20. (*A*) Simultaneous LV pressure tracing, pulmonary venous capillary (PVC) tracing, phonocardiogram, and M-mode echocardiogram of a patient with a Beall-Surgitool MV prosthesis and abnormal seating of the valve. The rhythm is atrial fibrillation. The A_2 to opening click (OC) interval is variable despite minimal variation of the RR interval. Degree of shortening of the A_2 to OC interval is proportional to the height of the V wave on the pulmonary venous capillary tracing. The tallest measured V wave of 98 mm Hg is associated with A_2 to OC interval of 0.02 second. A recording of the echo behind the suture ring in systole may represent cocking of the disc or apparent displacement of the disc behind the suture ring. A systolic murmur is recorded in each cycle length. (*B*) Cinefluoroscopic study during diastole (above) and systole (below). During diastole, the disc seats itself normally, but shrinks in size. During systole, the disc is in a stuck position, producing mitral regurgitation. (*C*) Surgical specimen from a patient with disc variance. The margins are irregular with swelling of the disc. HF = high frequency. (Reproduced by permission from Kotler MN, Segal BL, Parry WR. Echocardiographic and phonocardiographic evaluation of prosthetic heart valves. Cardiovasc Clin 1978;9:187–207.)

by excessive rocking motion beyond the normal range. However, an occasional dehiscence can be present in patients with paravalvular leaks with less than 20 degrees rocking motion. It should also be noted that not all valves with greater than 20 degrees rocking motion will have significant dehiscence. Valve dehiscence has also been reported by two-dimensional echocardiograms in patients with porcine biopros-

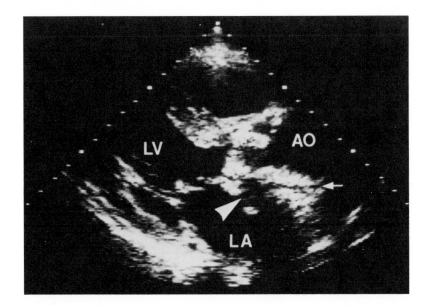

A

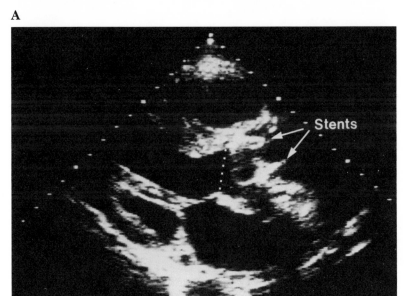

B

Figure 9.21. Valve dehiscence occurring in a drug addict with an aortic Carpentier-Edwards prosthetic valve. The change from diastole (*A*) to systole (*B*) and excessive rocking of posterior base of leaflet are evident. The diastolic position of the prosthetic valve is indicated by the dotted line. In addition, the leaflets are thickened and an echo-free space (*large and small white arrows*) is evident. Recent endocarditis with an annular and posterior aortic wall abscess was found at surgery. Ao = aorta.

theses (36). A diagnosis of ring dehiscence was made when the motion of the sewing ring was not consonant with the surrounding cardiac tissues. Parasternal long-axis and apical four-chamber views appear to be the best views for detecting MV dehiscence, while parasternal long-axis and short-axis views appear to be best for detecting aortic valve dehiscence. In patients with dehiscence, severe valvular regurgitation is present, which can be readily detected by Doppler echocardiography.

BACTERIAL ENDOCARDITIS

The differentiation between vegetation, clot, and normal metallic prosthetic valve is difficult by M-mode and two-dimensional echocardiography. Excessive reverberation and beam width artifacts with two-dimensional echocardiography may not allow precise definition of disc or ball valve motion (83). Two-dimensional echocardiography is particularly helpful in detecting vegetations and their complications in patients with bioprosthetic valves (Fig. 9.22A). Endocarditis of a bioprosthesis is a serious complication, with an annual incidence similar to that of mechanical valves, approximately 1 to 3 percent. However, a high mortality of approximately 33 percent has been reported (84, 85). Aortic valve endocarditis is generally more common than MV endocarditis. If infection is localized to the cusp or tissue, medical therapy may result in steriliza-

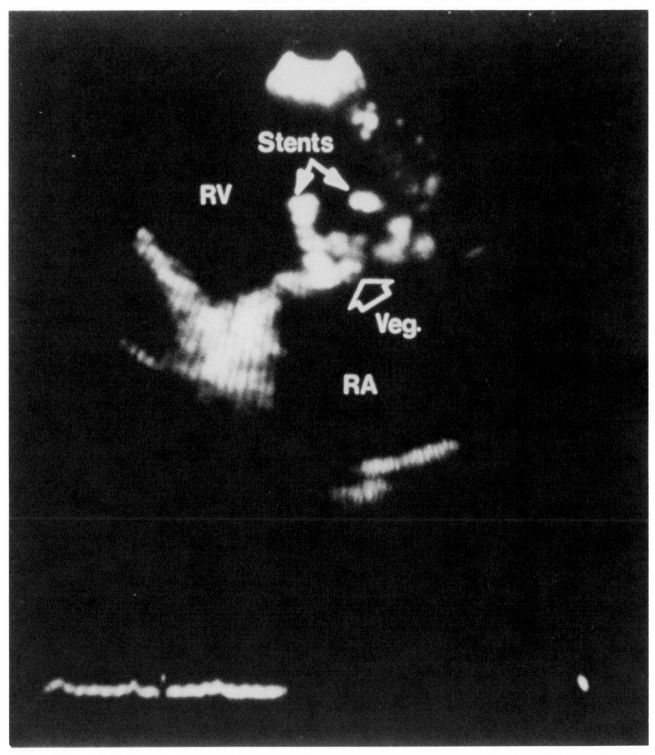

Figure 9.22. (*A*) Modified parasternal right ventricular (RV) inflow view in a drug addict with tricuspid valve endocarditis on a tissue valve. The large vegetations (Veg.) are attached to the individual leaflets (*white arrows*).

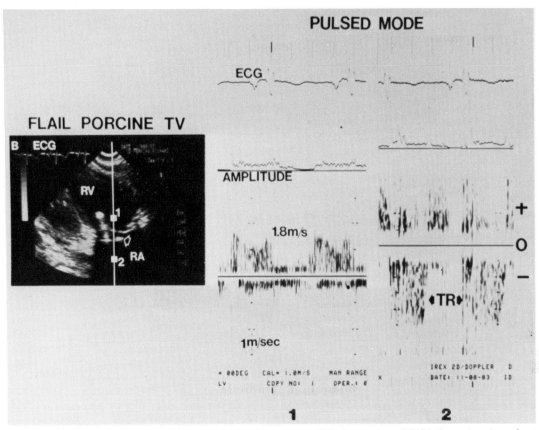

Figure 9.22. (*B*) Pulse mode Doppler recording obtained from a modified parasternal RV inflow view in a drug addict with bacterial endocarditis. Sample volumes were obtained from positions 1 and 2. Representative Doppler spectra of transtricuspid flow of the porcine heterograft were recorded in positions 1 and 2. A maximum gradient of 13 mm Hg (position 1) and significant tricuspid regurgitation (TR) were identified by Doppler. Position 2 was detected in the right atrium (RA). A flail tricuspid leaflet was detected by two-dimensional echocardiography (*large open arrow*). TV = tricuspid valve.

tion and cure the infection. If infection involves the sewing ring with valve ring abscess, significant paravalvular leaks, or dehiscence; surgery may be required. Distinction between a vegetation and a calcified or fibrotic nodule is not usually possible by echocardiography alone. The echogenic masses can be seen attached to and moving freely within the leaflet. On occasion, a flail leaflet can occur as a result of the destructive process. Valvular regurgitation can be detected by Doppler echocardiography (Fig. 9.22B). Generally, cinefluoroscopy is disappointing in detecting vegetations. However, if the vegetations are large enough to interfere with motion of the valve or produce an aortic root or annular abscess, decreased excursion of the disc or ball or excessive rocking motion may be recognized by cinefluoroscopy. Complications of endocarditis such as an aortic root abscess, mitral annular abscess, and intramyocardial abscess can be recognized by two-dimensional echocardiography (68, 69).

Primary Valve Degeneration of Bioprosthetic Valves

Primary valve failure is defined as valvular stenosis or insufficiency due to tissue degeneration without histologic or bacterial evidence of infection. Durability appears to be the greatest problem with all bioprosthetic valves (86–90). Degeneration of porcine valves in children is a more serious problem, occurring in up to 38 percent of pediatric patients 30 to 56 months following implantation (87–89). Other investigators have reported a 23 percent incidence of calcific stenosis with the Ionescu-Shiley valve, developing at a mean of 30 months post implantation in children under 17 years of age (90). Degeneration of bioprosthetic valves results from calcification in the commissural regions of the cusp, leading to calcific stenosis or tears in the cusp. Both M-mode and two-dimensional echocardiography can be used to measure cusp thickness and cusp excursion (Fig. 9.23). Leaflet tear can be detected by localized fluttering of the cusp recorded during systole

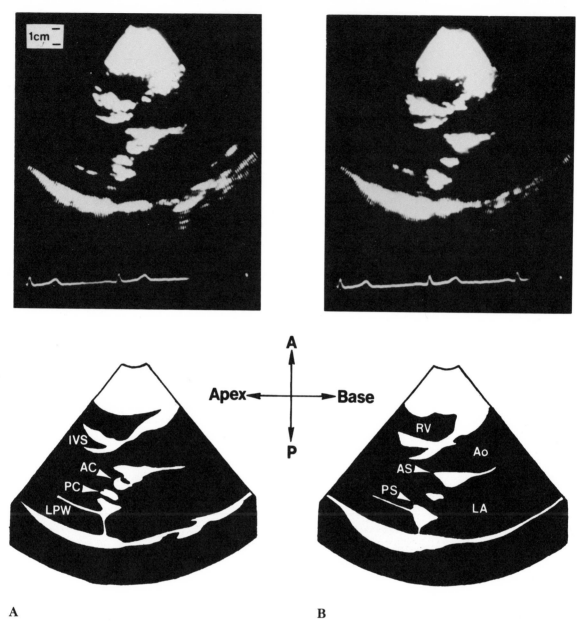

Figure 9.23. Two-dimensional echocardiogram obtained from the parasternal region of the LV long-axis in diastole (*A*) and in systole (*B*) in a patient with primary valve degeneration. The individual leaflets are thickened and restricted in motion. A = anterior; AC = anterior cusp; Ao = aorta; AS = anterior stent; IVS = interventricular septum; LPW = left ventricular posterior wall; P = posterior; PC = posterior cusp; PS = posterior stent; RV = right ventricle.

and diastole. Shown in Figure 9.24 is an example of leaflet tear that produced severe valvular insufficiency and was recognized by both M-mode and two-dimensional echocardiography. Diastolic fluttering of normal porcine valve leaflets in the mitral position has been reported in patients with aortic valve regurgitation (91). Doppler echocardiography is particularly useful in differentiating primary from secondary cusp fluttering. Calcification usually appears as focal deposits localized at the commissures next to the sewing ring.

As calcification progresses, it becomes more generalized and involves the body of the leaflets. This may result in stenosis of the bioprosthetic valves, and two-dimensional (Fig. 9.25) and Doppler echocardiography are extremely useful in assessing the degree of bioprosthetic stenosis (Fig. 9.15) (36, 58) or the degree of LV outflow obstruction following aortic valve replacement (92). The orifice size of the bioprosthetic valve in the mitral position can be determined by Doppler data using the pressure half-time measure-

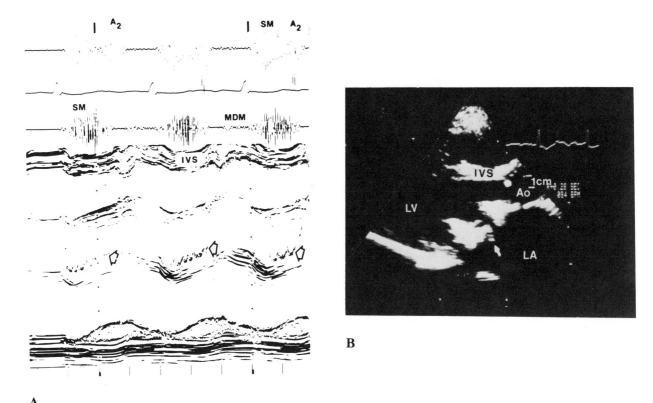

A

Figure 9.24. (*A*) Simultaneous phonocardiogram (above) and M-mode echocardiogram (below) of a patient with a flail porcine MV prosthesis. A loud crescendo-decrescendo systolic murmur (SM) as well as a mid-diastolic rumble (MDM) is recorded. In association with the systolic murmur, marked coarse fluttering of the posterior cusp is seen (*open arrows*). (*B*) Two-dimensional echocardiogram of same patient obtained in the parasternal long-axis view during systole. The white arrow depicts the flail cusp shown prolapsing beyond the plane of the prosthetic valve annulus into the LA. AO = aorta; IVS = interventricular septum.

ment (58). Again, baseline Doppler studies after surgery are extremely useful in following these patients.

Valve-heart mismatch can occur following the insertion of large, usually cage ball prostheses in the mitral position. Rahmitoola has drawn attention to obstruction to ventricular outflow or inflow due to reduced effective orifice size of the valve prosthesis (93). This may occur because the prosthetic valve area is smaller than that of a normal human valve area. Orifice size may be further reduced by tissue ingrowth or epithelialization. In addition, the size of the prosthesis that may be inserted may be limited by the size of the valve annulus. When a narrow LV outflow tract has been demonstrated by echocardiography, ball and cage valves should not be inserted (94). Bioprosthetic valves should not be inserted in the mitral position in the presence of a narrow LV outflow tract either (94, 95).

Mechanical Malfunction

On rare occasions, mechanical malfunction can occur in the absence of fibrous ingrowth, clot formation, paravalvular leak, or disc variance. Rare instances of

Bjork-Shiley and St. Jude MV malfunction have been reported (33). In one instance, one of the leaflets of the St. Jude mitral prosthesis suddenly embolized; the patient presented with acute pulmonary edema secondary to severe mitral regurgitation and underwent successful insertion of a second St. Jude MV prosthesis (96).

SUMMARY

Noninvasive techniques are particularly helpful in evaluating the function of mechanical prostheses and tissue valves. Combined phonocardiography with M-mode echocardiography, cinefluoroscopy, and Doppler echocardiography are the most useful noninvasive techniques in differentiating normal from abnormal metallic prosthetic valve function. The intensity of the opening and closing clicks and associated murmurs depends on the type of prosthetic valve, the heart rate, rhythm, and underlying hemodynamic status. Arrhythmias or conduction disturbances may produce motion patterns that mimic the echocardiographic signs of

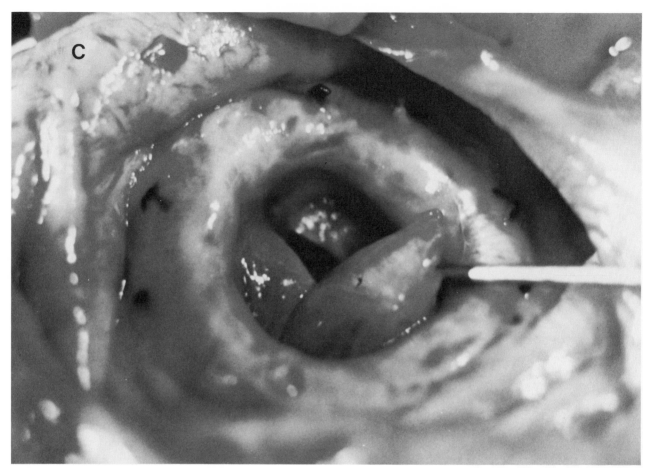

Figure 9.24. (*C*) Autopsy specimen demonstrates torn and avulsed leaflet as shown by the probe. (Reproduced by permission from Mintz GS, Kotler MN, Segal BL. The role of two-dimensional echocardiography in the non-invasive evaluation of prosthetic heart valve function. In: Giuliani E, ed. Two-dimensional real-time ultrasonic imaging of the heart. Boston: Martinus Nijhoff, 1985:115–23.)

malfunctioning prosthetic valves. Two-dimensional echocardiography is of limited help in assessing patients with metallic prosthetic valves due to reverberation artifacts and side-lobe echoes. However, two-dimensional echocardiography is extremely useful in excluding underlying LV dysfunction. In addition, two-dimensional echocardiography allows determination of the precise alignment of the prosthetic valves so that optimal M-mode evaluation of the disc or poppet motion can be undertaken. Two-dimensional echocardiography also allows diagnosis of pericardial effusion and exclusion of other valvular abnormalities. Differentiation of thrombus formation or tissue ingrowth from paravalvular regurgitation or dehiscence is possible by echophonocardiography, Doppler echocardiography, and cinefluoroscopy. Doppler echocardiography is the most sensitive noninvasive technique in diagnosing paravalvular leaks. In addition, significant obstruction across a prosthetic valve can be determined by

calculation of the maximal gradient across the obstructed orifice using Doppler echocardiography. In the mitral position, the effective valve orifice can be readily calculated. The differentiation between benign physiologic regurgitation and true pathologic regurgitation by Doppler is not always possible. Disc variance is a potentially serious and lethal problem with the older Beall-Surgitool valves, and can be readily detected by a combination of echophonocardiography, cinefluoroscopy, and Doppler echocardiography. With regard to bioprosthetic valves, two-dimensional echocardiography is superior to M-mode in detecting primary valve failure. In addition, detection of vegetations, valve alignment, and ring and individual leaflet motion can be readily accomplished by two-dimensional echocardiography. When considering the value of noninvasive techniques in prosthetic valve function, it is essential that the patient serve as his or her own control in the follow-up assessment.

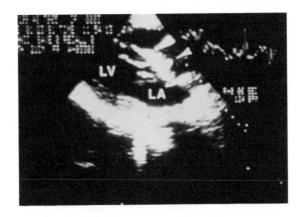

A

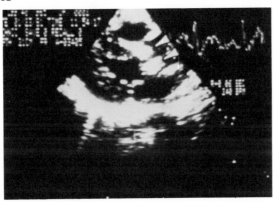

B

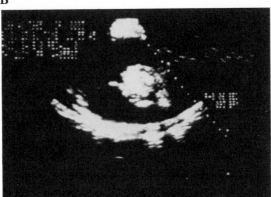

C

Figure 9.25. (*A*) and (*B*) Diastolic and systolic frames of a two-dimensional echocardiographic study in the parasternal long-axis view of a patient with calcified and stenotic bioprosthesis in the aortic position (*white arrowheads*). The systolic frame from the parasternal short-axis view (*C*) shows marked reduction in the orifice of the aortic bioprosthesis. The patient had a 100 mm Hg pressure gradient across the prosthesis.

D

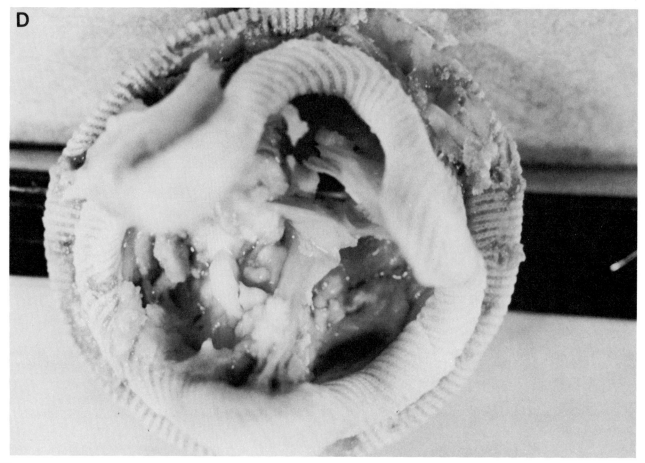

Figure 9.25.   (*D*) Surgically excised specimen showing extensive calcification and thickening of leaflets. (Reproduced by permission from Mintz GS, Kotler MN, Segal BL. The role of the two-dimensional echocardiography in the non-invasive evaluation of prosthetic valve function. In: Giuliani ER, ed. Two-dimensional real-time ultrasonic imaging of the heart. Boston: Martinus Nijhoff, 1985:115–23.)

REFERENCES

1. Harken DE, Soroff HS, Taylor WJ, Lefemine AA, Gupta SK, Lunzer S. Partial and complete prosthesis in aortic insufficiency. J Thorac Cardiovasc Surg 1960;40:744–62.
2. Kotler MN, Segal BL, Parry WR. Echocardiographic and phonocardiographic evaluation of prosthetic heart valves. Cardiovasc Clin 1978;9:187–207.
3. Felner JM, Miller DD. Echocardiographic characteristics of mechanical prosthetic heart valves. Echocardiography 1984;1:261–310.
4. Smith ND, Raizada V, Abrams J. Auscultation of the normally functioning prosthetic valve. Ann Intern Med 1981;95:594–8.
5. Cunha CLP, Giuliani ER, Callahan JA, Pluth JR. Echo-phonocardiographic findings in patients with prosthetic heart valve malfunction. Mayo Clin Proc 1980;55:231–42.
6. Simon EB, Kotler MN, Segal BL, Parry W. Clinical significance of multiple systolic clicks from Starr-Edwards prosthetic aortic valves. Br Heart J 1977;39:645–50.
7. Bjork VO, Holmgren A, Olin C, Ovenfors CO. Clinical and hemodynamic results of aortic valve replacement with the Bjork-Shiley tilting disc valve prosthesis. Scand J Thorac Cardiovasc Surg 1971;5:177–91.
8. Nitter-Hauge S, Semb B, Ahdelnoor M, Hall KV. A 5 year experience with the Medtronic Hall disc valve prosthesis. Circulation 1983;68(suppl II):169–74.
9. Starek PJK, Murray GF, Keagy BA, Wilcox BR. Clinical experi-
ence with the Hall pivoting disc valve. J Thorac Cardiovasc Surg 1983;31:II-66–8.
10. Beaudet RL, Poirier NL, Guerraty AJ, Doyle D. Fifty-four months experience with an improved tilting disc valve (Medtronic-Hall). J Thorac Cardiovasc Surg 1983;31:II-89–93.
11. Nitter-Hauge S. Echocardiographic and phonocardiographic characteristics of the Hall-Kaster aortic disc valve prosthesis. Life Support Systems 1983;1:165–72.
12. DePace N, Lichtenberg R, Kotler MN, Mintz GS, Segal BL, Goel I. Echocardiographic and phonocardiographic assessment of the St. Jude cardiac valve prosthesis. Chest 1981;80:272–7.
13. Raizada V, Smith ND, Hoyt TW, et al. Phonocardiographic characteristics of the St. Jude prosthesis in the aortic position. Chest 1982;81:95–6.
14. Nicoloff DM, Emery TW, Arom KV, et al. Clinical and hemodynamic results with the St. Jude medical cardiac valve prosthesis—a three year experience. J Thorac Cardiovasc Surg 1981;82:674–83.
15. Wortham DC, Tri TB, Bowen TE. Hemodynamic evaluation of the St. Jude medical valve prosthesis in the small aortic annulus. J Thorac Cardiovasc Surg 1981;81:615–20.
16. Mirro MJ, Pyhel J, Wann LS, Weyman AE, Tavel ME, Stewart J. Diastolic rumbles in normally functioning porcine mitral valves. Chest 1978;73:189–92.
17. Wiltrakis MG, Rahimtoola SH, Harlan BJ, DeMots H. Diastolic rumbles with porcine heterograft prosthesis in the atrioventricular position: normal or abnormal prosthesis. Chest 1978;74:411–3.

18. Horowitz MS, Goodman DJ, Hancock EW, Popp RL. Non-invasive diagnosis of complications of the mitral bioprosthesis. J Thorac Cardiovasc Surg 1976;71:450–7.

19. Gordon RF, Najmi M, Kingsley B, et al. Spectroanalytic evaluation of aortic prosthetic valves. Chest 1974;66:44–9.

20. Stein PD, Sabbah H, Lakier JB, Goldstein S. Frequency spectrum of the aortic component of the second heart sound in patients with normal valves, aortic stenosis and aortic porcine xenografts. Potential for detection of porcine xenograft degeneration. Am J Cardiol 1980;46:48–52.

21. Stein PD, Sabbah HN, Lakier JB, Kemp SR, Magilligan DJ. Frequency spectra of the first heart sound and of the aortic component of the second heart sound in patients with degenerated porcine bioprosthetic valves. Am J Cardiol 1984;53:557–61.

22. Foale RA, Joo TH, McClellan JH, et al. Detection of aortic porcine valve dysfunction by maximum entropy spectral analysis. Circulation 1983;68:42–9.

23. Brodie BR, Grossman W, McLaurin L, et al. Diagnosis of prosthetic valve malfunction with combined echo-phonocardiography. Circulation 1976;53:93.

24. Johnson ML, Paton BC, Holmes JH. Ultrasonic evaluation of prosthetic valve motion. Circulation 1970;42(suppl II):3.

25. Douglas JE, Williams GD. Echocardiographic evaluation of the Bjork-Shiley prosthetic valve. Circulation 1974;50:52–7.

26. Gibson TC, Starek PJK, Moos S, Craige E. Echocardiographic and phonocardiographic characteristics of Lillehei-Kaster mitral valve prosthesis. Circulation 1974;49:434–40.

27. Panidis IP, Ren JF, Kotler MN, et al. Clinical and echocardiographic evaluation of the St. Jude cardiac valve prosthesis: follow up of 126 patients. J Am Coll Cardiol 1984;4:454–62.

28. Amann FW, Burckhardt D, Hasse J, Gradel E. Echocardiographic features of the correctly functioning St. Jude medical valve prosthesis. Am Heart J 1981;80:278–84.

29. Feldman HJ, Gray RJ, Chaux A, et al. Noninvasive in vivo and in vitro study of the St. Jude mitral valve prosthesis: evaluation using two-dimensional and M-mode echocardiography, phonocardiography and cinefluoroscopy. Am J Cardiol 1981;49:1101–9.

30. Tri TB, Schatz RA, Watson TD, Bowen TE, Schiller NB. Echocardiographic evaluation of the St. Jude medical prosthetic valve. Chest 1981;80:278–84.

31. Horowitz MS, Tecklenberg PL, Goodman DJ, et al. Echocardiographic evaluation of the stent mounted aortic bioprosthetic valve in the mitral position. In vitro and in vivo studies. Circulation 1976;54:91–6.

32. Kotler MN, Mintz GS, Segal BL, Parry WR. Clinical uses of two-dimensional echocardiography. Am J Cardiol 1980;45:1061–82.

33. Kotler MN, Mintz GS, Panidis I, et al. Non-invasive evaluation of normal and abnormal prosthetic valve function. J Am Coll Cardiol 1983;2:151–73.

34. Schapiro JN, Martin RP, Fowles RE, et al. Two-dimensional echocardiographic assessment of patients with bioprosthetic valves. Am J Cardiol 1979;43:510–9.

35. Martin RP, French JW, Popp RL. Clinical utility of two-dimensional echocardiography in patients with bioprosthetic valves. Adv Cardiol 1980;27:294–304.

36. Usher BW. Echocardiographic assessment of patients with bioprosthetic valves. Echocardiography 1984;1:311–32.

37. Mehlman DJ, Resnekov L. A guide to the radiographic identification of prosthetic valves. Circulation 1978;57:613–23.

38. Mehlman DJ, Resnekov L. A guide to the radiographic identification of prosthetic heart valves. Circulation 1984;69:102–4.

39. White AJ, Dinsmore RE, Buckley MJ. Cineradiographic evaluation of prosthetic cardiac valves. Circulation 1973;48:882–9.

40. Gimenez JL, Soulen RL, Davile JC. Prosthetic valve detachment. Its roentgenographic recognition. Am J Radiol 1968;103:595–600.

41. Mintz GS, Carlson EB, Kotler MN. Comparison of noninvasive techniques in evaluation of the nontissue cardiac valves. Am J Cardiol 1982;49:39–44.

42. Sands MK, Lachman AS, O'Reilly DJ, Leach CN, Sappington JB, Katz AM. Diagnostic value of cinefluoroscopy in the evaluation of prosthetic heart valve dysfunction. Am Heart J 1982;104:622–7.

43. Castenada ZW, Nicoloff D, Jorgensen C, Nath PH, Zollikofer C, Amplatz K. In vivo radiographic appearance of the St. Jude valve prosthesis. Radiology 1980; 134:775–6.

44. Abbasi AS, Allen MW, DeChristofaro D, Ungor J. Detection and estimation of the degree of mitral regurgitation by range-gated pulsed Doppler echocardiography. Circulation 1980;61:143–7.

45. Hatle E, Angelsen B, eds. Doppler ultrasound in cardiology. Physical principles and clinical applications. Philadelphia: Lea and Febiger, 1985:188–205.

46. Holen J, Simonsen S, Froysaker T. An ultrasound Doppler technique for the non-invasive determination of the pressure gradient in the Bjork-Shiley mitral valve. Circulation 1979;59:436–42.

47. Weinstein IR, Marbarger JP, Perez JE. Ultrasonic assessment of the St. Jude prosthetic valve: M-mode, two-dimensional and Doppler echocardiography. Circulation 1983;68:897–905.

48. Veyrot C, Cholot N, Abitbol G, et al. Non-invasive diagnosis and assessment of aortic valve disease and evaluation of aortic prosthesis function using echo pulsed Doppler velocimetry. Br Heart J 1980;43:393–413.

49. Dellsperger KC, Wieting DW, Baehr DA, et al. Regurgitation of prosthetic heart valves: dependence on heart rate and cardiac output. Am J Cardiol 1983;51:321–8.

50. Gross CM, Wann LS. Doppler echocardiographic diagnosis of porcine bioprosthetic cardiac valve malfunction. Am J Cardiol 1984;53:1203–5.

51. Pearlman AS. Doppler echocardiography: a promising method for investigating prosthetic valve dysfunction. Echocardiography 1984;1:257–9.

52. Stamm RB, Martin RP. Quantification of pressure gradients across stenotic valves by Doppler ultrasound. J Am Coll Cardiol 1983;2:707–18.

53. Ramirez ML, Wong M, Sadler N, Shah PM. Doppler evaluation of 106 bioprosthetic and mechanical aortic valves, abstracted. J Am Coll Cardiol 1985;5:527.

54. Lillehei CW. Worldwide experience with the St. Jude mitral valve prosthesis. Clinical and hemodynamic results. Contemp Surg 1982;20:17–32.

55. Nicoloff DM, Emery RW, Arom KV, et al. Clinical and hemodynamic results with the St. Jude medical cardiac valve prosthesis: a three year experience. J Thorac Cardiovasc Surg 1981;82:674–83.

56. Wortham DC, Tri TB, Bowen TE. Hemodynamic evaluation of the St. Jude medical valve prosthesis in the small aortic annulus. J Thorac Cardiovasc Surg 1981;81:615–26.

57. Bjork VO, Henze A. Ten years experience with the Bjork-Shiley tilting disc valve. J Thorac Cardiovasc Surg 1979;78:331–42.

58. Ryan T, Armstrong WF, Dillon JC, Feigenbaum H. Doppler evaluation of patients with porcine mitral valves, abstracted. J Am Coll Cardiol 1983;5:526.

59. Comess KA, Beach KW, Janko CL, Reamer RP, Otto CM, Pearlman AS. Prevalence and factors influencing bioprosthetic regurgitation by Doppler, abstracted. J Am Coll Cardiol 1985;5:392.

60. Ramirez ML, Wong M. Reproducibility of stand alone continuous-wave Doppler recording of aortic flow velocity across bioprosthetic valves. Am J Cardiol 1985;55:1197–9.

61. Panidis IP, Morganroth J, David D, Chen CC, Kotler MN. Prosthetic mitral valve motion during cardiac dysrhythmias: an echocardiographic study. Am J Cardiol 1983;51:996–1004.

62. Zaky A, Steinmetz E, Feigenbaum H. Role of atrium in closure of mitral valve in man. Am J Physiol 1969;217:1652–9.

63. Laniado S, Yellin E, Kotler M, Levy L, Stadler J, Terdiman R. A study of the dynamic relations between the mitral valve echogram and phasic mitral flow. Circulation 1975;51:104–13.

64. Agnew TM, Carlisle R. Premature valve closure in patients with a mitral Starr-Edwards prosthesis and aortic incompetence. Br Heart J 1970;32:436–9.

65. Sands MJ, Kreulen TH, McDonough MT, Fadali MA, Spann IB. Pseudomalfunction of a Beall mitral valve prosthesis in the presence of paravalvular aortic regurgitation. Am J Cardiol 1975;36:88–90.

66. David D, Michelson EL, Naito M, Chen CC, Schaffenburg M, Dreifus LS. Diastolic "locking" of the mitral valve: the impor-

tance of atrial systolic and intraventricular volume. Circulation 1983;67:640–5.

67. Busch UW, Pechacek LW, Garcia E, Mathur VS, Hall RJ. Premature closure of prosthetic mitral valves as a consequence of gravity. Cathet Cardiovasc Diagn 1982;8:131–6.

68. Brandenburg RO, Giuliani ER, Wilson WR, Geraci JE. Infective endocarditis—a 25 year overview of diagnosis and therapy. J Am Coll Cardiol 1983;1:280–91.

69. Mardelli TJ, Ogawa S, Hubbard FE, Dreifus LS, Meixell LL. Cross-sectional echocardiographic detection of aortic ring abscess in bacterial endocarditis. Chest 1978;74:576–8.

70. Bendt TB, Goodman DJ, Popp RL. Echocardiographic and phonocardiographic confirmation of suspected mitral prosthetic valve malfunction. Chest 1976;70:221–30.

71. Pfeifer J, Goldschlager N, Sweatman T, et al. Malfunction of mitral ball valve due to thrombus. Report of two cases with notes on early clinical diagnosis. Am J Cardiol 1972;29:95–9.

72. Oliva PB, Johnson ML, Pomerantz M, et al. Dysfunction of the Beall mitral prosthesis and its detection by cinefluoroscopy and echocardiography. Am J Cardiol 1973;131:393–6.

73. Kawai N, Segal BL, Linhart JW. Delayed opening of Beall mitral valve detected by echocardiography. Chest 1975;67:239–41.

74. Moreno-Cabral RJ, McNamara JJ, Mamiya RT, et al. Acute thrombotic obstruction with Bjork-Shiley valves: diagnostic and surgical considerations. J Thorac Cardiovasc Surg 1978;75:321–30.

75. Bernal-Ramirez JA, Phillips JH. Echocardiographic study of malfunction of Bjork-Shiley prosthetic heart valve in the mitral position. Am J Cardiol 1977;40:449–53.

76. Copans H, Lakier JB, Kinsley RH, Colsen PR, Fritz VY, Barlow JB. Thrombosed Bjork-Shiley mitral prosthesis. Circulation 1980;61:169–74.

77. Chandraratna PAN, Lopez JM, Hildner FJ, Samet P, Ben-Zwi J. Diagnosis of Bjork-Shiley aortic valve dysfunction by echocardiography. Am Heart J 1976;91:318–24.

78. Kotler MN, Panidis I, Mintz GS, Ross J. Advances in cardiac valves. Clinical perspectives. DeBakey ME, ed. New York: Yorke Medical Books, 1983:213–28.

79. Pearlman AS, Scoblionko DP, Saal AK. Assessment of valvular heart disease by Doppler echocardiography. Clin Cardiol 1983;6:573–87.

80. Williams GA, Labovitz AJ. Doppler hemodynamic evaluation of prosthetic (Starr-Edwards and Bjork-Shiley) and bioprosthetic (Hancock and Carpentier-Edwards) cardiac valves. Valve function. Am J Cardiol 1985;56:325–32.

81. Hoit B, Dittrich H, Sahn D, Dalton N, Valdes-Cruz LM, Main J. Clinical studies of the efficacy of color flow mapping Doppler for evaluation of prosthetic heart valves, abstracted. J Am Coll Cardiol 1985;5:527.

82. Burggraff GW, Craige E. Echocardiographic studies of left ventricular wall motion and dimensions after valvular heart surgery. Am J Cardiol 1975;35:473–80.

83. Kotler MN, Mintz GS, Segal BL. Echophonocardiographic evaluation of normal and abnormal prosthetic valve function. Cardiovasc Clin 1983;13:117–45.

84. Rossiter SJ, Stimson EB, Oyer PE, et al. Prosthetic valve endocarditis. Comparison of tissue valves and mechanical valves. J Thorac Cardiovasc Surg 1978;76:795–803.

85. Ferrans VJ, Boyce SW, Billingham ME, et al. Infection of glutaraldehyde-preserved porcine valve heterografts. Am J Cardiol 1979;43:1123–36.

86. Oyer PE, Miller DC, Stinson EB, Reitz BA, Moreno-Cabra RJ, Shumway NE. Clinical durability of the (Hancock) porcine bioprosthetic valve. J Thorac Cardiovasc Surg 1980;80:824–33.

87. Magilligan DJ Jr, Lewis JW Jr, Java FM, et al. Spontaneous degeneration of porcine bioprosthetic valves. Ann Thorac Surg 1980;30:259–66.

88. Silver MM, Pollock J, Silver MD, et al. Calcification in porcine xenograft valves in children. Am J Cardiol 1980;45:685–9.

89. Sanders SP, Freed MD, Norwood WL, et al. Early failure of porcine valves implanted in children, abstracted. Am J Cardiol 1980;45:449.

90. Walker WE, Duncan JM, Frazier OH, et al. Early experience with the Ionescu-Shiley pericardial xenograft valve. J Thorac Cardiovasc Surg 1983;86:570-5.

91. Bloch WN Jr, Felner JM, Wickliffe C, et al. Echocardiogram of the porcine aortic bioprosthesis in the mitral position. Am J Cardiol 1976;38:293–8.

92. Wilkes HS, Berger M, Gallerstein PE, Berdoff RL, Goldberg E. Left ventricular outflow obstruction after aortic valve replacement: detection with continuous wave Doppler ultrasound recording. J Am Coll Cardiol 1983;1:550–3.

93. Rahimtoola SH. Valve replacement—a perspective. Am J Cardiol 1975;35:711–5.

94. Nanda NC, Gramiak R, Shah PM, et al. Echocardiographic assessment of left ventricular outflow width in the selection of mitral valve prosthesis. Circulation 1973;48:1208–14.

95. Denbow CE, Pluth JR, Giuliano ER. The role of echocardiography in the selection of mitral valve prosthesis. Am Heart J 1980;99:586–8.

96. Hasse J. Advances in cardiac valves. Clinical perspectives. DeBakey ME, ed. New York: Yorke Medical Books, 1983:115–23.

10
Ischemic Myocardial Disease

Natesa Pandian
Shan Shen Wang
Deeb Salem
John Funai

Coronary artery disease is the most common adult heart disease in the Western world. The hallmark of coronary artery disease is ischemia with resultant segmental left ventricular (LV) wall motion abnormalities. Ischemic myocardial disease is associated with transient and permanent anatomic and functional alterations of the myocardium and related valvular structures. A large body of work has established the increasing role of echocardiography in the evaluation of patients with ischemic heart disease. Since 1976, echocardiography has evolved from simple M-mode graphics to sophisticated imaging of the whole heart by two-dimensional echo and measurement of blood flow, hemodynamics, and cardiac output by Doppler techniques. Thus, echocardiography is uniquely suited to the study of structural and functional abnormalities in ischemic myocardial disease.

This chapter reviews the role of M-mode, two-dimensional, and Doppler echocardiographic techniques in the assessment of transient myocardial ischemia, acute myocardial infarction, and the complications of myocardial infarction. Furthermore, some innovative applications such as esophageal echocardiography, intraoperative epicardial imaging, and ultrasonic characterization of infarcted myocardium are discussed.

EFFECT OF ISCHEMIA AND INFARCTION ON MYOCARDIUM

Ischemia results in the rapid appearance of myocardial contraction and relaxation abnormalities, often within a few beats of reduction in coronary blood flow (1). The myocardium may regain normal function if the ischemia is transient. Persistent myocardial ischemia usually results in cell death within about 3 hours, and the resultant regional myocardial dysfunction persists. Myocardial territories are discretely supplied by the different coronary arteries; thus myocardial contractile dysfunction is usually focal. In the presence of such focal or regional myocardial dysfunction, other normally perfused regions of myocardium may contract more vigorously than normal, and global LV systolic function may be preserved. On the other hand, if the spatial extent of the myocardial dysfunction is initially large or enlarges, global LV function deteriorates, and pump failure may develop. In addition to systolic pump dysfunction, ischemia and infarction also decrease the diastolic compliance of the LV, which may impair LV filling. Thus, ischemia and infarction adversely affect the two critical functions of the LV: filling and pumping. Most of the clinical manifestations and prognostic consequences of ischemic myocardial disease are re-

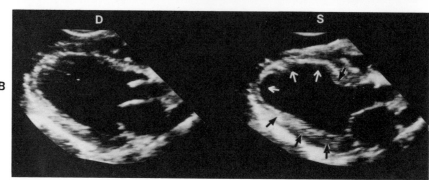

Figure 10.1. Effect of ischemia on regional myocardial contraction in a dog. (*A*) Long-axis two-dimensional echocardiographic views of the LV in diastole (D) and systole (S). All regions thicken and contract normally during systole, and the cavity becomes smaller. (*B*) After occlusion of the left anterior descending coronary artery, there is significant impairment of regional contraction. The mid and distal portions of the septum and the apex are akinetic while the basal septum and the posterior wall contract well. The LV cavity becomes dilated.

lated to these abnormalities. The impairment of regional and global function and the location and extent of myocardial damage may result in other complications such as ventricular aneurysm formation, papillary muscle injury leading to mitral regurgitation, and septal or free wall rupture.

Echocardiographic techniques provide unique noninvasive information concerning all of the anatomic and functional effects of ischemia and infarction. A two-dimensional echocardiogram, shown in Figure 10.1, illustrates the effect of acute occlusion of a coronary artery in a dog. In Figure 10.1A, the long-axis view shows that all regions of the LV myocardium, the septum, the apex, and the posterior wall, contract normally. Following occlusion of the proximal left anterior descending coronary artery (Figure 10.1B), the mid and apical portions of the septum and the LV apex become akinetic, while the unaffected basal portion of the septum and the posterior wall contract normally. Besides the regional contraction abnormality, the whole LV cavity is enlarged. Although coronary artery disease results in segmental wall motion abnormalities that may not be detected by M-mode echocardiography, all regions of the myocardium can be visualized with two-dimensional echocardiography by obtaining images from the conventional planes. In Figure 10.2, short-axis imaging of the LV allows detection of wall motion abnormalities of the inferoposterior wall and posterior portion of septum due to ischemia induced by circumflex coronary artery occlusion. In the following sections, the echocardiographic evalua-

tion of such myocardial abnormalities in humans following ischemia and infarction are reviewed.

IMAGING TECHNIQUES

M-Mode Echocardiography

Prior to the advent of two-dimensional echocardiography, M-mode echocardiography was used in the evaluation of the LV in ischemic heart disease (2). The value of the M-mode technique in this condition is limited because of the inherent inability of M-mode to examine the LV in its entirety. Coronary artery disease is a focal disease characterized by regional myocardial involvement during ischemia or infarction. Therefore, unless the narrow M-mode beam traverses the ischemic or infarcted muscle region, the abnormality may not be identified. Slow scanning of the whole LV with M-mode may permit detection of some of the abnormalities. However, the LV is a three-dimensional chamber, and even the most careful M-mode scanning cannot exclude major wall motion abnormalities. Furthermore, M-mode echocardiography cannot reliably estimate the extent of the regional abnormalities. Nevertheless, the M-mode technique does have a role, albeit small, in the evaluation of ischemic myocardium. Because of its excellent temporal sampling capability, changes in wall thickness, wall motion, and thickening can be depicted by M-mode echocardiography. Figure 10.3 shows a normal LV with the M-mode beam transecting the ventricular chamber at the level of the atrioventricular (AV) valve chordae. The interventricu-

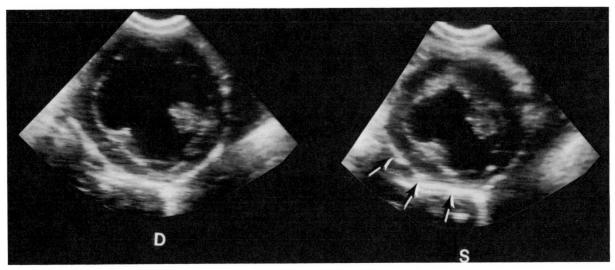

Figure 10.2.   Short-axis two-dimensional echocardiographic views showing the effect of circumflex coronary artery occlusion on regional LV myocardial contraction. The inferoposterior wall and the posterior portion of the septum exhibit systolic wall thinning and dyskinesis. D = diastole; S = systole.

lar septum (IVS) and the posterior wall are well defined, allowing accurate measurements of wall thickness and motion of the segment being examined. Inward endocardial motion and systolic wall thickening seen in Figure 10.3 are fundamental properties of the normal myocardium. Ischemia affects both of these characteristics, and Figure 10.4 illustrates the effect of

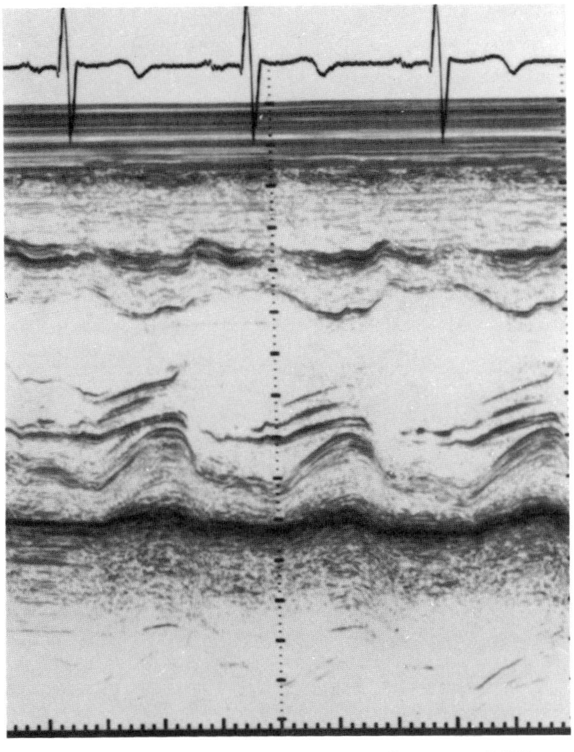

Figure 10.3.   M-mode echocardiogram of a normal LV. Both the IVS and the posterior wall (PW) exhibit normal systolic inward motion and thickening.

infarction on myocardial function. In this patient with a posterior myocardial infarction, the posterior wall fails to move inwardly and does not exhibit normal systolic thickening. This is in contrast to the IVS, which is of normal thickness, contracts with concentric inward wall motion, and displays normal systolic wall thickening. Similarly, M-mode studies obtained from patients with anteroseptal myocardial infarction display decreased septal thickening and excursion and normal posterior wall motion. An old transmural myocardial infarction results not only in reduced wall thickness but also scarring (3). Such a muscle region appears thinner and exhibits more intense echo reflectance due to the different acoustic properties of the myocardial fibrosis and the normal myocardium. Thus, abnormal regions of LV myocardium following infarction can only be imaged and defined if the M-mode beam is directed through them. During a conventional M-mode examination of the LV, the beam is directed through the IVS and the posterior wall. Such a beam orientation may not detect an abnormality occurring in an anterolateral wall region. Positioning the transducer laterally on the chest wall and directing the beam medially may allow definition of the structural and functional changes of the anterolateral wall. Although such approaches might be useful in selected cases, there are major limitations in the M-mode assessment of coronary disease. Because the M-mode technique samples only a relatively small portion of the LV at any moment, the translational and rotational motion of the heart is difficult to appreciate and may unduly influence wall motion analysis. Such difficulties in practical performance and interpretation limit the usefulness of the M-mode technique in coronary artery disease.

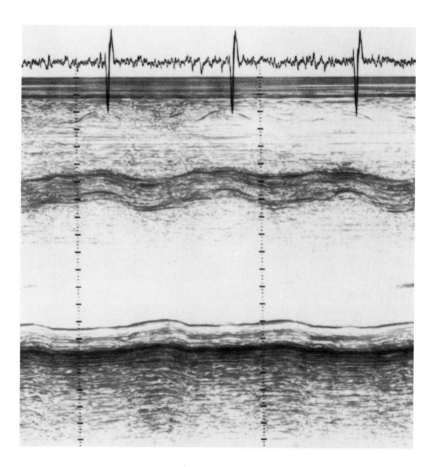

Figure 10.4. M-mode echocardiogram from a patient with posterior myocardial infarction. The diastolic thickness and systolic motion and thickening of the septum are in the normal range. By contrast, the posterior LV wall is thin, and its inward motion and thickening during systole are drastically reduced. The LV cavity is dilated.

Two-Dimensional Echocardiography

Two-dimensional echocardiography overcomes many of these difficulties. It is possible to obtain technically adequate two-dimensional echocardiographic studies in almost all patients with coronary artery disease. It allows examination of the whole LV chamber using the parasternal, apical, and subcostal approaches. Rotation of the transducer at these sites allows imaging of the LV in a number of different planes. Such an examination provides not only images at different levels in different planes, but enables three-dimensional representation of LV structure and function. This chapter concentrates primarily on the use of two-dimensional echocardiography in the evaluation of ischemic myocardial disease.

MYOCARDIAL INFARCTION

Millions of adult patients are hospitalized each year with acute myocardial infarction. A significant number of these patients die before receiving medical attention. The early survivors follow several different clinical courses. About 50 percent have an uncomplicated course, while 15 percent to 20 percent die in the hospital due to complications of myocardial ischemia. During the mid-1970s to mid-1980s, the management of patients with acute myocardial infarction changed from passive observation to active intervention in an attempt to arrest ongoing ischemia and to limit infarction size. The questions that arise in a patient admitted with suspicion of acute myocardial infarction concern the presence or absence of an acute myocardial infarction, the location and extent of infarction, the effect of infarction on global LV function, and the presence or absence of associated complications. Two-dimensional and Doppler echocardiographic techniques currently play a major role in the evaluation of the function and size of the infarcted myocardium (4, 5). In contrast to other methods such as electrocardiography (ECG), cardiac enzyme determinations, hemodynamic data, and radioisotope scans, echocardiography allows serial assessment of the anatomic changes occurring after an infarction, and the effects of myocardial infarction on LV and right ventricular (RV) functions.

Detection and Localization of Regional Myocardial Dysfunction

Abnormalities in regional LV wall motion occur very rapidly following ischemia, even before infarction develops. The affected myocardial region becomes thinner, and both wall motion and systolic wall thickening are reduced. The magnitude of such effects varies; the

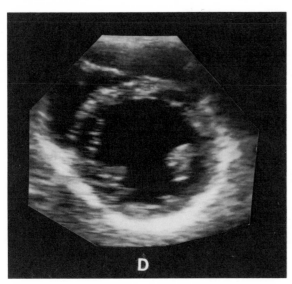 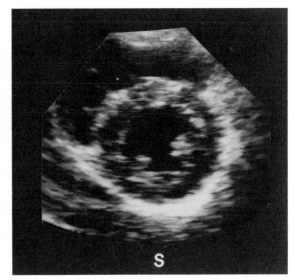

Figure 10.5. Short-axis two-dimensional echocardiogram from a patient with a normal ventricle without myocardial infarction. All regions of the myocardium contract normally. D = diastole; S = systole.

myocardium may exhibit decreased motion (hypokinesis) or thickening, absence of any significant motion (akinesis) or thickening, or systolic outward bulging (dyskinesis) with systolic thinning. These abnormalities are readily detected by two-dimensional echocardiography. Experimental studies have indicated that two-dimensional echocardiography correlates well with sonomicrometry and force-gauge mapping in detection of regional dyskinesis during ischemia and infarction (6, 7). Dyskinesis and increased brightness of the involved myocardium have been noted on echocardiograms following experimental myocardial infarction (8). In addition to endocardial motion, analysis of systolic wall thickening provides precise information regarding changes in myocardial contractility during ischemia (6). Previous studies have indicated that wall motion and wall thickening abnormalities measured by two-dimensional echocardiography correlate well with pathologic infarct size and location both in animal models and in humans (7–12). Further, they give an indication of the myocardial area at risk of infarction following occlusion (13). Thus, the presence of a regional wall motion abnormality in the setting of coronary artery disease indicates the presence of ischemia or infarction in most circumstances. If the infarction exceeds one-third of the transmural thickness of a myocardial region, systolic wall thinning results (12). However, the absence of regional wall motion abnormalities does not exclude acute myocardial infarction. Infarctions involving less than one-third of the transmural thickness of a myocardial segment or less than one-third of the circumferential extent of the segment may be associated with no changes in wall motion or in systolic wall thickening. Thus, a small

subendocardial infarction may not always be associated with wall motion or thickening abnormalities (14). Early clinical studies compared two-dimensional echocardiography to LV angiograms and demonstrated a good correlation between the two techniques in the detection of regional myocardial dysynergy (15). In the past decade it has become apparent that two-dimensional echocardiography is superior to contrast angiography because it enables a three-dimensional interrogation of the LV and detection of myocardial contractile abnormalities in areas that are not border-forming on the angiographic LV silhouettes. Figures 10.5 and 10.6 from two different patients illustrate the utility of short-axis imaging. Figure 10.5 is from a patient admitted with chest pain in whom a myocardial infarction was not detected. In this short-axis image, the entire circumference of myocardium contracts normally. By contrast, Figure 10.6 was obtained from a patient with a documented inferior myocardial infarction. The inferoposterior LV wall regions are akinetic while the anterior portion of the septum and the anterior and lateral wall regions contract normally. A parasternal long-axis view in this same patient (Fig. 10.7) discloses normal septal contraction but an akinetic posterior wall.

Old infarctions are characterized by muscle thinning, fibrosis, and scarring. Such areas appear thin with bright echoes on two-dimensional echocardiograms (2). Figure 10.8 shows such an image from a patient with old anteroseptal infarction. The septum is thin with high-intensity echoes; on real-time viewing, the septum exhibited akinesis and absence of systolic thickening.

A comprehensive two-dimensional echocardiographic

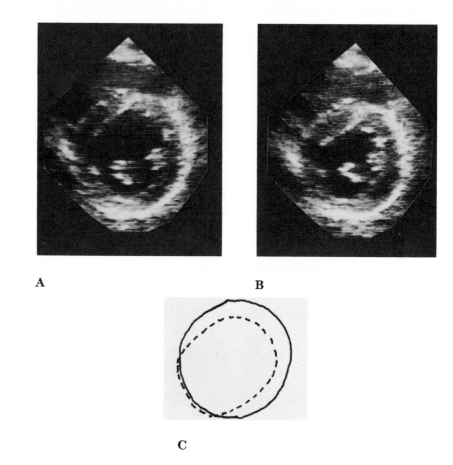

A   B

C

Figure 10.6. Short-axis two-dimensional echocardiogram from a patient with an inferior myocardial infarction. The inferoposterior wall regions are thin and dyskinetic (*C*), while the remainder of the myocardium contracts and thickens vigorously. (*A*) Diastolic image. (*B*) Systolic image.

examination of the heart in a patient with myocardial infarction should include imaging from many different views. Imaging from parasternal long- and multiple short-axis imaging planes and apical and subcostal imaging planes provides information concerning the location of myocardial dysynergy and the three-dimensional spatial extent of the infarcted area. In anterior myocardial infarctions in general, the anterior two-thirds of the IVS, the anterior wall and anterolateral wall, and the LV apical region are involved in regional dysfunction. Following inferior or posterior myocardial infarctions, the inferoposterior myocardial region be-

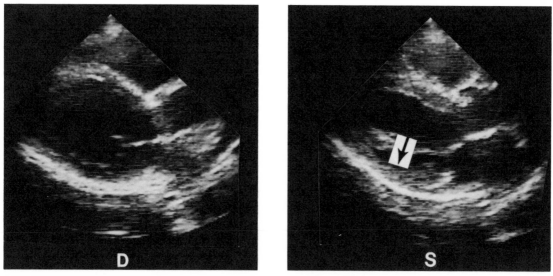

D   S

Figure 10.7. Parasternal long-axis view from the same patient shown in Figure 10.6, displaying impaired contraction of the posterior wall and normal contraction of the septum. D = diastole; S = systole.

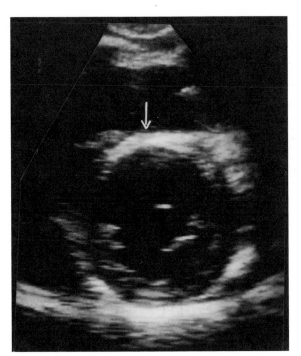

Figure 10.8. Two-dimensional echocardiogram in an old septal myocardial infarction. In this short-axis view, the scarred septum (*arrow*) appears thin with high-intensity bright echoes.

comes dysynergic, which additionally usually involves the posterior one-third of the IVS. Care should be exercised to ensure that all areas of the myocardium are imaged adequately using optimal image orientations. The LV apex, for example, is generally not well visualized in the conventional parasternal long-axis view. By moving the transducer lower and laterally on the chest, the long-axis plane of the LV apex can be imaged. This view should always be employed whenever apical dysynergy is suspected. Apical long-axis and four-chamber views should also be used to delineate the apex. The three-dimensional geometry of the apex resembles the tip of a cone, and this topography is greatly distorted by apical infarctions. Graded 180-degree rotation of the transducer at the apical region enables visualization of all aspects of the apex. Changing the depth of the image along with appropriate alterations in the ultrasound gain settings to "magnify" the apex should also be performed. The apical views, while unique among imaging techniques, are also associated with a problem inherent to echocardiography. Since the incident ultrasound beam is parallel to the walls of the LV, visualization and spatial resolution of these structures may be suboptimal. Careful adjustment of the ultrasound equipment settings and real-time viewing of the images unmask the regional abnormalities. Care should be exercised in the interpretation of wall motion in short-axis views. If only a suboptimal short-axis imaging plane is obtained, great care must

be taken during the interpretation of off-axis views since these may yield artifactual regional wall motion abnormalities. A tangential short-axis view at the mitral valve level is particularly troublesome where the motion of the posterior region of the AV groove or mitral annulus is sufficiently irregular in the normal heart to be mistaken for a dyskinetic LV posterior wall. Correcting the transducer angulation to avoid the annulus region and visualize the LV myocardium below it provides an optimal short-axis view.

Occasionally, an inferior infarction may extend into the RV free wall and compromise RV function. Since the inferior and lateral free wall regions of the RV are more often involved in infarction, the parasternal long-axis view may not provide sufficient information on RV infarction because this view primarily transects the RV outflow tract area. Lower level short-axis views, apical four-chamber views, and subcostal views are necessary to visualize the RV free wall adequately, and these views should be routinely employed in the examination of the RV when RV infarction is suspected. The entity of RV infarction is increasingly recognized. Early diagnosis of RV infarction is critical, particularly when associated with hypotension. This will dictate acute management that differs considerably from the conventional care of isolated LV infarction. This management involves the administration of fluids and cautious use of drugs such as nitroglycerin. Clinical features including jugular venous distention, elevated right heart pressures, and abnormalities in the right precordial ECG leads are useful in the recognition of RV infarction. The detection of regional RV wall motion abnormalities is often diagnostic. Hence, it is essential to employ the echocardiographic views described earlier to visualize all portions of the RV wall. Figure 10.9 is a subcostal four-chamber view recorded in a patient with RV infarction. It disclosed a dilated RV and an akinetic RV free wall.

Another important concern in the identification of regional contraction abnormalities of the LV or RV by two-dimensional echocardiography is the heterogeneity of normal myocardial function (12, 16, 17). While the absence of motion and thickening or the presence of frank systolic bulging and systolic thinning is clearly abnormal and indicates ischemia or infarction, reductions of normal thickening and motion (hypokinesis) may occur without ischemia. Experimental work has indicated that as blood flow progressively decreases in a region of myocardium, normal contraction is replaced initially by hypokinesis and later by akinesis and dyskinesis (18). Thus, hypokinesis is also an indicator of ischemic myocardium, but it can pose a problem in clinical interpretation because of heterogeneity in contraction within the normal ventricle. Thus,

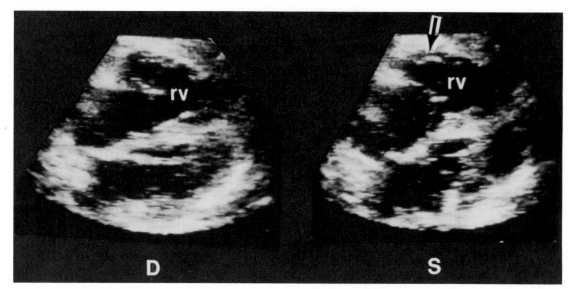

Figure 10.9. Subcostal four-chamber view from a patient with right ventricular (RV) infarction. The RV free wall (*arrow*) is akinetic, and the RV cavity is dilated. D = diastole; S = systole.

while hypokinesis is a sensitive indicator of abnormal myocardial perfusion, it is not highly specific.

Even dyskinesis, particularly of the IVS, may not be specific for ischemia occasionally. Left bundle branch block, altered conduction sequence due to RV pacing, and certain types of Wolff-Parkinson-White syndrome are associated with paradoxic septal motion. Similarly, RV volume overload or cardioplegic cardiac surgery results in paradoxic septal motion. The septum, however, is not thinner than normal and thickens during contraction, so that in these situations evaluation of the septal motion in the light of associated abnormalities prevents misinterpretation.

The ability to localize regional dyskinesis and thereby the infarction provides information on the coronary artery involvement. Correlative studies of two-dimensional echocardiography with ECG, LV cine-angiography, coronary arteriography, radionuclide ventriculography, and postmortem findings have shown excellent correspondence (9, 15, 19–22). The location of the infarct also offers information of prognostic value. Anterior myocardial infarcts are more frequently associated with complications than inferior myocardial infarcts. Inferolateral infarctions have a more serious prognosis than isolated inferior infarctions. Furthermore, delineation of the initial site and size of infarction permits recognition of the topographic changes that accompany the evolution or extension of an acute myocardial infarction.

Quantitation of Regional Myocardial Dysfunction and Infarction

A number of investigators have clearly demonstrated that the spatial extent of regional wall contraction abnormalities relates to the size of myocardial infarction. Experimental studies have shown that quantitation of regional dysfunction based on both endocardial motion and systolic wall thickening correlates well with pathologic infarct size (7, 10, 11). Analysis of systolic wall thickening abnormalities provides a more accurate index of the extent of regional dysfunction (12). As pointed out earlier, however, the absence of contraction abnormalities does not exclude infarction, but if an infarction is present in that setting, it is often very small and limited to the subendocardium (10, 12).

A number of approaches have been employed to quantify the spatial extent of myocardial infarction using two-dimensional echocardiography. One approach is to acquire multiple short-axis views from base to apex, then measure the circumferential extent of dysynergic myocardium at each level, and finally compute a total LV myocardial area that is involved in myocardial infarction, expressed as a percentage of the LV. Another approach is to employ apical long-axis or four-chamber views, define the extent of abnormally contracting myocardial segments, and compute the total LV area involved in regional dysfunction. Both these approaches can be combined to express a three-dimensional spatial extent of myocardial infarction. Often, the spatial extent of LV dysynergy may overestimate the size of myocardial infarction because the adjacent nonischemic myocardial segments also display wall motion abnormalities. Experimental work has shown that an area adjacent to an infarct, even when associated with normal blood flow, can exhibit regional dysynergy (23). This is probably due to a tethering effect. Nevertheless, the determination of the spatial extent of myocardial dysynergy does give information about the extent of ischemia or infarction in a given LV. This is particularly useful when serial studies are utilized to assess the course of myocardial infarction and its effects on LV chamber architecture and function.

Quantitative assessment of regional myocardial dysfunction and its consequent effects on LV function has played a major role in assessing the acute and chronic prognosis of patients who have suffered acute myocardial infarctions. Patients with a larger extent of regional dysfunction suffer more complications and have a higher mortality (24–26). Serial quantitation of regional myocardial dysfunction may also be of value in assessing the effect of interventions aimed at reducing infarct size (27). Animal investigations and human studies have indicated that the extent of regional myocardial dysfunction does not change from the first few hours to the first 2 days after the acute infarction. Thus, increases in the extent of regional dysfunction may indicate extension of myocardial injury. The relationships of coronary obstruction, infarct size, and the extent of regional myocardial function in humans, however, are complex. The presence of coronary collaterals, previous myocardial infarctions, and spontaneous myocardial reperfusion may alter these simple relationships. Further regional myocardial dysfunction may persist for hours following prolonged ischemia and "stunning" of the myocardium without definite infarction. These factors pose problems in using quantitative measurements of the extent of regional myocardial dyskinesis to assess the amount of myocardium salvaged following interventions. This limitation occurs not only with echocardiography but with all invasive and noninvasive imaging methods. A recent study indicated that reperfusion decreases the extent of regional myocardial dysfunction, but subsequently, the relationship between infarct size and myocardial dyskinesis becomes poorer (28).

Serial echocardiographic evaluations of infarcted myocardium indicate that the extent of regional LV wall motion abnormalities gradually decreases as the infarct scar contracts and becomes smaller (29). Myocardial infarction also results in certain topographic changes in the LV at and adjacent to the infarcted area. Regional cavity dilatation and a decrease in wall thickness occur in a considerable number of patients. In one clinical study that utilized two-dimensional echocardiography, eight of 28 patients with acute myocardial infarction demonstrated infarct expansion, and these patients were found to have a significantly greater 8-week mortality (30). Infarct expansion may be an important mechanism of the progressive LV dilatation, and detection of this abnormality may identify this high-risk group so that aggressive management can be instituted.

Evaluation of Global Left Ventricular Function

The integrated functional characteristics of the different myocardial regions constitute global LV function. When a sufficiently large amount of myocardium becomes dysfunctional, global LV function is impaired during both systole and diastole. Many studies have demonstrated unequivocally that global LV systolic function is an important determinant of morbidity and mortality. The theoretic aspects and practical applications of two-dimensional echocardiography in the assessment of global LV size and systolic function have been discussed in detail in Chapter 9. In general, two-dimensional echocardiography compares well with other invasive and noninvasive imaging techniques in providing information about global pump function. Doppler echocardiography is another technique that allows serial assessment of global LV function (31). Flow velocity across different valves can be recorded, and cardiac output can be calculated as the product of the flow velocity integral and great vessel or valve area. Aortic flow velocity recordings are particularly useful in the assessment of LV systolic performance. Figure 10.10 shows aortic flow velocity waveforms before and after a large infarction in a dog. The large infarction diminished the LV pump function, and consequently, there were reductions in the peak velocity, the velocity integral, and the rate of flow acceleration. Similar changes have been observed during transient ischemia in humans (32). Serial Doppler measurements of aortic flow velocities are useful to monitor the effect of interventions on cardiac output.

Left ventricular diastolic function is also impaired in ischemic heart disease (33). Myocardial relaxation is an energy-dependent process that can be significantly affected by ischemia. Relaxation abnormalities are associated with altered LV compliance, which results in impaired diastolic filling (34, 35). Analysis of the mitral flow velocity profile has shown that diastolic inflow changes are good indicators of filling dysfunction (36). Changes in mitral valve flow occur during both acute ischemia and infarction (37, 38). Figure 10.11 displays the effect of acute ischemia on mitral flow velocity. Compared to the normal flow pattern in the control state shown in Figure 10.11A, ischemia results in diminution of early filling velocity and accentuation of late filling velocity (during atrial contraction). Similar patterns have been demonstrated in patients with myocardial infarction (38). Furthermore, such clinical studies may lead to routine bedside protocols that will direct the management of acute myocardial infarction according to changes in diastolic filling patterns.

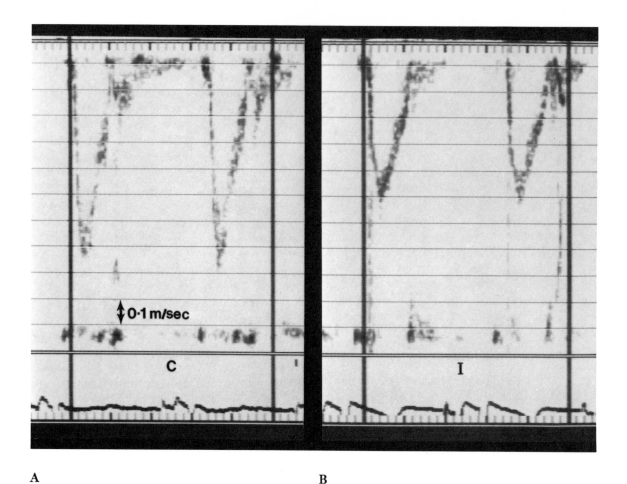

A   B

Figure 10.10. Doppler echocardiographic recording of aortic blood flow velocity portraying the effect of ischemia (I) and consequent depressed LV function on aortic flow in a dog. (*A*) Normal flow velocity with impaired LV function. (*B*) During ischemia, peak velocity, the velocity integral, and rate of flow acceleration are diminished. C = control.

Complications of Ischemic Myocardial Disease and Myocardial Infarction

The complications of myocardial infarction include extension of the infarct and severe LV dysfunction resulting in pump failure or severe ventricular tachyarrhythmias and fibrillation. Some patients who survive infarctions develop LV dilatation and permanent severe muscle dysfunction with marked reduction in cardiac output, so-called chronic ischemic cardiomyopathy. Other mechanical complications leading to severe hemodynamic deterioration are ventricular aneurysm formation, ventricular septal rupture, and papillary muscle dysfunction or rupture. Most of these entities are potentially treatable with surgery and the chances for survival can be dramatically improved by optimally timed surgical intervention. Hence, prompt diagnosis of the mechanical complications of myocardial infarction is of critical importance. All of these mechanical complications of myocardial infarction can be detected by echocardiographic techniques (39).

Ischemic Cardiomyopathy

Ischemic heart disease is the major cause of congestive heart failure in the mid-1980s. The use of the term "ischemic cardiomyopathy" is relatively recent. It describes patients with dilated hearts due to occlusive coronary artery disease. These patients may present without angina pectoris, and although a history of repeated myocardial infarction is often documented, there are a small percentage of patients with ischemic cardiomyopathy and no definitive history of myocardial infarction. The ventricular size, morphology, and function in these patients are indistinguishable from those in patients with idiopathic dilated cardiomyopathy.

The two-dimensional echocardiogram in Figure 10.12 illustrates a dilated LV with diffusely impaired function. Regional variability of myocardial dysfunction may be present and pronounced. More frequently, however, there is severe global depression in contraction with chamber dilatation, and thus, diagnosis of ischemic heart disease as the etiology of the dilated cardiomyopathy is not always possible. Mitral regurgi-

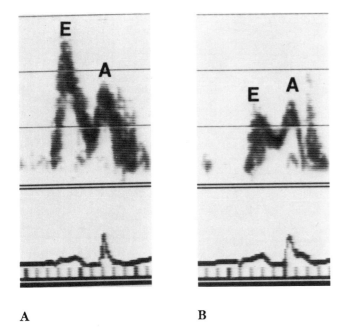

A   **B**

Figure 10.11.   Doppler echocardiographic recording of mitral blood flow velocity illustrating a normal filling pattern (*A*) and an altered filling pattern secondary to ischemia (*B*). During ischemia, the early filling velocity (E) is decreased relative to the late diastolic filling velocity during atrial contraction (A).

tation is often present due to inadequate coaptation of mitral leaflets, which is secondary to LV cavity dilatation. If the cardiomyopathy has been long-standing, then the right heart chambers may also be enlarged. Left ventricular thrombi may be present as the low flow state enhances clot formation.

Left Ventricular Aneurysm

Left ventricular aneurysm is a common complication among survivors of myocardial infarction. Infarct ex-

pansion and thinning of the infarcted muscle eventually result in an outpouching of the LV in that region. Aneurysms occur four times more commonly in the apex and anterior wall than in the posterior wall. Two-dimensional echocardiography is the technique of choice for the assessment of a ventricular aneurysm (40). It appears as an outpouching of the ventricular myocardium with usually well-defined borders. Occasionally, the margins may be less well demarcated. A fully developed aneurysm as shown in Figure 10.13 displays discrete borders even during diastole. Further expansion or bulging during systole occurs in the aneurysmal region as the rest of the unaffected myocardium contracts inward. Occasionally, the aneurysmal wall may exhibit akinesis rather than dyskinesis. A septal aneurysm is portrayed in Figure 10.14 with the previously described topographic abnormalities. Left ventricular aneurysms may be associated with continuing angina, arrhythmias, congestive heart failure, or embolic events from thrombi within an aneurysm. Figure 10.15 shows an apical aneurysm harboring a clot. Although aneurysms at other sites are less common, they do occur in inferior, posterior, or posterolateral myocardial regions (Figs. 10.16 and 10.17). Two-dimensional echocardiography accurately delineates the location and extent of LV aneurysms and the presence or absence of associated thrombi. Right ventricular aneurysms are rare but can occur following RV infarction (Fig. 10.18).

Pseudoaneurysm or False Aneurysm

Pseudoaneurysm or false aneurysm is a relatively uncommon complication following myocardial infarction. Pseudoaneurysm results when the myocardial infarction leads to perforation of the LV free wall and forms a localized hemopericardium limited by adher-

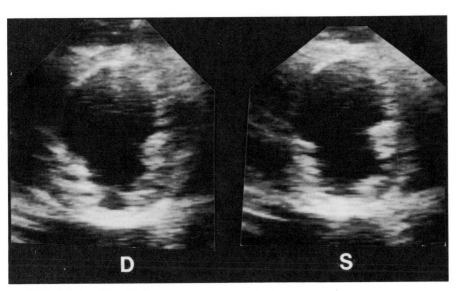

Figure 10.12.   Short-axis two-dimensional echocardiogram from a patient with ischemic cardiomyopathy. The ventricular cavity is dilated, and LV contraction is severely decreased in all myocardial segments. D = diastole; S = systole.

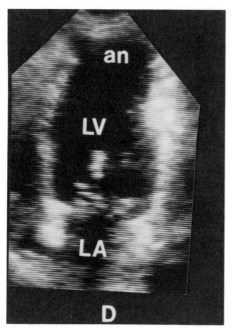
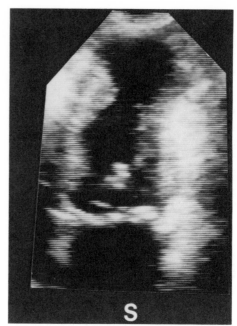

Figure 10.13.   Apical two-dimensional echocardiographic view of an apical LV aneurysm (an). Dilatation and outpouching of the apex are noted in diastole (D). With systole (S), the aneurysmal area is dyskinetic while the basal portions of the LV contract normally.

ent parietal pericardium instead of resulting in tamponade. Two-dimensional echocardiography shows a regional pouchlike configuration of the LV with discontinuity of the myocardial echoes at the neck of the pouch (Fig. 10.19). The differentiation of a true aneurysm from a pseudoaneurysm may be difficult and involves identifying the typically narrow neck of a pseudoaneurysm or a wide margin surrounding a true aneurysm (41). Pseudoaneurysms are commonly filled with thrombus. Two-dimensional echocardiography is superior to angiography in definitively diagnosing pseudoaneurysm since two-dimensional echocardiography

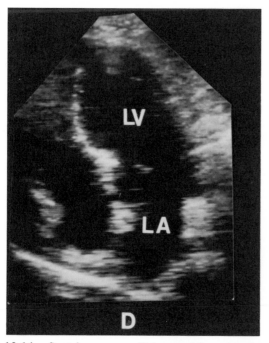
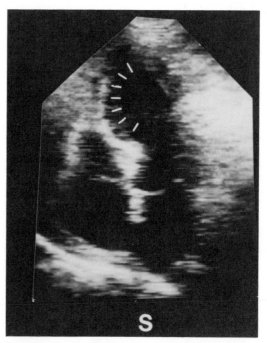

Figure 10.14.   Septal aneurysm. This apical four-chamber two-dimensional echocardiogram discloses thinning of the distal half of the IVS, along with regional dilatation and systolic dyskinesis. The apex is also involved in regional dysfunction. D = diastole, S = systole.

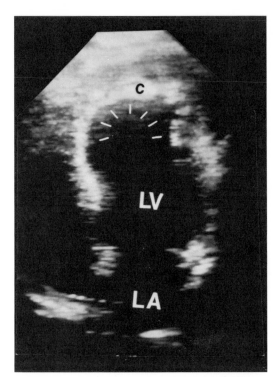

Figure 10.15. Apical LV aneurysm. Apical two-dimensional echocardiographic view demonstrates a dilated aneurysmal apex with a layered clot (C) in the aneurysm. The borders of the aneurysm are not as well demarcated as in Figures 10.13 and 10.14.

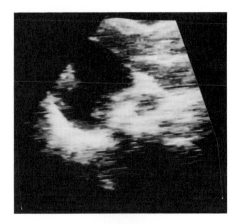

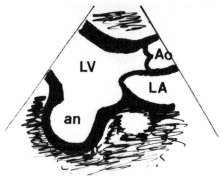

Figure 10.16. Parasternal long-axis two-dimensional echocardiogram depicting a posterior wall aneurysm (an). Posterior or inferior wall aneurysms are less common than apical aneurysms. Ao = aorta.

enables visualization of the entire extent of the abnormality while angiographic dye might not opacify a pseudoaneurysmal cavity if it is occupied by thrombus. Furthermore, flow within the pseudoaneurysm may be documented by Doppler.

Left Ventricular Thrombus

Left ventricular thrombus is common in myocardial infarction, particularly within LV aneurysms. Thrombus formation is more frequent following anterior myocardial infarction than inferior myocardial infarction. Ventricular thrombus is visualized by two-dimensional echocardiography as a distinct mass of echoes present in systole and diastole that appears to be discrete from the myocardial wall (Chap. 13) (42). Well-defined contraction abnormalities are usually present in the subjacent ventricular myocardium. Thrombi may appear as a single- or multilobed intracavitary mass. They may be layered, discrete, protuberant, mobile, or strandlike with smooth or irregular borders. A layered thrombus may not project into the LV cavity while globular and linear thrombi often do (Fig. 10.20). Thrombi have been visualized as early as 5 to 6 days after infarction, and the majority occur in the region of the cardiac apex adjacent to a dysynergic area (42).

Occasionally, the thrombus may be freely mobile, and the luminal aspect of the thrombus can exhibit motion independent of the adjacent wall motion. Recent work has suggested that thrombi of a protruding type embolize more frequently than layered thrombi. In one study, free intracavitary mobility of the thrombus was present in more than half of those patients with embolic events and virtually absent in the group without (43). Occasionally, echocardiographic artifact or noise may simulate a thrombus. Artifacts are usually less well defined than thrombi, do not move with the underlying myocardial wall, and are often present only in systole or diastole in a single echocardiographic view. Therefore, confirmation of a suspected thrombus requires visualization in multiple orthogonal views.

Ventricular Septal Rupture

Ventricular septal rupture is a well-recognized mechanical complication of myocardial infarction. Untreated, it is often fatal. Survival has been dramatically improved by appropriately timed surgical intervention. Hence, prompt diagnosis is critical. Ventricular septal rupture may complicate infarction of either anterior or inferior walls. When inferior LV infarction is associated

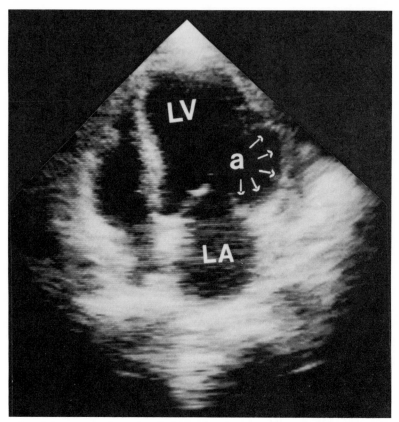

Figure 10.17.   Aneurysm involving posterolateral wall. Four-chamber two-dimensional echocardiographic view of a posterolateral wall aneurysm (*a with arrows*). (Reproduced courtesy of Dr. Edgar Schick, Boston University Medical Center.)

with RV infarction, the incidence of septal rupture is strikingly high. This high incidence of septal rupture occurs because the RV and the posterior IVS as well as the posterior LV free wall are all involved in the infarction. Rupture of the septum typically occurs at the junction of the infarcted necrotic myocardium and the noninfarcted myocardium within the first week of infarction. The rupture site and adjacent infarct are typically thinned and aneurysmal; indeed, regional infarct expansion may be a precursor of rupture. Two-dimensional echocardiography provides immediate and detailed information about the presence of a ventricular septal rupture (39, 44, 45). The presence, location, and size can be determined by two-dimensional echocardiography, and in addition to demonstrating the defect, the extent of underlying myocardial involvement can often be determined. Ventricular septal defects following anterior myocardial infarction usually occur in the anteroapical portion of the septum (Fig. 10.21). In patients with inferior myocardial infarction, the defect often occurs in the posterior half of the IVS. Careful two-dimensional echocardiographic examination of the septum reveals the defect in the septum. The myocardium at the site of the septal defect appears thinner than normal or even aneurysmal (Fig. 10.22). During systole, the septal aneurysm usually bulges into the RV with widening of the defect. Abnormalities of

mitral leaflets or papillary muscles are not generally seen in these patients. Often, however, because the anatomy of septal rupture is that of a serpiginous dissection tract rather than a stab wound, a large well-defined defect may not always be visualized. Off-axis images may be necessary to delineate the ventricular septal defect (5). While contrast echocardiography can be used in an attempt to identify a defect, absence of a positive or negative contrast crossover does not definitely exclude a shunt (Chap. 18).

Pulsed and color flow Doppler echocardiography aids in differentiating ventricular septal rupture from mitral regurgitation (Fig. 10.23) (5, 46). In the presence of a ventricular septal defect, Doppler examination usually reveals the presence of turbulent high-velocity left-to-right flow across the septal defect. Careful mapping of the entire IVS is required to delineate the location and direction of abnormal flow jets. Besides detecting the presence of a ventricular septal defect, Doppler echocardiographic quantitation of the pulmonary and aortic blood flows gives an indication of the severity of the left-to-right shunt.

Papillary Muscle Dysfunction and Rupture

Dysfunction of the mitral apparatus and support structures occurs in a number of patients with myocardial

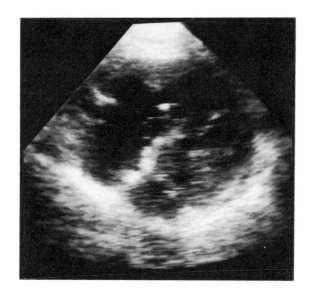

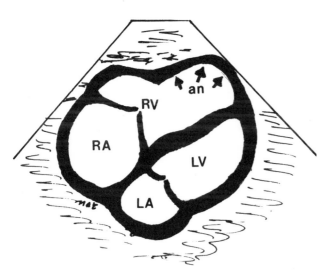

Figure 10.18. Right ventricular aneurysm. Subcostal four-chamber view showing an aneurysm (an with arrows) involving the RV free wall. This patient has sustained an inferior myocardial infarction with extensive RV infarction. The RV cavity is dilated as well. RA = right atrium.

infarction and can lead to worsening heart failure or angina. If there is active disruption of either the papillary muscle or of the other subvalvular apparatus such as tendinous chords, severe mitral regurgitation may occur suddenly, requiring surgical correction. More commonly, the papillary muscle involvement is less severe and is associated with only minimal mitral regurgitation due to improper coaptation of the mitral leaflets. Isolated papillary muscle necrosis alone does not always result in mitral regurgitation. The subjacent myocardium may also be ischemic or infarcted with resultant dysynergy. Such regional dyskinesis and cavity dilatation lead to apical displacement of the mitral valve coaptation and incomplete closure, which result in mitral regurgitation. The papillary muscle may ap-

pear small by two-dimensional echocardiography, with increasing echo brightness as the infarction organizes and becomes fibrotic. The subjacent myocardium is often thinned and dysynergic. The mitral leaflets, when closed in systole, are displaced apically instead of coapting at the level of the mitral annulus as in a normal ventricle (Fig. 10.24) (47). Occurrence of mitral valve prolapse is uncommon in the presence of simple papillary muscle dysfunction but does occur with papillary muscle rupture when the resultant flail leaflet prolapses into the left atrium (LA) during systole (Fig. 10.25). If there is transection of the papillary muscle (39), a discrete mass may be seen attached to the flailing anterior or posterior leaflet on the two-dimensional echocardiogram. Papillary muscle rupture is often associated with a new holosystolic murmur. This physical finding is not specific for mitral apparatus dysfunction because it also occurs following rupture of the ventricular septum. Both conditions may be associated with acute and profound hemodynamic collapse including severe pulmonary congestion. The murmurs in both entities are also typically associated with a palpable precordial thrill. While it has been alleged that papillary muscle rupture can be distinguished from ventricular septal rupture based on the location of the thrill and murmur (i.e., mitral regurgitation at the LV

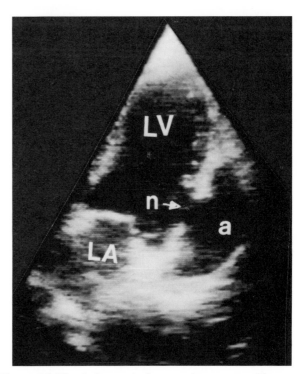

Figure 10.19. Left ventricular pseudoaneurysm. The pseudoaneurysm (a) is seen as an encapsulated cavity with communication to the LV cavity via a narrow neck (n). Pseudoaneurysms occur when a free wall rupture is sealed and loculated by the pericardium. They are often filled with clots. (Reproduced courtesy of Dr. Edgar Schick, Boston University Medical Center.)

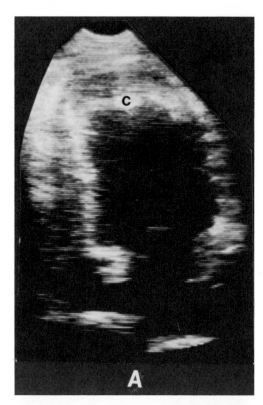

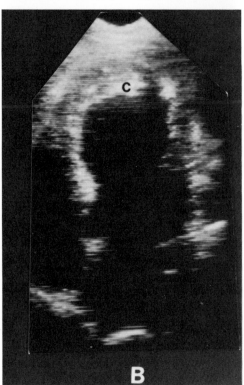

Figure 10.20. Left ventricular clot. Apical two-dimensional echocardiographic views from two different patients who had antero-apical myocardial infarction. The apexes are aneurysmal and filled with clots (C). (*A*) The clot is a layered type. (*B*) The clot is globular. Organized clots are generally brighter than the surrounding myocardium. An apical aneurysm is the most common site for LV clot formation. The subjacent myocardium is almost always dysynergic.

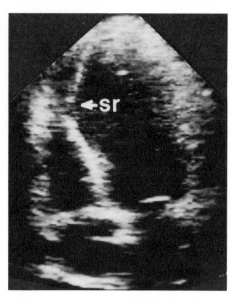

Figure 10.21. Ventricular septal rupture following myocardial infarction. This patient had sustained a large anteroseptal infarction and subsequently developed a septal rupture (sr).

apex versus septal rupture at the lower sternal border), such clinical differentiation is not always reliable. When mitral regurgitation results from rupture of the head of the posterior papillary muscle, the anterior direction of the regurgitant jet may result in the systolic thrill being maximal at the left sternal border, when it may be indistinguishable from that of ventricular septal rupture. Two-dimensional echocardiography is extremely valuable in differentiating ventricular septal rupture from papillary muscle dysfunction or rupture. The addition of pulsed Doppler echocardiography greatly aids differentiation by showing the presence or absence of mitral regurgitation. Not only can mitral regurgitation be detected, but the severity of mitral regurgitation can be semi-quantitated by pulsed and continuous wave Doppler echocardiography.

IMAGING OF CORONARY ARTERIES

Proximal portions of both right and left coronary arteries can be imaged by two-dimensional echocardiography (48, 49). The orifices of both coronary arteries can be visualized in the parasternal short-axis view of the aorta. The same view may not be optimal for simultaneous visualization of both coronary arteries, and separate views may be necessary for each vessel. Figure 10.26 shows the left main coronary artery and its bifurcation into left anterior descending and circumflex branches. Visualization of the bifurcation generally requires further transducer adjustment. In Figure 10.27, the right coronary artery is seen. Imaging of the coronary arteries is difficult because of their constant

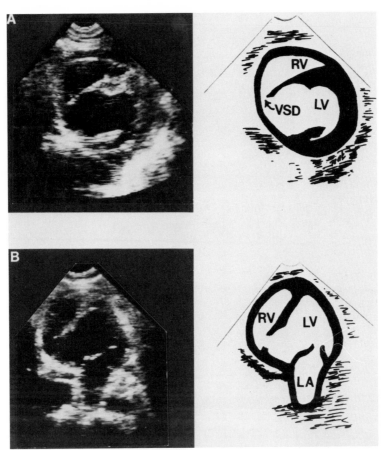

Figure 10.22. Ventricular septal rupture in a patient with inferior and septal myocardial infarction. (*A*) A short-axis two-dimensional echocardiographic view recorded slightly off-axis. A defect in the ventricular septum (VSD) at the junction with the posterior LV free wall is noted. The posterior half of the septum is aneurysmal. Thinning of the inferoposterior LV free wall and RV free wall is also noted. (*B*) A modified apical view demonstrating aneurysmal thinning and a defect in the basal septum. In this patient, the conventional views did not reveal the VSD clearly, and off-axis views were necessary to delineate it. (Reproduced with permission from Pandian NG, Isner JM, McInerney KP, et al. Non-invasive assessment of the complicated myocardial infarction: use of Doppler and two-dimensional echocardiography to differentiate ventricular septal rupture from rupture of mitral apparatus. Echocardiography 1985;2:329.)

motion in and out of the viewing plane with each cardiac cycle. Apical views have been used with some success to examine the proximal coronary arteries. An attempt must be made to record the coronary artery images in each patient. It is of special importance in children with possible coronary artery anomalies and those with coronary artery aneurysms secondary to mucocutaneous lymph-node syndrome. Occasionally, arteriovenous fistulas involving coronary arteries may be encountered in adults. With a strong index of suspicion, special off-axis views and use of pulsed wave Doppler echocardiography to evaluate flow abnormalities are required for an echocardiographic diagnosis. Coronary arteriosclerosis is associated with intimal thickening and plaque formation with or without coronary stenosis. Atherosclerotic plaques and obstructions produce high-intensity echoes. Figure 10.28 illustrates right coronary ostial obstruction. Although proximal atherosclerotic coronary artery obstructions can be successfully imaged in adults, the

sensitivity and specificity of echocardiographic diagnosis are not sufficiently high in adults to have a meaningful impact on management strategies. Further improvements in equipment and techniques may make it more useful.

STRESS ECHOCARDIOGRAPHY IN THE EVALUATION OF CHRONIC CORONARY ARTERY DISEASE

In patients with ischemic heart disease, selective coronary arteriography is required for the anatomic diagnosis and assessment of coronary artery disease. Many forms of stress testing are used to assess the physiologic significance of coronary artery lesions. Often these stress tests are employed to detect the presence of coronary artery disease prior to determining the need for invasive arteriography. As discussed earlier, an established infarction is associated with regional myocardial abnormalities that are present even in a

Figure 10.23. Doppler echocardiography in ventricular septal rupture. (*A*) Pulsed Doppler echocardiographic sampling in the RV cavity close to the posterolateral septum shows a high-velocity turbulent blood flow jet during systole. Sampling in different areas in both RV and LV in this patient demonstrated that the shunt direction was left to right. (*B*) Apical four-chamber view. Pulsed Doppler echocardiographic examination of the LA shows normal diastolic mitral flow and no mitral regurgitation. VS = ventricular septum. (Reproduced with permission from Pandian NG, Isner JM, McInerney KP, et al. Non-invasive assessment of the complicated myocardial infarction: use of Doppler and two-dimensional echocardiography to differentiate ventricular septal rupture from rupture of mitral apparatus. Echocardiography 1985;2:329.)

Parasternal Short-Axis

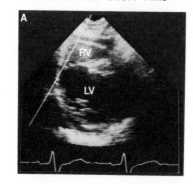

Apical 4-Chamber

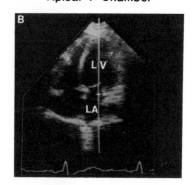

Sample Volume: RV-VS Junction

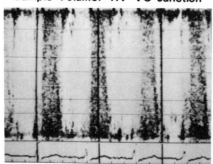

Sample Volume: LA

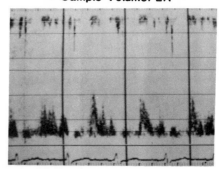

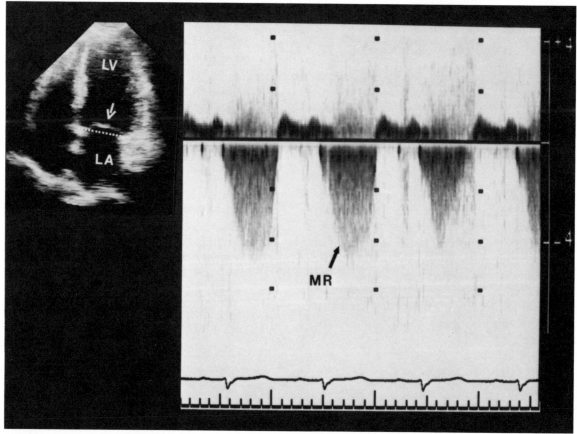

Figure 10.24. Papillary muscle dysfunction secondary to ischemic myocardial disease. In the apical four-chamber view at systole shown on the left, the mitral leaflet coaptation is displaced apically with the leaflets failing to reach the plane of the mitral annulus (*white dotted line*). As shown on the right, such incomplete closure causes mitral regurgitation (MR) in a continuous wave Doppler recording obtained from the apical window.

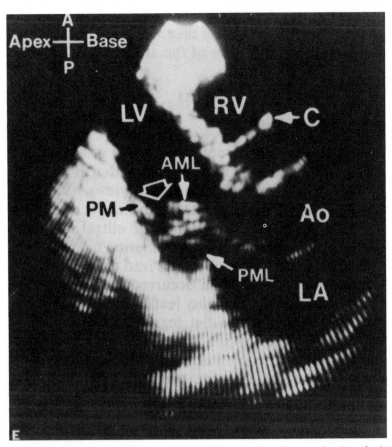

Figure 10.25. Papillary muscle rupture secondary to myocardial infarction. Long-axis view depicting ruptured papillary muscle mass attached to the anterior mitral leaflet (AML). The open arrow points to the site of rupture. A = anterior; Ao = aortic root; C = catheter; P = posterior; PM = base of the papillary muscle; PML = posterior mitral leaflet. (Reproduced by permission of the American Heart Association, Inc., from Mintz GS, Victor MF, Kotler MN, et al. Two-dimensional echocardiographic identification of surgically correctable complications of acute myocardial infarction. Circulation 1981;64:91.)

resting state. Many patients, however, have coronary arterial stenoses that are sufficiently severe to be clinically significant but do not reduce resting coronary blood flow. Accordingly, myocardial function at rest is preserved in these individuals, but it may deteriorate in the face of stresses that cause myocardial oxygen requirements to rise beyond the capability of the stenotic artery to supply nutrient flow to the affected area. Experimental studies have provided a rational basis for the clinical use of echocardiography during stress interventions (6, 50). M-mode echocardiography was originally employed during exercise to assess myocardial dysfunction in patients with coronary artery disease. However, exaggerated chest and lung movement during exercise obscured the echo window available in many subjects, and this problem greatly limited early studies using M-mode echocardiography. Furthermore, regional dysfunction that might occur in areas not examined by M-mode echocardiography can be missed. The use of two-dimensional echocardiography during exercise testing has greatly facilitated the utility of stress echocardiography in the detection and

assessment of ischemic heart disease (51–54). Nevertheless, satisfactory studies are not easily obtained when two-dimensional echocardiographic imaging is performed during exercise. Acquisition of two-dimensional echocardiographic images immediately after symptom-limited maximum exercise has allowed a notable improvement in the quality of images without significantly missing the effects of ischemia on regional wall motion or global LV function (53). The storage of appropriate images on floppy disks for subsequent review on computer-generated split screens has further improved the feasibility and utility of exercise echocardiography. In many laboratories, exercise echocardiography has become a routine test in the evaluation of patients with ischemic heart disease. Exercise echocardiography can be performed with either treadmill, supine, or upright bicycle exercise testing protocols. A variety of other forms of myocardial stress can also be used to provoke ischemic myocardial dysfunction. Pharmacologic agents such as isoproterenol, dobutamine or dipyridamole can be used to provoke regional ischemia, and echocardiographic imaging performed

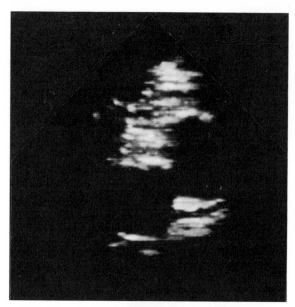

raphy is an ideal method with which to study myocardial mechanics during transient ischemia and reperfusion in patients. Two-dimensional echocardiography has been recently used during coronary angioplasty and has demonstrated that LV wall motion abnormalities develop almost immediately with balloon inflation, prior to ECG changes and frequently prior to the onset of symptoms (55). These studies have documented that clinically silent LV dysynergy is an early marker of acute transient ischemia in humans. Measurement of the extent of myocardium involved in regional dysfunction during balloon occlusion of the coronary artery provides information on the area of myocardium at risk (56). The contribution of coronary collaterals is indicated by the presence or absence of regional myocardial dysynergy during the angioplasty balloon inflation. Early experience suggests that myocardium not sup-

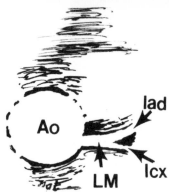

Figure 10.26.   Short-axis two-dimensional echocardiographic view at the level of the aortic root displaying the left coronary artery. Ao = aorta; lad = left anterior descending branch; lcx = left circumflex branch; LM = left main coronary artery.

following such pharmacologic interventions can delineate stress-induced ischemic myocardial dysfunction (54). This type of pharmacologic stress echocardiography circumvents the problems of chest wall movement (i.e., during exercise), which often interferes with adequate echocardiographic imaging.

Besides rendering information on the presence or absence of ischemia, stress echocardiography can also delineate the extent of ischemic myocardium and locate the diseased coronary arteries. Further, the effect of ischemia on global LV function can be simultaneously assessed with stress echocardiography.

ECHOCARDIOGRAPHY DURING PERCUTANEOUS TRANSLUMINAL CORONARY ANGIOPLASTY

Because of its capability to detect ischemic myocardial dysfunction promptly, two-dimensional echocardiog-

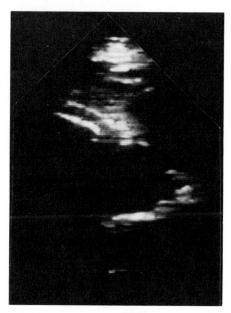

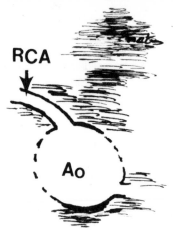

Figure 10.27.   Short-axis two-dimensional echocardiographic view depicting the right coronary artery (RCA). Ao = aorta.

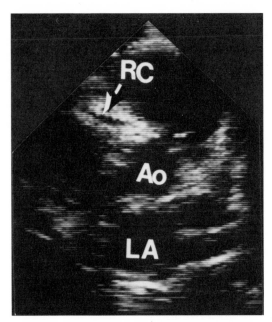

Figure 10.28.   Ostial obstruction of the right coronary artery (RC) is demonstrated in this short-axis view. Ao = aorta.

ported by coronary collaterals immediately becomes ischemic and dysfunctional. Conversely, in patients with coronary collaterals, such regional myocardial dysfunction does not occur promptly during balloon inflations. Since these transient episodes of myocardial ischemia during angioplasty are often accompanied by neither chest pain nor ECG changes, this technique is useful in the timing of the balloon inflations. After the first balloon inflation, subsequent balloon inflations are performed only after the regional myocardial dysynergy disappears and function reverts to control levels. Thus, two-dimensional echocardiography has a potential role in the catheterization laboratory during coronary angioplasty, providing valuable information in the assessment of myocardial function in these patients and also as a monitor of LV wall motion abnormalities during the procedure.

INTRAOPERATIVE ECHOCARDIOGRAPHY IN THE EVALUATION OF ISCHEMIC MYOCARDIAL DISEASE

Esophageal Echocardiography

An esophageal echocardiographic transducer was developed in the early 1980s to enable viewing of the cardiac structures from the esophagus. It comprises an ultrasound transducer fixed to the tip of a steerable endoscope. It can be introduced easily into the esophagus just as it is during an esophageal endoscopic procedure. The probe is then connected to a commercial ultrasound imaging system and can be moved up

and down and tipped anteriorly in the esophagus as necessary to obtain images of the cardiac chambers and valves from base to apex. A number of centers have used this approach to monitor cardiac function continuously in patients during cardiac and noncardiac surgery (57–60). After the patient has been intubated, it takes less than 20 seconds to introduce the probe into the esophagus. Since the source of imaging is the esophagus, all posterior structures will be seen in a reverse manner compared to the conventional anterior chest imaging (i.e., posterior strucures will be seen at the top of the image and anterior structures will be seen at the bottom of the image). Both short- and long-axis images of the LV and RV can be obtained using this method. Since no chest wall or lung tissue intervenes between the probe and the cardiac structures, high-resolution imaging can be obtained in the majority of patients. In patients with ischemic heart disease undergoing noncardiac surgical procedures such as vascular surgery, development of intraoperative ischemia has been successfully detected by the appearance of regional wall motion abnormalities, which often precede the ischemic ECG changes. Both regional and global systolic function can be continuously assessed by esophageal echocardiography. The development of hypotension in the patients undergoing surgery should indicate either a hypovolemic state or myocardial depression. If hypovolemia is the cause of hypotension, then esophageal echocardiographic images will reveal a small LV cavity, increased wall thickness, and enhanced wall motion. On the other hand, if myocardial depression is the cause of hypotension, myocardial contractility will be seen to be diminished. Thus, besides detecting intraoperative ischemia, esophageal echocardiographic monitoring provides information regarding the hemodynamic state. In patients undergoing cardiac surgery, monitoring of cardiac function before and after completion of cardiopulmonary bypass will indicate the state of regional and global LV function. After coronary bypass grafting and cessation of cardiopulmonary bypass, the cause of regional wall motion abnormalities can be directly assessed by examining the myocardial images from this approach. When there is development of intraoperative ischemia or infarction, localization of the regional wall motion abnormalities might indicate which coronary artery or graft might be responsible for such ischemia. Figure 10.29 was obtained from a patient who developed intraoperative ischemia involving the left anterior descending coronary artery distribution. The systolic images display dyskinesis of the lower IVS and the apex. Improving technology and growing experience with this approach indicate that esophageal echocardiography could play a major role in monitoring patients undergoing surgery.

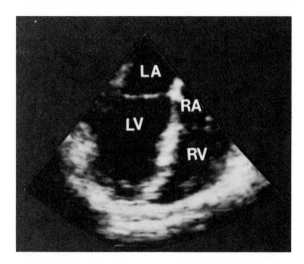

A

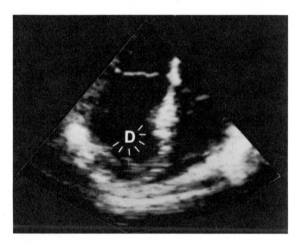

B

Figure 10.29.   Esophageal echocardiographic detection of intraoperative ischemia. This four-chamber view illustrates systolic dyskinesis (D) involving the LV apex and adjoining septum. (*A*) A diastolic image. (*B*) A systolic image. RA = right atrium.

Direct Epicardial Cardiac Imaging

Special transducer probes are also available for placement directly on the heart in patients undergoing open-heart surgery to delineate the cardiac anatomy and function (16, 61). These probes can be repeatedly sterilized or couched in a sterile sleeve. Direct epicardial imaging allows viewing the heart in many different planes. Using this approach, assessment of LV function before and after coronary bypass surgery has been performed and the immediate improvement in ventricular function has been noted after bypass grafting.

Direct Coronary Artery Imaging with High-Frequency Two-Dimensional Echocardiography

The ability to image the coronary arteries in a beating heart will have important clinical and experimental application. Toward this end, a new method for imaging coronary arteries in open-chested humans during surgery has been developed (62). Using a 9- or 12-megahertz transducer, coronary arterial obstructions in a beating heart can be recorded and localized during surgery. This method may allow intraoperative verification and localization of atherosclerotic lesions and aid in accurate saphenous vein bypass grafts. Transverse-axis views of normal and atherosclerotic human coronary arteries are shown in Figure 10.30. Bright, irregular atherosclerotic plaques are seen to protrude into the lumen, producing significant eccentric narrowing of the vessel. Experimental work in dogs and postmortem human hearts indicates that such imaging can not only assess the anatomic severity of coronary lesions accurately but can also give information about the functional significance of coronary stenotic lesions (63). Furthermore, vasomotor changes can be assessed by analyzing the changes in the diameter or cross-sectional area of the coronary artery (64), and miniaturized Doppler suction cups can measure the reactive hyperemic flow response, following temporary occlusion of native coronary arteries or bypass grafts. Another potential role for this technique is in the setting of intraoperative coronary angioplasty using either a balloon catheter or a laser probe (65), but its utility warrants further investigation.

MYOCARDIAL TISSUE CHARACTERIZATION BY ULTRASOUND

Ischemia and infarction result in certain characteristic structural abnormalities in the myocardium. Besides the identification of ischemic myocardium by contraction abnormalities, ultrasound is capable of directly identifying abnormal tissue regions based on altered acoustic properties. Ultrasound has been shown to interact differently with ischemic and infarcted muscle compared to interaction with the normal myocardium. Ultrasonic tissue characterization has been discussed in detail in Chapter 20. Since the mid-1970s, there has been a growing interest in the study of altered acoustic properties of abnormal cardiac tissue. Fundamental acoustic parameters studied include ultrasound velocity, attenuation, and backscatter. Changes in myocardial tissue architecture, elasticity, and relative content of collagen and water can alter its acoustic properties, and these changes can be assessed by three basic approaches: direct visualization, image-processing and pattern-recognition techniques, and quantitative mea-

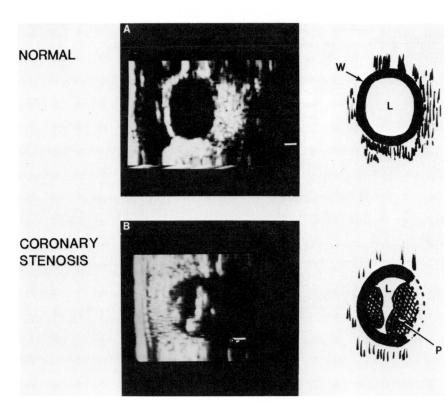

NORMAL

CORONARY STENOSIS

Figure 10.30. High-frequency two-dimensional echocardiographic images of human coronary arteries. Transverse views. (*A*) Depicts a normal coronary artery. (*B*) Discloses atherosclerotic plaques projecting into the arterial lumen. L = lumen; W = wall; P = plaque.

surement of acoustic parameters (8, 66–69). Direct visualization is a qualitative approach dependent on the observer's pattern-recognition abilities. A scar due to an old infarction appears as a thin wall of myocardium with extremely bright echoes (Fig. 10.8). Occasionally, even 5-day-old infarctions have been noted to show abnormal tissue texture on two-dimensional echocardiograms in some experimental studies. Computerized image and signal processing allows image enhancement and may render regions of abnormality more apparent. Slightly increased local echo amplitudes from infarct regions can be accentuated so as to allow clearer delineation of the area of brighter gray levels. Besides such visual appreciation of digitized echo forms, further numerical and statistical analyses can be performed in a multiparametric approach to define regions of ischemia and infarction. Investigations have also focused on the measurement of acoustic parameters by using both transmitted ultrasound in in vitro models to quantify signal attenuation and by using reflected ultrasound in in vivo models to measure integrated backscatter. These approaches have shown that not only old infarction but freshly ischemic myocardium can be reliably identified. Since analysis of reflected ultrasound is more likely to have clinical application, further work has centered on analysis of integrated backscatter. A number of such studies have shown that infarcted tissue exhibits increased levels of backscatter compared to normal myocardium (70, 71). Another ramification of this work has been the quanti-

tative analysis of texture of two-dimensional echocardiographic images (72). This involves analysis of the spatial distribution or pattern of regional echo intensities. Some of the quantitative texture measures include gray-level histogram statistics, edge count, gray-level run length statistics, and gray-level difference statistics. From these, measures of the heterogeneity or homogeneity of gray level, and of the size and spatial distribution of individual spots in the speckle pattern of the two-dimensional echocardiographic image can be derived. A number of other approaches such as polar texture analysis are being studied currently (73). Further studies are necessary before the clinical application of these quantitative tissue characterizations in ischemic heart disease.

EVALUATION OF PATIENTS WITH CHEST PAIN OR DYSPNEA

Chest pain and dyspnea are common symptoms. These often evoke great concern because of their well-known association with coronary artery disease. The differential diagnosis of these symptoms includes a wide variety of both cardiac and noncardiac conditions. Echocardiographic evaluation provides valuable information about many cardiac causes such as aortic stenosis, mitral valve prolapse and other valvular disorders, hypertrophic cardiomyopathy, aortic dissection, and pericarditis. Some patients may have more than one etiology for chest pain (i.e., patients with coronary artery disease may also have hypertrophic myopathy or aortic stenosis), and therefore, aggressive evaluation of patients with chest pain should not be curtailed after a single cause for the pain is identified and a single diagnosis made.

CONCLUSION

Ischemic heart disease, although its primary effect is on myocardium, often affects all of the structures of the heart. Echocardiography is ideally suited to examine all of the structural and functional consequences of ischemic heart disease. As a noninvasive technique, echocardiography can be performed serially in these patients not only in the laboratory but also at the bedside in the intensive care unit, catheterization laboratory, and the operating room. Improvements in technology continue with remarkable new developments such as two-dimensional flow mapping. Such technologic innovations have fostered an ever-increasing role for echocardiography in the evaluation of patients with ischemic heart disease.

REFERENCES

1. Tennant R, Wiggers CJ. The effect of coronary occlusion on myocardial contraction. Am J Physiol 1935;112:351.
2. Feigenbaum H. Echocardiography. 3rd ed. Philadelphia: Lea & Febiger, 1981.
3. Corya BC. Echocardiography in ischemic heart disease. Am J Med 1977;63:10.
4. Pandian NG, Skorton DJ, Kerber RE. Role of echocardiography in myocardial ischemia and infarction. Mod Concepts Cardiovasc Dis 1984;53:19.
5. Pandian NG, Isner JM, McInerney KP, et al. Non-invasive assessment of the complicated myocardial infarction: use of Doppler and two-dimensional echocardiography to differentiate ventricular septal rupture from rupture of mitral apparatus. Echocardiography 1985;2:329.
6. Pandian NG, Kerber RE. Two-dimensional echocardiography in experimental coronary stenosis. I. Sensitivity and specificity in detecting transient myocardial dyskinesis. Comparison with sonomicrometers. Circulation 1982;66:597.
7. Wyatt HL, Meerbaum S, Heng MK, Rit J, Gineret P, Corday E. Experimental evaluation of the extent of myocardial dysynergy and infarct size by two-dimensional echocardiography. Circulation 1981;63:607.
8. Skorton DJ, Melton H, Pandian NG, et al. Detection of acute myocardial infarction in closed-chest dogs by analysis of regional two-dimensional echocardiographic gray-level distributions. Circ Res 1983;52:36.
9. Weiss JL, Bulkley BH, Hutchins GM, et al. Two-dimensional echocardiographic recognition of myocardial injury in man: comparison with post-mortem studies. Circulation 1981;63:401.
10. Pandian NG, Koyanagi S, Skorton DJ, et al. Relations between two-dimensional echocardiographic wall thickening abnormalities, myocardial infarct size and coronary risk area in normal and hypertrophied myocardium in dogs. Am J Cardiol 1983;52:1318.
11. Nieminen M, Parisi A, O'Boyle J, et al. Serial evaluation of myocardial thickening and thinning in acute experimental infarction: identification and quantification using two-dimensional echocardiography. Circulation 1982;66:174.
12. Lieberman AN, Weiss JL, Jugdutt BI, et al. Two-dimensional echocardiography and infarct size: relationship of regional wall motion and thickening to the extent of myocardial infarction in the dog. Circulation 1981;63:739.
13. Kaul S, Pandian NG, Gillam L, et al. Contrast echocardiography in acute myocardial ischemia. III. An in vivo comparison of the extent of abnormal wall motion with the area at risk. J Am Coll Cardiol. 1986;7:383.
14. Pandian NG, Skorton DJ, Collins SM, et al. Myocardial infarct size threshold for two-dimensional echocardiographic detection. Sensitivity of wall thickening and endocardial motion abnormalities in small versus large infarction. Am J Cardiol 1985;55:551.
15. Kisslo JA, Robertson D, Gilbert BW, et al. The comparison of real-time two-dimensional echocardiography and cineangiography in detecting left ventricular asynergy. Circulation 1977;54:134.
16. Likoff M, Reichek N, St. John Sutton M, et al. Epicardial mapping of segmental myocardial function: an echocardiographic method applicable in man. Circulation 1982;66:1050.
17. Pandian NG, Skorton DJ, Collins S, et al. Heterogeneity of left ventricular segmental wall thickening and excursion in two-dimensional echocardiograms of normal humans. Am J Cardiol 1983;51:1667.
18. Pandian NG, Kieso RA, Kerber RE. Relationship between myocardial blood flow by layer and abnormalities of wall thinning on two-dimensional echocardiograms, abstracted. Am J Cardiol 1982;49:918.
19. Hegor JJ, Weyman AE, Wann LS, et al. Cross-sectional echocardiography in acute myocardial infarction: detection and localization of regional left ventricular asynergy. Circulation 1979;60:531.
20. Stamm RB, Gibson RS, Bishop HL, et al. Echocardiographic detection of infarct-localized asynergy and remote asynergy during acute myocardial infarction: correlation with the extent of angiographic coronary disease. Circulation 1983;67:233.
21. Van Reet RE, Quinones MA, Poliner LR, et al. Comparison of two-dimensional echocardiography with gated radionuclide ventriculography in the evaluation of global and regional left ventricular function in acute myocardial infarction. J Am Coll Cardiol 1984;3:243.
22. Nixon JV, Narahara KA, Smitherman TC. Estimation of myocardial involvement in patients with acute myocardial infarction by two-dimensional echocardiography. Circulation 1980;62:1248.
23. Kerber RE, Marcus ML, Ehrhardt J, et al. Correlation between echocardiographically demonstrated segmental dyskinesis and regional myocardial perfusion. Circulation 1975;52:1097.
24. Hegor JJ, Weyman AE, Wann LS, et al. Cross-sectional echocardiographic analysis of the extent of left ventricular asynergy in acute myocardial infarction. Circulation 1980;61:1113.
25. Gibson RS, Bishop HL, Stamm RB, et al. Value of early two-dimensional echocardiography in patients with acute myocardial infarction. Am J Cardiol 1982;49:1110.
26. Nishimura RA, Takik AJ, Shub C, et al. Role of two-dimensional echocardiography in the prediction of in-hospital complications after acute myocardial infarction. J Am Coll Cardiol 1984;4:1080.
27. Meltzer RS, Woythaler JT, Buda AJ, et al. Two-dimensional echocardiographic quantification of infarct size alteration by pharmacologic agents. Am J Cardiol 1979;44:257.
28. Taylor AL, Kieso RA, Melton J, et al. Echocardiographically detected dyskinesis, myocardial infarct size and coronary risk region relationships in reperfused canine myocardium. Circulation 1985;71:1292.
29. Gibbons EF, Hogan RD, Franklin TD, et al. The natural history of regional dysfunction in a canine preparation of chronic infarction. Circulation 1985;71:394.
30. Eaton LW, Weiss JL, Bulkley BH, et al. Regional cardiac dilatation after acute myocardial infarction: recognition by two-dimensional echocardiography. N Engl J Med 1979;300:57.
31. Hatle L, Angelsen B. Doppler ultrasound in cardiology. Philadelphia: Lea & Febiger, 1982.
32. Teague SM, Mark DB, Radford M, et al. Doppler velocity profiles reveal ischemic exercise responses, abstracted. Circulation 1984;70:II-185.
33. St. John Sutton MG, Frye R, Smith H, et al. Relation between left coronary artery stenosis and regional left ventricular function. Circulation 1978;58:491.
34. Grossman W, Mann T. Evidence for impaired left ventricular

relaxation during acute ischemia in man. Eur J Cardiol 1978;7: 239.

35. Hammermeister K, Warbasse J. The rate of change of left ventricular volume in man. II. Diastolic events in health and disease. Circulation 1974;49:739.

36. Rokay R, Kuo LC, Zoghbi WA, et al. Determination of parameters of left ventricular diastolic filling with pulsed Doppler echocardiography: comparison with cineangiography. Circulation 1985; 71:543.

37. Fisher DC, Voyles WF, Sikes W, Greene ER. Left ventricular filling patterns during ischemia: an echo/Doppler study in open-chest dogs, abstracted. J Am Coll Cardiol 1985;5:426.

38. Fujii J, Yazaki Y, Sawada H, et al. Non-invasive assessment of left and right ventricular filling in myocardial infarction with a two-dimensional Doppler echocardiographic method. J Am Coll Cardiol 1985;5:1155.

39. Mintz GS, Victor MF, Kotler MN, et al. Two-dimensional echocardiographic identification of surgically correctable complications of acute myocardial infarction. Circulation 1981;64:91.

40. Weyman AE, Peskoe SM, Williams ES, et al. Detection of left ventricular aneurysms by cross-sectional echocardiography. Circulation 1976;54:936.

41. Catherwood E, Mintz GS, Kotler MN, et al. Two-dimensional recognition of left ventricular pseudoaneurysm. Circulation 1980; 62:294.

42. Asinger RW, Mikell FL, Sharma B, et al. Observations on detecting left ventricular thrombus with two-dimensional echocardiography. Am J Cardiol 1981;47:145.

43. Meltzer RS, Visser CA, Kan G, Roelandt J. Two-dimensional echocardiographic appearance of left ventricular thrombi with systemic emboli after myocardial infarction. Am J Cardiol 1984;53:1511.

44. Scanlan JG, Seward JB, Tajik AJ. Visualization of ventricular septal rupture utilizing wide angle two-dimensional echocardiography. Mayo Clin Proc 1979;54:381.

45. Farcut JC, Borsante L, Rigaud M, et al. Two-dimensional echocardiographic visualization of ventricular septal rupture after acute anterior myocardial infarction. Am J Cardiol 1980;45:370.

46. Miyatake K, Okamoto M, Kinoshita N, et al. Doppler echocardiographic features of ventricular septal rupture in myocardial infarction. J Am Coll Cardiol 1985;5:182.

47. Godley RW, Weyman AE, Feigenbaum H, et al. Patterns of mitral leaflet motion in patients with probable papillary muscle dysfunction, abstracted. Am J Cardiol 1979;43:411.

48. Weyman AE, Feigenbaum H, Dillon JC, et al. Noninvasive visualization of the left main coronary artery by cross-sectional echocardiography. Circulation 1976;54:169.

49. Rogers EW, Feigenbaum H, Weyman AE, et al. Evaluation of left coronary artery anatomy in vitro using cross-sectional echocardiography. Circulation 1980;62:782.

50. Pandian NG, Kieso RA, Kerber RE. Two-dimensional echocardiography in experimental coronary stenosis. II. Relationship between systolic wall thinning and regional myocardial perfusion in severe coronary stenosis. Circulation 1982;66:603.

51. Wann LS, Faris JV, Childress RH, et al. Exercise cross-sectional echocardiography in ischemic heart disease. Circulation 1979;60: 1300.

52. Maurer G, Nanda NC. Two-dimensional echocardiographic evaluation of exercise-induced left and right ventricular asynergy: correlation with thallium scanning. Am J Cardiol 1981;48:720.

53. Robertson WS, Feigenbaum H, Armstrong WF, et al. Exercise echocardiography: a clinically practical addition in the evaluation of coronary artery disease. J Am Coll Cardiol 1983;2:1085.

54. Child JS. Stress echocardiography: a technique whose time has come. Echocardiography 1984;2:107.

55. Hanser AM, Gangadharan V, Ramos RG, et al. Sequence of mechanical, electrocardiographic and clinical effects of repeated coronary occlusion in human beings: echocardiographic observations during coronary angioplasty. J Am Coll Cardiol 1985;53: 193.

56. Pandian NG, Salem DN, Funai JT, et al. In vivo assessment of left ventricular risk area and coronary collateral function during acute temporary coronary occlusion in humans, abstracted. Circulation 1984;70:II-403.

57. Schliiter M, Langenstein BA, Polster JA, et al. Transesophageal cross-sectional echocardiography with a phased array transducer system. Technique and initial clinical results. Br Heart J 1982;48:67.

58. Kremer P, Cahalan M, Beaupre P, et al. Intra-operative myocardial ischemia detected by transesophageal two-dimensional echocardiography, abstracted. Circulation 1983;68(suppl III):332.

59. Pandian NG, England M, Hudson J, et al. Continuous monitoring of cardiac function by two-dimensional echocardiography using precordial and esophageal transducers. Ultrasonic Imaging 1984; 6:225.

60. Topol EJ, Weiss JL, Guzman PA, et al. Immediate improvement of dysfunctional myocardial segments after coronary revascularization: detection by intraoperative transesophageal echocardiography. J Am Coll Cardiol 1984;4:1123.

61. Spotnitz HM, Young CYH, Spotnitz AJ, et al. Intra-operative left ventricular performance evaluated by two-dimensional ultrasound. Circulation 1980;62:329.

62. Sahn DJ, Brandt PWT, Barratt-Boyes B, et al. Ultrasonic angiographic correlations for imaging coronary atherosclerotic lesions in open-chested humans during surgery. Circulation 1981;64:205.

63. Funai JT, Pandian NG, Salem DN, Lojeski EW. Can quantitative high-frequency two-dimensional echocardiography predict the physiologic significance of a coronary stenosis, abstracted. Circulation 1984;70:II-393.

64. Funai JT, Pandian NG, Lojeski EW, et al. Study of coronary artery vasomotion by high-frequency two-dimensional echocardiography: effects of nitroglycerin, alpha adrenergic stimulation and beta blockade on coronary artery cross-sectional area, abstracted. Circulation 1984;70:II-184.

65. Funai JT, Pandian NG, Isner JM, et al. Utility of high-frequency two-dimensional echocardiography in the performance of laser coronary angioplasty. Clin Res 1984;32:671.

66. Skorton DJ, Collins SM. Characterization of myocardial structure with ultrasound. In: Greenleaf J, ed. Tissue characterization with ultrasound. Boca Raton, FL: CRC Press, Inc. (in press).

67. Namery J, Lele PP. Ultrasonic detection of myocardial infarction in dogs. IEEE Ultrasonics Symposium, 1972, 72 CHO 708–854: 491.

68. Mimbus JW, Yuhas DE, Miller JG, et al. Detection of myocardial infarction in vitro based on altered attenuation of ultrasound. Circ Res 1977;41:192.

69. Gramiak R, Wang RC, Schenk EA, et al. Ultrasonic detection of myocardial infarction by amplitude analysis. Radiology 1979;130: 713.

70. Mimbus JW, Bauwens D, Cohen RD, et al. Effects of myocardial ischemia on quantitative ultrasonic backscatter and identification of responsible determinants. Circ Res 1981;49:89.

71. Mararas EI, Barzilai B, Perez JE, et al. Changes in backscatter throughout the cardiac cycle. Ultrasonic Imaging 1983;5:229.

72. Skorton DJ, Collins SM, Nichols J, et al. Quantitative texture analysis in two-dimensional echocardiograms: application to the diagnosis of experimental myocardial contusion. Circulation 1983;68:217.

73. McPhearson DD, Aylward PE, Knosp BM, et al. Ultrasound characterization of acute myocardial ischemia by polar texture analysis, abstracted. Circulation 1984;70:II-396.

11
Cardiomyopathy

Martin St. John Sutton

INTRODUCTION

Cardiomyopathy is a term used to describe a wide spectrum of heart muscle diseases predominantly involving the left ventricle, but frequently also involving the right ventricle, that results in progressive ventricular dysfunction and over time culminates in heart failure (1). Although the World Health Organization (WHO) has recommended cardiomyopathy be used to describe only primary myocardial disease of unknown etiology (1), it is currently used widely to describe left and right ventricular dysfunction resulting from a number of causes, including advanced coronary artery disease, infiltrative disorders, myocarditis, and cardiotoxic agents. Traditionally, cardiomyopathies have been classified into three major types—hypertrophic, dilated, and restrictive (1). This classification is based upon left ventricular chamber architecture and associated abnormalities of systolic ejection and diastolic filling.

Doppler echocardiography has a major diagnostic role to play in distinguishing among the three major types of cardiomyopathy. Symptoms of exercise intolerance and dyspnea develop in all three due to insidious left ventricular failure, which is their final common pathway. Recognition of each type of cardiomyopathy is important clinically because their pharmacologic management is different.

Hypertrophic cardiomyopathy is characterized by increased left ventricular mass with normal or decreased left ventricular cavity volume. The echocardiographic hallmarks are increased wall thickness, which may be concentric or asymmetric; normal or decreased left ventricular cavity diameter; and preserved systolic function. In dilated cardiomyopathy, left ventricular volume and mass are both increased, but the increase in volume is disproportionately greater than the increase in mass such that the left ventricular cavity is more spherical than elliptical in configuration. The characteristic echocardiographic stigmata are increased cavity diameter, normal or slightly increased wall thickness, and severely depressed contractile function. In restrictive cardiomyopathy, the left ventricular volume is usually normal and left ventricular mass may be normal, but is frequently increased. The echocardiographic features include normal left ventricular cavity diameter, increased or normal wall thickness, and decreased systolic function. There is overlap between the three types of cardiomyopathy, and especially between the hypertrophic and restrictive varieties. However, when the echocardiographic abnormalities are interpreted as an integral part of the clinical history, physical examination, chest radiograph, and electrocardiogram, there is usually little doubt as to which type of cardiomyopathy is present. This chapter describes the Doppler echocardiographic findings in the three major types of cardiomyopathy.

HYPERTROPHIC CARDIOMYOPATHY

Since the initial description of hypertrophic cardiomyopathy (HCM) as a discrete entity by Brock (2) and Teare (3), it has become evident that there is an obstructive variety, in which a resting or provokable left ventricular outflow tract gradient is present, and a variety in which obstruction to left ventricular ejection is not present at rest or provokable by physiologic or pharmacologic maneuvers. Early echocardiographic studies demonstrated that in the obstructive form of HCM, the left ventricular hypertrophy is invariably asymmetric (4, 5), whereas the nonobstructive form may be asymmetric but is more commonly characterized by concentric hypertrophy (6–11), which is indistinguishable echocardiographically from the concentric left ventricular hypertrophy that occurs in systemic hypertension. However, the increased left ventricular mass in nonobstructive HCM does not develop in

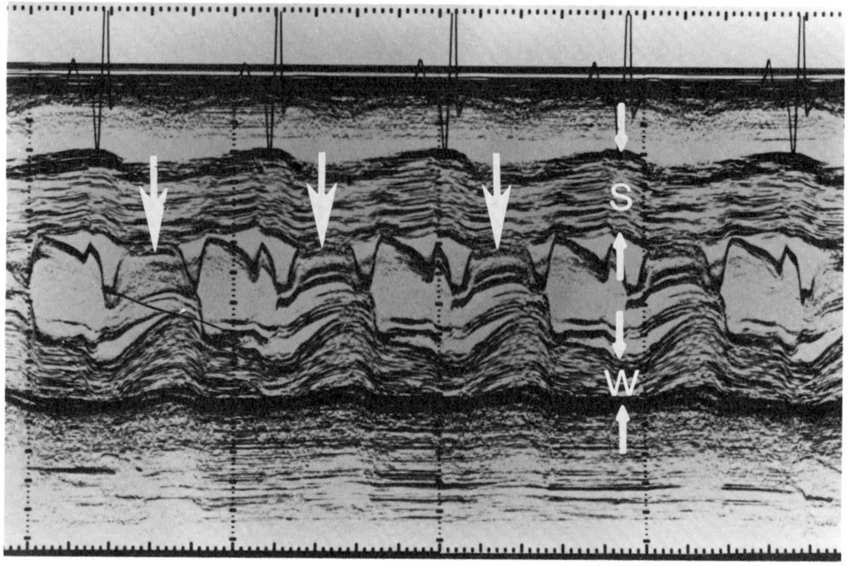

Figure 11.1. M-mode echocardiogram from a patient with HCM showing the characteristic asymmetrically hypertrophied septum (S) and the posterior LV wall (W) (the ratio of S/W was 2.7/1.3 = 2.1). In addition, there is SAM of the mitral valve (*large arrows*), a normal size left ventricle with mild septal hypomobility, but normal fractional LV shortening.

response to increased afterload, but is usually genetically determined.

Many hypotheses have been advanced as to the etiology of obstructive HCM, including derangement of the sympathetic innervation of the heart (12), dominant inheritance of an eccentric form of left ventricular hypertrophy (13, 14), prolonged isometric contraction due to the catenoid configuration of the interventricular septum (15), and recently an abnormal sensitivity to adenosine (16). The uncertainties regarding both the etiology and the mechanics of left ventricular ejection with regard to the presence of outflow tract obstruction (17–21) have been responsible for the plethora of terms used to describe this form of cardiomyopathy, which include idiopathic hypertrophic subaortic stenosis (IHSS), muscular subaortic stenosis (MSS), asymmetric septal hypertrophy (ASH), and hypertrophic obstructive cardiomyopathy (HOCM), etc. (22–24).

M-mode and two-dimensional echocardiography have been invaluable in HCM for establishing the diagnostic criteria (4, 5, 6, 25–36); characterizing the systolic ejection dynamics and the site of "obstruction" (25, 30, 37–46); assessing the efficacy of medical and surgical treatment with beta adrenergic receptor blockers (26), calcium channel antagonists (47–49), disopyramide (50), and myotomy-myectomy and mitral valve replacement, respectively (51–59); quantitating the changes in left ventricular geometry and function with time (21, 60–66); and elucidating the genetic pattern of inheritance (13, 14, 67–69). Recently Doppler has enabled quantitation of the left ventricular outflow tract gradients at rest and after provocation (20, 57, 70–72).

Figure 11.2. M-mode echocardiogram from a patient with HCM in whom it is difficult to identify the right side of the ventricular septum, even with variation in the gain settings, so that septal thickness cannot be determined. This patient has no SAM at rest. With two-dimensional echo, the right side of the septum is located, shown here by the arrows, indicating the presence of ASH with a septal/posterior ratio of 2.5.

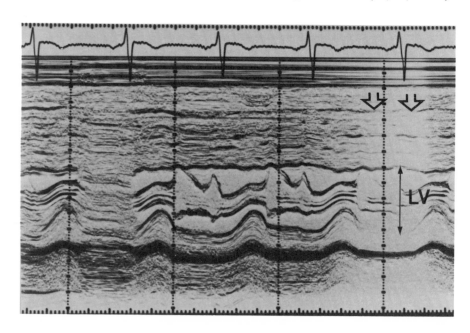

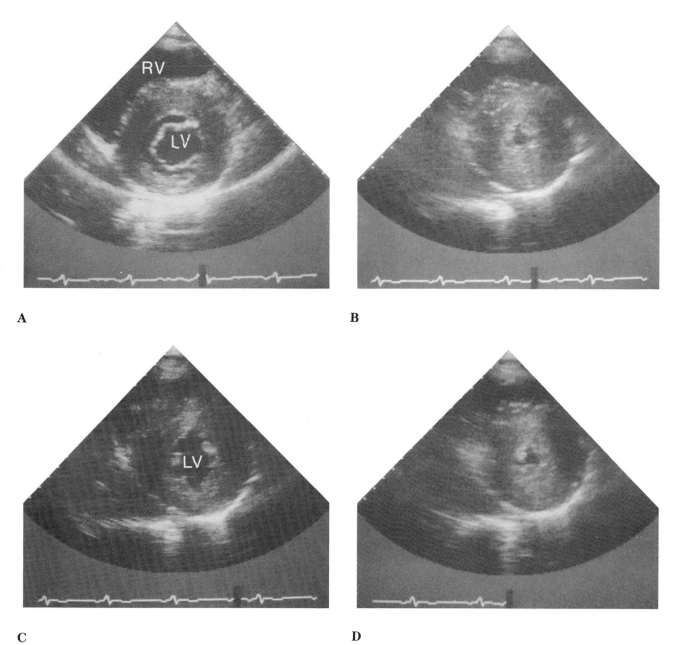

Figure 11.3. Two-dimensional echocardiogram from a patient with HCM showing short axis of the left ventricle in diastole (*A*) with ASH, and in systole, during which the cavity is almost completely obliterated (*B*). Short axis view at midcavity level in diastole (*C*) demonstrates that the ASH extends at least to midcavity level, and in systole the cavity is virtually shut down (*D*).

There is no other single cardiac abnormality in which ultrasound has been so useful as in HCM, and not surprisingly Doppler echocardiography is currently the diagnostic modality of choice.

The diagnostic criteria were initially described by M-mode echocardiography and consisted of asymmetric hypertrophy of the interventricular septum (ASH) (4–7, 73), systolic anterior motion of the mitral valve (SAM) (25–32), anterior dislocation of the mitral valve (33), septal hypomobility (29, 30), and premature closure of the aortic valve (34). Although none of these

individual echocardiographic abnormalities is specific for HCM (36, 73–82), their combined presence makes the diagnosis certain. Narrowing of the left ventricular outflow tract and left ventricular outflow tract gradients at cardiac catheterization corresponds with the presence of the ASH and the timing of SAM on M-mode LV echocardiograms (83, 84). Two-dimensional Doppler echocardiography has characterized the abnormalities in left ventricular chamber architecture, ejection dynamics, and diastolic filling patterns and, in addition, elucidated the site and mechanism of LV outflow obstruction as well as confirming the M-mode diagnostic criteria (20, 41–43, 46, 48, 49, 54, 62, 65, 71, 72, 85–96).

One of the first features of HCM recognized by M-mode echo was the disproportionately greater thickness of the proximal interventricular septum compared to the posterior left ventricular wall (4–7) (Fig. 11.1). This was termed *asymmetric septal hypertrophy* (ASH), and defined as the ratio of end-diastolic septal to posterior wall thickness of greater than 1.3:1 (4, 5, 7, 73). ASH was initially believed to be pathognomonic of HCM and was used as a noninvasive marker in assessing the first-degree relatives of probands with HCM, and demonstrated the dominant pattern of genetic inheritance (13, 64, 67). However, ASH has subsequently been described in a number of conditions involving the right and/or the left ventricle in which asymmetric rather than concentric hypertrophy develops, sometimes in response to increased afterload (76–79, 97–101).

The location of the asymmetric hypertrophy in HCM varies from patient to patient. It most commonly involves the basal and mid portions of the septum, but may extend throughout the septum from the base to the apex (8–11, 62, 65, 66, 102). ASH may also extend to the anterior or posterior left ventricular free wall, and on occasion completely encircle the left ventricular cavity so that on cross-section the ventricle appears concentrically hypertrophied (10, 11, 62, 65, 66). Alternatively, ASH may be confined to the proximal septum (8, 11), when it is termed *disproportionate upper septal thickening* (78) (DUST); to the posterior septum; or rarer still to the apical septum, resulting in obliteration of the apex of the left ventricular cavity (9, 11, 102–104).

ASH may be difficult to identify with M-mode echocardiography alone. This is due most commonly to technical problems in distinguishing the right ventricular surface of the septum from the tricuspid subvalve apparatus, so that septal thickness cannot be measured (Fig. 11.2), or due to unusual angulation of the ultrasound beam with respect to the interventricular septum (105). ASH may not be detected when it is confined to the posterior or apical septum because these regions are not interrogated by the M-mode echo beam (8). Two-dimensional echocardiographic imaging of the interventricular septum in patients with suspected HCM should be performed in orthogonal views to define the location and severity of ASH. This necessitates obtaining parasternal long and serial short axis views, as well as apical and subcostal four chamber views (Figs. 11.3–11.8). ASH may also be overlooked with two-dimensional echo, particularly from the apical four chamber view, when the gain settings are too low. This occurs because the right and left endo-

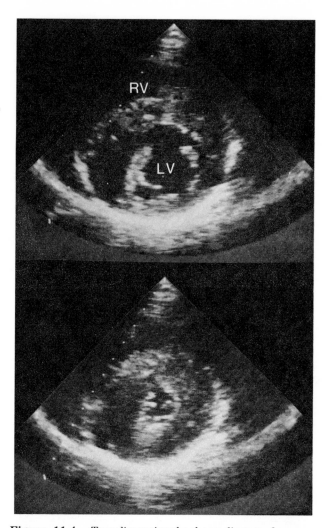

Figure 11.4. Two-dimensional echocardiogram from a patient with HCM showing the short axis view of the left ventricle. The anterior septal and inferior wall thicknesses are similarly increased, but of note is the extreme asymmetric hypertrophy involving the posterior septum in diastole (*A*) and in systole (*B*).

cardial surfaces of the septum are attenuated when the ultrasound beam is parallel to them, and the septum appears thinner than in reality. In patients after septal myotomy-myectomy, short axis views of the left ventricle at the base will also demonstrate the site of septal myotomy-myectomy as a wedge-shaped channel in the proximal anterior septum (Fig. 11.9).

When ASH occurs in the proximal septum, it usually encroaches upon, and may severely narrow, the left ventricular outflow tract (Fig. 11.10). In children, the ventricular chamber volumes are small and ASH may encroach upon both right and left ventricular outflow tracts, or predominantly narrow the right ventricular outflow tract so that the clinical, electrocardiographic, and hemodynamic findings lead to the clinical diagnosis of infundibular stenosis or dual-chambered right ventricle with intact septum (106–108). HCM should

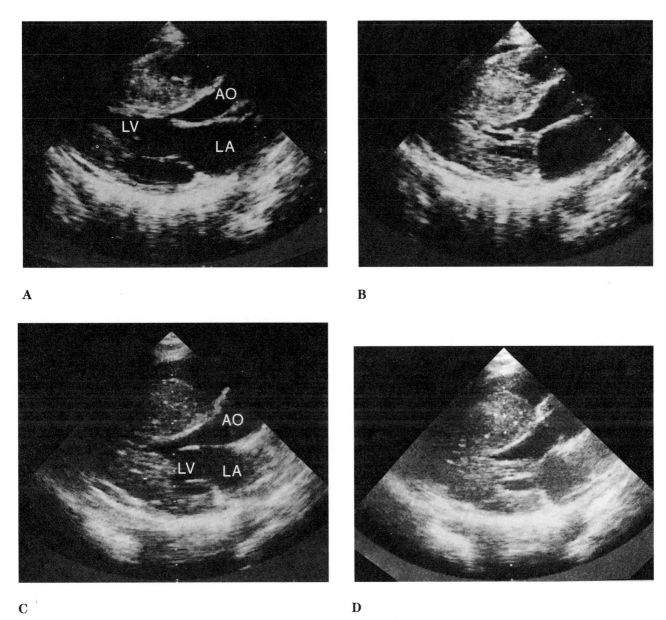

A

B

C

D

Figure 11.5. Two-dimensional echocardiogram from two patients with HCM. There is extreme asymmetric septal hypertrophy compared to the inferior wall in diastole (*A* and *C*), which is still apparent in systole (*B* and *D*). There are bright spots within the septum, which are specular reflections representing either fibrosis or myocardial fiber disarray.

therefore be included in the differential diagnosis of right ventricular outflow tract obstruction with intact septum in children.

The textural appearance by two-dimensional echocardiography of the region of the septum that is asymmetrically hypertrophied is often strikingly different from that of the myocardium composing the free left ventricular wall (Figs. 11.5, 11.11) (85). The ASH is brighter and has a speckled or granular appearance compared to the free left ventricular wall, which is less reflective and homogeneous. This increased specular reflectance and lack of homogeneity of ASH may be caused by the increased number of myocardial inter-

faces resulting from disarray of the myocardial fibers that predominate in the ventricular septum. However, the relationship between fiber disarray and echo reflectance has not been examined quantitatively.

Systolic Anterior Motion of the Mitral Valve

The resting left ventricular systolic pressure gradients in HCM were shown by echo to result from dynamic narrowing of the left ventricular outflow tract by abnormal systolic motion of the mitral valve (SAM) (11, 25–27, 37, 44, 84, 108). SAM consists of anterior movement of the mitral valve toward the septum in early

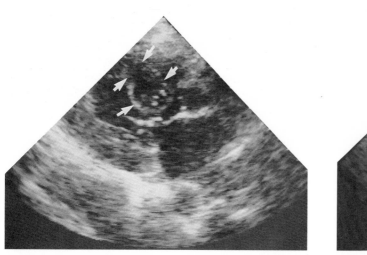
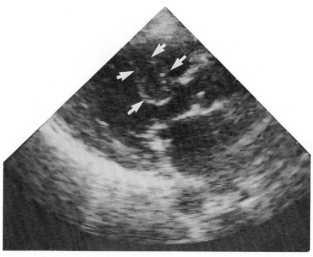

A   **B**

Figure 11.6. Two-dimensional echocardiogram from a patient with HCM showing the LV long axis with differential upper septal thickening (DUST), indicated by the arrows in diastole (*A*) and in systole (*B*). There are three large specular reflections from the upper septum.

systole, often with contact between the mitral valve leaflets themselves or the subvalve apparatus and the interventricular septum (Figs. 11.12, 11.13). In some patients, SAM results in complete obliteration of the left ventricular outflow tract due to rapid coaption of the mitral valve and septum in early systole, with the anterior mitral valve leaflet remaining in apposition with the septum until the end of systole, at which time it moves abruptly posteriorly prior to opening (Fig. 11.12). In some patients with SAM, the endocardial area of the left ventricular surface of the septum that makes

systolic contact with the mitral valve becomes thickened, and can be clearly visualized as a plaque or septal callous when the LV outflow tract is imaged from the left parasternal view (Fig. 11.14).

SAM is visualized optimally by two-dimensional echocardiography when the left ventricular outflow tract is imaged in the long axis view from the left parasternal region or from the apex (Figs. 11.15, 11.16). SAM may sometimes be difficult to identify with two-dimensional echo when the left ventricle is small because of severe asymmetric septal hypertrophy and

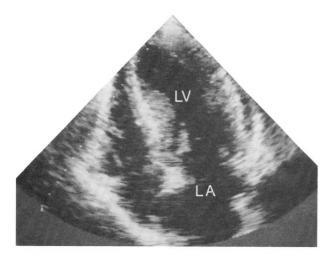
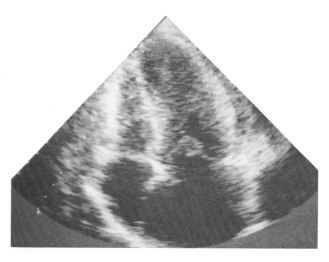

A   **B**

Figure 11.7. Two-dimensional echocardiogram of the apical four chamber view from a patient with HCM in whom marked asymmetric septal hypertrophy is seen easily in diastole (*A*). The LV free wall is hypertrophied and the left atrium is dilated, but the right heart chambers are of normal size. In systole (*B*), the LV cavity is almost completely obliterated, with the septum and free wall in apposition from midcavity level to the apex. The left atrium is enlarged and the interatrial septum bows toward the right atrium.

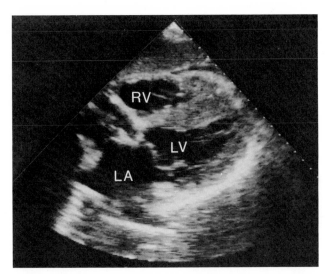

Figure 11.8. Two-dimensional echocardiogram from a patient with HCM, obtained via the subcostal route, showing ASH extending from the proximal septum and progressively increasing in thickness toward the apex.

hypertrophy of the papillary muscles, which displace the mitral valve apparatus anteriorly into a narrowed and crowded outflow tract (33). In such patients, SAM can be detected by carefully reviewing the two-dimensional images in slow motion, or by making use of the rapid repetition frequency of the M-mode and directing the M-mode echo cursor through the left ventricular outflow tract under two-dimensional echo guidance. SAM is present in the majority of patients with resting left ventricular outflow tract gradients (26, 27, 40, 41, 43, 44, 83, 84, 109, 110), and can be elicited in those with

only provokable gradients by physiologic maneuvers or pharmacologic interventions that either diminish left ventricular end-diastolic volume (Valsalva maneuver or nitrates) or augment left ventricular contractile state (isometric exercise and catecholamines). These maneuvers should be performed in all patients with ASH and no resting SAM whenever dynamic outflow tract obstruction is suspected clinically. SAM is not usually present when the left ventricular outflow tract has been enlarged and the gradient abolished by septal myotomy-myectomy, and is not present in patients with nonobstructive HCM (52–57, 111). Although SAM is not pathognomonic of HCM and has been reported in a number of unrelated conditions (36, 74–77, 80–82), the presence of combined SAM and ASH make the diagnosis of HCM almost a certainty.

The anatomic level in the left ventricular outflow tract at which SAM causes obstruction varies (11, 40, 41–43, 46, 84, 112–114), and should be determined in the left parasternal and apical long views of the left ventricle. SAM involves most commonly the mitral valve at the level of the junction of the chordae tendinae and the tips of the leaflets, but it may occur at the midchordal level, or the level at which the chordae insert into the papillary muscles (11, 40, 112). Not only is SAM of diagnostic value in HCM, but if the duration of contact between the mitral valve apparatus and the septum is measured on M-mode echocardiography, the magnitude of the left ventricular outflow tract gradient can be calculated (83). These noninvasive estimations have correlated with the gradients measured at cardiac

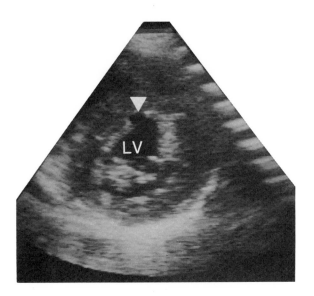

A

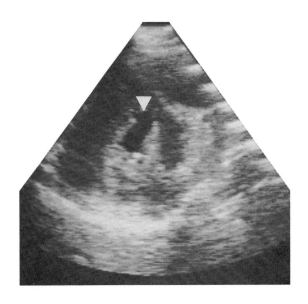

B

Figure 11.9. Two-dimensional echocardiogram of the LV short axis from a patient with HCM post–myectomy-myotomy. There is an anterior septal wedge-shaped channel visible, shown by the arrows, in diastole (*A*) and in systole (*B*). There was no postoperative SAM and LV outflow tract gradients.

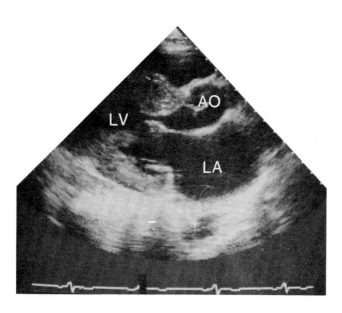

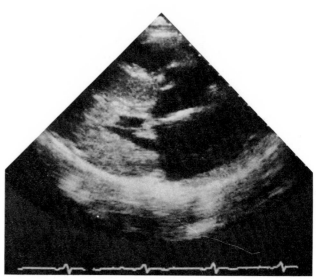

A   **B**

Figure 11.10. Two-dimensional echocardiogram of the LV long axis from a patient with HCM showing narrowing of the LV outflow tract due to extreme hypertrophy of the septum, which extends into the left ventricle in diastole (*A*) and virtually obstructs the egress of blood from the left ventricle in systole (*B*).

catheterization (83), but are now rarely used because left ventricular outflow tract gradients can be directly quantitated by Doppler.

Left Ventricular Architecture and Systolic Function

Left ventricular cavity size may be normal, but is usually small (Fig. 11.17). End-diastolic left ventricular shape varies with the extent and location of the ASH (3, 7–11, 62, 66, 102–104). When ASH extends circumferentially from the septum into the free wall, the cavity

shape may be indistinguishable from the concentrically hypertrophied left ventricle of severe idiopathic or reno-vascular hypertension. More commonly, ASH involves the proximal septum and extends for a variable distance down the long axis of the septum toward the apex (3, 7–11, 62, 66, 102–104), bulging into and indenting the cavity so that it becomes crescent-shaped rather than ellipsoidal. This can be seen easily in the apical two chamber view (Figs. 11.5, 11.15, 11.16). In

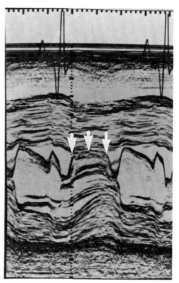

Figure 11.12. M-mode echocardiogram showing the early onset of SAM (*arrows*), with contact between the mitral valve on the left side of the septum extending for almost the complete duration of systole. SAM moves abruptly posteriorly prior to mitral valve opening.

Figure 11.11. A magnified view of the proximal septum in a patient with HCM showing the increased echo brightness or sparkling in the region of ASH, which differs from the adjacent myocardium with normal acoustic properties.

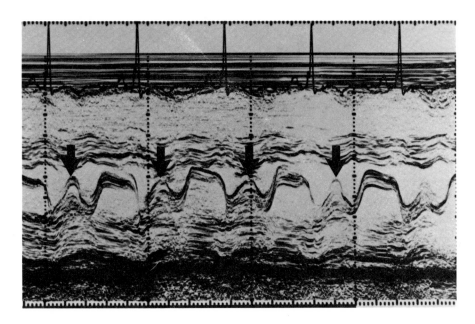

Figure 11.13. M-mode echocardiogram showing SAM with no or only minimal short duration contact between the mitral valve and the septum (*arrows*).

the apical and parasternal long axis views and in the apical five chamber view, ASH involving the proximal interventricular septum can be visualized narrowing the left ventricular outflow tract (Figs. 11.15, 11.16). By contrast, when ASH is confined to the apical septum, the left ventricular cavity is squared off at the apex as though there were an apical filling defect (9, 102–104).

In addition to the septum being asymmetrically hypertrophied, its systolic thickening and endocardial excursion is markedly reduced (29, 30, 87, 115, 116). This septal hypocontractility is best appreciated when the septum is visualized in profile from the parasternal long axis, or from the subcostal four chamber view

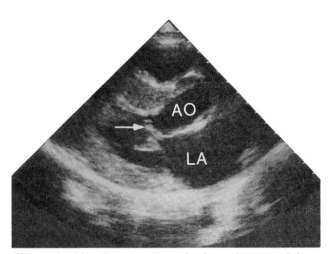

Figure 11.14. Two-dimensional echocardiogram of the LV long axis showing the callous or plaque on the left side of the septum in a patient with HCM. This echo brightness represents subendocardial fibrosis, which develops on the left side of the septum in HCM in response to systolic contact of the mitral valve. The arrow indicates SAM of the mitral valve.

where both the right ventricular and left ventricular endocardial surfaces can be clearly identified (Figs. 11.5, 11.17). This reduced systolic thickening does not indicate the presence of concomitant coronary artery disease. Reduced systolic septal thickening also occurs in severe concentric left ventricular hypertrophy due to systemic hypertension, and is not specific for HCM. The resultant effects of decreased septal thickening on left ventricular cavity function is twofold. First, the decreased septal excursion results in decreased inward wall motion during systole, which means that the septum makes little contribution to cavity emptying. However, this is compensated for by inward motion of the free left ventricular wall being more vigorous than normal (87, 115–118). This is well demonstrated on short axis sections of the left ventricle in real time. The augmented excursion of the left ventricular free wall is due to regional "unloading"—that is, the free wall contracts more vigorously because it shortens against less resistance since the septum does not shorten to an equivalent extent. Second, the left ventricular cavity does not reduce its length normally because the increased thickness of the septum splints the long axis of the left ventricle (119). This results in an incoordinate pattern of contraction (115, 118) that can be seen in orthogonal two-dimensional echo views of the left ventricular cavity. In short axis images of the left ventricle at midcavity level and at the apex, septal excursion is reduced, while excursion of the free wall is increased, resulting in coaption with the septum in early to mid-systole with near cavity obliteration (Figs. 11.3, 11.5, 11.17, 11.18). Similarly, in the apical four chamber view the septum is hypomobile, and the enhanced endocardial motion of the free wall in many patients obliterates the cavity initially at the mid-cavity

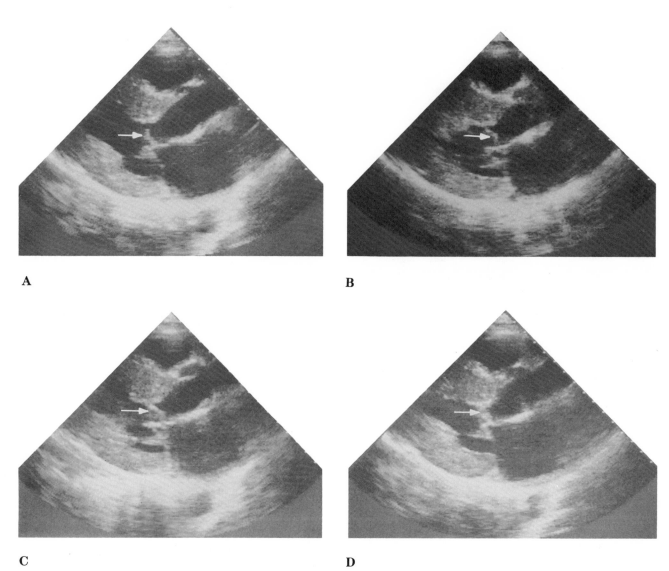

A

B

C

D

Figure 11.15. Serial two-dimensional echocardiographic frames of the LV long axis in HCM showing the development of SAM (*arrows*), which moves into the LV outflow tract obstructing left ventricular ejection.

level extending quickly downward toward the apex (119) (Figs. 11.7, 11.17, 11.18). This almost complete left ventricular cavity emptying is comparable to that seen on LV contrast angiography (17, 120).

Left ventricular pump function is characteristically normal or supranormal in HCM (120). The supranormal ejection phase indices of systolic pump function result from the small cavity size and its almost complete emptying (11). An additional reason for the increased left ventricular ejection fraction is the presence of mitral regurgitation in approximately 50% of patients (11, 86, 121, 122), as part of the stroke volume is ejected into the left atrium, which is a low resistance sink. The mitral regurgitation is probably secondary to the altered cavity geometry, with the mitral valve apparatus being displaced into a crowded left ventricular outflow tract. Furthermore, blood is ejected in the direction of

the mitral valve annulus, rather than along the long axis of the left ventricle toward the aorta as in the normal heart, because the ASH bulges into the LV outflow tract (11) (Fig. 11.19). Apart from the septal hypomobility, regional wall motion abnormalities in HCM are rare. However, regional wall motion should be carefully sought in serial short axis and in the apical four and two chamber views. Although the coronary arteries are characteristically large and normal, coronary disease and myocardial infarction have been reported in a proportion of patients at autopsy (123).

Left Ventricular Outflow Tract Obstruction

There is continuing debate about whether or not there is true obstruction to left ventricular ejection (18–21). Careful analysis of the systolic blood flow velocity

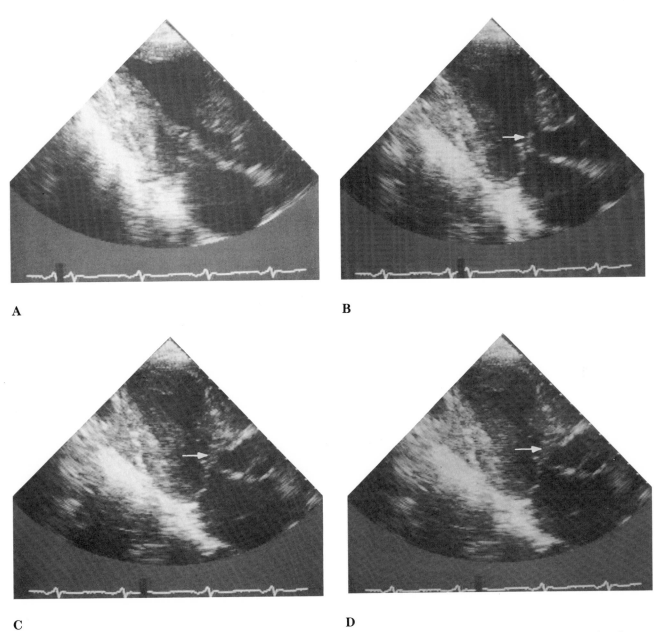

A   B

C   D

Figure 11.16. Serial two-dimensional echocardiographic frames of the LV long axis from the apex, demonstrating the onset of SAM (*arrows*) in early systole, and obstruction to left ventricular ejection.

spectra obtained invasively and noninvasively have not completely resolved this issue. Instantaneous blood flow velocity spectra recorded with catheter-tipped flow probes positioned in the ascending aorta revealed no consistent differences between obstructive and nonobstructive HCM (17). Pulsed- and continuous-wave Doppler velocity spectra, recorded from the left ventricular outflow tract, indicate that patients with left ventricular outflow tract gradients can be detected in the majority of cases (20, 46, 89, 93, 95). Doppler velocity spectra should be obtained from the left ventricular outflow tract in all patients with HCM (Fig. 11.20). The pulsed-wave Doppler sample volume

should be positioned first in the proximal left ventricular outflow tract from the apical five chamber or apical long axis view, and then advanced progressively toward and subsequently beyond the aortic valve, to detect the location of the step-up in velocity and also to exclude coexistent aortic stenosis, which has been described in association with HCM (97, 98, 108). Continuous-wave recordings should also be recorded routinely from the apex, suprasternal notch, and second right intercostal space to obtain the highest velocity amplitude (Fig. 11.21).

Recent Doppler studies have shown that obstructive and nonobstructive HCM can be differentiated by the

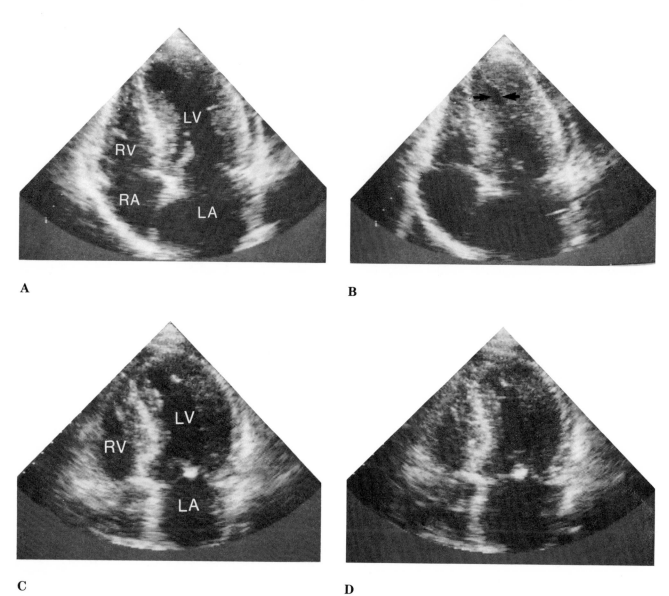

A   **B**

C   **D**

Figure 11.17. Two-dimensional echocardiogram of the apical four chamber view in two different patients with HCM. The massive asymmetric septal hypertrophy results in a crescent LV shape. There is indentation of the midcavity by septal bulging in diastole (*A*), with a bipartite cavity configuration at end-systole and blood trapped in the apex of the LV (*B, arrows*). There is hypertrophy of the septum, which has a dumbbell appearance and very abnormal diastolic cavity shape (*C*). During systole the LV cavity length changes little, but the inward motion of the free wall gives the LV cavity an almost cylindrical shape (*D*). Note that the septum varies little in thickness from diastole to systole.

morphology of the flow velocity spectra obtained from the ascending aorta (20, 57, 71, 93). In the nonobstructive type, there is a single peak in the velocity envelope similar to normal. In the obstructive type the velocity spectra are bifid, with an early high amplitude peak in midsystole and a second smaller later peak in late systole (Fig. 11.22) (20). From the left ventricular outflow tract peak and mean velocities, both peak and mean gradients can be calculated using the Bernoulli equation (20, 57, 71, 93).

The timing of the peak velocity in the left ventricular outflow tract and the onset of SAM establish their cause-and-effect relationship. The peak velocity occurs after the onset of systolic anterior motion of the mitral valve, suggesting that there is true obstruction to left ventricular ejection (20) (Fig. 11.23). The left ventricular outflow tract gradients in HCM calculated from Doppler blood flow velocities correlate closely with those measured at cardiac catheterization. In a minority of patients, most of whom are children or adolescents, the increased septal thickness and its encroachment on the right ventricular outflow tract result in right ventricular outflow tract obstruction, which may occasionally be severe, exceeding 100 mmHg (106,

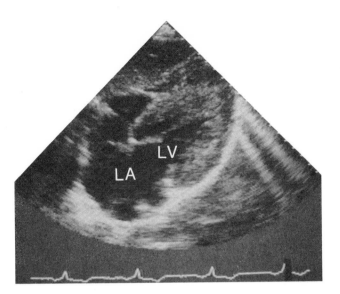

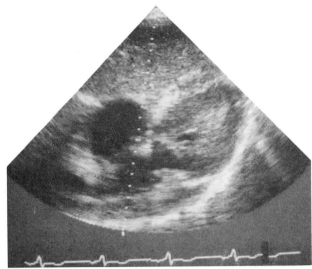

A   **B**

Figure 11.18.   Two-dimensional echocardiogram from the subcostal route showing a hypertrophic left ventricle and a large left atrium (*A*). In systole, the LV almost completely empties (*B*).

107). Blood flow velocity spectra should be recorded from the right ventricular outflow tract in these patients from the left parasternal short axis view, and from the subcostal route in which the right ventricular outflow tract and pulmonary artery are aligned parallel with the Doppler beam.

Left Ventricular Diastolic Function

While left ventricular systolic function is normal or even supranormal in HCM, diastolic function may be seriously impaired (48, 49, 87, 90–94, 115–117, 124). Great interest has been shown in left ventricular diastolic dysfunction in this disease because it is not known why a large proportion of patients with obstructive HCM develop congestive heart failure with supranormal systolic function, and also why there is a higher incidence of angina in patients with left ventricular diastolic dysfunction (119, 125).

The echocardiographic abnormalities suggesting left ventricular diastolic dysfunction have involved mostly the mitral valve, and consist of delayed mitral valve opening with respect to minimum left ventricular dimension, prolongation of the time period from atrial systole to mitral valve closure, and decreased maximum diastolic closing velocity (EF slope) of the anterior mitral valve leaflet (25, 115–118, 126–129). Normally the mitral valve opens within a few milliseconds of minimum left ventricular dimension (130), but in almost two-thirds of patients with HCM, mitral valve opening is delayed by up to 200 msec, indicating prolonged isovolumic relaxation due to decreased myocardial compliance and slowed release of systolic

wall tension (115). The time interval on the M-mode echo between the peak of the atrial systolic wave on the mitral valve to mitral valve closure is prolonged (prolonged AC segment or beta bump) in almost one-third of patients, indicating increased left ventricular diastolic pressure. In addition, the early maximal closing velocity of the anterior mitral valve leaflet (EF slope) is decreased, and this has been interpreted to reflect increased resistance to left ventricular filling due to decreased distensibility (115, 126, 129). However, the decreased maximal closing velocity of the anterior mitral valve leaflet probably results from its diastolic contact with the septum because the maximum closing velocity of the posterior leaflet is normal (129), and both should theoretically be similarly affected by alterations in left ventricular distensibility. Thus, the different closing velocities of the two leaflets more likely represent displacement of the mitral valve apparatus into the narrowed left ventricular outflow tract. Studies using computer analysis of M-mode echocardiograms reported delayed or slowed relaxation and decreased peak rates of left ventricular cavity filling (115–119) (Fig. 11.24). These observations of abnormal left ventricular diastolic filling characteristics have been confirmed by analysis of time activity curves derived from radionuclide angiograms (131, 132).

The presence of abnormal left ventricular diastolic function is also suggested by Doppler echocardiography (90–94). The antegrade transmitral or left ventricular inflow tract blood flow velocity profile differs from normal in the majority of patients (Fig. 11.25). The peak velocity during rapid diastolic filling (E wave) is re-

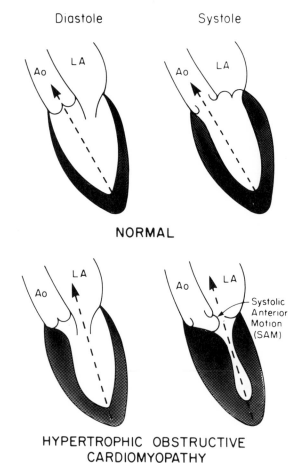

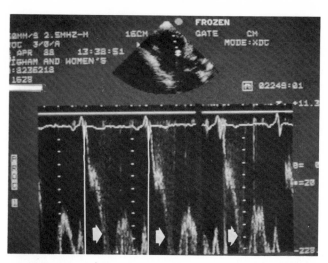

Figure 11.20. Blood flow velocity recordings from the LV outflow tract in HCM with pulsed-wave Doppler. Note the late systolic peaking (*arrows*) and increased velocity of blood flow with aliasing of the maximum velocity (greater than 2.2 m/sec).

Figure 11.19. In the normal heart the left ventricle contracts along its own long axis such that blood flow is directed toward the aortic valve and aorta. A tentative mechanism for the high incidence of mitral regurgitation (which approaches 50% in HCM) is that the ASH alters left ventricular chamber architecture and the position of the long axis of the left ventricular cavity. Thus, during systolic contraction, blood flow is directed toward the mitral valve annulus and left atrium, which, together with the left ventricular outflow tract obstruction from SAM, results in mitral regurgitation.

Almost 50% of the patients with HCM have mitral regurgitation (86, 121, 122, 136, 137), which varies from trivial to severe. Before Doppler was available, mitral regurgitation was suggested by an enlarged left atrium that expanded in systole. A large left atrium per se does not necessarily denote the presence of mitral regurgitation, since it may also occur in the presence of chronically elevated left ventricular end-diastolic pressure. However, Doppler can unequivocally document the presence of mitral regurgitation by detecting retrograde systolic flow across the mitral valve into the left atrium. The severity of mitral regurgitation should be

duced and its duration prolonged, indicating abnormally slow left ventricular filling. Furthermore, the peak velocity during atrial systole (A wave) is augmented. Thus the E/A ratio that has been advocated as an index of left ventricular diastolic properties is decreased. This ratio (133), reflects the interaction of ventricular mass, volume, and diastolic pressure, and is usually considerably diminished consistent with decreased compliance.

The abnormal position of the mitral valve apparatus and the altered left ventricular ejection dynamics may be important features in the genesis of calcification of the mitral valve annulus, which occurs more frequently than in an age-matched control population (30, 134, 135).

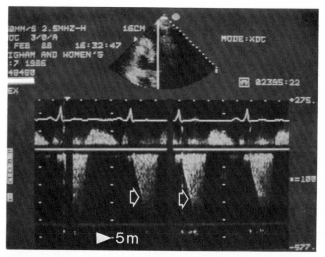

Figure 11.21. Continuous-wave Doppler recording from the left ventricular outflow tract in HCM shows a late peaking and a maximum velocity of 3.8 m/sec, consistent with an LV outflow tract gradient of between 55 and 60 mmHg.

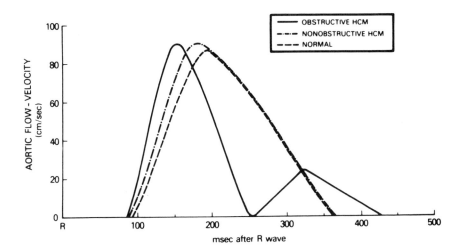

Figure 11.22. Doppler flow velocity signals recorded from the ascending aorta with respect to the timing of the R wave on the EKG. Hypertrophic cardiomyopathy characteristically peaks earlier than either the normal heart or the nonobstructive hypertrophic cardiomyopathy, and there is often a second velocity peak. (Reproduced with permission from Maron BJ, Gottsdiener JS, Arle J, Rosing DR, Wesley YE, Epstein SE. Dynamic subaortic obstruction in hypertrophic cardiomyopathy: Analysis by pulsed wave Doppler echocardiography. J Am Coll Cardiol 1985;6:1–15).

semiquantitated, by flow mapping with pulsed-wave Doppler (138), or with color-flow Doppler or quantitation of the mitral regurgitant fraction (139, 140) (see Chapter 7).

Occasionally, patients with HCM develop vegetative endocarditis involving the mitral valve and/or aortic valve (141, 142). This may relate to the high incidence of mitral regurgitation and the abnormal left ventricular systolic ejection dynamics.

Premature Aortic Valve Closure

An additional echocardiographic finding in HCM that has been interpreted as indicative of dynamic obstruction in the left ventricular outflow tract is the presence of premature or mid-systolic aortic valve closure (34, 143) (Fig. 11.26). This is best appreciated by dropping an M-mode line through the aortic valve leaflets under two-dimensional echo guidance. The aortic leaflets

open rapidly, and then in early systole the right and/or noncoronary cusp on M-mode drifts into the closed position in the center of the aortic root. This movement or centralization of the cusps is due to the Venturi effect of blood being ejected at high velocity such that much of the stroke volume has been evacuated within the first third of systole as the small hypertrophic ventricle contracts (109). This premature aortic valve closure at the end of left ventricular ejection occurs because the aortic valve leaflets have no tensor apparatus and once flow diminishes, the aortic leaflets close, although they may be reopened by blood egressing from the ventricle during the latter third of systole.

Doppler echocardiography has recently demonstrated the presence of mild aortic regurgitation (1+ to 2+) in between a quarter to one-third of patients (Fig. 11.27) (144). This mild aortic regurgitation has no hemodynamic importance, but may possibly explain why the aortic valve leaflets are involved in more than

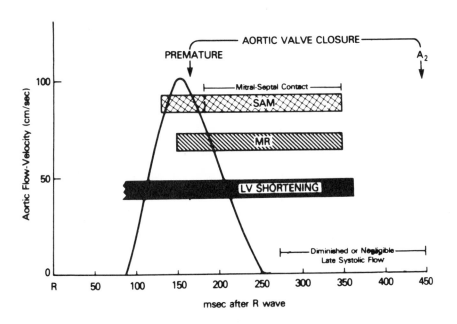

Figure 11.23. The relationship between the timing of the peak aortic flow velocity and the onset of SAM, mitral regurgitation, and left ventricular shortening in HCM. (Reproduced with permission from Maron BJ, Gottsdiener JS, Arle J, Rosing DR, Wesley YE, Epstein SE. Dynamic subaortic obstruction in hypertrophic cardiomyopathy: Analysis by pulsed wave Doppler echocardiography. J Am Coll Cardiol 1985;6:1–15).

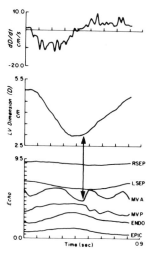

Figure 11.24. The bottom panel shows the computer output of a digitized M-mode echocardiogram from a patient with HCM. The XY coordinates of the right and left septal surfaces, the anterior and posterior mitral valve leaflets, and the posterior wall endocardium and epicardium are shown with time. The change in LV dimension with time is shown above. Mitral valve opening (*arrow*) normally coincides with minimal LV dimension, but is delayed by approximately 65 msec in this patient with HCM (normal = 10 ± 5 msec). The left ventricular dimension increases slowly throughout diastole so there is no discrete rapid filling phase. The peak rate of change of left ventricular dimension is shown at the top. (Reproduced by permission of the American Heart Association, Inc. from St. John Sutton M, Tajik JA, Gibson DG, Brown DJ, Seward JB. Echocardiographic assessment of left ventricular filling and septal and posterior wall dynamics in idiopathic hypertrophic subaortic stenosis. Circulation 1978;57:517.)

50% of the cases of vegetative endocarditis in this disease (144).

Other Conditions

Other conditions that have echocardiographic appearances similar to HCM include idiopathic chronic systemic and renovascular hypertension in which 10 to 15% may have ASH, but only very rarely are these conditions associated with SAM and outflow tract obstruction. Furthermore, reduction in afterload with blood pressure lowering agents usually results in regression of left ventricular hypertrophy, while left ventricular remodeling does not occur in HCM because the left ventricular hypertrophy is genetically determined. Other conditions that have echo features similar to HCM with SAM have been reported. They include Friedreich's ataxia (145–147), pheochromocytoma (148), Fabry's disease (149), and Pompe's disease (150).

HCM is occasionally associated with a number of developmental anomalies involving the neural crest tissue, such as tuberous sclerosis (151), pheochromocytoma (146), lentiginosis (107, 152, 153), and neurofibromatosis (154), and therefore when these conditions are present with clinical findings of left ventricular outflow obstruction, HCM should be excluded by Doppler echocardiography. HCM occurs sporadically in approximately 40% of patients, but is genetically determined by dominant inheritance in 60% (13, 14, 69). It has been reported in mono- and dizygotic twins, and in two successive generations of the same family. Thus, echo examination of first-degree relatives of probands with HCM should be attempted wherever possible.

Figure 11.25. Transmitral Doppler blood flow velocity signals in HCM (*A*) and normal (*B*). In HCM, the peak velocity during rapid filling (E wave) is decreased and the duration of filling prolonged, while the peak velocity during atriosystolic contraction (A wave) is greater than during rapid filling. Thus the E/A velocity ratio is less than unity; in normal hearts, the E/A ratio is greater than unity. LV early diastolic filling in HCM is often not only slow but prolonged.

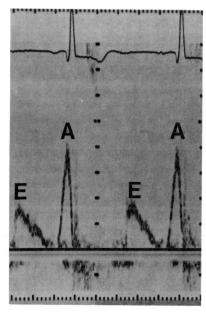
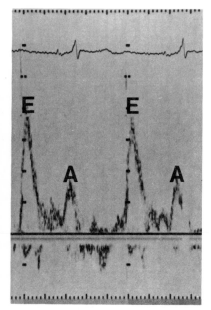

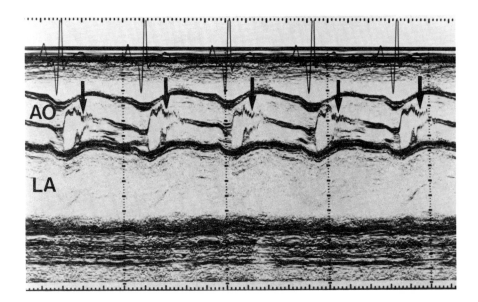

Figure 11.26. M-mode echocardiogram from a patient with HCM showing the aorta, aortic valve, and left atrium posteriorly. The aortic valve opens rapidly, but both the right and noncoronary cusps move briskly to the closed position (*arrows*), consonant with the end of left ventricular ejection. This premature or early AV closure is one of the M-mode echocardiographic diagnostic criteria for HCM.

DILATED CARDIOMYOPATHY

The diagnostic features of dilated cardiomyopathy (DCM) are increased left ventricular end-diastolic and end-systolic volumes, severely impaired global contractile function with an ejection fraction of less than 40%, and progressive symptomatic congestive heart failure (1, 148, 155–164). The pathoetiology in the majority of patients with DCM is unknown, but in a proportion there is growing evidence that viral myocarditis or immunologic abnormalities may be implicated (165–170). Whatever the etiology, the primary problem is that the myocardium fails to shorten normally—the relationship between load and the velocity of shortening is shifted leftward of normal, while the force-length relationship is shifted downward and to the right of normal. The diminished left and right ventricular contractile function is accompanied by ventricular dilatation, which by LaPlace's law results in a predictable increase in end-systolic wall stress (afterload), that is, an increase in the force that the myocardium must overcome to eject blood into the systemic circulation. This increase in wall stress is the stimulus to left ventricular hypertrophy; however, the increase in left ventricular volume in DCM is disproportionately greater than the increase in mass, so that wall stress is only rarely normalized (171). Wall stress is important because it is a major determinant, not only of myocardial oxygen consumption, but also of ventricular architecture (172–174). Furthermore, ejection phase indices of left ventricular pump function vary inversely with wall stress—the higher the stress, the lower the ejection fraction (175–177). The chronic elevation of wall stress results in left ventricular remodeling, but as the left ventricular volume insidiously increases, the hypertrophy becomes progressively more inadequate, the ventricle becomes more spherical, and contractile function further deteriorates (178).

Most patients with DCM have symptoms of congestive heart failure, and Doppler echocardiography simply confirms the clinical diagnosis. However, in some patients the diagnosis is made initially by Doppler echocardiography before symptoms develop, when cardiomegaly is discovered on routine physical examination or on chest x-ray. Doppler echocardiography has a prominent diagnostic role in DCM. Because the long-term prognosis of DCM is poor and cardiac transplantation is the only form of therapy that unequivocally prolongs survival (179), accurate serial assessment of cardiac function is essential not only to assess the response to pharmacologic agents but also to optimally time cardiac transplantation.

DCM was first diagnosed noninvasively by M-mode

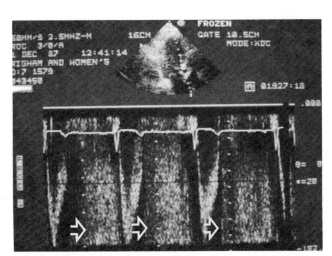

Figure 11.27. Pulsed-wave Doppler recording from the LV outflow tract in a patient with HCM, demonstrating a high-velocity holodiastolic signal (*arrows*) from retrograde blood flow due to aortic regurgitation.

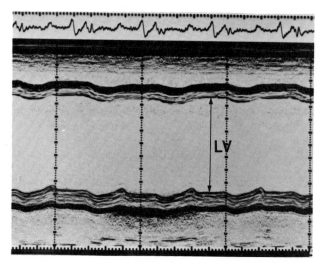

Figure 11.28. M-mode echocardiogram from a patient with DCM showing a dilated LV cavity, and LV end-diastolic dimension of 7.3 cm with mild concentric left ventricular hypertrophy and extremely poor systolic contractile function, indicated by fractional shortening of approximately 5%.

echocardiography by the presence of increased end-diastolic and end-systolic left ventricular dimensions, normal or slightly increased wall thickness, equivalent reduction in septal and posterior wall excursion, and severely decreased fractional shortening (Fig. 11.28). The mitral valve is anatomically normal, but the distance between the E point of the anterior mitral valve leaflet and the left side of the septum is increased (Fig. 11.29) (180, 181). Usually the time interval from the A point on the anterior mitral valve leaflet to mitral valve closure—the AC segment or B bump—is prolonged, indicating increased left ventricular end-diastolic pressure (182). Additional M-mode echocardiographic fea-

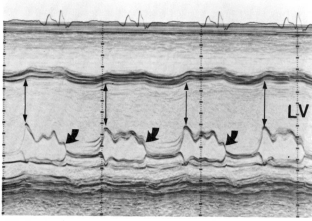

Figure 11.29. M-mode echocardiogram from a patient with DCM showing a dilated LV cavity with mitral E point–septal separation of 3.8 cm (normal is less than 0.8 cm), and a beta bump indicating elevation of LV end-diastolic pressure. The RV outflow tract is also dilated.

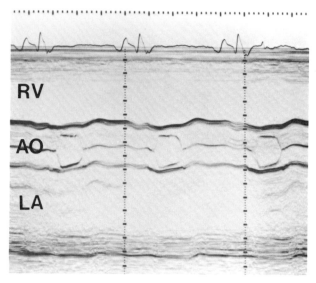

Figure 11.30. M-mode echocardiogram in DCM showing a dilated right ventricular outflow tract. The anterior motion of the aorta during systole is decreased, and the aortic valve leaflets drift slowly into the open position, rather than snapping open briskly, and then drift closed, suggesting decreased stroke volume. The left atrium is enlarged.

tures include an almost immobile aortic root with only minor anterior displacement during systole, and normal-appearing aortic valve leaflets that open slowly and having done so, begin to drift closed again, indicating diminished stroke volume and shortened ejection time (Fig. 11.30). The right ventricular outflow tract dimension is increased, and the left atrium enlarged because of elevated left ventricular diastolic pressure or secondary mitral regurgitation (183). Left ventricular dilatation and dysfunction due to severe triple coronary artery disease or anterior left ventricular aneurysm formation cannot be reliably differentiated from DCM by M-mode echocardiography because of its limited lateral resolution. This is especially important when septal motion is abnormal due to left bundle branch block.

Two-dimensional Doppler echocardiography enables the diagnosis to be confidently established, and cardiac architecture, contractile function, hemodynamics, semi-quantitation of right- and left-side atrioventricular valve regurgitation, and detection of intracardiac thrombus to be accurately assessed. Left parasternal long axis and the three conventional short axis sections of the left ventricle (the base, midcavity, and apex) demonstrate greatly enlarged end-systolic and end-diastolic chamber dimensions and usually normal absolute wall thickness (Figs. 11.31–11.33). Relative wall thickness, which is the ratio of end-diastolic wall thickness to end-diastolic cavity radius, is severely diminished. In real time, there is concentric inward wall motion during systole and outward wall motion in diastole, with severely reduced fractional shortening.

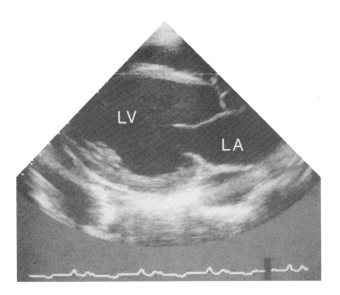

A

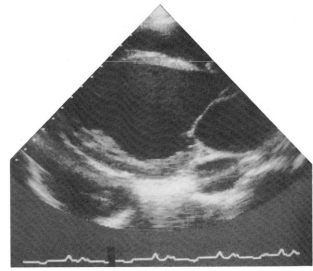

B

Figure 11.31.   Two-dimensional echocardiogram of the LV long axis in DCM showing a greatly enlarged chamber in diastole (*A*) and little change in size in systole (*B*). The mitral valve opens, but with a much increased distance between the anterior leaflet tip and the left side of the septum (increased E point–septal separation).

In severe DCM, the diameter of the midcavity short axis section is often larger than that at the base because of the change in left ventricular cavity shape to a more spherical configuration. In patients with DCM who develop left bundle branch block or intraventricular conduction defects, septal motion is usually abnormal. Although segmental wall motion abnormalities have been reported in DCM (184–186), they are rare and should suggest that the left ventricular dysfunction is due to coronary artery disease rather than primary myocardial disease especially when the electrical activation sequence is normal.

Cephalad angulation of the transducer along the left ventricular long axis from the left parasternal position brings the aortic valve into view (Fig. 11.34). Although the aortic valve leaflets are normal, their motion pattern is abnormal—the cusps move slowly to the open position and then drift instead of snapping back into apposition at end-systole similar to that in the M-mode echo (Fig. 11.30). This characteristic motion pattern and shortened ejection time indicate diminished left ventricular stroke volume (187). In the same imaging plane, the tricuspid and pulmonary valve leaflets are visualized (Fig. 11.34) and have similar leaflet motion patterns, suggesting decreased right ventricular inflow and outflow, respectively. The left atrium in this plane is posterior to the aorta, and is usually but not always dilated (Fig. 11.34).

The apical four chamber images of the heart usually demonstrate enlargement of all of the cardiac chambers (Fig. 11.33). The left ventricular cavity is enlarged and spherical because of the proportionately greater increase in the minor rather than in the major axis, with the ratio of short/long cavity axes approaching unity. Thus, the left ventricle in DCM resembles that of chronic volume overload due to mitral regurgitation; only the contractile function is severely reduced. Endocardial motion is greatly but equally diminished in the septum and the left ventricular free wall in the apical two and four chamber views, and in the left ventricular long axis view.

Since the left ventricle is dilated and wall motion severely reduced, blood flow within the left ventricle is greatly decreased and thrombus has an increased tendency to form within the left ventricular cavity, particularly at the apex (Fig. 11.35) (188). Because of the high incidence and devastating complications of systemic embolism of intracardiac thrombi, every effort must be made to detect intracardiac thrombus in all patients with DCM, whether or not they are taking anticoagulants. When the heart is enlarged, the left ventricular apex may not be visualized well in the apical four chamber view because it is in the near field of the transducer, and unless the transducer is moved more posteriorly and down an intercostal space, thrombus within the apex may be overlooked. Furthermore, in DCM, large muscular trabeculations develop on the endocardial surface of the left ventricle close to the apex as the left ventricle hypertrophies, and these may be confused with thrombus. Left ventricular thrombus should only be diagnosed when visualized in orthogonal views, that is, in the apical four and two chamber views and in short axis sections through the apex, when thrombus appears as a filling defect within

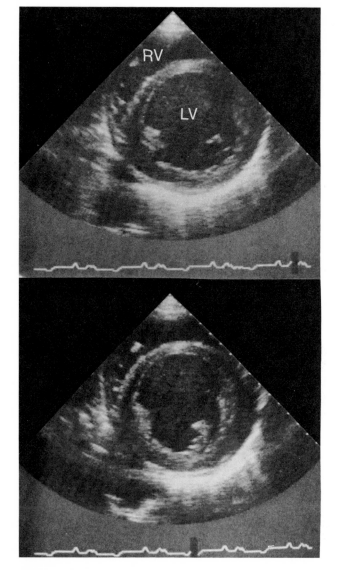

RV

LV

Figure 11.32. Two-dimensional echocardiogram of the LV short axis at high papillary muscle level, showing a greatly dilated left ventricle (*A*), with little reduction in cavity area in systole (*B*).

the cavity (189, 190) (Fig. 11.36). Thrombus may be flat, laminated, and immobile, or protuberant and very mobile, and it is the latter morphologic characteristics that are associated with an increased likelihood of embolization (191).

The mitral valve leaflets exhibit a characteristic motion pattern denoting diminished left ventricular contractile function and often increased LV end-diastolic pressure (182) (Fig. 11.29). This abnormal mitral valve leaflet motion may be due partly to the large end-systolic left ventricular cavity volume and the relatively small change in volume from systole through diastole, and partly due to the alteration in left ventricular geometry, such that papillary muscles and chordae tendinae subtend a greater than normal angle to the

mitral valve annulus. This angle increases progressively as the left ventricular chamber dilates (Fig. 11.37). The relative change in the position of papillary muscle, without any concomitant change in chordal length, results in improper coaptation between the anterior and posterior mitral valve leaflets, which with dilatation of the mitral valve annulus results in mitral regurgitation (192–195) of varying severity in 50 to 75% of patients with DCM.

The left atrium in the apical two and four chamber views is usually enlarged due to mitral regurgitation or to chronically elevated left ventricular diastolic pressure (Fig. 11.33). Three of the four pulmonary veins are visible from the apical four chamber view and they are usually dilated when there is severe mitral regurgitation. The presence and severity of mitral regurgitation should be assessed with pulsed-wave or Doppler color flow mapping of the left atrium (196) (see Chapter 7).

After flow mapping the left atrium with the pulsed-wave Doppler, the sample volume should be positioned in the left ventricle immediately subjacent to the mitral valve leaflets to obtain blood flow velocity spectra from the left ventricular inflow tract. The increased resistance to filling in DCM, resulting from diminished left ventricular compliance, might be expected to be discernible as a combination of diminished peak velocity during rapid early filling, prolongation of the rapid filling phase, and augmentation of the peak velocity during atrial systole (133). However, in patients with DCM and mitral regurgitation, the peak E wave velocity during rapid filling, peak A wave velocity during atrial systole, and the E/A velocity ratio are usually normal (Fig. 11.38) (197). By contrast, in patients without or with only trivial mitral regurgitation, the peak E wave velocity is diminished, the duration of rapid filling phase is prolonged, the A wave velocity is increased, and the E/A ratio is less than 1.0, indicating "diastolic myocardial dysfunction" and diminished compliance (Fig. 11.38) (197). In a proportion of these latter patients, however, the E/A ratio may be normal (198). Thus, the transmitral velocity signals in DCM may be modified by development of mitral regurgitation, and should therefore be interpreted with caution and with knowledge of left ventricular loading conditions.

The right ventricle is often dilated, and as it increases in size either as the result of primary failure of right ventricular myocardial shortening or secondary to pulmonary hypertension from elevated left ventricular diastolic pressure and tricuspid regurgitation, the moderator band takes off from the right side of the septum at closer to a right angle than normal. In addition, the right ventricle becomes apex-forming. The diminished right ventricular contractile function is apparent since end-systolic and end-diastolic cavity areas in the apical four chamber view are similar (Fig.

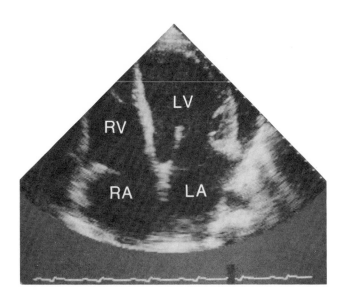
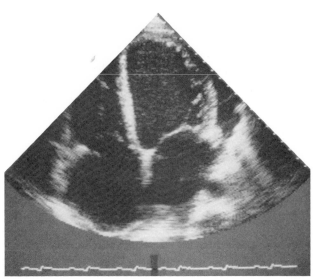

A   **B**

Figure 11.33. Two-dimensional echocardiogram of the apical four chamber view in DCM. Four chamber enlargement (*A*) with very poor RV and LV contractile function is evident from the minor change in ventricular areas from diastole to systole (*B*). The enlarged atria are due to both right and left atrioventricular valve regurgitation from the major architectural remodeling of the two ventricles.

11.33). Although the tricuspid valve leaflets are normal, the right ventricular dilatation, the concomitant increase in tricuspid valve ring circumference (199), and elevation of pulmonary artery pressure result in tricuspid regurgitation (200). The tricuspid regurgitation should be semiquantitated by flow mapping of the right atrium with pulsed-wave Doppler in the same way as in the assessment of mitral regurgitation, and graded

from 1+ to 4+. The peak velocity of the regurgitant tricuspid jet should be obtained with continuous-wave Doppler. From this the pressure difference between the right atrium and right ventricle can be calculated (200–202), from which pulmonary artery systolic pressure can be determined (see Chapter 7). The right atrium is usually enlarged either because of the elevated right ventricular diastolic pressure or the tricuspid regurgi-

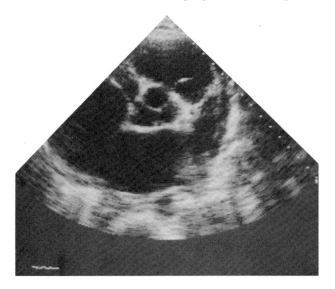
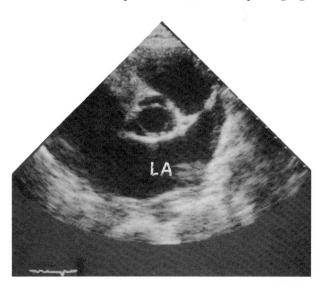

A   **B**

Figure 11.34. Two-dimensional echocardiogram of the short axis of the aorta in DCM showing the aortic valve, pulmonary valve, and tricuspid valves in diastole (*A*) and systole (*B*). The left atrium, right atrium, and right ventricular outflow tract are dilated. During systole, the aortic valve leaflets drift open with a motion pattern and orifice area consistent with decreased stroke volume.

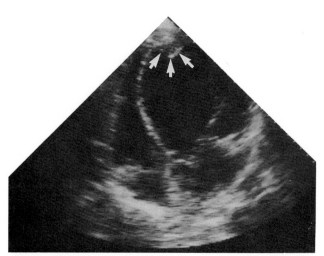

Figure 11.35. Two-dimensional echocardiogram of the four chamber view in DCM showing a greatly dilated and spherical-shaped left ventricle with thrombus in the LV apex (*arrows*).

tation. The inferior vena cava is often dilated; tricuspid regurgitation can be detected in either the inferior or the superior vena cava by positioning the pulsed-wave Doppler sample volume within the IVC or SVC from the subcostal and right supraclavicular approaches, respectively, and detecting reversed flow in systole (Fig. 11.39).

Three forms of dilated cardiomyopathy worthy of mention are familial or X-linked cardiomyopathy (203), peripartum cardiomyopathy (Fig. 11.40) (204, 205), and the unexplained left ventricular dysfunction/cardiomyopathy associated with acquired immunodeficiency syndrome (AIDS) (206–208) (Fig. 11.41). There are no distinguishing or specific echocardiographic features in any of these three types of myopathy, but they all result in dilated left ventricular cavities, severely depressed global contractile function with or without right heart dilatation, and right ventricular dysfunction. The clinical presentation of congestive heart failure and cardiomegaly within the last trimester or the first five months following parturition should suggest peripartum cardiomyopathy. Note that, in peripartum cardiomyopathy, when left ventricular function is assessed serially, reduction in left ventricular volumes and return to normal function occurs in 50% of the patients within six months (204, 205). Congestive heart failure in more than one young female member of the same family suggests X-linked cardiomyopathy (203), while cardiomegaly and left ventricular failure in the setting of AIDS should prompt careful two-dimensional echocardiographic assessment of cardiac size and function to detect the presence of AIDS cardiomyopathy.

RESTRICTIVE CARDIOMYOPATHY

The spectrum of left ventricular geometry in restrictive cardiomyopathy (RCM) is more varied than in either HCM or DCM. Although left ventricular chamber size is almost always normal, wall thickness may be decreased, normal, or increased, and these changes may occur throughout the ventricles or be localized to specific regions within the ventricles (1, 208). Those with increased wall thickness may appear both clinically and echocardiographically very similar to nonobstructive hypertrophic cardiomyopathy. Regardless of the ventricular chamber architecture, however, the physiologic commonality in RCM is the increased resistance to left ventricular filling (209). This increased resistance to filling is associated with elevated left ventricular diastolic pressure, left atrial hypertension and enlargement, and secondary pulmonary hypertension. There may also be increased resistance to filling of the right ventricle due to primary myocardial dysfunction and diminished distensibility, with concomitant increase in right ventricular diastolic pressure, right atrial dilatation, systemic venous hypertension, and, often, associated tricuspid regurgitation (209). The incidence of the different types of RCM varies geographically (210). In the eastern part of the African continent, endomyocardial fibrosis is reported to account for approximately one-quarter of all cardiovascular deaths. In the western world, RCM represents only between 5 and 10% of noncoronary cardiomyopathies, with amyloid heart disease being the most frequent form, occurring de novo, and in association with rheumatoid arthritis and multiple myeloma.

RCM may be arbitrarily divided into two major categories: 1) endomyocardial fibrosis, including Leoffler's fibroplastic endocarditis, and 2) infiltrative myocardial diseases, which include amyloid, sarcoid, hematochromatosis, and Pompe's and Fabry's diseases (1, 211).

Endomyocardial Fibrosis

In the majority of patients with endomyocardial fibrosis (EMF), sheets of fibrous tissue of varying thickness develop in the subendocardium, initially involving the apices of the ventricles and extending into the inflow tracts of the right and left ventricles (211–213). The distribution of this nondistensible endocardial fibrosis may be patchy or confluent, but it effectively forms a cardiac endoskeleton, which results in a marked increase in chamber stiffness and characteristic right and left ventricular filling patterns. The echocardiographic features of EMF are a normal size left ventricle, increased left ventricular wall thickness, and increased echo reflectance of the subendocardial surface consistent with fibrous replacement. Initially, sys-

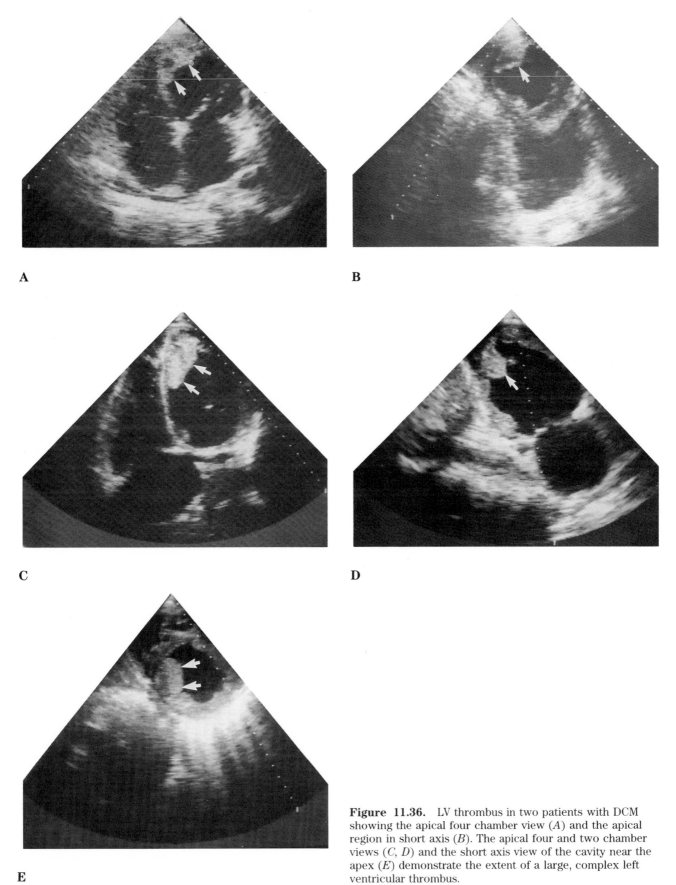

A

B

C

D

E

Figure 11.36. LV thrombus in two patients with DCM showing the apical four chamber view (*A*) and the apical region in short axis (*B*). The apical four and two chamber views (*C, D*) and the short axis view of the cavity near the apex (*E*) demonstrate the extent of a large, complex left ventricular thrombus.

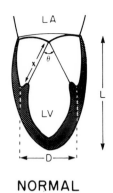

NORMAL

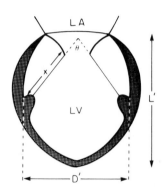

DILATED CARDIOMYOPATHY

Figure 11.37. The left ventricular remodeling that occurs in DCM as the LV dilates results in only a minor increase in LV length but a major increase in LV short axis diameter, so that the normal angle the papillary muscles subtend to the mitral valve annulus is greatly increased. Since the chordal and leaflet lengths do not change, the leaflets are unable to coapt normally and this, together with the minor increase in mitral valve ring circumference, are probably the major mechanisms for mitral regurgitation.

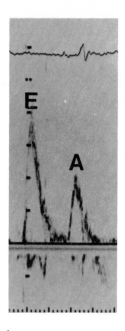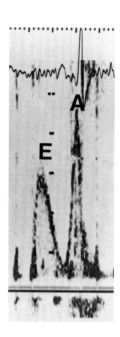

A   B

Figure 11.38. Doppler transmitral blood flow velocities from two patients with DCM. The peak velocity during rapid filling (E wave) exceeds the peak velocity during atriosystolic contraction when there is mitral regurgitation (*A*); but in patients with DCM and little or no mitral regurgitation, the peak E wave velocity is reduced and the peak A wave velocity increased, so that the E/A velocity ratio may be above or below unity (*B*). Thus, interpretation of the transmitral flow velocity signals should only be made with knowledge of the left ventricular loading conditions.

tolic contractile function is only mildly depressed and intracavity thrombus appears as filling defects in the apices of one or both ventricles (214–219). The left atrium is usually enlarged due to elevated left ventricular diastolic pressure rather than mitral regurgitation, although mitral regurgitation may be present, and should be assessed by pulsed-wave Doppler or color flow mapping. The right ventricular cavity is usually normal size or mildly enlarged, with increased right ventricular wall thickness and slightly decreased systolic function, all of which is visualized easily in the subcostal four chamber view. Tricuspid regurgitation may be present due to pulmonary hypertension secondary to elevated left-side pressures. In addition, if tricuspid regurgitation is present, pulmonary artery systolic pressure should be calculated from the peak velocity of the regurgitant jet obtained with continu-

ous-wave Doppler. The atrioventricular and semilunar valves may also be thickened in EMF, resulting in valvular regurgitation. Endomyocardial fibrosis is usually more extensive when it presents with symptoms in childhood, when it may involve the aortic valve, resulting in important aortic stenosis.

Fibroplastic endocarditis (Loeffler's syndrome) presents with physiologic, anatomic, and echocardiographic features similar to EMF, but is associated with peripheral blood hypereosinophilia of unknown cause. The left and right ventricular cavities are small and concentrically hypertrophied with extensive subendocardial fibrosis. The walls appear thick, hypokinetic, and highly echo-reflective particularly along the endocardium (220–222). The right and left ventricles may be filled with extensive thrombus, which adheres to the thickened endocardial surfaces and effectively obliterates the ventricular cavities (220–222). The thrombus-filled ventricular chambers and enlarged right and left atria can be clearly visualized in the apical four chamber view (Fig. 11.42). The mitral and tricuspid valves and both semilunar valves are intrinsically normal, but exhibit motion patterns consistent with decreased ventricular performance and diminished cardiac output.

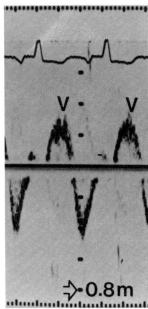

Figure 11.39. Doppler flow velocity recordings from the inferior vena cava in a patient with DCM shows dramatic systolic velocity signal (V), indicating the presence of tricuspid regurgitation. The calibration markers represent 20 cm/sec velocity.

Infiltrative Restrictive Cardiomyopathy

The most frequent forms of RCM encountered in the western world are those resulting from myocardial infiltration with substances ranging from elemental iron as in hemochromatosis (223–228), glycogen in Pompe's and Cori's diseases (150, 229–231), glycolipids in Fabry's disease (149, 232, 233), amyloid (101, 234–239), and sarcoid (240–243). The most common of these is amyloid. The intra- or intercellular deposition of noncontractile materials disrupts both myocardial contraction and relaxation either by myocyte injury and subsequent replacement fibrosis, or by development of an interstitial intercellular network that forms a mesoskeleton, which slowly but progressively impairs myocardial compliance. The change in left ventricular compliance is usually characterized by slowed myocardial relaxation and abnormally slow diastolic filling, which correlate with the dip and plateau in the left ventricular diastolic pressure contour. Typically there is preservation of near-normal systolic function (209).

Infiltration of the myocardium by amyloid may be patchy or homogenous, and is not confined to the left ventricular myocardium (101, 234). It may involve all four cardiac chambers, the atrioventricular and semilunar valves, the coronary arteries, and the specialized conducting tissue (234). There are no pathognomonic echocardiographic features of amyloid, although it can invariably be diagnosed confidently with Doppler echo-

cardiography by the presence of a constellation of abnormalities (235–239).

The left ventricular cavity size is normal or more commonly small, the septum and posterior left ventricular wall thicknesses are greatly increased (Fig. 11.43) (101, 238, 239). There is a direct relationship between wall thickness and survival—the greater the wall thickness, the shorter the survival (239). Between one-quarter and one-third of patients have asymmetric septal hypertrophy (ASH) (101, 239) (Fig. 11.44). The septum in those with ASH is hypomobile, but even in those with concentric hypertrophy, endocardial excursion and systolic thickening of the posterior wall and septum are strikingly reduced, and this can be appreciated in serial short axis sections of the left ventricle obtained from the left parasternal region. Several additional abnormalities, apparent on M-mode echocardiography, are helpful in establishing the diagnosis of amyloid (101, 235, 237). These include increased right ventricular free wall thickness (237) (Fig. 11.44), nonspecific mitral and/or aortic valve leaflet thickening (Fig. 11.45), pericardial effusions, and increased echo reflectance of the left ventricular myocardium, which is perhaps the most impressive feature (101) (Fig. 11.43). The increased myocardial reflectance is due to the changed acoustic properties of the myocardium, resulting from the intercellular deposition of amyloid. This is demonstrated as multiple-linear echoes within the septum and posterior left ventricular wall, which have the same locus of movement as the endocardial surfaces (Fig. 11.43) (101, 237). Computer processing of the M-mode echocardiograms in amyloid has demonstrated both regional and global left ventricular dysfunction, out of proportion to the increase in wall thickness or alteration in left ventricular geometry. These abnormalities include greatly reduced peak rate of left ventricular filling, prolonged isovolumic relaxation, and impaired regional left ventricular systolic and diastolic mechanics (244).

Two-dimensional echocardiography allows complete examination of the whole heart, and demonstrates that amyloid infiltration is not confined to the ventricular chambers (101, 238, 239, 245). In serial short axis and long axis views from the left parasternal region, left ventricular architecture resembles that of nonobstructive hypertrophic cardiomyopathy with a small cavity, usually with severe concentric left ventricular hypertrophy, decreased systolic function, and slowed left ventricular filling. From these views alone, amyloid may be difficult to distinguish from HCM (Figs. 11.46, 11.47). However, the left ventricular myocardium has a sparkling appearance by two-dimensional echocardiography (101, 239), which is even more striking than the M-mode appearance, and is due to the change in acoustic properties secondary to the altered composi-

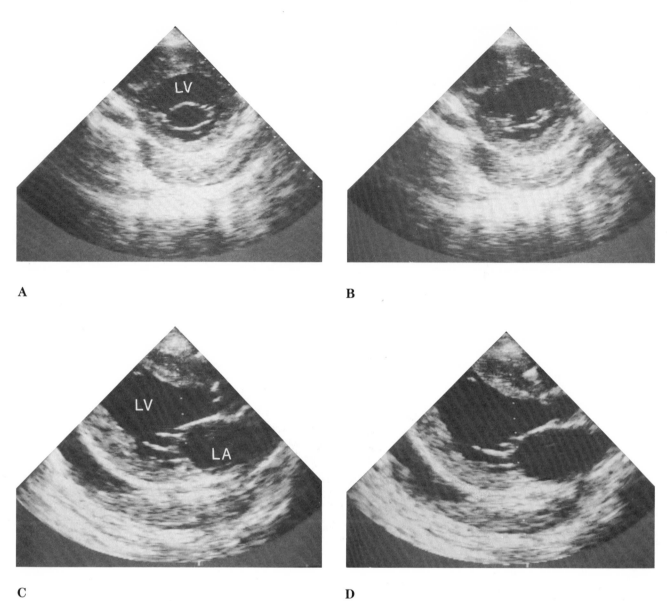

Figure 11.40. Two-dimensional echocardiogram from a patient with peripartum cardiomyopathy, showing the short axis of the left ventricle in systole (A) and diastole (B) with a mild left ventricular dilatation, severely impaired systolic function, and a moderate size posterior pericardial effusion. The left ventricular long axis also shows the minimal change in left ventricular size from diastole (C) to systole (D) and the moderate size pericardial effusion.

tion of the myocardium from amyloid deposition (246, 247). The right ventricle usually is similarly affected with markedly increased right ventricular free wall thickness (237), best seen in the subcostal four chamber view (Fig. 11.48) or in the subcostal view of both ventricles in short axis. Both right and left ventricular systolic function is seriously impaired in almost two-thirds of patients. Although the electrocardiogram in amyloid may suggest previous myocardial infarction (234, 248) usually in the anterior left ventricular wall, left ventricular segmental wall motion abnormalities are rare, in spite of the fact that amyloid deposits have been demonstrated histologically in the coronary arterial walls (234).

In the apical four chamber view, the enlarged right and left atria contrast with the small hypertrophic ventricular chambers (Fig. 11.49). The increased thickness of the interatrial septum, which occurs in one-third of patients, must be diagnosed in the subcostal four chamber view or in the left parasternal view of the short axis of aorta to exclude artefactual widening of this structure caused by divergence of the ultrasound beam in the far field, which occurs in the apical four chamber view. Additional two-dimensional echocardiographic findings in amyloid are nonspecific thickening of the mitral and tricuspid valves, which does not result in commissural fusion or in narrowing of the valve orifice areas. The decreased mitral and tricuspid valve

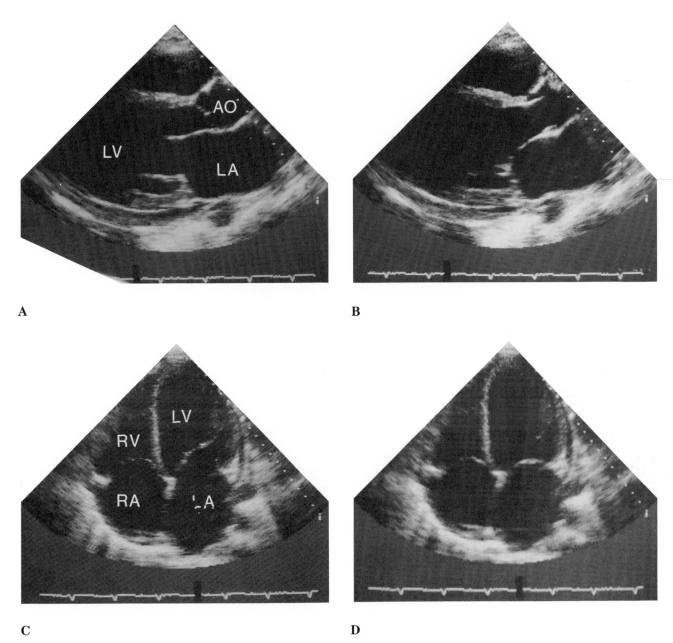

A

B

C

D

Figure 11.41. Two-dimensional echocardiogram from a patient with AIDS, showing the dilated poorly-contracting left ventricle in long axis in diastole (*A*) and in systole (*B*). The apical four chamber view shows that all four chambers are dilated in diastole (*C*) and in systole (*D*). A small pericardial effusion is present.

leaflet mobility partly reflects decreased ventricular performance, but also the restricted motion due to increased leaflet thickness, even though cusp coaption is usually normal. The semilunar valves may also be thickened with amyloid deposits, but this occurs less often than with the atrioventricular valves. The semilunar valve leaflets often appear bright, and their mobility is mildly reduced. These changes are not associated with valve stenosis, although regurgitation is common, occurring in approximately 90% of patients (245). The valvular regurgitation is usually mild, and its

frequency of occurrence by color-flow or pulsed Doppler is mitral (90%), tricuspid (70%), aortic (43%), and pulmonic (23%) (245). Between one-half and two-thirds of patients develop pericardial effusions, which range in size from small to very large (Figs. 11.46, 11.47) (101, 240, 241).

Sarcoid

Sarcoid is a rare form of infiltrative cardiomyopathy, occurring in less than 5% of patients with systemic

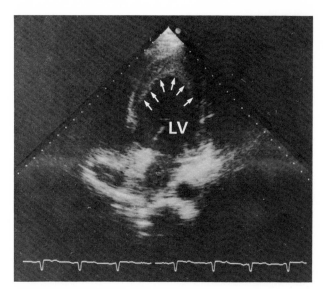

Figure 11.42. Two-dimensional echocardiogram of the left ventricle from the apex in a patient with Loeffler's RCM and eosinophilia, demonstrating the dilated left ventricle with laminated left ventricular thrombus at the apex (*arrows*).

sarcoid. It has a very poor prognosis, with a 50% mortality within two years of diagnosis, either from sudden death due to arrhythmia or from congestive heart failure (240, 241). The myocardium is infiltrated with noncaseating granulomata, which predominantly involve the left ventricle (240) and have a predilection for the anterolateral papillary muscle, the inlet portion of the interventricular septum, and the midventricular free wall (241). Although the infiltration is usually patchy, in isolated cases, granulomata may be distributed throughout both ventricles. The natural history of the intramural granulomatous infiltrates is to form fibrous tissue scars. When these involve the left ventric-

ular free wall, they result in thinning of the left ventricular wall and occasionally aneurysm formation, while those involving the papillary muscles cause contractile dysfunction and result in mitral regurgitation (240, 241). Thinning of the proximal septal myocardium following fibrous scarring of resolving granulomata frequently involves the conducting system and accounts for the abnormalities in electrical activation, syncope, and sudden death (241).

Echocardiographically, the left ventricular cavity is usually normal or slightly dilated, and left ventricular wall thickness is increased except for the echo bright areas of focal thinning and scarring (242, 243) (Fig. 11.50). These areas of scarring can be identified by their greater echo reflectance and diminished myocardial wall thickness, and because they are associated with marked segmental wall motion abnormalities. The fibrous tissue replacement increases myocardial stiffness and resistance to filling, so that ventricular filling is characteristically slow and prolonged, and in the late stages of the disease is accompanied by severe impairment of systolic function. In the four chamber view, the left atrium is invariably enlarged due to mitral regurgitation, which results from the propensity of the papillary muscles to be involved in sarcoid (241). The right heart chambers are usually dilated, and the passive right ventricular myocardial stiffness and resistance to filling are both increased. Tricuspid regurgitation may result directly from right heart involvement in sarcoid or it may result from pulmonary hypertension secondary to concomitant pulmonary parenchymal disease.

Myocardial Infiltration with Iron

There is a wide range of myocardial abnormalities in idiopathic hemochromatosis and in iron overload from

Figure 11.43. M-mode echocardiogram from a patient with RCM due to cardiac amyloid, showing increased septal (s) and posterior wall thicknesses (w), minor LV dilatation, and severely decreased contractile function. Note the linear intramyocardial echos in the septum and posterior wall, which are characteristic of amyloid.

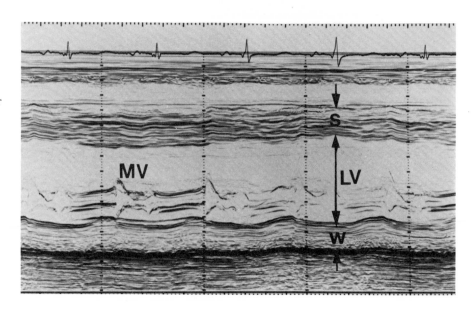

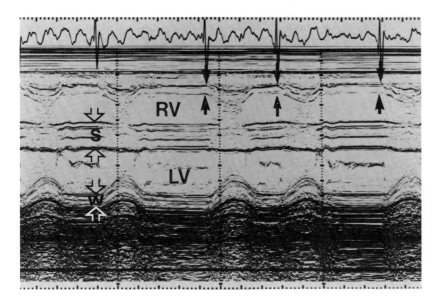

Figure 11.44. M-mode echocardiogram of the patient with amyloid RCM showing an asymmetrically hypertrophied septum (s) compared to the posterior LV wall (w) (s/w ratio = 1.6), and increased right ventricular wall thickness (*solid black arrows*).

multiple blood transfusions (greater than 100 units) for chronic anemia secondary to hemoglobinopathies (223, 228). Deposition of iron occurs more in ventricular than in atrial myocardium, and involves the epicardial or outer third of the ventricular wall more than the middle or endocardial thirds (223). Iron infiltration occurs in myocytes as well as in interstitial cells (223). The intracellular iron deposition in the myocytes is associated with degeneration of myocardial fibers, with consequent replacement fibrosis. These myocardial changes are accompanied by severe contractile dysfunction in 35 to 40% of patients (228). In patients with

hemochromatosis and clinical evidence of heart disease, M-mode and two-dimensional echocardiographic examination demonstrate a moderately dilated left ventricle with normal wall thickness, minimal increase in left ventricular mass, marked reduction in systolic thickening of the septum and free left ventricular wall, and moderate to severe global dysfunction, but no segmental wall motion abnormalities (Fig. 11.51) (224, 227–229). The atrioventricular and semilunar valves are normal. The right ventricular myocardium, although infiltrated, is usually of normal size and function; however, there is biatrial enlargement that is visualized best in the apical four chamber view (228). One important feature of the left ventricular dysfunction in idiopathic hemochromatosis is that the iron deposition, and to a variable extent the left ventricular dysfunction, can be reversed with iron chelation therapy, provided that the myocardium is not overwhelmingly replaced by fibrous tissue (226, 227).

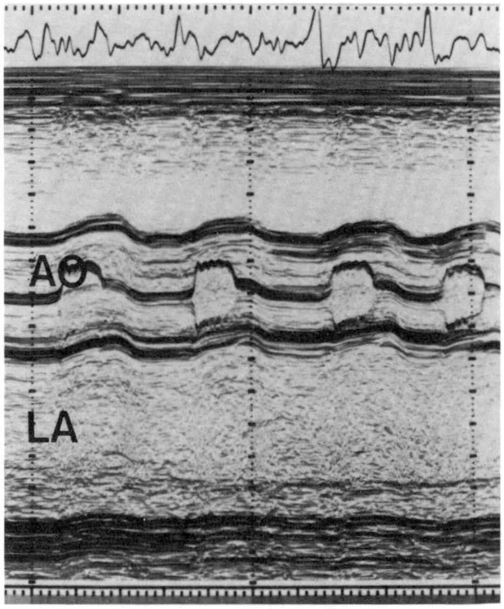

Pompe's, Cori's, and Fabry's Infiltrative Diseases

The glycogen and lipid storage diseases, including Pompe's, Cori's, and Fabry's diseases, are rare (149, 150, 229–233). There are, therefore, only a few echocardiographic reports that describe increased right and left ventricular wall thickness, which is usually concentric but may be assymetric with ASH (149), and ventricular systolic function varies from normal to reduced (Fig. 11.52). Pericardial effusions have also been described.

Idiopathic RCM

There is also a form of RCM in which the etiology cannot be determined, but is not due to infiltration of the myocardium. The clinical hemodynamic and Dopp-

Figure 11.45. M-mode echocardiogram from a patient with amyloid RCM showing thickened aortic valve leaflets, dilated right ventricular outflow tract, and left atrium with decreased excursion of the aortic root consistent with reduced stroke volume.

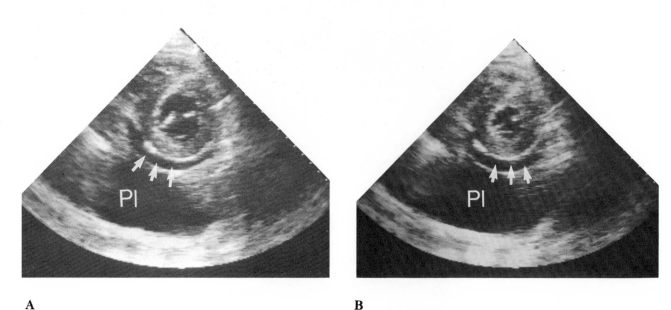

A   **B**

Figure 11.46. Two-dimensional echocardiogram of the LV short axis in diastole (*A*) and in systole (*B*) in a patient with amyloid RCM showing normal size LV cavity, increased wall thickness, increased echo brightness of the myocardium, decreased contractile function, a small pericardial effusion (*arrows*), and a large left pleural effusion (Pl).

ler echocardiographic findings are often indistinguishable from infiltrative RCM. Idiopathic noninfiltrative RCM is characterized echocardiographically by a normal size, hypertrophied LV and often hypertrophied RV with biatrial enlargement (Fig. 11.53), and usually moderate mitral and tricuspid regurgitation. The left ventricular filling patterns by pulsed-wave Doppler vary, and include those with decreased E wave and augmented A wave velocities, to those with normal or increased early rapid filling velocities (E wave) and decreased or normal atriosystolic (A wave) velocities.

Cardiomyopathy from Cardiotoxic Drugs

A number of pharmacologic agents are cardiotoxic. Two in particular, Adriamycin and Cyclophosphamide, when used in therapeutic doses, may result in severe depression of left ventricular function (249–254). The myocardial dysfunction resulting from Adriamycin is dose-related and irreversible, and usually results when the total dosage exceeds 450 mg/kg/m^2, but occasionally develops with a substantially smaller dosage (249). Echocardiography has been of greater value than elec-

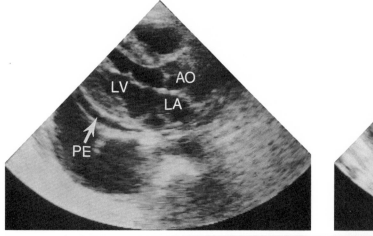

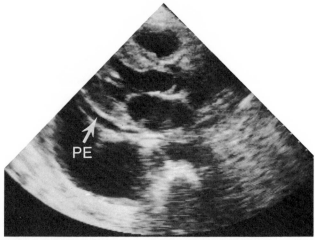

A   **B**

Figure 11.47. Two-dimensional echocardiogram of the LV long axis in amyloid RCM in diastole (*A*) and in systole (*B*) showing normal LV size, increased myocardial reflectance, decreased contractile function, a small pericardial effusion (*arrows*), and a large pleural effusion.

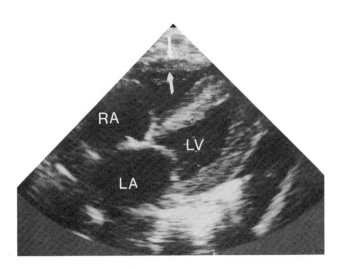

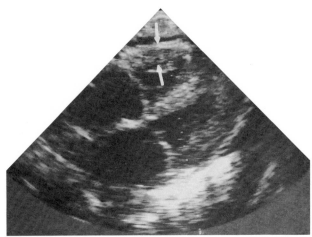

A   **B**

Figure 11.48. Two-dimensional echocardiogram of the subcostal four chamber view in diastole (*A*) and systole (*B*), showing the increased interatrial septum and increased right ventricular free wall thicknesses, which are characteristic findings in amyloid RCM.

trocardiography in detecting the early onset of myocardial damage and contractile dysfunction (251). The echocardiographic features of Adriamycin cardiomyopathy include a normal left ventricular end-diastolic dimension, increased end-systolic dimension, normal wall thickness, very poor contractile function, no segmental wall motion abnormalities, and a tendency to left ventricular dilatation with time (251, 252) (Figs. 11.54, 11.55).

Cyclophosphamide (cytoxan), in the dosage range used for immunosuppression prior to bone marrow transplantation, is accompanied by severe left ventricular contractile dysfunction within 72 hours of admin-

istration in approximately one-third of the patients (254). The incidence of left ventricular dysfunction following Cyclophosphamide is dose-related (Fig. 11.56). In severe cases, there is extensive interstitial myocardial hemorrhage, which results in sudden increase in left ventricular wall thickness developing within 72 hours of therapy, with concomitant dramatic reduction in ejection fraction. Often hemorrhagic pericarditis with effusion and occasionally tamponade develop concomitantly (255). However, the increase in wall thickness and the left ventricular dysfunction revert to normal at long term followup, unlike that due to Adriamycin.

Chloroquine, which is used extensively worldwide as an antimalarial agent, is the latest in a line of drugs that may result in dilated cardiomyopathy (256).

Neurocardiac Syndromes

There is an increasing number of genetically inherited neuromyelopathies that have a wide range of left ventricular contractile dysfunction, wherein myocardial involvement appears to be an integral part of the complete gene expression. The age at onset and rate of progression of the myocardial lesions appear to vary independently of the severity of the neurological involvement, and often determine the prognosis. The left ventricular dysfunction occurring in the neurocardiac syndromes can be divided into hypertrophic and dilated cardiomyopathies.

The Doppler echocardiographic findings in Friedreich's ataxia are a normal or small left ventricular chamber, usually with concentric left ventricular hypertrophy but occasionally with asymmetric hypertro-

Figure 11.49. Two-dimensional echocardiogram of the apical four chamber view of a patient with amyloid RCM in diastole, showing the small hypertrophied right and left ventricles, thickened mitral valve leaflets, and markedly dilated right and left atria.

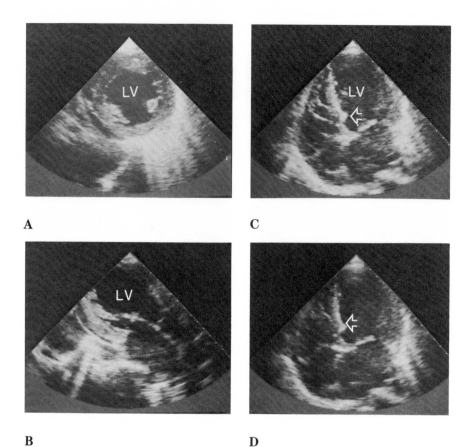

Figure 11.50. Two-dimensional echocardiographic parasternal short-axis (*A*), long-axis (*B*), and apical four-chamber views (*C, D*) of a patient with biopsy-proven cardiac sarcoid. There is increased echo brightness and fibrosis of the papillary muscle (*A, B*). The proximal interventricular septum is thin and scarred (*C, D*) with increased echo reflectiveness (*arrows*). The left ventricle is mildly dilated. The papillary muscle and proximal septal fibrosis are characteristic two-dimensional echocardiographic features of sarcoid.

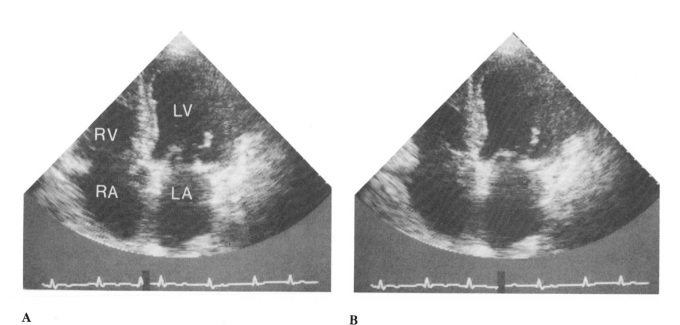

Figure 11.51. Two-dimensional echocardiogram of the apical four chamber views from a patient with hemochromatosis, showing minor right and left ventricular dilatation in diastole (*A*) and little change in ventricular chamber sizes from diastole (*A*) to systole (*B*). In this patient, there is additional biatrial dilatation.

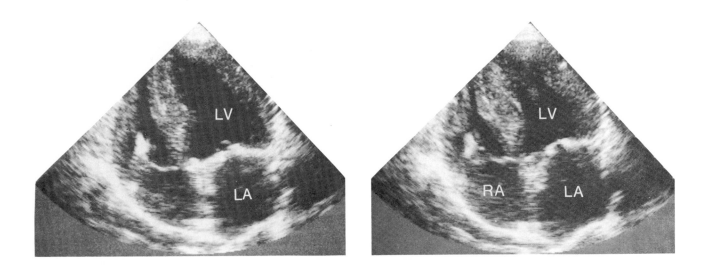

A   **B**

Figure 11.52. Two-dimensional echocardiogram of the apical four chamber views from a patient with biopsy-proven Fabry's cardiomyopathy in diastole (A) and systole (B), showing mild LV dilatation, severe LV hypertrophy, and ASH with only moderate contractile function.

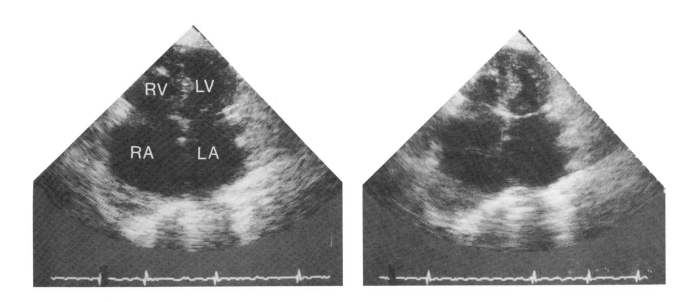

A   **B**

Figure 11.53. Two-dimensional echocardiogram of the apical four chamber view from a patient with idiopathic RCM, showing small hypertrophied right and left ventricles, biatrial dilatation, and moderately well-preserved LV systolic contractile function in diastole (A) and in systole (B).

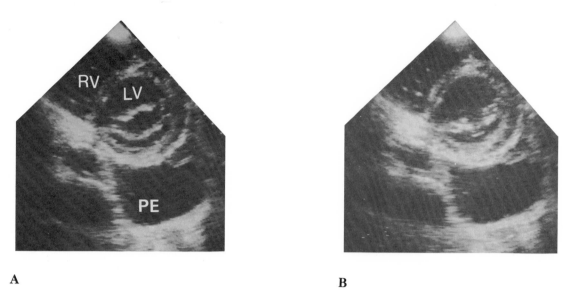

Figure 11.54. Two-dimensional echocardiogram from a patient with severe adriamycin cardiotoxicity, showing the LV in short axis in diastole (*A*) and in systole (*B*). There is a large left pleural effusion.

phy (ASH), and initially normal systolic contractile function (145–147, 257). In patients with ASH, systolic anterior motion of the mitral valve and left ventricular outflow tract gradients have been reported, suggesting that hypertrophic obstructive cardiomyopathy may occur on occasion (145, 146). The left ventricular hypertrophy in Friedreich's ataxia results initially only in diastolic dysfunction (147) but later in the course of the disease, progressive left ventricular systolic dysfunction develops with congestive heart failure resulting in death in the third or fourth decade (145).

Nemaline myelopathy is a form of muscular dystro-

phy characterized by generalized hypotonia, muscle weakness, and skeletal dysmorphism, which is associated with rapidly progressive biventricular dilatation and contractile dysfunction consistent with dilated cardiomyopathy, developing in the second or third decade (258). The echocardiographic features are those of severe four chamber enlargement; intrinsically normal atrioventricular and semilunar valve leaflets, with mitral and tricuspid regurgitation resulting from the major changes in ventricular chamber architecture; and dilatation of the atrioventricular valve rings (259) (Fig. 11.57).

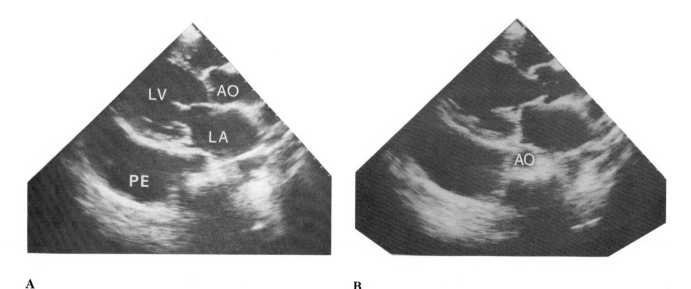

Figure 11.55. Two-dimensional echocardiogram of the LV long axis, in the same patient with adriamycin cardiomyopathy, in diastole (*A*) and in systole (*B*) with a large left pleural effusion.

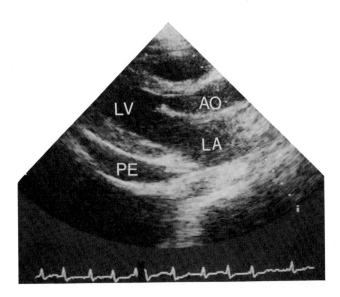 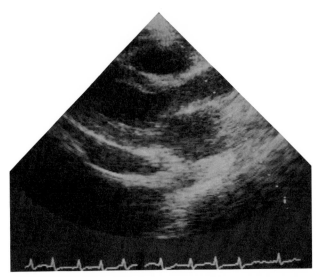

A   **B**

Figure 11.56. Two-dimensional echocardiogram of the LV long axis from a patient with cytoxan cardiotoxicity 72 hours after treatment in preparation for bone marrow transplantation. Note the posterior pericardial effusion due to myocardial hemorrhage, and the severe LV dysfunction demonstrated by the minimal change in LV cavity size from diastole (*A*) to systole (*B*).

Duchenne's progressive muscular dystrophy is associated with an unusual segmental form of cardiac involvement (260–263). Echocardiographically the left ventricular cavity is a normal size and, in the early stages of the disease, is associated with increased wall thickness and near normal function. In half of the patients and predominantly in the older ones, the epicardial half of the posterolateral left ventricular wall is progressively replaced with fibrous tissue (262–264). This causes dramatic segmental wall motion abnormalities, with hypokinesis or akinesis of this region, but sparing of the remainder of the heart (262).

Lastly, in approximately half of the patients with dystrophia myotonica (Steinert's disease), in which electrocardiographic abnormalities and disturbance of conduction are common, minor perturbations of systolic and diastolic dysfunction occur (265, 266). However, these are rarely severe enough to warrant the description of cardiomyopathy.

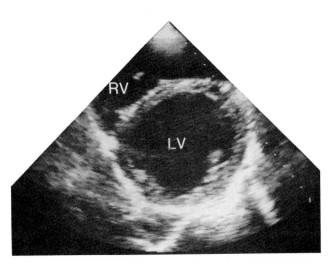 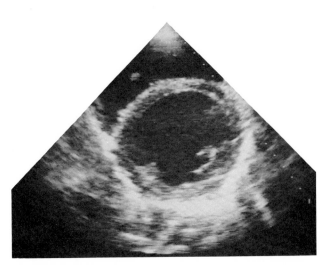

A   **B**

Figure 11.57. Two-dimensional echo of the LV short axis from a patient with nemaline cardiomyopathy. The left ventricle is extremely dilated with almost no change in chamber size from diastole (*A*) to end-systole (*B*).

REFERENCES

1. Report of the WHO/ISFC task force on the definition and classification of cardiomyopathies. Br Heart J 1980;44:672–673.
2. Brock R. Functional obstruction of the left ventricle (acquired aortic subvalve stenosis). Guy's Hosp Rep 1957;106:221–238.
3. Teare D. Asymmetrical hypertrophy of the heart in young adults. Br Heart J 1958;20:1–8.
4. Henry WL, Clark CE, Epstein SE. Asymmetric septal hypertrophy (ASH): Echocardiographic identification of the pathognomonic anatomic abnormality of IHSS. Circulation 1973;47:225–233.
5. Henry WL, Clark CE, Epstein SE. Asymmetric septal hypertrophy the unifying link in the IHSS disease spectrum: Observations regarding its pathogenesis, pathophysiology and course. Circulation 1973;47:827.
6. Abbasi AS, MacAlpin RN, Eber LM, Pearce ML. Echocardiographic diagnosis of idiopathic hypertrophic cardiomyopathy without outflow obstruction. Circulation 1972;46:897.
7. Henry WL, Clark CE, Roberts WC, Morrow AG, Epstein SE. Difference in distribution of myocardial abnormalities in patients with obstructive and non-obstructive asymmetric septal hypertrophy (ASH): Echocardiographic and gross anatomic findings. Circulation 1974;50:447.
8. Maron BJ, Gottdiener JS, Bonow RO, Epstein SE. Hypertrophic cardiomyopathy with unusual locations of left ventricular hypertrophy undetectable by M-mode echocardiography. Circulation 1981;63:409–418.
9. Yamaguchi H, Ishimura T, Nishiyama S. Hypertrophic non-obstructive cardiomyopathy with giant negative T waves (apical hypertrophy): Ventriculographic and echocardiographic features in 30 patients. Am J Cardiol 1979;44:401–412.
10. Shapiro LM, McKenna WJ. Distribution of left ventricular hypertrophy in hypertrophic cardiomyopathy: A two-dimensional echocardiographic study. J Am Coll Cardiol 1983;2:437–444.
11. Wigle ED, Sasson Z, Henderson MA, et al. Hypertrophic cardiomyopathy. The importance of the site and extent of hypertrophy. A Prog Review Cardiovasc Dis 1985;28:1–83.
12. Pearse AGE. Histochemical and electron microscopy of obstructive cardiomyopathy. In: Wolstenholme GEW, O'Connor M, eds. CIBA Foundation symposium on cardiomyopathy. London: Churchill Livingstone, 1964.
13. Clark CE, Henry WL, Epstein SE. Familial prevalence and genetic transmission of idiopathic hypertrophic subaortic stenosis. N Engl J Med 1973;289:709–714.
14. Maron BJ, Nichols PF, Pickle LW, Wesley YE, Mulvihill JJ. Patterns of inheritance in hypertrophic cardiomyopathy: Assessment by M-mode and two-dimensional echocardiography. Am J Cardiol 1984;53:1087–1094.
15. Hutchins GM, Buckley BH. Catenoid shape of the interventricular septum: Possible cause of idiopathic hypertrophic subaortic stenosis. Circulation 1978;58:392–397.
16. Watt A. Hypertrophic cardiomyopathy: A disease of impaired adenosine mediated autoregulation of the heart. Lancet 1984;1:1271–1273.
17. Murgo JP, Alter BR, Dorethy JF, Altobelli SA, McGranahan GM. Dynamics of left ventricular ejection in obstructive and non-obstructive hypertrophic cardiomyopathy. J Clin Invest 1980;66:1369.
18. Criley JM, Siegel RJ. Obstruction is unimportant in the pathophysiology of hypertrophic cardiomyopathy. Postgrad Med J 1986;62:515–529.
19. Criley JM, Siegel RJ. Has "obstruction" hindered our understanding of hypertrophic cardiomyopathy? Circulation 1985;72:1148–1154.
20. Maron BJ, Gottdiener JS, Arce J, Rosing DR, Wesley YE, Epstein SE. Dynamic subaortic obstruction in hypertrophic cardiomyopathy: Analysis by pulsed wave Doppler echocardiography. J Am Coll Cardiol 1985;6:1–15.
21. Wigle ED, Henderson M, Rakowski H, Wilansky S. Muscular (hypertrophic) subaortic stenosis (hypertrophic obstructive cardiomyopathy): The evidence for true obstruction of left ventricular outflow. Postgrad Med J 1986;62:531–536.
22. Goodwin JF, ?IHSS, ?HOCM, ?ASH. A plea for unity. Am Heart J 1975;89:269–277.
23. Shah PM. IHSS-HOCM-MSS-ASH? Circulation 1975;51:577–580.
24. Maron BJ, Epstein SE. Hypertrophic cardiomyopathy: A discussion of nomenclature. Am J Cardiol 1979;43:1242–1244.
25. Shah PM, Gramiak R, Kramer DH. Ultrasound localization of left ventricular outflow obstruction in hypertrophic obstructive cardiomyopathy. Circulation 1969;40:3–11.
26. Popp RL, Harrison DC. Ultrasound in the diagnosis and evaluation of therapy of idiopathic hypertrophic subaortic stenosis. Circulation 1969;40:905–914.
27. Shah PM, Gramiak R, Adelman AG, Wigle ED. Role of echocardiography in diagnostic and hemodynamic assessment of hypertrophic subaortic stenosis. Circulation 1977;44:891–898.
28. King JF, DeMaria AN, Reis RL, Bolton MR, Dunn MI, Mason DT. Echocardiographic assessment of idiopathic hypertrophic subaortic stenosis. Chest 1973;64:723–731.
29. Rossen RM, Goodman DJ, Ingham RE, Popp RL. Ventricular systolic septal thickening and excursion in idiopathic hypertrophic subaortic stenosis. N Engl J Med 1974;291:1317–1319.
30. Tajik AJ, Giuliani ER. Echocardiographic observations in idiopathic hypertrophic subaortic stenosis. Mayo Clin Proc 1974;49:89–97.
31. Feizi O, Emanuel R. Echocardiographic spectrum of hypertrophic cardiomyopathy. Br Heart J 1975;37:1286–1302.
32. Shah PM, Sylvester LJ. Echocardiography in the diagnosis of hypertrophic obstructive cardiomyopathy. Am J Med 1972;82:830–835.
33. Rodger JC. Motion of mitral apparatus in hypertrophic cardiomyopathy with obstruction. Br Heart J 1976;38:732–737.
34. Krajcer Z, Orzan F, Pechacek LW, Garcia E, Leachman RD. Early systolic closure of the aortic valve in patients with hypertrophic subaortic stenosis and discrete subaortic stenosis: Correlation with preoperative and postoperative hemodynamics. Am J Cardiol 1978;41:823–829.
35. Rossen RM, Goodman DJ, Ingham RE, Popp RL. Echocardiographic criteria in the diagnosis of idiopathic hypertrophic subaortic stenosis. Circulation 1974;50:747.
36. Maron BJ, Epstein SE. Hypertrophic cardiomyopathy. Recent observations regarding the specificity of three hallmarks of the disease: Asymmetric septal hypertrophy, septal disorganization and systolic anterior motion of the anterior mitral valve leaflet. Am J Cardiol 1980;45:141.
37. Cohen ML, Teichholz LE, Gorlin R. B-scan ultrasonography in idiopathic subaortic stenosis: Study of left ventricular outflow tract and mechanism of obstruction. Br Heart J 1976;38:595.
38. Maron BJ, Gottdiener JS, Roberts WC, Henry WL, Savage DD, Epstein SE. Left ventricular outflow tract obstruction due to systolic anterior motion of the anterior mitral valve leaflet in patients with concentric left ventricular hypertrophy. Circulation 1978;57:517–533.
39. Crawford MH, Groves BM, Horwitz LD. Dynamic left ventricular outflow tract obstruction and systolic anterior motion of the mitral valve in the absence of asymmetric septal hypertrophy. Am J Med 1978;65:703–708.
40. Gilbert BW, Pollick C, Adelman AG, Wigle ED. Hypertrophic cardiomyopathy: Subclassification of M-mode echocardiography. Am J Cardiol 1980;45:861–872.
41. Maron BJ, Harding AM, Spirito P, Roberts WC, Waller BF. Systolic anterior motion of the posterior mitral leaflet: A previously unrecognized cause of dynamic subaortic obstruction in patients with hypertrophic cardiomyopathy. Circulation 1983;68:282–293.
42. Spirito P, Maron BJ. Significance of left ventricular outflow tract cross-sectional area in hypertrophic cardiomyopathy: A two-dimensional echocardiographic assessment. Circulation 1983;67:1100–1108.
43. Spirito P, Maron BJ. Patterns of systolic anterior motion of the mitral valve in hypertrophic cardiomyopathy: Assessment by two-dimensional echocardiography. Am J Cardiol 1984;54:1039–1046.
44. Pollick C, Rakowski H, Wigle ED. Muscular subaortic stenosis: The quantitative relationship between systolic anterior motion and the pressure gradient. Circulation 1984;69:43–49.

45. Sheikhzadeh A, Eslami B, Stierle V, Langbehn AF. Mid-ventricular obstruction. A form of hypertrophic obstructive cardiomyopathy—And systolic anterior motion of the mitral valve. Clin Cardiol 1986;9:607–613.

46. Rakowski H, Sasson Z, Wigle ED. Echocardiographic and Doppler assessment of hypertrophic cardiomyopathy. J Am Soc Echo 1988;1:31–47.

47. Rosing DR, Condit JR, Maron BJ. Verapamil therapy. A new approach to the pharmacologic treatment of hypertrophic cardiomyopathy. III. Effects of long-term administration. Am J Cardiol 1981;48:545–553.

48. Iwase M, Sotobata I, Takagi S, Miyaguchi K, Jing HX, Yokota M. Effects of diltiazem on left ventricular diastolic behavior in patients with hypertrophic cardiomyopathy: Evaluation with exercise pulsed Doppler echocardiography. J Am Coll Cardiol 1987;9:1099–1105.

49. Suwa M, Hirota Y, Kanamura K. Improvement in left ventricular diastolic function during intravenous and oral diltiazem therapy in patients with hypertrophic cardiomyopathy: An echocardiographic study. Am J Cardiol 1984;54:1047–1053.

50. Pollick C. Muscular subaortic stenosis. Hemodynamic and clinical improvement after disopyramide. N Engl J Med 1982;307:997–999.

51. Shah PM, Gramiak R, Adelman AG, Wigle ED. Echocardiographic assessment of the effects of surgery and propranolol on the dynamics of outflow obstruction in hypertrophic subaortic stenosis. Circulation 1972;45:516–521.

52. Morrow AG, Reitz BA, Epstein SE, et al. Operative treatment in hypertrophic subaortic stenosis. Techniques and the results of pre- and postoperative assessments in 83 patients. Circulation 1975;52:88–102.

53. Maron BJ, Berrill WH, Freier PA, Kent KM, Epstein SE, Morrow AG. Long-term clinical course and symptomatic status of patients after operation for hypertrophic subaortic stenosis. Circulation 1978;57:1205–1213.

54. Schapira JN, Stemple DR, Martin RP, Rakowski H, Stinson EB, Popp RL. Single and two-dimensional echocardiographic visualization of the effects of septal myectomy in idiopathic hypertrophic subaortic stenosis. Circulation 1978;58:850–860.

55. Beahrs MM, Tajik AJ, Seward JB, Giuliani ER, McGoon DC. Hypertrophic obstructive cardiomyopathy: Ten to 21 years followup after partial septal myectomy. Am J Cardiol 1983;51:1160–1161.

56. Spirito P, Maron BJ. Morphologic determinants of hemodynamic state after ventricular septal myotomy-myectomy in patients with obstructive hypertrophic cardiomyopathy: M-mode and two-dimensional echocardiographic assessment. Circulation 1984;70:984–995.

57. Stewart WJ, Schiavone WA, Salcedo EE, Lever HM, Cosgrove DM, Gill CC. Intra-operative Doppler echocardiography in hypertrophic cardiomyopathy: Correlations with the obstructive gradient. J Am Coll Cardiol 1987;10:327–335.

58. Krajcer Z, Lufschanowski R, Angelini P, Leachman RD, Cooley DA. Septal myomectomy and mitral valve replacement for idiopathic hypertrophic subaortic stenosis. An echocardiographic and hemodynamic study. Circulation (Suppl I) 1980;62:158–164.

59. Fighali S, Krajcer Z, Leachman RD. Septal myomectomy and mitral valve replacement for idiopathic hypertrophic subaortic stenosis: Short and long term follow-up. J Am Coll Cardiol 1984;3:1127–1134.

60. Maron BJ, Bonow RO, Cannon RO, Leon MB, Epstein SE. Hypertrophic cardiomyopathy. Interrelations of clinical manifestations, pathophysiology, and therapy. N Engl J Med 1987;316:780–789, 844–852.

61. Shah PM, Adelman AG, Wigle ED. The natural and unnatural history of hypertrophic obstructive cardiomyopathy. Circ Res (Suppl II) 1974;34:179–195.

62. Maron BJ, Gottdiener JS, Epstein SE. Patterns and significance of distribution of left ventricular hypertrophy in hypertrophic cardiomyopathy. A wide-angle, two-dimensional echocardiographic study of 125 patients. Am J Cardiol 1981;48:418–428.

63. Maron BJ, Lipson LC, Roberts WC, Savage DD, Epstein SE. "Malignant" hypertrophic cardiomyopathy: Identification of a subgroup of families with unusually frequent premature death. Am J Cardiol 1978;41:1133–1140.

64. Ten Cate FJ, Roelandt J. Progression to left ventricular dilatation in patients with hypertrophic obstructive cardiomyopathy. Am Heart J 1979;97:762–765.

65. Louie EK, Maron BJ. Hypertrophic cardiomyopathy with extreme increase in left ventricular wall thickness, functional and morphologic features and clinical significance. J Am Coll Cardiol 1986;8:57–65.

66. Spirito P, Maron BJ, Bonow RO, Epstein SE. Severe functional limitation in patients with hypertrophic cardiomyopathy and only mild localized left ventricular hypertrophy. J Am Coll Cardiol 1986;8:537–544.

67. Van Dorp WG, Ten Cate FJ, Vletter WB, Dohmen H, Roelandt JS. Familial prevalence of asymmetric septal hypertrophy. Eur J Cardiol 1986;4:349–357.

68. Ten Cate FJ, Hugenholtz PG, Van Dorp WG, Roelandt JS. Prevalence of diagnostic abnormalities in patients with genetically transmitted asymmetric septal hypertrophy. Am J Cardiol 1979;43:731–737.

69. Maron BJ, Mulvihill JJ. The genetics of hypertrophic cardiomyopathy. Ann Intern Med 1986;105:610–613.

70. Hatle L, Angelsen B. Doppler ultrasound in cardiology. 2nd ed. Philadelphia: Lea & Febiger, 1985.

71. Yock PG, Hatle L, Popp RL. Patterns and timing of Doppler-detected intracavitary and aortic flow in hypertrophic cardiomyopathy. J Am Coll Cardiol 1986;8:1047.

72. Cogswell TL, Sagar KB, Wann LS. Left ventricular ejection dynamics in hypertrophic cardiomyopathy and aortic stenosis: Comparison with the use of Doppler echocardiography. Am Heart J 1987;113:110.

73. Epstein SE, Henry WL, Clark CE. Asymmetric septal hypertrophy. Ann Intern Med 1974;81:650–680.

74. Maron BJ, Gottdiener JS, Perry LW. Specificity of systolic anterior motion of the anterior mitral leaflet for hypertrophic cardiomyopathy: Prevalence in a large population of patients with other diseases. Br Heart J 1981;45:206–21.

75. Bulkley BH, Fortuin NJ. Systolic anterior motion of the mitral valve without asymmetric septal hypertrophy. Chest 1976;69:694–696.

76. Maron BJ, Verter J, Kapur S. Disproportionate ventricular septal thickening in the developing normal human heart. Circulation 1978;57:520–526.

77. Larter WE, Allen HD, Sahn DJ, Goldberg SJ. The asymmetrically hypertrophied septum. Further differentiation of its causes. Circulation 1976;53:19–27.

78. Maron BJ, Clark CE, Henry WL. Prevalance and characteristics of disproportionate ventricular septal thickening in patients with acquired or congenital heart disease: Echocardiographic and morphologic findings. Circulation 1977;55:489–496.

79. Abbasi AJ, Slaughter JC, Allen MW. Asymmetric septal hypertrophy in patients on long-term hemodialysis. Chest 1978;74:548–551.

80. Mintz GS, Kotler MN, Segal BL, Parry WR. Systolic anterior motion of the mitral valve in the absence of asymmetric septal hypertrophy. Circulation 1978;57:256–263.

81. Bougher DR, Rakowski H, Wigle ED. Mitral valve systolic anterior motion in the absence of hypertrophic cardiomyopathy. Circulation 1978;58:916.

82. Gardin JM, Talano JV, Stephanides L, Fizzano J, Lesch M. Systolic anterior motion in the absence of asymmetric septal hypertrophy. A buckling phenomenon of the chordae tendineae. Circulation 1981;63:181.

83. Henry WL, Clark CE, Glancy DL, Epstein SE. Echocardiographic measurement of the left ventricular outflow tract gradient in idiopathic hypertrophic subaortic stenosis. N Engl J Med 1973;288:989–993.

84. Pollick C, Rakowski H, Wigle ED. Muscular subaortic stenosis: The temporal relationship between systolic anterior motion of the anterior mitral valve leaflet and pressure gradient. Circulation 1982;66:1087–1093.

85. Martin RP, Rakowski H, French J, Popp RL. Idiopathic hypertrophic subaortic stenosis viewed by wide-angle, phased array echocardiography. Circulation 1979;59:1206–1217.

86. Kinoshita N, Nimura Y, Okamoto M, Miyatake K, Nagata S, Sakakibara H. Mitral regurgitation in hypertrophic cardiomyopathy. Non-invasive study by two-dimensional Doppler echocardiography. Br Heart J 1983;49:574–583.

87. Kaul S, Tei C, Shah PM. Interventricular septal and free wall dynamics in hypertrophic cardiomyopathy. J Am Coll Cardiol 1983;4:1024–1030.

88. Ciro E, Maione S, Giunta A, Maron BJ. Echocardiographic analysis of ventricular septal dynamics in hypertrophic cardiomyopathy and other diseases. Am J Cardiol 1984;53:187–193.

89. Jenni R, Ruffmann K, Vieli A, Anliker M, Krayenbuehl HP. Dynamics of aortic flow in hypertrophic cardiomyopathy. Eur Heart J 1985;6:391–398.

90. Takenaka K, Dabestani A, Gardin JM, et al. Left ventricular filling in hypertrophic cardiomyopathy: A pulsed Doppler echocardiographic study. J Am Coll Cardiol 1986;7:1263–1271.

91. Giddings SS, Snider AR, Rocchini AP, Peters J, Farnsworth R. Left ventricular diastolic filling in children with hypertrophic cardiomyopathy; assessment with pulsed Doppler echocardiography. J Am Coll Cardiol 1986;8:310–316.

92. Maron BJ, Spirito P, Green KJ, Wesley YE, Bonow RO, Arce J. Noninvasive assessment of left ventricular diastolic function by pulsed Doppler echocardiography in patients with hypertrophic cardiomyopathy. J Am Coll Cardiol 1987;10:733–742.

93. Bryg RJ, Pearson AC, Williams GA, Labovitz AJ. Left ventricular systolic and diastolic flow abnormalities determined by Doppler echocardiography in obstructive hypertrophic cardiomyopathy. Am J Cardiol 1987;59:925.

94. Sasson Z, Hatle LV, Appleton CP, Popp RL. Doppler ultrasound assessment of diastolic function in hypertrophic cardiomyopathy (abstr). Circulation (Suppl III) 1986;74:228.

95. Nishimura RD, Tajik AJ, Reeder GS, Seward JB. Evaluation of hypertrophic cardiomyopathy by Doppler colour flow imaging—Initial observations. Mayo Clin Proc 1986;61:631.

96. Mills TJ, Seward JB, Khanderia BK, Klein AL, Oh JK, Tajik AJ. Color flow imaging in cardiomyopathies: Observations and implications. Echocardiography 1987;4:527–534.

97. Dop YL, Deanfield JE, McKenna WJ, Dargie HJ, Oakley CM, Goodwin JF. Echocardiographic differentiation of hypertensive heart disease and hypertrophic cardiomyopathy. Br Heart J 1980;44:395.

98. Nanda NC, Gramiak R, Shah PM, Stewart S, DeWeese JA. Echocardiography in the diagnosis of idiopathic hypertrophic subaortic stenosis coexisting with aortic valve disease. Circulation 1974;50:752–757.

99. Hess OM, Schneider J, Turina M, Carroll JD, Rothlin M, Krayenbuehl HP. Asymmetric septal hypertrophy in patients with aortic stenosis, an adaptive mechanism or a coexistence of hypertrophic cardiomyopathy? J Am Coll Cardiol 1983;1:783.

100. Smolenskii AV. Asymmetric hypertrophy of the myocardium in patients with hypertension (echocardiographic data). Kardiologia 1983;23:69.

101. Siqueira-Filho AG, Cuhna LP, Tajik AJ, Seward JB, Schattenberg TT, Giuliani ER. M-mode and two-dimensional echocardiographic features in cardiac amyloidosis. Circulation 1981;63:188–196.

102. Sakamoto T, Tei C, Muramaya M, et al. Giant negative T wave inversion as a manifestation of asymmetric apical hypertrophy (AAH) of the left ventricle. Echocardiographic and ultrasonocardiotomographic study. Jpn Heart J 1976;17:611–629.

103. Maron BJ, Bonow RO, Seshagiri TNR, Roberts WC, Epstein SE. Hypertrophic cardiomyopathy with ventricular septal hypertrophy localized to the apical region of the left ventricle (apical hypertrophic cardiomyopathy). Am J Cardiol 1982;49:1838–1848.

104. Keren G, Belhassen B, Sherez J, et al. Apical hypertrophic cardiomyopathy: Evaluation by non-invasive and invasive techniques in 23 patients. Circulation 1985;71:45–56.

105. Fowles RG, Martin RP, Popp RL. Apparent asymmetric septal hypertrophy due to angled intraventricular septum. Am J Cardiol 1980;46:386.

106. Fiddler GI, Tajik AJ, Weidman WH, McGoon DC, Ritter DG,

Giuliani ER. Idiopathic hypertrophic subaortic stenosis in the young. Am J Cardiol 1978;42:793–799.

107. St. John Sutton MG, Tajik AJ, Giuliani ER, Gordon H, Su WPD. Hypertrophic obstructive cardiomyopathy and lentiginosis: A little known neural ectodermal syndrome. Am J Cardiol 1981;47:214–217.

108. Harrison EE, Sbar SS, Martin H, Pupello DF. Coexisting right and left hypertrophic subvalvular stenoses and apical left ventricular outflow obstruction due to aortic valve stenosis. Am J Cardiol 1977;40:133.

109. Wigle ED, Adelman AG, Silver MD. Pathophysiological consideration in muscular subaortic stenosis. In: Wolstenholme GEW, O'Connor M, eds. Hypertrophic obstructive cardiomyopathy. Ciba Foundation Study Group 47. London: Churchill, 1971.

110. Henry WL, Clark CE, Griffith JM, Epstein SE. Mechanism of left ventricular outflow tract obstruction in patients with obstructive asymmetric septal hypertrophy (idiopathic hypertrophic subaortic stenosis). Am J Cardiol 1975;35:337–345.

111. Bolton MR, King JF, Polumbo RD, et al. The effects of operation on the echocardiographic features of idiopathic hypertrophic subaortic stenosis. Circulation 1974;50:897–900.

112. Wigle ED, Rakowski H, Pollick C. Cardiomyopathy: Predicted for the foreseeable future. In: Yu P, Goodwin JF, eds. Progress in cardiology 10. Philadelphia: Lea and Febiger, 1981.

113. Rakowski H, Fulop J, Wigle ED. The role of echocardiography in the assessment of hypertrophic cardiomyopathy. Postgrad Med J 1986;62:557.

114. Nagata S, Nimura Y, Beppu S, Park Y-D, Sakakibara H. Mechanism of systolic anterior motion of the mitral valve and site of intraventricular pressure gradient in hypertrophic obstructive cardiomyopathy. Br Heart J 1983;49:234–243.

115. St. John Sutton MG, Tajik AJ, Gibson DE, Brown DJ, Seward JB, Giuliani ER. Echocardiographic assessment of left ventricular filling and septal and posterior wall dynamics in idiopathic hypertrophic subaortic stenosis. Circulation 1978;57:512–520.

116. Sanderson JE, Traill TA, St. John Sutton MG, Brown DJ, Gibson DG. Left ventricular relaxation and filling in hypertrophic cardiomyopathy; an echocardiographic study. Br Heart J 1978;40:596.

117. Hanrath P, Mathey DG, Siegert R, Bleifeld TW. Left ventricular relaxation and filling pattern in different forms of left ventricular hypertrophy: An echocardiographic study. Am J Cardiol 1980;45:15–23.

118. Gibson DG, Sanderson JE, Traill TA, Brown DJ, Goodwin JF. Regional left ventricular wall movement in hypertrophic cardiomyopathy. Br Heart J 1978;40:1327–1333.

119. St. John Sutton MG, Tajik AJ, Smith KC, Ritman E. Angina in idiopathic hypertrophic subaortic stenosis. A clinical correlate of regional left ventricular dysfunction. A videometric and echocardiographic study. Circulation 1980;61:561–568.

120. Grant C, Raphael MJ, Steiner RE, Goodwin JF. Left ventricular volume and hypertrophy in outflow obstruction. Cardiovasc Res 1968;4:346–355.

121. Dinsmore RE, Sanders CA, Hawthorne JW. Mitral regurgitation in idiopathic hypertrophic subaortic stenosis. N Engl J Med 1966;275:1225–1228.

122. Wigle ED, Adelman AG, Auger P, Marquis Y. Mitral regurgitation in muscular subaortic stenosis. Am J Cardiol 1969;24:698–706.

123. Maron BJ, Epstein SE, Roberts WC. Hypertrophic cardiomyopathy and transmural myocardial infarction without significant atherosclerosis of the extramural coronary arteries. Am J Cardiol 1979;43:1086–1102.

124. Lorell BH, Paulus WJ, Grossman W, Wynne J, Cohn PF. Modification of abnormal left ventricular diastolic properties by nifedipine in patients with hypertrophic cardiomyopathy. Circulation 1982;65:499–508.

125. Pitcher D, Wainwright R, Maisey M, Curry P, Sowton E. Assessment of chest pain in hypertrophic cardiomyopathy using exercise thallium-201 myocardial scintigraphy. Br Heart J 1980;44:650–656.

126. Moreyra E, Klein JJ, Shimada H, Segal BL. Idiopathic hypertrophic subaortic stenosis diagnosed by reflected ultrasound. Am J Cardiol 1969;23:32–37.

127. Quinones MA, Gaasch WH, Waisser E, Alexander JK. Reduction in the rate of diastolic descent of the mitral valve echogram in patients with altered left ventricular diastolic pressure–volume relations. Circulation 1974;49:246–254.

128. DeMaria AN, Miller RR, Amsterdam EA, Markson W, Mason DT. Mitral valve early diastolic closing velocity in the echocardiogram in relation to sequential diastolic flow and ventricular compliance. Am J Cardiol 1976;37:693–700.

129. Venco A, Recusani F, Sgalumbro A. Diastolic movement of mitral valve in hypertrophic cardiomyopathy: An echocardiographic study. Br Heart J 1980;43:159–163.

130. Upton MT, Gibson DG. The study of left ventricular function from digitized echocardiograms. Prog Cardiovasc Dis 1978;20:259–384.

131. Bonow RO. Left ventricular filling in ischemia and hypertrophic heart disease. In: Grossman WG, Lorell BH, eds. Diastolic relaxation of the heart. Boston: Martinus Nijhoff, 1987.

132. Bonow RO, Vitale DF, Maron BJ, Bacharach SL, Frederick TM, Green MV. Regional left ventricular asynchrony and impaired global left ventricular filling in hypertrophic cardiomyopathy: Effect of verapamil. J Am Coll Cardiol 1987;9:1108–1116.

133. Rokey R, Kuo LC, Zoghbi WA. Determination of parameters of left ventricular diastolic filling with pulsed Doppler echocardiography: Comparison with cineangiography. Circulation 1985;71:543.

134. Kronzon I, Glassman E. Mitral ring calcification in idiopathic hypertrophic subaortic stenosis. Am J Cardiol 1978;42:60–66.

135. Motamed HE, Roberts WC. Frequency and significance of mitral annular calcium in hypertrophic cardiomyopathy: Analysis of 200 necropsy patients. Am J Cardiol 1987;60:877–884.

136. Frank S, Braunwald E. Idiopathic hypertrophic subaortic stenosis: Clinical analysis of 126 patients with emphasis on the natural history. Circulation 1968;37:759–788.

137. Simon AL, Ross J Jr, Gault JH. Angiographic anatomy of the left ventricle and mitral valve in idiopathic hypertrophic subaortic stenosis. Circulation 1967;36:852–867.

138. Abbasi AS, Allen MW, DeCristofaro D, Ungar I. Detection and estimation of the degree of mitral regurgitant flow by range-gated pulsed Doppler echocardiography. Circulation 1980;61:143.

139. Rokey R, Sterling LL, Zoghbi WA, et al. Determination of regurgitant fraction in isolated mitral or aortic regurgitation by pulsed Doppler two-dimensional echocardiography. J Am Coll Cardiol 1986;7:1273–1278.

140. Blumlein S, Bouchard A, Schiller NB, et al. Quantitation of mitral regurgitation flow by Doppler echocardiography. Circulation 1986;74:306–314.

141. Linhart JW, Taylor WJ. Bacterial endocarditis in a patient with idiopathic hypertrophic subaortic stenosis. Circulation 1966;34:595–596.

142. Vecht RJ, Oakley CM. Infective endocarditis in three patients with hypertrophic obstructive cardiomyopathy. Br Med J 1968;2:455–459.

143. Pridie RB, Oakley CM. Mechanism of mitral regurgitation in hypertrophic cardiomyopathy. Br Heart J 1980;32:203–208.

144. Theard M, Bhatia SB, Plappert T, St. John Sutton M. Doppler echocardiographic study of the frequency and severity of aortic regurgitation in hypertrophic cardiomyopathy. Am J Cardiol 1987;60:1143–1147.

145. Van Der Hauwaert LG, Dumoulin M. Hypertrophic cardiomyopathy in Friedreich's ataxia. Br Heart J 1976;38:1291–1298.

146. Smith ER, Sangalang VE, Heffernan LP, Welch JP, Flemington CS. Hypertrophic cardiomyopathy. The heart disease of Friedreich's ataxia. Am Heart J 1977;428–434.

147. St. John Sutton MG, Olukotun AY, Tajik AJ, Lovett JL, Guiliani ER. Left ventricular function in Friedreich's ataxia: An echocardiographic study. Br Heart J 1980;44:309–316.

148. Goodwin JF. Prospects and predictions for the cardiomyopathies. Circulation 1974;50:210–219.

149. Colucci WS, Lorell BH, Schoen FJ, Warhol MJ, Grossman W. Hypertrophic obstructive cardiomyopathy due to Fabry's disease. N Engl J Med 1982;307:926–928.

150. Rees A, Elbl F, Minhas K, Solinger R. Echocardiographic evidence of outflow tract obstruction in Pompe's disease (glycogen storage disease of the heart). Am J Cardiol 1976;37:1103–1106.

151. Brandenberg RO, Tajik AJ, Giuliani ER. Congenital cardiovascular lesions associated with idiopathic hypertrophic subaortic stenosis (IHSS) (abstr). Circulation (Suppl II) 1972;46:134.

152. Polani PE, Moynahan EJ. Progressive cardiomyopathic lentiginosis. Q J Med 1972;41:205–225.

153. Somerville J, Bonham-Carter RE. The heart in lentiginosis. Br Heart J 1972;34:58–66.

154. Elliott CM, Tajik AJ, Giuliani ER, Gordon H. Idiopathic hypertrophic subaortic stenosis associated with cutaneous neurofibromatosis: Report of a case. Am Heart J 1976;92:368–372.

155. Goodwin JF. Congestive and hypertrophic cardiomyopathies. A decade of study. Lancet 1970;1:731–739.

156. Field BJ, Baxley WA, Russell RO Jr, et al. Left ventricular function and hypertrophy in cardiomyopathy with depressed ejection fraction. Circulation 1973;47:1022–1031.

157. Abbasi AS, Chahine RA, Macalpin RN, Kattus AA. Ultrasound in the diagnosis of primary congestive cardiomyopathy. Chest 1973;63:937–943.

158. Millward DK, McLaurin LP, Craige E. Echocardiographic studies of the mitral valve in patients with congestive cardiomyopathy and mitral regurgitation. Am Heart J 1973;85:413–421.

159. Corya BC, Feigenbaum H, Rasmussen S, Black MJ. Echocardiographic features of congestive cardiomyopathy compared with normal subjects and patients with coronary artery disease. Circulation 1974;49:1153–1159.

160. Ghafour AJ, Gutgesell HP. Echocardiographic evaluation of left ventricular function in children with congestive cardiomyopathy. Am J Cardiol 1979;44:1332–1338.

161. Goldberg SJ, Valdes-Cruz LM, Sahn DJ, Allen HD. Two-dimensional echocardiographic evaluation of dilated cardiomyopathy in children. Am J Cardiol 1983;52:1244.

162. DeMaria AN, Bommer W, Lee G, Mason DT. Value and limitations of two-dimensional echocardiography in assessment of cardiomyopathy. Am J Cardiol 1980;46:1224–1231.

163. Keren G, Billingham ME, Weintraub D, Stinson EB, Popp RL. Mildly dilated congestive cardiomyopathy. Circulation 1985;72:302–309.

164. Shah PM. Echocardiography in congestive or dilated cardiomyopathy. J Am Soc Echo 1988;1:78–87.

165. Obeyesekere J, Hermon Y. Arborvirus heart disease, myocarditis and cardiomyopathy following dengue and chikungunya fever—A follow-up study. Am Heart J 1973;85:186–194.

166. Cambridge G, MacArthur CGC, Waterson AP, Goodwin JF, Oakley CM. Antibodies to Coxsackie B viruses in congestive cardiomyopathy. Br Heart J 1979;41:692–696.

167. Fowles RE, Bieber CP, Stinson EB. Defective in vitro suppressor cell function in idiopathic congestive cardiomyopathy. Circulation 1979;59:483–491.

168. Sanderson JE, Koech D, Iha D, Ojiambo HP. T-lymphocyte subsets in idiopathic dilated cardiomyopathy. Am J Cardiol 1985;55:755–758.

169. Eckstein R, Mempel W, Bolte HD. Reduced suppressor cell activity in congestive cardiomyopathy and in myocarditis. Circulation 1982;65:1224–1229.

170. Anderson JL, Carlquist JF, Hammond EH. Deficient natural killer cell in patients with idiopathic dilated cardiomyopathy. Lancet 1982;2:1124–1127.

171. Laskey WK, St. John Sutton M, Zeevi G, Hirshfeld JW, Reichek N. Left ventricular mechanisms in dilated cardiomyopathy. Am J Cardiol 1984;54:620–625.

172. Weber KT, Janicki JS, Hefner LL. Left ventricular force-length relations of isovolumic and ejecting contractions. Am J Physiol 1976;33:231.

173. Yin FLP. Ventricular stress. Circ Res 1981;49:829.

174. Grossman W, Jones D, McLaurin LP. Wall stress and patterns of hypertrophy in the human left ventricle. J Clin Invest 1975;56:56.

175. Borow KM, Green LH, Grossman W, Braunwald E. Left ventricular end-systolic stress-shortening and stress-length relations in humans. Normal values and sensitivity to inotropic state. Am J Cardiol 1982;50:1301–1308.

176. St. John Sutton M, Plappert TA, Hirshfeld JW, Reichek N.

Assessment of left ventricular mechanics in patients with asymptomatic aortic regurgitation: A two-dimensional echocardiographic study. Circulation 1984;69:259–268.

177. St. John Sutton M, Plappert TA, Crosby L, Douglas P, Mullen J, Reichek N. Effects of reduced left ventricular mass on chamber architecture, load and function: A study of anorexia nervosa. Circulation 1985;72:991–1000.

178. Hirota Y, Shimizue G, Kaku K, Saito T, Kino M, Kawamura K. Mechanisms of compensation and decompensation in dilated cardiomyopathy. Am J Cardiol 1984;54:1030–1038.

179. Hassell LA, Fowles RE, Stinson EB. Patients with congestive cardiomyopathy as cardiac transplant recipients. Am J Cardiol 1981;47:1205–1209.

180. Massie BM, Schiller NB, Ratshin RA, Parmley WW. Mitral septal separation: New echocardiographic index of left ventricular function. Am J Cardiol 1977;39:1008–1016.

181. Child JS, Krovokapich J, Perloff JK. Effect of left ventricular size on mitral-E point to ventricular septal separation in assessment of cardiac performance. Am Heart J 1981;101:797–805.

182. Konecke LL, Feigenbaum H, Chang S, Corya BC, Fischer JC. Abnormal mitral valve motion in patients with elevated left ventricular diastolic pressures. Circulation 1973;47:989.

183. Levisman JA. Echocardiographic diagnosis of mitral regurgitation in congestive cardiomyopathy. Am Heart J 1977;93:33.

184. Takahashi M, Fujisawa A, Nakamura M, Kannagi T, Kawai C. Localized disorders of left ventricular wall motion in congestive cardiomyopathy. J Cardiogr 1981;11:1241.

185. Yazawa Y, Hayashi S, Hosokawa O, et al. Regional wall motion of the left ventricle in congestive cardiomyopathy: In comparison with progressive muscular dystrophy of Duchenne type. J Cardiogr 1981;11:1233.

186. Wallis DE, O'Connell JB, Henkin RE, Costanzo-Nordin MR, Scanlon PJ. Segmental wall motion abnormalities in dilated cardiomyopathies: A common finding and good prognostic sign. J Am Coll Cardiol 1984;4:674–679.

187. Pratt RC, Parisi AF, Harrington JJ, Sasahara AA. The influence of left ventricular stroke volume on aortic root motion: An echocardiographic study. Circulation 1976;53:947.

188. Gottdiener JS, Gay JA, Van Voorhees L, DiBianco R, Fletcher RD. Frequency and embolic potential of left ventricular thrombus in dilated cardiomyopathy: Assessment by 2-dimensional echocardiography. Am J Cardiol 1983;52:1281.

189. Asinger RW, Mikell FL, Sharma B, Hodges M. Observations on detecting left ventricular thrombus with two-dimensional echocardiography: Emphasis on avoidance of false positive diagnosis. Am J Cardiol 1981;47:145–146.

190. Reeder GS, Tajik AJ, Seward JB. Left ventricular mural thrombus: Two-dimensional echocardiographic diagnosis. Mayo Clin Proc 1981;56:82–86.

191. Hangland JM, Asinger RW, Mikell FL, Elsperger J, Hodges M. Embolic potential of left ventricular thrombi detected by two-dimensional echocardiography. Circulation 1984;70:588–589.

192. Ballester M, Jajoo J, Rees S, Rickards A, McDonald L. The mechanism of mitral regurgitation in the dilated left ventricle. Clin Cardiol 1983;6:333–338.

193. Boltwood CM, Dei C, Wong M, Shah PM. Quantitative echocardiography of the mitral complex in dilated cardiomyopathy: The mechanism of functional mitral regurgitation. Circulation 1983;68:498–508.

194. Pollick C, Pittman M, Filly K, Fitzgerald PJ, Popp RL. Mitral and aortic valve orifice area in normal subjects and in patients with congestive cardiomyopathy: Determinations by two-dimensional echocardiography. Am J Cardiol 1982;49:1191–1196.

195. Chandraratna PA, Aronow WS. Mitral valve ring in normal versus dilated left ventricle. Chest 1981;79:151–157.

196. Gardin JM, Seri LT, Elkayam N, et al. Evaluation of dilated cardiomyopathy by pulsed wave Doppler echocardiography. Am Heart J 1983;10:1057–1065.

197. Takenaka K, Dabestani A, Gardin JM, et al. Pulsed Doppler echocardiographic study of left ventricular filling in dilated cardiomyopathy. Am J Cardiol 1986;58:143–147.

198. Kenny J, Plappert T, St. John Sutton M. Relationship between instantaneous Doppler velocity across the mitral valve and instantaneous left ventricular volume in normal and hypertrophied hearts. Br Heart J, in press.

199. Tei C, Pilgrim JP, Shah PM, Ormiston JA, Wong M. The tricuspid valve annulus: Study of size and motion in normal subjects and in patients with tricuspid regurgitation. Circulation 1982;66:665–671.

200. Yock PG, Popp RL. Non-invasive estimation of right ventricular systolic pressure by Doppler ultrasound in patients with tricuspid regurgitation. Circulation 1984;70:657–662.

201. Currie PJ, Seward JB, Chan K-L, et al. Continuous wave Doppler determination of right ventricular pressure: A simultaneous Doppler-catheterization study in 127 patients. J Am Coll Cardiol 1986;6:750–756.

202. Chan K-L, Currie PJ, Seward JB, Hagler DJ, Mair DD, Tajik AJ. Comparison of three Doppler ultrasound methods in the prediction of pulmonary artery pressure. J Am Coll Cardiol 1987;9:549–554.

203. Berko BA, Swift M. X-linked dilated cardiomyopathy. N Engl J Med 1987;316:1186–1191.

204. Sanderson JE, Adesanya CO, Anjorin FP, Parry EH. Postpartum cardiac failure—Heart failure due to volume overload? Am Heart J 1979;97:613–621.

205. Cole P, Cook F, Plappert T, Saltzman D, St. John Sutton M. Longitudinal changes in left ventricular architecture and function in peripartum cardiomyopathy. Am J Cardiol 1987;60:871–876.

206. Fink L, Reichek N, St. John Sutton M. Cardiac abnormalities in acquired immune deficiency syndrome. Am J Cardiol 1984;54:1161–1163.

207. Cohen IS, Anderson DW, Virmani R, Reen BM, Macher AM, Sennesh J. Congestive cardiomyopathy in association with the acquired immunodeficiency syndrome. N Engl J Med 1986;315:628–630.

208. Siegel RJ, Shah PK, Fishbein MC. Idiopathic restrictive cardiomyopathy. Circulation 1984;70:165.

209. Benotti JR, Grossman W, Cohn PF. Clinical profile of restrictive cardiomyopathy. Circulation 1980;61:1206–1212.

210. Goodwin JF. Obliterative and restrictive cardiomyopathies. In: Hurst JW, Logue RB, Schlant RC, Wenger NK, eds. The heart. 4th ed. New York: McGraw Hill, 1978.

211. Waller BF. Pathology of the cardiomyopathies. J Am Soc Echo 1988;1:4–19.

212. Fauci AS, Harley JB, Roberts WC, Ferrans VJ, Gralnick HR, Bjornson BH. The idiopathic hypereosinophilic syndrome. Clinical, pathophysiologic and therapeutic considerations. Ann Intern Med 1982;47:780–792.

213. Roberts WC, Liegler DG, Carbone PP. Endomyocardial disease and eosinophilia. A clinical and pathologic spectrum. Am J Med 1969;46:28–42.

214. Hess OM, Turina M, Jenning A, Goebel NH, Scholer Y, Krayenbuehl HP. Pre and post-operative findings in patients with endomyocardial fibrosis. Br Heart J 1978;40:406.

215. George B, Gaba FE, Talabi AI. M-mode echocardiographic features of endomyocardial fibrosis. Br Heart J 1982;48:222.

216. Candell-Riera J, Permanyer-Meralda G, Soler-Soler J. Echocardiographic findings in endomyocardial fibrosis. Chest 1982;82:88.

217. Vijayaraghavan G, Davies J, Sadanandan S, Spry CJF, Gibson DG, Goodwin JF. Echocardiographic features of tropical endomyocardial disease in South India. Br Heart J 1983;50:450.

218. Acquatella H, Schiller NB, Puigbo JJ, Gomez-Mancebo JR, Suarez C, Acquatella G. Value of two-dimensional echocardiography in endomyocardial disease with and without eosinophilia. A clinical and pathologic study. Circulation 1983;67:1219.

219. Acquatella H, Schiller NB. Echocardiographic recognition of Chaga's disease and endomyocardial fibrosis. J Am Soc Echo 1988;1:60–68.

220. Davies J, Gibson DG, Foale R, et al. Echocardiographic features of eosinophilic endomyocardial disease. Br Heart J 1982;48:434.

221. Gottdiener JS, Maron BJ, Schooley RT, Harley JB, Roberts WC, Fauci AS. Two-dimensional echocardiographic assessment of the idiopathic hypereosinophilic syndrome. Anatomic basis of

mitral regurgitation and peripheral embolization. Circulation 1983;67:572–578.

222. Bletry O, Scheuble C, Careze P, Masquet C, Priollet P. Cardiac manifestations of the hypersinophilic syndrome. The value of 2-dimensional echocardiography. Arch Mal Coeur 1984;77:633.

223. Buja LM, Roberts WC. Iron in the heart etiology and clinical significance. Am J Med 1971;51:209–221.

224. Henry WL, Nienhuis AW, Wiener M, Miller DR, Canale VC, Piomelli S. Echocardiographic abnormalities in patients with transfusion dependent anemia and secondary myocardial iron deposition. Am J Med 1978;64:547.

225. Leon MB, Borer JS, Bacharach SL, et al. Detection of early cardiac dysfunction in patients with severe beta-tholassemia and chronic iron overload. N Engl J Med 1979;301:1143.

226. Short EM, Winkle RA, Billingham ME. Myocardial involvement in idiopathic hemachromatosis. Morphologic and clinical improvement following resection. Am J Med 1981;67:1275–1279.

227. Candell-Riera J, Lu L, Seres L, et al. Cardiac hemachromatosis: Beneficial effects of iron removal therapy—An echocardiographic study. Am J Cardiol 1983;52:824–829.

228. Olson LJ, Baldus WP, Tajik AJ. Echocardiographic features of idiopathic hemachromatosis. Am J Cardiol 1987;60:885–889.

229. Gussenhoven WJ, Busch HFM, Kleijer WJ, De Villeneuve VH. Echocardiographic features in the cardiac type of glycogen storage disease II. Eur Heart J 1983;4:41–43.

230. Hwang B, Meng CCL, Lin CY, Hsu HC. Clinical analysis of five infants with glycogen storage disease of the heart: Pompe's disease. Jpn Heart J 1986;27:25–34.

231. Olson LJ, Reeder GS, Noller KL, Edwards WD, Howell RR, Michels VV. Cardiac involvement in glycogen storage disease. III. Morphologic and biochemical characterization with endomyocardial biopsy. Am J Cardiol 1984;53:900–908.

232. Bass J, Shrivastava S, Grabowski G, Desnick RJ, Miller JH. The M-mode echocardiogram in Fabry's disease. Am Heart J 1980;100:807–812.

233. Cohen IS, Fluri-Lundeen J, Wharton TP. Two-dimensional echocardiographic similarity of Fabry's disease to cardiac amyloidosis: A function of ultrastructural analogy. JCU 1983;2:437–441.

234. Roberts WC, Waller BF. Cardiac amyloidosis causing cardiac dysfunction: Analysis of 54 necropsy patients. Am J Cardiol 1983;52:137–146.

235. Child JS, Levisman JA, Abbasi AS, Macalpin RN. Echocardiographic manifestations of infiltrative cardiomyopathy, a report of seven cases due to amyloid. Chest 1976;70:726–731.

236. Borer JS, Henry WL, Epstein SE. Echocardiographic observations in patients with systemic infiltrative disease involving the heart. Am J Cardiol 1977;39:184–188.

237. Child JS, Krivokapich AJ, Abbasi AS. Increased right ventricular wall thickness on echocardiography in amyloid infiltrative cardiomyopathy. Am J Cardiol 1979;44:1391–1395.

238. Cueto-Garcia L, Tajik AJ, Kyle RA, et al. Serial echocardiographic observation in patients with primary systemic amyloidosis: An introduction to the concept of early (asymptomatic) amyloid infiltration of the heart. Mayo Clinic Proc 1984;59:589–597.

239. Cueto-Garcia L, Reeder GS, Kyle RA, et al. Echocardiographic findings in systemic amyloidosis: Spectrum of cardiac involvement and relation to survival. J Am Coll Cardiol 1985;6:737–743.

240. Roberts WC, McAllister HA, Ferrans BJ. Sarcoidosis of the heart. A clinico-pathologic study of 55 necropsy patients (group I) and review of 78 previously described necropsy patients (group II). Am J Med 1977;63:86–108.

241. Silverman JK, Hutchins GM, Bulkley BH. Cardiac sarcoid. A clinicopathologic study of 84 unselected patients with systemic sarcoidosis. Circulation 1978;58:1204–1211.

242. Lewin RF, Mor R, Spitzer S, Arditti A, Hellman C, Agmon J. Echocardiographic evaluation of patients with systemic sarcoidosis. Am Heart J 1985;110:116–122.

243. Gregor P, Widimsky P, Sladkova T, Petrikova J, Cervenka V, Visek V. Echocardiography in sarcoidosis. Jpn Heart J 1984;25:499–508.

244. St. John Sutton M, Reichek N, Kastor JA, Giuliani ER. Computerized M-mode echocardiographic analysis of left ventricular dysfunction in cardiac amyloid. Circulation 1982;66:790–799.

245. Klein AL, Oh JK, Miller FA, Seward JB, Tajik AJ. Two-dimensional and Doppler echocardiographic assessment of infiltrative cardiomyopathy. J Am Soc Echo 1988;1:48–59.

246. Bhandari AK, Nanda NC. Myocardial texture characterization by two-dimensional echocardiography. Am J Cardiol 1983;50:817–825.

247. Skorton DJ, Collins SM. Clinical potential of ultrasound tissue characterization in cardiomyopathy. J Am Soc Echo 1988;1:69–77.

248. Carroll JD, Gaasch WH, McAdam KPWJ. Amyloid cardiomyopathy: Characterization by a distinctive voltage mass relationship. Am J Cardiol 1982;99:9–13.

249. Gottdiener JS, Mathison DJ, Borer JS, et al. Doxorubicin cardiotoxicity: Assessment of late ventricular dysfunction by radionuclide cineangiography. Ann Intern Med 1981;94:430–435.

250. Mimbs JW, O'Donnell M, Miller JG, Sobel BE. Detection of cardiomyopathic changes induced by doxorubicin based on quantitative analysis of ultrasonic backscatter. Am J Cardiol 1981;47:1056.

251. Hutter JJ, Sahn DJ, Woolfenden JM, Carnahan Y. Evaluation of the cardiac effects of doxorubicin by serial echocardiography. Am J Dis Child 135, 1981;35(7):653–7.

252. Borow KM, Henderson K, Newman A, et al. Assessment of left ventricular contractility in patients receiving doxorubicin. Ann Intern Med 1983;99:750.

253. Mills BA, Roberts RW. Cyclophosphamide-induced cardiomyopathy: A report of two cases and review of the English literature. Cancer 1979;43:2223–2226.

254. Gottdiener JS, Appelbaum FR, Ferrans VJ, Deisseroth A, Ziegler J. Cardiotoxicity associated with high dose cyclophosphamide therapy. Arch Intern Med 1981;141:758–763.

255. Appelbaum FR, Strauchen JA, Gram RG, et al. Acute lethal carditis caused by high dose continuation chemotherapy. Lancet 1976;2:58–62.

256. Estes ML, Ewing-Wilson D, Chou SM, et al. Chloroquine neuromyotoxicity. Clinical and pathologic perspective. Am J Med 1987;82(3):447–455.

257. Gottdiener JS, Hawley R, Maron BJ, Bertorini TF, Engle WK. Characteristics of the cardiac hypertrophy in Friedreich's ataxia. Am Heart J 1982;103:525.

258. Meier C, Gertsch M, Zimmerman A, Voellmy W, Geissbuhler J. Nemaline myopathy presenting as cardiomyopathy. N Engl J Med 1983;308:1536–1537.

259. Rosenson RS, Mudge GH, St. John Sutton M. Nemaline cardiomyopathy. Am J Cardiol 1986;58:175–177.

260. Goldberg SJ, Feldman L, Reinecke C, Stern LZ, Sahn DJ, Allen HD. Echocardiographic determination of contraction and relaxation of the left ventricular wall in normal subjects and patients with muscular dystrophy. Circulation 1980;62:1061–1069.

261. Farah MG, Evans EB, Vignos PJ. Echocardiographic evaluation of left ventricular function in Duchenne's muscular dystrophy. Am J Med 1980;69:248.

262. Goldberg SJ, Stern LZ, Feldman L, Allen HD, Sahn DJ, Valdes-Cruz LM. Serial two-dimensional echocardiography in Duchenne muscular dystrophy. Neurology 1982;32:1101.

263. Goldberg SJ, Stern LZ, Feldman L, Sahn DJ, Allen HD, Valdes-Cruz LM. Serial left ventricular wall measurements in Duchenne's muscular dystrophy. J Am Coll Cardiol 1983;2:136.

264. Perloff JK, Roberts WC, DeLeon AC, O'Doherty D. The distinctive electrocardiogram of Duchenne's progressive muscular dystrophy. Am J Med 1967;42:179–188.

265. Ahmad M, Sanderson JE, Dubowitz V, Hallidie-Smith KA. Echocardiographic assessment of left ventricular function in Duchenne's muscular dystrophy. Br Heart J 1978;40:734–740.

266. Venco A, Saviotti M, Besana D, Finardi G, Lanzi G. Noninvasive assessment of left ventricular function in myotonic muscular dystrophy. Br Heart J 1978;40:1262–1266.

12
Pericardial Disease

Pamela Douglas

Despite many recent advances in medical imaging, echocardiography remains the technique of choice for the diagnosis of pericardial effusion (1–5). Echocardiography is the only noninvasive means of quantitating the volume of pericardial fluid and provides information regarding the hemodynamic significance of pericardial effusions. Echocardiography has also been a useful tool in understanding the mechanisms of electrical alternans and pulsus paradoxus and in guiding pericardiocentesis (24–26, 44).

Imaging the pericardium itself is helpful in defining structural abnormalities such as focal and diffuse thickening and detecting the presence of cysts and tumors. In this chapter, the applications of echocardiography in the study of pericardial diseases are discussed, together with the limitations of the technique.

PERICARDIAL EFFUSION

In normal humans, the pericardial space is formed by reflection of the visceral pericardium back on itself to form the parietal pericardium (6). This space normally contains approximately 20 milliliters of serous fluid, an amount not reliably detected by any imaging technique. Larger collections, however, are readily identified by M-mode and two-dimensional echocardiography; the need for such identification and the ease and accuracy with which it can be performed contributed greatly to the development of these techniques (4, 5).

M-mode Echocardiography

Diagnosis of a pericardial effusion relies on the appearance of an echo-free space either posterior to the left ventricle (LV) or anterior to the right ventricle (RV). This echo-free space decreases in size or disappears at the left atrioventricular groove (Table 12.1; Fig. 12.1). The echo-free acoustic quality of the fluid distinguishes

it from myocardium and pericardium in most cases, although the increased acoustic impedance of intrapericardial masses and fibrinous organization of inflammatory exudates may make the diagnosis of pericardial effusion difficult.

The abrupt cessation of the echo-free space at the atrioventricular groove is best visualized with M-mode echocardiography by sweeping the ultrasound beam from the mid-LV cavity to the base of the heart, where the anterior mitral leaflet merges to become the posterior aortic root and the posterior LV wall is contiguous with the left atrial (LA) wall. This characteristic "disappearance" of the pericardial effusion is due to reflection of the pericardium onto the pulmonary veins so that there is no true pericardial space posterior to the LA. Instead, the pericardium forms an oblique sinus, which is separate from the LA wall. Although this space is continuous with the remainder of the pericardial sac, it only rarely becomes filled with fluid because the pericardium between the inferior vena cava and the left pulmonary veins is taut.

Another useful diagnostic M-mode echocardiographic sign in pericardial effusions is the loss of normal parietal pericardial motion, caused by damping of cardiac motion by the pericardial fluid so that normal epicardial motion is not transmitted to the parietal pericardium. Pericardial motion may be partially preserved, in small or loculated effusions or when the pericardial layers are thickened and adherent secondary to organization of exudative effusions.

Technical Considerations

Technical considerations are extremely important in the accurate diagnosis of pericardial effusion. Correct positioning of the beam is essential because too medial an orientation may image an artifactual border of a posterior echo-free space (5). Complete scanning of the LV makes this error much less likely.

Table 12.1.   Criteria for Diagnosis of Pericardial Effusion

Posterior echo-free space
Diminution of space at left atrioventricular groove
Loss of posterior pericardial motion

Optimal visualization of pericardial fluid requires recording over a range of gain settings (Fig. 12.2). Step-wise reductions and increases in the gain settings provide better definition of the posterior pericardial echo and the LV epicardium and endocardium, which minimizes the potential for false-positive diagnosis of pericardial effusion. It is essential that both the anterior and posterior epicardial borders (RV and LV) are well defined. Correct use of the reject, damping, depth compensation, and intensity controls reduces the incidence of both false-positive and false-negative diagnoses.

Serial echocardiographic studies may be especially useful in assessing changes in the size of pericardial effusions (7) following medical therapy and after pericardiocentesis.

Two-Dimensional Echocardiography

Much of the previous discussion of M-mode echocardiography applies to two-dimensional echocardiography, including the importance of technically adequate recordings. However, the ability to image the heart from several echographic windows and to view

its entire circumference in several planes is a substantial advantage (Figs. 12.3, 12.4, 12.5, 12.6, and 12.7). The tendency for small amounts of fluid to collect posteriorly when the patient is supine can be clearly demonstrated in the long- and short-axis parasternal views as a clear space behind the LV extending up to the posterior atrioventricular groove. The apical four-chamber view is less sensitive than the parasternal views for detecting pericardial effusion. However, the appearance of an echo-free space around the roof of the right atrium (RA) may be the earliest sign of a pericardial effusion. Quantitation of the volume of pericardial fluid depends on its pattern of distribution around the heart, and therefore, two-dimensional echocardiographic estimates of the volume of pericardial effusions are more accurate than those of M-mode echocardiography. Many false-positive reports of effusions by M-mode echocardiography can be clearly and correctly identified using two-dimensional techniques, which better define the size, shape, and extent of both normal and abnormal extracardiac structures.

Loculated pericardial effusions may be difficult to visualize with M-mode methods (Fig. 12.8). They occur commonly after cardiac surgery (8), when echographic imaging is often difficult, and frequently contain blood, making acoustic differentiation from surrounding tissues difficult. These fluid collections are commonly located posteriorly, either medially or laterally, and are often confined by adhesions between visceral and

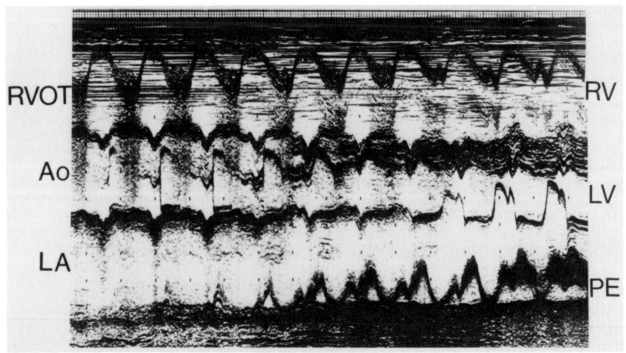

Figure 12.1.   M-mode echocardiogram of a patient with a small pericardial effusion. On the left are the right ventricular outflow tract (RVOT), aorta (Ao), and LA. On the right are the RV, septum, LV, and a small pericardial effusion (PE). Note the gradual diminution of the echo-free space toward the LA and enhanced motion of the RV free wall and LA wall.

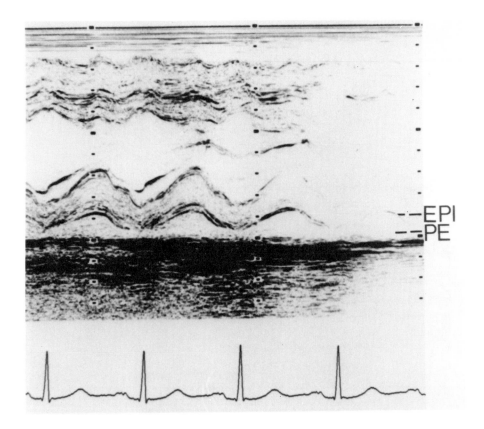

Figure 12.2. M-mode echocardiogram of a patient with a small pericardial effusion (PE). Towards the right of the scan, the gain is turned down so that the epicardium (EPI) is easily identified and the pericardial space becomes echo free.

parietal pericardium. Most importantly, postoperative pericardial effusions may cause tamponade, especially if they compress the low-pressure RA. If pericardial effusion is suspected following open heart surgery, two-dimensional echocardiography is the diagnostic modality of choice.

Quantitation of Fluid

Very small amounts of pericardial fluid are indistinguishable from the normal systolic separation of the visceral pericardial-epicardial echo from the parietal pericardial echo. As the volume of fluid increases, the separation persists longer through the cardiac cycle,

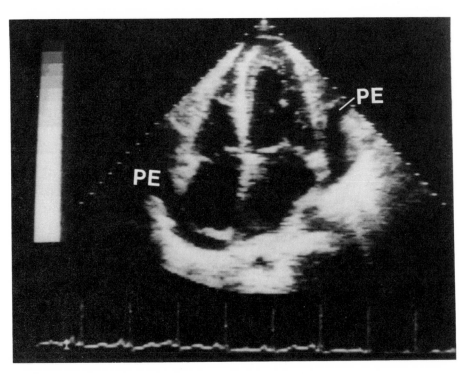

Figure 12.3. Two-dimensional echocardiogram in the apical four-chamber view demonstrating a pericardial effusion (PE) lateral to the LV and RV and above the dome of the RA.

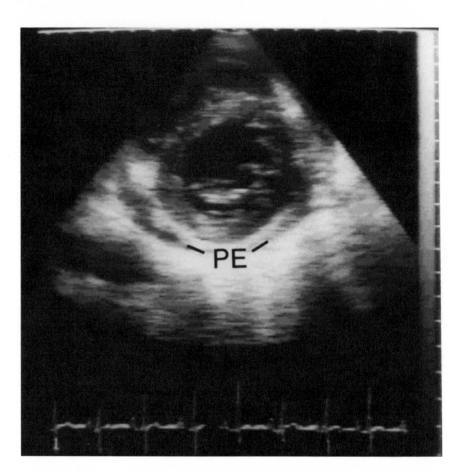

Figure 12.4. Two-dimensional echocardiogram of the parasternal short-axis view of the same patient as in Figure 12.3. The pericardial effusion (PE) is shown posterior to the LV.

and the parietal pericardial echo becomes flat relative to the epicardial echo (Fig. 12.9). The volume of pericardial fluid bears no relationship to the presence or absence of pericardial friction rubs (9).

Horowitz et al. (10) were able to identify effusions as small as 15 mL by subtracting calculated epicardial from pericardial volumes. However, this method is laborious and inaccurate (11), and effusions of less than 50 mL cannot be reliably detected. For larger effusions, most clinical laboratories rely on semiquantitative estimation only (2). Pericardial effusions that are only detectable posteriorly are small (<500 mL); when effusions are present both anteriorly and posteriorly, they are at least moderate (500–1000 mL); if the posterior clear space exceeds 1 centimeter, the effusions are generally large (>1000 mL). Assessment of the volume of pericardial effusions is at best only semiquantitative, depending on the size of the heart and the distribution of fluid around it (12), both of which are more readily appreciated by two-dimensional echocardiography. The absolute size of pericardial effusions often does not correlate with the clinical signs on physical examination.

Pitfalls in the Diagnosis of Pericardial Effusions

Many circumstances can create the echographic appearance of a pericardial effusion. These fall into four general categories (Table 12.2): misinterpretation of an anterior clear space; misinterpretation of noncardiac structures posterior to the heart; errors in identifying cardiac landmarks, especially posteriorly; and abnormal cardiac or pericardial structures in any region of the heart. Many of these false-positives can be correctly identified using either careful M-mode scanning or multiple two-dimensional views. However, some abnormalities of the pericardium can only be differentiated from juxtacardiac structures with difficulty, and the diagnosis of pericardial effusion may hinge on knowledge of the patient's clinical history.

Anterior pericardial fluid is usually seen only in moderate or large effusions but does occur in small loculated effusions. An anterior clear space is not always present, even in large effusions. In smaller effusions or even in the absence of a detectable posterior effusion, an echo-free area may be visualized anterior to the RV free wall (Fig. 12.10). This is generally due to epicardial fat or other mediastinal structures (e.g., foramen of Morgagni hernia, pericardial cyst, thrombus, thymoma, or lymphoma). Thus, diagnosis of anterior pericardial effusion in the absence of an obvious posterior effusion must be interpreted with caution (2).

Abnormal structures may occur adjacent to any of the cardiac chambers. Anterior masses are less readily

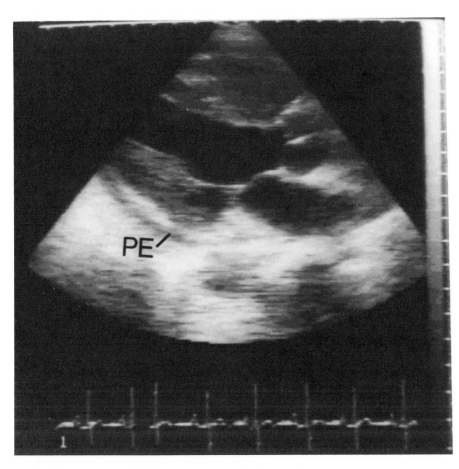

Figure 12.5. Two-dimensional echocardiogram in the same patient as in Figures 12.3 and 12.4. The pericardial effusion (PE) is shown posterior to the LV wall and disappears behind the LA.

misinterpreted as effusions because of the absence of a posterior clear space. Posterior structures, however, are more easily misinterpreted as the diagnosis does not depend on concomitant evidence of an effusion elsewhere. Perhaps the most common posterior struc-

ture mistaken for a pericardial effusion is a retrocardiac left pleural effusion (Figs. 12.11 and 12.12). Key features in differentiation are the large size of a pleural effusion in the absence of any anterior pericardial effusion, lack of characteristic gradual decrease in the

Figure 12.6. Two-dimensional echocardiogram of a patient with a larger pericardial effusion (PERI EFF) than in Figure 12.5.

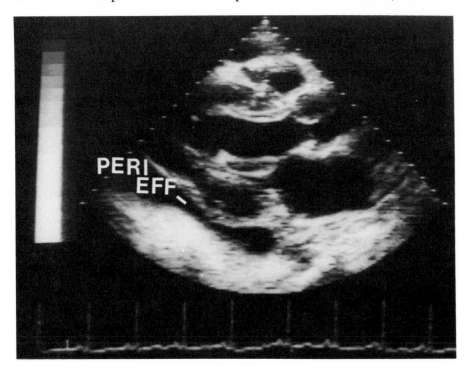

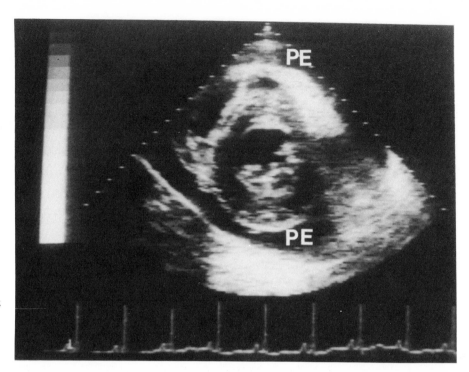

Figure 12.7. Two-dimensional echocardiogram of parasternal short-axis view of the same patient as in Figure 12.6. The pericardial effusion (PE) is clearly seen posterior to the LV and anterior to the RV free wall.

echo-free space from the LV to the LA, and position of the clear space posterior to the descending aorta rather than between it and the posterior LV wall. Coexistent pericardial and pleural effusions also occur and may be recognized by keeping in mind the characteristics of each abnormality and the position of the descending thoracic aorta, and by identifying the pericardium as the membrane separating the two echo-free spaces.

The descending aorta is readily visualized on several standard echocardiographic views and has been mistaken, especially with M-mode methods, for a posterior effusion. Similarly, a very large LA with portions ex-

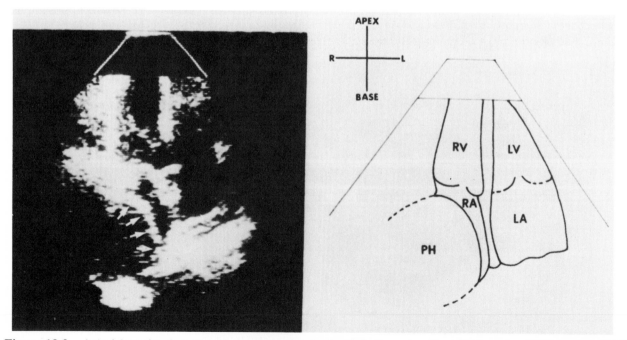

Figure 12.8. Apical four-chamber view of two-dimensional echocardiogram showing a large pericardial hematoma (PH) compressing the right side of the RA wall (*arrows*). Note the slitlike appearance of the RA cavity. L = left; R = right. (Reproduced by permission from Kronzon I, et al. Cardiac tamponade by loculated pericardial hematoma: limitations of M-mode echocardiography. J Am Coll Cardiol 1983;1(3):913–5.)

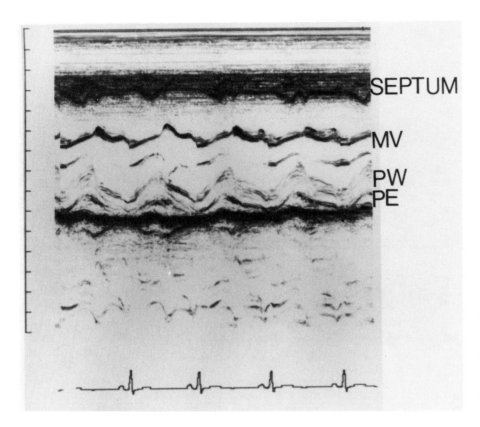

Figure 12.9. M-mode echocardiogram of a patient with a very small pericardial effusion (PE). The separation between the epicardium and the pericardium is maximal during systole and disappears at end diastole. MV = mitral valve; PW = left ventricular posterior wall.

tending posterior to the LV wall may simulate a pericardial effusion (13). Full visualization of the LV or two-dimensional echocardiographic views should clarify the true nature of both structures.

On occasion, the oblique sinus of the pericardium may fill with fluid in the presence of a large effusion and appear as an echo-free area posterior to the LA (Fig. 12.13). Careful scanning will demonstrate continuity between this space and the echo-free space behind the LV (14, 15).

Other extracardiac structures may have the echographic appearance of a loculated effusion. These include subphrenic effusions seen on subcostal views, cysts, tumors (both primary and metastatic), and malignancies infiltrating the pericardium such as lymphoma (16–19).

Errors in identification of the LV posterior wall can also create the appearance of an effusion. The mitral annulus, especially when calcified, may be mistaken for the myocardium; the basal portion of the LV cavity then appears to be an effusion. Similarly, an LV inferior wall aneurysm or pseudoaneurysm may create difficulty in

identifying true anatomic landmarks. The pericardium itself may become sufficiently thickened to mimic the appearance of an effusion. However, motion of the parietal pericardium is not flat but appears as a second line, parallel to the epicardium.

A few circumstances may produce a false-negative diagnosis; these are generally related to excess echoes within the effusion. The causes include excessive gain settings, causing echoes to fill in a normally clear space, and echoes produced by blood, thrombus, inflammatory tissue, or tumor in the effusion.

Effects of Effusions on Normal Cardiac Motion

Soon after echocardiography was first used to diagnose pericardial fluid, alteration of cardiac motion in the presence of an effusion was noted. Even in moderate-size effusions, the anterior RV and LA walls have an exaggerated motion pattern. In larger effusions, the heart behaves like a fluid-filled sac suspended by the great vessels. Abnormal cardiac motion is most easily seen with two-dimensional echocardiographic methods and is related to the size of the effusion, the absence of any restraining adhesions, and intrapericardial pressure. Thus, with any free effusion of sufficient volume, the heart may swing freely during the cardiac cycle in both the anteroposterior plane and with a counterclockwise rotational movement in the horizontal plane (20). Thus, different structures may be visu-

Table 12.2. Causes of False-Positive Diagnosis of Effusion

Anterior echo-free space without posterior effusion
Misreading of noncardiac structures
Errors in identifying cardiac landmarks
Other abnormal cardiac or pericardial structures

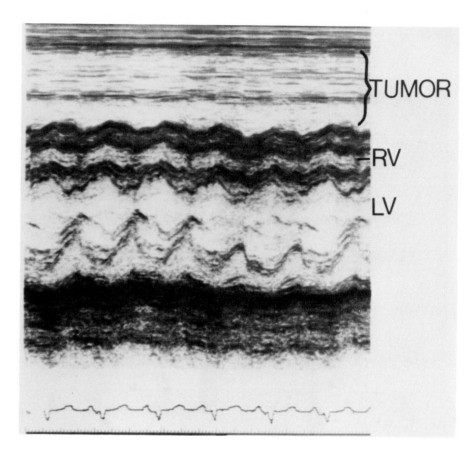

Figure 12.10. M-mode echocardiogram of a patient with a mediastinal tumor appearing as an echo-free space anterior to the RV. There is no posterior echo-free space.

alized at different times in the cardiac cycle. In addition, excessive cardiac motion may render imaging difficult.

Swinging of the heart may produce synchronous motion of the anterior and posterior walls, creating the appearance of abnormal wall motion. For example, if the entire heart moves anteriorly during systole, a normally contracting septum may appear dyskinetic. The echographic finding of the swinging heart has led to an understanding of the mechanism of electrical

Figure 12.11. M-mode echocardiogram of a patient with a small pericardial effusion (PERI EFF), a slightly thickened pericardium (PERICARD), and small retrocardiac pleural effusion (PLEURAL EFF). The pericardium is well defined by the presence of the two effusions; without the presence of the pericardial effusion, it would be easy to misconstrue the pleural fluid as being cardiac in origin. PW = posterior wall.

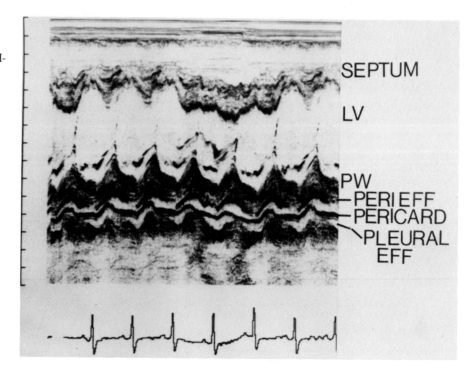

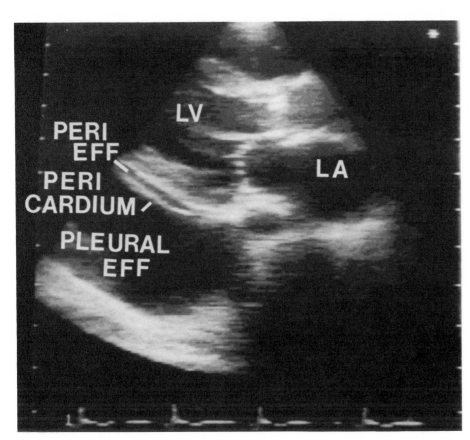

Figure 12.12. Two-dimensional echocardiogram of a patient with a small pericardial effusion (PERI EFF) and a much larger pleural effusion (PLEURAL EFF). As in Figure 12.11, the presence of the small PERI EFF aids in accurate identification of the pleural fluid.

alternans. If the excursion of the heart is substantial, it may not return to the same position at each time during the cardiac cycle. Sequential QRS complexes may be inscribed with the heart very near the chest wall, giving a normal amplitude, or separated from it by a large effusion, giving a relatively low QRS voltage. Thus, electrical alternans is closely related to the size of effusion and the mobility of the heart within it.

Motion abnormalities of each of the cardiac valves have been noted in the presence of large effusions (21–23). The most common is mitral valve prolapse, which may be either late or holosystolic; this has been attributed to systolic posterior motion of the heart (Fig. 12.14). Other abnormalities include tricuspid valve prolapse, systolic anterior motion of the mitral valve, early systolic closure of the aortic valve, and midsystolic notching of either the aortic or pulmonic valves. Diagnosis of any of these abnormalities cannot be made reliably in the presence of an effusion. Echocardiography should be repeated after reduction in the pericardial effusion or following pericardiocentesis to determine whether these abnormalities are genuine or simply resulting from the pericardial effusion.

CARDIAC TAMPONADE

While echocardiography is the method of choice for defining the anatomy of the pericardial space, it is less reliable in determining the hemodynamic significance of large pericardial effusions. Since size alone is of less importance than the rapidity of fluid accumulation, the echocardiographer must turn to additional features to establish the diagnosis of cardiac tamponade (Table 12.3). These features are abnormalities of atrial and ventricular wall motion, which are dependent on the volume of pericardial fluid and the relative intracardiac and intrapericardial pressures. Many of the M-mode findings of cardiac tamponade are also present in pulsus paradoxus associated with obstructive airway disease (24). However, more extensive use of two-dimensional echocardiography has shown it to be extremely sensitive and specific in the diagnosis of cardiac tamponade. Pericardial tamponade is a clinical syndrome whose recognition relies on the echographic abnormalities corroborating the clinical findings (25).

M-Mode Echocardiography

Several of the echographic findings in tamponade are related to cyclic respiratory changes in cardiac filling (24–27). Most prominent is the exaggeration of the normal inspiratory increase in RV dimension, which is followed by an expiratory decrease. Often, the LV displays reciprocal changes in dimension with respiration (Fig. 12.15 and 12.16). These findings are explained by the reduction in intrathoracic pressure with inspi-

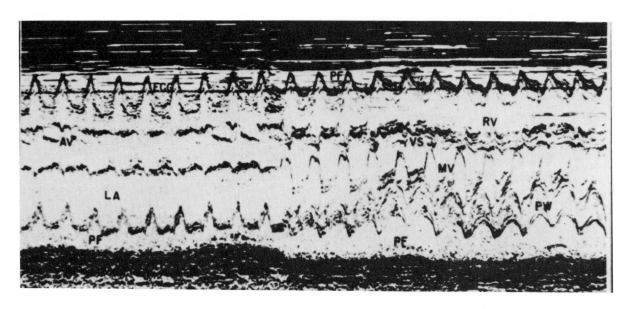

Figure 12.13. Echographic scan from aortic valve (AV) and LA to mitral valve (MV) and LV. There are large anterior and posterior echo-free spaces (PF = pericardial fluid), the posterior one being continuous behind LA posterior wall and left ventricular posterior wall (PW). Left atrial posterior wall motion is increased and abnormal (anteri- or during systole). ECG = electrocardiogram; VS = ventricular septum. (Reproduced by permission from Lemire F, Tajik AJ, Guiliani ER, et al. Further echocardiographic observations in pericardial effusion. Mayo Clin Proc 1976;51:16.)

Figure 12.14. M-mode echocardiogram of a patient with a large pericardial effusion (PE). The arrows demonstrate holosystolic mitral valve prolapse and middiastolic collapse or posterior motion of the RV free wall.

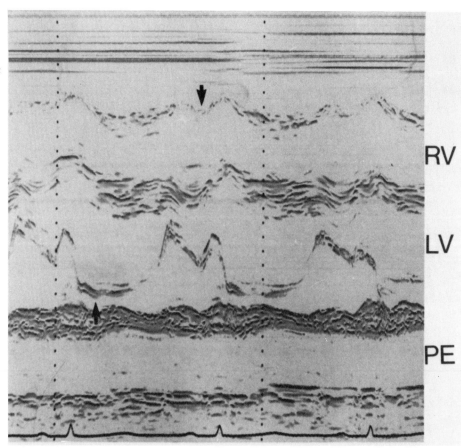

Table 12.3. Echocardiographic Findings Associated with Cardiac Tamponade

Marked respiratory variation in RV and LV dimensions
Decreased RA or RV sizes
Inspiratory decrease in mitral valve (EF) slope
Early systolic notching of RV free wall
Right ventricular collapse
Right atrial or LA inversion
Marked inspiratory increase in tricuspid and pulmonic flows

ration, which increases venous return to the right heart, and by the restraining pericardium, which limits ventricular filling.

The slope of the mitral valve (EF slope) and its anterior excursion in patients with pericardial tamponade have been reported to decrease with inspiration, presumably reflecting the decrease in LV stroke volume (Fig. 12.17) (26). Care must be taken in the interpretation of altered EF slope in tachycardia, as the shortened diastole may cause the mitral valve A wave to be superimposed on rapid filling.

The absolute sizes of both the RA and RV are usually decreased in tamponade, although this is rarely a useful diagnostic tool (Fig. 12.18). There is great variability in the size of right heart chambers, and this alone obscures separation of pathologic and normal states (27). However, if the RV dimension is extremely

small (M-mode diameter <2 millimeters at end expiration) (28) or if serial studies are available showing decreasing RV size, this finding may be useful.

Several studies have demonstrated abnormalities of RV wall motion in association with tamponade. Vignola et al. (22) noted early systolic notching of the RV free wall. Armstrong et al. (29) and Engel et al. (30) reported an early diastolic inward motion of the RV free wall, termed "diastolic collapse" (Fig. 12.14). Instead of moving anteriorly at end systole, the RV free wall continues to move posteriorly. Maximal posterior wall motion occurs up to 0.16 second after mitral valve opening, instead of 0.04 second or more before it. This abnormality may be due to pericardial pressure exceeding RV pressure during early diastole and causing indentation of the myocardium (31). With atrial systole, RV pressure exceeds pericardial pressure, and the chamber expands.

A "swinging heart" is frequently noted in patients with tamponade. While this abnormal motion pattern may bear some relationship to the size or etiology of the effusion (22), it is not useful in identifying tamponade.

Two-Dimensional Echocardiography

Many of the M-mode echocardiographic findings of tamponade may also be observed on two-dimensional

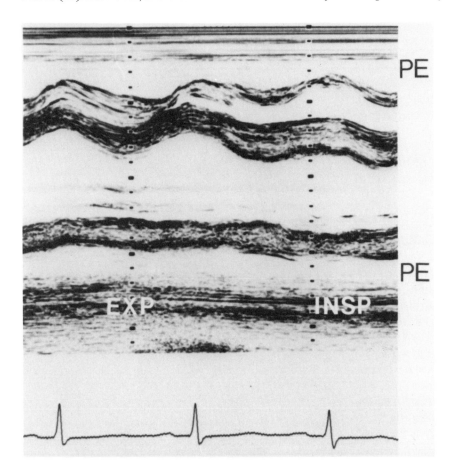

Figure 12.15. M-mode echocardiogram of a patient with a large pericardial effusion (PE) seen both anteriorly and posteriorly. There is reciprocal variation in RV and LV sizes with decreased RV size and increased LV size during expiration (EXP), with the reverse occurring during inspiration (INSP).

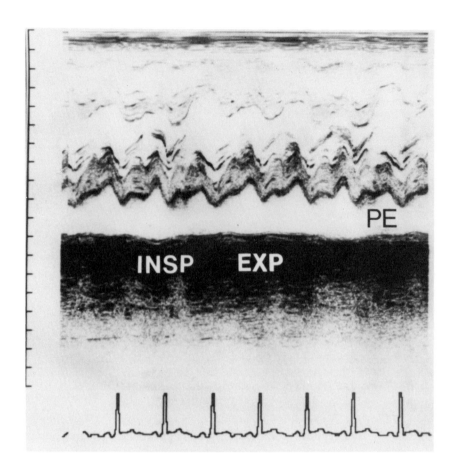

Figure 12.16. M-mode echocardiogram of a patient with a large pericardial effusion (PE) demonstrating reciprocal variability in RV and LV diameters during inspiration (INSP) and expiration (EXP).

echocardiographic recordings. Since the right-sided chambers are more extensively visualized with two-dimensional echocardiography, the utility of RV collapse (32–35) and the recognition of a similar pattern of RA wall motion (32, 36, 37) have recently been recognized as useful indicators of tamponade.

Right ventricular collapse is most easily seen in the parasternal short-axis views at the level of the aortic valve and appears as an early diastolic indentation of the anterior free wall and outflow tract (Fig. 12.19). This sign has been reported to have a sensitivity, specificity, and predictive accuracy of close to 100 percent for the hemodynamic changes associated with cardiac tamponade measured at cardiac catheterization (32). In both animal (33) and human studies (32, 34), RV collapse was associated with significant hemodynamic impairment (21% reduction in cardiac output in dogs), and it promptly disappeared following removal of even small amounts of pericardial fluid. Preliminary evidence suggests that RV collapse may be more sensitive to mild reductions in cardiac output caused by tamponade than pulsus paradoxus (35, 36).

Right atrial collapse presents a similar concave appearance, sometimes termed inversion of the atrial free wall (Fig. 12.20) (37). It occurs in late diastole and early systole, when the RV collapse is resolving; col-

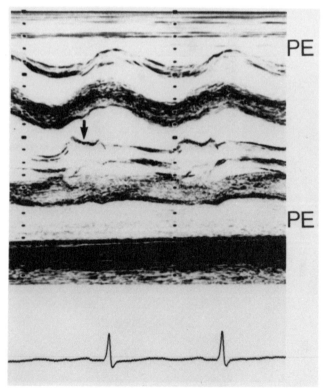

Figure 12.17. M-mode echocardiogram of a patient with a large pericardial effusion (PE) showing decreased EF slope of the anterior mitral leaflet (*arrow*).

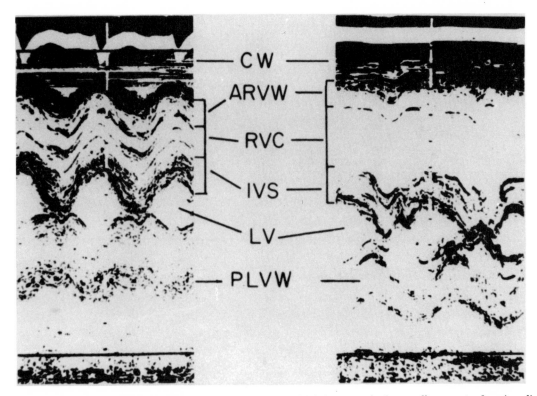

Figure 12.18. M-mode echocardiogram before (left) and after (right) removal of a small amount of pericardial fluid, showing expansion of the RV end-diastolic dimension after drainage. Along with this relative change in RV end-diastolic diameter, systolic pressure rose from 60 to 95 millimeters of mercury, and symptomatic improvement occurred. Although gains vary somewhat between studies shown, septal and anterior right ventricular wall (ARVW) thicknesses were measured and were confirmed on another record performed prior to pericardiocentesis, which showed LV anatomy in a less optimal manner. The calibration factor is the same for both studies. CW = chest wall; IVS = interventricular septum; PLVW = posterior left ventricular wall; RVC = right ventricular cavity. (Reproduced by permission from Schiller NB, Botvinick EH. Right ventricular compression as a sign of cardiac tamponade. Circulation 1977;56(5):774–9.)

lapse of the two chambers may have a reciprocal relationship as the stroke volume moves through the heart. Right atrial collapse is best recorded in the apical four-chamber view but may be seen whenever the RA is well visualized, including parasternal short-axis and subcostal four-chamber views. If the pericardial reflection behind the LA is sufficiently high to allow fluid accumulation, the LA may also demonstrate diastolic collapse (Fig. 12.21).

Right atrial collapse occurs earlier in tamponade than RV collapse because the atrial wall is more pliable, and it is not always associated with hemodynamic compromise. Similarly, it does not resolve as promptly as RV collapse following pericardiocentesis but requires removal of additional fluid (32). The sensitivity and specificity of this sign are dependent on its duration, since pericardial pressure may transiently exceed atrial pressure if atrial pressure is abnormally low, even in the absence of tamponade (e.g., hypovolemic states). Similarly, increasing intrapericardial pressure prolongs inversion. It has been suggested that in the presence of an effusion, more transient inversion

may be a helpful marker of impending tamponade (37). However, the usefulness of this sign remains controversial. The extent of inward motion seems unrelated to hemodynamic compromise.

Since the production of RA or RV collapse relies on both the flexibility of the chamber walls and the relative levels of intracavitary and intrapericardial pressures, patients with elevated right-sided pressures, tricuspid or pulmonic regurgitation, or RV hypertrophy may lack such findings in tamponade (38, 39). Knowledge of the patient's clinical history and attention to associated right-sided abnormalities, as well as the use of multiple diagnostic criteria for tamponade, obviate potentially false-negative diagnoses.

When a loculated effusion results in tamponade, the usual diagnostic echographic criteria for tamponade may be absent. Reciprocal changes in RV and LV sizes and right-sided chamber collapse are dependent on fluid moving freely within the pericardial space. Because two-dimensional echocardiography provides additional information compared to M-mode, it may be

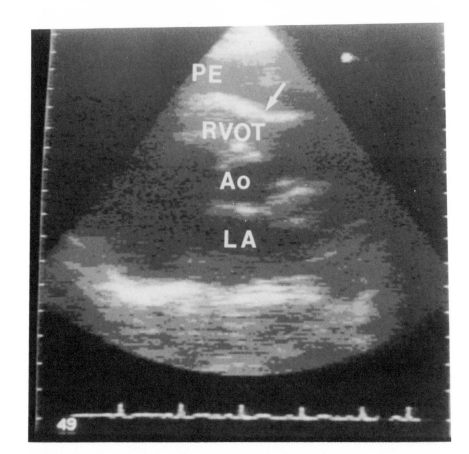

Figure 12.19. Two-dimensional echocardiogram of the parasternal short-axis view showing pericardial effusion (PE), left ventricular outflow tract, aortic root (Ao), and LA. The arrow demonstrates early diastolic indenting of the right ventricular outflow tract (RVOT).

Figure 12.20. Apical four-chamber view of a patient with large pericardial effusion. The arrow demonstrates RA collapse occurring during late diastole.

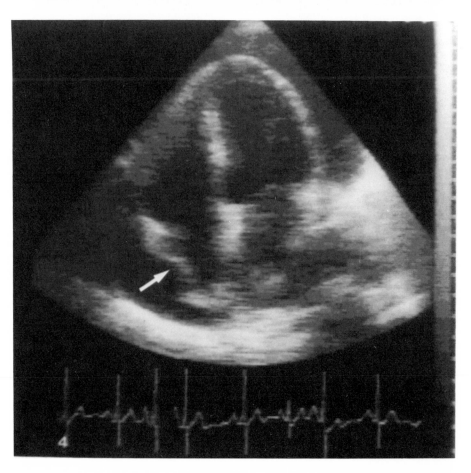

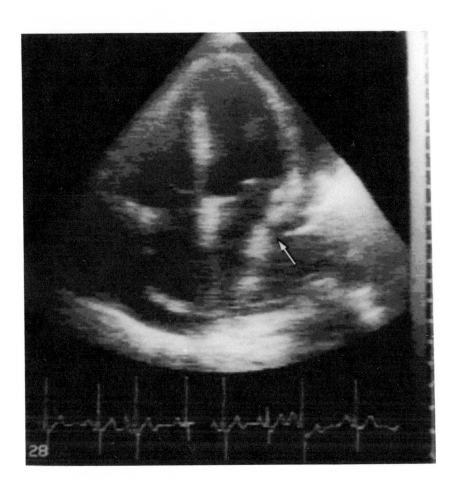

Figure 12.21. Apical four-chamber view of the same patient as in Figure 12.20, showing LA collapse, also in late diastole (*arrow*).

the only means of identifying the effusion and, therefore, is essential for diagnosis (40).

Doppler Echocardiography

In normal humans, there are small inspiratory increases in tricuspid and pulmonic peak flow velocities and stroke volumes and corresponding decreases in left-sided parameters. Pandian et al. (41, 42) have shown that this normal respiratory variation in velocities is increased markedly in tamponade. In tamponade, both the tricuspid and pulmonic valve peak velocities nearly double with inspiration, while both mitral and aortic valve velocities are halved. These observations, termed "flow velocity paradoxus," provide important insight into the mechanism of pulsus paradoxus. While these results are preliminary, quantiation of respiratory variation of transvalvular flow may prove clinically useful after more extensive investigation.

Pericardiocentesis

Two-dimensional echocardiography may be extremely valuable, if not indispensable, in guiding pericardiocentesis. Prior to the procedure, echocardiographic exam-

ination should be performed to confirm that fluid is present and whether or not it is loculated. Two-dimensional echocardiography identifies the optimal approach by defining the area of largest effusion (maximal myocardial-pericardial separation) most easily reached percutaneously, while avoiding abnormal structures and vital organs. Although the standard approach is subcostal, use of two-dimensional echocardiography to define anatomy has reduced the use of the subcostal approach to less than 30 percent of cases with few complications (43, 44). Two-dimensional echocardiography also identifies patients at higher risk of complications due to tumors, inflammatory stranding, etc.

Other investigators have used two-dimensional echocardiography during pericardiocentesis to determine the position of the needle or catheter within the pericardial space. The most successful approach uses contrast echocardiography (saline injection after 10-mL fluid withdrawal) to localize the needle tip in the pericardial space or in a cardiac chamber (Fig. 12.22) (45, 46). This technique is especially useful with bloody effusions when the appearance of the withdrawn fluid does not localize its origin. Direct imaging of the needle is difficult as the tip itself may not be in the image plane

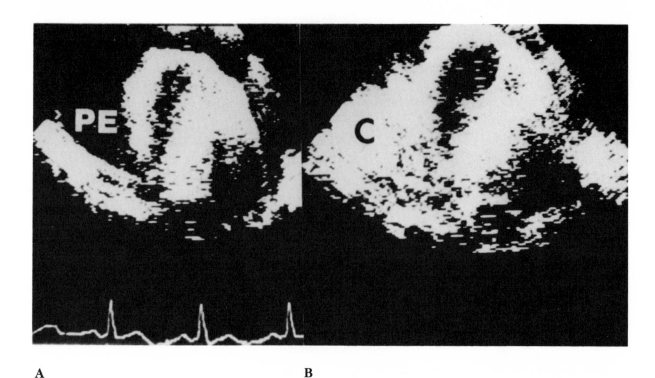

A   B

Figure 12.22. (*A*) Apical four-chamber two-dimensional echocardiographic view of a large pericardial effusion (PE). (*B*) Apical four-chamber view of the same patient after injection of saline solution through the pericardiocentesis needle. A contrast effect, *C*, is seen within the pericardial sac. (Reproduced by permission from Chandraratna PAN, Reid CL, Nimala-suriya A, et al. Application of two-dimensional contrast studies during pericardiocentesis. Am J Cardiol 1983;52:1121.)

or, due to ringing, may be visualized in an incorrect location.

PERICARDIAL THICKENING

M-Mode Echocardiography

The echocardiographic diagnosis of pericardial thickening is far less reliable than that of pericardial effusion (47, 48). At present, no systematic prospective study has been performed to determine the sensitivity and specificity of a positive echographic finding. A retrospective comparison of echocardiographic and surgical or autopsy findings (47) revealed an anatomic corroboration of pericardial disease in only 76 percent of patients. In addition, this study identified seven patterns with pericardial thickening, and these findings (Fig. 12.23) correlated with the anatomic appearances. A brief review of this classification demonstrates the variety of echographic appearances included under the diagnosis of pericardial thickening.

The first pattern was of two dense, parallel, but discrete echoes, which occurs in the absence of thickening, due to adhesions between the pericardial layers. The appearance of echoes between the pericardial layers (pattern 2) suggested denser adhesions. A double line composing the visceral but not parietal peri-

cardial echo (pattern 3) was often seen in the presence of an effusion and indicated thickening of the visceral layer with or without parietal layer involvement. Similarly, a thickened parietal pericardium (pattern 4) was often associated with fluid but variably associated with visceral pericardial thickening. Alternatively, both layers may appear thickened (pattern 5) with or without fluid. Thickening of both layers moving in a nonparallel fashion with an echo-dense space between them (pattern 6) failed to distinguish between thickening, adhesions, and effusion. If motion was parallel (pattern 7), however, fusion of thickened layers or a severely thickened parietal pericardium was found.

Clinically useful generalizations can be drawn from these results: 1) If the two pericardial layers are moving in an exactly parallel fashion, there is likely no effusion. However, even mild damping of parietal layer movement indicates the presence of fluid. 2) Dense echoes observed from either layer do not obviate thickening of the other layer. 3) The appearance of an echo-dense area between the pericardia is nonspecific, representing either fluid, adhesions, or thickening.

In most cases, echocardiographic studies tend to overestimate pericardial thickness, sometimes grossly (49). Usually more specific information may be obtained using serial studies, or if pericardial and pleural

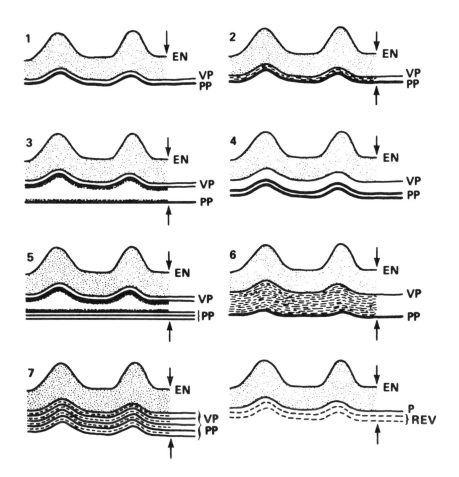

Figure 12.23. Diagrammatic representation of patterns of pericardial thickening. Patterns 1 through 7 are suggestive of pericardial thickening, adhesions, or effusion. The last diagram is not considered suggestive of pericardial disease. See text for description of the seven patterns. EN = endocardium; P = pericardium; PP = parietal pericardium; REV = intermittent reverberations; VP = visceral pericardium. (Reproduced by permission from Schnittger I, Bowden RE, Abrams J, et al. Echocardiography: pericardial thickening and constrictive pericarditis. Am J Cardiol 1978;42:388–95.)

effusions coexist, the pericardium may be well isolated acoustically by the two echo-free spaces. In general, however, other noninvasive techniques such as computed tomography are superior for the assessment of pericardial thickness (50).

Two-Dimensional Echocardiography

Two-dimensional echocardiographic methods are little better for measurement of pericardial thickness. However, localized abnormalities are more easily visualized, including structures within the effusion (e.g., fibrin stranding, metastases) as well as the pericardium itself. In some cases, this may give clues to the etiology of the pericardial disease and aid in its interpretation.

Technical Considerations

As with the imaging of effusions, technique is extremely important. Evaluation of the pericardium should be performed with variation in damping and gain controls. While these maneuvers help, they may not entirely eliminate confusing reverberations behind

a strong pericardial echo. Such echoes may mimic parallel lines, thereby simulating additional pericardial thickness, but should be ignored if occurring posterior to a dense parietal layer (47). An additional cause of a false-positive appearance of pericardial thickening is the presence of mass lesions, which are usually malignant, and are either adherent to, adjacent to, or infiltrating the pericardium.

CONSTRICTIVE PERICARDITIS

The echocardiographic diagnosis of constrictive pericarditis relies heavily on the appearance of a thickened pericardium. In addition, several intracardiac abnormalities have been associated with constriction (Table 12.4). However, none of them are diagnostic, and several are nonspecific. Thus, the recognition of constrictive pericarditis is often difficult and depends on the presence of several suggestive features. In patients with combined effusion and constrictive pericarditis (effusive-constrictive pericarditis), the echographic manifestations of constriction may be obscured, as are the clinical and hemodynamic manifestations (51).

Table 12.4. Echocardiographic Findings Associated with Constrictive Pericarditis

Thickened pericardium
Parallel but separated epicardial and pericardial echoes
Abnormal LV filling pattern
Abnormal septal motion
Abnormal pulmonic valve motion
Rapid mitral valve (EF) slope
Inspiratory leftward movement of atrial and ventricular septa
Dilated inferior vena cava and hepatic veins

Following pericardiocentesis, however, new findings characteristic of constriction may be noted.

M-mode Echocardiography

One of the first proposed and most common diagnostic criteria is flattening of the LV posterior wall motion in mid- to late diastole (Fig. 12.24) (52, 53). Normal diastolic endocardial motion consists of three phases: rapid posterior motion corresponding to rapid filling and ventricular relaxation, a longer middiastolic period of gradual posterior motion, and an additional small indentation corresponding to atrial systole. Patients with constriction have preserved, if not increased, early diastolic rapid filling, corresponding to the early dip in LV pressure. By contrast, in mid- and late diastole, there is little or no posterior endocardial movement (<1.0 mm throughout diastole) as compared to normals (1.5–4.0 mm), and the "a" wave is obliterated. The echographic finding of abrupt cessation of posterior motion of the endocardium and therefore of ventricular filling is synchronous with the early, sudden plateau of LV diastolic pressure and with the occurrence of the auscultatory finding of a pericardial knock (54). These findings graphically reflect the constraints of the diseased pericardium on ventricular filling.

The mitral valve may also display abnormal motion as a result of the altered LV filling pattern. A rapid EF slope has been described in constriction (47, 53) and has been attributed to the abrupt decrease in transmitral flow accompanying cessation of filling. This finding appears to be specific, but insensitive.

Several patterns of abnormal septal motion have been observed in constrictive pericarditis (Figs. 12.24 and 12.25) (55–57). These include paradoxic septal motion throughout systole as well as isolated brief anterior movements in early or late diastole. The paradoxic motion is unrelated to respiratory cycling and may be differentiated from an RV volume overload pattern because the greatest anterior motion occurs in late diastole, coincident with atrial systole and not with ventricular systole. While the cause of the paradoxic motion is unclear, an isolated, brief late diastolic anterior motion may be related to the accommodation of atrial filling volume, as the relatively fixed posterior wall can no longer serve this function. The septum may also show a short anterior motion in early diastole corresponding with a pericardial knock (57).

Premature pulmonic valve opening in middiastole has also been described in constriction, as well as in several other entities (58). This is a nonspecific finding that is believed to result from an early diastolic rise in

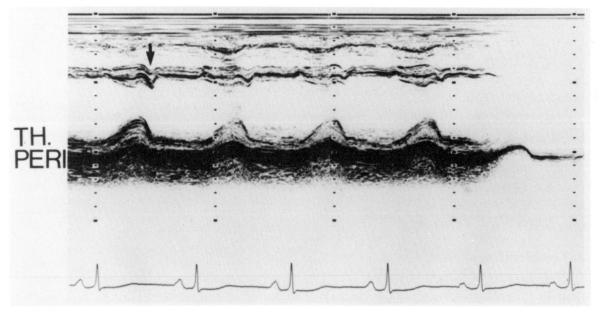

Figure 12.24.   M-mode echocardiogram of a patient with a thickened pericardium (TH. PERI) and probable constrictive pericarditis. Note the flat endocardial echo during diastole and the early diastolic posterior motion of the LV septum (*arrow*).

The differential diagnosis of constrictive pericarditis and restrictive cardiomyopathy may be difficult. These two disease entities can be differentiated indirectly because the LV cavity size is smaller and septal thickening is normal in constriction (60). Janos et al. (61) have used computerized analysis of M-mode echocardiograms with some success. Distinguishing features in constriction include a shorter rapid filling period and a higher peak rate of posterior wall thinning.

Two-Dimensional Echocardiography

Two-dimensional echocardiography, because of its lower sampling frequency and real-time display format, relies more on qualitative abnormalities in diagnosing constrictive pericarditis. Many of these, however, correspond to M-mode findings (62).

As with M-mode, two-dimensional methods overestimate pericardial thickness, a highly gain-dependent measurement. The heart is generally small or normal in size, although the atria may be enlarged. The pericardium is seen as a thickened single or double echo and may be rigid.

The LV filling pattern is usually abnormal in constrictive pericarditis with abrupt and premature cessation of rapid filling. This is followed by little or no increase in LV volume throughout the remainder of diastole. This finding corresponds to the endocardial flattening observed with M-mode, but the latter may be slight and easily overlooked by even experienced observers. This abnormality has been quantitated by frame-by-frame volumetric analysis and has been found to correspond to accelerated cavity expansion in early diastole (62). Thus, the majority of cavity filling occurs in the initial third of diastole. Other findings similar to M-mode include rapid closure of both atrioventricular valves after early diastolic filling and paradoxic septal motion.

Two-dimensional methods also provide additional information. Both the ventricular and atrial septa may demonstrate an inspiratory leftward bulge, probably related to an increase in right-heart filling (62). The immobility of the pericardium may be more easily observed in real time than on M-mode recordings. The inferior vena cava and hepatic veins are often markedly dilated due to high venous pressures. When pericardial calcification is present, it strongly suggests the diagnosis of constrictive pericarditis.

Doppler Echocardiography

The abnormal LV filling pattern characteristic of constrictive pericarditis can also be assessed with Doppler echocardiography. In 1984, Agatston et al. (63) reported a distinctive pattern of mitral valve flow consisting of increased early diastolic filling velocity, rapid

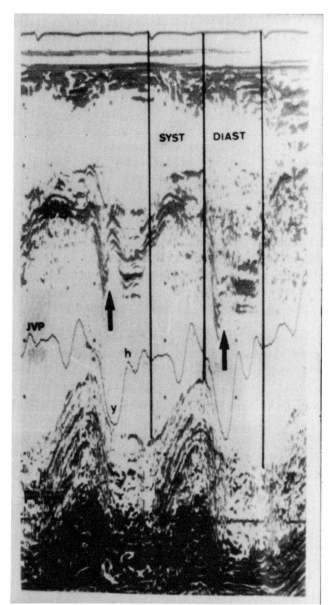

Figure 12.25. Echocardiogram of interventricular septum (IVS) and posterior left ventricular wall (PLVW) recorded simultaneously with jugular venous pulse (JVP). Simultaneous occurrence of abnormal early diastolic notch in IVS and deep "y" trough in JVP is shown. In addition, paradoxic systolic motion of IVS can be seen. The arrows point to the beginning of the abnormal early diastolic notch in IVS. DIAST = diastole; SYST = systole. (Reproduced by permission from Candell-Riera J, Del Castillo HG, Permanyer-Miralda G et al. Echocardiographic features of the interventricular septum in chronic constrictive pericarditis. Circulation 1978;57(6):1156.)

RV pressure so that it equals or exceeds pulmonary artery diastolic pressure and causes valve opening. Another abnormality seen in the pulmonic valve trace is extreme respiratory variation in "a" wave amplitude (59).

deceleration of velocity, and shortened filling period. These parameters reflect abnormal filling as seen in M-mode and two-dimensional echocardiography, with increased flow velocity and rapid posterior wall thinning correlating with the angiographic observation of accelerated cavity expansion, and rapid flow deceleration corresponding to increased EF slope and the premature cessation of cavity expansion. These findings and the 1985 report that flow analysis may be sensitive to LV compliance (64) indicate that Doppler methods may prove useful in differentiating constriction from restriction.

OTHER FORMS OF PERICARDITIS

There are many etiologies of pericardial effusion and constriction (65). In general, echocardiography is of little help in establishing the etiology. The finding of intrapericardial structures on two-dimensional echoes has been thought to indicate effusive-constrictive disease but occurs commonly in a wide variety of clinical entities. Most often, these are fibrin masses or stranding (Fig. 12.26). Bandlike intrapericardial echoes have been noted in patients with mediastinal radiation, renal disease, purulent pericarditis, and traumatic hemoperi-

cardium (66). Cauliflowerlike masses have been noted in both metastatic disease and tuberculous pericarditis (67, 68).

OTHER PERICARDIAL ABNORMALITIES

The normal pericardium serves to fix the heart partially within the chest as well as to prevent cardiac dilation. With congenital or surgical absence of the pericardium, there may be excessive cardiac motion, dilation of the RV, and paradoxic septal motion (68, 69). Differentiation from RV volume overload may be difficult, although echocardiographic detection of the absence of a pericardial echo has been described (70).

Congenital pericardial cysts most commonly occur at the right costophrenic angle and are therefore more readily noted on chest x-ray than routine echocardiography. However, two-dimensional echocardiography may assist in differentiating a cyst from a solid mass, while angiography may be necessary to exclude an aneurysm (71).

Trauma rarely involves the pericardium without affecting the heart or other mediastinal structures. Pericardial contusion or pericardial tears are common following nonpenetrating trauma, but unless the un-

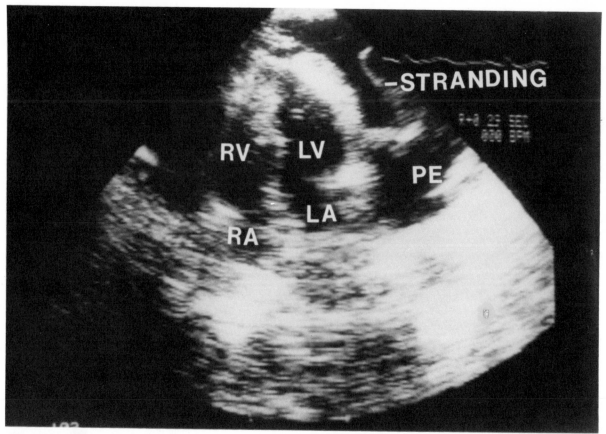

Figure 12.26.   Two-dimensional echocardiogram in the apical four-chamber view showing RV, LV, RA, LA, and a large pericardial effusion (PE). Within the pericardial effusion is shown fibrin stranding. The etiology of this patient's effusion was renal failure.

usual complication of cardiac herniation occurs (72), these entities generally have the echographic appearance of a nontraumatic effusion.

REFERENCES

1. Chandraratna PAN. Uses and limitations of echocardiography in the evaluation of pericardial disease. Echocardiography 1984;1(1):55–74.
2. Tajik AJ. Echocardiography in pericardial effusion. Am J Med 1977;63:29–40.
3. Popp RL. Echocardiographic assessment of cardiac disease. Circulation 1976;54(4):538–52.
4. Feigenbaum H, Waldhausen JA, Hyde LP. Ultrasound diagnosis of pericardial effusion. JAMA 1965;191(9):711–4.
5. Feigenbaum H. Echocardiographic diagnosis of pericardial effusion. Am J Cardiol 1970;26:475–9.
6. Spodick DH. The normal and diseased pericardium: current concepts of pericardial physiology, diagnosis and treatment. J Am Coll Cardiol 1983;1:240–51.
7. Allen JW, Harrison EC, Camp JC, Borsari A, Turnier E, Lau FYK. The role of serial echocardiography in the evaluation and differential diagnosis of pericardial disease. Am Heart J 1977;93(5):560–7.
8. Weitzman LB, Tinker WP, Kronzon I, Cohen ML, Glassman E, Spencer FC. The incidence and natural history of pericardial effusion after cardiac surgery—an echocardiographic study. Circulation 1984;69(3):506–11.
9. Markiewicz W, Brik A, Brook G, Edoute Y, Monakier I, Markiewicz Y. Pericardial rub in pericardial effusion: lack of correlation with amount of fluid. Chest 1980;77(5):643–6.
10. Horowitz MS, Schultz CS, Stinson EB, Harrison DC, Popp RL. Sensitivity and specificity of echocardiographic diagnosis of pericardial effusion. Circulation 1974;50:239–47.
11. Parameswaran R, Goldberg H. Echocardiographic quantitation of pericardial effusion. Chest 1983;83(5):767–70.
12. D'Cruz I, Prabhu R, Cohen HC, Glick G. Potential pitfalls in quantification of pericardial effusions by echocardiography. Br Heart J 1977;39:529–35.
13. Ratshin RA, Smith M, Hood WP. Possible false-positive diagnosis of pericardial effusion by echocardiography in presence of large left atrium. Chest 1974;65(1):112–4.
14. Greene DA, Kleid JJ, Naidu S. Unusual echocardiographic manifestation of pericardial effusion. Am J Cardiol 1977;39:112–5.
15. Lemire F, Tajik AJ, Giuliani ER, Gau GT, Schattenberg TT. Further echocardiographic observations in pericardial effusion. Mayo Clin Proc 1976;51:13–7.
16. Lin TK, Stech JM, Albert WG, Lin JJ, Farha SJ, Hagan CT. Pericardial angiosarcoma simulating pericardial effusion by echocardiography. Chest 1978;73(6):881–3.
17. Millman A, Meller J, Motro M, et al. Pericardial tumor or fibrosis mimicking pericardial effusion by echocardiography. Ann Intern Med 1977;86(4):434–6.
18. Foote WC, Jefferson CM, Price HL. False-positive echocardiographic diagnosis of pericardial effusion. Chest 1977;71(4):546–9.
19. Morales CE, Eng-Cecena L, Pechacek LW, de Castro CM, Garcia E. Echocardiographic mimic of loculated pericardial effusion due to fluid accumulation in the subphrenic space. Tex Heart Inst J 1984;11(4):392–4.
20. Matsuo H, Matsumoto M, Hamanaka Y, et al. Rotational excursion of heart in massive pericardial effusion studied by phased-array echocardiography. Br Heart J 1979;41:513–21.
21. Levisman JA, Abbasi AS. Abnormal motion of the mitral valve with pericardial effusion: pseudo-prolapse of the mitral valve. Am Heart J 1976;91(1):18–20.
22. Vignola PA, Pohost GM, Curfman GD, Myers GS. Correlation of echocardiographic and clinical findings in patients with pericardial effusion. Am J Cardiol 1976;37:701–7.
23. Nanda NC, Gramiak R, Gross CM. Echocardiography of cardiac valves in pericardial effusion. Circulation 1976;54(3):500–4.
24. Settle HP, Adolph RJ, Fowler NO, Engel P, Agruss NS, Levenson NI. Echocardiographic study of cardiac tamponade. Circulation 1977;56(6):951–9.
25. Pandian NG, Rifkin RD, Wang SS. Echocardiography in cardiac tamponade—current status. Echocardiography 1985;4:6–10.
26. D'Cruz IA, Cohen HC, Prabhu R, Glick G. Diagnosis of cardiac tamponade by echocardiography. Circulation 1975;52:460–5.
27. Martins JB, Kerber RE. Can cardiac tamponade be diagnosed by echocardiography? Circulation 1979;60(4):737–42.
28. Schiller NB, Botvinick EH. Right ventricular compression as a sign of cardiac tamponade. Circulation 1977;56(5):774–9.
29. Armstrong WF, Schilt BF, Helper DJ, Dillon JC, Feigenbaum H. Diastolic collapse of the right ventricle with cardiac tamponade: an echocardiographic study. Circulation 1982;65(7):1491–6.
30. Engel PJ, Hon H, Fowler NO, Plummer S. Echocardiographic study of right ventricular wall motion in cardiac tamponade. Am J Cardiol 1982;50:1018–21.
31. Fowler NO, Shabetai R, Braunstein JR. Transmural ventricular pressures in experimental cardiac tamponade. Circ Res 1959;7:733–9.
32. Singh S, Wann LS, Schuchard GH, et al. Right ventricular and right atrial collapse in patients with cardiac tamponade—a combined echocardiographic and hemodynamic study. Circulation 1984;70(6):966–71.
33. Leimgruber PP, Klopfenstein HS, Wann LS, Brooks HL. The hemodynamic derangement associated with right ventricular diastolic collapse in cardiac tamponade: an experimental echocardiographic study. Circulation 1983;68(3):612–20.
34. Armstrong WF, Helper DJ, Schilt BF, Dillon JC, Feigenbaum H. Diastolic collapse of the right ventricle: echocardiographic evidence of occult cardiac tamponade, abstracted. Am J Cardiol 1982;49:1010.
35. Palmer TE, Wann LS, Klopfenstein HS, Janzer DJ, Kalbfleisch JH. Right ventricular diastolic collapse is a more sensitive sign of cardiac tamponade than pulsus paradoxus, abstracted. Circulation 1983;68:III-334.
36. Klopfenstein HS, Schuchard GH, Wann LS, et al. The relative merits of pulsus paradoxus and right ventricular diastolic collapse in the early detection of cardiac tamponade: an experimental echocardiographic study. Circulation 1985;71(4):829–33.
37. Gillam LD, Guyer DE, Gibson TC, King ME, Marshall JE, Weyman AE. Hydrodynamic compression of the right atrium: a new echocardiographic sign of cardiac tamponade. Circulation 1983;68(2):294–301.
38. Kronzon I, Cohen ML, Winer HE. Diastolic atrial compression: a sensitive echocardiographic sign of cardiac tamponade. J Am Coll Cardiol 1983;2(4):770–5.
39. Gaffney FA, Keller AM, Peshock RM, Lin JC, Firth BG. Pathophysiologic mechanisms of cardiac tamponade and pulsus alternans shown by echocardiography. Am J Cardiol 1984;1662–6.
40. Kronzon I, Cohen ML, Winer HE. Cardiac tamponade by loculated pericardial hematoma: limitations of M-mode echocardiography. J Am Coll Cardiol 1983;1(3):913–5.
41. Pandian NG, Wang SS, McInerney K, et al. Doppler echocardiography in cardiac tamponade. Abnormalities in tricuspid and mitral flow response to respiration in experimental and clinical tamponade, abstracted. J Am Coll Cardiol 1985;5(2):485.
42. Pandian NG, Rifkin RD, Wang SS. Flow velocity paradoxus—a Doppler echocardiographic sign of cardiac tamponade: exaggerated respiratory variation in pulmonary and aortic blood flow velocities, abstracted. Circulation 1984;70(II):1524.
43. Callahan JA, Seward JB, Tajik AJ, et al. Pericardiocentesis assisted by two-dimensional echocardiography. J Thorac Cardiovasc Surg 1983;85:877–9.
44. Callahan JA, Seward JB, Tajik J. Cardiac tamponade: pericardiocentesis directed by two-dimensional echocardiography. Mayo Clin Proc 1985;60:344–7.
45. Chandraratna PAN, Reid CL, Nimalasuriya A, Kawanishi D, Rahimtoola SH. Application of 2-dimensional contrast studies during pericardiocentesis. Am J Cardiol 1983;52:1120–2.
46. Chandraratna PAN, First J, Langevin E, O'Dell R. Echocardiographic contrast studies during pericardiocentesis. Ann Intern Med 1977;87(2):199–200.
47. Schnittger I, Bowden RE, Abrams J, Popp RL. Echocardiography:

pericardial thickening and constrictive pericarditis. Am J Cardiol 1978;42:388–95.

48. Horowitz MS, Rossen R, Harrison DC. Echocardiographic diagnosis of pericardial disease. Am Heart J 1979;97(4):420–7.

49. Pandian NG, Skorton DJ, Kieso RA, Kerber RE. Diagnosis of constrictive pericarditis by two-dimensional echocardiography: studies in a new experimental model and in patients. J Am Coll Cardiol 1984;4(6):1164–73.

50. Isner JM, Pandian NG, McInerney KP, Caldeira ME, Funai JT, Bojar RM. The pericardial tourniquet: evaluation of the anatomic and physiologic features of constrictive pericarditis by combined use of computed tomography and cardiac ultrasound. Echocardiography 1985;2(2):197–205.

51. Hancock EW. Subacute effusive-constrictive pericarditis. Circulation 1971;43:183–92.

52. Voelkel AG, Pietro DA, Folland ED, Fisher ML, Parisi AF. Echocardiographic features of constrictive pericarditis. Circulation 1978;58(5):871–5.

53. Chandraratna PAN, Aronow WS, Imaizumi T. Role of echocardiography in detecting the anatomic and physiologic abnormalities of constrictive pericarditis. Am J Med Sci 1982;383(3):141–6.

54. Tyberg TI, Goodyer AVN, Langou RA. Genesis of pericardial knock in constrictive pericarditis. Am J Cardiol 1980;46:570–5.

55. Gibson TC, Grossman W, McLaurin LP, Moos S, Craige E. An echocardiographic study of the interventricular septum in constrictive pericarditis. Br Heart J 1976;38:738–43.

56. Pool PE, Seagren SC, Abbasi AS, Charuzi Y, Kraus R. Echocardiographic manifestations of constrictive pericarditis. Chest 1975;68(5):684–8.

57. Candell-Riera J, Del Castillo HG, Permanyer-Miralda G, Soler-Soler J. Echocardiographic features of the interventricular septum in chronic constrictive pericarditis. Circulation 1978;57(6):1154–8.

58. Wann LS, Weyman AE, Dillon JC, Feigenbaum H. Premature pulmonary valve opening. Circulation 1977;55(1):128–33.

59. Doi JL, Sugiura T, Spodick DH. Motion of pulmonic valve and constrictive pericarditis. Chest 1981;80(4):513–5.

60. Horowitz MS, Rossen RM, Harrison DC, Popp RL. Ultrasonic evaluation of constrictive pericardial disease, abstracted. Circulation 1974;49,50(suppl III):87.

61. Janos GG, Arjunan K, Meyer RA, Engel P, Kaplan S. Differentiation of constrictive pericarditis and restrictive cardiomyopathy using digitized echocardiography. J Am Coll Cardiol 1983;1(2):541–9.

62. Lewis BS. Real time two dimensional echocardiography in constrictive pericarditis. Am J Cardiol 1982;49:1789–93.

63. Agatston AS, Rao A, Price RJ, Kinney EL. Diagnosis of constrictive pericarditis by pulsed Doppler echocardiography. Am J Cardiol 1984;54:929–30.

64. Rokey R, Kuo LC, Zoghbi WA, Limacher MC, Quinones MA. Determination of parameters of left ventricular diastolic filling with pulsed Doppler echocardiography: comparison with cineangiography. Circulation 1985;71(3):543–50.

65. Guberman BA, Fowler NO, Engle PJ, Gueron M, Allen JM. Cardiac tamponade in medical patients. Circulation 1981;64(3):633–40.

66. Martin RP, Bowden R, Filly K, Popp RL. Intrapericardial abnormalities in patients with pericardial effusion. Circulation 1980;61(3):568–72.

67. Chandraratna PAN, Aronow WS. Detection of pericardial metastases by cross-sectional echocardiography. Circulation 1981;63(1):197–9.

68. Chia BL, Choo M, Tan A, Ee B. Echocardiographic abnormalities in tuberculous pericardial effusion. Am Heart J 1984;107(5):1034–5.

69. Payvandi MN, Kerber RE. Echocardiography in congenital and acquired absence of the pericardium. Circulation 1976;53(1):86–92.

70. Hermann H, Raizner AE, Chahine RA, Luchi RJ. Congenital absence of the left pericardium: an unusual palpation finding and echocardiographic demonstration of the defect. South Med J 1976;69(9):1222–5.

71. Rogers CI, Seymour EQ, Brock JG. Atypical pericardial cyst location: the value of computed tomography. J Comput Assist Tomogr 1980;48:683.

72. Christides C, Laskar M, Kim M, Grousseau-Renaudie D, Pouget X. Post traumatic rupture of the pericardium with cardiac luxation associated with myocardial infarction and a rupture of the aortic isthmus. J Chir (Paris) 1981;118:505.

13
Intracardiac Masses

Joel Raichlen

In the past, cardiac tumors, thrombi, and anatomic variants were interesting anomalies whose diagnosis was rarely made without autopsy (1). With the development of cardiac catheterization, angiographic techniques provided the first means of identifying these abnormalities ante mortem. The development of M-mode echocardiography permitted the noninvasive detection of cardiac masses, but its sensitivity was low; angiography was generally required to assess the size and location of the mass. These imaging modalities have now largely been replaced by two-dimensional echocardiography (2–8). By providing direct visualization of the heart in multiple planes, two-.dimensional echocardiography enables determination of the size, shape, and mobility of cardiac masses, their location and type of myocardial attachment, and their relation to surrounding cardiac structures. Guided by this information, surgeons can explore for cardiac tumors without the necessity of preoperative cardiac catheterization (2–4). In addition, the sensitivity and reliability of two-dimensional echocardiography has resulted in its being the study of choice for the diagnosis and monitoring of intracardiac thrombi and for the identification of chord and valvelike congenital anomalies.

PRIMARY CARDIAC TUMORS

Primary tumors of the heart are relatively rare, with a prevalence in autopsy series ranging from 0.0017 percent to 0.28 percent (9–11). Since they produce no characteristic signs or symptoms, cardiac tumors can be clinically diagnosed in only 5 to 10 percent of cases (12). When clinical findings are produced, they are the result of mass effects on cardiac hemodynamics, embolization, local tumor invasion, or constitutional symptoms (7). Clinical presentations vary widely: syncope, angina, dyspnea or edema due to valvular or outflow tract obstruction; acute systemic arterial ische-

mic events due to systemic embolization of tumor fragments; congestive heart failure due to myocardial tumor invasion; pulmonary hypertension due to pulmonary tumor emboli or obstruction to left heart filling; recurrent tachyarrhythmias or, more rarely, heart block presumably due to invasion of the conduction system; chest pain due to coronary tumor emboli and myocardial necrosis; hemolytic anemia or thrombocytopenia due to mechanical destruction of cells by tumor; constitutional symptoms such as fever, malaise, cachexia, and weight loss; pericarditis with effusion or tamponade due to pericardial involvement; arthralgias, hepatic dysfunction, or Raynaud's phenomenon presumably due to systemic or immune responses to tumor breakdown products; or signs and symptoms mimicking bacterial endocarditis such as fever, changing murmurs, skin lesions, clubbing, anemia, elevated erythrocyte sedimentation rate, and hyperglobulinemia (7, 12, 13). Diagnosing primary cardiac tumors from these signs and symptoms requires a high index of suspicion. When the possibility of a tumor is considered, two-dimensional echocardiography is the diagnostic modality of choice to identify, localize, and determine the characteristics of the tumor mass (2). In general, it is the only study required prior to surgical intervention (2, 3, 14).

When a cardiac tumor is detected with ultrasound, it is important to define its three-dimensional anatomy, especially if surgical excision is contemplated. Several echocardiographic features that help determine whether surgical excision is feasible should also be carefully examined. These include tumor morphology (e.g., the presence of stalk) and tumor location: Does it involve the myocardium? Does it span the atrioventricular (AV) groove? Does it include other organs juxtaposed to the heart? Does it involve valvular tissues? Does it obstruct ventricular inflow or outflow?

The most common primary tumors involving the endocardium and myocardium are myxomas, sarco-

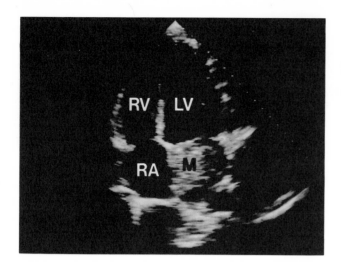

A

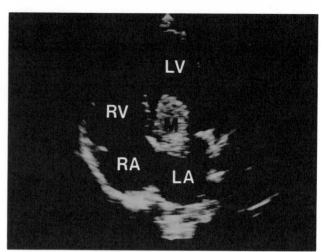

B

Figure 13.1. Left atrial myxoma (M) which prolapses from the LA into the LV in diastole. (*A*) Apical four-chamber view showing the large tumor mass filling the LA in systole. (*B*) Apical four-chamber view and (*C*) parasternal long-axis view showing the mass prolapsing across the mitral valve in diastole.

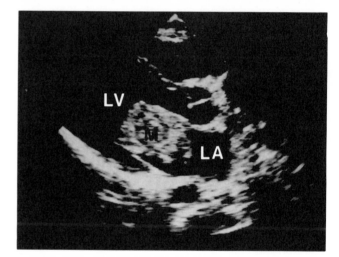

C

mas, rhabdomyomas, lipomas, and fibroelastomas, which together account for over 80 percent of all primary cardiac tumors in adults (11). The most common of these are myxomas, which constitute 30 to 50 percent of all primary tumors (Figs. 13.1, 13.2, 13.3, and 13.4) (10–12, 15, 16). These benign neoplasms occur predominantly in adults aged 30 to 60, with a 3:1 female predominance (1, 12, 15, 17). In a series of 130 myxoma patients, 65 percent presented with symptoms consistent with valvular heart disease, 36 percent with embolic phenomena (Fig. 13.2), 5 percent with sudden death, 4 percent with pericarditis, 3 percent with myocardial infarction, and 2 percent with a fever of unknown origin (11). Sixteen percent of patients were asymptomatic, with the myxoma an incidental finding.

Although myxomas may occur anywhere within the heart, over 90 percent are found in the atria, with 75 to 86 percent occurring in the left atrium (LA), 8 to 20

percent in the right atrium (RA), and 5 to 11 percent in the right or left ventricles (RV and LV, respectively) (11, 12, 18, 19). Rarely, myxomas may be multiple (Fig. 13.3), in which case biatrial involvement is most common (20, 21). Ninety percent of myxomas are pedunculated with a stalk that is attached most frequently to the left inter-atrial septum in the region of the oval fossa (14, 21–23) and may prolapse into the LV in diastole (Figs. 13.1 and 13.2). The remaining 10 percent are sessile and may be more difficult to identify, particularly when the tumors are small (14).

The specific site of tumor attachment is important in planning the approach to surgical resection. It can be accurately determined using two-dimensional echocardiography in over 80 percent of cases, with the greatest difficulty encountered in large atrial tumors that remain in contact with the surrounding myocardium (Fig. 13.4) (2). Definition of the attachment site generally

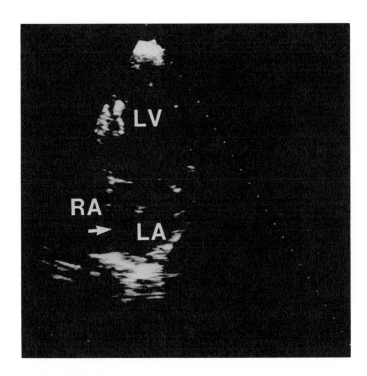

A

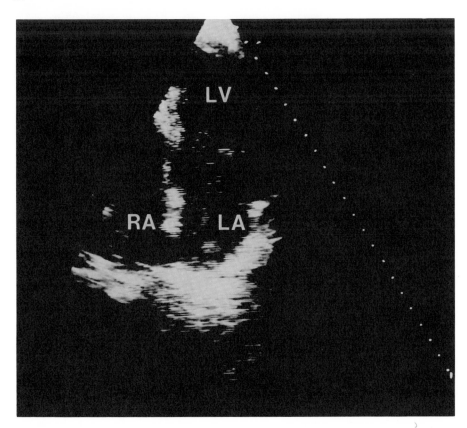

B

Figure 13.2. Mobile, compliant LA myxoma with an irregular shape imaged in the apical four-chamber view. (*A*) Systolic image demonstrating the point of attachment on the left interatrial septum (*arrow*). (*B*) Diastolic image showing the myxoma prolapsing into the LV.

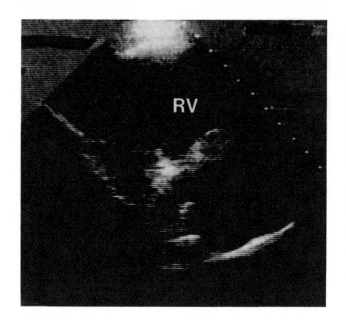

A

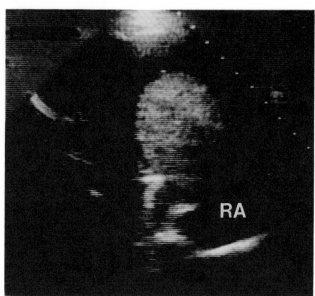

B

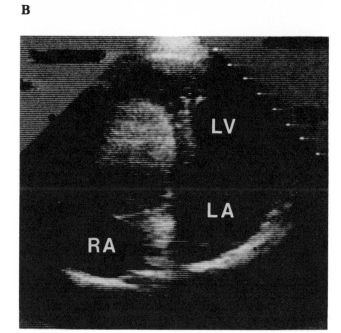

C

Figure 13.3. Right ventricular inflow view showing a large right atrial myxoma (*A*) in systole and (*B*) prolapsing into the RV in diastole. (*C*) Diastolic image of the apical four-chamber view showing attachment of the myxoma to the interatrial septum.

requires imaging the tumor in multiple views. In the case of an inter-atrial septal attachment, the subcostal and apical four-chamber views are most valuable. In difficult diagnostic cases, demonstrating that the mass is free of contact with the mitral valvular apparatus reduces possible confusion with mitral valvular vegetations, mitral annular calcification, and calcification of the mitral leaflets or chordae tendineae. It has been suggested that the identification and characterization of tumor masses may be enhanced by acoustic ampli-

tude processing techniques such as color two-dimensional imaging (24).

The echocardiographic appearance of atrial myxomas has been found to correlate with findings on gross inspection. Those that appear compliant and deformable on echocardiograms (Fig. 13.2) tend to be gelatinous, papillary, and friable when examined, while those that appear nondeformable (Figs. 13.3 and 13.4) are more apt to be firm, smooth, and nonfriable (2). This may be of clinical relevance: In one series of 30

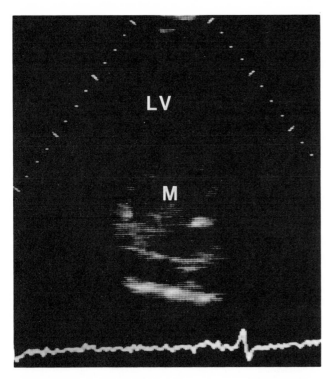

Figure 13.4.   Apical two-chamber view showing a large nondeformable left atrial myxoma (M) completely filling the LA and protruding through the mitral valve into the LV.

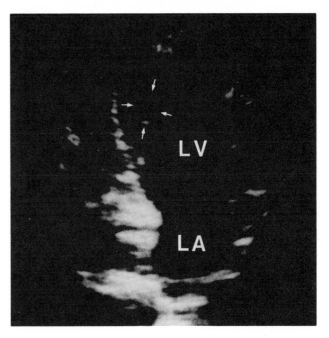

Figure 13.5.   Apical two-chamber view of a mobile ovoid thrombus (*arrows*) with a central echolucency adjacent to an akinetic segment of the LV. The thrombus subsequently disappeared without intervening anticoagulant or thrombolytic therapy.

patients with primary cardiac tumors, the six with evidence of systemic emboli all had tumors that were gelatinous in consistency (2). The tumors associated with embolic phenomena were smaller than those without evidence of emboli (Fig. 13.2 versus Figs. 13.1 and 13.4).

Two-dimensional echocardiographic demonstration of lucent areas within myxoma has been attributed to areas of hemorrhage or necrosis found pathologically (2, 25). The finding of such echolucencies within an atrial mass is believed to help differentiate atrial myxoma from atrial thrombus (26–29), but central echolucencies have also been encountered in thrombi, presumably due to clot lysis (Fig. 13.5) (25–30). Other studies have suggested a constellation of echocardiographic findings as favoring the diagnosis of myxoma over thrombus (31–33). Atrial myxoma is most likely when a mobile mass with a mottled, ovoid appearance and sharply demarcated borders is found, especially when attached to the interatrial septum in a heart with a normal-size atrium and a normal AV valve. Thrombus is favored by the appearance of an irregular, layered, immobile mass with a broad base located on the posterior atrial wall, especially in an enlarged atrium with a stenotic AV valve. The inability to demonstrate any site of mural attachment favors the diagnosis of thrombus rather than myxoma. Differentiation between tumors and thrombi may be aided by tissue

characterization techniques (34). Studies thus far have demonstrated that analysis of ultrasonic backscatter can often distinguish between intracardiac echos caused by thrombi and those attributable to tumors and artifacts (35).

Although primary benign tumors in adults more commonly occur in the LA than the RA, primary malignant tumors are more commonly found in the RA (10). Malignant primary neoplasms, which are almost always sarcomas (Fig. 13.6), are the second most common cardiac tumors, making up roughly 20 percent of all primary tumors (10, 11, 36). The most common of these malignant tumors is the angiosarcoma, which occurs in all age groups and is two to three times more common in males (11, 37, 38). Over 70 percent of angiosarcomas occur in the RA (11). They rapidly expand into the myocardium and pericardium and frequently metastasize to the lungs and mediastinal lymph nodes (7, 10).

Echocardiographic demonstration of RA tumors requires multiple tomographic orientations. Complete assessment necessitates examination of the parasternal RV inflow view, the parasternal short-axis view at the level of the aortic, tricuspid, and pulmonic valves, the apical and subcostal four-chamber views, and the subcostal view of the junction between the RA and the inferior vena cava (Fig. 13.7). Early identification of primary tumors is of great importance: It enables

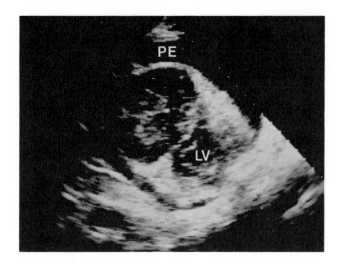

A

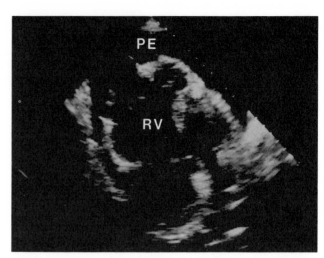

B

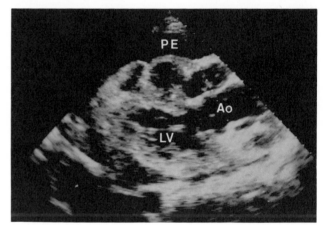

C

Figure 13.6. (*A*) Cross-sectional view at the midventricular level showing a large spindle cell sarcoma filling the RV cavity. (*B*) A more proximal section and (*C*) a parasternal long-axis view showing the sarcoma extending through the wall of the RV into the pericardial space and into the right ventricular outflow tract. PE = pericardial effusion.

surgical resection, which can be curative in benign neoplasms and prolong survival in malignant neoplasms (6).

The second most common benign tumor is the lipoma (11). Cardiac lipomas are found at all ages and are equally distributed between males and females (39). Most are sessile or polypoid, with half originating in the subendocardium, one-quarter in the subepicardium, and another quarter arise completely intramuscular (7, 40). These tumors most commonly affect the LV, RA, and the inter-atrial septum (Fig. 13.8).

When occurring in the LV or RV, myocardial tumors are best assessed using apical and subcostal views. While large tumors are easily distinguishable since they may fill the ventricular cavity (Fig. 13.6), small sessile or intramural tumors are more difficult to diagnose (Fig. 13.9). Because they may be of similar echodensity as the surrounding myocardium, it is important to

focus attention on areas with asymmetric thickening, especially when associated with hypokinesis.

Although myxomas are the most common tumors in adults, they are exceedingly rare in children and almost never occur in infants (11, 41). The most common tumor in the pediatric age group is the rhabdomyoma, which is probably a hamartoma rather than a true neoplasm (10, 11, 41–43). Forty percent of such tumors occur at younger than 6 months of age, with many present at birth (Fig. 13.10), suggesting it is a congenital tumor (44). Rarely, cardiac rhabdomyomas have been diagnosed on prenatal echocardiograms (45). These tumors are usually multiple (90 percent) and deeply embedded in the RV or LV wall, making surgical excision almost impossible (10, 46). However, there have been recent reports of successful resections (47–49). In an early series, only 15 percent of patients survived to age 5 (44). Rhabdomyomas are associated

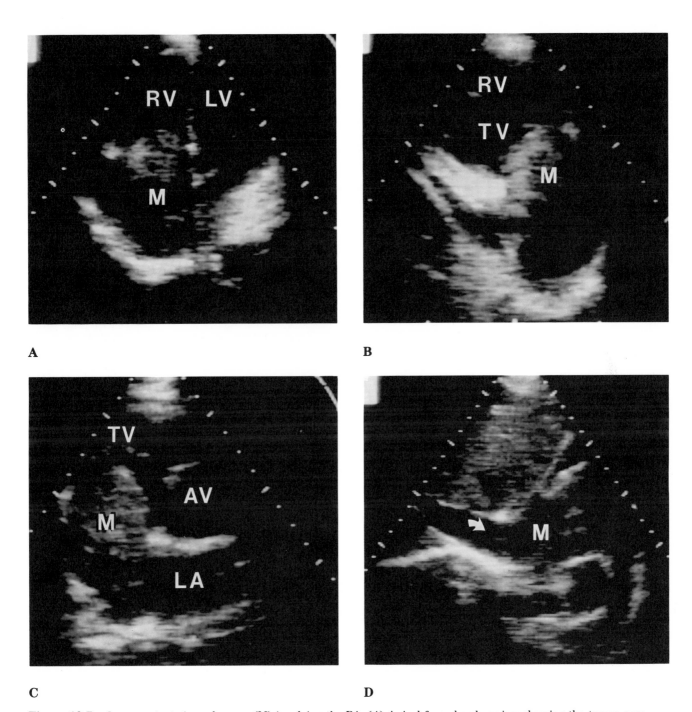

A

B

C

D

Figure 13.7.   Large metastatic melanoma (M) involving the RA. (*A*) Apical four-chamber view showing the tumor completely filling the RA. (*B*) Right ventricular inflow view in early diastole showing the mass abutting the tricuspid valve (TV). (*C*) Parasternal cross-sectional view at the level of the aortic valve (AV) showing the mass in early systole totally separated from the TV. (*D*) Subcostal view showing extension of the tumor into the inferior vena cava (*arrow*).

with tuberous sclerosis, which is inherited as an autosomal dominant. Two-dimensional echocardiograms are recommended for screening of fetuses and newborns with positive family histories for tuberous sclerosis (46, 47, 50).

Fibromas are the second most common primary tumor in children, are almost always single, and occur

in the ventricular myocardium (11). These benign tumors have been resected from the apex or ventricular free wall, but those involving the interventricular septum are frequently inoperable (11). Although successful resections have also been performed for other benign neoplasms, the prognosis for malignant or metastatic tumors in children is extremely poor (46,

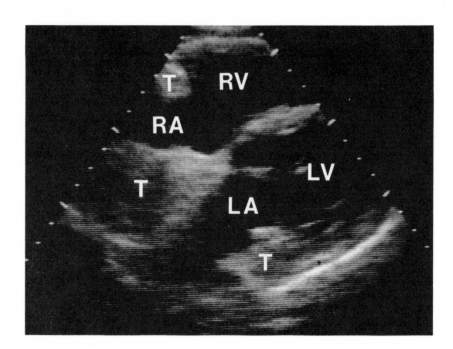

Figure 13.8. Cardiac lipomas presenting as multiple echodense tumors (T). The largest tumor mass involves the intra-atrial septum, with smaller tumors observed in the LA and RA.

51). As in adults, two-dimensional echocardiography is the study of choice for diagnosing and guiding the management of cardiac masses in the pediatric population (46–48, 52, 53).

METASTATIC CARDIAC TUMORS

In autopsy series, cardiac metastases are found 20 to 40 times more commonly than primary cardiac tumors, with a prevalence averaging 10 percent in patients with

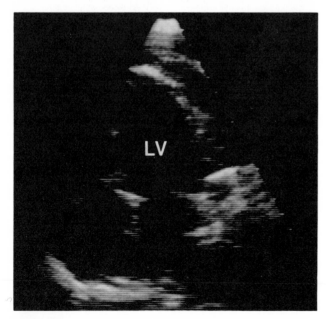

Figure 13.9. Apical four-chamber view showing intramural tumor (T) within the lateral wall of the LV in a patient with metastatic breast carcinoma.

malignant disease outside the heart (1, 11, 54, 55). Almost all malignant tumors have been found to metastasize to the heart, with the most common (in order of decreasing frequency) being bronchogenic carcinoma, carcinoma of the breast, malignant melanoma, leukemias, and lymphomas (56). Melanomas are the malignancies most likely to involve the heart, with metastases found in over 50 percent of cases (57, 58). Cardiac involvement is also found in up to half of patients with leukemia, one-quarter of patients with bronchogenic carcinoma, and one-sixth of patients with breast carcinoma or lymphoma (57, 59).

Metastatic disease may reach the heart by direct extension (Fig. 13.11) as in bronchogenic carcinomas, by embolic hematogenous spread as in malignant melanomas (Figs. 13.7 and 13.12) or via lymphatic channels as in breast carcinomas (Fig. 13.9), and lymphomas (60). Metastases from lung and breast carcinomas most commonly involve the pericardium, frequently without cardiac involvement, while melanoma and leukemia involve the heart with or without pericardial involvement. Cardiac metastases involving the pericardium may be associated with signs and symptoms of pericarditis including pericardial effusions, constrictive pericarditis, and cardiac tamponade (11). Since the presence of pericardial metastases may preclude operative intervention in otherwise resectable tumors, echocardiography may provide important clinical data in oncologic patients. Suggestive findings include diffuse pericardial thickening in the presence of externally compressing masses (Figs. 13.12 and 13.13) or irregularly appearing nodules attached to the visceral or parietal pericardium (Fig. 13.14). The finding of

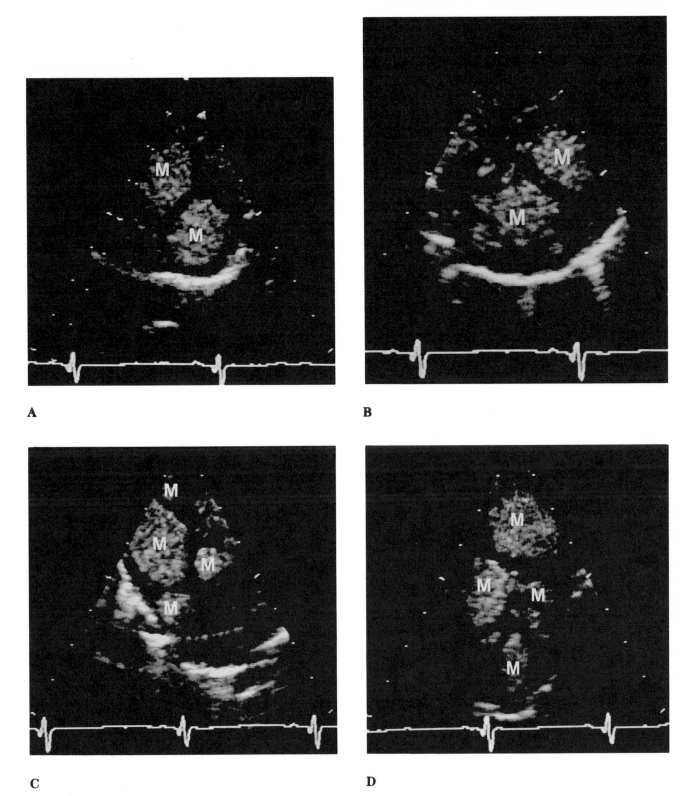

Figure 13.10.   Cardiac rhabdomyomas. (*A*) and (*B*) provide cross-sectional views through the ventricles showing large tumor masses (M) completely filling the RV and LV. (*C*) and (*D*) show the large number of tumor masses that were present in this newborn.

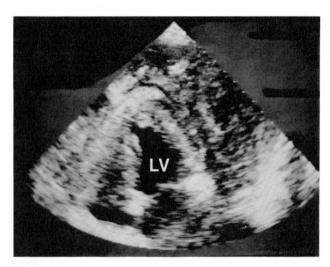

Figure 13.11. Large tumor mass (T) surrounding the ventricles and extending into the lateral wall of the LV.

discrete masses that move with the cardiac cycle and protrude into a pericardial effusion in a patient with a known primary malignancy is highly suggestive of pericardial metastases (61, 62). Non-discrete echo densities, lacelike echogenic structures, and intrapericardial bandlike echodensities are not diagnostic of malignant involvement and may represent a number of etiologies such as post-traumatic or post-inflammatory fibrinous strands, radiation-induced adhesions, or uremic pericarditis (62).

When metastatic tumor involves the cardiac chambers, the right heart is more frequently involved than the left (Figs. 13.7, 13.15 and 13.16) (1, 10). Although they are most often clinically silent, intracardiac metastases can manifest as follows: superior vena cava syndrome from tumor obstruction; supraventricular arrhythmias due to infiltration of the conduction system; myocardial infarction due to coronary artery compression or tumor emboli; cardiomegaly or congestive heart failure due to myocardial tumor infiltration; nonbacterial endocarditis due in part to immune complex reactions associated with the malignancy; and murmurs or hypotensive symptoms related to direct tumor obstruction (57, 63). Intracavitary cardiac tumors are usually primary malignancies. Intracavitary metastases, while relatively uncommon, are more likely to result in embolic phenomena or mechanical hemolysis (31, 64). Malignant melanomas are the tumors that most commonly metastasize to the endocardium. They appear echocardiographically as a mass extending into the intracavitary space and should be examined in multiple views to determine the full extent of tumor involvement (Fig. 13.7) (58, 61).

CARDIAC THROMBI

The development of ultrasound as a cardiac imaging technique was contingent on the echolucency of blood, which permitted the demonstration of cardiac structures in motion. With the development of higher frequency and higher resolution clinical ultrasound equipment, it was observed that echocardiographic contrast could be found within cardiac chambers in association with low cardiac output or regional blood stasis and in the inferior vena cava in both diseased and normal hearts (65–69). Investigations of this phenomenon have determined that blood echogenicity depends on such factors as blood velocity, erythrocyte aggregation, and the concentration of plasma proteins (70–73). While these dynamic intracavitary echos (sometimes referred to as "cardiac smoke") can be differentiated from cardiac thrombus (65, 74), the conditions with which they are associated predispose to the development of mural thrombi, and their demonstration should prompt a search for concurrent thrombus (Fig. 13.17) (75). Given the potentially devastating consequences of cardiac emboli, the identification of mural thrombi is of major clinical relevance. The ability of two-dimensional echocardiography to visualize noninvasively the cardiac chambers in multiple views makes it the diagnostic study of choice when a cardiac source of embolism is clinically suspected.

Left Ventricular Thrombi

Mural thrombus in the LV is found in the clinical setting of transmural myocardial infarctions, LV aneurysms, and cardiomyopathies (76). Autopsy studies of postinfarction patients have documented the incidence of thrombus to range from 17 to 66 percent (77–80). Initially, mural thrombi were only suspected following clinical embolic events. With the development of LV angiography, thrombi could be diagnosed ante mortem, but the sensitivity was low due to poor resolution and difficulty in distinguishing mural thrombi from adjacent myocardium (81–83). Since many thrombi occur within the cardiac apex, M-mode echocardiography has been of very limited value in detecting or characterizing these masses (84). The advent of two-dimensional echocardiography has greatly enhanced the ability to detect and characterize mural thrombi. Studies in animals with anatomic validation have shown that the acoustic properties of acute thrombi permit their detection (identification and differentiation from static blood and adjacent myocardium) within 45 minutes to 3 hours of the stimulus for formation, with thrombi as small as 6 mm being detectable (85). Studies in humans have demonstrated mural thrombi in the first day following infarction, with most occurring in the first 4 days (86).

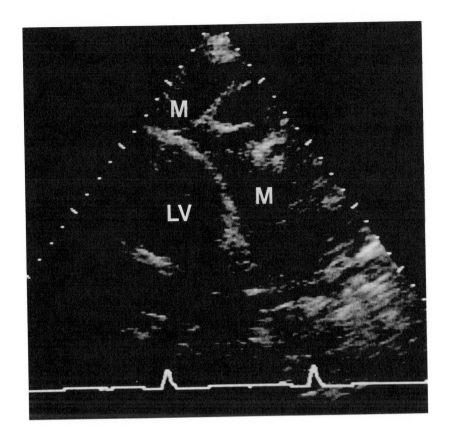

A

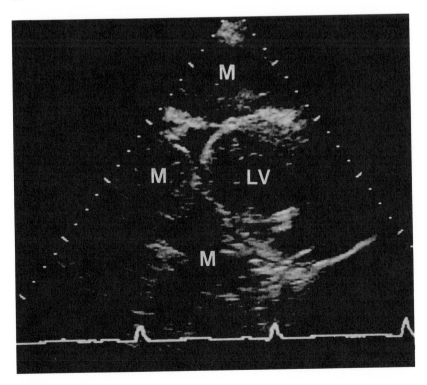

B

Figure 13.12.   Parasternal views of the LV showing large nonhomogeneous masses (M) surrounding the heart and compressing the LV in a patient with metastatic melanoma.

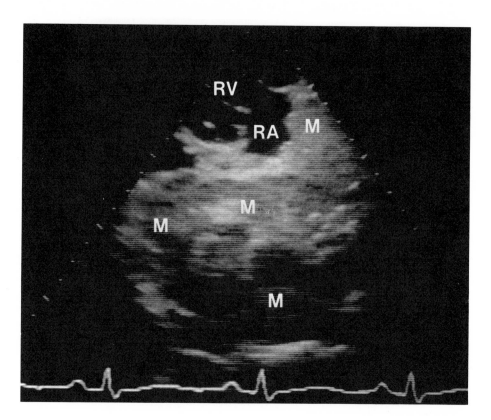

A

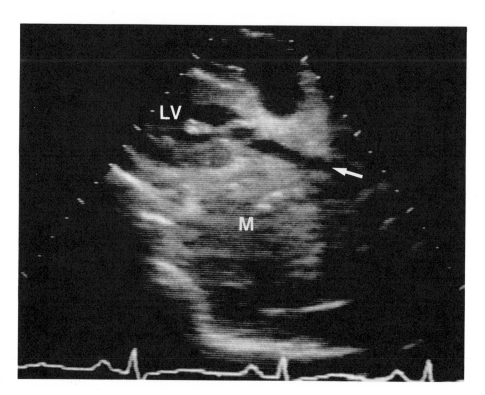

Figure 13.13. (*A*) Large tumor mass (M) surrounding the heart and infiltrating the wall of the RA in a patient with Ewing sarcoma. (*B*) The tumor compressed the LA leaving only a slitlike opening for the cavity (*arrow*).

B

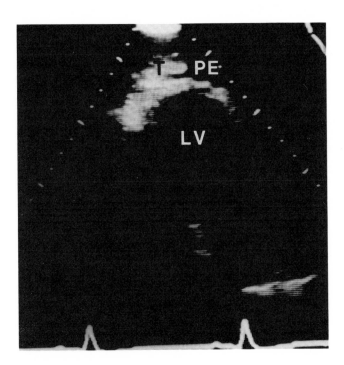

A

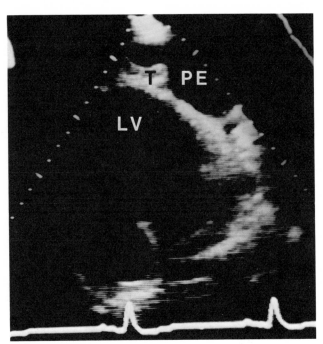

B

Figure 13.14. Metastatic tumor (T) attached to the epicardial surface of the LV in a patient with adenocarcinoma. (*A*) Tumor surrounding the ventricular apex showing its irregular border. (*B*) A slightly different view showing the T attached to the ventricular epicardium with a portion protruding into the pericardial effusion (PE).

The sensitivity and specificity of two-dimensional echocardiography in detecting LV thrombus approaches 90 percent (81, 87). Mural thrombus appears as a mass with distinct margins adjacent to the endocardium, which can be distinguished from the underlying myocardium by its increased acoustic density (Fig. 13.18). The thrombus can usually be identified due to disruption of the continuity of the ventricular wall, particularly when the mass protrudes into the ventricular cavity (Fig. 13.19). Mural thrombus may be freely mobile (Fig. 13.20) or move with the adjacent wall. In ischemic heart disease, mural thrombus is associated with akinesis or dyskinesis. These wall motion abnormalities are generally associated with areas of transmural infarction and myocardial thinning. Therefore, the finding of a relative increase in apparent wall thickness or of normal wall thickness in a region of dyskinesis or within an aneurysm is highly suggestive of underlying mural thrombus (88). Although infrequently found in association with inferior infarctions, mural thrombi occur in 30 to 40 percent of transmural anterior infarctions, more likely associated with large infarcts (high creatine phosphokinase levels), infarcts involving the apex, or those associated with ventricular aneurysms (86, 89–91). As a consequence, ventricular thrombi occur most commonly at the apex or along the anterior wall of the heart, and the search for them should focus on the apical views (Figs. 13.18 and 13.19).

The echodensity of protruding thrombi tends to be greater than that of the underlying myocardium, but mural thrombi that lie flat against the adjacent wall tend to be less echodense and therefore more difficult to identify (75). Occasionally, thrombi have a layered appearance with increased echodensity along the intracavitary margin and relative echolucency between the surface of the thrombus and the endocardium. Under some circumstances (e.g., with suboptimal image quality), it may be extremely difficult to identify an intracavitary mass as thrombus. In such instances, serial echocardiographic examinations may be valuable in making a definitive diagnosis. The identification of serial changes in a suspicious echodensity strongly favors the likelihood of thrombus. Over time, cardiac thrombi may develop a more characteristic appearance or may completely disappear, either spontaneously or on anticoagulant therapy (Fig. 13.5) (75, 92). This does not occur with papillary muscles, heavy muscular trabeculations (as occur at the apex in hypertrophied hearts), or aberrant chordal structures, all of which might on occasion be confused with ventricular thrombi. False-positive studies may also result from

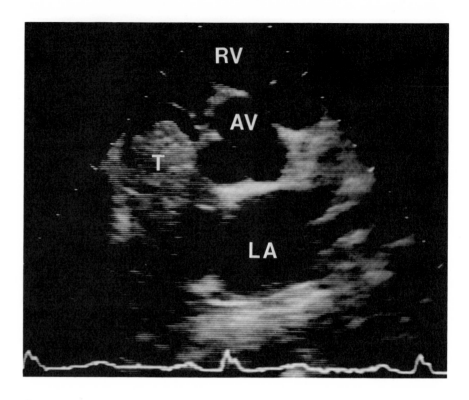

A

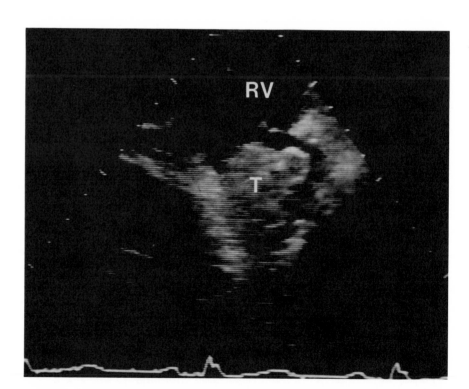

Figure 13.15. (*A*) Parasternal cross-sectional view at the level of the AV and (*B*) right ventricular inflow view showing a large nonhomogeneous tumor (T) filling the RA.

B

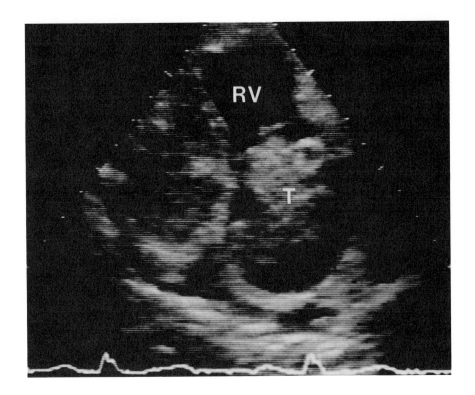

C

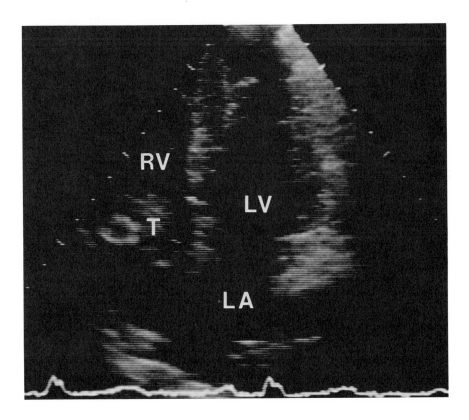

D

Figure 13.15 (cont'd.). (*C*) Slightly angulated right ventricular inflow view and (*D*) apical four-chamber view showing the multilobulated appearance of the tumor in a patient with a large hepatocellular carcinoma that extended from the right lobe of the liver into the inferior vena cava and into the RA.

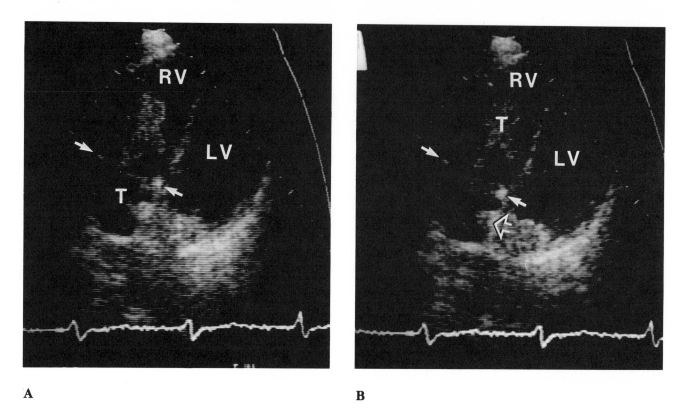

Figure 13.16.   Metastatic thyroid carcinoma involving the right heart. (*A*) In early diastole, the tumor (T) fills the RA and extends into the RV, filling a large portion of the cavity. (*B*) Later in diastole, the site of T attachment is demonstrated on the RA wall (*open arrow*), with a large stalk seen prolapsing across the tricuspid valve anulus (*solid arrows*) with the bulk of the tumor in the RV.

spurious intracavitary echos originating adjacent to the heart, from the chest wall, from the transducer casing, or occasionally from distant echodensities such as the spine. Many of these can be differentiated by their ill-defined irregular margins and their apparent lack of motion despite normal adjacent myocardial motion (93). In the case of apical artifacts, misinterpretations may be fostered by technical difficulties associated with the low near-field resolution of the echo transducer. In general, the likelihood of false-positive diagnoses can be minimized by optimizing gain attenuation settings and by requiring that mural thrombi be identified in the same anatomic location in a minimum of two sector orientations (75).

Systemic Emboli and Anticoagulation

Systemic emboli are clinically diagnosed in up to 12 percent of patients sustaining acute myocardial infarctions (94–96). Autopsy findings suggest that the incidence may range as high as 52 percent or 56 percent in patients with LV aneurysms or myocardial infarctions, with the emboli causing or contributing to death in 12 to 33 percent (76, 96, 97). The incidence of emboli in

patients with echocardiographically demonstrated ventricular thrombus ranges from 0 to 27 percent in large series (86, 91, 98, 99), with most embolic events occurring within 3 to 4 months of infarction (89, 90, 100). In some patients, emboli occur without evidence of mural thrombi (86, 101). These most likely result from small thrombi that are beyond the resolution of current equipment.

Echocardiographic studies of postinfarction patients have suggested that certain characteristics of LV thrombi predispose to the development of systemic emboli. The most important of these are protrusion of the thrombus into the ventricular cavity (Fig. 13.19) and free mobility of the thrombus (Fig. 13.20) (98, 99, 102, 103). In one study, the likelihood of embolization increased from 27 percent overall, to 40 percent when the thrombus protruded, to 60 percent when it displayed intracavitary motion (99). In that study, 85 percent of patients with freely mobile thrombi had embolic events. Characteristics that did not predispose to embolic events included the presence of swirling intracavitary echoes ("cardiac smoke") consistent with low flow, the relative echodensity of the thrombus, a layered or heterogenous appearance of the thrombus,

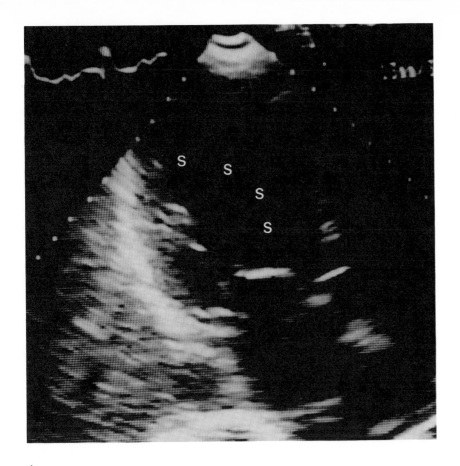

A

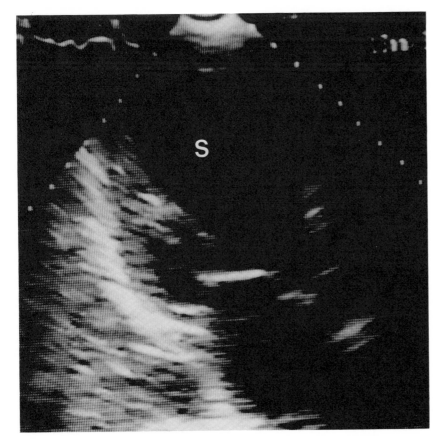

B

Figure 13.17. Dynamic intracavitary echos within the LV. (*A*) 'Cardiac smoke' (S) swirling within the LV. (*B*) A more circular cloud of echoes in the same patient.

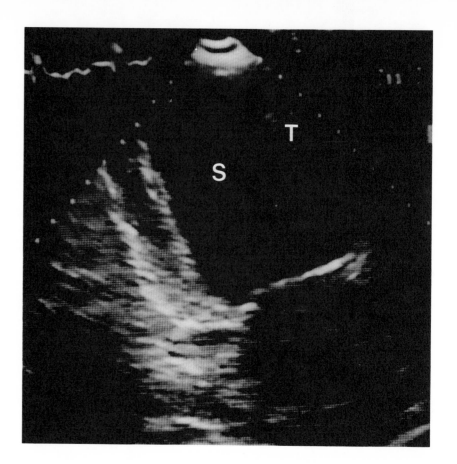

C

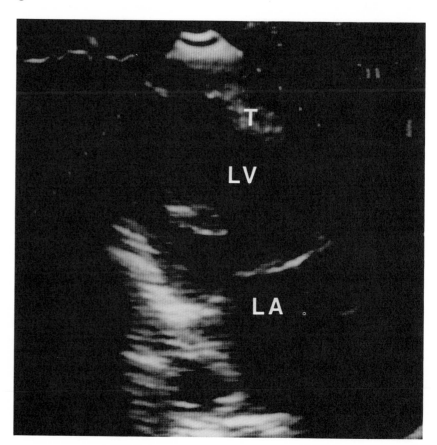

D

Figure 13.17 (cont'd.). (*C*)
Thrombus (T) adjacent to the myocardium with an echolucent area
separating it from the intracavitary
echoes. (*D*) Slightly different orientation showing the full length of
the T.

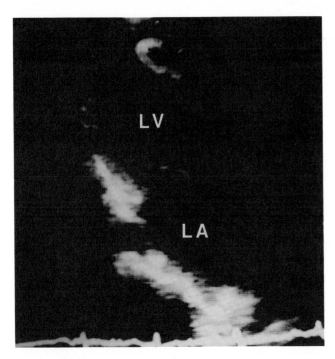

Figure 13.18. Apical long-axis view of the heart showing an echodense thrombus (T) with distinct margins near the LV apex.

or the presence of an associated aneurysm. A recent study of texture analysis of LV thrombi suggested that specific tissue characteristics may identify thrombi at high risk of embolization (104).

The effect of anticoagulant therapy on ventricular thrombi is variable: Most remain unchanged or resolve (89, 90, 98), while others may increase in size despite adequate anticoagulation (105). In some patients, thrombi resolve without anticoagulant therapy (Fig. 13.5) (106, 107). The utility of therapeutic anticoagulation lies in the prevention of systemic embolization. With few exceptions (98, 108), long-term studies have demonstrated significantly fewer embolic events in anticoagulated patients with echocardiographic evidence of mural thrombi than in those without anticoagulant therapy (82, 89, 90, 94, 109, 110).

The high incidence of LV thrombus formation in the first week following anterior infarction indicates that two-dimensional echocardiography should be obtained in all patients with acute transmural anterior wall myocardial infarctions. Initial examination should be performed on the third or fourth day following infarction and repeated 1 week later in negative studies. While anticoagulant therapy should be considered in all those with evidence of mural thrombus, attention should be focused on echocardiographic characteristics associated with particularly high risk of embolization. Patients with LV thrombi that protrude into the cavity, especially those that are freely mobile, warrant

therapeutic anticoagulation for 3 to 6 months. It is recommended that therapy can be discontinued thereafter, even if evidence of residual thrombus persists, since clot organization and endothelialization should have occurred by that time, making further fragmentation and embolization unlikely (111). This recommendation is supported by retrospective data demonstrating a very low incidence of systemic embolism in patients with chronic LV aneurysms (112). Since mural thrombus has been found to recur after discontinuation of anticoagulation (86), repeat echocardiograms are warranted in those patients whose thrombi shrink or resolve during therapy. Evidence of thrombus enlargement or recurrence on repeat examination warrants consideration of a protracted course of anticoagulation.

Echocardiographic findings have not proved as valuable for guiding anticoagulant therapy in patients with cardiomyopathies. A study of 123 men with dilated poorly contractile LVs on two-dimensional echocardiograms encountered mural thrombus in 36 percent (113), an incidence similar to that reported in autopsy series of cardiomyopathy patients (114, 115). The majority of thrombi were visualized in the apex of the LV. During the average 2-year follow-up, there was no difference in incidence of embolic events between those with and those without evidence of thrombus (13 percent and 10 percent, respectively). In addition, the likelihood of embolization in the former group did not differ when the thrombi were flat, pedunculated, or mobile (113).

Left Atrial Thrombi

Surgical and autopsy series of patients with mitral stenosis have encountered LA thrombi in 14 to 36 percent (116–119), with echocardiographic evidence being present in only 33 to 61 percent of those with documented thrombi (118, 119). In clinical studies of mitral stenosis patients, the echocardiographic diagnosis of LA thrombus is made in 5 to 14 percent (101, 118–120). Thrombi are most commonly encountered in association with an enlarged LA and atrial fibrillation (Fig. 13.21) (101, 120). During routine echocardiography, the presence of these conditions should prompt a careful examination of the LA for evidence of thrombus in two or more views.

Atrial thrombi appear echocardiographically as round or ovoid masses with clearly distinct borders, most often with a broad base of attachment to the atrial wall (Figs. 13.22 and 13.23). Although most are mobile homogenous echodensities, they may be small, flat and occasionally immobile masses that layer along the atrial wall, thus making identification difficult. Rarely, LA thrombi will appear as a free-floating ball

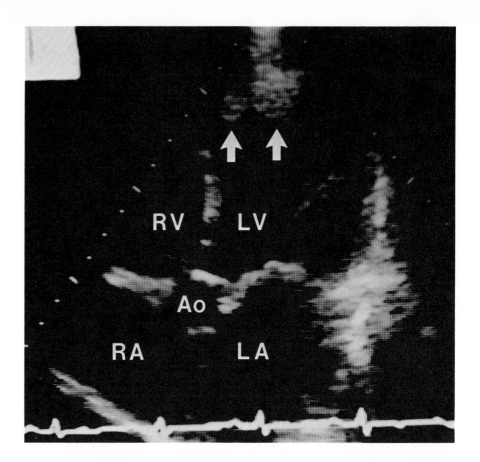

A

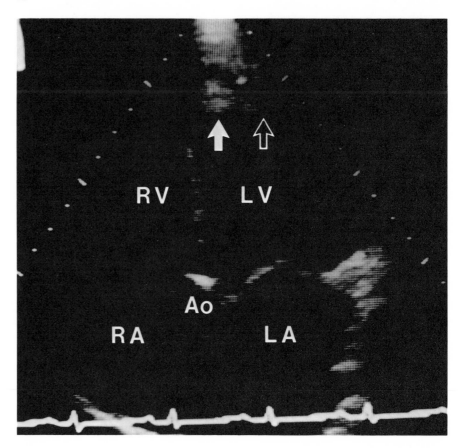

Figure 13.19. (*A*) Apical five-chamber view of the heart showing a bilobed apical thrombus (*solid arrows*) protruding into the cavity of the LV. (*B*) A slightly different projection showing an echolucent area within a portion of the thrombus (*open arrow*). Ao = aortic root.

B

422

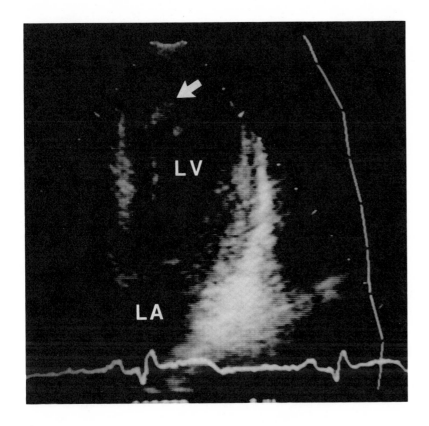

A

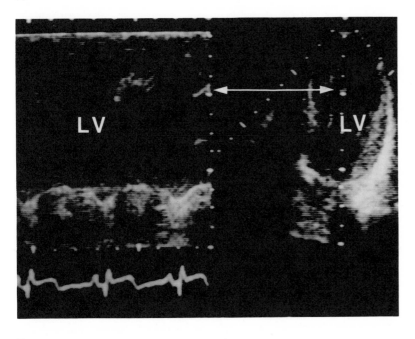

B

Figure 13.20. (*A*) Apical four-chamber view showing a mural thrombus (*arrow*) protruding into the LV. (*B*) The marked mobility of the mass is demonstrated by positioning an M-mode cursor through the end of the thrombus (*long arrow*).

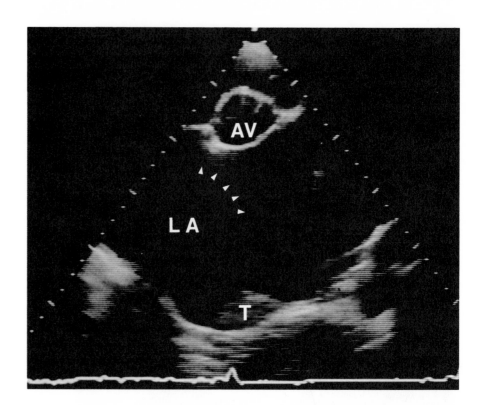

Figure 13.21. Parasternal cross-sectional view at the level of the AV showing a massively dilated LA with mural thrombus (T) along the posterior wall in a patient with a prosthetic mitral valve. Dynamic intracavitary echoes ("smoke") were faintly visualized (*triangles*).

(121–124). Thrombi diagnosed by echocardiography are usually attached to the posterior wall but may also be found on the septal, lateral, or upper atrial walls (31, 119). The vast majority that go unrecognized are in the LA appendage (118–120). In order to maximize visual- ization of thrombi, the LA should be examined in the standard parasternal, apical, and subcostal projections and in a modified short-axis parasternal view with angulation of the transducer to enhance imaging of the atrial appendage (125) (Fig. 13.24). The detection of

Figure 13.22. Apical four-chamber view showing a large thrombus (T) with a broad base of attachment along the LA wall in a patient with mitral stenosis, left atrial dilatation and atrial fibrillation.

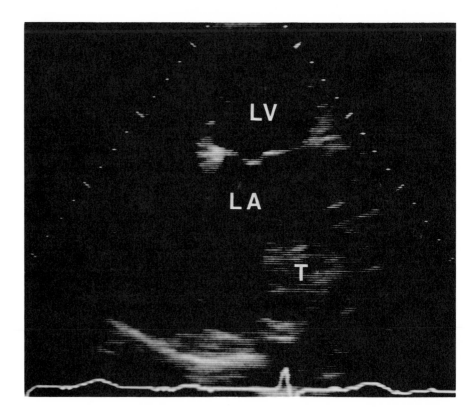

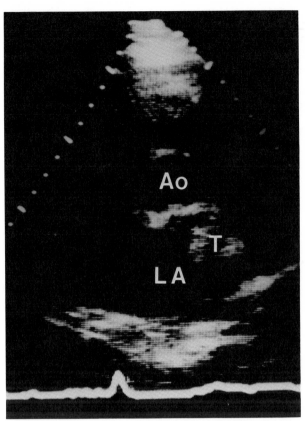

Figure 13.23. Cross-sectional image of the heart at the level of the proximal aorta (Ao) showing a thrombus (T) within the LA in a patient with mitral stenosis and atrial fibrillation.

LA appendage thrombi may further be enhanced by transesophageal two-dimensional echocardiography (126).

The frequency of thrombus involvement in the atrial appendage is likely related to its enclosed configuration, which predisposes to blood stasis in the presence of atrial fibrillation. The importance of blood stasis in atrial thrombus formation in rheumatic mitral valvular disease is supported by the demonstration of an inverse relationship between thrombus formation and the severity of accompanying mitral regurgitation (101). Even in the presence of atrial fibrillation and a "giant" LA, no patients with severe mitral regurgitation had evidence of LA thrombi, whereas the incidence was 50 percent in those without severe regurgitation.

Cardiac Source of Systemic Emboli

It is common for many neurologists to refer patients with transient ischemic events or completed strokes for echocardiography to "rule out cardiac source of embolus." This practice was encouraged by reports relating cerebral embolic events to various cardiac findings demonstrated by echocardiography such as mitral valve prolapse, mitral annular calcification, aortic sclerosis, hypertrophic cardiomyopathy, rheumatic heart disease, and atrial fibrillation (127–134). While a broad spectrum of cardiac disorders can be documented in patients sustaining acute cerebral events, the use of echocardiography in the routine screening of such patients cannot be supported. Several studies have shown that the likelihood of demonstrating a potential cardiac source of an embolic event is negligible in the absence of clinical evidence of heart disease (134–137). Therefore, echocardiographic examination of patients with evidence of cerebral ischemia should be limited to patients with historic, physical, or laboratory (i.e., electrocardiogram, chest x-ray) evidence of cardiovascular disease.

Right Heart Thrombi

Thrombi involving the RA or RV are rare findings that are usually unsuspected or may present clinically as outflow obstruction or pulmonary emboli. They may be formed primarily in the right heart or be secondary to thromboemboli. Primary thrombi are found in conditions associated with blood stasis due to low cardiac output states (e.g., cardiomyopathies, severe cor pulmonale, and occasionally myocardial infarctions) (18, 114, 138–141). They may also occur spontaneously, in association with intracardiac catheters, or following tissue injury (e.g., after transvenous catheter ablation of the AV node) (52, 138, 142, 143). Right heart thrombi are usually immobile and appear echocardiographically as heterogeneous, layered masses with distinct margins extending into the intracavitary space. Occasionally, they may calcify and appear as very bright echodensities (144). In the RA they may appear as a curvilinear band of echoes crossing the chamber (32). Thrombi involving the right heart are best demonstrated in RV/RA views from the apical, subcostal, and left parasternal windows. Imaging of RA thrombi may be enhanced by off-axis views from the parasternal cross section at the level of the aortic valve or by imaging from the RV apex by positioning the transducer a few centimeters medial to the usual apical window. In cardiac enlargement, examination from the right parasternal acoustic window may be required (145).

Secondary thrombi are the result of peripheral embolization with trapping of thromboemboli in the right heart. They are rare occurrences, with an autopsy incidence of 0.7 percent involving the RA and 0.4 percent involving the RV (146). In patients with deep venous thrombosis, the incidence may be as high as 9 percent (147). Enroute to the lungs, thromboemboli may become entrapped in the tricuspid valve apparatus (occasionally resulting in tricuspid regurgitation) or

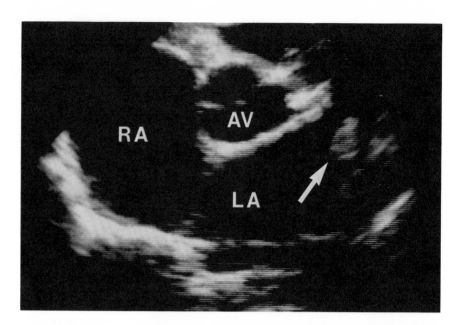

A

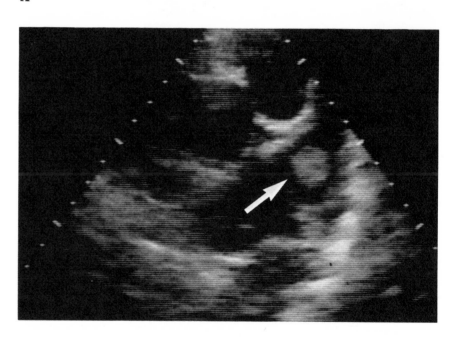

Figure 13.24. (*A*) Parasternal cross-sectional view at the level of the AV showing a thrombus in the LA appendage (*arrow*). (*B*) Modified short-axis view more clearly demonstrating the thrombus within the LA appendage.

B

more rarely at the eustachian valve or in the interatrial septum across a patent foramen ovale (138, 148–151). On two-dimensional echocardiography, they appear as irregular, curvilinear, often serpentine masses. They tend to be highly mobile and may float freely in the RA or RV with or without a demonstrable site of endocardial attachment or may prolapse across the tricuspid valve in diastole or into the RV outflow tract in systole (Fig. 13.25) (138, 145, 150, 152–154). The chaotic pattern of motion seen in mobile thrombi has been sug-

gested as a differentiating feature from other RA masses such as myxomas (148). When RA thrombi are thin, they may be difficult to differentiate from normal structures such as eustachian valve remnants and the Chiari network.

Echocardiography has documented partial or total dissolution of thrombi during anticoagulant or thrombolytic therapy (148, 149, 155), but the latter has also been implicated in the promotion of pulmonary emboli (149, 156). Because freely mobile thrombi have been

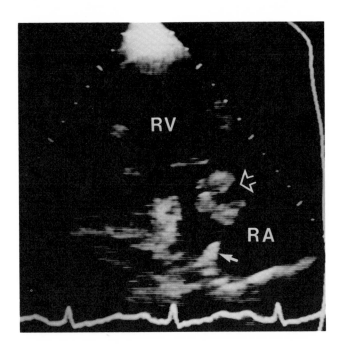

A

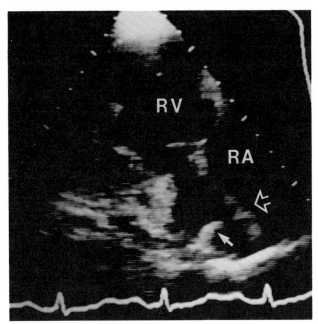

B

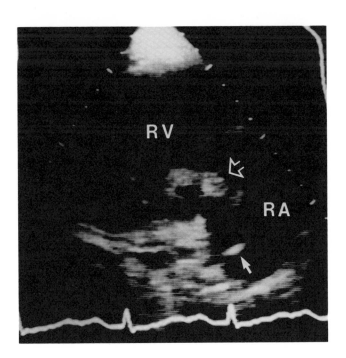

C

Figure 13.25. Highly mobile, deformable RA thromboembolus (*open arrow*) in a patient with metastatic carcinoma of the lung. (*A*) A ball-like appearance of the thrombus within the dilated RA. (*B*) An uncoiled, more linear appearance of the thrombus extending from the eustachian valve to the tricuspid valve. (*C*) Extension of the thrombus through the tricuspid valve, into the RV. Solid arrows point to transvenous pacing catheter.

associated with massive pulmonary emboli and death (Fig. 13.26) (145, 148–150, 152, 157), surgical embolectomy should be strongly considered when such masses are encountered (32, 152, 155, 158). Anticoagulant therapy is appropriate for patients with laminar thrombi, with surgical intervention reserved for those in whom medical therapy is unsuccessful or contraindicated. Since pulmonary emboli have also been associated with catheter-related thrombi (159–161), prophylactic anticoagulation has been suggested in patients with permanent catheters and conditions associated with low cardiac output such as congestive heart failure (154).

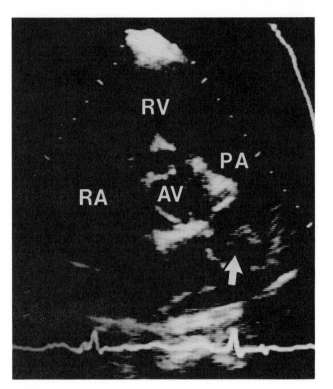

A

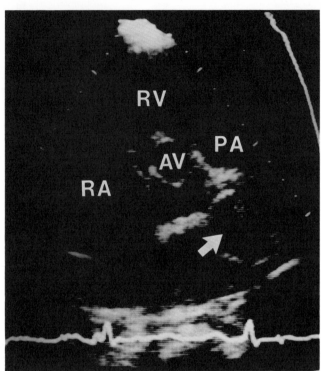

B

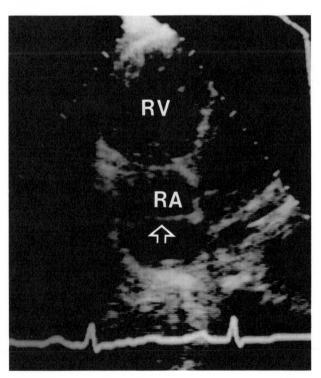

C

Figure 13.26.   Same patient as in Figure 13.25, 1 week later, during a sudden episode of severe dyspnea. Cross-sectional views at the level of the aortic valve (AV) in systole (*A*) and in diastole (*B*), showing a mobile thromboembolus (*arrow*) in the proximal right pulmonary artery (PA). The RA appears free of thrombus. (*C*) A dense band of organized thrombus (*open arrow*) is observed within the RA in the apical view. The mobile RA thrombus in Figure 13.25 was most likely wound around this structure.

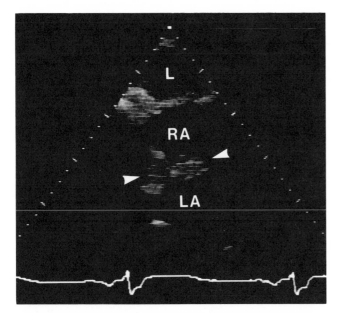

Figure 13.27. Subcostal view showing lipomatous hypertrophy of the intra-atrial septum. The lack of adipose tissue in the region of the foramen ovale results in the bilobed appearance of the mass (*arrowheads*). L = liver.

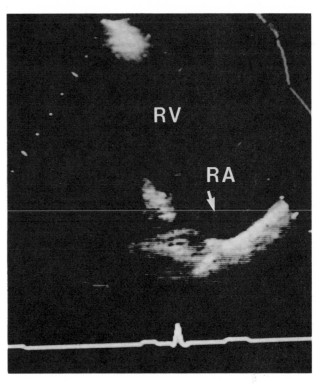

Figure 13.28. Right ventricular inflow view showing a eustachian valve (*arrow*) within the RA.

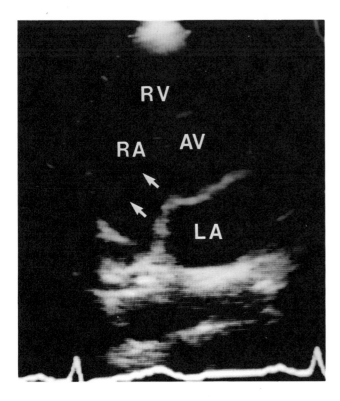

A

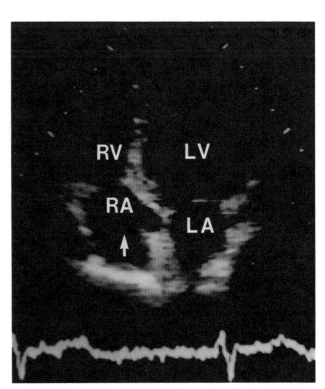

B

Figure 13.29. (*A*) Cross-sectional view at the level of the aortic valve (AV) showing a Chiari network (*arrows*) extending across the RA. (*B*) Apical four-chamber view showing a Chiari network attached to the walls of the RA.

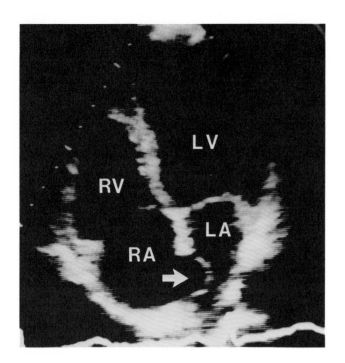
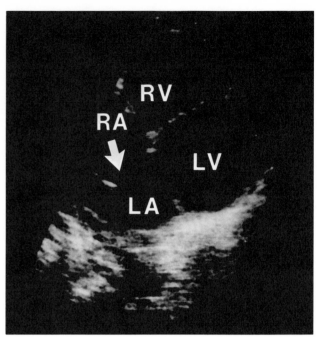

A   B

Figure 13.30. (*A*) Apical and (*B*) subcostal four-chamber views of hearts showing an atrial septal aneurysm (*arrow*) bulging from the RA into the LA.

MISCELLANEOUS MASSES

A number of congenital and acquired conditions may be manifest as anomalous masses on two-dimensional echocardiograms. These generally represent incidental findings whose significance lies in possible confusion with clinically important intracardiac masses. Recognition of the echocardiographic characteristics of these conditions, therefore, is important to prevent the incorrect diagnosis of intracardiac tumors or thrombi.

The most clinically significant of these anomalies is lipomatous hypertrophy of the atrial septum, an excessive accumulation of adipose tissue in the interatrial septum that generally spares the region of the foramen ovale. As a consequence, when imaged from the subcostal view, it has a bilobed or dumbbell-shaped appearance with globular thickening posterosuperior and anteroinferior to the membrane of the oval fossa (Fig. 13.27) (162). In one echocardiographic series, the atrial thickness ranged from 1.5 to 3 cm (162), but tumors as large as 7 or 8 cm have been documented in autopsy series (11). These generally occur in elderly patients and have been associated with obesity. While often an incidental finding, this abnormality is frequently associated with atrial arrhythmias and abnormal P-wave morphology on electrocardiogram and has on occasion been associated with sudden death (11, 162–164).

Congenital remnants of the sinus venosus may appear as echodensities within the RA. These include the Chiari network and the eustachian valve. The eustachian valve is a not uncommon echocardiographic finding, which is easily recognized due to its location at the junction of the inferior vena cava and the RA. It appears as an echodense rim of tissue within the RA, which is best visualized in the parasternal RV inflow view (Figs. 13.25 and 13.28). The Chiari network is a thin, fenestrated, weblike membrane that appears as a highly reflective, freely mobile, filamentous echodensity within the RA (Fig. 13.29). Its clinical relevance lies in its relative frequency and its potential for confusion with tricuspid valve abnormalities (e.g., flail leaflets or vegetations, RA thromboemboli, or possibly pedunculated tumors). This congenital remnant has an autopsy incidence in 2 to 3 percent and has been encountered in 1 to 1.5 percent in large echocardiographic series (165, 166). The membrane generally originates at the junction of the RA and inferior vena cava, extends across the chamber toward the tricuspid ring, and inserts into the interatrial septum or RA wall. Depending on its course, it may be imaged best in the parasternal short-axis view at the aortic valve level, the RV inflow view, the apical or subcostal four-chamber view, or the subcostal inferior vena cava–RA view.

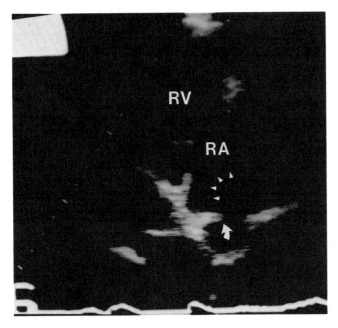

A

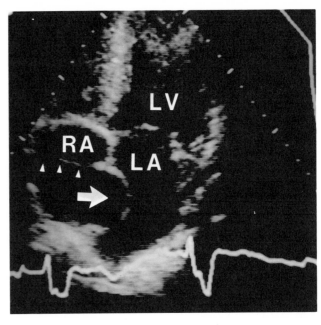

B

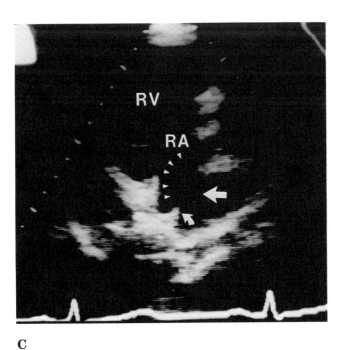

C

Figure 13.31. Multiple congenital anomalies involving the RA. (*A*) Right ventricular inflow view showing a Chiari network (*arrowheads*) and a prominent eustachian valve (curved arrow). (*B*) Apical four-chamber view showing a Chiari network and an atrial septal aneurysm (*straight arrow*). (*C*) Right ventricular inflow view showing a Chiari network, a eustachian valve, and an atrial septal aneurysm.

Aneurysms of the interatrial septum are outpouchings in the region of the oval fossa that may be confused with atrial masses. At autopsy, the incidence is 1 percent, and it has been detected in 0.2 percent to 0.6 percent of routine echocardiograms (167–170). While isolated reports have associated this anomaly with various cardiac pathologies, larger series suggest

that atrial septal aneurysms in adults represent incidental findings without associated symptoms (170–173). Rarely, this condition has been associated with a midsystolic click and, when large in size, may be a potential cause of embolic phenomena or ventricular inflow obstruction (169, 171, 174). When the aneurysm involves the entire atrial septum, there appears to be a

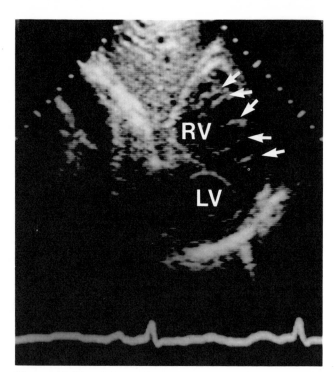

Figure 13.32. Subcostal cross section at the level of the LV showing multiple echodense bands within a dilated RV in a patient with recurrent pulmonary emboli. At autopsy, these were shown to be bands of organized thrombus.

high frequency of complex congenital cardiac anomalies (167).

Echocardiographically, atrial septal aneurysms appear as thin curvilinear echodensities localized to the midportion of the interatrial septum. They bulge into the RA (most often) or LA, often undulating between the two, with the motion fluctuating with the cardiac cycle and less frequently with respiration (168, 175). They are best imaged in the subcostal or apical four-chamber views and can frequently be seen in the parasternal basal cross section (Fig. 13.30). The characteristic location and motion pattern enable differentiation of an atrial septal aneurysm from a tumor mass, mobile thrombus, prominent eustachian valve, or Chiari network. Atrial size and Doppler echocardiographic findings are useful in excluding the presence of an atrial septal defect and can help prevent confusion with atrial septal enlargement and bulging secondary to AV valvular regurgitation (167, 176–178). When difficult to identify, imaging may be facilitated by use of echocardiographic contrast techniques (172). Occasionally, these congenital anomalies may be seen in combination (Fig. 13.31).

Hypertrophied ventricular trabeculations and aberrant fibrous bands are generally incidental echocardiographic findings. Their importance lies in possible confusion with or masking of more significant intra-

ventricular echodensities (e.g., mural thrombi) (Fig. 13.32). They may also be misinterpreted as part of the adjacent wall, resulting in the spurious diagnosis of asymmetric hypertrophy. In hearts removed during transplantation, thickened trabeculae were encountered in 43 percent of LVs and 28 percent of RVs (179). Two-dimensional echocardiograms were able to identify them with a sensitivity and specificity of 80 percent and 85 percent in the LV, and 60 percent and 72 percent in the RV. Hypertrophic trabeculations appeared as endocardial prominences in the parasternal short-axis or apical views. These are best differentiated from intracavitary thrombi by demonstrating normal wall motion adjacent to the echodensity, movement of the structure in a constant pattern with the cardiac cycle and finding echo-free areas on each side of the echodensity (179). Multiple standard and off-axis imaging planes may be required to separate these from mural thrombus or from adjacent myocardium.

Aberrant fibrous bands or "heart strings" (false tendons, ectopic chordae) are benign, more frequently left-sided structures that extend between papillary muscles, from papillary muscles to ventricular walls, or between two endocardial surfaces (Fig. 13.33). In unselected or healthy adults, echocardiographic evidence of false tendons are encountered in 0.5 to 6.4 percent (180–183). However, an incidence of 37 percent has been documented in severely diseased hearts (179). One reason for this difference may be that marked ventricular dilatation as in aneurysm formation may stretch muscular trabeculations into false tendons (Fig. 13.34) (183). Though occasional associations have been reported with premature ventricular contractions (182, 184), aberrant bands are generally believed to represent incidental findings of no clinical significance.

Catheters passing into or through the right heart are common causes of intracavitary echodensities that are easily recognized by their characteristic location and appearance. Swan-Ganz catheters are typically encountered passing through the RV from the parasternal window. They appear as linear echodensities that move with the cardiac cycle (Fig. 13.35). Transvenous pacing catheters are much brighter echodensities that are usually best visualized in the apical or subcostal four-chamber views (Fig. 13.36). Other tomographic views are often useful in demonstrating aberrant positioning or dislodgment of a pacemaker or catheter. Two-dimensional echocardiography can also be used to guide catheter placement, as in pericardiocentesis, or to demonstrate complications of invasive procedures, as may occur with pacemakers, left or right heart catheterization, or pericardiocentesis (Fig. 13.37) (185). Other foreign bodies such as needles, nails, and bullets have been successfully identified or localized using two-dimensional echocardiography (18, 186, 187).

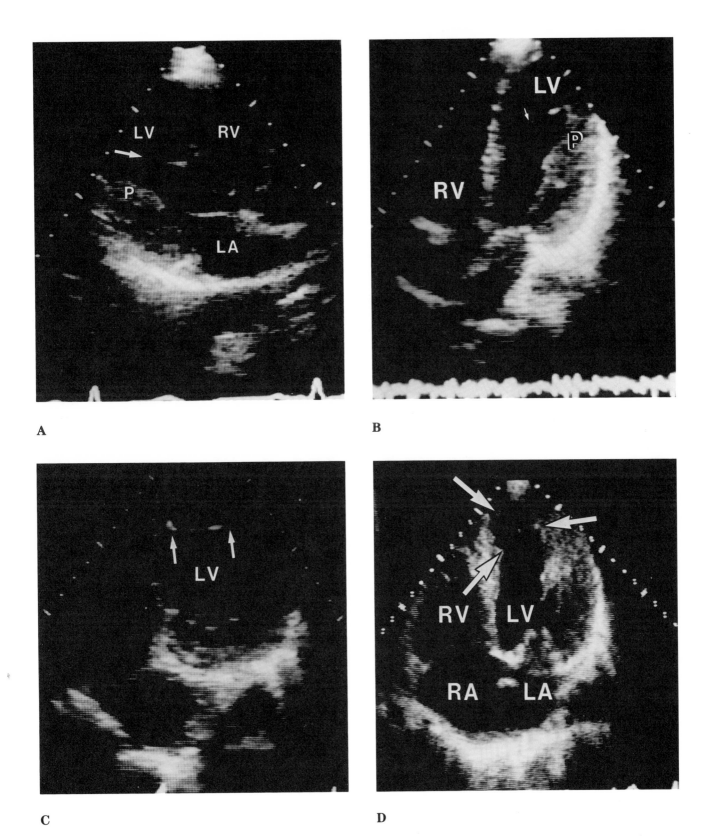

A

B

C

D

Figure 13.33.   (*A*) Parasternal view of the LV showing an aberrant fibrous band (*arrow*) inserting into the ventricular septum. (*B*) Apical four-chamber view showing an ectopic chorda extending from the base of a papillary muscle (P) to the septum. (*C*) Apical view of the ventricles showing a false tendon extending between two endocardial surfaces (*arrows*). (*D*) Apical four-chamber view showing a network of three false tendons meeting in the apex of the LV.

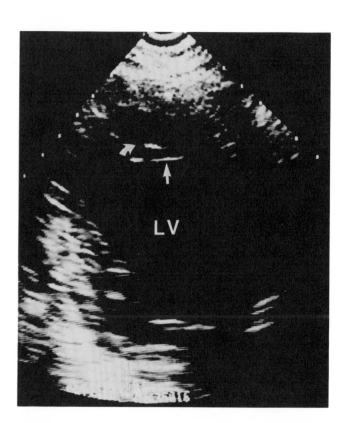

A   B

Figure 13.34.   (*A*) Apical view of the LV showing a muscular trabeculation (*curved arrow*) stretching across an area of aneurysmal dilatation. A second, more faint linear echodensity (*straight arrow*) is seen proximal to the first. (*B*) In a slightly different projection, these appear as two fibrous bands near the apex of the LV.

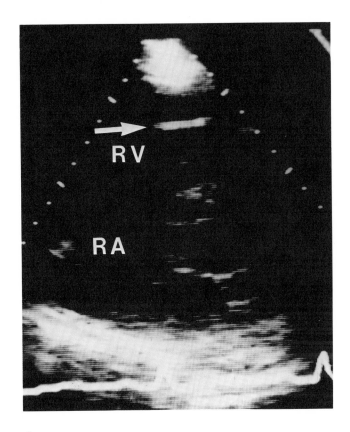

A

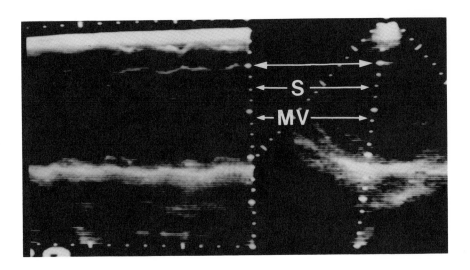

B

Figure 13.35. (*A*) Parasternal
cross section showing a Swan-Ganz
catheter (*arrow*) traversing the RV.
(*B*) Parasternal long-axis view of
the heart showing an M-mode cursor through the catheter, which lies
in the RV outflow tract. The
M-mode tracing shows the motion
of the catheter (*long arrow*) during
the cardiac cycle. MV = mitral
valve; S = interventricular septum.

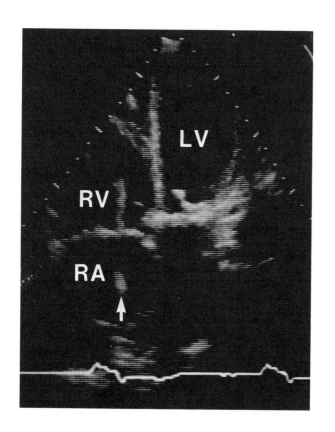

A

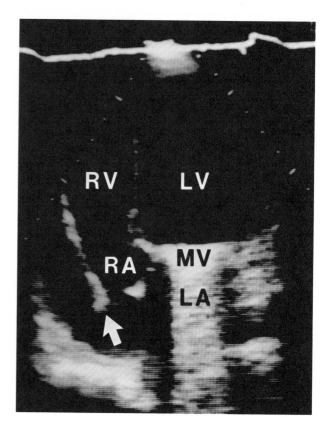

B

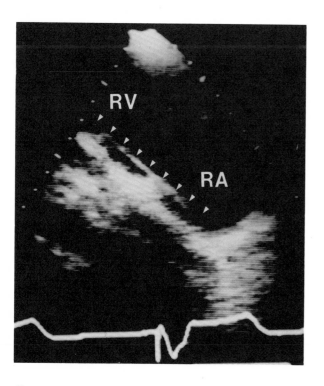

C

Figure 13.36. (*A,B*) Apical four-chamber views of patients with pacing catheters (*arrows*) extending from RA into RV. (*C*) Right ventricular inflow view showing a pacing catheter lying along the wall of the RA and RV (*arrowheads*). MV = prosthetic mitral valve.

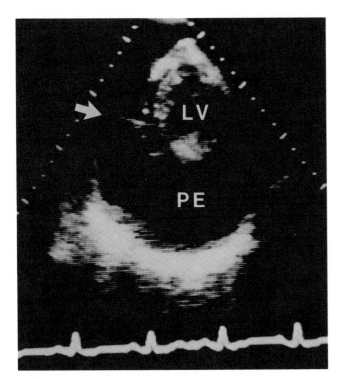

Figure 13.37. Parasternal cross section at the level of the LV showing a large pericardial effusion (PE) and a pericardiocentesis needle (*arrow*) impinging on the epicardium of the heart.

REFERENCES

1. Prichard RW. Tumors of the heart. Review of the subject and report of one hundred and fifty cases. Arch Pathol 1951;51:98–128.
2. Fyke FE, Seward JB, Edwards WD, et al. Primary cardiac tumors: experience with 30 consecutive patients since the introduction of two-dimensional echocardiography. J Am Coll Cardiol 1985;5:1465–73.
3. Donahoo JS, Weiss JL, Gardner TJ, Fortuin NJ, Brawley RK. Current management of atrial myxoma with emphasis on a new diagnostic technique. Ann Surg 1979;189:763–7.
4. Dunnigan A, Oldham HN, Serwer GA, Benson DW. Left atrial myxoma: is cardiac catheterization essential?. Am J Dis Child 1981;135:420–1.
5. St John Sutton MG, Mercier LA, Giuliani ER, Lie JT. Atrial myxomas: a review of clinical experience in 40 patients. Mayo Clin Proc 1980;55:371–6.
6. Larrieu AJ, Jamieson WRE, Tyers GF, et al. Primary cardiac tumors: experience with 25 cases. J Thorac Cardiovasc Surg 1982;83:339–46.
7. Silverman NA. Primary cardiac tumors. Ann Surg 1980;191:127–38.
8. Sicart M, Roudaut R, d'Agata P, et al. The contribution of bidimensional echocardiography in the diagnosis of cardiac tumours, based on 25 observed cases. Eur J Radiol 1981;1:241–4.
9. Straus R, Merliss R. Primary tumors of the heart. Arch Pathol 1945;39:74–8.
10. Heath D. Pathology of cardiac tumors. Am J Cardiol 1968;21:315–27.
11. McAllister HA, Fenoglio JJ. Tumors of the cardiovascular system. In: Armed Forces Institute of Pathology, ed. Atlas of Tumor Pathology. Washington, DC: 1978. Facs. 15. 2nd series.
12. Bloor CM, O'Rourke RA. Cardiac tumors: clinical presentations and pathologic correlations. Curr Probl Cardiol 1984;9:1–48.
13. Goodwin JF. The spectrum of cardiac tumors. Am J Cardiol 1968;21:307–14.
14. Salcedo EE, Adams KV, Lever HM, Gill CC, Lombardo H. Echocardiographic findings in 25 patients with left atrial myxoma. J Am Coll Cardiol 1983;1:1162–6.
15. Bulkley BH, Hutchins GM. Atrial myxomas: a fifty year review. Am Heart J 1979;97:639–43.
16. Griffiths GC. A review of primary tumors of the heart. Prog Cardiovasc Dis 1965;7:465–79.
17. Nasser WK, Davis RH, Dillon JC, et al. Atrial myxoma: clinical and pathologic features in nine cases. Am Heart J 1972;83:694–704.
18. Felner JM, Knopf WD. Echocardiographic recognition of intracardiac and extracardiac masses. Echocardiography 1985;2:3–55.
19. Meller J, Teichholz LE, Pichard AD, Matta R, Herman MV. Left ventricular myxoma: echocardiographic diagnosis and review of the literature. Am J Med 1977;63:816–23.
20. Dashkoff N, Boersma RB, Nanda NC, Gramiak R, Andersen MN, Subramanian S. Bilateral atrial myxomas: echocardiographic considerations. Am J Med 1978;65:361–6.
21. Tway KP, Shah AA, Rahimtoola SH. Multiple biatrial myxomas demonstrated by two-dimensional echocardiography. Am J Med 1981;71:896–9.
22. Kronzon I, Rosenzweig B, Dack S. Diagnosis of a large left atrial myxoma: the role of two-dimensional echocardiography. J Clin Ultrasound 1982;10:39–41.
23. Perry LS, King JF, Zeft HJ, Manley JC, Gross CM, Wann LS. Two-dimensional echocardiography in the diagnosis of left atrial myxoma. Br Heart J 1981;45:667–71.
24. Allan LD, Joseph MC, Tynan M. Clinical value of echocardiographic colour image processing in two cases of primary cardiac tumour. Br Heart J 1983;49:154–6.
25. Bhandari AK, Nanda NC, Hicks DG. Two-dimensional echocardiography of intracardiac masses: echo pattern–histopathology correlation. Ultrasound Med Biol 1982;8:673–80.
26. Thier W, Schluter M, Krebber HJ, et al. Cysts in left atrial myxomas identified by transesophageal cross-sectional echocardiography. Am J Cardiol 1983;51:1793–5.
27. Bryhn M, Gustafson A, Stubbe I. Two-dimensional echocardiography in the diagnosis of hemorrhages in a left atrial myxoma. Acta Med Scand 1982;212:433–5.
28. Rahilly GT, Nanda NC. Two-dimensional echocardiographic identification of tumor hemorrhages in atrial myxomas. Am Heart J 1981;101:237–9.
29. Sharma S, Munsi SC, Bhattacharya SB. Value of echo-lucent areas detected by real-time two-dimensional echocardiography in differentiation of intracardiac mass lesions. J Cardiovasc Ultrasonography 1982;1:59–63.
30. Reeder GS, Tajik AJ, Seward JB. Left ventricular mural thrombus: two-dimensional echocardiographic diagnosis. Mayo Clin Proc 1981;56:82–6.
31. DePace NL, Soulen RL, Kotler MN, Mintz GS. Two-dimensional echocardiographic detection of intraatrial masses. Am J Cardiol 1981;48:954–60.
32. Panidis IP, Kotler MN, Mintz GS, Ross J. Clinical and echocardiographic features of right atrial masses. Am Heart J 1984;107:745–58.
33. Liu HY, Panidis I, Soffer J, Dreifus LS. Echocardiographic diagnosis of intracardiac myxomas. Chest 1983;84:62–7.
34. Thijssen JM. Ultrasonic characterization: prospects of tumour diagnosis. Eur J Radiol 1984;4:312–7.
35. Green SE, Joynt LF, Fitzgerald PJ, Rubenson DS, Popp RL. In vivo ultrasonic tissue characterization of human intracardiac masses. Am J Cardiol 1983;51:231–6.
36. Sanoudos G, Reed GE. Primary cardiac sarcoma. J Thorac Cardiovasc Surg 1972;63:482–6.
37. Glancy DL, Morales JB, Roberts WC. Angiosarcoma of the heart. Am J Cardiol 1968;21:413–9.
38. Panella JS, Paige ML, Victor TA, Semerdjian RA, Hueter DC. Angiosarcoma of the heart, diagnosis by echocardiography. Chest 1979;76:221–3.
39. Colucci WS, Braunwald E. Primary tumors of the heart. In:

Braunwald E, ed. Heart disease—a textbook of cardiovascular medicine. Philadelphia: WB Saunders, 1988:1476.

40. Fine G. Neoplasms of the pericardium and heart. In: Gould SE, ed. Pathology of the heart and blood vessels. Springfield, Ill.: Charles C Thomas, 1968:851.
41. Nadas AS, Ellison RC. Cardiac tumors in infancy. Am J Cardiol 1968;21:363–6.
42. Fenoglio JJ, McAllister HA, Ferrans VJ. Cardiac rhabdomyoma: a clinicopathologic and electron microscopic study. Am J Cardiol 1976;38:241–51.
43. Gasul BM, Arcilla RA, Lev M. Heart disease in children. Philadelphia: JB Lippincott, 1966:1086.
44. Bigelow NH, Klinger S, Wright AW. Primary tumors of the heart in infancy and early childhood. Cancer 1954;7:549–63.
45. Birnbaum SE, McGahan JP, Janos GG, Myers M. Fetal tachycardia and intramyocardial tumors. J Am Coll Cardiol 1985;6:1358–61.
46. Bini RM, Westaby S, Bargeron LM, Pacifico AD, Kirklin JW. Investigation and management of primary cardiac tumors in infants and children. J Am Coll Cardiol 1983;2:351–7.
47. Marx GR, Bierman FZ, Matthews E, Williams R. Two-dimensional echocardiographic diagnosis of intracardiac masses in infancy. J Am Coll Cardiol 1984;3:827–32.
48. Duncan WJ, Rowe RD, Freedom RM, Izukawa T, Olley PM. Space-occupying lesions of the myocardium: role of two-dimensional echocardiography in detection of cardiac tumors in children. Am Heart J 1982;104:780–5.
49. Arciniegas E, Hakimi M, Farooki ZQ, Truccone JN, Green EW. Primary cardiac tumors in children. J Thorac Cardiovasc Surg 1980;79:582–91.
50. Fowler RS, Keith JD. Cardiac tumors. In: Keith JD, Rowe RD, Vlad P, eds. Heart disease in infancy and childhood. New York: Macmillan, 1978:1040–5.
51. Schmaltz AA, Apitz J. Primary heart tumors in infancy and childhood—report of four cases and review of literature. Cardiology 1981;67:12–22.
52. Riggs T, Paul MH, DeLeon S, Ilbawi M. Two-dimensional echocardiography in evaluation of right atrial masses: five cases in pediatric patients. Am J Cardiol 1981;48:961–6.
53. Grenadier E, Lima CO, Barron JV, et al. Two-dimensional echocardiography for evaluation of metastatic cardiac tumors in pediatric patients. Am Heart J 1984;107:122–6.
54. DeLoach JF, Haynes JW. Secondary tumors of heart and pericardium; review of the subject and report of one hundred thirty-seven cases. Arch Intern Med 1953;91:224–49.
55. Goudie R. Secondary tumours of the heart and pericardium. Br Heart J 1955;17:183–8.
56. Rosenthal DS, Braunwald E. Hematological-oncological disorders and heart disease. In: Braunwald E, ed. Heart disease, a textbook of cardiovascular medicine. Philadelphia: WB Saunders, 1988:1744–69.
57. Applefeld MM, Pollock SH. Cardiac disease in patients who have malignancies. Curr Probl Cardiol 1980;4:1–37.
58. Glancy DL, Roberts WC. The heart in malignant melanoma: a study of 70 autopsy cases. Am J Cardiol 1968;21:555–71.
59. Roberts WC, Glancy DL, DeVita VT Jr. Heart in malignant lymphoma (Hodgkin's disease, lymphosarcoma, reticulum cell sarcoma and mycosis fungoides): a study of 196 autopsy cases. Am J Cardiol 1968;22:85–107.
60. Hanfling SM. Metastatic cancer to the heart: review of the literature and report of 127 cases. Circulation 1960;22:474–83.
61. Kutalek SP, Panidis IP, Kotler MN, Mintz GS, Carver J, Ross JJ. Metastatic tumors of the heart detected by two-dimensional echocardiography. Am Heart J 1985;109:343–9.
62. Friedman TD, Kotler MN, Victor MF, Mintz GS. Two-dimensional echocardiographic detection of pericardial and pleural metastases. J Cardiovasc Ultrasonography 1982;1:205–9.
63. Johnson MH, Soulen RL. Echocardiography of cardiac metastases. Am J Radiol 1983;141:677–81.
64. Goodwin JF. The spectrum of cardiac tumors. Am J Cardiol 1968;21:307–14.
65. Mikell FL, Asinger RW, Elsperger KJ, Anderson WR, Hodges M. Regional stasis of blood in the dysfunctional left ventricle:

echocardiographic detection and differentiation from early thrombosis. Circulation 1982;66:755–63.
66. Sigel B, Coelho JCU, Spigos DG, et al. Ultrasonography of blood during stasis and coagulation. Invest Radiol 1981;16:71–6.
67. Garcia-Fernandez MA, Moreno M, Banuelos F. Two-dimensional echocardiographic identification of blood stasis in the left atrium. Am Heart J 1985;109:600–1.
68. Vandenbossche J, Van Kuyk M, Englert M. Echocardiographic detection of blood stasis pattern in the left atrium. J Cardiovasc Ultrasonography 1983;2:341–2.
69. Meltzer RS, Klig V, Visser CA, Teichholz LE. Spontaneous echocardiographic contrast in the inferior vena cava. Am Heart J 1985;110:826–30.
70. Wolverson MK, Nouri S, Joist JH, Sundaram M, Heiberg E. The direct visualization of blood flow by real time ultrasound: clinical observations and underlying mechanisms. Radiology 1981;140:443–8.
71. Sigel B, Machi J, Beitler JC, Justin JR, Coelho JC. Variable ultrasound echogenicity in flowing blood. Science 1982;218:1321–3.
72. Machi J, Sigel B, Beitler JC, Coelho JCU, Justine JR. Relation of in-vivo blood flow to ultrasound echogenicity. J Clin Ultrasound 1983;11:3–10.
73. Shung KK. Physics of blood echogenicity. J Cardiovasc Ultrasonography 1983;2:401–6.
74. Iliceto S, Antonelli G, Sorino M, Biasco G, Rizzon P. Dynamic intracavitary left atrial echoes in mitral stenosis. Am J Cardiol 1985;55:603–6.
75. Asinger RW, Mikell FL, Sharma B, Hodges M. Observations on detecting left ventricular thrombus with two dimensional echocardiography: emphasis on avoidance of false positive diagnoses. Am J Cardiol 1981;47:145–56.
76. Nixon JV. Left ventricular mural thrombus. Arch Intern Med 1983;143:1567–71.
77. Parkinson J, Bedford DE. Cardiac infarction and coronary thrombosis. Lancet 1928;1:4–11.
78. Jordan RA, Miller RD, Edwards JE, Parker RL. Thromboembolism in acute and in healed myocardial infarction: intracardiac mural thrombosis. Circulation 1952;6:1–6.
79. Bean WB. Infarction of the heart: III. Clinical course and morphological findings. Ann Intern Med 1938;12:71–94.
80. Garvin CF. Mural thrombi in the heart. Am Heart J 1941;21:713–20.
81. Visser CA, Kan G, David GK, Lie KI, Durrer D. Two dimensional echocardiography in the diagnosis of left ventricular thrombus: a prospective study of 67 patients with anatomic validation. Chest 1983;83:228–32.
82. Takamoto T, Kim D, Urie PM, et al. Comparative recognition of left ventricular thrombi by echocardiography and cineangiography. Br Heart J 1985;53:36–42.
83. Reeder GS, Lengyel M, Tajik AJ, Seward JB, Smith HC, Danielson GK. Mural thrombus in left ventricular aneurysm: incidence, role of angiography, and relation between anticoagulation and embolization. Mayo Clin Proc 1981;56:77–81.
84. Ports TA, Cogan J, Schiller NB, Rappaport E. Echocardiography of left ventricular masses. Circulation 1978;58:528–36.
85. Mikell FL, Asinger RW, Elsperger KJ, Anderson WR, Hodges M. Tissue acoustic properties of fresh left ventricular thrombi and visualization by two dimensional echocardiography: experimental observations. Am J Cardiol 1982;49:1157–65.
86. Visser CA, Kan G, Meltzer RS, Lie KI, Durrer D. Long-term follow-up of left ventricular thrombus after acute myocardial infarction: a two-dimensional echocardiographic study in 96 patients. Chest 1984;86:532–6.
87. Stratton JR, Lighty GW, Pearlman AS, Ritchie JL. Detection of left ventricular thrombus by two-dimensional echocardiography: sensitivity, specificity and causes of uncertainty. Circulation 1982;66:156–66.
88. DeMaria AN, Bommer W, Neumann A, et al. Left ventricular thrombi identified by cross-sectional echocardiography. Ann Intern Med 1979;90:14–8.
89. Weinreich DJ, Burke JF, Pauletto FJ. Left ventricular mural

thrombi complicating acute myocardial infarction. Ann Intern Med 1984;100:789–94.

90. Keating EC, Gross SA, Schlamowitz RA, et al. Mural thrombi in myocardial infarctions: prospective evaluation by two-dimensional echocardiography. Am J Med 1983;74:989–95.

91. Asinger RW, Mikell FL, Elsperger J, Hodges M. Incidence of left ventricular thrombosis after acute transmural myocardial infarction. N Engl J Med 1981;305:297–302.

92. Frandsen EH, Egeblad H, Mortensen SA. Transience of left ventricular thrombosis. Br Heart J 1983;49:193–4.

93. Visser C, Roelandt J. Left ventricular thrombus. Echocardiography 1985;2:245–55.

94. VA Cooperative Clinical Study Group: Anticoagulants in acute myocardial infarction. JAMA 1973;225:724–9.

95. Miller RD, Jordan RA, Parker RI, Edwards JE. Thromboembolism in acute and in healed myocardial infarction. II. Systemic and pulmonary arterial occlusion. Circulation 1952;6:7–15.

96. Hellerstein HK, Martin JW. Incidence of thromboembolic lesions accompanying myocardial infarction. Am Heart J 1947;33:443–52.

97. Dubnow MH, Burchell HB, Titus JL. Postinfarction ventricular aneurysm: clinicopathologic and electrocardiographic study of 80 cases. Am Heart J 1965;70:753–60.

98. Visser CA, Kan G, Meltzer RS, et al., Embolic potential of left ventricular thrombus after myocardial infarction: a two-dimensional echocardiographic study of 119 patients. J Am Coll Cardiol 1985;5:1276–80.

99. Haugland JM, Asinger RW, Mikell FL, Elsperger J, Hodges M. Embolic potential of left ventricular thrombi detected by two-dimensional echocardiography. Circulation 1984;70:588–98.

100. Kinney EL. The significance of left ventricular thrombi in patients with coronary heart disease: a retrospective analysis of pooled data. Am Heart J 1985;109:191–4.

101. Beppu S, Park Y, Sakakibara H, Nagata S, Nimura Y. Clinical features of intracardiac thrombosis based on echocardiographic observation. Jpn Circul J 1984;48:75–82.

102. Meltzer RS, Visser CA, Kan G, Roelandt J. Two-dimensional echocardiographic appearance of left ventricular thrombi with systemic emboli after myocardial infarction. Am J Cardiol 1984;53:1511–3.

103. Stratton JR, Resnick AD. Increased embolic risk in patients with left ventricular thrombi. Circulation 1987;75:1004–11.

104. Lloret RL, Cortada X, Bradford J, Metz MN, Kinney EL. Classification of left ventricular thrombi by their history of systemic embolization using pattern recognition of two-dimensional echocardiograms. Am Heart J 1985;110:761–5.

105. Arvan S. Persistent intracardiac thrombi and systemic embolization despite anticoagulant therapy. Am Heart J 1985;109:178–81.

106. Spirito P, Bellotti P, Chiarella F, Domenicucci S, Sementa A, Vecchio C. Prognostic significance and natural history of left ventricular thrombi in patients with acute anterior myocardial infarction: a two-dimensional echocardiographic study. Circulation 1985;72:774–80.

107. Arvan S. Left ventricular mural thrombi secondary to acute myocardial infarction: predisposing factors and embolic phenomenon. J Clin Ultrasound 1983;11:467–73.

108. Simpson MT, Oberman A, Kouchoukos NT, Rogers WJ. Prevalence of mural thrombi and systemic embolization with left ventricular aneurysm: effect of anticoagulation therapy. Chest 1980;77:463–9.

109. Chalmers TC, Matta RJ, Smith H, Kunzler A-M. Evidence favoring the use of anticoagulants in the hospital phase of acute myocardial infarction. N Engl J Med 1977;297:1091–6.

110. Arnott WM, Biggs R, Gilchrist AR, Hunter RB, Pickering G, Reid DD, Wright JH, Douglas AS. Assessment of short-term anticoagulant administration after cardiac infarction: report of the working party on anticoagulant therapy in coronary thrombosis to the medical research council. Br Med J 1969;1:335–42.

111. Arvan S. Mural thrombi in coronary artery disease: recent advances in pathogenesis, diagnosis, and approaches to treatment. Arch Intern Med 1984;144:113–6.

112. Lapeyre AC, Steele PM, Kazmier FJ, Chesebro JH, Vlietstra RE, Fuster V. Systemic embolism in chronic left ventricular aneurysm: incidence and the role of anticoagulation. J Am Coll Cardiol 1985;6:534–8.

113. Gottdiener JS, Gay JA, VanVoorhees L, DiBianco R, Fletcher RD. Frequency and embolic potential of left ventricular thrombus in dilated cardiomyopathy: assessment by 2-dimensional echocardiography. Am J Cardiol 1983;52:1281–5.

114. Roberts WC, Ferrans VJ. Pathologic anatomy of the cardiomyopathies: idiopathic dilated and hypertrophic types, infiltrative types and endomyocardial disease with and without eosinophilia. Hum Pathol 1975;6:287–342.

115. Fowler NO, Gueron M, Rowlands DT. Primary myocardial disease. Circulation 1961;13:498–508.

116. Nichols HT, Blanco G, Morse DP, Adam A, Baltazar N. Open mitral commissurotomy: experience with 200 consecutive cases. JAMA 1962;182:268–70.

117. Wallach JB, Lukash L, Angrist AA. An interpretation of the incidence of mural thrombi in the left auricle and appendage with particular reference to mitral commissurotomy. Am Heart J 1953;45:252–4.

118. Shrestha NK, Moreno FL, Narciso FV, Torres L, Calleja HB. Two-dimensional echocardiographic diagnosis of left atrial thrombus in rheumatic heart disease: a clinicopathologic study. Circulation 1983;67:341–7.

119. Schweizer P, Bardos P, Erbel R, et al. Detection of left atrial thrombi by echocardiography. Br Heart J 1981;45:148–56.

120. Masuda Y, Morooka N, Yoshida H, Watanabe S, Inagaki Y. Noninvasive diagnosis of thrombus in the heart and large vessels: usefulness of two-dimensional echocardiography and X-ray CT. Jpn Circul J 1984;48:83–9.

121. Warda M, Garcia J, Pechacek LW, Massumkhani A, Hall RJ. Auscultatory and echocardiographic features of mobile left atrial thrombus. J Am Coll Cardiol 1985;5:379–82.

122. Tabak SW, Maurer G. Echocardiographic detection of free-floating left atrial thrombus. Am J Cardiol 1984;53:374–5.

123. Gottdiener JS, Temeck BK, Patterson RH, Fletcher RD. Transient ("hole-in-one") occlusion of the mitral valve orifice by a free-floating left atrial ball thrombus: identification by two-dimensional echocardiography. Am J Cardiol 1984;53:1730.

124. Sunagawa K, Orita Y, Tanaka S, Kituchi Y, Nakamura M, Hirata T. Left atrial ball thrombus diagnosed by two-dimensional echocardiography. Am Heart J 1980;100:89–94.

125. Herzog CA, Bass D, Kane M, Asinger R. Two-dimensional echocardiographic imaging of left atrial appendage thrombi. J Am Coll Cardiol 1984;3:1340–4.

126. Aschenberg W, Schluter M, Kremer P, Schroder E, Siglow V, Bleifeld W. Transesophageal two-dimensional echocardiography for the detection of left atrial appendage thrombus. J Am Coll Cardiol 1986;7:163–6.

127. Barnett HJM, Jones MW, Boughner DR, Kostuk WJ. Cerebral ischemic events associated with prolapsing mitral valve. Arch Neurol 1976; 33:777–82.

128. Barnett HJM, Boughner DR, Taylor PW, Cooper PE, Kostuk WJ, Nichol PM. Further evidence relating mitral valve prolapse to cerebral ischemic events. N Engl J Med 1980;302:139–44.

129. DeBono DP, Warlow CP. Mitral-annulus calcification and cerebral or retinal ischaemia. Lancet 1979;2:383–5.

130. Ridolfi RL, Hutchins GM. Spontaneous calcific emboli from calcific mitral annulus fibrosus. Arch Pathol Lab Med 1976;100:117–20.

131. Nishide M, Irino T, Gotoh M, Naka M, Tsjui K. Cardiac abnormalities in ischemic cerebrovascular disease studied by two-dimensional echocardiography. Stroke 1983;14:541–5.

132. Wolf PA, Dawber TR, Colton T, Thomas E. Epidemiologic assessment of atrial fibrillation as a risk factor for stroke: the Framingham study. Neurology (Minneap) 1976;26:359.

133. Hinton RC, Kistler JP, Fallon JT, Friedlich AL, Fisher CM. Influence of etiology of atrial fibrillation on incidence of systemic embolism. Am J Cardiol 1977;40:509–13.

134. Bergeron GA, Shah PM. Echocardiography in patients with acute cerebral events. Clin Cardiol 1982;5:637–9.

135. Come PC, Riley MF, Bivas NK. Roles of echocardiography and arrhythmia monitoring in the evaluation of patients with suspected systemic embolism. Ann Neurol 1983;13:527–31.

136. Greenland P, Knopman DS, Mikell FL. Asinger RW, Anderson DC, Good DC. Echocardiography in diagnostic assessment of stroke. Ann Intern Med 1981;95:51–3.

137. Donaldson RM, Emanuel RW, Earl CJ. The role of two-dimensional echocardiography in the detection of potentially embolic intracardiac masses in patients with cerebral ischaemia. J Neurol Neurosurg Psychiatry 1981;44:803–9.

138. Felner JM, Churchwell AL, Murphy DA. Right atrial thromboemboli: clinical, echocardiographic and pathophysiologic manifestations. J Am Coll Cardiol 1984;4:1041–5.

139. Manno BV, Panidis IP, Kotler MN, Mintz GS, Ross J. Two-dimensional echocardiographic detection of right atrial thrombi. Am J Cardiol 1983;51:615–6.

140. Stowers SA, Leiboff RH, Wasserman AG, Katz RJ, Bren GB, Hsu I. Right ventricular thrombus formation in association with acute myocardial infarction: diagnosis by 2-dimensional echocardiography. Am J Cardiol 1983;52:912–3.

141. Come PC. Transient right atrial thrombus during acute myocardial infarction: diagnosis by echocardiography. Am J Cardiol 1983;51:1228–9.

142. Schuster AH, Zugibe F Jr, Nanda NC, Murphy GW. Two-dimensional echocardiographic identification of pacing catheter-induced thrombosis. Pace 1982;5:124–8.

143. Kunze KP, Schluter M, Costard A, Nienaber CA, Kuck KH. Right atrial thrombus formation after transvenous catheter ablation of the atrioventricular node. J Am Coll Cardiol 1985;6:1428–30.

144. Patel AK, Kroncke GM, Heltne CE, Kosolcharoen PK, Thomsen JH. Multiple calcified thrombi (rocks) in the right ventricle. J Am Coll Cardiol 1983;2:1224–7.

145. Rosenzweig MS, Nanda NC. Two-dimensional echocardiographic detection of circulating right atrial thrombi. Am Heart J 1982;103:435–6.

146. Wartmann WB, Hellerstein HK. The incidence of heart disease in 2000 consecutive autopsies. Ann Intern Med 1948;28:41–65.

147. Havig O. Deep vein thrombosis and pulmonary embolism. Acta Chir Scand 1977;Suppl 478:1–120.

148. Saner HE, Asinger RW, Daniel JA, Elsperger KJ. Two-dimensional echocardiographic detection of right sided cardiac intracavitary thromboembolus with pulmonary embolism. J Am Coll Cardiol 1984;4:1294–301.

149. Starkey IR, deBono DP. Echocardiographic identification of right-sided cardiac intracavitary thromboembolus in massive pulmonary embolism. Circulation 1982;66:1322–5.

150. Panidis IP, Manno BV, Kotler MN, Mintz GS. Right atrial thromboembolus: echocardiographic detection in patient with fatal pulmonary embolism. J Cardiovasc Ultrasonography 1983;2:337–9.

151. Nellessen U, Daniel WG, Matheis G, Oelert H, Depping K, Lichtlen PR. Impending paradoxical embolism from atrial thrombus: correct diagnosis by transesophageal echocardiography and prevention by surgery. J Am Coll Cardiol 1985;5:1002–4.

152. Redish GA, Anderson AL. Echocardiographic diagnosis of right atrial thromboembolism. J Am Coll Cardiol 1983;1:1167–9.

153. Kachel RG. Prolapsing right atrial thrombus and deep venous thrombosis despite systemic coagulopathy. Am Heart J 1985;109:595–6.

154. Woolridge JD, Healey J. Echocardiographic diagnosis of right ventricular thromboembolism. Am Heart J 1983;106:590–1.

155. Cameron J, Pohlner PG, Stafford EG, O'Brien MF, Bett JHN, Murphy AL. Right heart thrombus: recognition, diagnosis and management. J Am Coll Cardiol 1985;5:1239–43.

156. Goldsmith JC, Lollar P, Hoak JC. Massive fatal pulmonary emboli with fibrinolytic therapy. Circulation 1982;64:1068–9.

157. Goldberg SM, Pizzarello RA, Goldman MA, Padmanabhan VT. Echocardiographic diagnosis of right atrial thromboembolism resulting in massive pulmonary embolization. Am Heart J 1984;108:1371–2.

158. Kinney EL, Zitrin R, Kohler KR, Cortada X, Varzaly LJ. Sudden appearance of a right atrial thrombus on two-dimensional echocardiogram: significance and therapeutic implications. Am Heart J 1985;110:879–81.

159. Schmaltz AA, Huenges R, Heil RP. Thrombosis and embolism complicating ventriculoatrial shunt for hydrocephalus: echocardiographic findings. Br Heart J 1980;43:241–3.

160. Prozan GB, Shipley RE, Madding GF, Kennedy PA. Pulmonary thromboembolism in the presence of an endocardial pacing catheter. JAMA 1968;206:1564–5.

161. Kinney EL, Allen RP, Weidner WA, Pierce WS, Leaman DM, Zeli RF. Recurrent pulmonary emboli secondary to right atrial thrombus around a permanent pacing catheter: a case report and review of the literature. Pace 1979;2:196–202.

162. Fyke FE, Tajik AJ, Edwards WD, Seward JB. Diagnosis of lipomatous hypertrophy of the atrial septum by two-dimensional echocardiography. J Am Coll Cardiol 1983;1:1352–7.

163. Isner JM, Swan CS, Mikus JP, Carter BL. Lipomatous hypertrophy of the interatrial septum: in vivo diagnosis. Circulation 1982;66:470–3.

164. Hutter AM, Page DL. Atrial arrhythmias and lipomatous hypertrophy of the cardiac interatrial septum. Am Heart J 1971;82:16–21.

165. Werner JA, Cheitlin MD, Gross BW, Speck SM, Ivey TD. Echocardiographic appearance of the Chiari network: differentiation from right-heart pathology. Circulation 1981;63:1104–9.

166. Cloez JL, Neimann JL, Chivoret G, et al. Echographic rediscovery of an anatomical structure: the Chiari network: apropos of 16 cases. Arch Mal Coeur 1983;76:1284–92.

167. Hanley PC, Tajik AJ, Hynes JK, et al. Diagnosis and classification of atrial septal aneurysm by two-dimensional echocardiography: report of 80 consecutive cases. J Am Coll Cardiol 1985;6:1370–82.

168. Longhini C, Brunazzi MC, Musacci G, et al. Atrial septal aneurysm: echopolycardiographic study. Am J Cardiol 1985;56:653–6.

169. Gallet B, Malergue MC, Adams C, et al. Atrial septal aneurysm—a potential cause of systemic embolism: an echocardiographic study. Br Heart J 1985;53:292–7.

170. Silver MD, Dorsey JS. Aneurysms of the septum primum in adults. Arch Pathol Lab Med 1978;102:62–5.

171. Wysham DG, McPherson DD, Kerber RE. Asymptomatic aneurysm of the interatrial septum. J Am Coll Cardiol 1984;4:1311–4.

172. Hauser AM, Timmis GC, Stewart JR, et al. Aneurysm of the atrial septum as diagnosed by echocardiography: analysis of 11 patients. Am J Cardiol 1984;53:1401–2.

173. Iliceto S, Papa A, Sorino M, Rizzon P. Combined atrial septal aneurysm and mitral valve prolapse: detection by two-dimensional echocardiography. Am J Cardiol 1984;54:1151–3.

174. Alexander MD, Bloom KR, Hart P, D'Silva F, Murgo JP. Atrial septal aneurysm: a cause for midsystolic click. Circulation 1981;63:1186–8.

175. Gondi B, Nanda NC. Two-dimensional echocardiographic features of atrial septal aneurysms. Circulation 1981;63:452–7.

176. Lin CS, Chen HY, Jan YI. The interatrial septal echocardiogram: relationship to left atrial volume change in the normal and diseased heart. Am Heart J 1984;107:519–25.

177. Percy RF, Conetta DA, Geiser EA, Bass TA, Conti CR, Miller AB. Correlation of paradoxical atrial septal motion and an interatrial pressure gradient in severe tricuspid regurgitation. Am J Cardiol 1985;55:1431–3.

178. Tei C, Tanaka H, Kashima T, Yoshimura H, Minagoe S, Kanehisa T. Real-time cross-sectional echocardiographic evaluation of the interatrial septum by right atrium–interatrial septum–left atrium direction of ultrasound beam. Circulation 1979;60:539–46.

179. Keren A, Billingham ME, Popp RL. Echocardiographic recognition and implications of ventricular hypertrophic trabeculations and aberrant bands. Circulation 1984;70:836–42.

180. Nishimura T, Kondo M, Umadome H, Shimono Y. Echocardiographic features of false tendons in the left ventricle. Am J Cardiol 1981;48:177–83.

181. Vered Z, Meltzer RS, Benjamin P, Motro M, Neufeld HN. Prevalence and significance of false tendons in the left ventricle as determined by echocardiography. Am J Cardiol 1984;53:330–2.

182. Suwa M, Hirota Y, Nagao H, Kino M, Kawamura K. Incidence of

the coexistence of left ventricular false tendons and premature ventricular contractions in apparently healthy subjects. Circulation 1984;70:793–8.

183. Friart A, Vandenbossche JL, Hamdan BA, Deuvaert F, Englert M. Association of false tendons with left ventricular aneurysm. Am J Cardiol 1985;55:1425–6.

184. Perry LW, Ruckman RN, Shapiro SR, Kuehl KS, Galioto FM, Scott LP. Left ventricular false tendons in children: prevalence as detected by 2-dimensional echocardiography and clinical significance. Am J Cardiol 1983;52:1264–6.

185. Iliceto S, Antonelli G, Sorino M, Calabrese P, Biasco G, Rizzon P. Two-dimensional echocardiographic recognition of complications of cardiac invasive procedures. Am J Cardiol 1984;53:846–8.

186. Hsiung MC, Chen CC, Wei J, et al. Two-dimensional echocardiographic demonstration of multiple needles in the heart. Am J Cardiol 1985;55:1245.

187. Sakai K, Hoshino S, Osawa M. Needle in the heart: two-dimensional echocardiographic findings. Am J Cardiol 1984;53:1482.

14
Extracardiac Vascular Abnormalities

Morris Kotler
Wayne Parry
Anthony Goldman

The aorta is recognized by M-mode echocardiography as two parallel echoes that move anteriorly with systole and posteriorly with diastole. The amplitude of motion of the anterior wall can be slightly greater than that of the posterior wall. Therefore, aortic root measurements are obtained in diastole. Generally, the aortic root is measured from the anterior edge of the anterior wall echo (leading edge) to the anterior edge of the posterior wall echo (leading edge). The echocardiographic measurements of the aortic root diameter correlate well with the angiographic measurements (1, 2). The normal aortic root dimension by M-mode echocardiography is 2.0 to 3.7 centimeters with a mean of 2.7 cm (3). The "ice-pick" view of the ascending aorta obtained by M-mode echocardiography limits its usefulness in assessing the aortic arch and descending aorta. Two-dimensional echocardiography allows the entire aorta to be evaluated from a variety of views and image planes (Table 14.1; Figs. 14.1 and 14.2). The ascending thoracic aorta and descending thoracic aorta (DTA) can be identified from the left parasternal long- (Fig. 14.3) and short-axis views (4). The aortic root can be measured at various levels in the parasternal long-axis views (5). Thus, the proximal aorta can be measured at the level of the aortic annulus, aortic sinuses, sinotubular junction, and proximal ascending aorta (Fig. 14.4). Therefore, considerable variation in the aortic root diameter can be obtained, depending on how the independent M-mode ultrasonic beam traverses the aortic root. The variation in aortic root diameters obtained by two-dimensional echocardiography may help explain why Doppler cardiac output determinations are dependent upon precise measurements obtained in a standardized fashion (6). Using the second right intercostal space, long- and short-axis views of the ascending thoracic aorta can be accomplished (Fig. 14.5). In order to evaluate the aortic arch, the suprasternal notch view is employed (Fig. 14.6A), and the curve of the aortic arch, the descending aorta, and the brachiocephalic vessels can be visualized. By rotating the transducer 90 degrees, a short-axis view of the aorta is obtained (Fig. 14.6B); the superior vena cava confluence of the right and left innominate veins and the right pulmonary artery are visualized. The subcostal long- and short-axis views can be useful in evaluating the distal DTA and abdominal aorta (Fig. 14.7). However, in order to visualize the entire DTA, a modified apical approach must be used (7, 8). The transducer is placed in the proximity of the apex of the left ventricle (LV), and the plane of the sector is primarily directed perpendicular to the sternum to image the short axis of the DTA. The sector plane is then rotated 90 degrees clockwise and directed medially to visualize the lower part of the DTA in a longitudinal fashion (Fig. 14.8). Identifying the DTA in the parasternal position is important to avoid confusing it with a dilated coronary sinus or pericardial effusion. In the parasternal long-axis view, the DTA is visualized as a circular, echo-free space behind the junction of the LV and left atrium (LA). To demonstrate that this structure is indeed the DTA and not a dilated coronary sinus, the transducer beam is rotated 90 degrees so that the long axis of the aorta and the entire descending aorta are visualized; the latter can be

Table 14.1. Echocardiographic Views in Aortic Aneurysms

1. Left parasternal long- and short-axis views of the proximal ascending aorta and DTA
2. Right parasternal long- and short-axis views of the ascending thoracic aorta
3. Suprasternal notch view of the aortic arch
4. Apical view of the DTA
5. Subcostal long- and short-axis views of the distal DTA and abdominal aorta
6. On- and off-axis views

followed superiorly until it curves and forms the aortic arch.

The DTA in the parasternal long- and short-axis views is a useful landmark in differentiating pericardial and pleural effusions (Fig. 14.9) (9). With pericardial effusions, the effusion separates the descending aorta from the posterior cardiac structures, whereas with pleural effusions, there is no separation between the descending aorta and posterior LV wall.

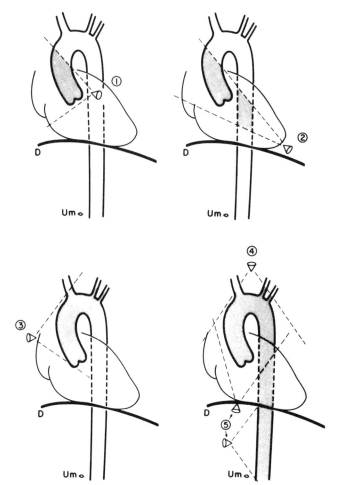

Figure 14.2. Various aortic segments imaged from transducer positions shown in Figure 14.1. 1 = precordial; 2 = apical; 3 = right parasternal including infraclavicular; 4 = suprasternal and supraclavicular; 5 = subcostal and abdominal; D = diaphragm; Um = umbilicus. (Reproduced by permission from Mathew T, Nanda NC. Two-dimensional and Doppler echocardiographic evaluation of aortic aneurysms and dissection. Am J Cardiol 1984;54:379–85.)

DILATATION OF THE AORTA AND ANEURYSMS

A dilated ascending aorta can be recognized by M-mode echocardiography, especially when the M-mode beam is directed superiorly and cephalad to visualize the aorta above the aortic leaflets (Fig. 14.10). In this patient, the aortic root measured 5.5 cm, whereas at the level of the aortic leaflets the aortic root diameter measured 3.7 cm. In patients with true aneurysms, paradoxic or posterior expansion of the posterior aortic wall during systole has been reported (3).

DeMaria and coworkers (10) were able to identify the type and localization of aneurysms of the ascending aorta by two-dimensional echocardiography. Thus, true saccular aneurysms (Fig. 14.11) can be differentiated from fusiform and dissecting aneurysms.

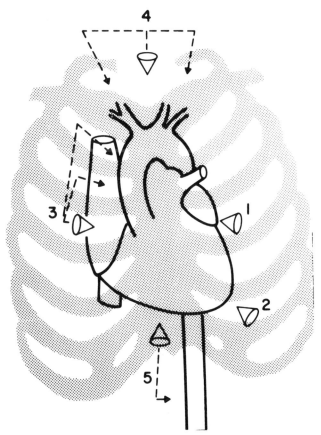

Figure 14.1. Various transducer positions used to examine the aorta. 1 = precordial; 2 = apical; 3 = right parasternal including infraclavicular; 4 = suprasternal and supraclavicular; 5 = subcostal and abdominal. (Reproduced by permission from Mathew T, Nanda NC. Two-dimensional and Doppler echocardiographic evaluation of aortic aneurysms and dissection. Am J Cardiol 1984;54:379–85.)

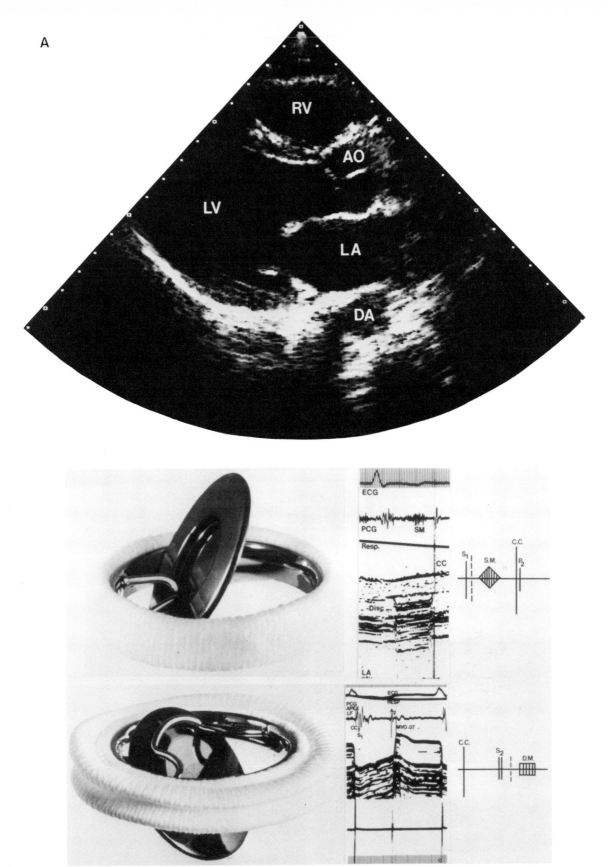

Figure 14.3. (*A*) Two-dimensional echocardiogram obtained from the parasternal long-axis view in a normal subject. (*B*) Two-dimensional echocardiogram obtained from the parasternal long-axis view in a patient with a dilated aorta (Ao). The descending aorta (Desc. Ao.) is enlarged and is seen as a circular structure at the artioventricular junction. The LA is compressed. AML = anterior mitral leaflet; AO = aortic root; DA = descending aorta; IVS = interventricular septum; LPW = left ventricular posterior wall; PML = posterior mitral leaflet.

NORMAL ADULT CROSS-SECTIONAL ECHOCARDIOGRAPHIC VALUES

Parasternal Long Axis View	N	Mean ± SD*	Range
Aorta (end-diastole): *Figure 1*			
1. Aortic annulus	68	1.9 ± 0.2	1.4–2.6
2. Sinus of Valsalva	68	2.8 ± 0.3	2.1–3.5
3. Sinotubular junction	64	2.4 ± 0.4	1.7–3.4
4. Ascending aorta	44	2.6 ± 0.3	2.1–3.4

Values are expressed in cm except where otherwise specified

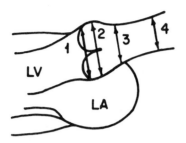

Figure 14.4. Normal adult cross-sectional echocardiographic values for the aorta obtained at four imaging planes. (Reproduced by permission from Triulzi M, Gilliam LD, Gentile F, Newell JB, Weyman AE. Normal adult cross-sectional echocardiographic values: linear dimensions and chamber areas. Echocardiography 1984;1:403–26.)

The ability to visualize an intimal flap by two-dimensional echocardiography in patients with dissecting aneurysms is based on several criteria (Table 14.2) (11, 12). The criteria are as follows: 1) The intimal flap should be seen in more than one view; 2) the intimal flap should have defined motion that is not parallel to the motion of any other cardiac structures such as the walls of the aorta or aortic valves: 3) the echogenic recorded intimal flap should not be confused by an extension or reverberation from any other cardiac structure: and 4) a reproducible echogenic interface should separate the true and false lumens. To increase the sensitivity and specificity of two-dimensional echocardiography in the diagnosis of aortic dissection, optimal visualization of the entire aorta is required, and multiple on- and off-axis views should be obtained. The

M-mode criteria for aortic root dissection are outlined in Table 14.2. A variety of conditions potentially give rise to false-positive diagnoses: calcific aortic valvular disease with a thickened or calcified aortic root, a catheter in the right ventricular (RV) outflow tract or pulmonary artery, and fluid in the transverse pericardial sinus (13, 14). Other disorders that may mimic aortic root dissection by M-mode echocardiography include intramural aortic abscess or abscess within the ventricular septum and a dilated aortic sinus (15, 16).

Although several investigators have described the M-mode echocardiographic findings in aortic root and ascending aortic dissecting aneurysms, the technique is limited by the inability to visualize the entire aorta and the high incidence of false-positive and false-negative studies (17–19). The intimal flap may mimic the motion

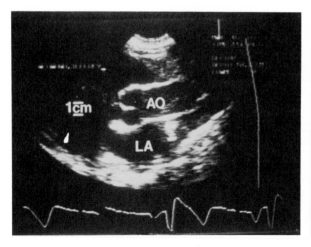 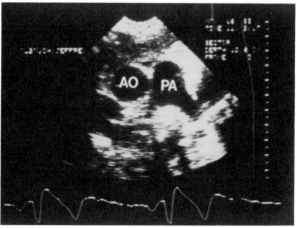

A **B**

Figure 14.5. (*A*) The ascending aorta is visualized from the second right intercostal space. A long-axis view where a long segment of the ascending aorta (AO) can be visualized. (*B*) The AO and pulmonary artery (PA) in cross section. The PA bifurcation can be seen in the high second right intercostal short-axis view.

and appearance of cardiac structures such as the aortic valve (19). In some patients, the intimal flap can be recognized by M-mode echocardiography (Fig. 14.12). In this patient, the midsystolic click was thought to be due to mitral valve prolapse but was actually a result of deceleration of blood flow occurring as a result of abrupt posterior motion of the intimal flap (20). To minimize the potential for false-positive diagnoses, M-mode echocardiography should be used to complement two-dimensional echocardiography in differentiating reverberation artifact from an intimal flap.

Type I dissecting aneurysms can be clearly visualized by a combination of on- and off-axis views, using the parasternal long-axis and the second right intercostal short- and long-axis views of the ascending thoracic aorta (Fig. 14.13) (21). In addition, type III dissecting aneurysms can be approached by using the modified apical approach, or the suprasternal view of aortic arch but angulating inferiorly and in a caudal direction. Extensive involvement of the ascending thoracic aorta and DTA by dissecting aneurysm can be recognized with both M-mode and two-dimensional echocardiography (Fig. 14.14). Complications of dissecting aneurysms can be detected by echo and Doppler echocardiography (Table 14.3). These complications include rupture into the right atrium (RA), which has been recognized by two-dimensional echocardiography (22). In addition, a to-and-fro motion of the intimal flap prolapsing into the LV during diastole has been reported (23, 24). During systole, the flap was thrust back into the aorta. In our original study using two-dimensional echocardiographic techniques for detecting aortic dissection, the sensitivity was 91 percent and the specificity was 94 percent (11). However, with greater experience and additional patients, the sensitivity and specificity have decreased. There are several reasons for these decreases: 1) the inability to perform complete studies of the entire thoracic and abdominal aorta in some patients, 2) the suboptimal studies frequently obtained in critically ill patients who are in intensive care unit settings and frequently on ventilators, and 3) the high number of false-positive echocardiographic studies that can occur as a result of an extension of a reverberation from other cardiac structures (Fig. 14.15). Listed in Table 14.4 are some of the causes of false-positive echocardiographic criteria for dissection. Atherosclerotic plaques attached to the aortic wall can also simulate an intimal flap (15, 25).

In a study of 13 patients with ascending aortic dissecting aneurysms, two-dimensional echocardiography yielded a sensitivity of 100 percent, a specificity of 88 percent, and overall diagnostic accuracy of 91 percent (26). However, its role in diagnosing distal aortic dissection was limited. In that particular study, the diagnosis of aortic dissection by two-dimensional echocardiography was made if any two of the following criteria were met: 1) aortic root dimension of at least 42 millimeters, 2) detection of an intraluminal structure within the proximal aorta consistent with an intimal flap that appeared to define a false channel (26), and 3) the presence of high-frequency oscillations of the intimal flap (27, 28). The inability to detect distal aortic dissecting aneurysms in that study may have been technical, since apical, parasternal, and subcostal views were not routinely employed. In the same study, the detection of pericardial fluid by two-dimensional echocardiography was associated with a poor prognosis (75% of patients dying) compared to an insignificant mortality in those without pericardial effusions (26).

Additionally, two-dimensional echocardiography provided useful information such as new wall motion abnormalities and valvular disease in a group of patients with chest pain and true negative studies for dissecting aneurysms.

McLeod and coworkers (29) reported on two-dimensional echocardiographic findings in 21 patients with confirmed ascending aortic aneurysms with a specificity of 93 percent and overall predictive accuracy of 90 percent. They relied heavily on two diagnostic criteria, namely, an aortic root enlargement of at least 42 mm and reduplication of wall echoes. An oscillating flap was visualized in only three patients. McLeod et al. also had disappointing results with DTA aneurysm, probably because a systematic method for visualizing the DTA was not utilized.

Conflicting findings have been reported when comparing the value of two-dimensional echocardiography and computed tomography in the diagnosis of aortic dissection. In Come's series (8), the results obtained by two-dimensional echocardiography and computed tomography were similar, whereas in other series, discrepancies were noted (14). In one patient, two-dimensional echocardiography failed to reveal an intramural thrombus noted on computed tomography; in two other patients with type I aortic dissecting aneurysms, the intimal flap was successfully imaged by two-dimensional echocardiography, whereas computed tomography failed to demonstrate the flap in either patient.

In 1986 we reported that magnetic resonance imaging is extremely useful in visualizing the entire DTA and seems to be reliable in detecting distal dissections (30). For the ascending aorta, two-dimensional echocardiography seems to be superior to non-gated magnetic resonance imaging in detecting the intimal flap and predicting complications such as acute aortic regurgitation and pericardial effusions.

Dynamic intracavitary echoes have been recorded in the aortic arch in type III aortic dissection (31). The intracavitary echoes continuously changed shape and motion and were smokelike in appearance. The pres-

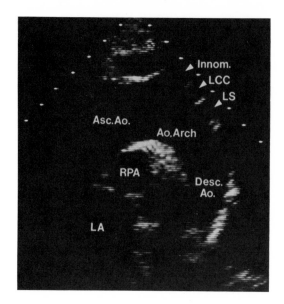

A

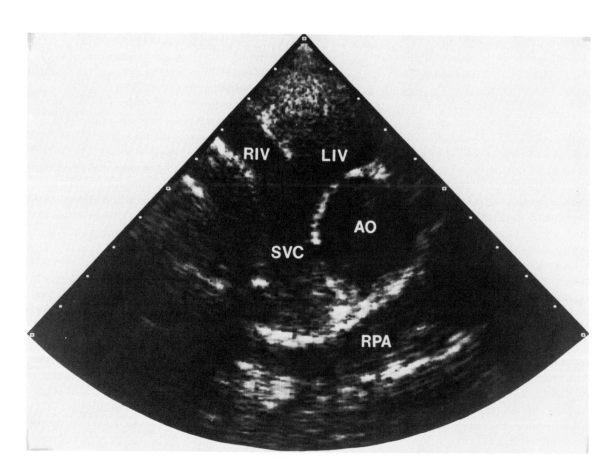

B

Figure 14.6. (*A*) Suprasternal view of the ascending aorta (Asc.Ao.) and aortic arch (Ao.Arch) demonstrating the origin of the brachiocephalic vessels. (*B*) Suprasternal view of the ascending aorta in short-axis view. The origin of the superior vena cava (SVC) is seen to arise from the drainage of the right (RIV) and left (LIV) innominate veins. The right pulmonary artery (RPA) is now seen on long-axis view. Innom. = innominate artery; LCC = left common carotid; LS = left subclavian.

ABDOMINAL AORTA

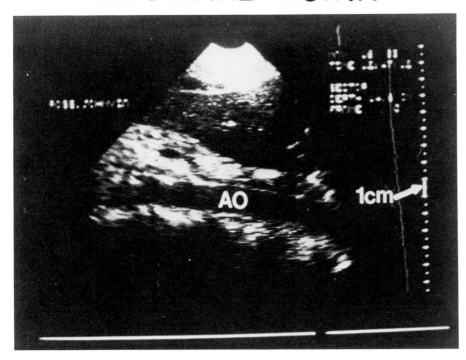

A

Figure 14.7. (*A*) A long-axis view of the abdominal aorta obtained from the subcostal position. The aorta (AO) is clearly seen and measures about 2 to 2.5 cm in diameter.

ence of smokelike moving echoes in the aortic arch proximal to the thrombosed false lumen (Fig. 14.16) is consistent with previous observations that spontaneous dynamic echoes can occur in association with disorders that produce blood stasis and thrombosis. These low-intensity spontaneous echoes have also been described in the LV in patients with LV dysfunction and in the LA in patients with mitral valve disease and associated thrombus (32, 33).

Although intimal flaps may oscillate, suggesting differential rates of filling of the false and true lumens, blood-flow patterns can be more reliably assessed by pulsed wave Doppler echocardiography (Fig. 14.16) (34). Documentation of flow in aortic dissection within both the true and false channels has been reported (12). Generally, the peak velocity is faster and the duration of forward flow phase is greater in the true lumen than in the false lumen. In addition, absence of flow may be detected by pulsed wave Doppler echocardiography in the false lumen in patients with a clotted false lumen.

Prominent venous valves within large innominate veins may be mistaken for an intimal flap within the aortic arch in patients in whom adequate quality suprasternal two-dimensional echocardiographic examinations are not obtained. By using Doppler echocar-

diography, the flow patterns within the vessel lumen can be clearly characterized as venous rather than arterial.

Some investigators suggest that the presence or absence of flow in the false lumen has both prognostic and therapeutic significance (35). Active flow within the false channel appears to have a poor prognosis.

Mathew and Nanda (12) have used Doppler echocardiography to follow patients with aortic dissection who have undergone surgical repair. Reappearance of flow signals noted in the false lumen would indicate reopening of the dissection. Postoperative leakage at the site of aortic root graft has also been documented by Doppler echocardiography (12). Mathew and Nanda (12) have observed Doppler flow signals within the native aorta in the area of a prosthetic graft during the immediate postoperative period. Persistence of flow beyond a few days is regarded as abnormal and implies leakage.

In a study using continuous wave Doppler ultrasound for diagnosis of aortic dissection, several investigators found a characteristic flow pattern in the aortic arch (36). An early systolic notch with a second acute peak was found in those patients with pulses present and an enlarged hump if pulses were absent. It was postulated that the early systolic notch resulted from

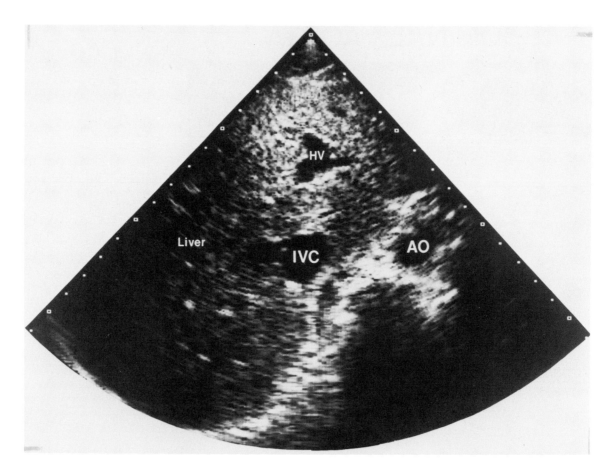

B

Figure 14.7, (cont'd.) (*B*) Short-axis view of the aorta (AO) and inferior vena cava (IVC) from the subcostal position. The liver and portions of the hepatic vein (HV) are seen. The normal relationship of AO to IVC is seen.

Figure 14.8. Thoracic aorta (T. AORTA) obtained from the apical position where the aorta is seen in longitudinal fashion. ANT. = anterior; MV = mitral valve; POS. = posterior.

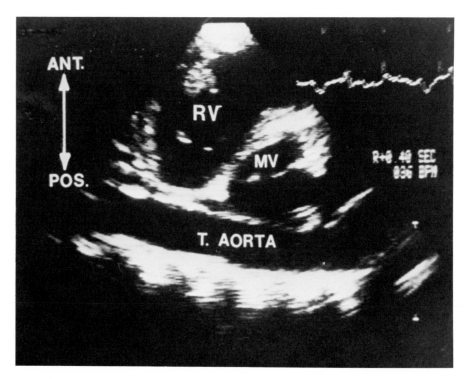

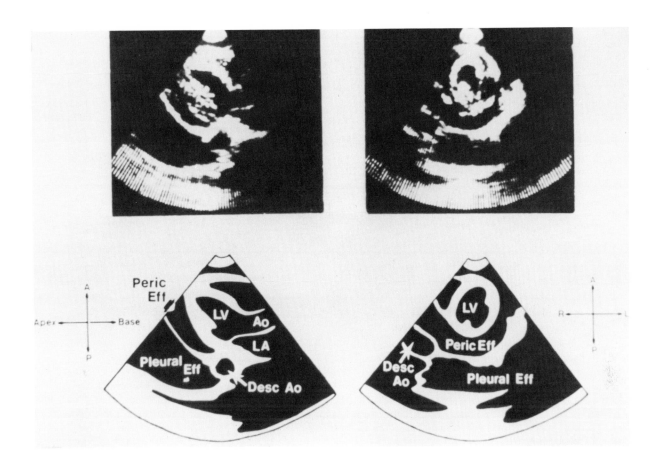

A   **B**

Figure 14.9.   Parasternal long-axis view (A) and parasternal short-axis view (B) in a patient with combined pericardial and pleural effusions. The normal intimate relationship of the descending aorta (Desc Ao) to the posterior wall of the ventricle is displaced by a moderate pericardial effusion (Peric Eff). Isolated pleural effusion (Pleural Eff) does not affect this relationship. A = anterior; AO = aorta; P = posterior.

transient dynamic obstruction of blood flow caused by the hernia of the false lumen in the true channel. It disappeared in cases of false lumen thrombosis. In patients with significant aortic regurgitation, diastolic backflow was also observed.

A new real-time two-dimensional color flow Doppler imaging system has been used in assessment of valvular lesions (37), and its potential and value in aortic dissecting aneurysms seem promising. Precise flow patterns in true and false lumens, site of entrance and exit tears, and assessment of surgical repair results would be possible with color Doppler angiocardiograms.

MARFAN'S SYNDROME AND ANNULOAORTIC ECTASIA

Patients with Marfan's syndrome and annuloaortic ectasia may have aneurysmal dilatation of the ascending thoracic aorta, beginning at the aortic valve annulus and terminating proximally at the innominate artery

(38). In a study comparing 14 patients with annuloaortic ectasia and 12 patients with secondary cause of aortic root dilatation, the aortic root diameter at the level of the aortic valve and 2 cm above the aortic valve was significantly larger in the annuloaortic ectasia patients (Fig. 14.17) (39). In contrast, the diameter of the DTA was greater in the second group of patients. The importance of recognizing patients with annuloaortic ectasia is that they are at risk for aortic root dissection or severe aortic regurgitation. In our series, a high percentage required surgery for either one or both indications (39). Because of the high incidence of spontaneous dissection in such patients, echocardiography should prove to be useful in the diagnosis and follow-up of these patients. In addition, it has been suggested that some patients with aortic root diameters exceeding 5 cm should be considered for prophylactic beta-blocker therapy in order to prevent dissection (40, 41). A large number of patients and more prolonged follow-up data are necessary to decide whether prophylactic betablockers have a role in pre-

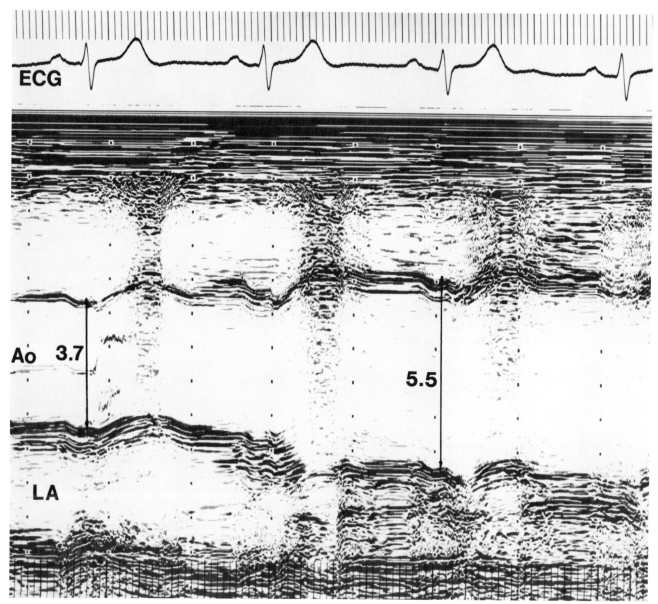

Figure 14.10. M-mode sweep of aorta (Ao) showing aneurysmal dilatation of the Ao above the aortic leaflets. ECG = electrocardiogram.

venting dissection in these patients. An association between annuloaortic ectasia and bicuspid aortic valve has been reported (42).

Aortic Sinus Aneurysm

Aneurysmal enlargement of the aortic sinuses has been reported in patients with Marfan's syndrome and annuloaortic ectasia (Fig. 14.18) (38). Aortic sinus aneurysms can be congenital or due to acquired lesions. The echocardiographic appearance can vary markedly, depending on the location of the aneurysm and on whether the aneurysm has ruptured. If it has ruptured, its appearance will vary depending into what chamber of the heart it ruptures (3).

The M-mode echocardiographic findings in a patient with an aortic sinus aneurysm displayed a peculiar pattern of echoes in the LV outflow tract, expanding during diastole as the aneurysm filled with blood (43). During systole, the aneurysm moved back into the aorta and out of the outflow tract. Aortic sinus aneurysms can rupture into a variety of places but are more prone to rupture into the right heart chambers (Fig. 14.19) (44). In ruptures into the right heart, fluttering of the tricuspid valve or interventricular septum has also been reported (44). Doppler echocardiography should be especially useful in locating abnormal flow patterns in patients with ruptured aortic sinus aneurysms. Aortic sinus aneurysm rupture less commonly

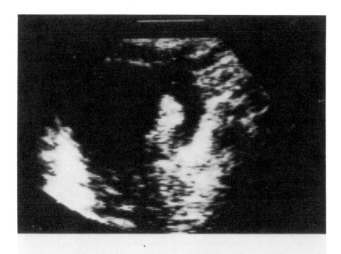

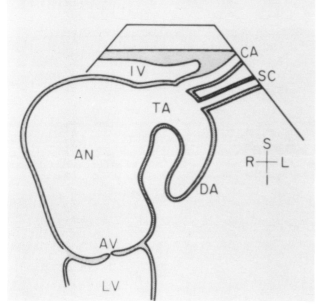

Figure 14.11. Ascending aortic aneurysm (AN). The suprasternal transducer position was used to visualize virtually the full extent of the AN. Note that the transverse arch (TA), brachiocephalic branches, and proximal thoracic descending aorta (DA) are not involved. AV = aortic valve; CA = carotid artery; I = inferior; IV = innominate vein; L = left; R = right; S = superior; SC = subclavian artery. (Reproduced by permission from Mathew T, Nanda NC. Two-dimensional and Doppler echocardiographic evaluation of aortic aneurysms and dissection. Am J Cardiol 1984;54:379–85.)

into the LV cavity, the interventricular septum (45), and the LA.

In rare situations when there is free communication between the aorta and RV, premature opening of the pulmonic valves has been reported as a result of high end-diastolic RV pressure (46).

Several reports have described the usefulness of

Table 14.2. Doppler Echocardiographic Criteria for Diagnosis of Aortic Dissection

1. Recognition of intimal flap as an oscillating two-dimensional structure within the aorta is best visualized by two-dimensional echocardiography, but precise motion can be evaluated by M-mode echocardiography
   a. Intimal flap should be seen in more than one view
   b. The intimal flap should have defined motion that is not parallel to the motion of any other cardiac or aortic root structure
   c. The echogenic recorded intimal flap should not be confused by an extension or reverberation from any other cardiac structure
   d. A repeatable echogenic interface should separate the true and false lumens
2. Aortic root dilatation (>42 mm)
3. Widening of anterior (16–21 mm) or posterior (10–13 mm) aortic root walls*
4. Maintenance of parallel motion of aortic root walls
5. Preservation of aortic leaflet motion†
6. Differential rates of filling of false and true lumens by Doppler or demonstration of absence of flow pattern in patients with thrombosed false lumen.

*May also occur in patients with advanced atherosclerosis or hypertension.
†Rarely, aortic valve motion is abnormal in proximal type I aortic root dissection, but may be "duplicated" and the intimal flap may prolapse into the LV outflow tract during diastole.

two-dimensional echocardiography in the diagnosis of aortic sinus aneurysms (44, 47).

Aortic Root Abscess

Several reports describe the value of echocardiography in the diagnosis of root abscesses (48–50). The original M-mode description included reduplication of the anterior aortic wall in the presence of large echocardiographic aortic valve vegetations (48). Two-dimensional echocardiography seems better suited to localize the precise site and extent of aortic root abscesses and is highly sensitive (Fig. 14.20) (49, 50).

Congenital Disorders of the Aorta Encountered in the Adult

A review of all the congenital disorders affecting the aorta is beyond the scope of this chapter. Huhta and coworkers (51) described aortic examinations by two-dimensional echocardiography in 255 children and infants with a variety of congenital abnormalities of the aorta. A high degree of sensitivity was obtained with this technique in such diverse conditions as hypoplasia of the aorta, truncus arteriosus, aortopulmonary window, Marfan's syndrome, anomalous origin of the left pulmonary artery, right aortic arch, anomalous right and left subclavian arteries, double arch, patent ductus arteriosus, aortic isthmus interruption, coarctation of the aorta, and obstruction of right descending aorta.

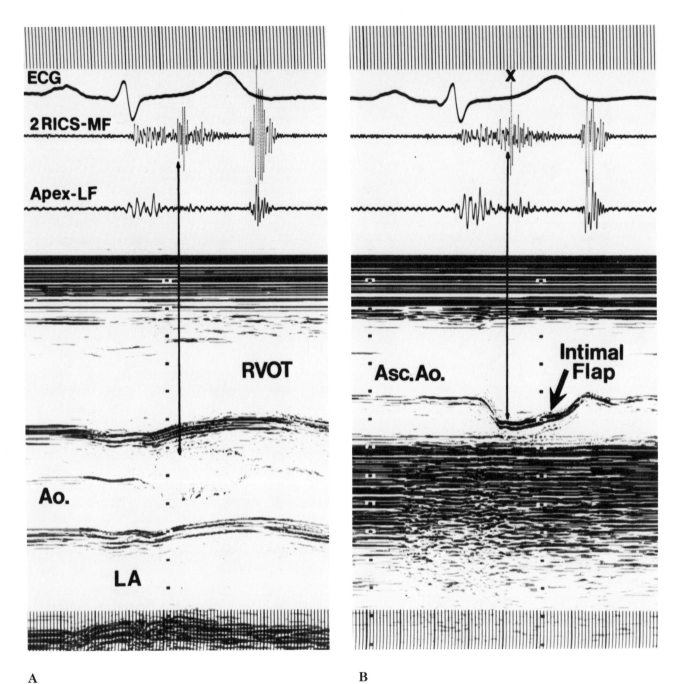

A

B

Figure 14.12.   (*A*) Simultaneous electrocardiogram (ECG), phonocardiogram, and echocardiogram obtained from standard parasternal view. Phonocardiogram recorded at second right intercostal space (2RICS) with medium-range filter (MF) shows midsystolic crescendo-decrescendo murmur with midsystolic click. Click was not recorded at apex with low-frequency filter (LF). Click does not coincide with maximal aortic valve opening. (*B*) Simultaneous ECG, phonocardiogram, and echocardiogram obtained at 2RICS, with transducer angulated slightly inferiorly and medially. Ascending aorta (Asc.Ao.) is visualized as is intimal flap. Midsystolic click is maximally recorded at 2RICS. X indicates click. Ao. = aorta; RVOT = right ventricular outflow tract. (Reproduced by permission from Victor MF, Mintz GS, Kotler MN, Parry WR, Wilson AR. Dissecting aneurysm associated with a midsystolic click. Arch Intern Med 1981;141:255–7.)

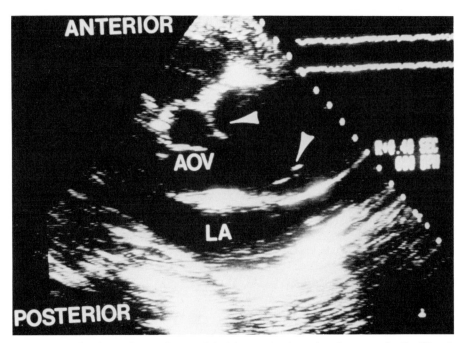

Figure 14.13. Two-dimensional echocardiographic modified long-axis view showing a markedly dilated aortic root (measuring 6 cm) and intimal flaps (*white arrows*). The LA is compressed. The intimal flaps did not oscillate in real time, suggesting no differential in filling of false and true lumens. AOV = aortic valve. (Reproduced by permission from Mattleman S, Panidis I, Kotler MN, Mintz GS, Victor M, Ross J. Dissecting aneurysm in a patient with Marfan's syndrome: recognition of extensive involvement of the aorta by two-dimensional echocardiography. J Clin Ultrasound 1984;12:219–21.)

In adults with coarctation, two-dimensional echocardiography is extremely useful in visualizing the coarcted segment (52) as well as the dilated proximal aorta or left subclavian artery and post-stenotic dilatation of the aorta. The precise gradient across the coarcted segment can also be calculated by Doppler echocardiography (Fig. 14.21) (53).

In patients undergoing repair of the coarcted segment, two-dimensional and Doppler echocardiography are extremely useful in following these patients to detect restenosis.

VENOUS ANOMALIES ENCOUNTERED IN THE ADULT

A persistent left superior vena cava draining to the coronary sinus occurs in approximately 0.5 percent of the normal population and in approximately 3 percent to 10 percent of patients with congenital heart disease (54).

The enlarged coronary sinus due to increased blood flow can be readily detected by two-dimensional echocardiography in the standard left parasternal long-axis view and on- and off-axis views (Fig. 14.22) (55). It is generally visualized as a discrete circular structure slightly superior to the posterior mitral valve leaflet. It

must be differentiated from the DTA. In the parasternal short-axis views, the coronary sinus is visualized at the level of the anterior mitral valve leaflet and is seen as a crescent-shaped structure posterior to the LA and continuous with the RA. In the apical four-chamber view, the coronary sinus appears as an oval-shaped structure along the lateral border of the LA. In order to differentiate between a persistent superior vena cava draining into the coronary sinus and the descending aorta, a contrast study can be performed. Following peripheral hand-agitated saline injection into a left-arm vein, the coronary sinus will opacify with contrast echoes. In addition, the RA and RV will eventually opacify. In some patients, the left superior vena cava can be visualized directly by the suprasternal short-axis view (Fig. 14.6*B*).

In patients with both right and left superior venae cavae, these vessels may be seen along both sides of the transverse aorta. In patients with a left superior vena cava and absence of right superior vena cava, the superior vena cava is seen along the left side of the transverse aorta (Fig. 14.23) (56). The usual pattern of a left innominate vein, coursing from left to right and superior to the transverse aorta, is absent.

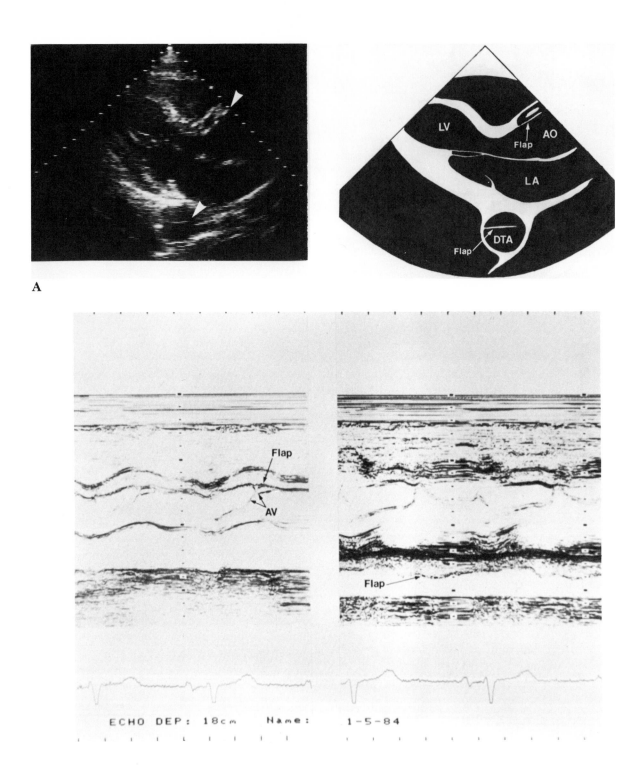

A

B

Figure 14.14. (*A*) Two-dimensional echocardiogram obtained in the parasternal long-axis view of an extensive type I dissecting aneurysm. The upper white arrow points to an intimal flap that is minimally separated from the anterior aortic wall. The lower white arrow depicts the intimal flap seen in the DTA. (*B*) M-mode echocardiogram of same patient obtained from the proximal aorta. The intimal flap is separated from the anterior aortic wall and interferes with the excursion of the right coronary aortic cusp. M-mode cursor (right) obtained from the parasternal long-axis view and directed through the DTA, demonstrating independent motion of the intimal flap. AO = aorta; AV = aortic valve. (Reproduced by permission from Goldman AP, Kotler MN, Scanlon MH, Ostrum BJ, Parameswaran R, Parry WR. Magnetic resonance imaging and two-dimensional echocardiography: an alternative approach to aortography in the diagnosis of aortic dissecting aneurysm. Am J Med 1986;80:1225–9.)

Table 14.3. Detection of Complications of Aortic Dissection by Doppler Echocardiography

1. Aortic regurgitation
   a. Disturbed flow pattern in LV outflow tract by Doppler
   b. Diastolic fluttering of anterior mitral valve leaflet or interventricular septum
   c. Left ventricular enlargement or LV wall motion suggestive of volume overload
2. Pericardial effusion or tamponade
   a. Right ventricular compression
   b. Right atrial inversion
3. Left pleural effusion
4. Compression of cardiac structures: external compression of LA or compression of mitral valve orifice with disturbed mitral valve flow pattern

Table 14.4. Causes of False-Positive Echocardiographic Criteria for Aortic Dissection

Extension or lateral resolution problem from thickened or calcified aortic valve

Reverberating echoes from another cardiac structure recorded within the aortic lumen

Spurious echoes recorded within aortic lumen due to excessive gain setting

Atherosclerotic plaques in aortic wall

Intima may be visualized as widely separated from the outer wall in patients with excessively thickened aortic walls

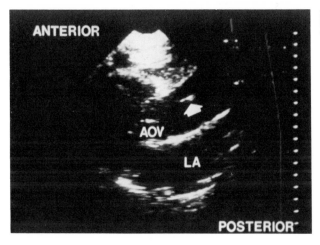
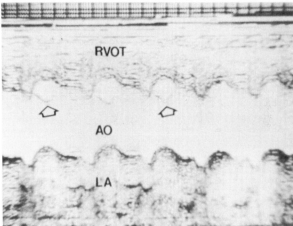

A

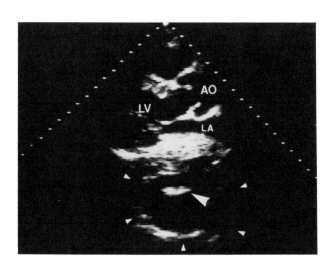
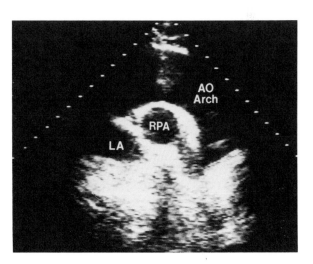

B

Figure 14.15. (*A*) Parasternal long-axis view of a two-dimensional echocardiogram. Left shows two-dimensional echocardiogram and right M-mode echocardiogram in a patient with proved type III dissecting aneurysm on angiography. An artifact (*solid white arrow*) is seen in the ascending aorta and is also visualized on M-mode cursor (*open arrow*). At surgery, no evidence of type I dissecting aneurysm was found. (*B*) Parasternal long-axis view (left) and suprasternal notch view (right) in a patient with a large hiatal hernia (*small arrows*). Initial impression by two-dimensional echocardiography was thought to be a distal dissecting aneurysm with intimal flap (*large arrow*) and secondary LA compression. The mass disappeared after surgical excision of the hiatal hernia. AO Arch = aortic arch; AOV = aortic valve; RPA = right pulmonary artery; RVOT = right ventricular outflow tract.

A

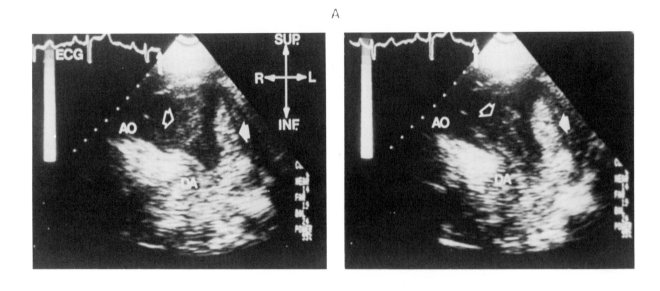

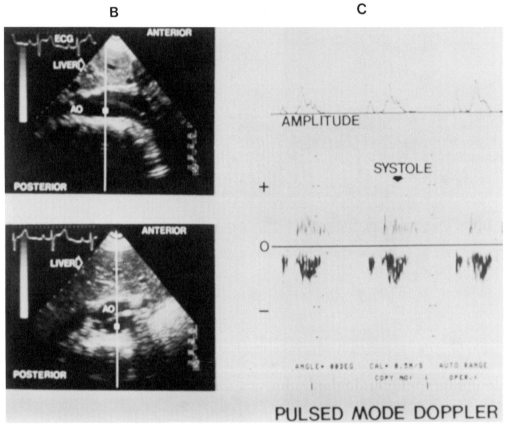

PULSED MODE DOPPLER

Figure 14.16. (*A*) Two-dimensional echocardiographic suprasternal notch view showing an echo mass involving the DTA distal to the origin of the left subclavian artery and probably representing a thrombosed false lumen (*solid arrowheads*). The true lumen of the descending aorta (DA) is compressed by a false lumen. In addition, intracavitary echoes with changing shapes and motion (*unfilled arrowheads*) are seen in the aortic arch (AO). (*B*) The two-dimensional echocardiogram of abdominal aorta (long-axis view, above and short-axis view, below) obtained from the subcostal view in same patient. The intimal flap separating true lumen from false lumen is evident. (*C*) Pulsed mode Doppler reveals flow signal recorded in distal channel only, which probably represents the true lumen. ECG = electrocardiogram; INF. = inferior; L = left; R = right; SUP. = superior. (Reproduced by permission from Panidis IP, Kotler MN, Mintz GS, Ross J. Intracavitary echoes in the aortic arch in a type III aortic dissection. Am J Cardiol 1984;54:1159–60.)

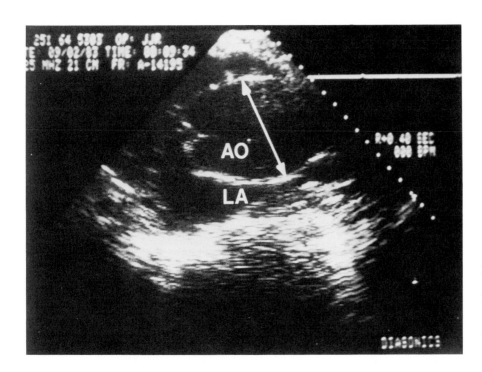

Figure 14.17. Two-dimensional echocardiogram obtained in the parasternal long-axis view. The ascending aorta (AO) is markedly dilated with compression of the LA. The aortic root (*arrow*) measures 7 cm.

TOTAL ANOMALOUS PULMONARY VENOUS RETURN ENCOUNTERED IN THE ADULT

In patients with total anomalous pulmonary venous return, the pulmonary veins usually converge to form a common pulmonary venous chamber posterior to the LA. Most often, the common pulmonary venous chamber drains into the coronary sinus or the superior vena cava by way of a left vertical vein and innominate vein. Less often, the common pulmonary venous chamber drains directly into the RA or to the hepatic-portal system. The two-dimensional echocardiographic features of the common pulmonary venous chamber have been described (57).

The common pulmonary venous chamber is visualized in the parasternal long-axis and apical four-chamber views. It is frequently visualized posteriorly and superiorly to the LA (Fig. 14.24). It is crucial to visualize the thin wall separating the common pulmonary venous chamber from the LA. Additional findings include enlarged RA, RV, and pulmonary arteries. In those patients where the common pulmonary venous chamber drains into the coronary sinus and RV, the connection can be visualized (Fig. 14.25).

In rarer instances where pulmonary venous return to the superior vena cava occurs by way of the left vertical vein and innominate vein to the superior vena cava, a dilated innominate vein or collar surrounding the transverse aorta can be visualized (56). In patients with total anomalous pulmonary venous return to the hepatic-portal system, the common pulmonary vein can often be followed in the subcostal views to its site of drainage below the diaphragm (56).

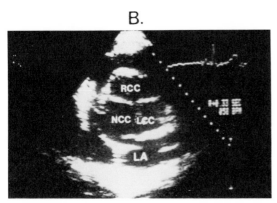

Figure 14.18. Parasternal long-axis view (*A*) and short-axis view (*B*) in a patient with aneurysmal dilatation of aortic sinuses (*large white arrows*). Ao = aorta; LCC = left coronary cusp; NCC = noncoronary cusp; RCC = right coronary cusp; RVOT = right ventricular outflow tract.

A

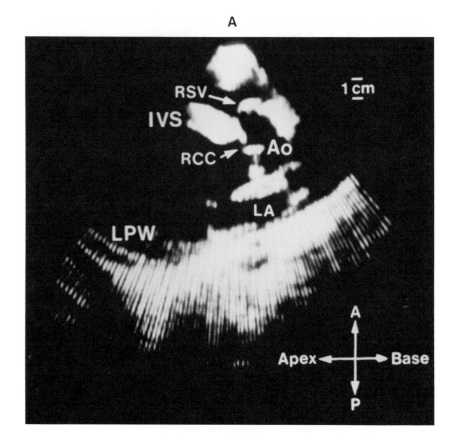

Figure 14.19. (*A*) A two-dimensional long-axis view of the heart. The right coronary cusp (RCC) is aneurysmal and the right aortic sinus (RSV) bulges into the right ventricular outflow tract. (*B*) Preoperative M-mode expanded scale echocardiogram recorded at paper speed of 100 mm per second. Diastolic fluttering of right side of interventricular septum (IVS) is demonstrated (*open arrows*). A = anterior; Ao = aorta; LPW = left ventricular posterior wall; LSB-HF = left sternal border–high frequency; P = posterior; RVAW = right ventricular anterior wall. (Reproduced by permission from Haaz WS, Kotler MN, Mintz GS, Parry WR, Spitzer S. Ruptured sinus of Valsalva aneurysm. Diagnosed by echocardiography. Chest 1980; 78:781–4.)

B

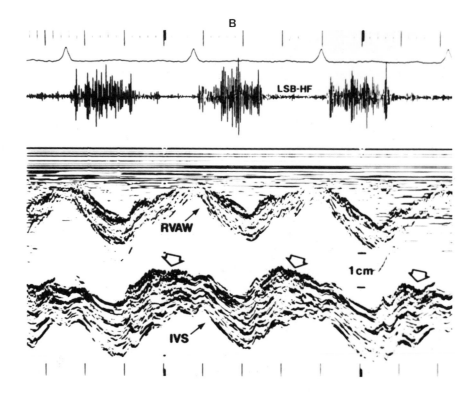

Infradiaphragmatic total anomalous pulmonary venous connection has been accurately diagnosed by a combination of two-dimensional and pulsed wave Doppler echocardiography (58).

SUMMARY

In summary, patients with dissecting aneurysms or saccular aneurysms can be readily identified by two-dimensional echocardiography provided complete evaluation of the entire thoracic aorta and abdominal aorta is performed. There are some patients in whom false-positive studies can occur as a result of extension of reverberation of echoes from another cardiac structure or as a result of spurious echoes seen in the aortic lumen caused by too high a gain setting. On rare occasions, a mobile atherosclerotic plaque in the aortic wall may simulate an intimal flap. Doppler echocardiography appears to offer a promising role in evaluating patients with dissecting aneurysms. Flow patterns in true and false lumens can be assessed. In addition, the results of surgery can be evaluated by paying attention to flow patterns in the graft and native vessel. Marfan's syndrome and the entity of annuloaortic ectasia can be readily recognized by two-dimensional echocardiography. The technique may allow follow up evaluation in assessing response to therapy as well as defining the natural history of these disorders. Additional disorders affecting the aorta such as aortic sinus aneurysms, aortic root abscesses, and coarctation of the aorta can be reliably diagnosed by two-dimensional echocardiography. Anomalous left subclavian vein drainage into the coronary sinus can be confirmed by contrast echocardiography with injection into a left peripheral arm vein.

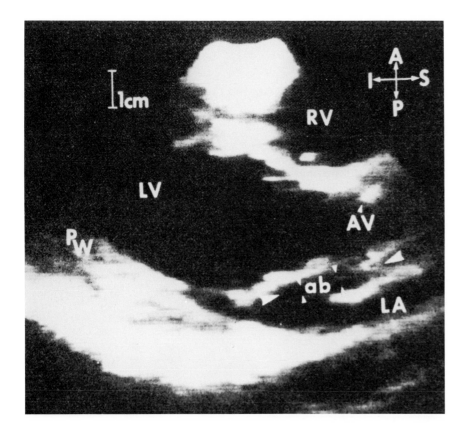

Figure 14.20. Still frames of the long-axis view of the left side of the heart in a young patient with aortic valve (AV) endocarditis whose complication of aortic root abscess (ab) involved the posterior aortic root and dissected down into the anterior mitral leaflet (*arrows*). PW = posterior wall. (Reproduced by permission from Brandenburg RO, Giuliani ER, Wilson WR, Geraci JE. Infective endocarditis—a 25 year overview of diagnosis and therapy. J Am Coll Cardiol 1983; 1:280–91.)

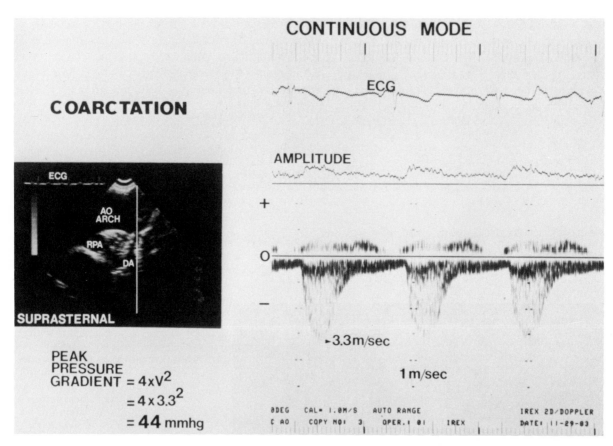

Figure 14.21. Two-dimensional echocardiogram (left) and continuous wave Doppler recording (right) from the suprasternal notch in a patient with coarctation of the aorta. On the left, the aortic arch (AO ARCH) is dilated, and the descending aorta (DA) is narrowed just distal to the origin of the left subclavian artery. The white line indicates the position of the Doppler beam. On the right, a peak systolic velocity of 3.3 meters per second is recorded from the DA, indicating a peak systolic pressure drop of 44 mm of mercury across the coarctation. ECG = electrocardiogram; RPA = right pulmonary artery.

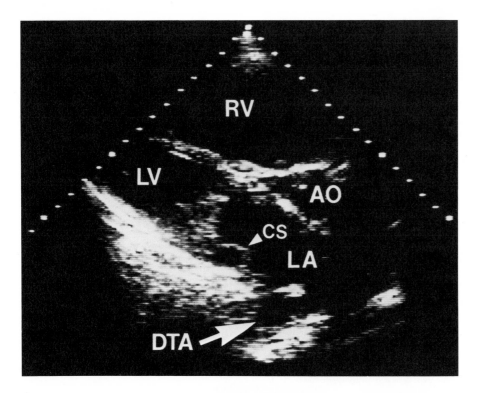

A

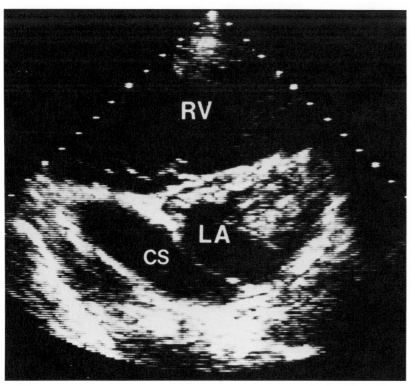

B

Figure 14.22. (*A*) Parasternal long-axis view of a patient with an atrial septal defect and persistent left superior vena cava draining into the coronary sinus (CS). Note the relationship of the CS to the DTA. The RV is markedly dilated. (*B*) Off-axis short-axis view of same patient showing the dilated CS in relationship to the LA. The exact connection and drainage into the RA are not visualized. AO = aorta.

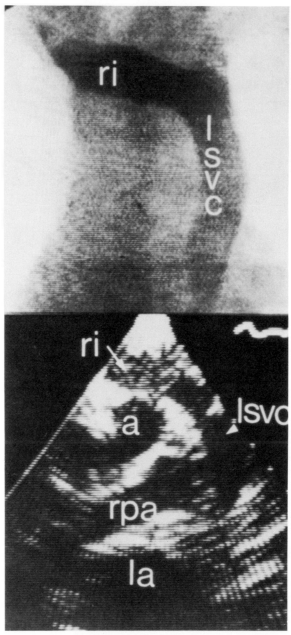

Figure 14.23. Frame from a cineangiogram (top) and suprasternal notch short-axis view (bottom) of a patient with absence of the right superior vena cava and a persistent left superior vena cava (lsvc) connecting to the coronary sinus. The right innominate vein (ri) courses from right to left superior to the transverse aorta (a). rpa = right pulmonary artery. (Reproduced by permission from Silverman NH, Snider AR, eds. Two-dimensional echocardiography in congenital heart disease. Norwalk, Conn.: Appleton-Century-Crofts, 1982:139.)

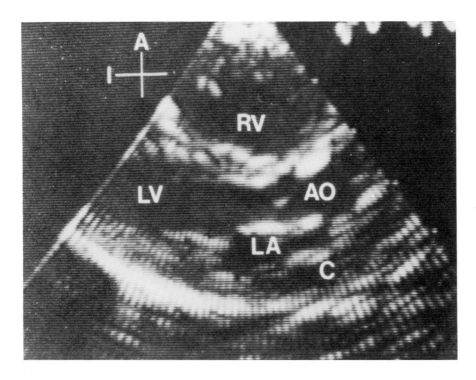

Figure 14.24.   Parasternal long-axis view of an infant with total anomalous pulmonary venous return to the coronary sinus. The common pulmonary venous chamber (C) is seen posterior and superior to the LA and separated from it by a thin wall. The RV is enlarged. A = anterior; AO = aorta; I = inferior. (Reproduced by permission from Silverman NH, Snider AR, eds. Two-dimensional echocardiography in congenital heart disease. Norwalk, Conn.: Appleton-Century-Crofts, 1982:206.)

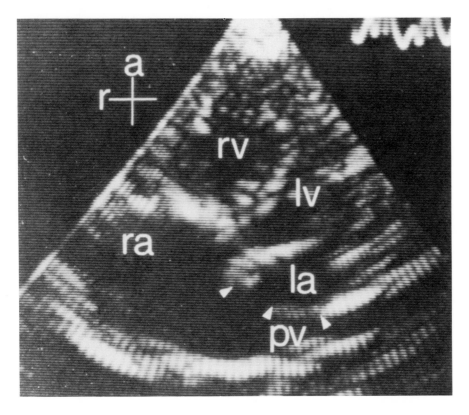

Figure 14.25.   Apical four-chamber view from same patient as in Figure 19-24. The pulmonary venous confluence (PV) is connected to the RA by a dilated coronary sinus. It is not possible to determine with certainty where the PV ends and the coronary sinus begins. The RA and RV are enlarged, and the RV is apex forming. A = apex; R = right. (Reproduced by permission from Silverman NH, Snider AR, eds. Two-dimensional echocardiography in congenital heart disease. Norwalk, Conn.: Appleton-Century-Crofts, 1982:206.)

REFERENCES

1. Gramiak R, Shah PM. Echocardiography of the aortic root. Invest Radiol 1968;3:356–66.
2. Francis GS, Hagan AD, Oury J, O'Rourke RA. Accuracy of echocardiography for assessing aortic root diameter. Br Heart J 1975;37:376–8.
3. Feigenbaum H. Echocardiography. 3rd ed. Philadelphia: Lea & Febiger, 1981:528–48.
4. Mintz GS, Kotler MN, Segal BL, Parry WR. Two-dimensional echocardiographic recognition of the descending thoracic aorta. Am J Cardiol 1979;44:232–8.
5. Triulzi M, Gillam LD, Gentile F, Newell JB, Weyman AE. Normal adult cross-sectional echocardiographic values: linear dimensions and chamber areas. Echocardiography 1984;1:403–26.
6. Ihlen H, Amilie JP, Dale J, et al. Determination of cardiac output by Doppler echocardiography. Br Heart J 1984;51:54–60.
7. Iliceto S, Antonelli G, Biasco G, Rizzon P. Two-dimensional echocardiographic evaluation of aneurysms of the descending thoracic aorta. Circulation 1982;66:1045–9.
8. Come PC. Improved cross-sectional echocardiographic technique for visualization of the retrocardiac descending aorta in its long axis. Am J Cardiol 1983;51:1029–32.
9. Haaz WS, Mintz GS, Kotler MN, Parry WR. Two-dimensional echocardiographic recognition of the descending thoracic aorta: value in differentiating pericardial from pleural effusions. Am J Cardiol 1980;46:739–43.
10. DeMaria AN, Bommer W, Neumann A, Weinert L, Bogren H, Mason DT. Identification and localization of aneurysms of the ascending aorta by cross-sectional echocardiography. Circulation 1979;59:755–79.
11. Victor MF, Mintz GS, Kotler MN, Wilson AR, Segal BL. Two-dimensional echocardiographic diagnosis of aortic dissection. Am J Cardiol 1981;48:1155–9.
12. Mathew T, Nanda NC. Two-dimensional and Doppler echocardiographic evaluation of aortic aneurysms and dissection. Am J Cardiol 1984;54:379–85.
13. Nanda NC, Gramiak R, Shah PM. Diagnosis of aortic root dissection by echocardiography. Circulation 1973;48:506–13.
14. Miller JL, Nanda NC, Singh RP, Mathew T, Iliceto S, Rizzon P. Echocardiographic diagnosis of aortic aneurysms and dissection. Echocardiography 1984;1:507–19.
15. Krueger SK, Starke H, Forker AD, Eliot RS. Echocardiographic mimics of aortic root dissection. Chest 1975;67:441–4.
16. Hirschfeld DS, Rodriguez HJ, Schiller NB. Duplication of aortic wall seen by echocardiography. Br Heart J 1976;38:843–50.
17. Moothart RW, Spangler RD, Blount SG Jr. Echocardiography in aortic root dissection. Am J Cardiol 1975;36:11–6.
18. Brown OR, Popp RL, Kloster FE. Echocardiographic criteria for aortic root dissection. Am J Cardiol 1975;36:17–22.
19. Stever SW, Parameswaran R, Goldslack P, Goldberg H. Unusual echocardiographic findings in aortic dissection. Arch Intern Med 1982;142:2221–3.
20. Victor MF, Mintz GS, Kotler MN, Parry WR, Wilson AR. Dissecting aortic aneurysm with a midsystolic click. Arch Intern Med 1981;141:255–7.
21. Mattleman S, Panidis I, Kotler MN, Mintz G, Victor M, Ross J. Dissecting aneurysm in a patient with Marfan's syndrome: recognition of extensive involvement of the aorta by two-dimensional echocardiography. J Clin Ultrasound 1984;12:219–21.
22. Nicod P, Firth BG, Pshock RM, Gaffney A, Hillis LD. Rupture of dissecting aortic aneurysm into the right atrium: clinical and echocardiographic recognition. Am Heart J 1984;107:1276–8.
23. Sraow JS, Desser KB, Benchimol A, De Sa'Neto A, Peebles S. Two-dimensional echocardiographic recognition of an aortic intimal flap prolapsing into the left ventricular outflow tract. J Am Coll Cardiol 1984;4:180–2.
24. Cohen ISH, Wharton T. "Duplication" of aortic cusp: new M-mode echocardiographic sign of intimal tear in aortic dissection. Br Heart J 1982;47:173–6.
25. Smuckler AL, Nomeir AM, Watts LE, Hackshaw BT. Echocardiographic diagnosis of aortic root dissection by M-mode and two-dimensional techniques. Am Heart J 1982;103:897–904.
26. Granato JE, Dee P, Gibson RS. Utility of two-dimensional echocardiography in suspected ascending aortic dissection. Am J Cardiol 1985;56:123–9.
27. Nicholson WJ, Cobbs BW. Echocardiographic oscillating flap in aortic root dissecting aneurysm. Chest 1976;76:305–7.
28. Curate WL, Peticlerc R, Dyrada F, Winsberg F. Echocardiographic demonstration of mobility of the dissecting flap of an aortic aneurysm. Radiology 1977;123:173–4.
29. McLeod AA, Monaghan MJ, Richardson PJ. Diagnosis of acute aortic dissecting by M-mode and cross-sectional echocardiography: a five year experience. Eur Heart J 1983;4:196–202.
30. Goldman AP, Kotler MN, Scanlon MH, Ostrum BJ, Parameswaran R, Parry WR. Magnetic resonance imaging and two-dimensional echocardiography: an alternative approach to aortography in the diagnosis of aortic dissecting aneurysm. Am J Med 1986;80:1225–9.
31. Panidis IP, Kotler MN, Mintz GS, Ross J. Intracavitary echoes in the aortic arch in type III aortic dissection. Am J Cardiol 1984;54:1159–60.
32. Mikell FL, Asinger RW, Elsperger J, Anderson WR, Hodges M. Regional stasis of blood in the dysfunctional left ventricle; echocardiographic detection and differentiation from early thrombosis. Circulation 1982;66:755–63.
33. Beppu S, Nimura Y, Sakakibara H, Nagata S, Park YD, Izumi S. High prevalence of left atrial thrombosis in cases of mitral valve disease with dynamic intracavitary echoes, abstracted. Circulation 1983;68(suppl III):335.
34. Okamoto M, Kinoshita N, Miyatabe K, Sakakibara H, Nimura Y. Blood flow analysis in dissecting aneurysms with two-dimensional echo-Doppler technique, abstracted. Circulation 1982;66(suppl II):91.
35. Dinsmore RE, Willerson JT, Buckley MJ. Dissecting aneurysm of the aorta: aortographic features affecting prognosis. Radiology 1972;105:567–72.
36. Dany F, Bensaid J, Blanc P, Virot P, Christides C, Kim M. Contribution of continuous wave Doppler ultrasound to the diagnosis of aortic dissection, abstracted. Circulation 1984;70(suppl II):395.
37. Miyatake K, Okamoto M, Kinoshita N, et al. Clinical applications of a new type of real-time two-dimensional Doppler flow imaging system. Am J Cardiol 1984;54:857–68.
38. Lemon DK, White W. Annuloaortic ectasia: angiographic, hemodynamic and clinical comparison with aortic valve insufficiency. Am J Cardiol 1978;41:482–6.
39. Fox R, Ren JF, Panidis IP, Kotler MN, Mintz GS, Ross J. Annulo-aortic ectasia: a clinical and echocardiographic study. Am J Cardiol 1984;54:177–81.
40. Ose L, McKusick VA. Natural history of specific birth defects. New York: Alan R. Liss, 1976:163–9.
41. Pyeritz RE. Propranolol retards aortic root dilatation in the Marfan syndrome, abstracted. Circulation 1983;68(suppl III):365.
42. McKusick VA, Logue RB, Bahnson HT. Association of aortic valvular disease and cystic medial necrosis of the ascending aorta; report of four instances. Circulation 1957;16:188–94.
43. Rothbaum DA, Dillon JC, Chang S, Feigenbaum H. Echocardiographic manifestation of right sinus of Valsalva aneurysm. Circulation 1974;49:768–71.
44. Haaz WS, Kotler MN, Mintz GS, Parry WR, Spitzer S. Ruptured sinus of Valsalva aneurysm. Diagnosis by echocardiography. Chest 1980;78:781–4.
45. Engel PJ, Held JS, vander Bel-Kahn J, Spitz H. Echocardiographic diagnosis of congenital sinus of Valsalva aneurysm with dissection of the interventricular septum. Circulation 1981;63:705–11.
46. Weyman AE, Dillon JC, Feigenbaum H, Chang S. Premature pulmonic valve opening following sinus of Valsalva aneurysm rupture into the right atrium. Circulation 1975;57:556–60.
47. Nishimura K, Hibi N, Kato T, et al. Real-time observation of ruptured sinus of Valsalva aneurysm by high speed ultrasonocardiotomography; report of a case. Circulation 1976;53:732–5.
48. Fox S, Kotler MN, Segal BL, Parry WR. Echocardiographic diagnosis of aortic valve endocarditis and its complications. Arch Intern Med 1977;137:85–9.
49. Brandenburg RO, Giuliani ER, Wilson WR, Geraci JE. Infective

endocarditis—a 25 year overview of diagnosis and therapy. J Am Coll Cardiol 1983;1:280–91.

50. Ellis SG, Goldstein J, Popp RL. Detection of endocarditis-associated perivalvular abscesses by two-dimensional echocardiography. J Am Coll Cardiol 1985;5:647–53.

51. Huhta JC, Gutgesel HP, Latson LA, Huffines FD. Two-dimensional echocardiographic assessment of the aorta in infants and children with congenital heart disease. Circulation 1984;70:417–24.

52. Weymann AE, Caldwell Rl, Hurwitz RA, Girod DA, Dillon JC, Feigenbaum H. Cross-sectional echocardiographic detection of aortic obstruction. 2. Coarctation of the aorta. Circulation 1978;57:498–502.

53. Hatle L, Angelsen IN. Doppler ultrasound in cardiology. 2nd ed. Philadelphia: Lea & Febiger, 1985:217–20.

54. Mantini E, Grondin CM, Lillehei CW, Edwards JE. Congenital anomalies involving the coronary sinus. Circulation 1966;33:317–27.

55. Snider AR, Ports TA, Silverman NH. Venous anomalies of the coronary sinus: detection by M-mode, two-dimensional and contrast echocardiography. Circulation 1979;60:721–7.

56. Silverman NH, Snider AR. Two-dimensional echocardiography in congenital heart disease. Norwalk, Connecticut: Appleton-Century-Crofts, 1982:135–9, 205–8.

57. Sahn DJ, Allen HD, Lange LW, Goldberg SJ. Cross-sectional echocardiographic diagnosis of the sites of total anomalous pulmonary venous drainage. Circulation 1979;60:1317–25.

58. Cooper MJ, Teitel DF, Silverman NH, Enderlein MA. Study of the infradiaphragmatic total anomalous pulmonary venous connection with cross-sectional and pulsed Doppler echocardiography. Circulation 1984;78:412–6.

15
Echo Doppler Assessment of The Transplanted Heart

Satinder Bhatia
Martin St. John Sutton

Cardiac transplantation is a therapeutic alternative for patients with severe congestive heart failure refractory to medical therapy (1). As a result, the number of cardiac transplants has escalated in the last five years. Thus, it is important to be familiar with the echocardiographic appearances of the transplanted heart, which may be regarded as a six-chamber organ.

ATRIA

The right and left atria consist of a portion of the recipient atria and the majority of the donor atria. The anastomoses between the donor and recipient atria result in large composite right and left atria, which have a slight hourglass shape (2, 3). The anastomoses between donor and recipient atria are identifiable as regions of increased echo-brightness, visualized best in the parasternal and apical views (Figs. 15.1, 15.2). Although the anastomoses usually appear as a region of increased echo intensity in the middle of the atrial free walls and interatrial septum, the interatrial anastomoses may occasionally protrude into the atrial cavity, suggesting thrombus or vegetations. The two atria are usually in normal sinus rhythm but on occasion develop atrial fibrillation. Although composite atria are potential sources of thrombus formation because of their large size and occasional development of atrial fibrillation, intra-atrial thrombus in the transplanted heart is rare.

The transmitral and transtricuspid Doppler blood flow velocity profiles may demonstrate two atrial systolic signals related to the asynchronous contractions of the recipient and donor atria (4). In the transplanted heart, early diastolic left ventricular filling predomi-nates, and atriosystolic filling is small due to the combination of enlarged atrial size and diminished force of atrial contraction (2).

VENTRICLES

In the early postoperative period, the right ventricle remodels in response to the increased pulmonary vascular resistance, with resultant cavity dilatation, systolic dysfunction (5–7), increased wall thickness, and tricuspid regurgitation (Fig. 15.3). Although pulmonary artery and right atrial pressures decrease by the end of the second week after surgery (Fig. 15.4), the right ventricle usually remains dilated and the increase in right ventricular wall thickness is unchanged during late follow-up (Fig. 15.5). Tricuspid regurgitation of varying severity persists in approximately two-thirds of patients, with regurgitant fractions as high as 60 percent in some patients (5, 7, 8). This early right ventricular pressure and volume overload frequently responds to diuretic therapy, so that right ventricular systolic function returns toward normal during the initial hospitalization.

The transplanted left ventricle also remodels in the early postoperative period but does so differently from the normal left ventricle (9). Cyclosporine produces hypertension that is refractory to medical therapy in 60 to 95 percent of cases (10, 11). During the first postoperative month, the left ventricular wall thickness and mass increase. After the first postoperative month, the left ventricle is characterized by reduced cavity dimensions and volume, abnormal septal motion, and increased wall thickness, but normal total muscle mass (9) (Fig. 15.5). End-diastolic relative wall thickness,

469

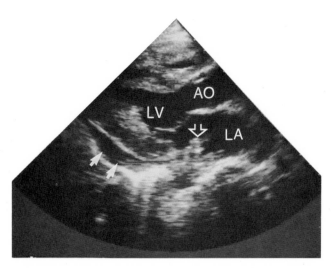

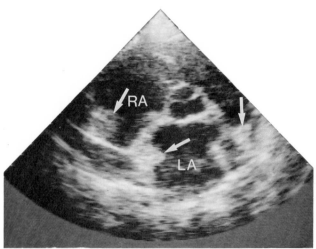

A   **B**

Figure 15.1. Two-dimensional echocardiogram of the long-axis view of the left ventricle from the parasternal region, showing a small pericardial effusion posteriorly (*A, white arrow*) and the left atrial anastomosis (*open arrow*) as an echobright structure in close proximity to the posterior atrioventricular groove (*A*). Two-dimensional echocardiogram of the short axis of the aorta at the aortic valve level showing the recipient-donor anastomosis in the free wall of the right atrium at left, in the interatrial septum, and in the free left atrial wall (*B, arrows*).

which is the ratio of end-diastolic wall thickness and left ventricular radius, is significantly increased, and consequently the end-diastolic volume-to-mass ratio is reduced. However, left ventricular shape described as the ratio of long and short cavity axes is normal. Left ventricular end-systolic meridional and circumferential wall stresses are significantly reduced because of the decreased volume-to-mass ratio. Ejection phase indexes of left ventricular pump function, including ejection frac-

tion, fractional shortening, and mean velocity of circumferential fiber shortening, are normal (12–14). In addition, load-independent indexes of contractility assessed as the slopes of the end-systolic wall stress versus end-systolic volume, and end-systolic stress versus fractional shortening relations are within the normal range.

Left ventricular diastolic function is usually normal in the transplanted heart, but occasionally elevated diastolic filling pressures, prolonged isovolumetric relaxation, and increased transmitral pressure half-times occur, suggesting restrictive physiology (15–17).

PERICARDIUM

Pericardial effusions occur frequently in the postoperative period (Fig. 15.6) and may occasionally result in tamponade. Cyclosporine has recently been suggested to induce pericardial effusions, since the reported incidence of effusions and tamponade is greater than in patients treated with azathioprine (18). Right atrial pressure is often elevated in the transplanted heart, and the usual echocardiographic findings of tamponade, including right atrial and right ventricular collapse, may be absent. However, cardiac tamponade should be suggested by the presence of increased flow velocity paradox in the great arteries and by markedly increased respiratory variation in the Doppler blood flow velocity signals obtained from the superior and inferior cavae.

ATRIOVENTRICULAR VALVES

The mitral and tricuspid valves are echocardiographically normal. However, tricuspid regurgitation of vary-

Figure 15.2. Two-dimensional echocardiogram of the apical four-chamber view showing anastomoses as echobright regions in the free right atrial wall, the interatrial septum, and the free left atrial wall (*arrows*). The composite right and left atria are enlarged and the anastomoses give them a slight hourglass configuration.

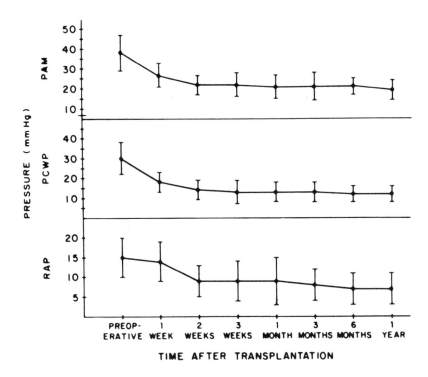

Figure 15.3. Mean pulmonary arterial (PAM), pulmonary capillary wedge (PCWP), and right atrial (RAP) pressures fall by the first week postoperatively and continue to fall over the second week after cardiac transplantation. (Reproduced with permission of the American Heart Association from Bhatia SJS, Kirshenbaum JM, Shemin RJ, et al: Time course of resolution of pulmonary hypertension and left ventricular remodelling after orthotopic cardiac transplantation. Circulation 76:819–826, 1987.)

ing severity is detectable by pulsed wave and colorflow Doppler in approximately two-thirds of patients at follow-up (5, 7, 8). Measurement of the velocity of the regurgitant jet by continuous wave Doppler after localizing the jet with Doppler color flow enables accurate noninvasive calculation of pulmonary artery pressures from the Bernoulli equation (19).

A recent study reported mitral regurgitation in the majority of transplant recipients, which was suggested to be related to the abnormal atrial contribution to mitral valve leaflet coaptation (3). However, other investigators have detected only mild to moderate regurgitation in a minority of patients using pulsed and color Doppler (7). A preliminary report has suggested that the new development or increase in severity of mitral regurgitation corresponds to rejection on endomyocardial biopsy (20).

SEMILUNAR VALVES AND GREAT ARTERIES

Although the pulmonic valve appears anatomically normal echocardiographically, mild pulmonic insufficiency is frequently detected by color flow Doppler, with a similar incidence in normal patients (21). Severe pulmonic insufficiency is rare, even in the early postoperative period, in our experience.

Aortic regurgitation occurs sporadically early after transplantation, even when the aortic valve appears normal echocardiographically, but it diminishes in incidence and severity at serial postoperative follow-up. The anastomoses between the donor and recipient

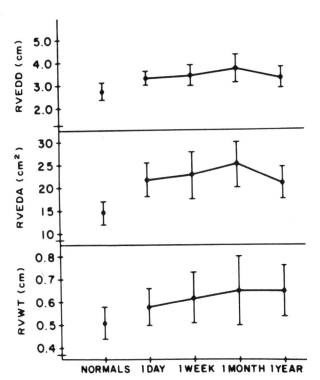

Figure 15.4. Right ventricular diastolic diameter (RVEDD), right ventricular end-diastolic cavity area (RVEDA), and right ventricular wall thickness (RVWT) all increase above normal over the course of the first month following transplantation.

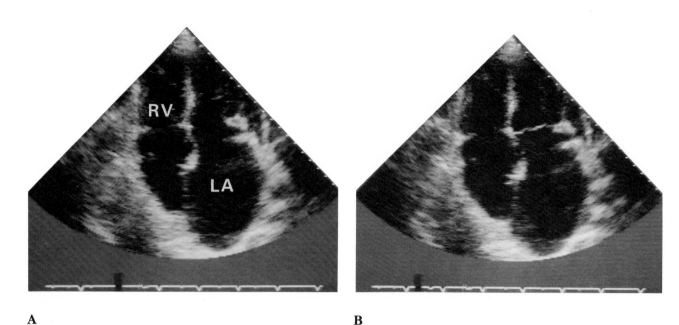

A   **B**

Figure 15.5. Two-dimensional echocardiogram of the apical four-chamber view in diastole (*A*) and in systole (*B*) from a patient one month following cardiac transplantation. The right ventricle is enlarged and the right ventricular volume changes little from systole to diastole. Septal motion is markedly abnormal in diastole, and the right and left atria are dilated.

great arteries appear normal by two-dimensional echocardiography, and flow across them is invariably normal by Doppler. We have detected by Doppler echocardiography only one case of mild stenosis across a pulmonary artery anastomosis, with a transanastomotic gradient of 15 mm Hg.

CARDIAC REJECTION

A major aim in the management of cardiac transplant patients has been the development of a specific, non-invasive diagnostic marker of moderate to severe rejection. Left ventricular diastolic function has been reported to be abnormal during rejection, manifested by shortened isovolumetric relaxation time, decreased mitral pressure half-time, and increased transmitral blood flow velocity during the rapid filling phase. However, these measurements of diastolic function are difficult to interpret because they are altered by variations in recipient atrial contraction, heart rate, and left ventricular loading conditions (16, 22, 23). Rejection episodes in patients maintained on cyclosporine in contrast to azathioprine are not associated with interstitial myocardial edema, and therefore are not associated with changes in left ventricular wall thickness or mass (24–26).

Left ventricular systolic function assessed by ejection phase indexes and load-independent indexes often remains unchanged during episodes of moderate to even severe rejection (13, 26, 27) (Figs. 15.7, 15.8). Thus, rejection in patients on cyclosporine is not characterized

by any consistent alteration in left ventricular (LV) architecture, hemodynamics, or systolic function, although LV diastolic compliance may be reduced (26).

SUMMARY

We have described the echocardiographic assessment of the transplanted heart based on experience with 50 patients. The composite atria are dilated and remain so, while the two ventricles adapt differently to their respective circulations. Tricuspid and pulmonary regurgitation are common, whereas left-sided valvular regurgitation is comparatively uncommon. In the early postoperative period, the right ventricle is dilated and contractile function is seriously impaired. However, as the pulmonary artery pressure falls, the tricuspid regurgitation diminishes in severity and right ventricular function improves. Left ventricular size is invariably normal, and septal motion is consistently abnormal, but contractile function is usually excellent throughout the early postoperative period, provided severe rejection causing hemmorhagic myocardial necrosis does not supervene. The majority of patients maintained on cyclosporine develop hypertension, which is associated with development of increased LV wall thickness. Accelerated atherosclerosis in the coronary arteries of the transplanted heart may result in important coronary arterial stenoses, regional myocardial ischemia, and development of regional wall motion abnormalities detectable by two-dimensional echocardiography.

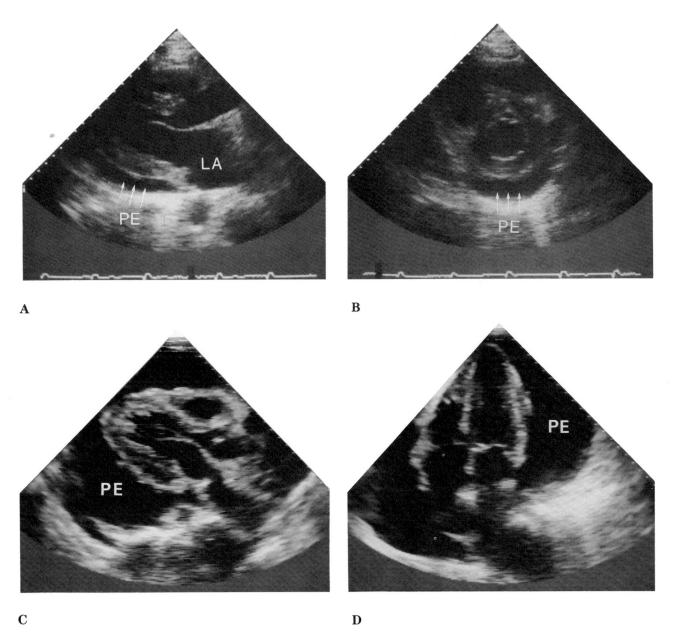

A

B

C

D

Figure 15.6. Two-dimensional echocardiogram from two patients three months after cardiac transplantation with pericardial effusions. On the left, a moderate-size pericardial effusion is visible posteriorly in the long-axis view (*A*) and short-axis view (*B*) of the left ventricle from the left parasternal region. On the right is a large circumferential pericardial effusion in the long-axis view (*C*) and in the apical four-chamber view (*D*).

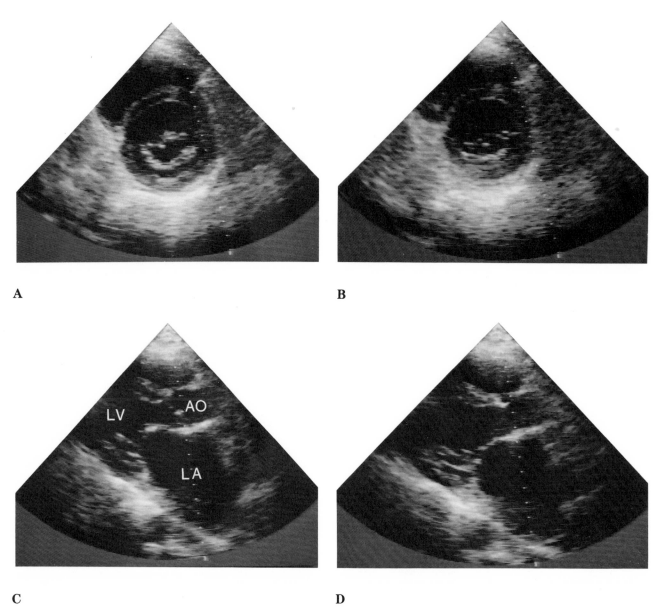

A

B

C

D

Figure 15.7. Two-dimensional echocardiogram from a patient with an acute rejection episode following cardiac transplantation. Immunosuppression therapy included prednisone and cyclosporine. Two-dimensional short-axis views of the left ventricle at mitral valve level in diastole (*A*) and in systole (*B*), and in the long axis in diastole (*C*) and in systole (*D*) show normal left ventricular wall thickness but very poor contractile function.

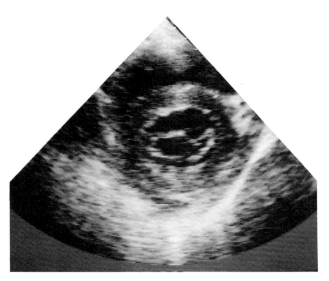

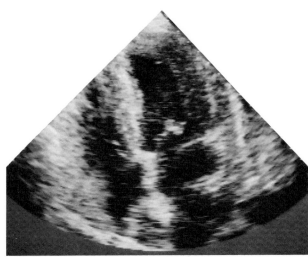

A   **B**

Figure 15.8.   Two-dimensional echocardiogram from a patient with chronic rejection following noncompliance with anti-rejection and antihypertensive therapy. The left ventricle is visualized in short axis in diastole (A) and in the apical four-chamber view (B), showing severe left ventricular hypertrophy and only moderately impaired contractile function.

REFERENCES

1. Fowler MB, Schroeder JS. Current status of cardiac transplantation. Mod Concepts Cardiovasc Dis 1986;55:37–41.
2. Suarez JM, Zoghbi WA, Leon CA, et al. Left ventricular filling dynamics in the transplanted heart: Assessment by Doppler echocardiography, abstracted. J Heart Transplant 1986;5:379.
3. Stevenson LW, Dadourian BJ, Kobashigawa J, et al. Mitral regurgitation after cardiac transplantation. Am J Cardiol 1987;60:119–122.
4. Valantine HA, Appleton CP, Hatle LK, et al. Influence of recipient atrial contraction on left ventricular filling dynamics of the transplanted heart assessed by Doppler echocardiography. Am J Cardiol 1987;59:1159–1163.
5. Bhatia SJS, Kirshenbaum JM, Shemin RJ, et al. Time course of resolution of pulmonary hypertension and right ventricular remodeling after orthotopic cardiac transplantation. Circulation 1987;76:819–826.
6. Hosenpud JD, Normal DJ, Cobanoglu A, et al. Serial echocardiographic findings early after heart transplantation: Evidence for reversible right ventricular dysfunction and myocardial edema. J Heart Transplant 1987;6:343–347.
7. Suarez JM, Leon CA, Zoghbi WA, et al. Valvular dysfunction in the transplanted heart, abstracted. J Heart Transplant 1986;5:392.
8. Lewen MK, Bryg RJ, Miller LW, et al. Tricuspid regurgitation by Doppler echocardiography after orthotopic cardiac transplantation. Am J Cardiol 1987;59:1371–1374.
9. Bhatia SJS, Schoen FJ, Shemin RJ, et al. Left ventricular architecture load and contractility after orthotopic cardiac transplantation, abstracted. Clin Res 1988; in press.
10. Thompson ME, Shapiro AP, Johnsen A-M, et al. The contrasting effects of cyclosporine-A and azathioprine on arterial blood pressure and renal function following cardiac transplantation. Int J Cardiol 1986;11:219–229.
11. Greenberg ML, Uretsky BF, Reddy PS, et al. Long-term hemodynamic follow-up of cardiac transplant patients treated with cyclosporine and prednisone. Circulation 1985;71:487–494.
12. Frist WH, Stinson EB, Oyer PE, et al. Long term hemodynamic results after cardiac transplantation. J Thorac Cardiovasc Surg 1987;94:685–693.
13. Corcos T, Tamburino C, Leger P, et al. Early and late hemodynamic evaluation after cardiac transplantation: A study of 28 cases. J Am Coll Cardiol 1988;11:264–269.

14. Lang RM, Borow KM, Neumann A. Systemic vascular resistance: An unreliable index of left ventricular afterload. Circulation 1986;74:1114–1123.
15. Valantine H, Appleton C, Hatle L, et al. Doppler echocardiographic evaluation of restrictive cardiomyopathy in heart transplant recipients, abstracted. J Heart Transplant 1986;5:374.
16. Valantine H, Fowler MB, Hunt SA, et al. Changes in Doppler echocardiographic indexes of left ventricular function as potential markers of acute cardiac rejection. Circulation (Suppl V) 1987;76:86–92.
17. Humen DP, McKenzie FN, Kostuk WJ. Restricted myocardial compliance one year following cardiac transplantation. Heart Transplant 1984;3:341–345.
18. Hastillo A, Thompson JA, Lower RR, Szentpetery S, Hess MC. Cyclosporine-induced pericardial effusion after cardiac transplantation. Am J Cardiol 1987;59:1220–1222.
19. Hsiung MC, Nanda NC, Kirklin J, et al. Value of color Doppler assessment of pulmonary artery pressure in cardiac transplant patients. J Am Coll Cardiol 1986;7:140A.
20. Hsiung MC, Nande NC, Kirklin JK, et al. Usefulness of color Doppler in the early detection of cardiac allograft rejection, abstracted. Circulation (Suppl II) 1986;74:180.
21. Kostucki W, Vandenbossche J-L, Friar TA, Englert M. Pulsed Doppler regurgitant flow patterns of normal valves. Am J Cardiol 1986;58:309–314.
22. Pope JC III, Zumbro GL, Battey LL, et al. Isovolumetric relaxation period as an indication of cardiac allograft rejection, abstracted. J Heart Transplant 1986;5:380.
23. Dawkins KD, Oldershaw PJ, Billingham ME, et al. Changes in diastolic function as a noninvasive marker of cardiac allograft rejection. Heart Transplant 1984;3:286–294.
24. Sagar KB, Hastillo A, Wolfgang TC, et al. Left ventricular mass by M-mode echocardiography in cardiac transplant patients with acute rejection. Circulation (Suppl II) 1981;64:216–220.
25. Dubroff JM, Clark MB, Wong CYH, et al. Changes in left ventricular mass associated with the onset of acute rejection after cardiac transplantation. Heart Transplant 1984;3:105–109.
26. Bhatia SJS, Schoen FJ, Shemin RJ, et al. Effects of moderate to severe rejection on left ventricular function after orthotopic cardiac transplantation, abstracted. Clin Res 1988;in press.
27. Paulsen W, Magid N, Sagar K, et al. Left ventricular function of heart allografts during acute rejection: An echocardiographic assessment. Heart Transplant 1985;4:525–529.

16

Echophonocardiography and Phonocardiography

Aubrey Leatham
Peter Mills
Paul Oldershaw

ECHOPHONOCARDIOGRAPHY

Echoes taken simultaneously with phonocardiograms have been invaluable in determining or confirming the origin of heart sounds (1, 2) because no other timing device can display the exact moment of valve opening and closing.

First Heart Sound

The mechanism of physiologic splitting of the first heart sound has been confirmed to be due to asynchronous closure of the mitral and tricuspid valves (1–3) (Fig. 16.1). The application of echophonocardiography to analysis of the first heart sound in bundle branch block has demonstrated that right bundle branch block may be divided into proximal block when tricuspid closure is delayed and peripheral block (occurring at arborization level and more likely to be associated with cardiac pathology) when there is little or no delay of tricuspid closure (4, 5). In left bundle branch block mitral closure is seldom delayed, suggesting that the block is peripheral.

Ejection Sounds

Echophonocardiography has demonstrated that the aortic ejection sound in a normally functioning bicuspid aortic valve is due to the final abrupt halt of the opening of the aortic valve (Fig. 16.2) (6). In the presence of clinical left ventricular outflow tract stenosis, an ejection sound indicates that the site of

obstruction is at the valvar level and that the aortic valve leaflets are mobile.

Second Heart Sound

The second heart sound, like the first, has two components—the aortic (A_2) and pulmonary (P_2)—caused by asynchrony between right and left ventricular contraction and thus right- and left-sided semilunar valve closure. The aortic component normally precedes pulmonary closure, and there is increased separation on inspiration mainly because of delay of the pulmonary component (7). By recording A_2 and P_2 clearly, the duration of right and left ventricular systole in the same heart cycle can be compared, the effect of respiration on the loading of the right and left ventricles can be estimated, and the intensity of the two components can be compared to assist in establishing the diagnosis of pulmonary hypertension.

Opening Snaps

Opening snaps of the mitral and tricuspid valve leaflets can be identified by their synchrony with the final halt of the opening of the anterior leaflets of these valves on the echocardiogram and thus may be differentiated from third heart sounds, which occur later.

Ventricular Filling Sounds

In addition to valve sounds, ventricular filling sounds can also be recorded. Approximately 150 ms after the

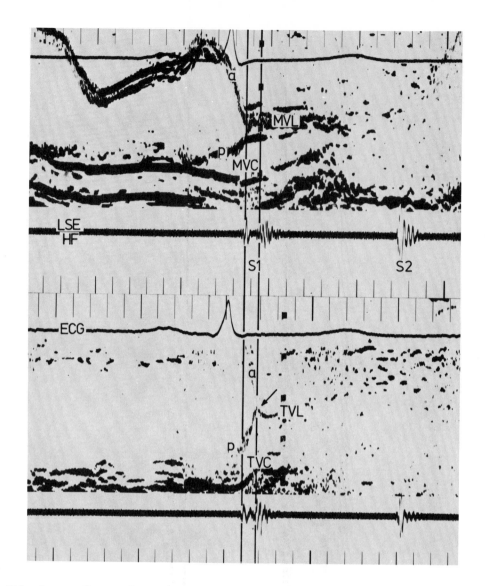

Figure 16.1. Echophonocardiogram demonstrating physiologic splitting of the first heart sound. The onset of the first component of the first sound coincides with the final halt of the closing mitral valve (MVC) and the second component with the final halt of a closing tricuspid valve (TVC). ECG = electrocardiogram; MVL = mitral valve leaflet; p = posterior mitral valve leaflet; LSE = left sternal edge; HF = high-frequency recording; TVL = tricuspid valve leaflet; a = anterior mitral valve leaflet; S1 = first heart sound; S2 = second heart sound. (From Sleight P, Van Jones J. Scientific Foundations of Cardiology. Portsmouth, NH: Heinemann, 1984. Used with permission.)

second heart sound, rapid ventricular filling may cause vibrations of sufficient intensity to be audible as the third heart sound. A third heart sound may be heard in healthy children and young adults but rarely in healthy subjects over 40 years; its presence in such subjects usually indicates ventricular disease.

Contraction of the atria may produce an atrial sound, fourth heart sound, in late diastole from vibrations caused by the resultant ventricular filling. In patients with left ventricular hypertrophy, atrial contraction is often more vigorous than normal, and the resultant increased ventricular filling may be associated with an audible fourth heart sound. Such vibrations may occasionally be audible in healthy patients.

Thus, heart sounds can be classified echophonocardiographically as 1) valve sounds (first sounds, ejection sounds, second sounds, or opening snaps, all of which are sharp high-frequency sounds) or 2) ventricular filling sounds (third and atrial, or fourth, sounds, which are dull low-frequency sounds that differ in quality on auscultation to the valve sounds).

CLINICAL USEFULNESS OF PHONOCARDIOGRAPHY

Phonocardiography can still make an important contribution to noninvasive diagnosis. The minimal number of simultaneous information channels is four; the most

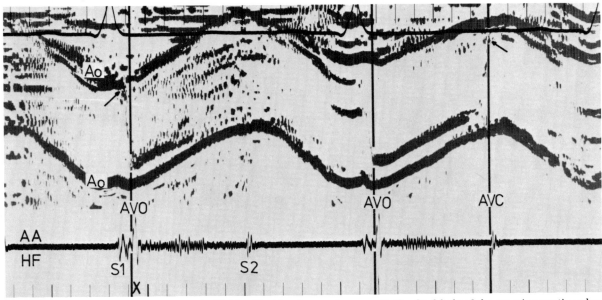

Figure 16.2. Aortic (Ao) ejection sound (X) identified by its synchrony with the final halt of the opening aortic valve (AVO). It is associated with a normally functioning but bicuspid aortic valve. AA = aortic area; HF = high-frequency recording; AVC = aortic valve closure; S1 = first heart sound; S2 = second heart sound. (From Sleight P, Van Jones J. Scientific Foundations of Cardiology. Portsmouth, NH: Heinemann, 1984. Used with permission.)

useful combination for diagnosis is two phonocardiograms, a carotid pulse tracing, and an electrocardiogram. A simultaneous echocardiogram may be necessary to identify the origin of a heart sound, but thus far the importance of echophonograms has been mainly as a research tool. The paper speed should be 100 mm/s, with good definition of frequencies between 30 and 400 cycles. With suitable recording apparatus, the following clinical problems can be resolved by phonocardiography.

Differentiation of Atrial Sounds from Physiologic Splitting of the First Sound

Differentiation of atrial sounds from physiologic splitting of the first heart sound can be clinically difficult, particularly when the first component of the first sound (mitral closure) is soft, which occurs if the PR interval is long enough to allow atrial contraction and relaxation to cause apposition of the mitral valve leaflets before ventricular contraction. In this situation the first component of the first sound normally has a low frequency. Such a low-frequency component has no clinical significance per se, but identification of an audible atrial sound is important because it always denotes abnormal left ventricular function from hypertrophy or fibrosis. Simultaneous low-frequency and high-frequency phonocardiograms and electrocardiograms demonstrate the relations of such vibrations to the P and QRS waves of the electrocardiogram (Fig. 16.3). Alternatively, an apex cardiogram may be used to show an abnormally large A wave.

Identification of Ejection Sounds

Aortic ejection sounds coincide with peak opening of aortic valve leaflets (see Fig. 16.2). If an echocardiographic channel is not available, a simultaneous indirect carotid pulse recording will show the ejection sound coinciding with the moment of the carotid upstroke. An isolated aortic ejection sound indicates that the aortic valve is bicuspid and a potential site for bacterial endocarditis and calcification in later life, leading to aortic stenosis (6).

Pulmonary ejection sounds may be difficult to differentiate from the second component of the split first sound. High-frequency phonocardiograms will show that the ejection sound follows tricuspid closure and dramatically diminishes or disappears during inspiration when the pulmonary valve is forced upward in presystole by vigorous atrial contraction (Fig. 16.4). An early pulmonary ejection sound that disappears on inspiration indicates pulmonary valve stenosis.

Second Heart Sound

An understanding of the second heart sound (8) is the key to determining the significance of heart murmurs, which may be present in approximately 90 percent of children younger than 15 years of age. Physiologic or innocent murmurs are usually soft but may occasionally be moderately loud (3/6) and thus cause diagnostic difficulties. These are invariably midsystolic ejection murmurs, and a phonocardiogram will immediately disclose this pattern and differentiate them from pansystolic murmurs, which always have a pathologic cause.

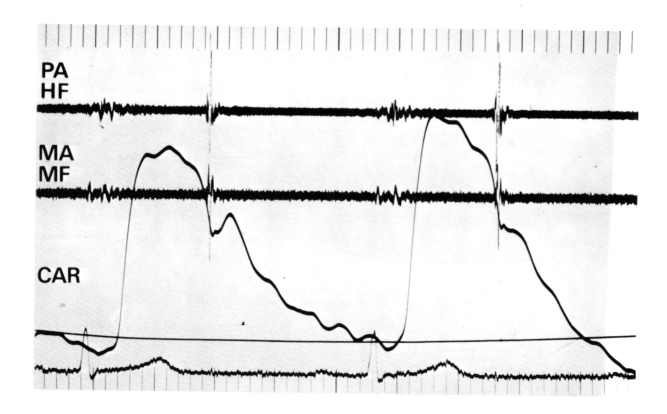

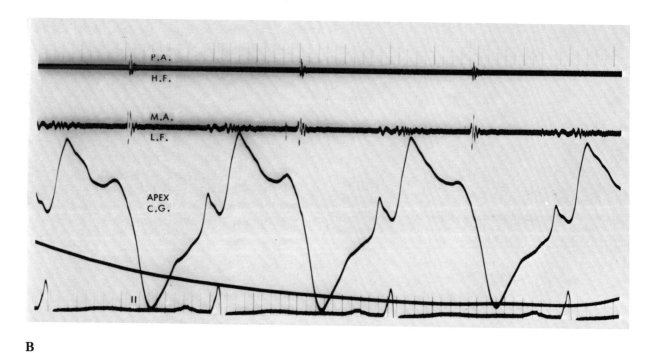

B

Figure 16.3. (A) Low-frequency mitral component of a physiologically split first sound. (B) Atrial sound and abnormal A wave of apex cardiogram (APEX CG) preceding ventricular systole is always abnormal. PA = pulmonary area; MA = mitral area; HF = high-frequency recording; LF = low-frequency recording; MF = medium-frequency recording; CAR = carotid-arterial tracing.

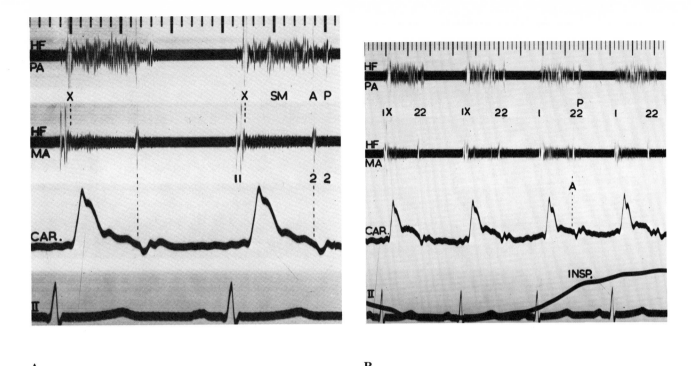

A

B

Figure 16.4. (A) Pulmonary ejection sound (X) occurring soon after the tricuspid component of the first sound in a patient with pulmonary valve stenosis. (B) Identification of a pulmonary ejection sound by its disappearance on inspiration. HF = high-frequency recording; PA = pulmonary area; MA = mitral area; S1 = first heart sound; S2 = second heart sound; SM = systolic murmur; A = aortic component of second heart sound; P = pulmonary component of second heart sound; CAR = carotid arterial tracing; INSP = inspiration. (From Leatham A. Auscultation of the Heart and Phonocardiography (2nd edition). London: Churchill Livingstone, 1975. Used with permission.)

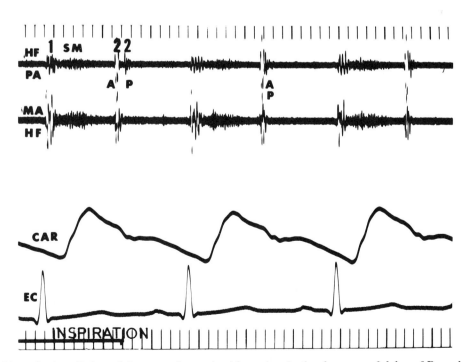

Figure 16.5. Physiologic splitting of the second sound, wide on inspiration because of delay of P_2 and nearly fused in expiration excluding atrial septal defect and pulmonary stenosis in this child with an ejection systolic murmur. HF = high-frequency recording; PA = pulmonary area; MA = mitral area; 1 = first heart sound; SM = systolic murmur; 2 = second heart sound; A = aortic component of second heart sound; P = pulmonary component of second heart sound; CAR = carotid arterial tracing; EC = echocardiogram. (From Leatham A. Auscultation of the Heart and Phonocardiography (2nd edition). London: Churchill Livingstone, 1975. Used with permission.)

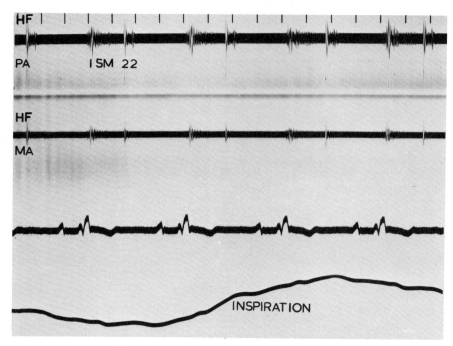

Figure 16.6. Wide splitting of the second sound because of nearly equal inspiratory delay of both A_2 and P_2 in a patient with atrial septal defect. HF = high-frequency recording; PA = pulmonary area; MA = mitral area; 1 = first heart sound; 2 = second heart sound; SM = systolic murmur. (From Leatham A. Auscultation of the Heart and Phonocardiography (2nd edition). London: Churchill Livingstone, 1975. Used with permission.)

Physiologic (innocent) ejection murmurs are maximal over the right ventricular outflow tract at the left sternal edge and are thought to be simply physiologic right ventricular outflow ejection vibrations. Although these murmurs may often be identified because they have a low-frequency grunting vibratory quality, they may sometimes be confused with ejection murmurs from increased right ventricular stroke volume (as in left to right shunts at atrial level) or from right ventricular outflow tract obstruction. In either case careful analysis of respiratory splitting of the second sound will establish, with few exceptions, whether the murmur is normal or abnormal. While inspiratory splitting of the second heart sound in normal subjects may be very wide, in the expiratory phase of continuous respiration with the subject reclining 30 to 40 degrees, splitting is barely discernible, or the two components are coincident (Fig. 16.5). This difference is particularly evident during slow, deep breathing. Splitting of the second heart sound in atrial septal defects is wide throughout the respiratory cycle (Fig. 16.6); in right ventricular outflow tract obstruction P_2 is late (Fig. 16.7), and the width of splitting is closely related to the severity of obstruction (Figs. 16.7, 16.8) (9). Phonocardiography is helpful in these respects for all but the most practiced auscultators and renders diagnostic cardiac catheterization unnecessary in most cases. Echocardiography has no comparable role in assessing pulmonary stenosis, but it is invaluable in diagnosing atrial septal defect.

In an acyanotic infant with a loud, long systolic murmur and no symptoms, the diagnosis often rests between a small hemodynamically unimportant ventricular septal defect and right ventricular outflow tract obstruction, either at a valvar or infundibular level. A late pulmonic component of the second heart sound (P_2) will immediately indicate pulmonary stenosis, but in tetralogy of Fallot P_2 is usually absent. Thus, before diagnosing a relatively unimportant ventricular septal defect and ruling out tetralogy of Fallot, it is essential to identify both components of the second heart sound. This is usually easier in the pulmonary area at a distance from the loud ventricular septal defect murmur. A high-speed phonocardiogram recorded at 100 to 200 mm/s may be necessary (Fig. 16.9). This differentiation is particularly useful in the very young patient when the electrocardiogram and x-ray film may be difficult to interpret and when a small ventricular septal defect may be difficult to detect on standard echocardiography.

In pulmonary hypertension P_2 is abnormally loud, and this is disclosed by an abnormal A_2/P_2 ratio in the pulmonary area and transmission of P_2 to the apex (Fig. 16.10). Normally even in the pulmonary area P_2 is dwarfed by the preceding A_2, and P_2 is seldom obvious at the apex in a normal subject, even in infancy. It

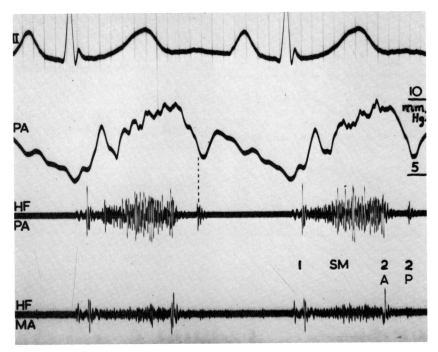

Figure 16.7. Pulmonary stenosis. Delay of P_2 is in proportion to the severity of the stenosis. HF = high-frequency recording; PA = pulmonary area; MA = mitral area; 1 = first heart sound; SM = systolic murmur; 2 = second heart sound; A = aortic component of second heart sound; P = pulmonary component of second heart sound. (From Leatham A. Auscultation of the Heart and Phonocardiography (2nd edition). London: Churchill Livingstone, 1975. Used with permission.)

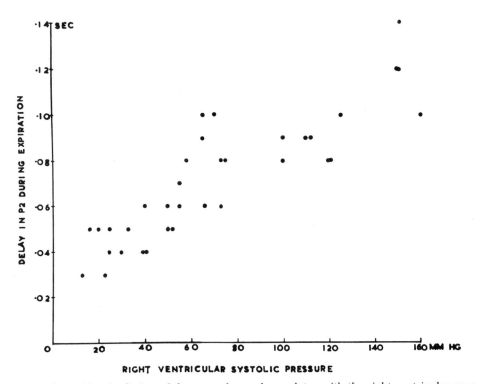

Figure 16.8. Delay of P_2 width of splitting of the second sound correlates with the right ventricular pressure and thus indicates the severity of the obstruction. (From Leatham A. Auscultation of the Heart and Phonocardiography (2nd edition). London: Churchill Livingstone, 1975. Used with permission.)

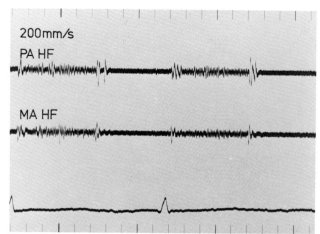

Figure 16.9. Ventricular septal defect with left to right shunt. Pulmonary stenosis, including tetralogy of Fallot, is excluded by the physiologic splitting of the second sound. PA = pulmonary area; MA = mitral area; HF = high-frequency recording. (From Leatham A. Auscultation of the Heart and Phonocardiography (2nd edition). London: Churchill Livingstone, 1975. Used with permission.)

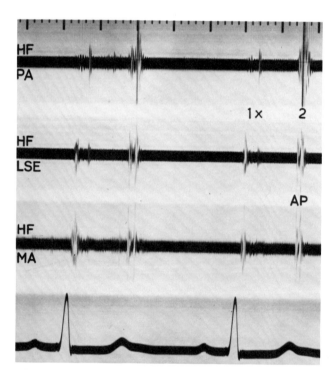

Figure 16.10. Pulmonary hypertension (Eisenmenger patent ductus arteriosus). Abnormal A_2/P_2 ratio and P_2 is transmitted to the mitral area. Also delayed ejection sound (X). HF = high-frequency recording; PA = pulmonary area; LSE = left sternal edge; MA = mitral area; 1 = first heart sound; 2 = second heart sound; A = aortic component of second heart sound; P = pulmonary component of second heart sound (From Leatham A. Auscultation of the Heart and Phonocardiography (2nd edition). London: Churchill Livingstone, 1975. Used with permission.)

should be remembered that the only other cause of a truly loud P_2 is an atrial septal defect, even with normal pulmonary pressures, when the hyperkinetic right ventricle produces a very sharp pulmonary artery pressure pulse with a rapid increase and decrease. In mitral regurgitation, however, A_2 may be abnormally soft when P_2 may become the louder component in the pulmonary area, even in the absence of pulmonary hypertension.

Systolic Murmurs

Because apical systolic murmurs may originate from the left ventricular outflow tract (ejection systolic murmur) or the mitral valve (regurgitant systolic murmur), some method of differentiation is needed (10). Ejection systolic murmurs are always midsystolic, finishing before the aortic component of the second sound (Fig. 16.11), whereas mitral systolic murmurs are almost always pansystolic, often with a late systolic crescendo and the murmur continuing up to and engulfing the aortic component of the second sound (Fig. 16.12). With mild mitral regurgitation, the murmur may be confined to late systole, but it invariably continues through and engulfs A_2. In mitral regurgitation there is shortening of left ventricular systole and A_2 may occur early. Thus, the murmur may appear short, and if P_2 is the dominant component of the second sound, the murmur may appear to stop before the second sound. A phonocardiogram from the apex with a simultaneous tracing from the pulmonary area and a simultaneous carotid pulse, or aortic valve echo, is needed to identify A_2 under these circumstances.

Thus, phonocardiography is very useful for differen-

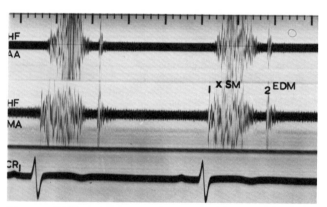

Figure 16.11. Aortic stenosis. Ejection systolic murmur finishing before A_2 at both aortic (AA) and mitral (MA) areas. Also ejection sound (X). HF = high-frequency recording; 1 = first heart sound; 2 = second heart sound; SM = systolic murmur; EDM = early diastolic murmur. (From Leatham A. Auscultation of the Heart and Phonocardiography (2nd edition). London: Churchill Livingstone, 1975. Used with permission.)

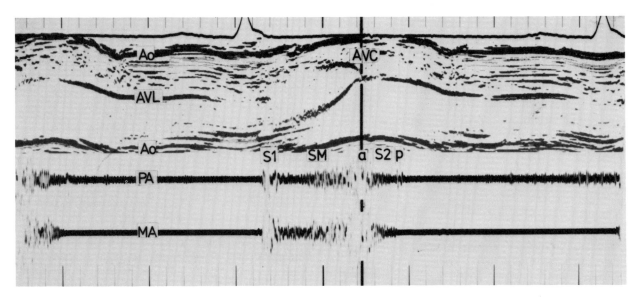

Figure 16.12. Mitral regurgitation pan (sometimes late) systolic murmur engulfing A_2, identified by a simultaneous phonocardiogram in the aortic (Ao) or pulmonary areas (PA) or an aortic valve echo. AVL = aortic valve leaflet; AVC = aortic valve closure; MA = mitral area; S1 = first heart sound; S2 = second heart sound; SM = systolic murmur; a = aortic component of second heart sound; p = pulmonary component of second heart sound. (From Leatham A. Auscultation of the Heart and Phonocardiography (2nd edition). London: Churchill Livingstone, 1975. Used with permission.)

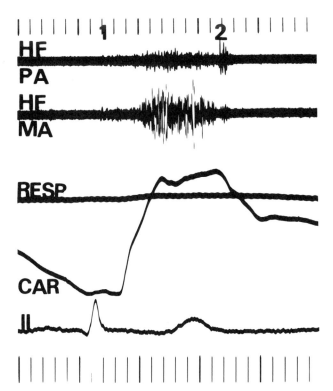

Figure 16.13. Hypertrophic obstructive cardiomyopathy with ejection systolic murmur shifted to the right but stopping before A_2. HF = high-frequency recording; PA = pulmonary area; MA = mitral area; RESP = respiratory murmur; CAR = carotid arterial tracing. (From Leatham A. Auscultation of the Heart and Phonocardiography (2nd edition). London: Churchill Livingstone, 1975. Used with permission.)

tiating aortic stenosis and mitral regurgitation, two common conditions in middle and old age. Echocardiography by itself may occasionally be misleading, particularly in the presence of aortic stenosis without heavy calcification or nonrheumatic mitral regurgitation when mitral leaflet prolapse may not be recognized. Left ventricular outflow tract obstruction from hypertrophic cardiomyopathy may be misdiagnosed as mitral regurgitation, but the phonocardiogram will show that the systolic murmur, though shifted to the right, stops before A_2 (Fig. 16.13).

SYSTOLIC TIME INTERVALS

Measurement of systolic time intervals is a method of assessing left ventricular function in terms of the timing of well-defined events in the cardiac cycle. It is entirely noninvasive and therefore has the advantage that repeated measurements can be made either in the basal state or after interventions. This technique has been used extensively to investigate clinical left ventricular disease and has been the subject of several reviews (11–13). The ability to express left ventricular function in terms of single numbers has advantages, but it must be stressed that this simplicity may conceal complex underlying changes in the circulatory state. Systolic time intervals have largely been superceded by two-dimensional Doppler echocardiography.

Measurement of Systolic Time Intervals

Three systolic time intervals are commonly measured (Chapter 5) (14):

1. left ventricular ejection time (LVET) (the time interval over which blood is ejected into the aorta);
2. electromechanical systole (Q-A$_2$) (the time from the onset of electrical activation of the left ventricle until the start of relaxation);
3. the pre-ejection period (PEP) (the interval between the onset of electromechanical systole and the onset of ejection).

These time intervals are based on the following measurements (see Fig. 16.1):

1. The electrocardiogram is used to determine the time of onset of electrical activation of the left ventricle. In most subjects this is the beginning of the Q wave in lead II or V$_6$, but not in patients with left bundle branch block and Wolff-Parkinson-White syndrome where there is a delta wave or during right ventricular pacing. In all these conditions the start of left ventricular activation is delayed with respect to the onset of the QRS complex by an unknown duration.
2. The phonocardiogram is used to determine the timing of aortic valve closure from the aortic component of the second heart sound (A$_2$). Phonocardiograms should be recorded from the region of the precordium where splitting of the second heart sound is clinically most obvious, which is usually the second left intercostal space. Normally, A$_2$ is the first component of the second sound. However, in patients with left bundle branch block, left ventricular disease, or severe hypertension, splitting may be reversed such that P$_2$ precedes A$_2$. In severe calcific aortic valve stenosis, the aortic component (A$_2$) of the second sound may be absent. Recordings should be obtained with a high-frequency filter (greater than 100 Hz). Measurement of the timing of heart sounds is, by convention, from the onset of the first high-frequency component.
3. The indirect carotid pulse is used to measure left ventricular ejection time. Recordings are usually obtained from the right carotid artery. The onset of left ventricular ejection corresponds with the start of the rapid upstroke of the carotid pulse; this is frequently preceded by a small upward displacement during isovolumetric contraction, so that ideally the record should show both events. The end of ejection corresponds to the dicrotic notch or incisura, whose nadir in the central aortic trace is synchronous with A$_2$. Transmission of the pulse to the carotid artery takes approximately 20 ms, but during this interval there is no significant change in the waveform (13). This is not the case for indirect pulses recorded from more peripheral arteries, which are not therefore suitable for measuring the systolic time intervals. The specifications of the transducer are important because if the time constant is less than 2.5 s, partial differentiation of the record may occur, causing significant errors in the timing.

General Points

Records are made photographically at a paper speed of 100 mm/s. To minimize the effects of respiration, measurements should be made over at least 10 successive beats and the results averaged.

Determinants of the Systolic Time Intervals

Heart Rate

Heart rate was recognized as a determinant of the ejection time as long ago as 1874 by Garrod (15). Exact relations between heart rate and the different systolic time intervals have not been defined in physical terms and thus regression equations must be used to compensate for variation in heart rate (Table 16.1). The most commonly used regression equations are those proposed by Weissler and colleagues (16), which form the basis of a "correction" for heart rate and consist of expressing values as those predicted to occur at zero heart rate. Left ventricular ejection time index (LVETI) is defined as:

$$LVETI = LVET + 1.7 \times heart\ rate,$$

and the normal mean value is 413 ± 14 ms (17). PEP is significantly less dependent on heart rate than either ejection time or Q-A$_2$ interval (see Table 16.1). Additional minor differences exist in children (18) and adults older than 65 years (19). The conventionally used regression equations were derived from a large population of normal subjects and are based on spontaneous variation in heart rate, recorded fasting between 0800 and 1000 hours. Other workers (20) also established regression equations using exercise to vary heart rate, but the slope of the regression lines differed from that of Weissler and associates (16). Harley and

Table 16.1. Calculation of Systolic Time Index Values from Resting Regression Equation

Sex	Equation	Normal index	Standard deviation
M	QS$_2$I = 2.1 HR + QS$_2$	546	14
F	QS$_2$I = 2.0 HR + QS$_2$	549	14
M	LVETI = 1.7 HR + LVET	413	10
F	LVETI = 1.6 HR + LVET	418	11
M	PEPI = 0.4 HR + PEP	131	10
F	PEPI = 0.4 HR + PEP	133	10

I = index; HR = heart rate; M = male; F = female; LVET = left ventricular ejection time; PEP = pre-ejection period.

co-workers (21) studied patients with complete heart block in whom the heart rate was varied using a ventricular pacemaker. These workers found yet another relation between heart rate and ejection time. It follows, therefore, that any correction for heart rate is arbitrary and limited to the conditions from which the regression equation is generated. A spontaneous increase in heart rate is brought about by a combination of parasympathetic withdrawal and sympathetic stimulation (22), of which the latter might have a separate effect on left ventricular contraction independent of any change resulting from the increase in heart rate. If a similar change in heart rate was brought about by parasympathetic withdrawal alone, the effects on left ventricular contraction may not necessarily be identical to those predicted by the standard regression equation. This possibility must be borne in mind when interpreting the results of any study in which drug-induced changes in heart rate occur.

A number of workers avoided the application of population regression equations by correcting for heart rate in individual subjects. This has been done by either pre-testing individuals with graded exercise tests and atrial pacing (23, 24) or using increasing doses of atropine (25). Interestingly in this latter study, the regression relationships showed little intra-subject variability but a larger degree of inter-subject variability.

Left Ventricular Filling

Head-up tilt or the application of venous tourniquets prolong PEP and LVETI (26). It is difficult to determine the mechanism of such changes because a number of alterations in central hemodynamics occur. These include a reduction in venous return and stroke volume as well as in left ventricular end-diastolic pressure and volume. These changes are inter-related although in no predictable way. Thus, a reduction in end-diastolic pressure is associated with a corresponding decrease in volume, the exact relation depending on the range of pressures involved and the nonlinear left ventricular pressure-volume curve of the individual patient. A reduction in end-diastolic volume may be associated with a reduction in the force of left ventricular contraction owing to Starling's law, whereas a reduction in end-diastolic pressure is associated with an increased pressure gradient across the aortic valve and, thus, with prolongation of PEP (27), unrelated to any separate change in left ventricular function that it might cause.

Peripheral Resistance

The effects of major changes in peripheral resistance can be detected with systolic time intervals. An in-

crease in aortic pressure induced by methoxamine or angiotensin (28, 29) prolongs ejection time and PEP, whereas a reduction in aortic pressure by amyl nitrate administration shortens both (30).

Inotropic State

Systolic time intervals are altered by administration of drugs with a positive inotropic effect. Such a positive inotropic effect implies one or more of a number of changes in left ventricular function occurring independently of any alteration in left ventricular filling. Such changes include increases in the rate of tension and pressure development, peak wall tension, and peak rate of wall movement during ejection. The effects of positive inotropic drugs on the systolic time intervals, however, are consistent and show a reduction in the pre-ejection period and in the Q-A_2 interval. A reduction in ejection time usually occurs because associated hemodynamic changes such as an increase in stroke volume (31) may have the opposite effect. Similar changes in humans occur during erect exercise (32). Ahmet and associates (33) demonstrated a close relation between changes in PEP in humans and a variety of indexes of contractility, including peak left ventricular dP/dt and peak dP/dt divided by developed pressure, known as V_{max}. A reduction in PEP occurs after intravenous administration of 10 percent calcium gluconate (34) or isoproterenol (28). PEP is prolonged by beta-blocking drugs (28), which may also result in a reduction in ejection time. Thus, positive and negative inotropic drugs have predictable effects on PEP and Q-A_2 interval but not on ejection time.

Left Ventricular Disease

Left ventricular disease has significant and consistent effects on the systolic time intervals. The characteristic abnormality is a delay in the onset of ejection (35), which causes prolongation of PEP, shortening of ejection time, and thus, an increase in the ratio PEP/LVET. These effects are independent of heart rate (36). The duration of electromechanical systole is usually unaltered, unless increased adrenergic activity is present, when it is shortened. This frequently occurs after acute myocardial infarction (37) and the extent to which this occurs correlates with urinary catecholamine excretion provided renal function is normal (38).

The mechanism by which the onset of ejection is delayed in left ventricular disease is obscure. The lack of prolongation of Q-A_2 suggests that it is not due to any negative inotropic effect in such patients. This difference from any acute, drug-induced alteration in left ventricular function is confirmed by other studies that have demonstrated that indexes of contractility are often sensitive in detecting clinical left ventricular disease (39). The ratio PEP/LVET has been shown to be related to ejection fraction (36), which is also dimensionless. A second factor that may prolong PEP and thus delay the onset of ejection is the presence of incoordinate left ventricular wall movement during isovolumetric contraction. This has been shown to relate closely to reduced peak left ventricular dP/dt (40).

Validation of Systolic Time Intervals

Estimates of ejection time derived from the indirect carotid pulse are virtually identical with those measured by micromanometer in the aortic root (41, 42). Estimates of PEP have been similarly validated against the interval between the Q wave of the electrocardiogram and the onset of the upstroke of the central aortic pressure trace. Although there has been considerable discussion as to the exact mechanism of production of the second heart sound, the coincidence in time of A_2 with aortic valve closure has been confirmed by echocardiography to within 5 to 10 ms (43, 44).

INDIRECT CAROTID ARTERIAL PULSE TRACINGS

The indirect carotid arterial pulse tracing reflects changes in carotid pressure and volume following slight compression of the artery by a recording device. The resultant tracing is very similar to a direct intra-arterial record and is used as a timing reference for hemodynamic events (see Systolic Time Intervals) (Chapter 5).

The carotid pulse is used most commonly to detect the aortic component of the second heart sound. Because of transmission delay the aortic component of the second sound occurs 0.01 to 0.05 seconds before the dicrotic notch and, hence, can be reliably identified if an indirect carotid tracing and a phonocardiogram are recorded simultaneously. In progressively severe aortic stenosis, the aortic component of the second heart sound becomes increasingly difficult to hear or record by phonocardiography, but its position on the phonocardiogram can be inferred from the dicrotic notch of a carotid tracing. In the absence of left bundle branch block, reversed splitting of the second heart sound, so detected, is one of the best indicators of increasing severity of stenosis. If the recorded second heart sound is greater than 0.05 seconds before the notch, the sound probably represents the pulmonary and not the aortic component of the second heart sound.

The other main use of indirect carotid arterial tracings is an evaluation of the upstroke of the carotid pulse. This is usually slow in patients with aortic stenosis, and several authors attempted to predict the severity of aortic stenosis by analysis of the indirectly recorded pulse contour. The parameter most commonly used is the arterial half-rise time (i.e., the time required for the pulse to reach one-half of its total height). Correlations have been made between prolonged arterial half-rise time and the severity of aortic stenosis in groups of subjects (45). However, the measurements are rarely diagnostic in the individual because the half-rise time depends on other factors, mainly myocardial contractility and vessel stiffness.

REFERENCES

1. Leatham A. Auscultation of the heart and phonocardiography (2nd edition). London: Churchill Livingstone, 1975.
2. Burggraf GW, Craig E. The first heart sound in complete heart block: phonoechocardiographic correlations. Circulation 1974; 50:17.
3. Brooks N, Leech G, Leatham A. Factors responsible for normal splitting of first heart sound, high speed echophonocardiographic study of valve movement. Br Heart J 1979;42:695.
4. Brooks N, Leech G, Leatham A. Complete right bundle branch block. Br Heart J 1979;41:637.
5. Dancy M, Leech G, Leatham A. Significance of complete right bundle branch block when an isolated finding. Br Heart J 1982;48: 217.
6. Leech G, Mills P, Leatham A. The diagnosis of a non-stenotic bicuspid aortic valve. Br Heart J 1978;40:941.
7. Leatham A. Splitting of the first and second heart sounds. Lancet 1954;2:607.
8. Leatham A. The second heart sound, key to auscultation of the heart. Acta Cardiol 1964;19:395.
9. Leatham A, Weitzman D. Auscultatory and phonocardiographic signs of pulmonary stenosis. Br Heart J 1957;19:303.
10. Leatham A. Systolic murmurs. Circulation 1958;17:601.
11. Weissler AM, Harris WS, Schoenfeld CD. Bedside techniques for the evaluation of ventricular function in man. Am J Cardiol 1969;23:577–583.
12. Harris WS. Systolic time intervals in the non-invasive assessment of left ventricular performance in man. In: Mirsky I, Ghista DN, Sandler H, eds. Cardiac mechanics. New York: Wiley, 1974:233.
13. Lewis RP, Rittgers SE, Forrester WF, Boudoulas H. A critical review of the systolic time intervals. Circulation 1977;56:146–158.
14. Wiggers CJ. Studies on the consecutive phases of the cardiac cycle and criteria of their precise determination. Am J Physiol 1921;56:415–438.
15. Garrod AH. On some points connected with the circulation of the blood, arrived at from a study of the sphygmograph trace. Proc R Soc 1874–1875;23:140.
16. Weissler AM, Harris WS, Schoenfeld CD. Systolic time intervals in heart failure in man. Circulation 1968;37:149–159.
17. Weissler AM, Harris LC, White GD. Left ventricular ejection time index in man. J Appl Physiol 1963;18:919–923.
18. Harris LC, Weissler AM, Manske AO, Danford BH, White GD, Hammill WA. Duration of the phases of mechanical systole in infants and children. Am J Cardiol 1964;14:448–452.
19. Willems JL, Roelandt J, De Geest H, Kesteloot H, Joosens JV. The left ventricular ejection time in elderly subjects. Circulation 1970;42:37–42.
20. Jones WB, Forster GL. Determinants of the duration of left ventricular ejection in normal young men. J Appl Physiol 1964;19: 279–283.
21. Harley A, Starmer CF, Greenfield JC Jr. Pressure-flow studies in man. An evaluation of the phases of systole. J Clin Invest 1969;48: 895–905.
22. Robinson BF, Epstein EF, Beiser CD, Braunwald E. Control of the heart rate by the autonomic nervous system: studies in man

between baroreceptor mechanisms and exercise. Circulation Res 1966;19:400–411.

23. Kelman AW, Sumer DJ, Lonsdale M, Laurence JR, Whiting B. Comparative pharmacokinetics and pharmacodynamics of cardiac glycosides. Br J Clin Pharmacol 1980;10:135–143.

24. Mertens HM, Mannebach H, Trieb G, Gleichmann U. Influence of heart rate on systolic time intervals. Effects of atrial pacing versus dynamic exercise. Clin Cardiol 1981;4:22–27.

25. Kelman AW, Sumner DJ. Systolic time interval v. heart rate regression equations using atropine reproducibility studies. Br J Clin Pharmacol 1981;12:15–20.

26. Stafford RW, Harris WS, Weissler AM. Left ventricular systolic time intervals as indices of postural circulatory stress in man. Circulation 1970;41:485–492.

27. Agress CM, Wegner S, Forrester JS, Chatterjee K, Swan HJG. An indirect method for evaluation of left ventricular function in acute myocardial infarction. Circulation 1972;46:291–297.

28. Harris WS, Schoenfeld CD, Weissler AM. Effects of adrenergic receptor activation and blockade on the systolic pre-ejection period, heart rate and arterial pressure in man. J Clin Invest 1967;46:1704–1714.

29. Shaver JA, Kroetz FW, Leonard JJ. The effect of steady state increases in systemic arterial pressure on the duration of left ventricular ejection time. J Clin Invest 1968;47:217–230.

30. Sawayama T, Ochiai M, Marumoto S. Influence of amyl nitrite inhalation on the systolic time indices in normal subjects and in patients with ischaemic heart disease. Circulation 1969;40:327–335.

31. Weissler AM, Schoenfeld CD. Effect of digitalis on systolic time intervals in heart failure. Am J Med Sci 1970;259:4–20.

32. Pigott VM, Spodick DH, Recta EH, Khan AH. Cardiocirculatory responses to exercise: physiologic study by non-invasive techniques. Am Heart J 1971;82:632–641.

33. Ahmet SS, Levinson GE, Schwarz CJ, Ettinger PO. Systolic time intervals as measures of the contractile state of the left ventricular myocardium in man. Circulation 1972;46:559–571.

34. Shiner PT, Harris WS, Weissler AM. Effects of acute changes in serum calcium levels on the systolic time intervals in man. Am J Cardiol 1969;24:42–48.

35. Jezek V. Clinical value of the polygraphic tracing in the study of the sequence of events during cardiac contraction. Cardiologica 1963;43:298–316.

36. Garrard CL Jr, Weissler AM, Dodge HT. The relationship of alterations in systolic time intervals to ejection fraction in patients with cardiac disease. Circulation 1970;42:455–462.

37. Toutouzas P, Gupta D, Samson R, Shilingford JP. Q-second sound interval in acute myocardial infarction. Br Heart J 1969;31:462–467.

38. Lewis RP, Boudoulas H, Forrester WF, Weissler AM. Shortening of electromechanical systole as a manifestation of excessive adrenergic stimulation in acute myocardial infarction. Circulation 1972;46:856–862.

39. Peterson KL, Skloven D, Ludbrook P, Utmer JB, Ross J Jr. Comparison of isovolumic and ejection phase indices of myocardial performance in man. Circulation 1974;49:1088–1101.

40. Gibson DG, Brown D. Assessment of left ventricular systolic function from simultaneous echocardiographic and pressure measurements. Br Heart J 1976;38:8–17.

41. Bush CA, Lewis RP, Leighton RT, Fontana ME, Weissler AM. Verification of systolic time intervals and the isovolumic contraction time from the apex cardiogram by micromanometer catheterisation of the left ventricle and the aorta. Circulation 1970;42:111–121.

42. Martin CE, Shaver JA, Leonard JJ. Direct correlation of systolic time intervals with internal indices of left ventricular function in man. Circulation 1971;44:419–431.

43. Anastassiades PC, Quinones MA, Gaasch WH, Adyanthaya AV, Waggoner AD, Alexander JK. Aortic valve closure: echocardiographic, phonocardiographic and haemodynamic assessment. Am Heart J 1976;91:228–232.

44. Sabbah NH, Stein PD. Valve origin of the aortic incisura. Am J Cardiol 1978;41:32–38.

45. Epstein EJ, Coulshed N. Assessment of aortic stenosis from external carotid pulse wave. Br Heart J 1964;26:84.

17
Digitized M-Mode Echocardiograms

Rex Dawson

The high repetition rate of M-mode echocardiograms (1000 s^{-1}) enables the position of various cardiac structures such as the endocardium, epicardium, and mitral valve to be identified accurately and their motion during the cardiac cycle defined. Conventional M-mode echocardiographic tracings can be used to measure left ventricular dimensions at end-diastole and end-systole, and specific patterns of abnormality can be recognized in a variety of cardiac diseases. Digitization of M-mode echocardiograms allows entry of the XY coordinates of cardiac structures of interest into a computer usually at 10-ms intervals so that these structures can be followed throughout the cardiac cycle. Dimension and the rate of change of dimension can be measured continuously, and the time relations between endocardial and valvular motion can be investigated, thus providing information about cardiac function that is not accessible when M-mode echocardiograms are analyzed by conventional methods. During the past decade the digitizing method has been used to study a wide variety of cardiac diseases. This technique has proved to be of clinical value and in many instances has also provided insight into the various mechanisms of impairment of cardiac function.

TECHNIQUE AND COMPUTING METHODS

It must be emphasized from the outset that the digitizing method can be applied only to M-mode echocardiograms that are of the highest technical quality. Traces must clearly show the exact position of the cardiac structures of interest throughout the cardiac cycle and must be recorded, together with an electrocardiogram, at a rapid paper speed (50–200 mm/s). To facilitate the timing of events a phonocardiogram and an apexcardiogram may be recorded simultaneously (Fig. 17.1).

The process of digitization is the derivation of a string of coordinate points that represent in digital form the position of echoes of interest at intervals throughout the cardiac cycle (1). The coordinate points are entered into a computer program along with depth and time calibration factors. Coordinate strings may be generated from echoes arising from both endocardial surfaces of the interventricular septum, endocardial and epicardial surfaces of the posterior left ventricular wall, cusps of the mitral valve, and posterior wall of the aorta. Similarly, strings of coordinates may also be generated from other continuous signals, such as the apexcardiogram or left ventricular pressure trace, which have been recorded together with the echocardiogram. The timing of aortic valve closure (A_2) and mitral valve opening can be accurately identified. The beginning and end of the cardiac cycle to be studied are taken as the times of onset of the successive electrocardiographic Q waves. Digitization of echocardiographic and simultaneous pulse or pressure records may be performed in a variety of ways. The simplest method (2–4) involves positioning the echocardiogram to be analyzed on a digitizing table and manually tracing the echoes of interest throughout the cardiac cycle using a hand-held cross-wire cursor. This method is fast, inexpensive, and relatively simple, but may introduce errors because the cursor may not always follow the echocardiographic structure of interest exactly as a result of hand movement or operator bias. Griffith and Henry (5) described a video scanner–analog computer system in which the echoes of interest were first traced manually onto transparent paper and then processed automatically by a television camera. The method allows the movement of up to eight cardiac structures to be studied, but these must be nonoverlapping; therefore, simultaneously recorded

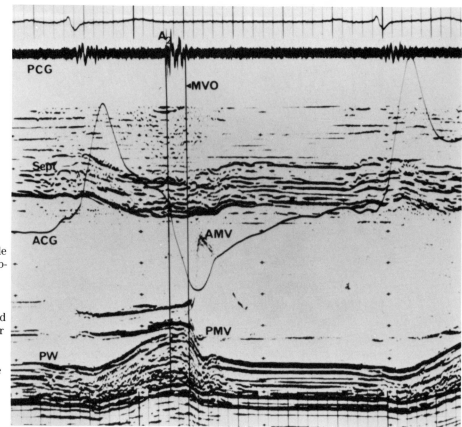

Figure 17.1. High-quality M-mode echocardiogram from a normal subject showing the left ventricle at the level of the tips of the mitral valve leaflets recorded together with an apexcardiogram (ACG) and phonocardiogram (PCG) at a paper speed of 100 mm/s. The vertical lines mark the timing of aortic valve closure (A$_2$) and mitral valve opening (MVO). PW = posterior wall; AMV = anterior mitral valve leaflet; PMV = posterior mitral valve leaflet.

traces of left ventricular pressure or the apexcardiogram cannot be analyzed. A similar method was described by van Zweiten and co-workers (6) in which the echoes to be analyzed are first traced with a lead pencil. The records are then transilluminated to increase the contrast for television scanning and subsequent conversion to digital form. Fully automatic methods for digitizing echocardiographic data have been described (7), but these require expensive complex equipment such as high-speed analog to digital converters and mass memory. Furthermore, pattern recognition algorithms are needed to extract the echoes arising from a structure of interest from other surrounding echoes. Van Zweiten and associates (6) reported that, in large series of average quality echocardiograms, attempts at digital processing using a fully automatic technique lead to a high failure rate.

These various digitizing methods generate a stream of coordinate points that are then reduced by interpolation to a fixed number of data points, usually 129 or 256 per beat (2, 8), which are used for all subsequent calculations. This step is necessary because the points comprising the original strings of coordinates for each structure of interest may not be synchronous with one another. The frequency response of the systems described is adequate to record accurately the motion of cardiac structures because Fourier analysis of left ventricular wall movement in humans shows that 90 percent of the information is contained in frequencies below 10 Hz and that no more than 1 percent of information is present in frequencies greater than 30 Hz (9). After digitization the strings of echocardiographic coordinates contain noise as well as useful information. It is customary to reduce or eliminate this using some form of filtering procedure. A simple moving average filter that does not cause a phase shift and produces only a 5 percent reduction in signal amplitude at 10 Hz is satisfactory for this purpose (2, 9).

After the strings of coordinates have been generated by the digitizing process, they can be stored by computer and further manipulations can be performed subsequently. For example, the coordinates of the left ventricular posterior wall endocardium can be instantaneously subtracted from the coordinates of the endocardium on the left side of the septum to give continuous left ventricular cavity dimension as a function of time. Similarly, the coordinates of the posterior wall epicardium can be subtracted from the coordinates of the posterior wall endocardium to give a continuous measure of left ventricular posterior wall thickness. Coordinate strings or the differences between them may be differentiated to derive rates of change with time. This can be achieved by digital differentiation using a central difference formula (9):

$$(X_{n+1} - X_{n-1})/2DT,$$

where X is the magnitude of the variable at points $n-1$ and $n+1$ and DT is the time interval between two successive data points. Records of rates of change allow peak values to be determined and patterns of change to be identified such as those occurring during left ventricular ejection or filling. Time-independent functions may be generated by plotting the coordinate strings of continuous left ventricular dimension against the coordinate strings of left ventricular pressure trace or the apexcardiogram, thus producing a pressure-dimension or apex-dimension loop, respectively. Finally, information contained in the strings of coordinates may be combined to produce complex quantities such as myocardial wall stress, work, and power.

REPRODUCIBILITY

Several authors reported the variability and reproducibility of measurements made from digitized echocardiograms (2, 10, 11). Potential sources of variability are: 1) interobserver (differences between readers digitizing the same echo trace), 2) intraobserver (differences between digitized traces made from the same echocardiogram by one observer on more than one occasion), 3) beat-to-beat variation caused by the effects of respiration or changes in cardiac cycle length, 4) day-to-day variation caused by differences in the body position of the subject being studied or in transducer angulation or by variations in the autonomic tone of the subject.

Pollick and colleagues (10), in a study of normal subjects using complex statistical analysis, assessed both inter- and intraobserver (technical) variability of observers digitizing the same cardiac cycles and also the biologic variability between beats, days, and subjects. It was found that technical variability was small for both measures of cavity dimension and wall thickness (correlation coefficient r values; 0.82–1.00) and rates of change of cavity dimension and wall thickness (correlation coefficient r values: 0.70–0.98). In contrast, biological variability was large with wide 95 percent confidence limits between measurements with respect to both dimension and, particularly, rates of change of dimension. However, the 95 percent confidence limits for these measurements could be substantially reduced by averaging values from at least five beats digitized on two separate occasions. Hall and co-workers (11) also found that interobserver variability was small, but they reported a much larger intraobserver variability, although the variance could be reduced by performing multiple measurements on the same beat. Gibson and Brown (2) assessed reproducibility by calculating the root mean square difference between pairs of determinations of dimension and rate of change of dimension. Intraobserver variability was smaller than day-to-day variability; the respective root mean square differences were 1.6 mm and 2.0 mm for end-diastolic dimension, 1.7 mm and 1.9 mm for end-systolic dimension, and 1.5 cm/s and 1.8 cm/s for peak rate of increase of left ventricular dimension. Virtually identical values for intraobserver variability are reported by St John Sutton (12) and Combellas (13) and their colleagues.

All reports show that the variance in measurements of dimension is substantially smaller than the variance in measurements of rates of change of dimension. This is probably explained by hand-eye incoordination preventing the observer from accurately tracing the often rapid slopes of the posterior wall and septum. Such errors may be minimized by recording the echocardiograms on a large scale and at a fast paper speed.

LEFT VENTRICULAR DIMENSION AND RATE OF CHANGE OF DIMENSION

Using the digitizing technique, a display is produced of left ventricular dimension and the rate of change of dimension as a function of time (Fig. 17.2). The rate of change of dimension may be normalized by dividing its value by the instantaneous dimension. The normalized rate of ventricular dimension decrease during systole with dimensional units of s^{-1} is equivalent to the velocity of circumferential fiber shortening (VCF). Gibson and Brown (14) demonstrated a close correlation between peak VCF derived from digitized M-mode echocardiograms and the peak rate of increase of ventricular pressure (peak dP/dt), providing there is no mitral regurgitation and that ventricular contraction is coordinate, indicating that peak VCF may be used as an index of ventricular systolic function.

The changes in left ventricular dimension during the cardiac cycle resemble those in left ventricular volume observed in humans (15). During diastole there is an initial rapid filling period followed by a mid-diastolic period of diastasis and culminating with a small increase in filling rate as a result of atrial systole. The period of rapid filling may be defined as beginning with mitral valve opening and ending either when the ventricular dimension or cavity volume diastolic filling curve shows a marked discontinuity or, alternatively, when the value for rate of dimension or volume increase has decreased to 20 percent of its peak value (9). Estimates using dimension or volume traces of the duration of rapid filling are identical.

Caution must be exercised if conclusions about ventricular volume changes are extrapolated from the continuous left ventricular dimension trace because, although ventricular volume approximates to the cube

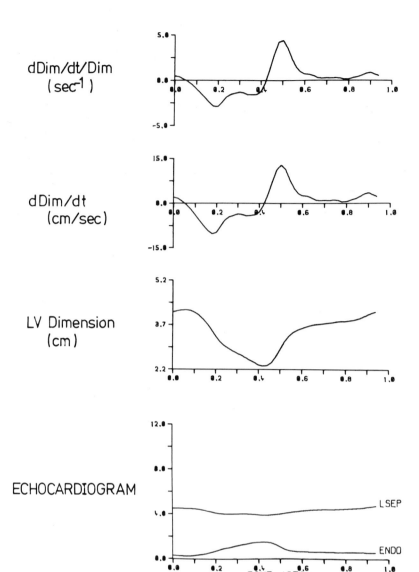

Figure 17.2. A digitized M-mode echocardiogram from a normal subject showing (from bottom to top) the XY coordinates of the endocardium of the septum and posterior left ventricular wall, continuous left ventricular (LV) dimension during the cardiac cycle, the rate of change of dimension with time (dDim/dt), and the normalized rate of change of dimension with time (dDim/dt/Dim).

of dimension when volume is small, this relationship is prone to considerable error when regional wall motion abnormalities are present or when the ventricle has enlarged and becomes more spherical as may occur in patients with heart disease. Upton and Gibson (9) examined in detail the relation between dimension and volume using cineangiography. In normal subjects the onset of systolic reduction in dimension and volume are synchronous, and there are no consistent differences in the timing of peak rates of decrease of dimension and volume. During diastole significant discrepancies become apparent. Peak rate of increase of dimension consistently precedes the peak rate of increase of volume by 40 to 60 ms. This may be because during early rapid filling there is a change in cavity shape toward a more spherical configuration as a result of a preferential increase in the transverse axis (16). Finally, the effect of left atrial systole on the left ventricular dimension trace is normally less marked

than its effect on the left ventricular volume trace. This is because contraction of the left atrium results in upward movement of the mitral valve ring, which encloses blood within the ventricle, thus increasing ventricular volume with only minor changes in left ventricular transverse dimension. A comparative echocardiographic and angiographic study showed a satisfactory agreement between the two methods with respect to estimates of both peak and mean rates of change of dimension (17).

Several authors (2, 12, 13, 18–24) measured end-diastolic and end-systolic dimensions derived from digitized M-mode echocardiograms in normal subjects. Mean values for end-diastolic dimension range from 4.7 to 5.1 cm, and for end-systolic dimension, 2.6 to 3.7 cm. These values correspond closely with published normal values derived from echocardiograms analyzed by conventional methods. The reported (12, 18, 20–24) mean values for normalized peak rates of dimension

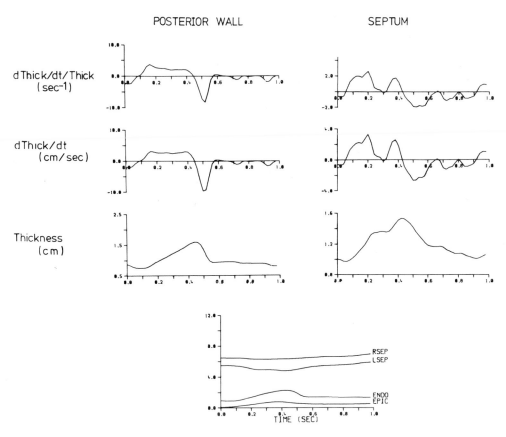

Figure 17.3. A digitized M-mode tracing from a normal subject showing (from bottom to top) the original data, continuous wall thickness, the rate of change of wall thickness (dThick/dt) and normalized rate of change of wall thickness (dThick/dt/Thick) for the left ventricular posterior wall (left) and intraventricular septum (right).

decrease during left ventricular ejection (peak VCF) range from 2.4 to 3.2 s^{-1}. During early left ventricular filling, the rate of increase in dimension is rapid; reported peak rates ranged from 11 to 19 cm/s (2, 12, 13, 18, 21–27) or from 2.5 to 5.7 s^{-1} when normalized (2, 20, 25). Bahler and associates (25) showed that in normal subjects heart rate and systolic function (peak VCF) are important variables in determining the value of normalized peak rate of ventricular dimension increase during diastole. This finding implies that both variables must be taken into account if normalized peak rate of dimension increase is used to compare diastolic function in groups of patients. Reported mean values for the duration of the rapid filling period ranged from 110 to 210 ms (2, 12, 13, 18, 19, 22, 24–27).

LEFT VENTRICULAR WALL THICKNESS AND RATE OF CHANGE OF THICKNESS

Continuous ventricular septal and posterior left ventricular wall thickness can be obtained by digitizing the endocardial surfaces of the septum and the endocardial and epicardial surfaces of the posterior wall throughout the cardiac cycle (Fig. 17.3). A continuous

measure of the rate of change of septal and posterior wall thicknesses (cm/s) and a normalized rate of change of septal and posterior wall thicknesses (s^{-1}) may also be derived. In normal subjects mean values for posterior wall end-diastolic and end-systolic thicknesses range from 0.7 to 0.9 cm and 1.5 to 1.7 cm, respectively. Mean values for septal end-diastolic and end-systolic thicknesses range from 0.7 to 1.0 and 1.2 to 1.5 cm, respectively. Estimates of end-diastolic wall thickness made by the digitizing method agree closely with angiographic estimates, but measurements of end-systolic wall thickness correlate less well. This discrepancy probably reflects the limitation of angiography in estimating wall thickness, particularly during systole, where endocardial infolding may cause a separation between radio-opaque endocardial markers and the boundary of the ventricular cavity identified by contrast medium, thus resulting in an overestimation of wall thickness.

The rate of change of thickness of the posterior left ventricular wall during the cardiac cycle is characteristic. During ejection there is a rapid increase in wall thickness; peak values range from 4.7 to 9.0 cm/s (9, 28). Maximum wall thickness occurs synchronously with mitral valve opening (29). During diastole the pattern of posterior wall movement resembles that of the left ventricular dimension trace; the peak rate of posterior wall thinning occurs synchronously with the peak rate of cavity dimension increase, and there is a clearly defined rapid thinning period of approximately the same duration as the ventricular rapid filling period. Mean values for peak thinning rates in normal subjects range from 6.7 to 10.7 cm/s (13, 22, 28, 29). The pattern of change in thickness of the septum during the cardiac cycle is less characteristic than that of the left ventricular posterior wall; there is no clearly defined rapid thinning period. The normalized peak septal thickening rates range from 3.0 to 4.7 s^{-1} (18). The peak normalized rate of septal thinning occurs later than the peak rate of posterior wall thinning; values range from a reported mean value of 3.4 ± 0.9 s^{-1} or 2.5 to 4.4 s^{-1} (18).

RELATION BETWEEN ENDOCARDIAL MOTION AND CARDIAC EVENTS

The digitizing method provides a means of assessing the relations between timing of endocardial motion and other events occurring during the cardiac cycle, particularly when an apexcardiogram and phonocardiogram are recorded simultaneously. In normal subjects a close time relation exists during early diastole between movement of the anterior leaflet of the mitral valve and changes in left ventricular posterior wall movement, suggesting that the forces acting on the valve are closely related to the pattern of ventricular filling (30). The onset of forward movement of the anterior mitral leaflet occurs synchronously with the onset of outward wall motion. The timing of peak mitral opening velocity and peak velocity of outward wall motion are also synchronous (Fig. 17.4) (31).

The first high-frequency component of the second heart sound recorded using a phonocardiogram, positioned on the precordium of the left upper sternal border, precisely identifies the timing of aortic valve closure (A_2) and the end of left ventricular ejection (32). In normal subjects aortic valve closure precedes the time of minimum cavity dimension; mean values range from 40 to 50 ms (13, 20, 27, 33). The duration of the time interval between the electrocardiographic Q wave and minimum dimension similar to the Q-A_2 interval varies with heart rate (34). The point of initial separation of the mitral valve cusps, which is used to time mitral valve opening, occurs within 10 ms of minimum cavity dimension in normal subjects (13, 19–23, 27, 33). The time period between aortic valve closure and mitral valve opening represents the isovolumetric relaxation time, which can be measured. Left ventricular dimension changes during this period can

be quantitated. Isovolumetric relaxation time in normal subjects ranges from 56 to 72 ms (13, 20, 22, 23, 25, 33, 35). The duration of isovolumetric relaxation has several determinants; there is an inverse correlation with heart rate (33) and left ventricular end-diastolic pressure (35) and a positive correlation with left ventricular posterior wall thickness (20) and mass (22). During isovolumetric relaxation, there is a small increase (0 percent to 5 percent) in transverse ventricular dimension (13, 20, 22, 23, 25, 33).

The timing of the upstroke and downstroke of the apexcardiogram is similar to that of the high-fidelity left ventricular pressure pulse (36, 37). The time interval between the onset of the upstroke and the E point of the apexcardiogram approximates the period of isovolumetric contraction. In normal subjects a small decrease in cavity dimension is observed; values (13, 27, 38, 39) range from -7 to -3 percent (expressed as a percentage of the total change in dimension during the cardiac cycle), because the E point of the apexcardiogram corresponds to the timing of maximal separation and not to the timing of opening of the aortic valve cusps. The O point of the apexcardiogram occurs almost synchronously with the nadir of the left ventricular pressure pulse (36, 37) and the timing of peak rate of left ventricular diastolic dimension increase (40). There is a close time relationship between the rapid filling wave of the apexcardiogram and the discontinuity on the continuous left ventricular dimension trace during diastole (40), which represents the end and not the peak of rapid ventricular filling. Apexcardiogram–echo dimension relations can be best displayed by the construction of a loop (Fig. 17.5), which in normal subjects has approximately square shape exhibiting little change in ventricular dimension during the upstroke and downstroke of the apexcardiogram.

SIMULTANEOUS ECHOCARDIOGRAPHIC AND PRESSURE MEASUREMENTS

Left ventricular wall stress is an important determinant of cardiac function, and its value closely reflects myocardial oxygen demand (41). There are two components of wall stress—longitudinal and circumferential—acting perpendicular to each other. For a spherical model the two are equal, but for an ellipsoid model the circumferential stress is greater (42). Wall stress is traditionally measured by combined hemodynamic and angiographic methods (42), but if continuous dimension and wall thickness are measured by echocardiographic methods, it is possible to derive values for both circumferential and longitudinal wall stress without recourse to angiography (14, 43, 44). Methods based on echocardiography are advantageous

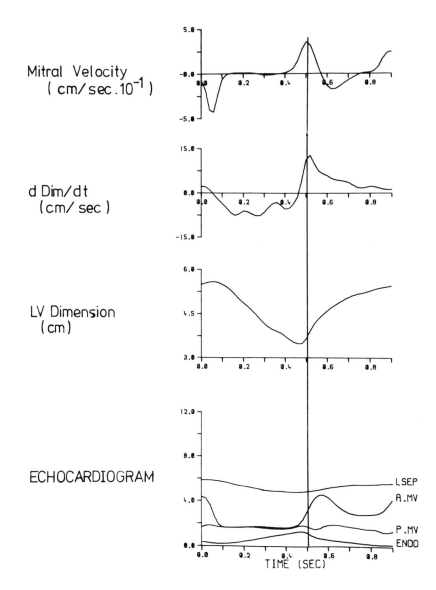

Figure 17.4. Display of digitized M-mode tracing from a normal subject showing (from bottom to top) the anterior and posterior leaflets of the mitral valve, continuous left ventricular (LV) dimension, rate of change of dimension (dDim/dt), and velocity of motion of the anterior leaflet of the mitral valve. The vertical line illustrates that the peak opening velocity of the mitral anterior leaflet and peak left ventricular dimension increase during diastole are virtually synchronous.

in that multiple determinations of stress can be made in a single patient (i.e., before, during, and after an intervention that might be expected to alter stress). When the left ventricular cavity is dilated, wall stress is usually increased, whereas wall stress is normal or even reduced when there is left ventricular hypertrophy and normal cavity size. Figure 17.6 illustrates a plot of continuous circumferential wall stress from a patient with normal left ventricular function. Peak stress occurs early in systole, diminishing later as cavity dimension decreases and the left ventricular wall thickens (9).

Myocardial power is a measure of the rate at which work is performed by the whole heart on the circulation. Alternatively, the power of a unit volume of the posterior left ventricular wall studied by echocardiography may be derived from the product of wall stress and the circumferential shortening rate (see Fig. 17.6). Gibson and Brown (14) reported values for peak power

of 46 ± 16 mW·cm^{-3} in subjects with normal left ventricular function and reduced levels in patients with ventricular dilatation and in those with increased wall thickness. Using the same data the work performed by the segment of posterior wall studied by the ultrasound beam can be derived from the time integral of power.

Simultaneous left ventricular pressure and echocardiographic left ventricular dimension measurements may be displayed in the form of a pressure-dimension loop (Fig. 17.7). The loop from a normal subject is approximately rectangular; there is little change in dimension during the periods of isovolumetric contraction and relaxation and in pressure during ventricular ejection and filling. The integral area of the pressure-dimension loop is an index of the mechanical work performed by the segment of the ventricle studied with the ultrasound beam. The ratio of the area of the pressure-dimension loop to the area of a rectangle that just encloses the loop is termed the "cycle efficiency"

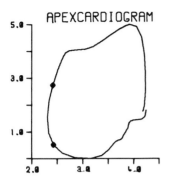

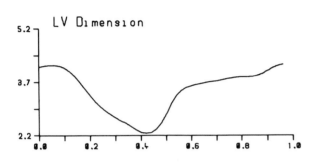

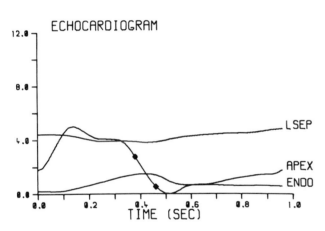

Figure 17.5. Display showing construction of a left ventricular (LV) dimension-apexcardiogram loop. The two timing marks on the apexcardiogram trace indicate the times of aortic valve closure and mitral valve opening.

and expresses the efficiency of energy transfer from the heart to the circulation (84 ± 4 percent in normal subjects) (14). Valvular heart disease, myocardial ischemia, and ventricular ectopic beats may distort the pressure-dimension loop and therefore reduce cycle efficiency.

DIGITIZED ECHOCARDIOGRAMS IN HEART DISEASE

Valvular Heart Disease

Digitization of M-mode echocardiograms with simultaneous recordings of phonocardiograms and apexcar-

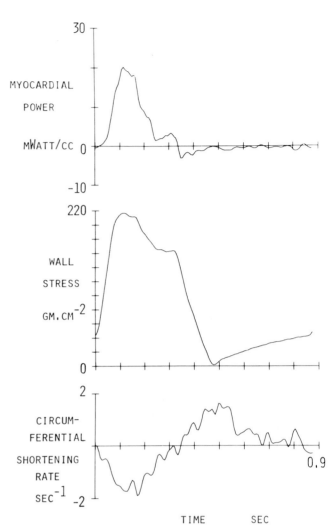

Figure 17.6. Display derived from a digitized M-mode tracing showing (from bottom to top), for the region of myocardium studied by the ultrasound beam, continuous velocity of circumferential shortening, wall stress, and myocardial power during the cardiac cycle.

diograms provides a powerful noninvasive tool for investigating the physiologic consequences of valvular heart disease and assessing the results of surgical treatment.

Mitral Valve Disease

The most striking abnormality observed in patients with mitral stenosis is derangement of the normal pattern of left ventricular dimension increase during diastole (Fig. 17.8). In patients with mitral stenosis, unlike normal subjects, there is no discrete rapid filling phase, and left ventricular dimension increases slowly and continues throughout diastole. The period of isovolumetric relaxation is shortened (33) (40 ± 20 ms), and the peak rate of left ventricular dimension increase

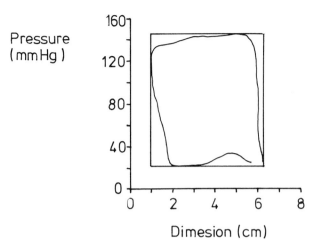

Figure 17.7. A left ventricular dimension-pressure loop. The area of the loop is an index of left ventricular stroke work. Efficiency (see text) is the ratio, expressed as a percentage, of the area of the loop to the area of the rectangle that just encloses the loop.

conventional variables that describe valve motion did not consistently distinguish between mild and severe stenosis, whereas variables related to left ventricular filling derived from the digitized M-mode echocardiogram reliably separated mild from severe disease. No patient with severe disease had a discrete rapid filling period. Peak rate of left ventricular dimension increase during diastole was less than 10 cm/s in all patients with severe stenosis. However, the peak rate of dimension increase was greater than 10 cm/s in all but six of the patients with mild stenosis.

Analysis of the pattern of left ventricular diastolic dimension increase and its rate of change allows examination of the functional effects of mitral valve surgery and allows comparisons between different surgical procedures and prostheses. In 14 patients undergoing closed mitral valvotomy, the mean peak rate of left ventricular diastolic dimension increase before operation was 7.2 cm/s, which increased significantly to a mean of 10.4 cm/s postoperatively (26). The effects of mitral valve replacement with a variety of prostheses upon the pattern of left ventricular filling has also been examined (26, 46). Mean values for peak rate of increase of dimension during diastole are 10.5 ± 4.2 cm/s in patients with Björk-Shiley prostheses, 10.3 ± 3.7 cm/s with Hancock xenograft prostheses, 13.2 ± 3.4 cm/s with the St Jude prosthesis, and 7.4 ± 3.0 cm/s

is reduced; values range from 6.9 to 7.2 cm/s (2, 26). Hall and colleagues (45) compared the digitized M-mode echocardiogram with conventional echocardiographic measurements in terms of diastolic closure rate, amplitude of anterior cusp motion, mitral valve closure index, and their respective abilities to distinguish between mild and severe mitral stenosis. The

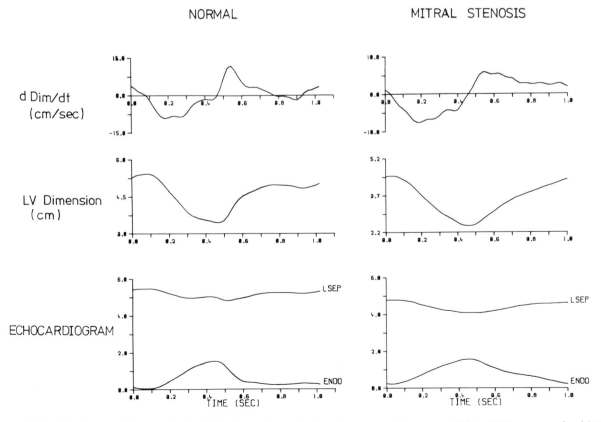

Figure 17.8. Continuous left ventricular (LV) dimension and rate of change of dimension (dDim/dt) in a normal subject (left) and in a patient with mitral stenosis (right).

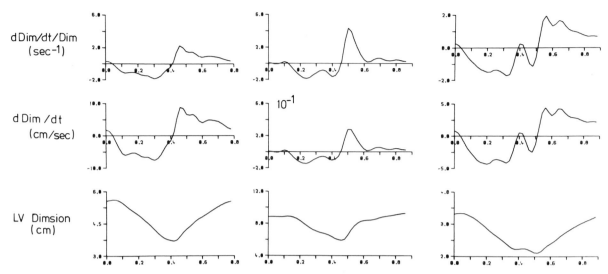

Figure 17.9. Continuous left ventricular (LV) dimension, rate of change of dimension (dDim/dt) and normalized rate of change of dimension (dDim/dt/Dim) in patients with a normally functioning mitral Björk-Shiley prosthesis (left), incompetent prosthesis (center), and obstructed mitral Björk-Shiley prosthesis.

with Starr-Edwards prostheses. These relative values demonstrate the hemodynamic advantages of replacing the mitral valve with a tilting disc prosthesis rather than a cage and ball device. If the 95 percent confidence limits for peak rate of diastolic dimension increase are known for each specific type of valve prosthesis, then postoperative valve malfunction may be detected by alterations in filling rate (26, 47). In a group of patients with Starr-Edwards prostheses and paraprosthetic leaks, the peak rate of increase of dimension was 17 ± 2 cm/s, which is significantly higher than the value for normally functioning prostheses of that type (26). Similarly, the peak rate of dimension increase during diastole was found to be greatly increased (25 ± 7 cm/s) in a group of patients with Björk-Shiley prostheses and paraprosthetic leaks (Fig. 17.9) (47). In contrast, patients with obstructed Björk-Shiley prostheses have values for peak rate of dimension increase below the 95 percent confidence limits for the normally functioning valve (26). Effects of prosthetic valve malfunction on systolic function have also been observed (47); increases in peak rates and normalized peak rates of left ventricular dimension decrease occur in patients with paraprosthetic leaks.

In mitral regurgitation the ventricular end-diastolic dimension is increased, reflecting the presence of a large stroke volume. Peak rate of left ventricular dimension increase during diastole is increased in comparison with normal subjects (22 cm/s) (2), and the period of rapid filling is reduced. If the mitral regurgitation is severe, then the apexcardiogram-dimension loop shows a significant reduction in dimension during the apex upstroke (36). Surgical correction of mitral regurgitation by repair of the valve is associated with a reduction in the peak rate of dimension increase during

diastole to within the normal range and normalization of the apex-dimension relations (26).

Aortic Valve Disease

Hemodynamically important aortic regurgitation is associated with a high end-diastolic volume, reflecting the presence of an increased stroke volume, and end-systolic volume is often also increased. The peak rate of increase of left ventricular dimension during diastole in patients with aortic regurgitation does not differ significantly from that of normal subjects, but as the cavity is dilated, values for normalized peak rate of increase in dimension may show a significant reduction from normal (2, 39). In comparison with normal subjects, end-systolic meridional wall stress is substantially elevated in patients with aortic regurgitation if the ejection fraction is reduced, but it is not increased if ejection fraction is normal (44). Apex-dimension loops have a characteristic shape (Fig. 17.10) in patients with aortic regurgitation; only small changes in dimension occur during isovolumetric contraction, but considerable increases occur during early relaxation, which results in loss of cycle efficiency. Digitized echo and apexcardiograms have been used to study the acute effects of aortic valve replacement on left ventricular function in patients with aortic regurgitation, and they reveal a complex pattern (39). Following operation left ventricular systolic dimension remains unchanged, but a reduction in end-diastolic dimension suggesting an improvement in left ventricular function becomes apparent in most patients within seven days after surgery. In contrast, the normalized peak rate of dimension decrease during systole (peak VCF) decreases, suggesting a deterioration in left ventricular

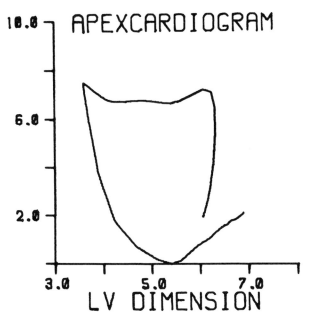

Figure 17.10. Left ventricular (LV) dimension-apexcardiogram loop in a patient with severe aortic regurgitation. The large increase in dimension during the apexcardiogram downstroke is characteristic.

systolic performance. Postoperatively, striking changes in the apex-dimension loops have been reported; dimension changes occur during the period of upstroke of the apexcardiogram, indicating incoordinate left ventricular contraction. These changes regress in most patients.

Left Ventricular Hypertrophy

Digitized echocardiograms have been used extensively to study the physiologic effects of left ventricular hypertrophy in systemic hypertension, aortic valve disease, and hypertrophic cardiomyopathy (18, 21, 48) and in various types of athletes (20–22, 27). Left ventricular hypertrophy may be considered as a beneficial homeostatic process in which wall thickness and mass increase to normalize peak systolic wall stress.

Secondary Left Ventricular Hypertrophy

In all groups of patients with secondary left ventricular hypertrophy, posterior wall and septal thickness are increased, but ventricular dimensions and systolic function, assessed in terms of peak VCF, usually remain within the normal range (20–23, 27). In contrast, ventricular diastolic function is abnormal in all groups of patients with left ventricular hypertrophy, except athletes with physiologic hypertrophy in whom diastolic function is invariably normal (22). Peak rate of dimension increase during diastole is reduced and the period of rapid filling prolonged, and these abnormali-

ties become more pronounced with increasing wall thickness (21, 22, 24) or with the presence of a "strain pattern" on the electrocardiogram (23). The reduced rate of left ventricular dimension increase during the early diastolic filling period is compensated by a greater dimension increase in late diastole as a result of atrial contraction, thus resulting in a normal end-diastolic dimension (19). The peak rate of posterior wall thinning is reduced in patients with secondary hypertrophy, and this abnormality correlates with the degree of wall thickening (22) and the presence of an electrocardiographic strain pattern (23). The period of isovolumetric relaxation is prolonged in comparison with normal subjects (20, 22, 27, 33), and there is a positive correlation between duration of isovolumetric relaxation and left ventricular posterior wall thickness, septal thickness, and mass (20, 22). Minimum cavity dimension and mitral valve opening normally occur almost synchronously (13, 20–22, 27). A disturbance of these time relations with delay in the timing of mitral valve opening relative to minimum cavity dimension is associated with incoordinate ventricular relaxation, manifest as outward wall motion during the period of isovolumetric relaxation. When the time relations between minimum cavity dimension and mitral valve opening are examined in patients with secondary left ventricular hypertrophy, a bimodal distribution is observed (20, 21). In one group of subjects, the normal time relations are preserved, and dimension changes during isovolumetric relaxation are minimal. In a second group, the time relations between minimum dimension and mitral valve opening are abnormal, and large changes in left ventricular dimension occur during isovolumetric relaxation, indicating incoordinate ventricular relaxation. In patients with systemic hypertension, the presence of abnormal dimension changes during isovolumetric relaxation is associated with a high incidence of concomitant coronary artery disease which may be occult (20). Abnormal dimension changes during the periods of inscription of the upstroke of the apexcardiogram and isovolumetric relaxation, indicating incoordinate contraction and relaxation, respectively, have been observed in patients with untreated malignant hypertension (27). These abnormal features, which may represent the effect of ischemia in uncontrolled malignant hypertension, resolve after control of blood pressure (27).

Hypertrophic Cardiomyopathy

A number of investigators have digitized M-mode echocardiograms from patients with hypertrophic cardiomyopathy to evaluate left ventricular function (18, 19, 21, 48, 49). The characteristic abnormality found in hypertrophic cardiomyopathy is a profound disruption of the normal pattern of left ventricular filling. Wide variability is found in both the peak rate of left ventricular dimension increase during diastole and the duration of rapid filling (9, 18, 19, 49). In most patients, the rapid filling period is decreased, suggesting restriction (9, 19). Propranolol prolongs the rapid filling period in a proportion of patients with hypertrophic cardiomyopathy, suggesting that its beneficial effects may result from increased time available for ventricular filling.

The asynchronous timing of peak septal and peak posterior wall thickness and minimum cavity dimension (Fig. 17.11) contributes to the disorganized pattern of relaxation (9, 18). A negative correlation has been described (18) between the peak rate of ventricular dimension increase during diastole and the delay in the timing of peak septal thickness and peak posterior wall thickness. The normalized septal thickening and thinning rates are reduced in comparison with normal subjects, but the normalized posterior wall thinning rate varies widely and may be increased, decreased, or unchanged, whereas normalized posterior wall thickening is unchanged or increased (18, 29). The peak rate of dimension increase during diastole is directly related to the normalized peak rate of posterior wall thinning, and patients with the lowest peak rates of ventricular dimension increase and wall thinning have the highest incidence of angina. A possible explanation for this finding is that tension decay is prolonged in slowly thinning myocardium, which compromises subendocardial blood flow. Isovolumetric relaxation is substantially prolonged (18, 49) in patients with hypertrophic cardiomyopathy (Fig. 17.12), and the normal close time relations between minimum cavity dimension and mitral valve opening is lost (Fig. 17.12); delay in mitral valve opening ranges from 70 to 93 ms (9, 19, 21). Left ventricular apexcardiogram dimension relations are also altered; abnormal dimension changes occur during the periods of upstroke and downstroke of the apexcardiogram, indicating ventricular incoordination during both isovolumetric contraction and early relaxation (Fig. 17.12) (9, 18, 21).

Left Ventricular Disease

Both structural and physiologic information can be derived from digitized echocardiograms, and the method has proved helpful in characterizing the abnormalities in a number of myocardial diseases, including dilated cardiomyopathy (2, 9, 44), amyloid heart (12), eosinophilic heart disease (50), Chagas' disease (13), and a variety of neurocardiac diseases (51–54).

In patients with dilated cardiomyopathy, end-diastolic and end-systolic dimensions are increased and peak VCF is reduced, indicating reduced ventricular systolic function. No specific pattern of diastolic ab-

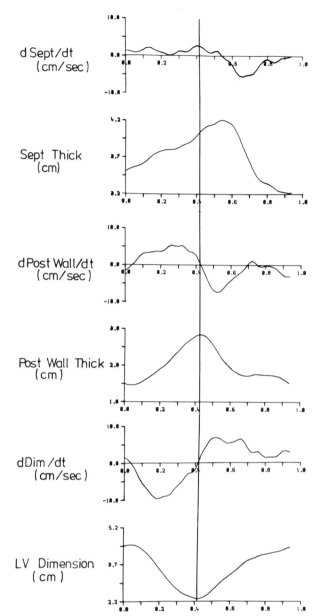

Figure 17.11. From bottom to top, continuous left ventricular (LV) dimension, its rate of change (dDim/dt); posterior wall thickness, its rate of change (dPost Wall/dt); septal thickness, its rate of change (dSept/dt) in a patient with hypertrophic cardiomyopathy. It is clear from inspection of the tracing that the normal synchronous relations between minimum cavity dimension (marked by the vertical line) and peak septal and peak posterior wall thickness are lost.

normality is observed, although the duration of isovolumetric relaxation is shortened if the left ventricular end-diastolic pressure is greatly elevated (35). The duration of isovolumetric relaxation detected noninvasively can thus be used to assess response to treatment. Left ventricular end-systolic stress, calculated using M-mode echocardiograms and cuff systolic arterial pressure, is increased three-fold in patients with dilated cardiomyopathy (44).

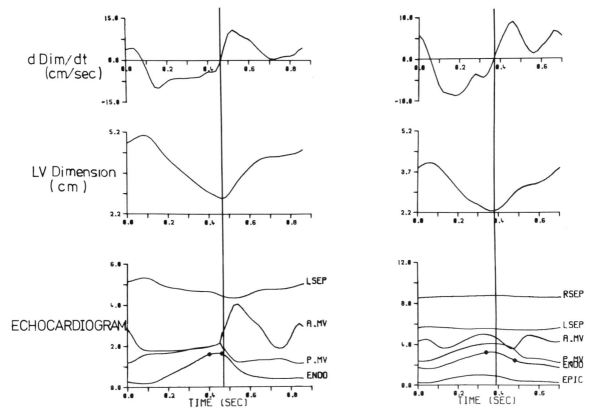

Figure 17.12. Display of digitized M-mode echocardiograms recorded from a normal subject (left) and from a patient with hypertrophic cardiomyopathy (right). The vertical line marks the timing of minimum cavity dimension. Aortic valve closure and mitral valve opening are indicated by the timing marks. In hypertrophic cardiomyopathy, isovolumetric relaxation (A_2-MVO) is prolonged and the normally synchronous relation between minimum cavity dimension and mitral valve opening is lost.

Study of patients with cardiac amyloid using digitized echocardiograms reveals characteristic abnormalities (12) that are principally disorders of left ventricular diastolic function. In comparison with that of normal subjects, left ventricular septal and posterior wall thicknesses in cardiac amyloid patients are increased, and peak systolic thickening and diastolic thinning rates are reduced for both the septum and posterior wall. Left ventricular dimension is usually normal or decreased, peak rate of cavity dimension increase during diastole is reduced, isovolumetric relaxation time is prolonged, and systolic function, assessed as peak VCF, is reduced. In eosinophilic endomyocardial disease (50), in contrast to amyloid heart disease, no specific pattern of abnormalities can be identified. Systolic function is normal and, although both the peak rate of diastolic dimension increase and period of rapid filling may be either increased or decreased, the presence of these abnormalities appears to be determined by whether there is associated mitral regurgitation.

Ischemic Heart Disease

Because M-mode echocardiography visualizes only a very small part of the left ventricle, it is of little value in the study of ventricular function in patients with coronary artery disease where the characteristic abnormality is incoordinate wall motion caused by regional differences of ventricular function. To overcome this limitation partially, the digitizing method can be applied to M-mode traces recorded not in isolation but simultaneously with left ventricular pressure or the apexcardiogram to produce a pressure-dimension or apex-dimension loop. In patients in whom wall motion is coordinate, the pressure- or apex-dimension loop has an approximately rectangular configuration. However, in patients in whom wall motion is incoordinate, the loops become distorted; dimension changes occur principally during the periods of isovolumetric contraction and relaxation (Fig. 17.13). Ventricular dimension changes during isovolumetric contraction and relaxation illustrated by using an apex-dimension loop can be used to detect but not to quantify incoordination, because the relation of the apexcardiogram to left ventricular pressure is undefined during ejection and filling. In a comparative angiographic study, apex-dimension loops have greater than 80 percent specificity and sensitivity in detecting regional abnormalities of wall movement wherever they are located within the

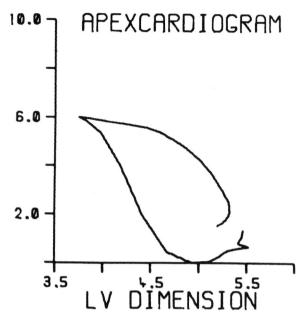

Figure 17.13. Left ventricular (LV) dimension-apexcardiogram loop in a patient with coronary artery disease. The shape of the loop, sloping to the left, is characteristic of abnormal wall motion in the region of myocardium under study occurring secondary to delayed inward wall motion in a distant region of the ventricle.

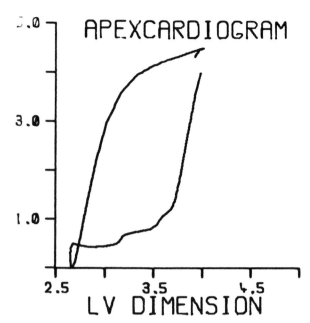

Figure 17.14. Left ventricular (LV) dimension-apexcardiogram loop in a patient with coronary artery disease. The shape of the loop, sloping to the right, is characteristic of a primary abnormality of wall motion occurring in a region of ischemic myocardium.

left ventricle (38). Because blood is incompressible, inward or outward wall movement during the isovolumetric period in one region of the ventricle must be associated with a net equal and opposite movement elsewhere in the ventricle. Therefore, dimension changes detected during the periods of isovolumetric contraction and relaxation using apex-dimension loops may be either primary abnormalities of wall motion or secondary compensatory abnormalities reflecting abnormal wall movement elsewhere in the ventricle. Distortion of the apex-dimension loop suggests a reduction in the efficiency of energy transfer from the myocardium to the circulation.

In patients with coronary artery disease, a common abnormality is a reduction in ventricular dimension during the upstroke of the apexcardiogram that approximates to the period of isovolumetric contraction (Fig. 17.13). Such a dimension change is a secondary abnormality in normal myocardium reflecting abnormal early systolic outward movement in a distant region of the ventricle not visualized by the M-mode ultrasound beam. Similarly, an increase in ventricular dimension during isovolumetric relaxation or the downstroke of the apexcardiogram is frequently observed (Fig. 17.13). This is a secondary event in normal myocardium resulting from premature thinning of the posterior wall and reflects prolonged or late onset of inward movement of myocardium in a distant region of the ventricle. Primary abnormalities of wall movement

are less commonly observed with increase in dimension during isovolumetric contraction and reduction in dimension during isovolumetric relaxation (Fig. 17.14). Reduction in dimension during isovolumetric relaxation has been demonstrated angiographically to be due to an abnormal increase in posterior wall thickness (28). Analysis of regional wall movement in patients with coronary artery disease using angiographic methods confirms that ventricular shape changes during the period of isovolumetric relaxation result from abnormal inward movement of myocardium supplied by a diseased coronary vessel and compensatory abnormal outward movement of nonaffected areas of myocardium (55).

A change in left ventricular shape during isovolumetric relaxation is related to loss of the normal well-defined relations between aortic valve closure, minimum cavity dimension, and mitral valve opening. It has been shown that in patients with coronary artery disease who exhibit features of incoordination the time intervals between the Q wave on the electrocardiogram and aortic valve closure (A_2) and Q to mitral valve opening remain constant, but that the time interval Q to minimum dimension is shortened (34). Shortening of Q to minimum dimension is closely associated with the presence of abnormal wall movement during isovolumetric contraction and is probably a manifestation of asynchronous termination of systole (33).

Apex-ventricular dimension loops and the time interval Q to minimum dimension have been used to investigate the effects of a variety of interventions in patients with chronic stable angina (34, 56, 57) and have also been applied to the study of patients with acute myocardial infarction (58, 59).

The effects of acute administration of nitroglycerin are complex (35, 56, 57). The time interval Q to minimum left ventricular dimension is reduced by nitroglycerin if this time interval is within the normal range in the control state, but it increases if the time interval is below the normal range in the control state. Nitroglycerin prolongs isovolumetric relaxation time and exacerbates abnormal dimension changes during the period of isovolumetric relaxation whether or not wall motion in the control state is coordinate. Effects similar to those of nitroglycerin are seen in patients with coronary artery disease following acute oral administration of propranolol (34). Although apparently exacerbating or provoking incoordinate left ventricular wall movement, both nitroglycerin and propranolol have potent antianginal effects. An explanation for this incongruity might be that by shortening the time interval Q to minimum dimension both drugs cause premature onset of posterior wall thinning (57). Thus, the time during which tension is developed in the ventricular wall is reduced (a major determinant of myocardial oxygen consumption) and the diastolic period augmenting coronary flow is prolonged. These advantages must outweigh the disadvantage of increased ventricular incoordination and associated reduction in cycle efficiency. The effects of coronary artery bypass grafting on indexes of coordinate left ventricular wall motion have also been studied. Revascularization does not alter wall motion if it was coordinate preoperatively. However, if wall motion was incoordinate preoperatively, it will considerably reduce the magnitude of abnormal dimension change during isovolumetric contraction and restores the time interval Q to minimum dimension to within the normal range (56).

In a serial study of patients with first myocardial infarction, incoordinate wall movement was detectable in all patients immediately after infarction and became most marked two to three days after the acute event (58). In those patients with Q wave infarction, the features of incoordinate wall movement persisted throughout the recovery period. By contrast, in patients with non–Q wave infarction, the features of incoordinate wall motion gradually resolved, and the apex-dimension loops returned to normal within eight weeks of infarction.

CONCLUSION

The digitizing method extends conventional M-mode echocardiography and provides information that can be used as a frame for analytical study of normal and abnormal cardiac structure and function. In addition to continuous left ventricular cavity dimension and wall thickness, their respective rates of change can be determined, the relations between endocardial movement and other physiologic events occurring during the cardiac cycle can be investigated, and characteristic abnormalities can be identified in a number of cardiac diseases. The normalized peak rate of dimension decrease during systole (peak VCF s^{-1}) can be used to assess ventricular contractile function and, when combined with continuous determinations of wall stress, can be used to calculate power. Finally, the technique has proved to be of particular value in the study of diastolic events and has highlighted the important role of abnormalities of diastolic function in many cardiac diseases.

REFERENCES

1. Logan-Sinclair RB, Oldershaw PJ, Gibson DG. Computing in echocardiography. Prog Cardiovasc Dis 1983;25:465.
2. Gibson DG, Brown DJ. Measurement of instantaneous left ventricular dimension and filling rate in man, using echocardiography. Br Heart J 1973;35:1141.
3. de Coodt PR, Mathey DG, Swan HJC. Automated analysis of the left ventricular diameter time curve from echocardiographic recordings. Comput Biomed Res 1976;9:549.
4. Saffer SI, Nixon JV, Mishelevick DJ. Simple method for computer aided analysis of echocardiograms. Am J Cardiol 1976;38:34.
5. Griffith JM, Henry WL. Video-scanner computer system for semiautomatic analysis of routine echocardiograms. Am J Cardiol 1973;32:961.
6. van Zweiten G, Bastiaans OL, Honkoop J, Vogel JA. Video tracing of M-mode echocardiograms. In: Lancee C, ed. Echocardiology. The Hague, Netherlands: Martinus-Nijhoff, 1976;469.
7. Hirsch M, Sanders WJ, Popp R. Computer processing of ultrasonic data from the cardiovascular system. Comput Biomed Res 1973;6:336.
8. Aubert AE, Denys BG, Denef B, Van de Werf F, De Geest H, Kesteloot H. Computer processing of echo-mechanocardiograms: methods and results. Comput Biomed Res 1982;15:57.
9. Upton MT, Gibson DG. The study of left ventricular function from digitized echocardiograms. Prog Cardiovasc Dis 1978;20:359.
10. Pollick C, Fitzgerald PJ, Popp RL. Variability of digitized echocardiography: size, source, and means of reduction. Am J Cardiol 1983;51:576.
11. Hall R, Bullock RE, Amer H, Griffiths C, Appleton D. Sources of error in digitizing M-mode echocardiograms. Ultrasonar Bull 1983; 5th Symposium on Echocardiology. p 107.
12. St John Sutton MG, Reichek N, Kastor JA, Giuliani ER. Computerized M-mode echocardiographic analysis of left ventricular dysfunction in cardiac amyloid. Circulation 1982;66:790.
13. Combellas I, Puigbo JJ, Acquatella H, Tortoledo F, Gomez JR. Echocardiographic features of impaired left ventricular function in Chagas's heart disease. Br Heart J 1985;53:298.
14. Gibson DG, Brown DJ. Assessment of left ventricular systolic function in man from simultaneous echocardiographic and pressure measurements. Br Heart J 1976;38:8.
15. Sandler M, Alderman EL. Determination of left ventricular size and shape. Circ Res 1974;34:1.
16. Gibson DG, Brown DJ. Continuous assessment of left ventricular shape in man. Br Heart J 1975;37:907.
17. Gibson DG, Brown DJ. Measurements of peak rate of left ventricular wall movement in man. Comparison of echocardiography and angiocardiography. Br Heart J 1975;37:677.

18. St John Sutton MG, Tajik AK, Gibson DG, Brown DJ, Seward JB, Giuliani ER. Echocardiographic assessment of left ventricular filling and septal and posterior wall dynamics in idiopathic hypertrophic subaortic stenosis. Circulation 1978;57:512.

19. Hanrath P, Mathey DG, Siegert R, Bleifeld W. Left ventricular relaxation and filling pattern in different forms of left ventricular hypertrophy: an echocardiographic study. Am J Cardiol 1979;45: 15.

20. Dawson JR, Sutton GC. Detection of clinically significant coronary artery disease in hypertensive patients. Echocardiographic study. Br Heart J 1981;46:595.

21. Gibson DG, Traill TA, Hall RJC, Brown DJ. Echocardiographic features of secondary left ventricular hypertrophy. Br Heart J 1979;41:54.

22. Shapiro LM, McKenna WJ. Left ventricular hypertrophy. Relation of structure to diastolic function in hypertension. Br Heart J 1984;51:637.

23. Moore RB, Shapiro LM, Gibson DG. Relation between electrocardiographic repolarisation changes and mechanical events in left ventricular hypertrophy. Br Heart J 1984;52:516.

24. Topol EJ, Traill TA, Fortuin NJ. Hypertensive hypertrophic cardiomyopathy of the elderly. N Engl J Med 1985;312:277.

25. Bahler RC, Vrobel TR, Martin P. The relation of heart rate and shortening fraction to echocardiographic indexes of left ventricular relaxation in normal subjects. J Am Coll Cardiol 1983;2:926.

26. St John Sutton MG, Traill TA, Ghafour AS, Brown DJ, Gibson DG. Echocardiographic assessment of left ventricular filling after mitral valve surgery. Br Heart J 1977;39:1283.

27. Shapiro LM, Beevers DG. Malignant hypertension: cardiac structure and function at presentation and during therapy. Br Heart J 1983;49:477.

28. Gibson DG, Traill TA, Brown DJ. Changes in left ventricular free wall thickness in patients with ischaemic heart disease. Br Heart J 1977;39:1312.

29. Traill TA, Gibson DG, Brown DJ. Study of left ventricular wall thickness and dimension changes using echocardiography. Br Heart J 1978;40:162.

30. Upton MT, Gibson DG, Brown DJ. Instantaneous mitral leaflet velocity and its relation to left ventricular wall movement in normal subjects. Br Heart J 1976;38:51.

31. Upton MT, Gibson DG, Brown DJ. Echocardiographic assessment of abnormal left ventricular relaxation in man. Br Heart J 1976;38:1001.

32. Hirschfield S, Lietman J, Boshat G, Borsmith C. Intracardiac pressure sound correlates of echocardiographic aortic valve closure. Circulation 1977;55:602.

33. Chen W, Gibson DG. Relation of isovolumic relaxation to left ventricular wall movement in man. Br Heart J 1979;42:51.

34. von Bibra H, Gibson DG, Nityanandan K. Effects of propranolol on left ventricular wall movement in patients with ischaemic heart disease. Br Heart J 1980;43:293.

35. Mattheus M, Shapiro E, Oldershaw PJ, Sacchetti R, Gibson DG. Noninvasive assessment of changes in left ventricular relaxation by combined phono-, echo- and mechanocardiography. Br Heart J 1982;47:253.

36. Venco A, Gibson DG, Brown DJ. Relation between apex cardiogram and changes in left ventricular pressure and dimension. Br Heart J 1977;39:117.

37. Willems JL, DeGeest H, Kesteloot H. On the value of apex cardiography for timing intracardiac events. Am J Cardiol 1971; 28:59.

38. Doran JH, Traill TA, Brown DJ, Gibson DG. Detection of abnormal left ventricular wall movement during isovolumic contraction and early relaxation. Comparison of echo- and angiocardiography. Br Heart J 1978;40:367.

39. Venco A, St John Sutton MG, Gibson DG, Brown DJ. Noninvasive assessment of left ventricular function after correction of severe aortic regurgitation. Br Heart J 1976;38:1324.

40. Prewitt T, Gibson DG, Brown DJ, Sutton GC. The "rapid filling wave" of the apex cardiogram. Its relation to echocardiographic and cineangiographic measurements of ventricular filling. Br Heart J 1975;37:1256.

41. Graham TP Jr, Covell JW, Sonnenblick EH. Control of myocardial oxygen consumption. J Clin Invest 1968;47:375.

42. Sandler H, Dodge HT. Left ventricular tension and stress in man. Circ Res 1963;13:91.

43. Brodie BR, McLaurin LP, Grossman W. Combined haemodynamic-ultrasonic method for studying left ventricular wall stress. Am J Cardiol 1976;37:864.

44. Reichek N, Wilson J, St John Sutton M, Plappert TA, Goldberg S, Hirshfield JW. Noninvasive determination of left ventricular end-systolic stress: validation of the method and initial application. Circulation 1982;65:99.

45. Hall R, Austin A, Hunter S. M-mode echogram as a means of distinguishing between mild and severe mitral stenosis. Br Heart J 1981;46:486.

46. St John Sutton MG, Roudaut R, Oldershaw P, Bricaud H. Echocardiographic assessment of left ventricular filling characteristics after mitral valve replacement with the St Jude medical prosthesis. Br Heart J 1981;45:365.

47. Dawkins KD, Cotter L, Gibson DG. Assessment of mitral Björk-Shiley prosthetic dysfunction using digitised M-mode echocardiography. Br Heart J 1984;51:168.

48. Sanderson JE, Gibson DG, Brown DJ, Goodwin JF. Left ventricular filling in hypertrophic cardiomyopathy. An echocardiographic study. Br Heart J 1977;39:661.

49. Alvares RF, Goodwin JF. Noninvasive assessment of diastolic function in hypertrophic cardiomyopathy on and off beta adrenergic blocking drugs. Br Heart J 1982;48:204.

50. Davies J, Gibson DG, Foale RA, et al. Echocardiographic features of eosinophilic heart disease. Br Heart J 1982;48:434.

51. St John Sutton MG, Olukotun AY, Tajik AJ, Lorett JL, Giuliani ER. Left ventricular function in Freidrich's ataxia. An echocardiographical study. Br Heart J 1980;44:399.

52. Ahmad M, Sanderson JE, Dubowitz V, Hallidie-Smith KA. Echocardiographic assessment of left ventricular function in Duchenne's muscular dystrophy. Br Heart J 1978;40:734.

53. Goldberg SJ, Feldman L, Reinecke C, Stern LZ, Sahn DJ, Allen HD. Echocardiographic determination of contraction and relaxation measurements of the left ventricular wall in normal subjects and patients with muscular dystrophy. Circulation 1980;62: 1061.

54. Venco A, Sariotti M, Besana D. Noninvasive assessment of left ventricular function in myotonic muscular dystrophy. Br Heart J 1978;40:1262.

55. Gibson DG, Prewitt TA, Brown DJ. Analysis of left ventricular wall movement during isovolumic relaxation and its relation to coronary artery disease. Br Heart J 1976;38:1010.

56. Wong P, Gibson DG. Effect of sublingual nitroglycerin on left ventricular wall movement in patients with coronary artery disease. Comparison with propranolol and saphenous bypass grafting. La Nouvelle Presse Medicale 1980;34:2393.

57. Gibson DG, Doran JH, Traill TA, Brown DJ. Regional abnormalities of left ventricular wall movement during isovolumic relaxation in patients with ischaemic heart disease. Eur J Cardiol 1978;7(suppl):251.

58. Dawson JR, Sutton GC. Incoordinate wall motion after acute myocardial infarction. Serial echocardiographic assessment. Br Heart J 1984;51:545.

59. Pierard LA, van Meurs-van Woezik H, Roelandt J. Left ventricular apex-dimension loops in acute myocardial infarction. Am J Cardiol 1984;54:526.

18
Contrast Echocardiography

Rodney Foale

INTRODUCTION

Contrast echocardiography is the production of a transient increase in echo intensity within an echocardiographic image. Echocardiographic contrast can be produced by a variety of interventions, all of which induce a change in the physical composition of blood by increasing the density of ultrasound targets. In routine clinical practice, these targets are gaseous bubbles (referred to as microbubbles) of approximately 15 to 40 μm in diameter. The clinical utility of contrast echocardiography derives from the scattered specular echoes that arise from these target particles within the path of the ultrasound beam. The contrast echo effect thus created is carried in the bloodstream and displays the blood flow patterns within the heart.

Among the first to report this phenomenon were Gramiak, Shah, and Kramer (1), who with Feigenbaum et al. (2) described the production of echocardiographic contrast effect within intracardiac chambers during cardiac catheterization. This technique has been used to study the abnormal blood flow in intracardiac shunts by assessing the timing and location of contrast appearance during M-mode echo recordings of right and left heart chambers. Figure 18.1 shows the sequence of contrast appearance from the right to the left side of the interventricular septum below the mitral valve, confirming a ventricular septal defect as the cause of the right-to-left shunt. The spatial orientation provided by two-dimensional contrast echocardiography has supplemented these observations by the direct visualization of abnormal blood flow between the cardiac chambers. The improvement in resolution of newer generation ultrasound systems has greatly facilitated the demonstration of abnormal cardiac connections, intracardiac shunts, and valvular regurgitation.

The introduction of Doppler ultrasound has challenged the role of two-dimensional contrast echocardiography in the detection of abnormal intracardiac blood flow patterns. Furthermore, the recent advent of color-flow cardiac Doppler provides the potential for simultaneous display of functional and anatomic information in an easily recognizable and completely noninvasive format. Nonetheless, contrast echocardiography remains a valuable adjunct to echocardiographic technique.

Recently, interest has focused on the development of polysaccharide or sonicated human serum albumen contrast agents consisting of particles small enough to traverse pulmonary or myocardial capillary beds. These developments herald an expansion in echocardiographic contrast techniques in two main areas. First, by transpulmonary passage of contrast injected into the right side of the circulation, an alternative to left heart angiography may be provided. Second, myocardial blood flow may be quantified in vivo by measuring the rate of contrast passage through the myocardium as the contrast traverses the capillary bed. Animal models have already been researched, but many problems remain, the most important of which is the need for a safe, nontoxic contrast-producing agent that does not interfere with regional blood flow.

MECHANISMS AND TECHNIQUES IN THE PRODUCTION OF CONTRAST ECHOCARDIOGRAPHIC EFFECT

Mechanisms of Contrast Production

Many techniques have been advocated for producing contrast echocardiographic effect (Table 18.1) (3–10). Two basic mechanisms that rely on different principles are involved. The first, used in the diagnosis of abnormal communications between pulmonary and systemic circulations, depends on the microbubbles that are filtered by the pulmonary capillary bed but are *not* reaching the left heart. The second depends on the contrast agent's traversing the capillary beds. Contrast

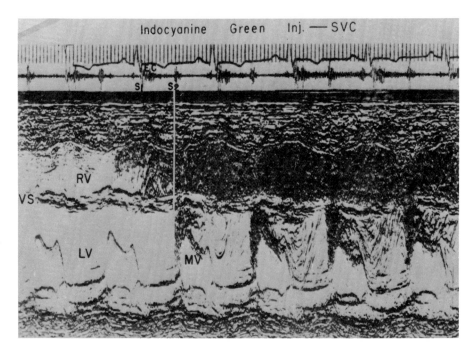

Figure 18.1. M-mode echocardiogram with contrast injection from a patient with a right-to-left shunt at ventricular level. Contrast echo appearance within the right heart is followed by contrast entering the left ventricle (LV) (below mitral valve [MV]) during isovolumetric relaxation. SVC = superior vena cava; VS = ventricular septum. (Reproduced from Tajik AJ, Seward JB. Contrast echocardiography. Cardiovasc Clin 1979;9:2.)

may, therefore, appear within the left heart from a right-sided injection or follow blood flow through myocardium when injected into the left heart (usually aorta).

In standard clinical practice, gaseous microbubbles are introduced as a bolus to the venous circulation. Earlier studies support the role of microbubbles as ultrasonic targets rather than turbulence induced at the cannula tip by the velocity of injection (11). It is generally believed that microbubbles are suspended in the solution in the syringe prior to injection. Support for this belief comes from the empirical observation that improved contrast effect follows vigorous hand agitation of the syringe. This enhancement of the contrast effect is probably due to further dispersion of atmospheric microbubbles (O_2, CO_2, and N_2) within the injectate (12). Microbubbles may also be produced at the cannula tip following a forceful injection since, according to Bernoulli's principle, dissolved gas in the blood condenses and forms microbubbles due to reduction in the partial pressure that occurs in the high-velocity bloodstream produced by pressure injection.

Whatever the mechanisms involved in their production, microbubbles remain in solution by the surface tension properties of the injectate. The dispersion of the bolus of ultrasonic targets depends on a number of factors, all of which are influenced by the injection technique. These factors include the length and tortuosity of the systemic venous route to the heart, the velocity of venous return, and the surface tension of the injectate, which should retard the dissolution of the small gaseous elements.

Ideally, the contrast material arrives in the right atrium (RA) as a discrete bolus, which in normal individuals passes through the right ventricle, pulmonary artery, and pulmonary capillary bed. In this passage through the right heart, the microbubbles travel

Table 18.1. Agents Used in Contrast Echocardiography

Contrast Agent	Authors	Condition
Indocyanine green	Gramiak et al. (1)	Validation of M-mode
	Feigenbaum et al. (2)	Anatomy
Saline	Duff, Gutgesell (3)	Right-to-left shunts after congenital heart surgery
Dextrose and dextrose/saline	Seward et al. (4)	Intracardiac shunts
Patient's own blood	Pieroni et al. (5)	Intracardiac shunts; valvular regurgitation
CO_2 gas	Reale (6)	Transpulmonary contrast
Hydrogen peroxide	Armstrong et al. (7)	Myocardial perfusion
Renograffin and saline	Tei et al. (8)	Myocardial perfusion
Polysaccharide complexes	Smith et al. (9)	Myocardial perfusion
Sugar/saline sonicated combinations (e.g., sorbitol, sorbitol/dextrose, carbonated saline, mannitol/dextrose, dextrose 50%, dextrose 70%)	Feinstein et al. (10)	Myocardial perfusion

with much the same velocity as the accompanying blood elements (13). Gaseous microbubbles used in routine clinical practice are too large to pass through the capillary bed and are filtered from the circulation and diffused across alveolar membranes to the alveoli. Thus, contrast effect is normally never observed in the left side of the heart, but is observed in anomalous systemic venous connections, abnormal intracardiac communications, or pulmonary arteriovenous shunts. The last may occur congenitally but also may occur in patients with pneumonic collapse and postoperative atelectasis.

Contrast agents under development for left heart studies and the study of myocardial blood flow are discussed in later sections of this chapter.

Practical Aspects of Contrast Technique

Venous Access

Adequate contrast echocardiographic studies can be obtained with appropriate peripheral venous access. Considering the minimally invasive nature of the technique, an antecubital vein is preferred, although the use of a central cannula positioned in the vena cava or RA results in a greatly enhanced contrast effect. With peripheral venous access, the left arm should be used because one of the most common congenital heart abnormalities is persistence of the left superior vena cava, which most frequently drains into the RA via the coronary sinus (CS) (14). This anomaly of systemic venous return will not be detected unless a left-arm vein is used.

An antecubital vein draining to the medial aspect of the arm is the best choice as its connections to axillary and subclavian veins are larger and less tortuous than its laterally draining counterpart. The size of the vein selected should permit the widest of standard intravenous cannulae to be inserted (in an adult, French gauge 17, 19, or 21; in an infant or child, a French gauge 21, 23, or 25). In neonates, venous access is less easily achieved. Nevertheless, satisfactory contrast effect can be obtained by injecting into a scalp vein needle or via an umbilical catheter or a previously positioned venous cannula.

Most of the various syringe attachments to the intravenous cannula owe their use to local prejudice and habit. The contrast effect can be enhanced if the injectate is rapidly followed by an equal volume of dextrose saline flush, which may accelerate the bolus of injectate to the venae cavae. This necessitates the connection of two syringes to the cannula by means of a three-way tap, which in turn is fitted to flexible tubing.

Injectate

The type and volume of injectate recommended vary among experienced ultrasound laboratories. Hand-agitated 5 percent dextrose for both injectate and flush is preferable for neonatal, pediatric, and adult populations. This solution avoids sodium load, which may be an important consideration in sick neonates, whose own blood may be withdrawn into the syringe and then quickly reinjected. Indocyanine green results in superior echocardiographic contrast effect and may be preferred in adult patients who present technical difficulties in obtaining adequate echocardiographic images. The superiority of this agent in producing contrast effect is probably due to its surface tension properties, which favor the persistence of suspended microbubbles.

Five to 10 ml of injectate in a 10-ml syringe, followed by injection of a similar volume of flush solution, is suitable for adult contrast echocardiographic examinations. In the neonate and infant, 1 to 5 mL is appropriate.

The force of injection appears to be one determinant of a satisfactory contrast effect. While this may relate to rapid delivery of the bolus to the right heart, the formation of microbubbles within the high velocity, low partial pressure jet may also contribute to this contrast effect. Injections of the selected agent and flush should be given as rapidly as the stability of venous access and manual dexterity will allow.

Precautions and Adverse Effects

Various precautions must be observed when undertaking contrast echocardiographic studies. First, a secure position for the intravenous cannula should be ensured so as to minimize the possibility of painful local extravasation of injectate into the tissues following a forceful bolus injection. Second, care should be taken to ensure sterility of the procedure so that the possibility of infective complications is minimized. Third, all visible bubbles must be carefully removed from the syringe and its connections since even in large left-to-right intracardiac shunts there may be transient shunt reversal from right to left with potential systemic embolism (15).

Despite the widespread use of the contrast echocardiographic method, the reported side effects are few. In more than 1000 contrast echocardiographic studies undertaken at our laboratory, no adverse systemic effects have been recorded. A survey undertaken by the American Society of Echocardiography reported the incidence of transient side effects, including neurologic and respiratory symptoms, as less than 0.1 percent, and no lasting adverse effects were reported (16). Nevertheless, the *potential* for systemic embolism must always be guarded against by the practice of meticulous technique.

Spontaneous Echoes and Other Mechanisms

Spontaneous Contrast Effect

Isolated contrast echoes that pass through systemic veins and the right side of the heart are common observations in subjects with indwelling intravenous cannulae and slow, even intravenous infusions. These echoes enter the venous circulation as microbubbles in the infusion.

Occasionally, isolated contrast echoes may be observed passing through the innominate vein or superior vena cava when a suprasternal view is employed in subjects without indwelling intravenous cannulae. The origin of these echoes is unexplained. One possibility is the entry of lipid particles, chylomicrons from the common bile duct. The particles approximate contrast microbubble size and should theoretically present as echo targets.

The high-resolution cardiac ultrasound systems now available often demonstrate spontaneous contrast echo effect within the heart and distended venae cavae in low blood flow states. This effect is subjectively different from the discrete targets that result from injections of standard contrast agents and appears as a cloud of small echo targets within dilated cardiac chambers where blood flow velocity is decreased (Fig. 18.2). This appearance has been reported in the left ventricle adjacent to akinetic infarcted regions (17, 18) and in patients with advanced cardiomyopathy and congestive heart failure. We have also observed this effect in massively distended left atria (LA) of patients with severe mitral stenosis. In this case, the echoes appear to pass into the left ventricle (LV) within the diastolic flow jet. Spontaneous contrast echoes can also be observed within dilated venae cavae and the hepatic venous radicles in pericardial constriction (19) and in severe right heart heart failure. A similar, although perhaps nosologically different, effect has been described using M-mode and two-dimensional echocardiography on the ventricular side of a prosthetic mitral valve (MV) (20–22).

Endocavitary Ablation

Contrast echoes identical to those produced with standard contrast agents were demonstrated after a direct-current (DC) discharge within the right side of the heart (23). This therapeutic procedure, termed *endocavitary ablation*, is used for the interruption of atrioventricular (AV) nodal conduction in patients who present with drug-resistant supraventricular arrhythmia. Following DC discharge of even small amounts,

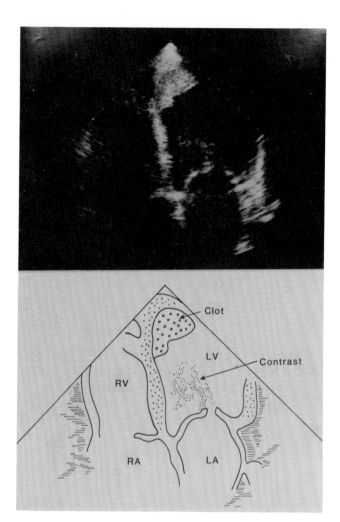

Figure 18.2. Spontaneous contrast echoes within the LV (apical four-chamber view) of a patient with dilated cardiomyopathy (and biventricular thrombus). The echoes (arrows) appear to swirl toward the apex with early diastolic filling following mitral valve opening.

great quantities of contrast echoes are seen in the right and occasionally the left heart chamber (Fig. 18.3). The contrast effect is due to gaseous release and not blood element destruction, and therefore, no threat is posed to the right- or left-sided circulations from particulate embolism (24). Nevertheless, embolism of small gaseous particles to end capillaries (e.g., in the brain) may have adverse consequences that do not manifest as gross neurologic defects, and small gaseous embolism may underlie subtle neurologic complications seen following cardiopulmonary bypass (25).

Quantification of Two-Dimensional Contrast Echocardiographic Effect

The maximum amplitude of the contrast echo signal and the rate of appearance and decay of the contrast

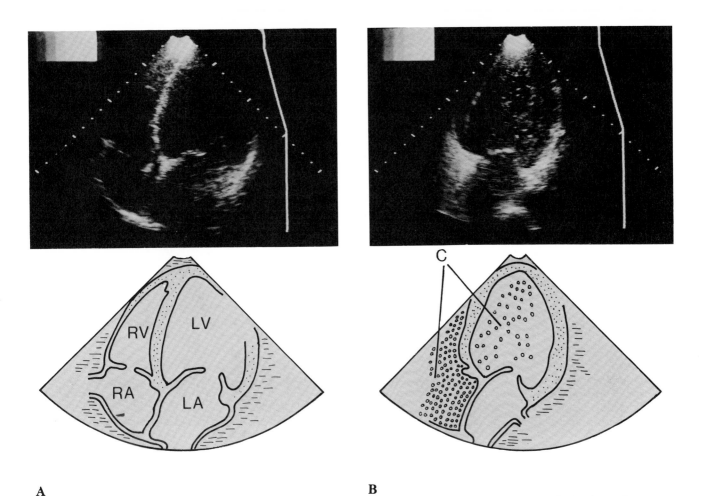

A   **B**

Figure 18.3. Intense contrast echo effect within the right heart and LV following direct current (DC) discharge in a patient undergoing His bundle ablation. (*A*) Control apical four-chamber view. (*B*) Following DC current discharge. C = contrast. (Reproduced with permission from Rowland E, Foale R, et al. Intracardiac contrast echoes during transvenous His bundle ablation. Br Heart J 1985;53:240.)

effect (time activity curve) are two features considered in any subjective assessment of contrast echocardiographic studies. Various reports have attempted to quantify the contrast detected by eye (26–30). Quantification of temporal changes in contrast echo amplitude is a complex task that at present requires sophisticated computer image-processing techniques.

The quantification of contrast echo effect began with the use of computer-aided video-densitometry. By sampling intensity within selected regions of interest (e.g., left and right outflow tracts, LV), it was shown that a computer-generated time intensity curve of contrast echo amplitude could be used to assist recognition of the left-to-right component of an intracardiac shunt (26, 27). This technique, however, has not gained widespread acceptance because the information obtained cannot distinguish artifact from true contrast signal.

The time course of the passage of echo contrast through the right heart has been used to derive an indicator-dilution curve from which cardiac output can be estimated (28). However, there have been major methodologic problems with this technique, including the constraints of background noise, motion artifact, and the unpredictable behavior exhibited by the contrast agents.

The problems of measuring myocardial perfusion by contrast echocardiography were addressed in an experimental model of myocardial ischemia (29). These authors ignored the necessity of direct intracoronary contrast echo injection and derived a correlation between the washout rate of contrast material and myocardial perfusion.

One major constraint of the method relates to the attenuation of ultrasound by its passage through microbubble contrast and the resulting distortion of intensity profiles when the contrast-filled myocardium presents a strong specular target. The potential for comparing myocardial perfusion in neighboring LV regions may also be restricted by nonuniform attenuation of the

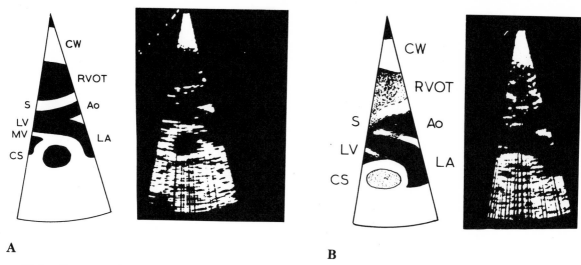

A   **B**

Figure 18.4.   Contrast echo effect within CS following a left-arm peripheral venous injection confirms drainage of a persistent left superior vena cava to dilated CS. (*A*) Control parasternal long-axis view. (*B*) Following contrast injection from a left arm. Ao = aorta; CW = chest wall; RVOT = right ventricular outflow tract; S = septum. (Reproduced with permission from Foale R, Bourdillon PDV, et al. Persistant left superior vena cava with coronary sinus and left atrial connections. Eur J Cardiol 1980;11:227.)

ultrasound sector as the beam traverses unequal tissue densities (29, 30). However, the measurement of myocardial blood flow by contrast echocardiography remains dependent on the validation of reliable time activity curves of myocardial contrast washout. Much active research is under way in contrast agent development and in signal processing, which may overcome many of the present constraints of quantitation.

THE DIAGNOSIS OF ABNORMAL VENOUS CONNECTIONS, INTRACARDIAC SHUNTS, AND VALVULAR REGURGITATION

Assessment of Anomalous Systemic and Pulmonary Venous Return

Anomalies of systemic venous return are frequently associated with other intracardiac abnormalities and are important if cardiac catheterization or surgery is contemplated (14). The most common abnormal venous connection is persistence of a left-sided superior vena cava. In this condition, both superior venae cavae return to the RA, the left via the CS, which dilates to accommodate the increased venous return from the left hemithorax. Less commonly, the left superior vena cava drains directly into the LA. Other abnormal systemic venous connections exist, including inferior vena caval drainage to abnormal azygous or hemiazygous systems.

The improvement in ultrasound technology and the experience gained from the use of suprasternal views as part of a standardized echocardiographic protocol have facilitated the visualization of superior venae cavae and innominate connections. Suspected abnormalities of the central venous connections may be

confirmed by M-mode and two-dimensional contrast echocardiographic studies (31, 32).

The presence of a dilated CS that appears to lie within the LA in the region of the posterior AV junction raises the possibility of a persistent left superior vena caval connection. Other causes of such dilatation should be considered, such as an RA pressure or volume overload or anomalous pulmonary venous return to the CS. This dilatation should not be confused with that of the descending aorta, which may be seen in a similar location in the parasternal long-axis view but lies outside the LA boundary. Contrast echocardiographic study via a left-arm vein will confirm the return of blood to the RA via the abnormal CS connection when the dilated sinus opacifies prior to the right-sided appearance of contrast agent (Fig. 18.4). Contrast echocardiography performed from the left arm has shown the rare abnormality of persistent left superior vena caval connection to the CS, whose course behind the LA is unroofed with a resulting right-to-left shunt at CS level (33). In this report, contrast appeared in the CS and LA simultaneously (Fig. 18.5).

The direct connection of left superior vena cava to LA results in opacification of only the atrial chamber following a left-arm injection; in the presence of an interatrial connection, the LA is opacified before the contrast appears in the RA. With persistence of the left superior vena cava, there is usually little or no functional venous connection between left and right hemithoraxes, and the normal right-sided superior vena cava drains into the RA. Therefore, injection of contrast from this side alone will confirm normal superior vena caval–RA connections by the opacification of the

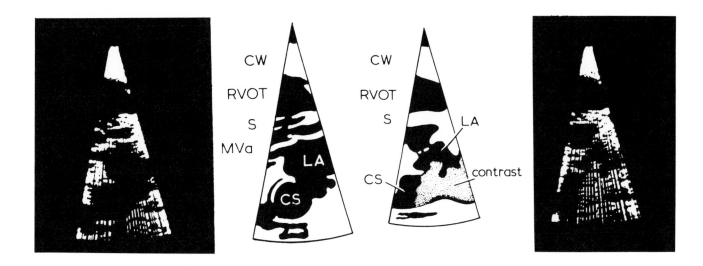

A   **B**

Figure 18.5. Contrast effect passing from CS to LA in a patient with an unroofed CS draining a persistent left superior vena cava. (*A*) Control parasternal long-axis view. (*B*) Following contrast injection. CW = chest wall; MVa = mitral valve; RVOT = right ventricular outflow tract; S = septum. (Reproduced with permission from Bourdillon PDV, Foale R, et al. Persistant left superior vena cava with coronary sinus and left atrial connections. Eur J Cardiol 1980;11:227.)

RA but will not determine the abnormalities of left vena caval drainage.

Anomalies of inferior vena caval connection may be demonstrated by injecting contrast into the femoral vein and timing the appearance of contrast in the LA and RA. Femoral venous catheterization, however, contradicts the essential minimally invasive advantages of contrast echocardiographic technique.

Anomalous pulmonary venous return to the CS may occur, in which case there is a dilatation of CS and a right-to-left shunt across atrial septum. Contrast injected via the left or right arm will result in the opacification of RA, then LA, thus displaying the obligatory right-to-left shunt at atrial level. The CS will remain unopacified, suggesting that it receives drainage from the pulmonary veins.

The Diagnosis of Interatrial Communications

The atrial septum may be viewed with two-dimensional echocardiography from parasternal and apical four-chamber positions but is best visualized from the subcostal position, where the target faces the ultrasound beam.

The interatrial septum can usually be imaged adequately in children and adults from all three transducer locations (i.e., parasternal, apical, and subcostal positions). However, the incidence of false-positive diagnoses for the condition in adults is high (34). Developments in two-dimensional ultrasound technology have improved resolution of the atrial septum, and contrast echocardiography remains a useful adjunct in those patients in whom an atrial septal defect is suspected.

Anatomy

Von Rokitansky elegantly described the anatomy of atrial septal defects in 1875 (35), but the nomenclature continues to evolve based on the defect's position in the atrial septum (36) and is described in detail in Chapter 25. For the purpose of contrast echo studies, these defects will be divided into four groups by their position in the interatrial septum: 1) high in the posterosuperior part of the septum (sinus venosus defect) and close to the orifices of the right superior vena cava and right upper pulmonary veins, 2) in the middle part of the atrial septum in the region of the fossa ovalis (ostium secundum defect), 3) in the lower part of the atrial septum at the crux of the heart (ostium primum or AV canal defect), and 4) in the region of the CS as part of a developmental complex that includes drainage of persistent left superior vena cava to LA directly. Other anatomic varieties exist, including a virtual total absence of the septum (common atrium) and defects that, although large, are fenestrated and may give a strong echocardiographic signal despite allowing considerable interatrial blood flow. Furthermore, under conditions of high LA pressure with distention, the foramen ovale, usually anatomically and functionally closed, may stretch, resulting in a left-to-right shunt. Under normal conditions, however, no blood flow in either direction occurs across a foramen ovale even if probe patent.

Physiologic Considerations

The physiology of blood flow across the interatrial septum depends on 1) the size of the defect, 2) the

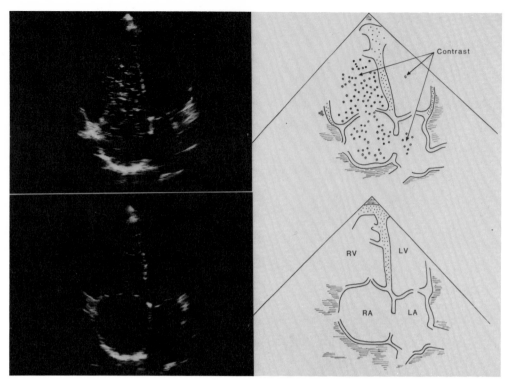

Figure 18.6. Contrast echocardiographic study of a patient with a 1.9:1.0 left-to-right shunt at atrial level. In this patient, a sinus venosus defect was demonstrated. Note that contrast appears within the LA and LV (arrows) and that the demonstration of only one microbubble in the LA and LV was sufficient to justify the diagnosis of an interatrial communication. (*Upper panel*) Following peripheral venous contrast injection. (*Lower panel*) Control apical four-chamber view.

distensibility of right ventricle (RV) and LV, and 3) the pressure and resistance of the pulmonary vascular tree. In diastole, with the two AV valves open, there is unhindered communication between the four cardiac chambers. Therefore, blood flows via the path of least resistance. Most often, no pressure difference exists across an atrial septal defect. The greater distensibility (or compliance) of the RV, therefore, allows for the left-to-right component of the atrial shunt. In the first instance, this will be limited simply by the anatomic size of the defect.

In small defects that allow a relatively small left-to-right shunt and in large defects, RV distensibility lessens exponentially throughout the diastolic filling period so that vena caval return to RA in later diastole is in part directed across the interatrial septum to LA. In older patients who develop changes in RV compliance or in patients who have a pressure load on the RV because of either RV outflow obstruction or a change in pulmonary vascular resistance, shunt reversal from right to left may increase significantly. The bidirectional nature of all dominant left-to-right shunting at atrial level has been demonstrated in a number of studies (37–40).

Right-to-left shunting across an isolated atrial septal defect is uncommon and results from pulmonary hypertension. In the neonate, the right-to-left shunt is obligatory when anomalous pulmonary venous return is to the RA rather than the LA chamber.

Contrast Echocardiography

In patients with a dominant left-to-right shunt, a peripheral venous contrast injection will result in the immediate opacification of the RA and RV, with transient appearance of contrast within the LA at end diastole and early systole (Fig. 18.6). Several authors have demonstrated this finding, which is seen even with anatomically small defects (41–46). The demonstration of LA contrast in subjects with uncomplicated atrial septal defects, however, is very dependent on obtaining technically high-quality images of the heart from any or all of the three transducer positions (parasternal, apical, and subcostal). Good contrast effect is mandatory for the demonstration of blood flow across the atrial septal defect. Failure to fulfill these requirements accounts for virtually all false-negative results. Paradoxically, an intense contrast effect tends to obscure the subtle change in echo intensities that indicates the presence of the transatrial blood flow from right to left. Experience has shown the value of a deliberately weak contrast effect (Fig. 18.6).

"Negative contrast effect" (Fig. 18.7) is the demonstration of unopacified blood within the RA from LA

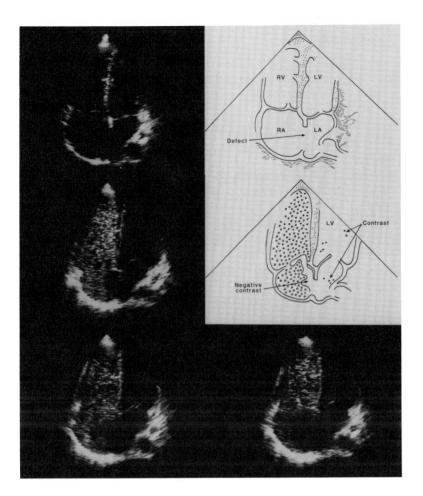

Figure 18.7. Sequential frames of negative echocardiographic effect (*arrows*) in a patient with ostium secundum atrial septal defect and a 2:1 left-to-right shunt. Note additional left heart contrast echo appearance. (Top panel) Control apical four-chamber view. (Lower panels) Expanding region of negative contrast.

blood flow across the atrial septal defect. This finding has been useful in the diagnosis of atrial septal defect when direct visualization of the defect is unclear or ambiguous (47). However, others have found limitations in detecting a negative contrast effect (48), which is often small and may be masked by the brightness of surrounding contrast effect. Furthermore, unopacified blood is seen within the RA from CS and vena caval return. Therefore, unless clearly observed as originating from the LA, this negative contrast effect is not specific for interatrial flow.

In patients with balanced shunts due to associated RV outflow obstruction or pulmonary hypertension and in patients with obligatory right-to-left shunts as in total anomalous pulmonary venous return, full opacification of LA can be seen across the defect following the appearance of RA contrast effect (41). It should be stressed that in such individuals absolute attention must be paid to the contrast technique so as to avoid any risk of systemic embolism.

The Diagnosis of Ventricular Shunts

Early reports of success in visualizing ventricular septal defects by two-dimensional echocardiography cor-

rectly predicted its present value in the diagnosis of ventricular shunts (49, 50). Defects of the membranous septum can now be readily detected, and the direct imaging of all but the smallest of muscular septal defects is possible using present-generation, high-resolution two-dimensional imaging systems. The advent of Doppler echocardiography has facilitated the noninvasive determination of a ventricular site for an intracardiac shunt by detecting abnormal interventricular blood flow patterns.

Pathophysiologic Considerations

The physiologic principles underlying the detection of atrial septal defects by contrast echocardiography are manifestly different for left-to-right shunts at ventricular level. Even in small atrial septal defects, there is some bidirectional shunt. In ventricular septal defects, shunt blood flow is unidirectional unless the defect is anatomically large or is complicated by either RV outflow tract obstruction or severe pulmonary vascular disease.

A small ventricular septal defect causes little or no functional disturbance to the left or right heart. In systole, there is restriction of left-to-right blood flow, so that the potential force of systemic pressure is not felt in the RV or the pulmonary circulation. Throughout diastole, the differences between RV and LV distensibilities maintain these pressure differences (51). The protection of the pulmonary circulation lessens as the size of the defect increases. With a moderate-size defect, there is substantial volume loading of both the LV *and* the RV. At this point, RV distensibility can diminish so that diastolic right-to-left shunting may occur. There is also the potential for a right-to-left shunt in moderate-size defects when RV pressure transiently exceeds that of the LV in late ejection and during isovolumetric relaxation.

Large ventricular septal defects are not restrictive of left-to-right flow, so that the LV and RV are both at systemic pressure. Thus, the pulmonary circulation is exposed to systemic pressure, and pulmonary hypertension may result.

Pulmonary vascular resistance or RV outflow obstruction determines the volume of left-to-right shunt. As RV distensibility approaches its limit, the opportunity for diastolic right-to-left shunting will increase. Eisenmenger's complex occurs when pulmonary vascular resistance increases so as to cause a reduction and then a reversal of left-to-right blood flow at ventricular level. Reversal of the left-to-right shunt may also be caused by RV outflow obstruction, which may occur as an accompanying congenital anomaly or may

develop at infundibular level as the RV hypertrophies. In these circumstances, right-to-left systolic shunting is obligatory when the obstruction causes suprasystemic RV pressure. Diastolic shunt reversal also occurs when secondary RV hypertrophy has prematurely limited RV distensibility.

Contrast Echocardiography

The aforementioned physiologic considerations determine the results of contrast echocardiographic study in ventricular septal defects. Thus, in small defects, no contrast will be seen within the LV at any time during the cardiac cycle after a right-sided injection. When the defect (and the shunt) become larger and have caused a substantial increase in RV systolic pressure and a change in diastolic distensibility, contrast will cross the defect into the left heart in late systole and early diastole (52, 53). Therefore, from this point (usually reached when the RV systolic pressure is 70 mm Hg or greater), a peripheral venous contrast injection will help confirm the presence of the septal defect (Fig. 18.8).

In ventricular septal defect complicating myocardial infarction, RV systolic pressures do not appear to permit a systolic right-to-left shunt. Right-to-left shunting then, when it occurs, is usually a diastolic event and is reflective of the relative diastolic dysfunction of RV and LV. Therefore, on occasion, the appearance of

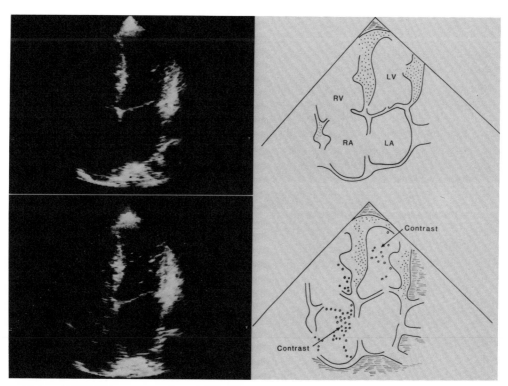

Figure 18.8.   Contrast effect within the right heart and LV (*arrows*) in a patient with a ventricular septal defect. In this patient, RV pressure was 50 percent of systemic pressure. (*Upper panel*) Control. (*Lower panel*) Following contrast injection.

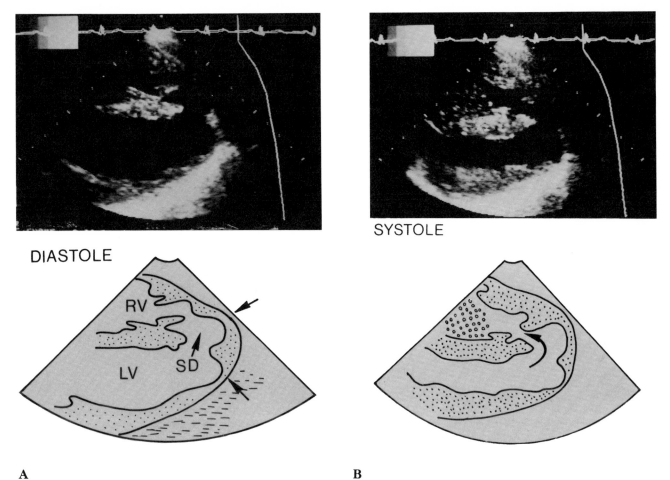

A   **B**

Figure 18.9. Subcostal four-chamber view in a patient with an apical myocardial infarction complicated by ventricular septal defect (SD). Note the defect (*arrows*), the regional systolic wall thinning with apical dyskinesis of the cardiac apex (*A*), and the washout of contrast from the apex (*B*) of the RV from the systolic left-to-right shunt. (Reproduced from Doble N, Smith G, Foale RA. Clin Cardiol [in press].)

left-sided contrast may aid in the confirmation of the diagnosis. More commonly, however, a systolic washout effect of negative contrast can be seen as the left-to-right systolic shunt occurs (Fig. 18.9).

With RV pressure load from RV outflow tract obstruction, such as in tetralogy of Fallot and Eisenmenger's complex (high pulmonary vascular resistance complicating ventricular septal defect), right-to-left passage of contrast is observed in systole and diastole. Thus, peripheral venous injection of contrast will result in the complete opacification of the LV after right heart contrast echoes appear. In RV outflow obstruction, the position of the defect in relation to the outflow vessels may determine the timing and pattern of the right-to-left shunt as illustrated in Fig. 18.10.

The Presence of Extracardiac Shunts: Patent Ductus Arteriosus

An extracardiac shunt through a patent ductus arteriosus is common in sick neonates, and M-mode echo-

cardiography has an established role in the diagnosis and follow-up of this condition (54, 55). The serial determinations of LA size and LA–aortic root ratio are useful noninvasive tools in assessing the magnitude of a left-to-right shunt through the duct.

Two-dimensional echocardiography has been used to visualize the patent ductus arteriosus directly, although obtaining unambiguous images of the region not infrequently poses a considerable technical challenge simply because of the anatomic location of the duct. Contrast injection performed during echocardiographic study adds considerably to the diagnosis of patent ductus arteriosus and establishes the direction of the shunt (56). In the sick neonate with an indwelling umbilical catheter positioned in the descending thoracic aorta, a left-to-right ductal shunt can be deduced from opacification of both aorta and pulmonary artery. Peripheral venous injection while imaging the area will provide an index of right-to-left shunting by the opacification of the descending aorta.

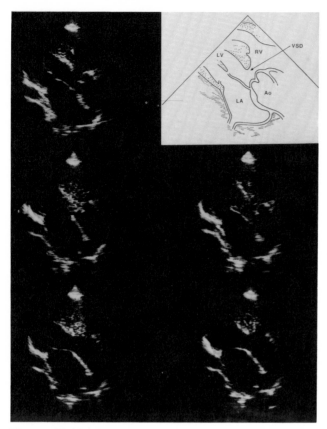

Figure 18.10. Tetralogy of Fallot with pulmonary stenosis. The relationship of aorta (Ao) to ventricular septal defect (VSD) is displayed in this modified apical two-chamber view. (*Upper panel*) Control. In subsequent frames (left to right, middle to lower panels), contrast is observed to fill the ventricle throughout diastole (*middle panel*), confirming the right-to-left diastolic shunt. (*Lower panel*) In systole, Ao receives exclusive LV blood flow. On other projections in this patient, systolic filling of pulmonary artery from contrast in RV blood was demonstrated.

The Detection of Valvular Regurgitation

Peripheral venous injection of contrast may identify right-sided valvular regurgitation when undertaken during two-dimensional echocardiographic study. In tricuspid regurgitation, persistence of contrast within the RA or its vena caval connections can be observed as the regurgitant tricuspid jet delays the clearance of the microbubbles from the atrial chamber.

Similarly, in pulmonary regurgitation, there is marked persistence of the contrast effect within the RV, and occasionally, individual microbubbles can be traced across the valve within the regurgitant bloodstreams.

False-positive diagnoses of valvular regurgitation, however, are frequent in low cardiac output states and in occasional patients in whom the delivery of a *discrete* bolus of contrast is not successful. Microbubbles whose appearance in the right heart is delayed cannot be reliably distinguished from the contrast effect of regurgitant flow. These factors and the advent of Doppler echocardiography have limited the application of the contrast echo technique in valvular regurgitation.

Contrast echocardiography to demonstrate mitral regurgitation during left heart study has been successfully substituted for conventional angiographic agents in reports of pacing-induced regional wall motion abnormalities and in the evaluation of MV competence following MV repair (57, 58). In the growing area of conservative MV procedures, contrast echocardiography from a direct LV injection may prove useful in the assessment of mitral competence *during* repair of the abnormal MV and, therefore, may aid in the operative assessment of repair adequacy. Similarly, in the assessment of percutaneous mitral valvuloplasty procedures, a considerable angiographic contrast load, which is mandatory for the proper evaluation of such procedures, might be avoided in the assessment of valve competence after balloon valvuloplasty (59). Expanding practical experience with both operative and percutaneous procedures will help determine the role of contrast echocardiography in these settings.

MYOCARDIAL CONTRAST ECHOCARDIOGRAPHY

In canine models of myocardial infarction, perfusion defects resulting from *total* coronary occlusion can be demonstrated by injecting a variety of newly developed contrast agents into the aortic root or coronary circulation (7, 8, 60–62). The area of infarction, or the area at risk for infarction (62), can be visualized from serial short-axis sections of the LV and can appear as non-contrast-enhanced regions (Fig. 18.11). The perfusion defects have been quantified for both the entire LV and for single tomographic planes using computer-assisted digitizing or digital subtraction methods. Independent groups (60–62) have demonstrated strong correlations with established methods for identifying infarct size (or areas at risk), such as staining autopsy specimens with nitro-blue tetrazolium, technetium autoradiography, and microsphere estimations of blood flow.

Preliminary evidence suggests that myocardial contrast echocardiography can localize and quantify the region of underperfused myocardium resulting from a *subtotal* occlusion of a coronary artery (63, 64). Using computer-assisted methods, time activity curves have been generated for normal, underperfused, and hyperemic myocardium (rendered hyperemic with dipyridamole infusion), which appear to correlate with myocardial blood flow (64).

The success of these developments and their application to humans will lie with the ease of transition

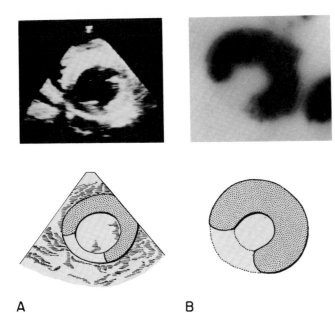

A   **B**

Figure 18.11. (*A*) Myocardial contrast echocardiography of a short-axis view at caudal level shows an area at risk in the posterior wall of the LV after left circumflex coronary artery occlusion. (*B*) Technetium autoradiography shows a risk area (cold spot) at the same level of the LV corresponding to the echocardiographic short-axis view in (*A*). (Reproduced from Kaul S, Pandian NG, Okada RD, et al. Contrast echocardiography in acute myocardial ischaemia: I. In vivo determination of total left ventricular "area at risk." J Am Coll Cardiol 1984;4(6):1272–82.)

from animal models to safe human study. This will be determined primarily by the development of contrast agents that can pass through the myocardial capillary network safely without altering regional circulation and have no deleterious effect on myocardium or systemic organs such as brain and kidney. Development of agents capable of passing through the pulmonary capillaries may provide myocardial contrast enhancement following injection from a peripheral vein. While the necessity for intra-arterial cannulation imposes some restriction on the method's wide application, this tool will be of such value if quantification of time activity curves for myocardial contrast effect proves reliable, safe, and reproducible that the constraints of intra-arterial investigation will be proportionately lessened. The value of a method that enables quantification of regional myocardial contractility and regional blood flow will be immeasurable.

REFERENCES

1. Gramiak R, Shah PM, Kramer DH. Ultrasound cardiography: contrast studies in anatomy and function. Radiology 1969;92:934.
2. Feigenbaum H, Stone JM, Lee DA, Nasser WK, Chang S. Identification of ultrasound echoes from the left ventricle using intracardiac injections of indocyanine green. Circulation 1970;41:615.
3. Duff DF, Gutgesell HP. The use of saline for the ultrasonic detection of a right-to-left shunt in the post-operative period, abstracted. Am J Cardiol 1976;37:132.
4. Seward JB, Tajik AJ, Spangler JG, Ritter DG. Echocardiographic contrast studies: initial experience. Mayo Clin Proc 1975;50:163.
5. Pieroni D, Varghese P, Rowe R. Echocardiography to detect shunt and valvular incompetence in children, abstracted. Circulation 1973;48:81.
6. Reale A. Contrast echocardiography: transmission of echoes to the left heart across the pulmonary vascular bed. Am J Cardiol 1980;45:401.
7. Armstrong W, Mueller T, Kinnei E, Tiekner G, Dillon J, Feibenbaum H. Assessment of myocardial perfusion abnormalities with contrast enhanced two-dimensional echocardiography. Circulation 1982;66:164–6.
8. Tei C, Sakamaki T, Shah P, et al. Myocardial contrast echocardiography. Circulation 1983;67:585–93.
9. Smith M, Kwan OL, Reiser J, Demaria AN. Superior intensity and reproducibility of SHU-454, a new right heart contrast agent. J Am Coll Cardiol 1984;3(4):992–8.
10. Feinstein S, Tencate FJ, Zwehl W, Ong J, Maurer G, Tei C, Shah PM, Meerbaum S, Corday E. Two-dimensional contrast echocardiography: in vitro development and quantitative analysis of echo contrast agents. J Am Coll Cardiol 1984;3(1):14–20.
11. Kremkau FW, Gramiak R, Carstensen EL, Shah PM, Kramer DH. Ultrasonic detection of cavitation at catheter tips. Am J Radiol 1970;110:117–83.
12. Corday E, Shah PM, Meerbaum S. Seminar on contrast two-dimensional echocardiography: applications and new developments. Part I. J Am Coll Cardiol 1984;3(1):1–5.
13. Levine RA, Techolz LE, Goldman ME, Steinmetz CY, Baker M, Meltzer RS. Microbubbles have intracardiac velocities similar to those of red blood cells. J Am Coll Cardiol 1984;3(1):28–33.
14. Mantin E, Grondin CM, Lillehei CW, Edwards JE. Congenital anomalies involving the coronary sinus. Circulation 1979;60:721.
15. Levine AR, Spach MS, Boineau JP, Canent RV, Capp MP, Jewett PH. Atrial pressure-flow dynamics in atrial septal defect (secundum type). Circulation 1968;37:476–88.
16. Bommer WJ, Shah PM, Allen H, Meltzer R, Kisslo JK. The safety of contrast echocardiography. J Am Coll Cardiol 1984;3(1):6–13.
17. Visser CA, Kan G, Ten Cate FJ, Lie KL, Roelandt J, Durrer D. Spontaneous intraventricular echoes in acute and chronic myocardial infarction, abstracted. Circulation 1983;68(suppl III):109.
18. Mikell FL, Asinger RS, Elsperger KJ, Anderson WR, Hodges M. Regional stasis of blood in the dysfunctional left ventricle: echocardiographic detection and differentiation from early thrombosis. Circulation 1982;66:755–63.
19. Hjemdahl-Monsen CE, Daniels J, Kaufman D, Stern EH, Teicholz LE, Meltzer RS. Spontaneous contrast in the inferior vena cava in a patient with constrictive pericarditis. J Am Coll Cardiol 1984;4(1):165–7.
20. Schuchman H, Feigenbaum H, Dillon JC, Chang S. Intracavitary echoes in patients with mitral prosthetic valves. J Clin Ultrasound 1975;3:107–10.
21. Martin RP, Preis LK Jr. Spontaneous left ventricular microbubbles in patients with metallic mitral prosthetic valves. In: Meltzer RS, Roelandt J, eds. Contrast echocardiography. The Hague, the Netherlands: Martinus Nijhoff, 1982:59–71.
22. Beppu S, Nimura Y, Sakakibaraih M, Nagata S, Park Y, Izumi S. High prevalence of left atrial thrombosis in cases of mitral valve disease with dynamic intracavitary echoes, abstracted. Circulation 1983;68(suppl III):335.
23. Foale RA, Rowland E, Nihoyannopoulos P, Perelman M, Krikler DM. Intracardiac contrast echoes during transvenous His bundle ablation. Br Heart J 1985;53,240–2.
24. Foale R, Rowland E, Nihoyannopoulos P, Webb S, Perelman M, Taylor KM, Krikler DM. Contrast effect after endocavitary ablation, abstracted. J Am Coll Cardiol 1985;5(2):454.
25. Henriksen L. Evidence suggestive of diffuse brain damage following cardiac operations. Lancet 1984;1:816–20.
26. Hagler DJ, Tajik AJ, Seward JB, Ritman EL. Videodensitronic quantification of left-to-right shunts with contrast echocardiography. In: Meltzer RS, Roelandt J, eds. Contrast echocardiog-

raphy. The Hague, the Netherlands: Martinus Nijhoff, 1982:298–303.

27. DeMaria AN, Bommer W, Rasor J, Tickner EG, Mason DT. Determination of cardiac output by two-dimensional contrast echocardiography. In: Meltzer RS, Roelandt J, eds. Contrast echocardiography. The Hague, the Netherlands: Martinus Nijhoff, 1982:289–97.

28. Roelandt J. Contrast echocardiography. Ultrasound Med Biol 1982;8:471–92.

29. Ong K, Maurer G, Feinstein S, Zwehl W, Meerbaum S, Corday E. Computer methods for myocardial contrast two-dimensional echocardiography. J Am Coll Cardiol 1984;3(5):1212–8.

30. Zwehl W, Areda J, Schwartz G, Feinstein S, Ong K, Meerbaum S. Physical factors affecting quantification of two-dimensional contrast echo amplitudes. J Am Coll Cardiol 1984;4(1):157–64.

31. Snider AR, Ports TA, Silverman NH. Venous anomalies of the coronary sinus: detection by M-mode, two-dimensional and contrast echocardiography. Circulation 1979;60:721.

32. Foale RA, Bourdillon PDV, Somerville J, Richards AF. Echocardiographic features of anomalous systemic and coronary venous return, abstracted. Br Heart J 1979;381.

33. Bourdillon PDV, Foale RA, Somerville J. Persistent left superior vena cava with coronary sinus and left atrial connections. Eur J Cardiol 1980;11:227–34.

34. Schapira JN, Martin RP, Fowles RE, Popp RL. Single and two-dimensional echocardiographic features of the interatrial septum in normal subjects and patients with an atrial septal defect. Am J Cardiol 1979;43:816.

35. von Rokitansky C. Die Defecte der Schedewande des Herzens: Pathologichanatomische Abhandlung Viena W Braumuller, 1875.

36. Perloff JK. In: The clinical recognition of congenital heart disease. Philadelphia: WB Saunders, 1978:277–87.

37. Levin AR, Spach MS, Boineau JP, Canent RV, Capp MP, Jewet PH. Atrial pressure flow dynamics in atrial septal defect (secundum type). Circulation 1968;37:476–88.

38. Kalmanson D, Veyrat C, Deraic L, Savier CH, Berkman M, Chiche P. Non-invasive technique for diagnosing atrial septal defect and assessing shunt volume using directional Doppler ultrasound. Br Heart J 1972;34:981.

39. Alexander JA, Rembert JC, Sealy WC, Greenfield JC. Shunt dynamics in experimental atrial septal defects. J Appl Physiol 1975;39:281.

40. Rasmussen K, Simonsen S, Storstein O. Quantitative aspects of right to left shunting in uncomplicated atrial septal defects. Br Heart J 1973;35:894.

41. Bourdillon PDV, Foale RA, Richards AF. Identification of atrial septal defects by cross-sectional contrast echocardiography. Br Heart J 1980;44:401–5.

42. Valdes-Cruz LM, Pieroni DR, Roland JM, Shematek JP. Recognition of residual post-operative shunts by contrast echocardiographic techniques. Circulation 1977;55:148–52.

43. Fraker TD, Harris PJ, Behar VS, Kisslo JA. Detection and exclusion of interatrial shunts by two-dimensional echocardiography and peripheral venous injection. Circulation 1979;59:379–84.

44. Valdes-Cruz LM, Pieroni DR, Roland JM, Varghese PJ. Echocardiographic detection of intracardiac right-to-left shunts following peripheral venous injections. Circulation 1976;558–62.

45. Pieroni DR, Varghese PJ, Rowe RD. Echocardiography to detect shunt and valvular incompetence in infants and children, abstracted. Circulation 1973;47/48 (suppl IV):81.

46. Sahn D. Application of contrast echocardiography for analysis of complex congenital heart disease in newborns. In: Meltzer RS, Roelandt J, eds. Contrast echocardiography. The Hague, the Netherlands: Martinus Nijhoff, 1982:214–34.

47. Weyman AE, Wann LS, Caldwell RL, Hurwitz RA, Dillon JC, Feigenbaum H. Negative contrast echocardiography: a new method for detecting left to right shunts. Circulation 1979;59:498–505.

48. Valdes-Cruz LM, Sahn DJ. Ultrasonic contrast studies for the detection of cardiac shunts. J Am Coll Cardiol 1985;3(4):978–85.

49. King DL, Steeg CN, Ellis K. Visualisation of ventricular septal defects by cardiac ultrasonography. Circulation 1973;48:1215.

50. Seward JB, Tajik AJ, Hagler DJ, Mair DD. Visualisation of isolated ventricular septal defect with wide angle two-dimensional sector echocardiography, abstracted . Circulation 1978;58(suppl II):202.

51. Tikoff G, Kuida H. Pathophysiology of heart failure in congenital heart disease. Mod Concepts Cardiovasc Dis 1972;41:1.

52. Serwer GA, Armstrong BE, Anderson PAW, Sherman D, Benson DW, Edwards SB. Use of contrast echocardiography for evaluation of right ventricular hemodynamics in the presence of ventricular septal defects. Circulation 1978;58:327–36.

53. Serruys PW, Vanden Brand M, Hugenholtz PG, Roelandt J. Intracardiac right to left shunts demonstrated by two-dimensional echocardiography after peripheral vein injection. Br Heart J 1979;42:429.

54. Silverman NH, Lewis AB, Heyman MA, Rudolph AM. Echocardiographic assessment of ductus arteriosus shunt in premature infants. Circulation 1974;50:821.

55. Bloom KR, Rodriques L, Swan EM. Echocardiographic evaluation of left-to-right shunt in ventricular septal defect and persistent ductus arteriosus. Br Heart J 1977;39:260.

56. Sahn DJ, Allen HD. Real time cross sectional echocardiography imaging and measurement of the patent ductus arteriosus in infants and children. Circulation 1978;58:343–54.

57. Maurer G, Torres MAR, Corday E, Haendlhen RV, Meerbaum S. Two-dimensional echocardiographic contrast assessment of pacing-induced mitral regurgitation. Relation to altered regional left ventricular function. J Am Coll Cardiol 1984;3(4):986–91.

58. Goldman ME, Mindich BP, Teichholz LE, Burgess N, Staville K, Fuster V. Intraoperative contrast echocardiography to evaluate mitral valve operations. J Am Coll Cardiol 1984;4(5):1035–40.

59. Zaibag M. (Personal Communication) Division of Cardiology, Riyadh Al Kharj Hospital, Saudi Arabia.

60. Armstrong WF, West SR, Mueller TM, Dillon JC, Feigenbaum H. Assessment of location and size of myocardial infarction with contrast-enhanced echocardiography. J Am Coll Cardiol 1983;67:585–93.

61. Armstrong WF, West SR, Mueller TM, Dillon JC, Feigenbaum H. Assessment of location and size of myocardial infarction with contrast-enhanced echocardiography. J Am Coll Cardiol 1983;2:63–9.

62. Kaul S, Pandian NG, Okada RD, Pomost GM, Weyman AE. Contrast echocardiography in acute myocardial ischaemia: I. In vivo determination of total left ventricular "area of risk." J Am Coll Cardiol 1984;4(6):1272–82.

63. Tei C, Kondo S, Meerbaum S, Ong K, Maurer G, Wood F, Sakamaki T, Shimoura K, Corday E, Shah PM. Correlation of myocardial echo contrast disappearance rate ("washout") and severity of experimental coronary stenosis. J Am Coll Cardiol 1984;3:39–46.

64. Ten Cate FO, Drury JK, Meerbaum S, Noordsy J, Feinstein S, Shah PM, Corday E. Myocardial contrast two-dimensional echocardiography: experimental examination at different flow levels. J Am Coll Cardiol 1984;3(5):1219–26.

19
Two-Dimensional Echocardiographic Image Analysis by Computer

Edward Geiser

Echocardiography has been widely accepted as a valuable tool in the qualitative assessment of patients with cardiac disease. This is due, in part, to the safety, portability, and low cost and the fact that it is the only technique providing real-time beat-to-beat tomographic images of the heart and its valvular structures. Other techniques such as rapid computed tomographic (CT) (Imatron) scanning do provide tomographic images at approximately 40-millisecond intervals. However, this imaging technique is limited by the orientation to its scan planes and by its size and cost.

The limitation of echocardiography is that it is a long-wavelength, low-energy technique. Penetration capabilities are far below those of other imaging modalities. Another limitation is the fact that two-dimensional echocardiographic images are formed using a coherent ultrasound beam as an energy source.

Since 1976, many papers have been written on measurements and calculations from two-dimensional echocardiography. These papers are directed toward all aspects of quantitation of left ventricular size and function. Early papers were directed at mass (1) while others looked at systolic (2, 3) and diastolic (4) function. Estimates of left ventricular volume have been a necessary part of the quantitation for evaluation of ejection fraction (EF). The accuracy with which left ventricular volume can be predicted in patients has been explored in simple to complex models (3, 5–10). Quantitation of regional wall motion as a marker of ischemic disease continues to be explored (11–14).

Other cardiac chambers have also received attention with respect to quantitation. Quantitation of right atrial volume has been used to evaluate the severity of tricuspid disease (15).

Digital computer processing of electrocardiograms has been pursued for many years. Crevasse and Ariet (16) give three major motivations for this computerization: 1) The electrocardiogram is a biologic signal that can be detected noninvasively; 2) the interpretation of the electrocardiogram requires a significant effort on the part of the cardiologist; and 3) the criteria for specific diagnoses consist of numerous detailed measurements that must be applied in a logical manner. In addition, the electrocardiogram is frequently obtained during exercise or patient movement, as in the case of Holter monitoring, causing artifacts to appear as noise in the electrocardiographic signal. Thus, the electrocardiogram lends itself to digital filtering in the computer and cycle averaging to improve its quality (i.e., improve its signal-to-noise ratio). These techniques are helpful, which is evidenced by the computer components of modern exercise-stress testing equipment (17).

It comes as no surprise that the digital computer has found its way into the analysis of two-dimensional echocardiograms. The test is performed frequently and noninvasively. Diagnosis or assessment of patient status requires that detailed measurements be obtained from the image. In the case of M-mode echocardiography, these measurements are linear. In the two-dimensional image, however, these measurements are largely areas. A stimulus to perform measurements in two-dimensional echocardiographic images is the fact that area changes appear to be less variable than linear measures (12, 18). This is particularly true in clinical situations where regional wall motion abnormalities that may not be detected by the M-mode studies are present.

In these settings, the computer is used as a measurement tool. It is usually interfaced to a digitizing-tablet, light-pen, or sonic-pen system, which allows points and traced borders to be entered from a display screen. Once the data are entered, the computer is used as a calculator. Areas, volumes, and regional radius or area change are produced. This would be very complex if done manually or without specific equipment.

Because of the low energy and coherent ultrasound used to form the two-dimensional image, two problems arise: First, a significant portion of the clinical studies are poor and do not lend themselves well to quantitation, and second, the accuracy and precision with which measurements can be made from echocardiography tend to decrease as the quality of the image decreases. This is very important when looking at secondary estimates of left ventricular function. These estimates are calculated from the raw data entered into the computer from the display screen (i.e., the borders). Therefore, estimates of stroke work, velocity of circumferential fiber shortening, or cardiac output depend on the accuracy of these initial borders or distances. In other words, the data obtained will only be as accurate or precise as the initial borders entered.

Therefore, it is not surprising that digital computer processing of two-dimensional echocardiographic images has received more and more attention (19–21). The American Society of Echocardiography has published a glossary of frequently used terms in digital-image processing as they relate to ultrasound (22). (While we have tried to avoid complex terminology in this chapter, the referenced glossary [22] is recommended for those with more than a casual interest in the subject.) This aspect of digital computer processing in two-dimensional echocardiograms is the subject of this chapter. Various methods for improving image quality are addressed. These digital techniques are largely time consuming and cannot be implemented easily in real time or as the patient study is being performed. Therefore, we usually discuss off-line processing from studies recorded on videotape. As such, it is important to realize that these images have already been heavily processed. The actual data obtained for the two-dimensional scan were obtained along a limited number of scan lines, usually between 100 and 200. The remainder of the image, especially in the far field, is interpolated by various techniques. The most frequent technique for filling gaps between the original

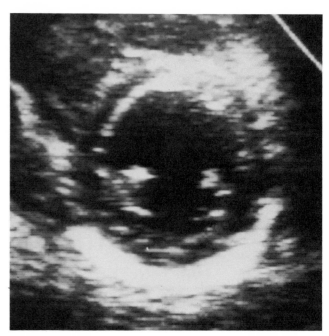

Figure 19.1. Good quality short-axis two-dimensional echocardiographic image obtained at the level of the papillary muscles.

scan lines in the digital scan converter is the ρ Θ technique (23). Figure 19.1 is a good quality image that has been digitized from videotape. Originally obtained along 200 scan lines, some of these data have been removed or compressed in the near field. Some missing data between scan lines have been filled by interpolation in the far field. Throughout this chapter, Figure 19.1 is used as an example on which to perform image-processing operations.

The purpose of quantitation in echocardiography is to improve the ability to detect change or deviation from normal objectively. Quantitation has been shown to be more objective in the evaluation of angiography (24). For the purpose of diagnosis, this objectivity means the ability to detect small changes in left ventricular diastolic volume, systolic volume, or small decreases in the fractional change in left ventricular size. In the case of ischemic heart disease, it means the ability to detect small regional abnormalities in function. In the case of hypertension or aortic stenosis, it means the ability to detect small increases in left ventricular wall area or mass. In the case of right-sided disease, it may mean the ability to detect small changes in the size of the right ventricle or atrium. In evaluating patients with already diagnosed disease, we again seek to detect small changes in chamber size or contractility reliably, to determine both disease progression and the results of therapy. Methods are needed to detect small changes in ventricular function in order to research and evaluate new medications or interventional treatments. The purpose of computer image processing in all of these situations is to improve data extraction from the images. This may be as simple as reformatting the images so that studies can be viewed side by side for better qualitative evaluation and thus can facilitate comparison. Images can be processed in an attempt to improve them, so that better sensitivity and specificity can be obtained from quantitation. Finally, the computer can help detect changes in brightness associated with echocardiographic contrast agents for the evaluation of myocardial perfusion or valvular regurgitation.

MANUAL BORDER TRACING AND CALIPER FUNCTIONS

There are commercial systems that can perform linear measurements from either a cursor on the video screen or a digitizing tablet. Many ultrasound machines incorporate such functions into the scanning equipment. Measurements such as wall thickness and chamber diameter can be made from two-dimensional parasternal long-axis views, where actual dimensions of the ventricle perpendicular to the wall at the tip of the mitral valve can be obtained. Thus, true perpendicular diameters can be measured along lines that are not available from a simple M-mode echocardiogram. In addition, measurements of septal and posterior wall thicknesses can be made perpendicular to their surfaces. Aortic root diameter, left atrial dimensions, and right-sided chamber dimensions can also be obtained.

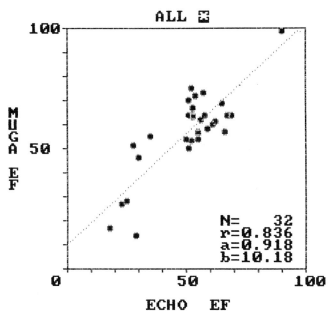

Figure 19.2. Correlation between multigated nuclear EFs (MUGA EF) and EFs calculated from two-dimensional echocardiographic short- and long-axis views (ECHO EF). The only criterion for inclusion in this graph was that the two-dimensional echocardiographic examination and the radionuclide study be performed during the same hospitalization. *a* is the regression slope and *b* is the *y* intercept.

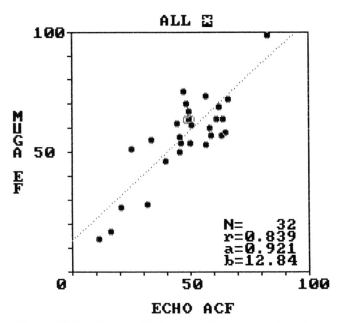

Figure 19.3. Relationship between the multigated nuclear EFs (MUGA EF) shown in Figure 19.2 and the area change fraction (ECHO ACF) calculated from the short-axis view alone of the two-dimensional echocardiographic study. *a* is the regression slope and *b* is the *y* intercept.

Areas can be measured by tracing the borders along the area of interest. After the system is calibrated, the enclosed area is converted into square centimeters. Short-axis area change fractions appear to be good indicators of left ventricular function, although normal values may vary at different levels in the ventricle (25). Areas can also be traced and calculated from the apical and subcostal views. Once these areas and a long-axis length from the apex to the midpoint of the mitral valve plane are determined, numerous formulas are available for calculating left ventricular volume. Once end-systolic and end-diastolic volumes are known, EF can be calculated (2, 3, 18). Figure 19.2 shows the relationship between multigated radionuclide EFs and EFs calculated from two-dimensional echocardiography in our laboratory. The echocardiographic volumes were calculated using a bullet formula (i.e., 5/6 × area × length). Figure 19.3 shows the correlation between the same multigated EFs and the area change fraction calculated from the short axis at the mid–papillary muscle level. It is obvious that the relationship is nearly identical. Figure 19.4 shows the regression of only the good and excellent quality two-dimensional echocardiographic studies with the corresponding EFs from the respective multigated scans. The correlation is much better: When only the poor quality studies are regressed on their corresponding radionuclide ejection fractions, the correlation coefficient is 0.514. This evidence further supports the fact that quantitations per-

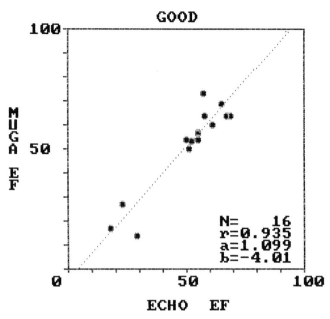

Figure 19.4. Regression of multigated nuclear EFs (MUGA EF) and the EFs (ECHO EF) calculated from the two-dimensional echocardiographic studies when only those patients with good and excellent quality two-dimensional echocardiographic studies are included.

formed on two-dimensional echocardiograms generally lose accuracy as the quality of the image decreases.

Throughout this chapter, reference is made to good quality and poor quality images. It seems appropriate to define these terms at this point.

Excellent quality studies are exceptionally good with good definition of both the endocardium and epicardium. Borders can be traced easily by the observer on all frames in the cardiac cycle.

Good quality studies are of somewhat poorer quality than the excellent quality studies, but the endocardium and epicardium are still well visualized. There are more areas of dropout, and in several frames, larger gaps may appear. However, borders are easily drawn, and the observer is not hesitant in filling regions of dropout.

Poor quality studies have more regions of dropout, which may occur in more than several frames. Occasionally, noise covers larger portions of the endocardium and epicardium. Borders can be drawn, but the observer is hesitant in filling either regions of dropout or regions obscured by noise.

Technically inadequate studies are of poor enough quality that the observer can only grossly identify walls and boundaries. The observer believes that digitization of borders from the image would be largely guesswork.

In summary, commercially available quantitation computers for echocardiography facilitate caliper measurements and border tracing. From these borders and distances, areas and numerous indexes of ventricular function are calculated. The utility of these data is

discussed in Chapter 9. Our purpose here is to review the utility of the computer with respect to its ability to improve the quality of the borders that go into these calculations.

DIGITIZATION OF TWO-DIMENSIONAL ECHOCARDIOGRAPHIC IMAGES

Videotape is the standard method of recording and archiving two-dimensional echocardiographic studies. It is convenient, many studies can be preserved on one tape, and the cost is fairly low. Still, this storage medium is cumbersome. A busy laboratory will have many tapes with old patient files and studies. If one is to be reviewed, the tape must be found and then serially scanned. In other words, if a patient study is to be reviewed, one must forward or reverse the tape until the study is reached. In many ways, it is more convenient to have the pertinent portions of a patient's two-dimensional study available for review almost on request. Most computers have a digital-disk operating system; that is, programs and data are stored on either floppy or hard disks. Digital disks have the advantage of being a random access medium. Any portion of the disk can be accessed without delay. A series of frames stored in digital format on disks can also be displayed over and over in a loop. Thus, the same cycle can be viewed continuously and without degradation. While most videotape players have some jitter or instability when placed in freeze frame, the digital image in the computer will be stable.

Because of the continuous loop and the stable freeze frame, the drawing of borders from digital images is preferable. The disadvantage is that significant computer time is required to read the image from the disk and display it on the image monitor. This delay causes a 25 percent to 50 percent reduction in the rate of playback of the cardiac cycle of interest. An alternative is to digitize the images directly from the videotape into random access memory (RAM) in the computer. Images available in the computer's memory can be displayed in real time and manipulated much faster than those that must be accessed and read from disks prior to display. The disadvantage of storing the images in RAM is the size of the computer memory required. Since the same factors determine either how large a disk is necessary or how much memory is needed, the following discussion applies to both.

The image, as it exists on videotape, is in analog form. In other words, it is a continuous voltage recorded on the magnetic tape. These voltages determine the brightness displayed as each line sweeps along horizontally on the television screen. The digital computer, however, cannot work with this analog voltage. The image itself must be converted into discrete num-

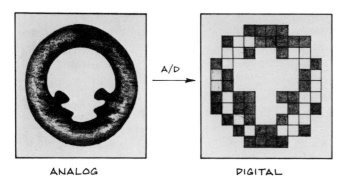

ANALOG   DIGITAL

Figure 19.5. Schematic diagram of ADC of an echocardiographic image. The gray level in each small region of the digital image is equal to the average voltage in the same region of the original analog image. (Reproduced with permission from Use of computer as an aid to the cardiologist. Cardiac Imaging: New Technologies and Clinical Applications 1986, pp 161–78. Used with permission of Albert Breast, Publisher, Cardiovascular Clinics of North America.)

bers (i.e., digits). This process is called "digitization" or "analog-to-digital conversion" (ADC). During this process, the average voltage describing the amplitude of the ultrasound within this region of the image is converted to a discrete number proportional to the voltage. Figure 19.5 is a schematic representation of this process. Each small section of the image for which a digital gray level is assigned is called a picture element, or "pixel." The digital image then is a matrix of pixels, each describing numerically the gray level in a small region of the image. Two factors determine the memory requirements for this digitized image: the number of pixels needed to describe the image accurately and the number of gray levels with which each pixel must be described.

In order to estimate the number of pixels needed, we should consider first the resolution of the ultrasound techniques. For a 3.25-megahertz transducer, the wavelength is approximately 0.5 millimeter. The resolution of the system will be approximately two wavelengths in the axial direction, or roughly 1 mm. Theoretically, in order to make measurements to this same resolution, there should be two pixels per mm. Since most adult two-dimensional echocardiograms are recorded at 14 to 16 centimeters in depth in the short-axis view, a pixel density of 256 by 256 nearly supplies the two pixels per mm and is probably adequate in most cases. As the depth of the scan increases to 20 or 22 cm, pixel densities of 512 by 512 may be necessary. Because of the presence of acoustic speckle and the lack of knowledge concerning the intervening tissues, it is doubtful that the theoretic resolution is achieved in patient scanning. Therefore, in most situations, 256 by 256 pixel images is probably adequate, and pixel densities above 512 by 512 provide additional advantage.

The second factor in determining the memory requirement of the computer is the number of gray levels with which each pixel is to be described. This quantization level is expressed in bits of computer memory. Thus, within four bits of computer memory, the number 0 to 15 can be represented in binary form. If the image was digitized then to four-bit gray scale resolution, the image could have 16 levels of gray. If each pixel was digitized with a one-byte (eight-bit) gray scale resolution, then each pixel could be quantized to one of 256 gray levels. Little information is available on how many gray levels are optimal for defining cardiac structure in echocardiographic images. Certainly the dynamic range of the ultrasound returning to the transducer easily warrants 256 gray levels. However, a trained observer looking at the display on a black and white television can only define between 16 and 32 shades of gray (26). Since a trained observer in echocardiography makes decisions concerning the position of structures and is able to digitize these identified structures manually, it is likely that no more than 32 levels of gray are necessary to describe the image. It is certainly difficult to envision a situation in which one pixel could be correctly picked as an edge point because its brightness was 1/64th or 1/256th different from its neighboring pixels. If four-bit resolution is used, then two pixels can be stored in one byte of computer memory. If five-bit or 32-level resolution is desired, then three pixels could be stored in each 16-bit word in memory. Once one chooses to digitize at 64 or 256 gray levels, the advantages in saving computer storage space are lost, and one pixel requires one byte of memory.

A third factor in determining hardware storage requirements is the speed with which one wishes to carry out the digitization. If one chooses to digitize 256 by 256 pixels and digitizes with 16 levels of gray so that two pixels occupy each byte of memory, then digitizing in real time at 30 video frames per second requires digitization and storage of approximately 2 million pixels per second or use of one megabyte of storage per second. This is about the maximum rate at which images can be digitized and directly stored on digital disks with inexpensive equipment. If one wishes to digitize images at 512 by 512 pixel densities and store 64 or 256 levels of gray, this transfer rate rises to nearly eight megabytes per second, which can only be maintained by storing directly in RAM.

REFORMATTING OF IMAGES FOR REVIEW

The situation frequently arises in clinical echocardiography when a patient's old study must be compared to a new study or when a study done before intervention must be compared to one after an intervention such as nitroglycerin or exercise. In these situations, side-by-side, or parallel, review for qualitative evaluation of change is preferable to serial review of the studies. Side-by-side review can be easily accomplished with digital memory.

The majority of information in the two-dimensional echocardiographic image occupies the central portion of the field. If we assume for a moment that the image has been digitized at 512 by 512 pixels, then the outer 128 columns on the left and right of the image can be discarded without sacrificing the image. The central 256 columns can then be stored in the left-hand portion of a new 512 by 512 frame. The corresponding central portion from a second, new study can then be placed in the right 256 columns. Both the old and new studies can be viewed simultaneously when this 512 by 512 image is displayed.

For purposes of comparison, the temporal sequence of the cardiac cycle can also be modified. The study performed immediately prior to exercise will ordinarily have a different heart rate than the study at the conclusion of exercise. Comparison of the two studies for wall motion abnormalities can best be accomplished if end diastole and end systole occur at the same time on both halves of the displayed screen. This is done by deleting frames from the longer cycle, usually near end diastole, or by duplicating frames from the shorter cycle. Various conventions to accomplish this cycle-length matching are used by different manufacturers.

Let us now return to the task of placing patient studies on digital disk. An image digitized at 256 by 256 has approximately 65,000 pixels. Thus, about eight images can be stored on a 5.25-inch floppy disk. This by itself would not make image storage on floppy disk attractive. However, if the image memory is segmented so that half of one image is occupied by parasternal long-axis view, the other half occupied by short-axis view, and the cycle compressed to eight pertinent points in time, then floppy-disk storage becomes attractive. To carry this further, systems are available commercially that can place four images of 128 by 128 resolution in the four corners of a 256 by 256 memory. Thus, four major views, each from eight points in time, can be stored on a single floppy disk. This is still more helpful, but whether the convenience of digital-disk storage warrants the expense has yet to be determined.

COMPUTER PROCESSING FOR IMAGE ENHANCEMENT

Noise and the Two-Dimensional Echocardiographic Image

We have previously stated that the purpose of processing echocardiographic images in the computer is to try to improve the image quality. This assumes an enhanced ability on the part of the observer to define structures of interest with the ultimate goals of increased accuracy and precision of measurements. In order to understand the effects of certain enhancement or image-processing techniques, it is necessary to understand the nature of the image we are trying to improve. Chapter 1 described the aspects of image formation and the fact that these images have a poor signal-to-noise ratio. What we wish to accomplish is a decrease in the noise and an increase in the signal. What are the properties of the signal we wish to preserve? What are the properties of the noise we wish to suppress?

When ultrasound is injected into the body and encounters tissue, one of two interactions occurs. The first is reflection from a specular (mirrorlike) target. This interaction involves large, planar surfaces with minor irregularities that are much smaller than the wavelengths of the ultrasound being used. In the specular case, usual reflection and refraction occur at the interface. The ultrasound is reflected back to the transducer and received. In this case, the larger, relatively smooth target produces a wave of sound returning to the transducer, which is in phase. In other words, the phase of the reflected sound is dominated, indeed determined for the most part, by the encounter with this large surface. However, even large specular targets such as the aorta have gaps at times (27). This is a result of reflections occurring from two different levels in the structure, either because of layers or because of the curvature of the structure. These two reflections arrive simultaneously at the face of the transducer but *out of phase* so that there is cancellation of their amplitudes, and no returning sound is perceived at that depth along that particular scan line. Thus, in the resultant image, although we know the aorta is generally circular and does not have holes, there may be portions of the wall that are missing.

This dropout is due to phase cancellation, which is due to ultrasound being used to derive the image of a single frequency. It is not difficult to understand that there would be no dominant wavelength or phase if a diffuse spectrum of sound were used. Waves that are predominantly of a single frequency and are capable of interfering with themselves are called "coherent" (28).

The second interaction involves an encounter with small discrete targets such as cellular structures. These targets are smaller than half a wavelength of the ultrasound. When such coherent waves encounter the small scattering targets, they are dispersed in all directions. These spheric wave fronts from the individual tiny scatterers can sum or cancel at the particular time that they encounter the receiving transducer. This produces a very fine texture, a salt and pepper pattern superimposed on the image. This pattern is commonly known as speckle and results from the interference of these dephased but coherent wavelets from the scattering targets (29). Speckle is considered an undesirable phenomenon (28). There is also good evidence that speckle reduces the measurement resolution of echocardiographic images (28, 30). This is not difficult to understand. The interference pattern resulting in speckle is a random phenomenon, described by negative exponential statistics (28, 29) and present to some degree at every point in the image. The gray scale seen at each point in the ultrasound image is not necessarily a true representation of the reflected amplitude from that position in the sample volume of the two-dimensional beam (28). In other words, the speckle modulates the image. Because of this and phase cancellations previously described for specular targets, the image displayed is not a true representation of the structures in the two-dimensional echocardiographic beam. It follows then, that to some extent, the edges of specular targets are blurred by this superimposed speckle and the resolution of the image is impaired. In laser images, experiments have shown that speckle degrades the resolution by a factor of five or more (31).

Since speckle is a random process, the standard deviation (SD) of the brightness of speckle in an image is equal to its mean (M). In other words, the speckle contrast c = SD/M = 1. Methods for improving ultrasound image quality are frequently measured in terms of their ability to reduce this speckle contrast, that is, their ability to fade the speckle into a homogenous gray tone superimposed on the image.

It is important to understand that while speckle noise in ultrasound images is random, it is *not* random in the same sense as electronic noise. The speckle pattern is random in the sense that the exact positions of regions of brightness cannot be predicted. However, for any given image geometry (i.e., transducer position and target position), the speckle pattern remains constant. If a transducer is used to image a tissue phantom, the pattern of speckle displayed will not change as long as the transducer is held in the same position. Either the transducer or the object must move in order for the speckle pattern to change. Electronic noise, on the other hand, is a completely random phenomenon and is different on every sequential frame in spite of the fact that the transducer and target position remain constant. Therefore, the amount of electronic noise in an image can be decreased by a factor of $1/\sqrt{n}$ by averaging sequential frames, where n is the number of frames averaged. On the other hand, averaging frames where the transducer and target remain in the same relationship will not change speckle contrast.

Speckle contrast in images can be reduced. One method employed in all ultrasound machines is low-pass filtration. Since speckle seems to be of a fine texture (of a high spatial frequency), some reduction in speckle can be achieved by low-pass filtration. However, the average speckle size is roughly equal to the resolution cell of the ultrasound machine (32). Therefore, a compromise must be reached between speckle reduction by low-pass filtration and degradation of the resolution of the instrument.

In seeming contradiction, we must state that speckle can also be decreased by image averaging. The condition, however, is that the images to be averaged must contain independent or uncorrelated speckle patterns. This effect of averaging uncorrelated speckle patterns accounts in part for the observer's ability to define structures better in echocardiographic images when the structures are in motion. The objects of interest in the study have a nonrandom and generally slower motion pattern, which allows their recognition. If multiple images during the cardiac cycle are averaged and viewed as a single image, not only is the speckle pattern "faded" but the structures of interest are blurred. In order to implement image averaging as a means of reducing speckle in the ultrasound machine, multiple images with independent speckle patterns must be obtained at close to the same time. Since speckle is dependent on the frequency of the transducer, obtaining images with transducers of different frequencies will produce images with independent speckle patterns. When these are summed on a nonphased sensitive basis, the resultant image will have a decrease in speckle contrast. Alternatively, two scans can be obtained from about the same time, with the same frequency transducer, but from different points of view. This technique is known as "compound scanning" and can be implemented in phased-array systems (28, 32). Both of these techniques are currently under investigation. When images with independent and uncorrelated cycle patterns are averaged, the speckle contrast is also reduced by the factor $1/\sqrt{n}$.

With this basic understanding of speckle, dropout, and specular target representation, we now explore postprocessing computer methods designed either to reduce noise (speckle) or enhance the signal (specular targets).

SINGLE PIXEL OPERATIONS

Thresholding

Thresholding is simply the operation of subtracting a background gray level from the image, assuming that the undesirable portions of the image occupy a lower gray level than signals of interest. This method does not exclude removing very high-level intensities, and indeed, thresholding may be accomplished at both ends of the gray-level spectrum.

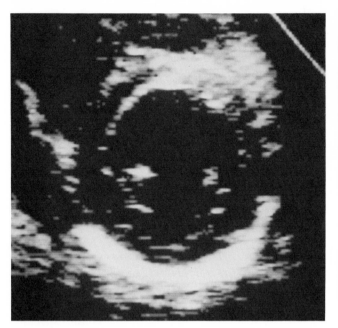

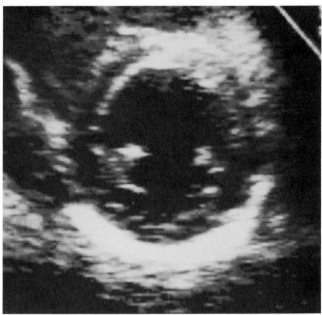

Figure 19.6. Effect of thresholding Figure 19.1 at a gray level of five. While much of the background has been removed, some of the echos representing endocardium in the posterior portion of the ventricle have also been deleted.

Figure 19.7. Results of regional thresholding where individual thresholds have been applied in eight equiangular portions of the ventricle extending from a point at the center of the cavity.

The method for selecting the background level to be removed is also a matter of choice. Frequently, the average gray level of the image is calculated, and any gray level below this is removed as background. Another method is to assume that the undesirable gray levels occupy a certain percentage of the pixels. In other words, all pixels whose gray levels are in the lower 40 percent of gray levels in the image could be removed. More complicated methods of choosing a threshold level have been devised such as in the temporal co-occurrence method (33). This method sets increasing gray levels as thresholds in two sequential images and then subtracts the thresholded images from each other. The gray level threshold that maintains the highest number of changing pixels between frames is the one chosen for the images. This thresholding method aims to preserve the motion information associated with cardiac structures.

In general, thresholding by itself is not a very successful technique for improving ultrasound images. Speckle, as we know, can have any brightness. Specular targets, on the other hand, can have low gray levels, depending on the depth, angle of incidence of the primary beam, and attenuation path traversed by the ultrasound. Therefore, selecting a single threshold level for the image may tend to remove noise from the near field of the image, but at the same time subtract wanted signal from the far-field wall where the gray level of desired structures tends to be lower. This can be seen in Figure 19.6, where the image of Figure 19.1 has been

thresholded at a gray level of five. One way of avoiding this problem is to assume that at any given region of the image, the brightness of the speckle is likely to be less than that of the specular targets. Thus, if an individual threshold is selected in various regions of the image, noise may be removed while the signal of interest is preserved. Figure 19.7 shows the results of regional thresholding applied in equiangular segments of the image that extend outward from the center of the ventricle.

Thresholding, while not sufficient by itself in most cases, is an important tool to be applied along with other operations. We refer to it subsequently with other image-processing techniques.

Histogram Modification

For a digital two-dimensional image, a gray level histogram can be constructed, showing the number of pixels in the image at each gray level. Figure 19.8 shows the histogram obtained from the central region of the left ventricle in our original image (Fig. 19.1). Most histograms of echocardiographic images are bimodal. In other words, there are a large number of low gray levels associated with the chambers and another peak occurrence at a higher gray level associated with the walls and specular targets.

One method of histogram modification is implemented in ultrasound machines and is usually referred to as "postprocessing." Postprocessing allows the user

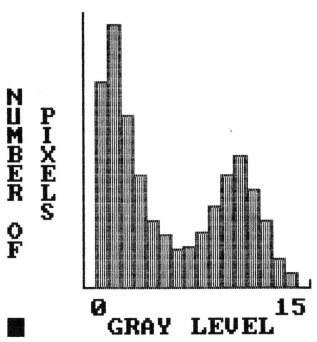

Figure 19.8. Histogram of the relative number of pixels at each gray level in the central portion of Figure 19.1.

to remap the gray levels in the image according to a set of predetermined curves. If this curve, for example, remaps low gray levels to higher levels to bring out some low-intensity feature, the histogram will shift and show a higher content of intermediate or high gray levels. One classic postprocessing technique is histogram equalization. This technique levels out the histogram so that each gray level occurs with equal frequency. Therefore, structures represented with very low intensity and associated with the endocardium or epicardium can be brought into the display range. However, low-level signals including speckle will also be enhanced. Therefore, histogram modification is sometimes used in association with thresholding. In this way, background can be removed and the remaining pixels distributed equally in gray levels over the full dynamic range. It is obvious that any relationship can be established for remapping gray levels. Those that have been found most useful are included as the postprocessing curves in ultrasound equipment. Processing echocardiographic images in the computer allows the user to apply virtually any relationship and combine histogram modification techniques with other enhancement procedures.

Image Averaging

In signal processing, as in electrocardiography, if one chooses the same RR cycle length during exercise and registers the cycles to be averaged on the peak of the R wave, then the signal-to-noise ratio will be improved by a factor of $1/\sqrt{n}$. This is because the noise or muscle artifact is truly random. Recall that while speckle pattern on any given image is random, for the same imaging geometry the speckle pattern is not random and will not change. Thus, speckle is not random in the same sense. The creation of an independent and uncorrelated speckle pattern demands some change. The important conclusion is that even though the speckle contrast is decreased by $1/\sqrt{n}$, the signal of interest is decreased by some other factor that cannot be predicted. An independent speckle pattern can be produced only if the transducer or the heart change position. Therefore, if the heart returned to exactly the same position in the chest at end diastole, if the patient's phase of respiration were exactly the same, and if the technician's hand did not move the transducer, then the positions both of the specular targets and the acoustic speckle in the image would be exactly the same. Image averaging of frames at the same time in the cardiac cycle tends to improve structure definition because there is change. Not only will speckle be decreased in contrast, but this movement between frames will cause misregistration of the specular targets of interest so that they will also be blurred. If the specular targets have moved too much, then their signal intensity will also be reduced by $1/\sqrt{n}$. Therefore, the degree of enhancement or improvement in the images cannot be predicted but is dependent on the degree of overlap or lack of overlap between the specular targets (still assuming that the geometry has changed enough for the speckle pattern in each of these images to be independent). Because of this, it is unlikely that any more cosmetic improvement will take place after the averaging of three or four frames from the same point in the cardiac cycle. It should also be noted that because of the movement of the specular targets, measurements made from these images could be less accurate. The same misregistration that causes gaps to be filled and the background texture to be more continuous also results in loss of definable edges. There is some evidence, however, that if gap filling does result so that edges are more continuous, the result may be decreased variability and increased consistency of measurements in poor quality images (34). Figure 19.9 is an example of frame averaging of four frames where the registrations have been well controlled. Figure 19.10 shows the average of four images where there is misalignment.

MULTIPLE PIXEL OPERATIONS

In the preceding sections, all calculations performed on images were done in single pixel locations. Even in the case of image averaging, the gray levels at the same relative pixel position in each image were averaged.

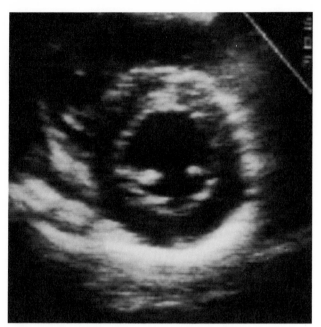

Figure 19.9. Resultant image from averaging four end-diastolic frames with good registration; that is, the positions of the endocardium and epicardium are nearly the same at end diastole in these four frames.

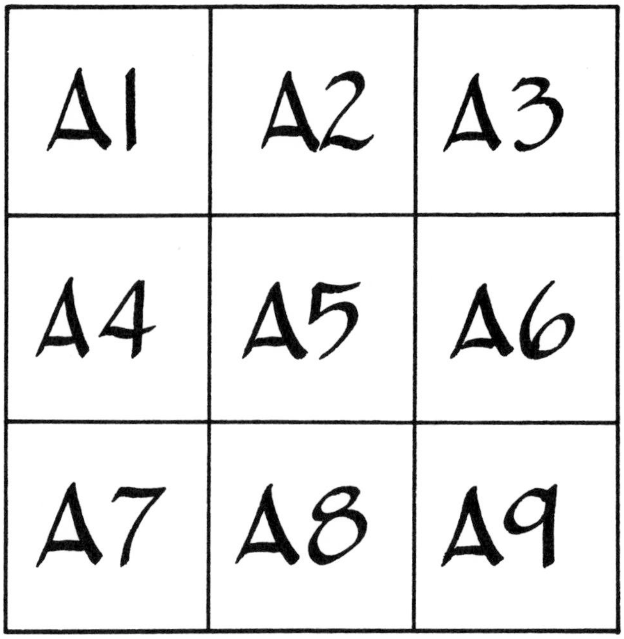

Thus, small regions of dropout were filled by the temporal variation in the gray level at that pixel location. Another method for filling these small regions on a single image is called "smoothing". In this case, the gap is filled using the spatial brightness level in the image around the gap. We refer to such operations as

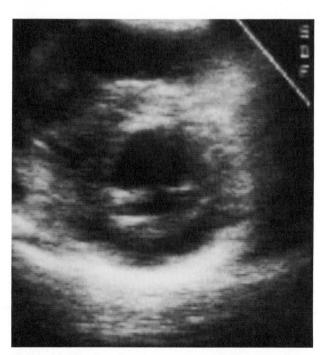

Figure 19.10. Results of averaging four frames with poor registration. This image shows a decrease in the speckle contrast similar to that seen in Figure 19.9, but the endocardial and epicardial information has also been degraded.

A1	A2	A3
A4	A5	A6
A7	A8	A9

Figure 19.11. Diagrammatic representation of a three-element by three-element mask, where A represents the amplitude of the gray level in each of the nine elements.

"mask operations." A mask image operation is a spatial formula that uses the gray level of surrounding pixels in order to modify the brightness of the pixel at the center of the mask.

Smoothing Operations

The most uncomplicated of the smoothing operations is simply spatial averaging. Figure 19.11 shows the 3 by 3 matrix, with the amplitudes of the gray levels in the pixels being labeled A_1 to A_9. For simple averaging, these amplitude values are added together and divided by 9. This value replaces the value in pixel A_5. The mask is then shifted one column and the process repeated. In this way, the mask is moved through each row and column, and the central gray level is replaced by the average of the neighborhood. The resultant image is shown in Figure 19.12. Variations of this are possible. Weighted averaging can be accomplished by multiplying pixels A_2, A_4, A_6, and A_8 by 2 and the central pixel A_5 by 3. The sum of the nine pixels will then be divided by 15, and this average will replace the value of A_5. This process can be represented by this equation

$$A_5 =$$

$$\frac{A_1 + A_3 + A_7 + A_9 + 2(A_2 + A_4 + A_6 + A_8) + 3A_5}{15}$$

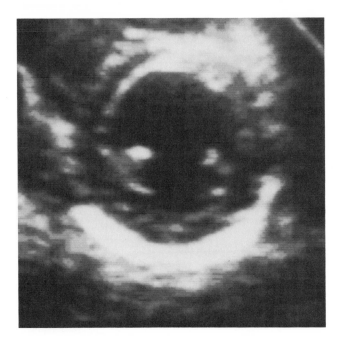

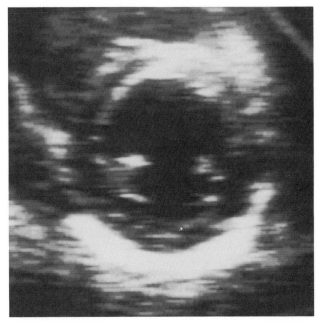

Figure 19.12. Results of a 3 by 3 smoothing operation in which the central pixel of the mask has been replaced by the average of the nine pixels within the mask.

A

For the sake of simplicity, we will express such an operation in the following form:

$$A_5 = \begin{vmatrix} 1 & 2 & 1 \\ 2 & 3 & 2 \\ 1 & 2 & 1 \end{vmatrix} \div 15$$

Such weighted operations provide less smoothing since the majority of the "weight" is placed on the nearest neighbors. Therefore, the blurring effect on the images is less. Gap filling and decrease in speckle contrast, however, will also be decreased.

In the previous examples, smoothing masks have been applied over symmetric regions. In other words, there are three units in both the X and Y direction. We know, however, that the echocardiographic image has an asymmetric resolution cell. In general, as pointed out, the axial resolution is roughly one to two wavelengths, while the azimuthal resolution is five to six wavelengths. To take advantage of this, Parker et al. (35) developed a method called "lateral filtration." Because of the type of system available to him, the exact form of his lateral filtration cannot be duplicated in our computer. Figure 19.13 thus applies similar asymmetric masks to the original image. In Figure 19.13A, the asymmetric averaging is accomplished with the three pixels on each side of the central pixel. In Figure 19.13B, a 3 by 7 weighted mask is utilized. While gaps are filled, it is apparent that the image information is greatly blurred.

Smoothing can also occur in the temporal dimension as noted with frame averaging. Garcia et al. (36) have implemented space-time smoothing for the filling of

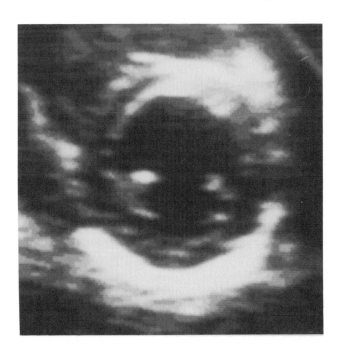

B

Figure 19.13. Results of lateral filtration. (*A*) The results of smoothing with a weighted 1 by 7 mask. (*B*) The results of smoothing with a weighted 3 by 7 mask.

gaps and removal of noise prior to edge detection. The mechanics involve replacing the pixel of interest with a weighted average of its eight neighbors in the present image, its three nearest neighbors in the previous image, and its three nearest neighbors in the succeeding image in time.

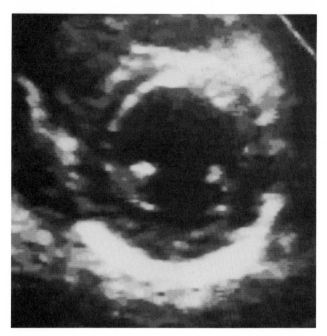

Figure 19.14.   Results of 3 by 3 median filtration on Figure 19.1.

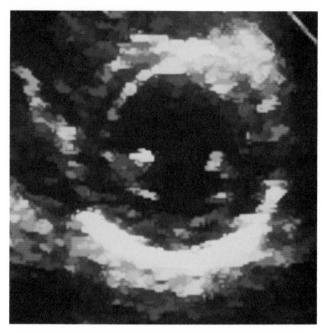

Figure 19.15.   Results of performing extremum sharpening on Figure 19.14.

Other modifications of smoothing have also been described. In one of these applications, the central pixel is replaced by the average of its k nearest neighbors in gray level within the 3 by 3 pixel region. The k can be chosen as any number between one and eight. If k is set to three, the central pixel will be averaged with the three pixels surrounding it that are nearest to its gray level. When k is eight, the results are the same as simple smoothing described previously. The effect of this operation is also to perform some gap filling and decrease speckle contrast while creating less blurring of the image.

Median filtering involves replacing the central pixel with the median value of its eight surrounding pixels. Figure 19.14 shows the effect of median filtration on the original image (Fig. 19.1). Since there is no set mathematical relationship that can restore the original image, operations of this type are called "nonlinear smoothing operations."

One method for increasing the contrast of images is termed "extremum sharpening." In this process, the mean gray level of the nine pixel neighborhood is calculated. If the central pixel falls above this mean, then the central pixel value is set equal to the highest gray level in the region; if the value of the central pixel is below the mean, then its value is set to the lowest gray level of the region. The combination of median filtration and extremum sharpening is useful in preprocessing of images before edge-enhancement operations are applied (20, 37). Figure 19.15 shows the result of applying extremum sharpening to the median filtering image of Figure 19.14.

Edge-Enhancement Masks

An edge in a picture is a change from one color or gray level to another. For instance, the edge of a building is seen and appreciated because it is a sharp change from one brightness or color to another. The sharpness of the edge depends on how rapidly the change in brightness occurs. It is not surprising that methods have been developed to search for a change of brightness. Gradient operators perform a discrete differentiation at each pixel in the image; looking for the rate of change in gray level. This type of edge detector has been reviewed by Abdou and Pratt (38).

A classic example is the discrete differential set of masks referred to as the Prewitt operation. This method of processing the images calculates the magnitude and direction of the gray level gradient at each pixel in the image and is given by the following expression:

$$ P = \left(\left| \begin{array}{ccc} -1 & 0 & 1 \\ -1 & 0 & 1 \\ -1 & 0 & 1 \end{array} \right|^2 + \left| \begin{array}{ccc} 1 & 1 & 1 \\ 0 & 0 & 0 \\ -1 & -1 & -1 \end{array} \right|^2 \right)^{1/2} $$

It can be seen that this is a discrete approximation of the partial differential of the image in the x and y directions.

That this differentiation does indeed take place can be demonstrated by a simple example in the x direction. The following three rows of numbers represent

gray level amplitude of 7 and 8 on the right. The 10 amplitudes across row two are plotted in Figure 19.16B. These x components calculated from the left-hand mask in the previous equation are

$$0 \quad 2 \quad 15 \quad 26 \quad 10 \quad -5 \quad -2 \quad 1$$

These values are plotted in Figure 19.16A. The peak of the Prewitt x component occurs at the maximum slope of the rising gray level, and a negative value is obtained at the later falloff in gray level from 10 to 8. Thus, the edge has been differentiated and enhanced. The results of applying this operation to Figure 19.1 are shown in Figure 19.17.

The LaPlacian operation is a simpler version of this in which the central pixel is multiplied by eight, and the surrounding eight pixels are subtracted from the total. This can be thought of as a differentiation in all directions. The LaPlacian values calculated for the eight pixels in row two of the example above are

$$0 \quad -2 \quad -8 \quad 9 \quad 22 \quad -4 \quad 1 \quad -7$$

These are plotted in Figure 19.16C. This function reaches a maximum at the peak gray level of the edge. The LaPlacian operation then gives us an enhanced local maximum.

The Sobel operation is very similar to the Prewitt operation:

$$S = \left(\begin{vmatrix} -1 & 0 & 1 \\ -2 & 0 & 2 \\ -1 & 0 & 1 \end{vmatrix}^2 + \begin{vmatrix} 1 & 2 & 1 \\ 0 & 0 & 0 \\ -1 & -2 & -1 \end{vmatrix}^2 \right)^{1/2}$$

The weight of the nearest neighbor in both the x and y positions now assumes the value of two. This operation is frequently referred to and its results appear to be nearly identical to Figure 19.17. Note that with both the Prewitt and Sobel operations, the edges of all targets are enhanced. The operations do not selectively enhance the edges of the ventricle.

Another family of operations is known as "compass gradient operations," or "template-matching operations." The positive and negative values, as seen in the Prewitt and Sobel operations, rotate 45 degrees in each sequential mask. A set of masks for a simple three-level operation is as follows:

$$\begin{vmatrix} -1 & 0 & 1 \\ -1 & 0 & 1 \\ -1 & 0 & 1 \end{vmatrix} \begin{vmatrix} -1 & -1 & 0 \\ -1 & 0 & 1 \\ 0 & 1 & 1 \end{vmatrix} \begin{vmatrix} -1 & -1 & -1 \\ 0 & 0 & 0 \\ 1 & 1 & 1 \end{vmatrix} \begin{vmatrix} 0 & -1 & -1 \\ 1 & 0 & -1 \\ 1 & 1 & 0 \end{vmatrix}$$

$$\begin{vmatrix} 1 & 0 & -1 \\ 1 & 0 & -1 \\ 1 & 0 & -1 \end{vmatrix} \begin{vmatrix} 1 & 1 & 0 \\ 1 & 0 & -1 \\ 0 & -1 & -1 \end{vmatrix} \begin{vmatrix} 1 & 1 & 1 \\ 0 & 0 & 0 \\ -1 & -1 & -1 \end{vmatrix} \begin{vmatrix} 0 & 1 & 1 \\ -1 & 0 & 1 \\ -1 & -1 & 0 \end{vmatrix}$$

The resultant image is produced by keeping the maximum value of these eight masks. The direction of

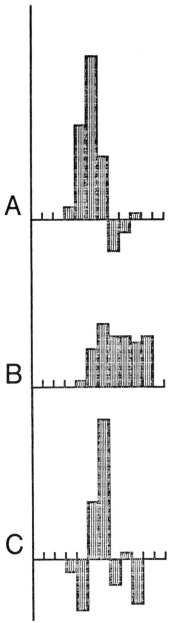

Figure 19.16. Plot of the resultant amplitudes from two gradient calculations across an edge in the original image (Fig. 19.1). (A) The calculated x component amplitude from the Prewitt operation. (B) The plot of the gray level amplitudes across a hypothetic edge. (C) A plot of the amplitudes obtained from a LaPlacian mask operation across the edge.

gray level amplitudes in a portion of the ultrasound image:

$$
\begin{array}{cccccccccc}
0 & 0 & 0 & 0 & 5 & 9 & 8 & 7 & 8 & 8 \\
0 & 0 & 0 & 1 & 6 & 10 & 8 & 8 & 7 & 8 \\
0 & 0 & 0 & 1 & 4 & 9 & 9 & 8 & 8 & 8 \\
\end{array}
$$

The amplitude of the gray level goes from 0 on the left to an edge with a somewhat higher amplitude at 9, 10, and 9, respectively, in column six, and then to a stable

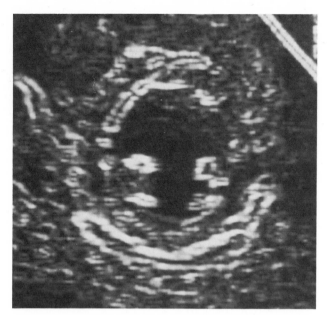

Figure 19.17. Results of the Prewitt gradient operation on Figure 19.1.

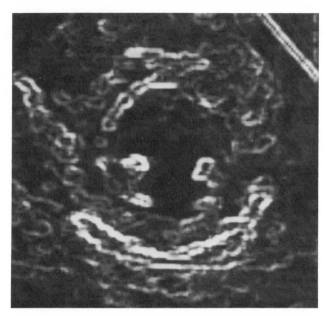

Figure 19.18. Results of performing the Prewitt gradient operation on the image with median filtration and extremum sharpening preprocessing (Fig. 19.15).

the gradient is the direction corresponding to that mask. The results obtained are comparable to those obtained with either the Prewitt or Sobel operation (38).

As mentioned previously, the results of image processing can be improved by using several operations in sequence on the same image. Figure 19.15 shows the results of median filtration and extremum sharpening on the image. Figure 19.18 shows the result of performing the Prewitt operation on Figure 19.15 and can be compared to performing the Prewitt operation on the original image as shown in Figure 19.17. Once the enhancement has been performed, image segmentation (i.e., identification of borders) is performed by thresholding the enhanced image and, if need be, histogram modification of the result.

ASYMMETRIC OPERATIONS

The work of Parker et al. (35) has been discussed in reference to lateral filtration. Realizing that the resolution cell of ultrasound is not symmetric, it seems reasonable to apply methods analogous to those listed previously. Our laboratory has explored asymmetric analogies to many of the operations described, including nonlinear smoothing operations and gradient operations. Certain advantages are also possible because the acoustic speckle in the image extends over fewer scan lines than does the reflection from a specular target. In examining speckle in laser images, Goodman (29) concluded that large fluctuations in size occur in the speckle pattern but that "no scale sizes are present beyond a certain small size cutoff." This same phenom-

enon seems to be true of the speckle in echocardiographic images. This small size cutoff, however, has been found to be approximately the same size as the resolution cell of the echocardiographic equipment (27, 28). Using this information, response filters can be designed that will enhance regions of brightness above this size limit to a greater extent than others. Figure 19.19 shows the results with one of these asymmetric mask operations.

Edge Detection

The areas derived from manually traced borders on good or excellent quality echocardiograms appear to have a intraobserver variability of about 8 percent to 10 percent (13, 25, 39). The least variable method of identifying endocardial borders for the purpose of quantitation appears to be drawing the border at the inner black-white interface of the achieved endocardium (39, 40). The most accurate method, however, seems to be drawing the borders through the center of the leading edge of the specular targets representing the endocardium in the image (39, 40). In an experiment in our laboratory, five expert observers were asked to define endocardial borders on every other frame of 30 cardiac cycles, six of which had been supplied from each of their own laboratories. They were asked to draw the inner black–white interface in order to keep the interobserver variation as low as possible. However, the studies were clinical studies, and certain time constraints were placed on the observers to simulate the setting of clinical quantitation.

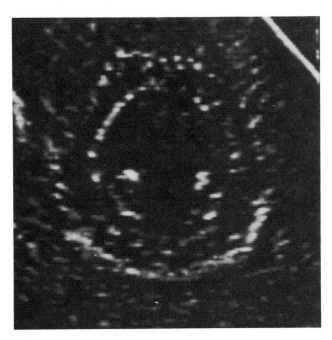

Figure 19.19. Results of forming an asymmetric gradient operation on Figure 19.1.

In this situation, the interobserver variability was found to be 13 percent in good quality studies and 9.9 percent in excellent quality studies.

The purpose of image-processing operations is to decrease speckle contrast or enhance edges so that better quantitative data can be obtained from echocardiograms. Collins et al. (37) have shown that computer processing of the images may improve the observer's ability to define the endocardium to some extent but does not markedly improve the results. Image averaging can produce some degree of gap filling depending on the registration of the images. The results may decrease variability and increase consistency in measurements from poor quality images (34).

This variability of 8 percent to 13 percent is not excessive and indeed is quite similar to that encountered with other techniques. In a 1985 review (41), calculations of ventricular volume from three-dimensional reconstructions of two-dimensional echocardiograms were compared to cardiac volumes calculated from x-ray techniques when both were applied to the same gold standards in vitro. For inanimate specimens and isolated contracting hearts, both angiographic and echocardiographic techniques have nearly identical correlation coefficients.

Then, how accurate should we strive to be in calculating volumes and EFs? The answer can be illustrated in a simple example. Assume that a patient has left ventricular dysfunction, with end-diastolic diameter of 6.0 cm and end-systolic diameter of 4.3 cm. The overall ventricular long-axis length from the center of the mitral valve plane to the apex is 8.8 cm, and this shortens by 10 percent during systole. If the patient's heart rate is 60, then an additional 1 mm of inward motion during systole in each wall results in a 12 percent increase in cardiac output. A 1.5-mm increase in wall motion (i.e., a 3-mm decrease in systolic dimension) will result in a 20 percent increase in cardiac output. If we assume that the entire increase in cardiac output results from a decrease in the end-systolic chamber size and that the heart rate stays constant, the end-systolic short-axis endocardial area needs only to decrease by 7 percent in order for there to be a 20 percent increase in cardiac output. Thus, while a 20 percent increase in cardiac output represents an important change in systolic function, it is below the interobserver variability.

From this example, it is not hard to understand that when the inter- and intraobserver variabilities decrease, the chances for detecting a change in function or size increase. The true accuracy or ability to measure volume and area compared to the known true volume and area may never be known with certainty because there is at present no absolute method for measuring cardiac volume in vivo. Remember that biplane angiography has the same variability in estimating volume as echocardiography in good and excellent quality studies in vitro. The precision with which we measure areas and volumes can be investigated, however, and the more reproducible and less variable these estimates are, even though they may not be absolutely accurate, the more they enable us to detect change.

Newly published evidence shows that both investigation of early ischemic disease (14) and detection of diastolic abnormalities (4, 42–44) require the assessment of frame-by-frame analysis of global or regional areas. Accurate manual digitization on a frame-by-frame basis of these borders is a tedious and time-consuming task. In addition, the frame-to-frame variability encountered requires rather elaborate smoothing of the defined borders (14).

It is not surprising that many groups have placed concentrated effort into programming unbiased objective computers to extract borders of interest from two-dimensional echocardiograms. The majority of this work is centered around the endocardium of the left ventricular cavity. While all of these techniques use similar parts, the way in which these parts are put together to arrive at a final algorithm for choosing the borders varies considerably. For a detailed discussion, the reader is referred to the original papers (36, 49–51). However, some common aspects of processing deserve further comment.

In general, search for the endocardial border is carried out in a radial direction. In most instances, an observer must define the center of the left ventricular cavity. From this point, rays are constructed outward, and the gray level along each of these rays is examined. Edges are best detected when the search is conducted perpendicular to the expected orientation of the edge. Generally, the maximum gradient occurs when the edge is approached directly, as opposed to obliquely. In spite of the fact that this geometric relationship is less optimum in apical views, satisfactory results with radial search have also been obtained from long-axis echocardiograms (45).

In the work of Garcia et al. (36), gaps were filled and noise removed from the image by the previously discussed space-time smoothing. Radial search for a maximal gradient was then employed along multiple radial lines. The edges produced from this method were evaluated by Zwehl et al. (46). Both computer- and manually defined endocardial borders were compared to the borders traced from the anatomic specimens. The correlation for both manually and computer-defined borders versus the anatomy was 0.95.

Delp et al. (47) and Buda et al. (48) have described an acquisition system and digital-processing technique for two-dimensional echocardiograms. After investigation of edge-enhancement routine, they concluded that axial gradient edge detection seemed simplest and most accurate. A systematic validation study of the borders obtained has not been reported to our knowledge.

Grube et al. (45) have reported on a system for detecting edges in apical long-axis views. Results obtained with this algorithm have been compared to manually defined borders from the apical echocardiograms following saline contrast injections during cardiac catheterization. The manually defined borders showed a correlation of 0.97 with those extracted automatically by the computer. The interobserver variability of manually defined borders was found to be 8.7 percent.

Robison et al. (49) also developed a method for identifying endocardial borders in sequences of images. In order to initiate this algorithm, the observer had to identify the endocardial border on the first frame. After this, the computer program predicted the most likely location for the border on sequential images, depending on the border chosen on the previous image. This algorithm did not search radially but searched moving along the border. Search was conducted in a limited angle of view as the decision-making process moved around the endocardial contour. Validation of the results was not vigorously pursued.

However, problems experienced by the other algorithms considered previously were partially obviated in the approach taken by Robison. The major problem was the presence of intracavitary structures. Obvi-

ously, the radial search cannot be undertaken with hope of detecting accurate borders if mitral valve and papillary muscle structures are present within the ventricle. By beginning the process of searching for the borders with an observer-identified endocardial contour on the first frame, the algorithm was directed toward the region of high probability for finding the borders and away from intracavitary structure.

The algorithms developed in our laboratory (50, 51) have also required tracing of initial borders by the observer. Thus, borders chosen by the algorithm are not completely objective. On the other hand, we have found that attempts at complete automation for endocardial and epicardial edge detection in multiple views lead to erroneous borders because of predictable confounding structures, unpredictable noise, and unpredictable translation. Thus, our present algorithms compromise between accuracy, complete automation and objectivity. The algorithm reported in our papers (50, 51) required the observer to define the opening end-diastolic endocardium, end-systolic endocardial border, and the closing end-diastolic border for the cycle to be studied. These three borders provide five important pieces of a priori knowledge: 1) the general size and shape of borders to be searched for, 2) the range of motion of the borders over the cycle, 3) the range of translation of the heart during the cycle, 4) the length of the cardiac cycle, and 5) the length of systole. This information is needed when one considers the complexity of searching for endocardial borders in a full range of clinical situations. Consider that the left ventricular wall can be moving inward toward the cavity, akinetic, not moving at all, or dyskinetic (i.e., moving outward). Depending on which cycle the observer chooses to process, translation can occur due to respiration or movement of the transducer on the chest wall. Because of this, the closing end-diastolic frame may not be in the same position as the opening end-diastolic frame for the cycle. For this reason, we have found it necessary for the operator to draw both of these frames. Finally, one cannot count on the position of the systolic border. The most extreme situation that we have encountered was a young patient with an atrial septal defect, paradoxic septal motion, and marked swinging of the heart due to a large pericardial effusion. In this study, the end-systolic endocardium fell almost completely outside of either end-diastolic endocardial border. Because of this, we find it necessary to know where the ventricle is at three points in the cardiac cycle.

Using the three borders, a large region of search is constructed that includes all three. This large search region is then superimposed on all of the frames in the cardiac cycle. The observer's borders are then thrown away, and a new search for the endocardium carried out on each frame but only within the superimposed region of interest. For a more detailed discussion of this algorithm, the reader is referred the original papers (50, 51).

Validation

At this point, it is appropriate to discuss validation of these computer-defined borders for clinical use. No matter which algorithm is employed, the cardiologist must ask, Are the borders accurate? Are they less variable than manually defined borders? Do they provide a saving in time? Static comparisons can be used as indirect validation of the accuracy of the detected borders. In several of the previously discussed reports, validation was carried out in this manner. Manually defined borders with contrast in the image were compared to those extracted by the edge detection algorithm (45). In this situation, there is still a question as to the accuracy of manually defined borders. This points out, however, a problem that exists with validation of all in vivo techniques. Simply stated, there is not a truly objective manner for carrying out validation of edges detected from images obtained in the intact human being. We do not have the capability to observe a slice of human heart directly during contraction. Therefore, validation studies to evaluate the correctness of the shape of borders must use borders drawn by trained expert observers as a gold standard (52).

Our algorithm was tested against five expert observers. Each observer sent six studies from his or her clinical laboratory as described before. The correlation between expert-drawn and computer-drawn borders was calculated for only the excellent quality studies since in these studies, by definition, the expert was confident of the position of the borders on each frame in the cardiac cycle. The correlation coefficient for areas enclosed by observer- versus computer-defined borders was 0.985. A statistically significant decrease in the interobserver variability was noted, with the computer-drawn borders having a 6.9 percent and 8.7 percent variability for excellent and good quality studies, respectively. The intraobserver variability of borders defined on two consecutive days was decreased from 6.5 percent to 4.5 percent and from 10.8 percent to 7.0 percent in excellent and good quality studies, respectively (53–55). In order to look at the reliability of the detection of wall motion defects, correlations were also carried out between each of the 64 radii comprising the individual borders. The correlation between the computer-defined and observer-defined radii describing each border was 0.909. This suggests that the automated borders could not only define the overall area of the ventricle, but could also describe the shape of the border. The implication is that wall motion

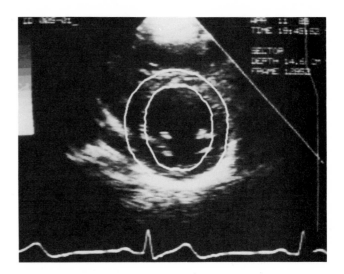

A

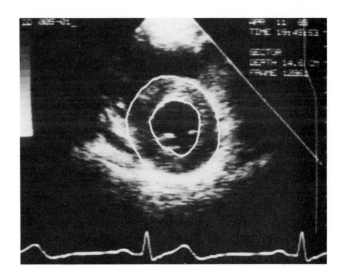

B

Figure 19.20. The end-diastolic (*A*) and end-systolic (*B*) frames from a cardiac cycle are shown. The computer-defined endocardial and epicardial borders are superimposed on Figure 19.1.

defects can be described by the computer-defined borders. There is continued variability even in the computer-defined borders because the region of interest is defined from the observer-identified borders. Thus, different thresholds may be selected depending on what each observer included in his or her drawn borders.

Another aspect of having the computer define the borders, however, is the time factor. In the previous studies, the length of time required for the computer to define all the frames in the cardiac cycle was 3 to 4 minutes or approximately 8 to 9 seconds per frame once the observer had defined the two end-diastolic and one end-systolic borders. The five observers, on

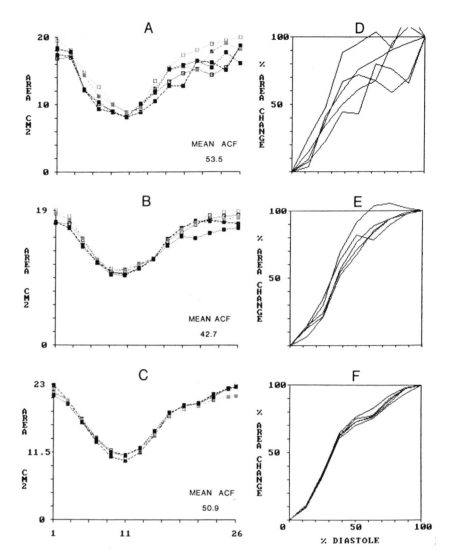

Figure 19.21. Results of manual border definition in two algorithms for automated endocardial border detection over one cardiac cycle. (*A*) A plot of the area enclosed by borders defined by five experts on every other frame of one cardiac cycle. (*B*) The areas enclosed by endocardial borders chosen by an automatic border detection algorithm. (*C*) Again, the areas enclosed by a second-generation algorithm, which uses information in both the endocardial and epicardial borders to choose the final endocardial edges. (*D*, *E*, and *F*) The diastolic filling characteristics obtained from the respective sets of borders. ACF = area change fraction.

the other hand, required a mean of nearly 50 seconds per frame to define the endocardial border. Another aspect to be considered is observer fatigue. Observers defining endocardial borders over a long period of time in the same day tend to grow lax and fatigued. While data are not available concerning the increase in variability as the day goes on, it is expected that the fatigue encountered by an observer drawing only three borders would be much less.

Epicardial Edge Detection

Computer-automated definition of the epicardial border also deserves mention at this time. Generally, detection of the epicardium presents more problems than that of the endocardium. Because of the pericardial echos and lung interface, more confusing noise and structure are present. However, calculation of wall stress (56) appears useful but variable (57), again suggesting that computer identification of the epicardium would be worthwhile.

Since 1984, we have approached the problem of epicardial edge detection as a "coupled" border definition problem. This approach has several advantages. The first and foremost advantage is that the wall thickness seems to be the most consistent single expected parameter during the cardiac cycle. Recall that the endocardial border can move inward, not move, or move outward. On top of this motion, external translation induced by breathing or transducer movement and unpredictable translation from other causes such as pericardial effusion can be superimposed. The wall thickness, however, between end diastole and end systole changes in a very consistent pattern. We know, for instance, that in a region of normal myocardium where the wall thickness goes from 10 to 16 mm, this thickening occurs in a fairly consistent pattern with little more than 1 mm in thickening on any single frame. We can also be sure that once thickening is started, there is virtually no possibility that any thinning will take place before the end-systolic thickness is reached. On the other hand, if the wall thins in a certain region, as may be seen with acute ischemia, it is unlikely that it will thicken at any portion of the cycle. Again, the thinning from end diastole to end systole will be very consistent in its pattern. Therefore, knowing the thickness at end diastole and the thickness at end systole, we can predict what the wall thickness is likely to be on any intervening frame. With this knowledge, we know that we should be searching for two borders that can be found at a known distance apart, no matter where they have translated on the screen.

The second advantage comes in regions of dropout. Gaps in either the endocardium or epicardium are produced by the constructive-destructive interference phenomenon described with speckle, or occur because of lack of a reflecting site perpendicular to the propagation of the ultrasound at this point in the wall. Because of the marked difference of the geometric surface of the endocardium and epicardium adjacent to each other, it is not unusual to find that the epicardial echo will still be present even though there is dropout in the endocardial contour. The reverse is also true. Therefore, we can use information regarding the wall thickness to interpolate or fill the gaps in the other border more accurately.

The final advantage is an improved ability of the algorithm to avoid intracavitary structures. One of the problems with the earlier algorithm defining endocardial borders alone was that it frequently latched on to the posterior portion of the papillary muscle instead of the endocardium in this region. Definition of two edges in this region or definition of the epicardium alone allows one either to evaluate the wall thickness or to set a maximum limit for the upper bound of the wall thickness accepted on a particular frame. Therefore, a decision can be made as to the likelihood of whether another border or structure found is beyond the allowable thickness and therefore inside the cavity.

Figure 19.20 shows end-diastolic and end-systolic endocardial and epicardial borders superimposed on Figure 19.1. Notice that the papillary muscles have been avoided successfully. Figure 19.21 shows areas defined by observers and the two algorithms as well as the diastolic filling characteristics of the ventricle plotted from each set of data. Figure 19.21A plots the areas of manually traced borders by the five expert observers. The mean area change fraction calculated between the first end diastole and end systole is 53.5 percent. Figure 19.21B is a plot of the areas over the cardiac cycle as defined by the first algorithm, which defines the endocardial border alone. The variability on each frame is decreased in the curves, and the curves are more grouped together. End diastole is slightly smaller than that traced by the observers, whereas end systole is slightly larger, accounting for a significantly

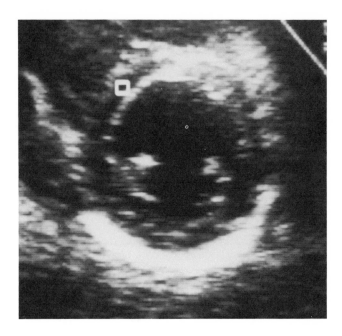

A

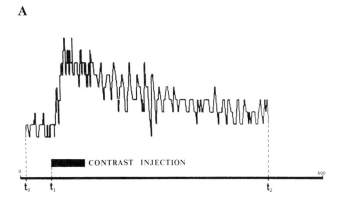

B

Figure 19.22. (*A*) A short-axis two-dimensional echocardiogram prior to injection of contrast agent into the coronary artery. The small box over the ventricular septum is the region of interest in which the brightness is to be studied over the course of the contrast injection. (*B*) The time versus brightness curve in this region following injection of contrast material.

different mean area change fraction of 42.7 percent. These differences are due in part to problems with intracavitary structure as previously described. Figure 19.21C is a plot of the endocardial areas obtained with the new algorithm, which employs information on both the epicardium and endocardium to detect borders. The variability is more markedly reduced, and the curves are slightly more together. Both the end-diastolic and end-systolic areas are slightly larger than those defined by the observers, with a mean area change fraction now calculated as 50.9 percent. Figure 19.21D, E, and F show the corresponding diastolic filling characteristics for these three sets of areas. This

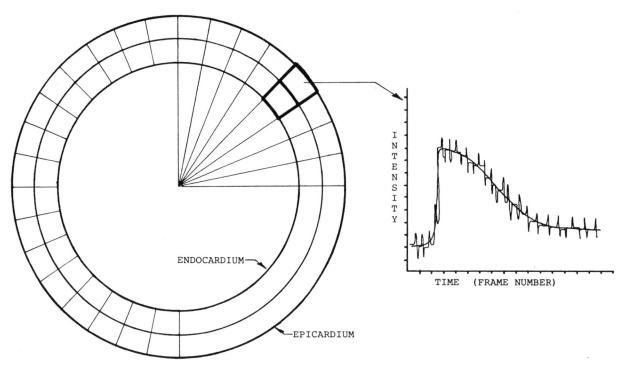

Figure 19.23.   Schema for dividing the myocardium into 32 subendocardial and 32 subepicardial regions. The brightness versus time curves from each of these regions can then be studied individually.

presentation of percentage of area versus percentage of diastole was chosen because it illustrates a potentially clinically useful datum for identification of myocardial constriction, which requires frame-by-frame analysis (4). The marked sequential reduction and variability are obvious. It should be pointed out that the manual borders traced were not traced for research purposes but were traced in a setting similar to that encountered in clinical practice. The manually defined borders were not manipulated or smoothed in any way. However, it seems obvious that a large amount of smoothing would have to be applied to each of the observers' curves in order to accomplish a marked reduction in the variability seen in Figure 19.21C.

Coronary Perfusion and Video Densitometry

Echocardiographic contrast agents and their applications have been discussed in Chapter 18, and we should include a brief discussion of the utility of computer processing in assessing these data. Various methods for approaching the problem of extracting the physiologic data from the echocardiographic images have been published (58–60). Again, the data to be extracted from the myocardial contrast studies are of two types: spatial and temporal. The spatial information shows the region perfused by the echocardiographic contrast material. The temporal information shows the rate of appearance and disappearance of the contrast agent.

The latter information is thought to contain relevant information regarding the degree of perfusion. By entering the video images from a contrast study into the computer, the gray level in any small region of myocardium can be examined sequentially over time. In Figure 19.22, this small region of myocardium over the septum is examined in sequential frames, and the increase in brightness and its decay are shown in Figure 19.22B. One of the problems encountered is that the myocardium moves. In order to obtain good temporal curves over many cardiac cycles, respirations must be held, and either frames in one portion of the cardiac cycle are processed or the region must be translated as the left ventricle contracts and relaxes. If a large region of the myocardium is to be studied over many cycles and during different phases of the cardiac cycle, then multiple endocardial and epicardial borders must be drawn. With the ability to define the endocardial and epicardial borders on multiple frames automatically comes the ability to study both the extent and time course of the brightness changes over the entire myocardium. Cardiac motion during systole can be accounted for by dividing the myocardium into equiangular segments from a central point defined as the center of mass of the epicardium on each individual frame. The average gray level within each of these equiangular regions should then be roughly comparable, except for the rotation of the heart during systole. The amount of data obtained for such an analysis

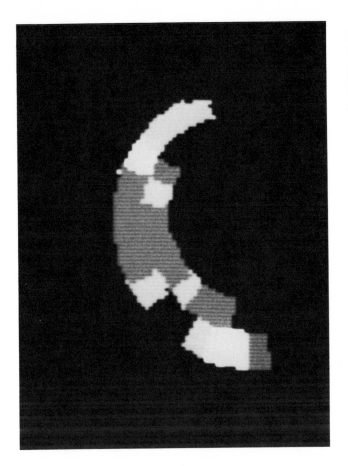

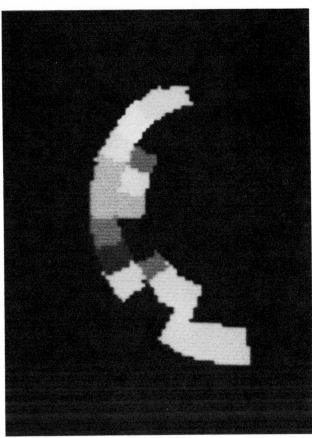

A

B

Figure 19.24.   Parametric images obtained from injection of contrast agent into the right coronary artery. (*A*) An image in which the brightness in the 64 regions is proportional to the maximum brightness achieved minus the average background brightness prior to contrast injection. (*B*) Each of the 64 regions has been assigned a gray level proportional to the length of time that the brightness in the region was above the background gray level prior to injection.

involving multiple frames and multiple cycles over 10 to 20 seconds is staggering. Computer processing can also help the observer to interpret this large amount of information. Where the observer would have difficulty in comparing the curves of brightness versus time over many regions, displays of certain parameters of these curves can facilitate rapid recognition of areas that differ considerably. This method of displaying various parameters of the regional brightness curves in their relative anatomic position is referred to as "parametric imaging." Similar methods have been used in phase analysis with radionuclide angiography for several years. Figure 19.23 shows a schematic representation in which the myocardial area on a short-axis view of the left ventricle has been divided into 32 equiangular segments and each of these segments divided into an endocardial and epicardial portion. The mean gray level in each of these areas is then followed over time. These regions can be displayed in the position of a representative end-diastolic frame and the gray level in each region given a brightness proportional to the relative magnitude of the parameter being measured. Figure 19.24 shows the parametric image in which each region is coded to the maximum brightness achieved after contrast was injected. Figure 19.24B shows a parametric image in which the gray level of each region is proportional to the length of time that the brightness was above background. Thus, differences between two important features of the 64 regional brightness curves can be appreciated. Many other features of the curves can be displayed such as the slope or time constant of the brightness decay. Which of these are important must still be decided by research. This method is another example in which the computer can serve as a powerful tool in reducing the information to a level easily implemented in a clinical setting.

SUMMARY

Ultrasound is a valuable qualitative tool. More and more attention is being placed on the value of quantitations obtained from two-dimensional echocardiography. Measurements and indexes of function obtained from good and excellent quality two-dimensional echocardiographic studies are comparable to those obtained from other imaging techniques. The variability in echocardiographic measurements is likely due to an interaction between an observer defining the borders and the image quality. Echocardiographic images have a poor signal-to-noise ratio. While many factors contribute to this, a major feature of the image is acoustic speckle and dropout due to the use of coherent ultrasound.

Many image-processing operations can be performed on these images in the computer. We have reviewed the most frequently applied operations. Examples have been shown in order to give the reader an idea of the obtained image. While one can calculate a decrease in the speckle contrast after performing these operations, the real test of whether the image has been improved depends on the qualitative assessment of a trained observer.

The current status of automated border detection algorithms has also been reviewed. Many of these algorithms preprocess the echocardiographic images using one or more of the operations illustrated. While the end product of such detection algorithms is a set of borders and measurements on the cardiac cycle, we believe the reader should have some understanding and knowledge of the intermediate processing techniques prior to border definition.

The accuracy and precision of indexes of left ventricular function calculated from echocardiographic data are dependent on the quality of the borders derived from the images. It seems safe to conclude that computer-assisted border definition algorithms provide an improvement in terms of reducing variability. This reduction in variability directly affects the sensitivity of echocardiographic measurements in detecting either changes in left ventricular function or small deviations from normal.

REFERENCES

1. Wyatt HL, Heng MK, Meerbaum S, et al. Cross-sectional echocardiography. I. Analysis of mathematic models for quantifying mass of the left ventricle in dogs. Circulation 1979;60(2):1104–13.
2. Parisi AF, Moynihan PF, Feldman CL, Folland ED. Approaches to determination of left ventricular volume and ejection fraction by real-time two-dimensional echocardiography. Clin Cardiol 1979; 2:257–63.
3. Schiller NG, Acquatella H, Ports TA, et al. Left ventricular volume from paired biplane two-dimensional echocardiography. Circulation 1979;60(5):647–55.
4. Pandian NG, Skorton DJ, Kieso RA, Kerber RE. Diagnosis of constrictive pericarditis by two-dimensional echocardiography: studies in a new experimental model and in patients. J Am Coll Cardiol 1984;4(6):1164–73.
5. Wyatt HL, Heng MK, Meerbaum S, et al. Cross-sectional echocardiography. II. Analysis of mathematic models for quantifying volume of the formalin-fixed left ventricle. Circulation 1980; 61(6):1119–25.
6. Folland ED, Parisi AF, Moynihan PF, Jones DR, Feldman CL, Tow DE. Assessment of left ventricular ejection fraction and volumes by real-time two-dimensional echocardiography. Circulation 1979;60(4):760–6.
7. Geiser EA, Lupkiewicz SM, Christie LG, Ariet M, Conetta DA, Conti CR. A framework for three-dimensional time-varying reconstruction of the human left ventricle: sources of error and estimation of their magnitude. Comput Biomed Res 1980;13:225–41.
8. Ariet M, Geiser EA, Lupkiewicz SM, Conetta DA, Conti CR. Evaluation of three-dimensional reconstruction to compute left ventricular volume and mass. Am J Cardiol 1984;54(3):415–20.
9. Nixon JV, Saffer SI, Lipscomb K, Blomqvist CG. Three-dimensional echoventriculography. Am Heart J 1983;105(3):435–43.
10. Moritz WE, Pearlman AS, McCabe DH, Medema DK, Ainsworth ME, Boles MS. An ultrasonic technique for imaging the ventricle in three dimensions and calculating its volume. IEEE Trans Biomed Eng 1983;BME-30(9):482–92.
11. Heger JJ, Wayman AE, Wann LS, Rogers EW, Dillon JC, Feigenbaum H. Cross-sectional echocardiographic analysis of the extent of left ventricular asynergy in acute myocardial infarction. Circulation 1980;61(6):1113–8.
12. Moynihan PF, Parisi AF, Feldman CL. Quantitative detection of regional left ventricular contraction abnormalities by two-dimensional echocardiography. I. Analysis of methods. Circulation 1981;63(4):752–60.
13. Parisi AF, Moynihan PF, Folland ED, Feldman CL. Quantitative detection of regional left ventricular contraction abnormalities by two-dimensional echocardiography. II. Accuracy in coronary artery disease. Circulation 1981;63(4):761–7.
14. Weyman AE, Franklin TD, Hogan RD, et al. Importance of temporal heterogeneity in assessing the contraction abnormalities associated with acute myocardial ischemia. Circulation 1984;70(1):102–12.
15. DePace NL, Ren JF, Kotler MN, Mintz GS, Kimbiris D, Kalman P. Two-dimensional echocardiographic determination of right atrial emptying volume: a noninvasive index in quantifying the degree of tricuspid regurgitation. Am J Cardiol 1983;52(5):525–9.
16. Crevasse L, Ariet M. Current status of computerized electrocardiography. In: Hurst JW, ed. Update III, the heart. New York: McGraw-Hill, 1980.
17. Sheffield LT. Quantitative approach to exercise testing for ischemic heart disease. In: Inelle HA et al., eds. Quantitatives in cardiology. Leiden, The Netherlands: Proceedings of the Boerhaave Courses, 1972.
18. Moynihan PF, Parisi AF, Folland ED, Jones DR, Feldman CL. A system for quantitative evaluation of left ventricular function with two-dimensional ultrasonography. Med Instrum 1980;14(2): 111–16.
19. Waag RC, Gramiak R, Lee PPK, Astheimer J. Digital processing of ultrasound images. IEEE Ultrasonics Symposium Proceedings 1976;163–7.
20. Skorton DJ, Collins SM. Digital computer image analysis in echocardiography. Echocardiography 1984;1(1):15–43.
21. Geiser EA, Oliver LH. Echocardiography: image processing in two-dimensional echocardiographic images. In: Geiser EA, guest ed. Automedica-computerized cardiac assessment procedures and techniques. London: Gordon & Breach, 1984.
22. Skorton DJ, Collins SM, Garcia E, et al. Digital signal and image processing in echocardiography: a glossary. Echocardiography 1985;11(1):5–8.
23. Leavitt SC, Hunt BF, Larsen HG. A scan conversion algorithm for displaying ultrasound images. Hewlett-Packard J 1983;October: 30–34.
24. Chaitman BR, DeMots H, Bristow JD, Rosch J, Rahimtoola SH. Objective and subjective analysis of left ventricular angiograms. Circulation 1975;52:420–5.
25. Haendchen RV, Wyatt HL, Maurer G, et al. Quantitation of regional cardiac function by two-dimensional echocardiography. I. Patterns of contraction in the normal left ventricle. Circulation 1983;67(6):1234–45.

26. Graham C. Vision and visual perception. New York: John Wiley & Sons, 1978.
27. Entrekin R, Melton HE. Real time speckle reduction in B-mode images. IEEE Ultrasonics Symposium Proceedings 1979;169–74.
28. Abbott JG, Thurstone FL. Acoustic speckle: theory and experimental analysis. Ultrasonic Imaging 1979;1:303–24.
29. Goodman JW. Some fundamental properties of speckle. J Opt Soc Am 1976;66(11):1145–50.
30. Kozma A, Christensen CR. Effects of speckle on resolution. J Opt Soc Am 1976;66(11):1257–60.
31. Young M, Faulkner B, Cole J. Resolution in optical systems using coherent illumination. J Opt Soc Am 1980;70:137–9.
32. Magnin PA. Coherent speckle in ultrasound images. Hewlett-Packard J 1983;October:39.
33. Zhang LF, Geiser EA. An approach to optimal threshold selection on a sequence of two-dimensional echocardiographic images. IEEE Trans Biomed Eng 1982;29(8):577–81.
34. Petrovic O, Feigenbaum H, Armstrong WF, et al. Digital averaging to facilitate 2D echocardiographic measurements. Circulation 1984;70(II):397.
35. Parker DL, Pryor TA, Ridges JD. Enhancement of two-dimensional echocardiographic images by lateral filtering. Comput Biomed Res 1979;12:265–77.
36. Garcia E, Gueret P, Bennett M, et al. Real time computerization of two-dimensional echocardiography. Am Heart J 1981;101(6):783–92.
37. Collins SM, Skorton DJ, Geiser EA, et al. Computer-assisted edge detection in two-dimensional echocardiography: comparison with anatomic data. Am J Cardiol 1984;53(9):1380–7.
38. Abdou IE, Pratt WK. Quantitative design and evaluation of enhancement/thresholding edge detectors. Proceedings of the IEEE 1979;67(5):753–63.
39. Conetta DA, Geiser EA, Skorton DJ, Pandian NG, Kerber RE, Conti CR. In vitro analysis of boundary identification techniques used in quantitation of two-dimensional echocardiograms. Am J Cardiol 1984;53(9):1374–9.
40. Wyatt HL, Haendchen RV, Meerbaum S, Corday E. Assessment of quantitative methods for 2-dimensional echocardiography. Am J Cardiol 1983;52(3):396–401.
41. Geiser EA. Three-dimensional echocardiographic reconstruction: how does it stack up? Int J Cardiol 1985;7(1):77–81.
42. Meaney E, Shabetai R, Bhargava V, et al. Cardiac amyloidosis, constrictive pericarditis and restrictive cardiomyopathy. Am J Cardiol 1976;38(5):547–56.
43. Tyberg TI, Goodyer AVN, Hurst VW, Alexander N, Langou RA. Left ventricular filling in differentiating restrictive amyloid cardiomyopathy and constrictive pericarditis. Am J Cardiol 1981;47(4):791–6.
44. Voelkel AG, Pietro DA, Folland ED, Fisher ML, Parisi AF. Echocardiographic features of constrictive pericarditis. Circulation 1978;58(5):871–5.
45. Grube E, Nitsch J, Backs B, Simon H. Automatic border extraction from 2-D echocardiograms. Circulation 1983;68(III):330.
46. Zwehl W, Levy R, Garcia E, et al. Validation of a computerized edge detection algorithm for quantitative two-dimensional echocardiography. Circulation 1983;68(5):1127–35.
47. Delp EJ, Buda AJ, Swastek MR, Smith JM, Meyer CR. The analysis of two-dimensional echocardiograms using a time-varying image approach. Comput Cardiol 1983;10:391–3.
48. Buda AJ, Delp EJ, Meyer CR, et al. Automatic computer processing of digital 2-dimensional echocardiograms. Am J Cardiol 1983;52(3):384–9.
49. Robison EP, Pryor TA, Wellard SJ, Jones DS, Ridges, JD. Recognition of left ventricular borders using two-dimensional echocardiographic images. Comput Biomed Res 1976;9:247.
50. Geiser EA, Oliver LJ, Zhang LF, Fu JK, Buss DD, Conti CR. An approach to endocardial boundary detection from sequential real time validation. In: Deconinck F, ed. Information processing in medical imaging. The Hague, The Netherlands: Martinus Nijhoff, 1984.
51. Zhang LF, Geiser EA. An effective algorithm for extracting serial endocardial borders from 2-dimensional echocardiograms. IEEE Trans Biomed Eng 1984;31(6):441–7.
52. Ritman EL, Sturm RE, Wood EH. Biplane roentgen videometric system (60/sec) studies of the shape and size of circulatory structures, particularly the left ventricle. Am J Cardiol 1973;32:180–7.
53. Oliver LH, Geiser EA, Zhang LF, et al. Evaluation of an automated border detection algorithm in 2D echo images of varying quality: observer vs computer. J Am Coll Cardiol 1984;3(2):564.
54. Geiser EA, Oliver LH, Gardin JM, et al. Computer automated endocardial edge detection from 2D echocardiograms: effective reduction in sequential area and shape variability for wall motion analysis. Clin Res 1984;32(2):167.
55. Geiser EA, Oliver LH, Zhang LF, et al. Quantitative and qualitative evaluation of an automated edge detection algorithm. Clin Res 1984;32(2):167.
56. Reichek N, Wilson J, St. John Sutton M, Plappert TA, Goldbert S, Hirshfeld JW. Noninvasive determination of left ventricular end-systolic stress: validation of the method and initial application. Circulation 1982;65(1):99–108.
57. Pandian NG, Skorton DJ, Collins SM, Falsetti HL, Burke ER, Kerber RE. Heterogeneity of left ventricular segmental wall thickening and excursion in 2-dimensional echocardiograms of normal human subjects. Am J Cardiol 1980;51(10):1667–73.
58. Ong K, Maurer G, Feinstein S, Zwehl W, Meerbaum S, Corday E. Computer methods for myocardial contrast two-dimensional echocardiography. J Am Coll Cardiol 1984;3(5):1212–8.
59. Maurer G, Ong K, Haendchen R, et al. Myocardial contrast two-dimensional echocardiography: comparison of contrast disappearance rates in normal and underperfused myocardium. Circulation 1984;69(2):418–29.
60. Geiser EA, Oliver HL, Buss DD, Pidgeon CV, Conti CR. Echocardiographic parametric images for visualization of echo contrast studies. Circulation 1984;70(1):11–15.

20
Ultrasonic Tissue Characterization of Myocardium

Derek Gibson

The aim of echocardiographic tissue characterization is to use ultrasound to gain information about the physical properties of targets within the tissues and to correlate this information with that derived from more established methods such as histology or biochemical analysis. In cardiology the technique is particularly applicable to detecting abnormalities within the myocardium, and it is with this field that the present account is concerned. Ultrasonic examination is not unique in giving information about the physical properties of the tissues; there has been a trend for information of this sort to become available from other recently introduced imaging methods such as computed tomographic or magnetic resonance imaging. Ultrasound has the advantages of 1) operating in real time, 2) avoiding electromagnetic radiation, and 3) low cost. This last, while to be greatly commended on social grounds, appears to be associated with ideas of financial parsimony. It has thus failed to attract the substantial funding available for developing other, more expensive, imaging techniques, and may well have contributed to the relatively slow progress in the development of ultrasonic tissue characterization.

INTERACTION OF ULTRASOUND WITH TISSUES

Ultrasonic tissue characterization depends as much as imaging on the interaction of ultrasound with the tissues. In both procedures the tissue is interrogated by the transducer, and in both information is extracted from the returning signal. The most important information necessary to build up an image comes from the position of targets within the heart. With tissue characterization the aim is to extract additional quantitative information from the returning echoes to make deductions about the physical or chemical constitution of the tissues giving rise to them. Indeed, it might be said that a better name for the procedure is not "tissue" but "echo" characterization.

If this characterization is not to be a wholly empirical procedure, it must be based on an understanding of the interactions between incident ultrasound and targets within the heart (1). These interactions are complex and at present are not completely understood. Specular reflection, upon which ultrasound images are classically said to depend, occurs when the target is large compared with the wavelength of the incident ultrasound, and so is seen in reflections from valve cusps or the endocardial surface of the septum. The proportion of incident ultrasound reflected depends on the difference in specific impedance of the two materials meeting at the interface (see Chapter 1). As with optical reflection, the angle of incidence equals the angle of reflection, so that the proportion of energy returning to the transducer depends critically on the angle of the interface to the ultrasound beam and is greatest when the two are perpendicular. Although specular reflections form the basis of cardiac imaging using ultrasound, they have proved much less informative for tissue characterization.

A second important process underlying image generation is backscattering. This occurs when the target is small compared with the wavelength of incident ultrasound, and it gives rise to the structural echoes between the main specular reflections (e.g., those arising from myocardium). The interaction depends on local inhomogeneities in physical properties, particularly in density and compressibility with their associated variation in the velocity of sound. The extent and direction of the scattered energy depends not only on the constitution of these inhomogeneities but also critically on their size and distribution within the tissue. Backscattered ultrasound energy is spread over a wide angle rather than in a uniform direction, so the amplitude of the returning signal depends less on the relative orientation of the structure and the incident beam. This is particularly the case when the scatterers are uniformly distributed. When distribution varies with direction, backscattering also occurs in preferential directions in a manner that depends on the underlying structure. The physical basis of backscattering is further complicated by the generation of new wave fronts by each of the numerous individual targets. These new wave fronts interfere with one another, affecting local amplitude and image texture in a manner again determined by the complex underlying structure. These ultrasound diffraction patterns potentially contain information about the arrangement of scatterers within the tissue and have been used to assess changes in myocardial fiber angle with depth across the ventricular wall (2).

When all these interactions are considered, it is clear that any information obtained about the tissues and, in particular, the myocardium will be fundamentally different from that derived from histology or biochemistry. The world displayed by ultrasonic characterization is concerned mainly with the structural members of tissues, their material properties, and their distribution. Its scale is based on that of the wavelength of interrogating ultrasound, approximately 0.5 mm at 3 MHz, and so is that of the hand lens rather than the microscope.

EXPERIMENTAL APPROACHES TO TISSUE CHARACTERIZATION

There have been many experimental approaches to ultrasonic tissue characterization based on studying the acoustic properties of isolated tissues. These have shed much light on one of the basic processes involved: the interaction of incident ultrasound with the tissue itself.

Detection of Collagen

It has been recognized for many years that collagen is likely to be a major determinant of echo generation by tissues. Collagen is approximately 1000 times less extensible than muscle, fat, or endothelium. In liver and breast, reflectivity is strongly related to the presence of fibrosis (3). O'Donnell and colleagues (4)

investigated backscattering by isolated myocardium, integrating it over the whole frequency range and eliminating phase cancellation effects. This quantity, integrated backscatter, derived from the myocardium was compared with that from a "perfect" reflector. The signal was gated, so that specular echoes were rejected and only those from myocardium studied. After experimental myocardial infarction, backscattering amplitude was considerably increased, particularly after four weeks, as fibrosis developed. At the same time, the frequency dependence of backscattering was reduced, so that the difference between normal and abnormal tissue became greater at lower (2 MHz) frequencies. Similar correlations have also been demonstrated between collagen content, estimated chemically as hydroxyproline concentration and backscattering in daunorubicin-induced cardiomyopathy in rabbits (5) and in spontaneously occurring cardiomyopathy in Syrian hamsters (6). Backscattering, however, does not depend simply on collagen content, because after experimental myocardial infarction reflectivity continues to increase after four weeks; hydroxyproline content, however, remains constant. During this later period, the collagen is thought to age when its structure and hence its mechanical properties change. In addition, when the tissue is treated with collagenase, reflectivity decreases but hydroxyproline content remains unaltered. When the acoustic fine structure of tissues is studied at much higher frequencies of ultrasound, in the range of 10 to 100 MHz, using the acoustic microscope, normal myocardium shows striking anisotropy, apparently because of muscle fiber orientation (7). Infarcted regions show marked nonuniformity of both attenuation and velocity possibly as a result of fibrosis within a matrix of myocardium. These results suggest that fibrosis might be a major determinant of backscattering amplitude by tissues, and that observed values are likely to depend on its distribution as well as its content.

Myocardial Ischemia and Water Content

Myocardial backscattering is increased in experimental myocardial ischemia. Within two hours of coronary occlusion, integrated backscatter can be shown to have increased by approximately 6 dB in comparison with control regions (8). This increase is not apparent until flow decreases below 20 percent of control, so it is not the flow reduction per se that causes the increased reflectivity but rather the effects of ischemic injury. Ultrasonic backscatter is also related to regional blood volume, because substitution of Krebs-Hensleit solution as perfusate increases backscatter without detectable increase in water content. Increasing myocardial water by hypertonic perfusate, however, leads to a

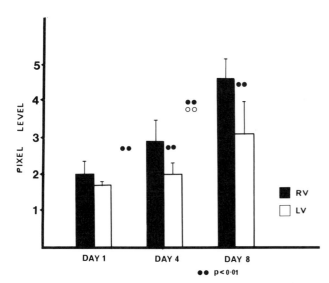

Figure 20.1. Changes in right (RV) and left ventricular (LV) myocardial echo amplitudes after heterotopic cardiac transplantation in the dog.

corresponding increase in backscatter of up to 12 dB (up to 400 percent).

Myocardial Inflammation

A relation between myocardial water content and echo backscattering must raise the possibility of detecting inflammation from measurements of myocardial echo amplitude. To test this hypothesis, cross-sectional echocardiograms with standardized gain settings were recorded over eight days in dogs after cardiac transplantation using a heterotopic abdominal model. Dur-

ing this period right and left ventricular myocardial pixel count increased in parallel with the severity of rejection as assessed from simultaneous ventricular biopsy (Fig. 20.1) (9). These results suggest another field of potential clinical application for ultrasonic tissue characterization.

PHASIC CHANGES IN BACKSCATTERING INTENSITY

Myocardial backscattering intensity changes during the cardiac cycle with an increase in reflected amplitude during ventricular ejection of approximately 4 to 5 dB and a corresponding increase during filling (Fig. 20.2) (10). These changes are abolished along with mechanical activity by coronary artery occlusion. From their timing they appear to be more closely related to changes in cavity volume rather than in wall tension and so are perhaps the result of changing myocardial fiber orientation. They are more obvious toward the apex than at the base of the heart and are compatible with regional variation in myocardial fiber structure. The existence of such changes makes it essential that the time during the cardiac cycle is specified for observations of myocardial acoustic properties. They might form the basis for methods of studying regional ventricular function.

TRANSMISSION OF ULTRASOUND BY TISSUES

To reach a target within the heart, ultrasound leaving the transducer must have traveled through the chest wall and the proximal tissues. The same applies to

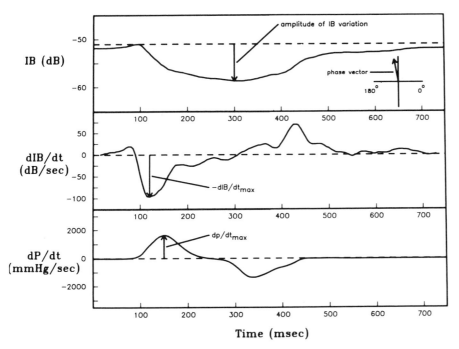

Figure 20.2. Changes in regional echo amplitude (IB) with time and its rate of change during the cardiac cycle. Note that the timing of these changes approximates those of dimension or volume. (From Wickline SA, Thomas LJ III, Miller JG, Sobel BE, Perez JE. The dependence of myocardial ultrasonic integrated backscatter on contractile performance. Circulation 1985;72: 183–192. Used with permission.)

echoes returning so that the effects of passage in both directions must be added to those of interaction with the target itself. As ultrasound passes through a homogeneous medium, it undergoes a process of attenuation, the extent of which is directly proportional to path length. This attenuation is in part the result of frictional forces between the longitudinal vibration and the medium itself, causing energy to be dissipated as heat. It is also due to scattering within the tissues or at specular reflections, so that the same processes that give rise to image generation also cause attenuation of the ultrasound reaching deeper structures. Strongly reflecting structures may intercept a significant proportion of the incident ultrasound, so that the intensity of the beam reaching those behind them is correspondingly reduced.

It is not only the amplitude of the ultrasound that changes as it passes through the tissues. Attenuation is greater at higher frequencies, which are thus selectively filtered out with increasing path length. Transmission of ultrasound by myocardium is altered in disease; in ischemic myocardium, for example, its dependence on frequency is significantly reduced (11), becoming dependent on its square rather than its cube. Interaction of ultrasound with proximal targets, particularly those within the myocardium, will distort the wave front by diffraction and interference. Even if it were possible, therefore, to define the nature of the ultrasound leaving the transducer in detail, by the time it reaches the tissues this pure signal would have been corrupted to a significant and undetermined extent. This effect is compounded by the backscattered signals arising from the tissues being further corrupted on their return to the transducer.

PROCESSING OF ULTRASOUND SIGNALS BY ECHOCARDIOGRAPHY

Echoes returning to the transducer must be processed to give rise to a useful image. These procedures are shown in Figure 20.3. They are potentially important because they further modify the information on which tissue characterization is based. Returning ultrasound leaving the tissues interacts with the transducer to give rise to an electrical output of the type shown in Figure 20.4, which is referred to as radio frequency (RF) signal. These signals are complex and depend on the overall amplitude, frequency content, and phase of the returning echo as well as on the properties of the transducer itself. In a commercial imaging apparatus, this signal is usually rectified and filtered so as to obtain its mean amplitude. Information about frequency content and phase is lost so that mean amplitude and arrival time alone are used to generate the image.

This initial step has therefore involved a considerable degree of data reduction. Even so, the range of amplitude arising from cardiac structures is very wide, spanning approximately 50 dB. It must be compressed if gray scale is to be displayed in the final image. This is normally achieved using a logarithmic amplifier whose exact characteristics will thus have a profound effect on recorded amplitude. In addition, receiver amplification is subject to depth compensation. Echoes arising from deeper structures are likely to be of lower amplitude than those arising more superficially even if the properties of the target are the same, because the path length of the ultrasound is longer and so attenuation is greater. This effect is compensated for by the use of swept gain, which makes use of the later arrival at the transducer of echoes from deeper structures in comparison with those from more superficial ones. If the gain of the transducer is rapidly increased after each pulse is released, echoes arising from deeper structures, arriving later, are subject to greater amplification and so give rise to comparable deflection on the final display. Such depth compensation is essential if a clinically useful image is to be generated, but it must be allowed for if amplitude is being measured.

The next stage is to convert the radial scan line system arising from a mechanical or phased array transducer into the standard horizontal raster using a scan converter (see Chapter 1). Because there is no one-to-one relation between individual points on these two coordinate systems, some method of interpolation must be used to fill those pixels that are not directly determined from the radial display. The exact method by which this interpolation is performed affects the distribution of amplitude across the image and its apparent texture. The image is then subject to postprocessing in which further changes are made to its subjective qualities by altering the gamma function of the system and adjusting the relative prominence given to low compared with higher amplitude signals. Partial differentiation of the image may also be performed to increase the prominence of endocardial boundaries. Such postprocessing can be implemented relatively simply, so that many options are supplied on commercially available machines whose use introduces major and unrecorded changes in the texture and amplitude distribution of the image.

The chain of events between backscattering or reflection of an ultrasonic pulse within the heart and its display on an image is thus long and complex, and underlying mechanisms are not well understood. Although some of these factors still cannot be controlled, others, particularly those related to machine design, could readily be standardized. In spite of this, ultrasonic apparatus is rarely calibrated, nor is its transfer function determined, although such steps would be

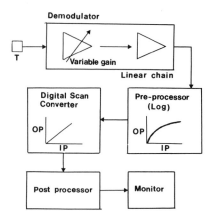

Figure 20.3. Block diagram showing image processing by a typical echocardiograph in clinical use. T = target; IP = input; OP = output.

regarded as routine in other branches of experimental physics.

CLINICAL TISSUE CHARACTERIZATION BASED ON ECHO AMPLITUDE

If quantification of characteristics of returning echoes is indeed the basis of tissue characterization, then assessment of regional amplitude might appear to be a promising approach. A number of observations in humans support this idea. Increased echo amplitude from calcium, particularly in valves, has frequently been documented. Some years ago, an increase in the amplitude of septal echoes with scarring was noted on M mode (12). Before these subjective observations can be converted into quantitative or semiquantitative estimates of echo intensity, the receive gain of the echocardiograph must be standardized.

In clinical use this variable is arbitrarily controlled by the operator to give optimal image quality. It is not an adequate criterion for absolute determinations because it lacks objectivity and is likely to depend

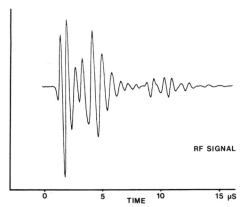

Figure 20.4. Recording of radio frequency (RF) signal from the transducer of a mechanical Advanced Technology Laboratories (ATL) sector scanner in the receive mode.

directly on the amplitude of the returning ultrasound itself. Alternatively, gain could be preset to some standard level, but this would be impractical in view of the well-known differences between patients in the settings required to obtain images of diagnostic quality. The exact basis of these differences is not clearly known, but they are due in part to energy loss across the chest wall, the presence or absence of lung disease, and path length within the thorax. One compromise has been to use the posterior pericardial echo as an internal standard (13). The constitution of pericardium is similar from patient to patient; it is approximately 50 percent collagen. Use of the pericardial echo in this way compensates for losses in the chest wall and variation in path length.

Other structures within the mediastinum such as aortic root or even material introduced surgically might be available in postoperative patients. In this way the upper end of the amplitude scale can be fixed. It cannot be assumed that zero deflection on the final record corresponds to zero echo amplitude unless the performance of the instrument has been specifically checked. If this assumption cannot be made, one possible standard is to use the amplitude of echoes from blood within the left ventricular cavity. Echo amplitude across the image will be materially affected by the depth compensation. It may be possible to dispense with this altogether, but this usually cannot be done without sacrificing image quality. A compromise has been to adopt a standardized linear setting, so that the initial echoes at the anterior part of the display are also set just to the highest gray scale level. An alternative but more complex method would be to adopt a "smart" display, so that gain settings are allowed for when measurements of regional intensity are made.

None of these approaches allows for the complex nature of the interaction between the ultrasound and proximal tissue. Greater proximal backscattering causes greater attenuation of the transmitted signal in both directions and hence a corresponding decrease in the amplitude of echoes returning from deeper targets. This effect must also be allowed for if gain settings are to be standardized completely. Such a procedure would be complex because the pattern of attenuation can potentially vary along each of the 100 or more lines making up the standard two-dimensional frame. One approach, termed rational gain compensation, has been to identify boundaries between blood and myocardium along each line of sight and, knowing the corresponding attenuation coefficients determined in vitro, to vary gain accordingly (14). In formalin-fixed hearts, this approach allows some improvement in the detection of small areas of scar tissue. Yet it still fails to correct for the effects of proximal tissue with abnormal acoustic properties, such as when posterior wall amplitude must be measured in the presence of an abnormally reflecting septum.

Although a qualitative estimate of regional echo amplitude can be gained from direct inspection of a gray scale display, a more satisfactory method is required if any quantification is to be achieved. Up to 256 gray scale levels are available on current equipment, yet the eye cannot distinguish more than a dozen, particularly at the brighter levels. Perception of gray scale levels depends not only on the absolute level, but also on the rate of amplitude change across the display. If this psychologic effect is not taken into account, major errors in interpretation can occur.

One method of avoiding these problems, suggested by Tanaka and Terasawa (13), is to record a series of images starting with high attenuation and increasing gain in a stepwise manner. The amplitude of any structure can thus be estimated from the gain setting of the image in which it first appears. Color has also been used, because it can be appreciated more easily than gray scale levels (except by color-blind individuals), it is not subject to the psychologic problems besetting gray scale interpretation, and a wider dynamic range is possible on both a screen and hard copy. Simple conversion of gray scale to color degrades the image, and it appears preferable to use a system of encoding such that gray scale and color can be combined. This system runs in real time, and it has proved useful in allowing instrument gain settings to be standardized at the time the recording is taken (15). Color substitution has been used to detect the effects of experimental myocardial infarction in dogs (16) and color-amplitude encoding to detect ventricular disease in humans (15).

These approaches allow semiquantitative estimates of regional amplitude to be made. However, even with such systems, problems remain. There is considerable variation between the amplitude of neighboring pixels representing a single structure in the display. This variation may result in part from real heterogeneities within the target caused by, for example, patchy fibrosis or infiltration. Superimposed on these, however, are the effects of speckle and interlacing and infilling from the scan converter, whose overall effects may be greater than those of any biologic variation. Again, a number of approaches are possible. The distribution of gray scale values can be described in relation to anatomic features such as the endocardial or epicardial surface of the venticle or the distribution of any apparent abnormalities of texture described. Alternatively, an area of interest can be identified, and a histogram of pixel intensity within it constructed so that median values can be calculated (Fig. 20.5, Plate IX). Provided that the area of interest is of a size comparable to that of the resolution cell, such median values will be relatively unaffected by speckle or other machine-dependent variables. Attempts to quantify the scatter of pixel gray scale levels or their spatial distribution fall into the category of texture analysis and are described later.

TISSUE CHARACTERIZATION IN HUMANS

The methods described previously, particularly those based on a subjective appreciation of changes in regional myocardial echo amplitude, have been applied to the diagnosis of heart muscle disease in humans. A "granular sparkling" of the myocardium in 12 of 13 cardiac amyloid disease patients has been described (17). In six patients these hyper-refractile areas were generalized throughout the myocardium, and in six they were localized to either the septum or the posterior wall. These changes were not apparent on M mode. Similar observations were made by Bhadari and Nanda (18), who described in four patients multiple discrete hyper-refractile areas within the myocardium whose distribution was either generalized or localized. In contrast, Hind and associates (19), in their study of eight patients, using color-amplitude encoding with a calibrated echocardiograph, found an abnormal increase in myocardial echo intensity in only a minority. Similarly, Chandrasekaran and colleagues (20), using more formal texture analysis, were unable to detect any significant abnormality between normal subjects and patients with amyloid disease, either in terms of amplitude or run-length nonuniformity because of considerable scatter of values in the group with amyloid disease. The cause of these discrepancies is not clear. In all groups myocardial thickness was greatly increased and characteristic M-mode appearances obtained. It is possible that the discrepancy might relate to heterogeneity between cases in the nature of the involvement by amyloid, possibly dependent on whether patients were identified from cardiac symptoms or other manifestations of paraproteinemia.

Abnormalities in myocardial echo amplitude have also been identified in patients with hypertrophic cardiomyopathy. These were described by Martin and co-workers (21) using phased array equipment. They noted that two layers could characteristically be identified within the septum, the thicker on the left ventricular sides. The latter was found to have multiple speckled echoes of higher amplitude within it, giving the myocardium a characteristic ground glass appearance. Transitional areas and the remainder of the myocardium were normal. Tanaka and associates (22) also noted high-amplitude echoes within the myocardium in patients with hypertrophic cardiomyopathy but were unable to confirm their strict localization to the left side of the intraventricular septum. These echoes were described as irregular in distribution and of large or medium amplitude. Using stepwise gain changes, Tanaka and colleagues identified their amplitude as having a mean value of approximately 15 dB above that of normal myocardium, although there was considerable scatter between cases. Bhandari and Nanda (18) observed discrete highly refractile areas, localized to part of the myocardium in 18 cases of hypertrophic cardiomyopathy, whereas in 7 myocardial echo intensity was normal. In a more general study of left ventricular hypertrophy, Shapiro and associates (23) noted septal myocardial echo intensity to be significantly increased by an average of 5 dB in 16 patients with hypertrophic cardiomyopathy in comparison with normal subjects. Smaller increases were present in the posterior wall. Although these changes were not seen in athletes with physiologic left ventricular hypertrophy, virtually identical changes occurred in patients with fixed left ventricular outflow obstruction (Fig. 20.6, Plate IX), and to a lesser extent in those with hypertension. The presence of increased myocardial echo intensity was found to correlate strongly with abnormal diastolic function, including prolongation of isovolumetric relaxation time and a reduced rate of dimension increase during filling and also with the presence of T-wave changes on the electrocardiogram characteristic of "left ventricular strain." An increase in left ventricular myocardial echo intensity appeared characteristic of pathologic left ventricular hypertrophy of any cause and not specific for hypertrophic cardiomyopathy.

Coronary artery disease is another common condition characterized by abnormalities of regional echo amplitude. Such changes were originally reported on the basis of the M-mode echocardiogram by Rasmussen and co-workers (12) and have frequently been observed on two-dimensional echocardiography, particularly following septal infarction. They may also involve the posterior wall, particularly in the subendocardial region, and the papillary muscles, when their presence often correlates with a systolic murmur and Doppler evidence of mitral regurgitation (Fig. 20.7, Plate IX) (18, 24, 25). Less common conditions in which an increase in myocardial echo intensity has been observed include Pompe's disease, hemochromatosis, chronic renal failure, endocardial fibroelastosis, endomyocardial fibrosis, and eosinophilic heart disease (Fig. 20.8, Plate IX) (18, 26, 27).

From these clinical correlations, it would seem likely that fibrosis is an important cause of increased myocardial echo intensity in humans, as would be predicted from experimental work. Direct evidence for this contention was obtained by Tanaka and associates (22), who, in cases of cardiomyopathy, correlated echocardiograms with autopsy findings and demon-

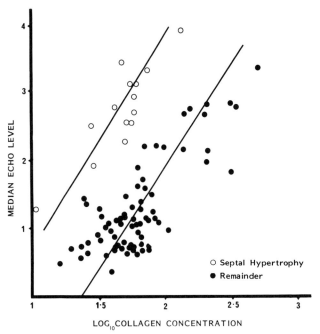

Figure 20.9. Relation between regional echo amplitude determined during life and local collagen concentration for septum and posterior left ventricular wall. (From Shaw TRD, Logan-Sinclair RB, Surin C, et al. Relation between regional echo intensity and myocardial connective tissue in chronic left ventricular disease. Br Heart J 1984;51:46–53. Used with permission.)

strated a strong association with myocardial fibrosis and degeneration, particularly at the boundary between normal and abnormal regions. Similar correlations between fibrosis and postmortem echocardiography in 36 cases were found Bhandari and colleagues (18). In a quantitative comparison between myocardial echo intensity derived from echocardiograms recorded within a week of death and autopsy material, Shaw and associates (24) found a correlation with myocardial echo intensity in a series of 20 patients with chronic left ventricular disease. The correlation with fibrosis detected histologically was weak, but the correlation with tissue hydroxyproline concentration was significantly better; it was 0.76 for posterior wall and papillary muscle and 0.86 for the septum. Doubling of the collagen content caused an increase in reflected amplitude of approximately 6.5 dB over the range of abnormalities studied (Fig. 20.9).

It seems likely that there are other clinically important causes of abnormal myocardial echo intensity in humans. Werner and co-workers (28) briefly recorded the appearance of sonolucent regions appearing in the septum in elderly patients with massive infarction. These observations have yet to be confirmed, because other authors noted no significant change in acute myocardial infarct patients (18). The possibility that myocardial inflammation is also a significant cause of increased myocardial echo intensity should be considered. Preliminary observations in humans have shown significant changes during episodes of acute rejection following heart transplantation, and transient increases associated with eosinophilic heart disease, acute rheumatic fever, and infective endocarditis have also been recorded.

TEXTURE ANALYSIS

Texture analysis is a means of extracting more information from the image than simple mean values of gray scale. Echocardiographic images are presented as arrays of units 256 × 256 on the screen; each unit is referred to as a pixel or single picture unit. Each pixel is recorded in one of a number of shades of gray, usually 64 on modern machines. Ultrasonic images have a characteristic granular or mottled texture. This appearance is determined in part by the characteristics of the targets within the structure being examined. The main factor determining image texture, however, is termed speckle after its equivalent optical phenomenon. Speckle arises directly from the use of coherent radiation for imaging when the targets are too small to be demonstrated separately. When the number of targets within the resolution cell is large, the pattern is referred to as "fully developed speckle." Its mean and modal amplitude values are determined by the strength of the scattering, but other features are largely independent of the target and are determined instead by the properties of the transducer and the instrument; such features include gray level probabilities and speckle cell size. The nature of the speckle varies over the image. When a phantom containing scatterers of uniform properties and distribution is used, the pattern changes from sharply granular close to the midfield in the region near the transducer to a smoother, coalescent appearance toward the periphery both in depth and laterally (azimuthally) (29). Speckle is thus a major feature determining the final texture of ultrasonic images, and its presence must be taken into account in any attempt at clinical texture analysis. In addition, its presence degrades resolution and interferes with appreciation of fine details of gray scale.

One approach to textural analysis has been to describe the scatter of gray scale values around the mean value as well as the mean itself. This can be done statistically by calculating skewness and kurtosis, a measure of the "peakedness" of the distribution. Decreased kurtosis implies that the distribution curve of gray scale values is broadened, indicating the presence of greater heterogeneity of values within the area sampled. This approach was effective in detecting regional abnormalities two days after experimental

myocardial infarction in dogs (30). Although there was also some increase in amplitude, it was not significant under the conditions of the experiment; neither did the skewness of the distribution change significantly. Our own experience has been consonant with this. An increase in regional amplitude occurring within the myocardium in humans is nearly always accompanied by increased spread of gray scale values. Documenting the spread has the advantage that absolute standardization is not required, and indeed Skorton and associates (30) were able to retrieve the information from Polaroid films.

More complex methods may also be used to detect this increased heterogeneity of gray scale values occurring in disease, and a number of algorithms have been developed, some of which are based on differences in gray scale levels between pixels separated on the image by predetermined amounts and in specified directions. Run length, the number of adjacent pixels with gray scale values within a specified range, can also be used in this way. These methods have been used to detect experimental myocardial contusion in dogs (31). Preliminary reports suggest that the method will detect abnormalities of the septum in patients with hypertrophic cardiomyopathy, although it may fail to detect significant change in those with myocardial amyloid (21).

A similar increase in gray scale values can be detected from direct observation of the RF signal. This approach avoids information loss associated with processing by the echocardiograph. Schnittger and colleagues (32) studied the effects of acute ischemia on the left ventricular myocardium of dogs as reflected in changes in the amplitude domain. A statistical approach was used based on the ratio of mean amplitude to standard deviation. This ratio increased by approximately 25 percent within one hour of the onset of ischemia. These results were achieved without absolute calibration of the equipment.

These results quantify the subjective observation that a regional increase in echo intensity occurring within the myocardium is seldom uniform; rather, close examination of the image indicates that an increase in the average value within a region is due to the appearance of a relatively small number of brighter pixels. The extent to which such observations on the image correlate with changes in the structure of the myocardium itself is far from clear because of the superimposition of the machine-dependent component of speckle. Future progress seems likely only when this component can be recognized and removed from the image. Promising approaches are already being developed in this direction. The pattern of fully developed speckle can often be identified from local features of the image and described in statistical terms, such as the ratio of local variance to local mean. Filtering the image in this way leads to substantial reduction of speckle with preservation of biologic features and enhanced recognition of small discrete changes (33). This is a field that is likely to develop rapidly in the future.

PROBLEMS IN CLINICAL TISSUE CHARACTERIZATION

Clinical echocardiographic tissue characterization is a relatively new field of investigation, and many problems remain to be solved. It has already become apparent that estimates of even simple variables such as myocardial amplitude have relatively poor reproducibility. These are due in part to machine gain, patient orientation, and path length. Even when determinations are compared in which these variables are fixed, however, considerable variation persists; the standard deviation between duplicate determinations is approximately 25 to 30 percent of the mean value for normal myocardium. Other uncontrolled factors must include motion of the heart with the cardiac cycle or respiration. Minor variation in the position of the transducer can lead to failure to sample identical regions of myocardium.

A second set of problems arise when it becomes necessary to define tissue abnormalities unambiguously. At first sight, it would appear that fibrosis of the myocardium is a clearly defined entity, but it has become apparent that wide differences exist between histologic and biochemical estimates. If such difficulties arise with fibrosis, the possibilities for uncertainty in defining entities such as ischemia or infarct size are obviously considerable. It may well transpire that the abnormalities delineated by ultrasound, which depend mainly on the mechanical properties of the tissue and the spatial distribution of the scatters within it, will never correlate precisely with those identified by tinctorial, physiologic, or biochemical methods.

In spite of these problems, considerable progress has already been made in this difficult field from a combination of theoretical, experimental, and clinical approaches. One factor favoring success has probably been the large difference in physical properties between normal myocardium and collagen, which allows significant results to be obtained even in the absence of rigorous quantification. Future progress will require action in a number of directions. Methods of standardization of echocardiographic equipment will be necessary both to increase the precision of measurement and to improve agreement between observations made in different centers. More precise quantification will lead to more exact echo characterization and will thereby enhance understanding of the processes un-

derlying image generation within the tissues. Finally, more extensive clinical correlations may lead to the definition of new and unexplored fields where the technique does more than simply reproduce the results of other, older established ones but uniquely increases knowledge of the natural history of disease and expands the possibilities of improved patient care.

BIBLIOGRAPHY

Chivers RC. Tissue characterization. Ultrasound Med Biol 1980;7:1–20.

Hill CR. Tissue characterization. In: Kurjak A, ed. Progress in medical ultrasound, vol 1. Amsterdam: Excerpta Medica, 1980;11–18.

Miller JG, Perez JE, Sobel BE. Ultrasonic characterization of myocardium. Prog Cardiovasc Dis 1985;28:85–110.

Skorton DJ, Collins SM. Digital computer image analysis in echocardiography. Echocardiography 1984;1:15–43.

REFERENCES

1. Chivers RC. Some scientific and technical aspects of medical ultrasonics. J Med Eng Technol 1981;5:128–133.
2. Nicholas D, Nicholas AW, Greenbaum R. An ultrasonic determination of cardiac muscle structure. Acous Imag 1982;11:95–107.
3. Fields S, Dunn F. Correlation of echocardiographic visibility of tissue with biological composition and physiological state. J Acoust Soc Am 1973;54:809–812.
4. O'Donnell M, Mimbs JW, Miller JG. Relationship between collagen and ultrasonic backscatter in myocardial tissue. J Acoust Soc Am 1981;69:580–588.
5. Mimbs JW, O'Donnell M, Miller JG, Sobel BE. Detection of cardiomyopathic changes induced by doxorubicin based on quantitative analysis of ultrasonic backscatter. Am J Cardiol 1981;47:1056–1060.
6. Perez JE, Barzilai B, Madaras EI, et al. Applicability of ultrasonic tissue characterization for longitudinal assessment and differentiation of calcification and fibrosis in cardiomyopathy. J Am Coll Cardiol 1984;4:88–95.
7. Yuhas DE, Kessler LW. Acoustic microscopic analysis of myocardium. National Bureau of Standards Spec Pub 525, Washington, DC, 1979;73–79.
8. Mimbs JW, Bauwens D, Cohen RD, O'Donnell M, Miller JG, Sobel BE. Effects of myocardial ischemia on quantitative ultrasonic backscatter and identification of responsible determinants. Circ Res 1981;49:89–96.
9. Dawkins KD, Haverich A, Aziz S, Billingham M, Jamieson SW, Gibson DG. Detection of acute cardiac rejection using color echocardiography. Circulation 1985;72:III-207.
10. Wickline SA, Thomas LJ III, Miller JG, Sobel BE, Perez JE. The dependence of myocardial ultrasonic integrated backscatter on contractile performance. Circulation 1985;72:183–192.
11. Mimbs JW, Yuhas DE, Miller JG, Weiss AN, Sobel BE. Detection of myocardial infarction in vitro based on altered attenuation of ultrasound. Circ Res 1977;41:192–198.
12. Rasmussen S, Corya BC, Feigenbaum H, Knoebel SB. Detection of myocardial scar tissue by M-mode echocardiography. Circulation 1978;57:230–237.
13. Tanaka M, Terasawa H. Echocardiography: evaluation of tissue character in myocardium. Jpn Heart J 1979;43:367–376.
14. Melton HE, Skorton DJ. Rational gain compensation for attenuation in cardiac ultrasonography. Ultrason Imag 1983;5:214–228.
15. Logan-Sinclair RB, Wong CM, Gibson DG. Clinical application of amplitude processing of echocardiographic images. Br Heart J 1981;45:621–627.
16. Parisi AF, Nieminen M, O'Boyle JE, et al. Enhanced detection of the evolution of tissue changes after acute myocardial infarction using color-encoded two-dimensional echocardiography. Circulation 1982;44:764–770.

17. Sequiera-Filho AG, Cunha CLP, Tajik AJ, Seward JB, Schattenberg IT, Guiliani ER. M-mode and two dimensional echocardiographic features in cardiac amyloidosis. Circulation 1981;63:188–196.
18. Bhandari AK, Nanda NC. Myocardial texture characterization by two-dimensional echocardiography. Am J Cardiol 1983;51:817–825.
19. Hind CRK, Gibson DG, Lavender JP, Pepys MB. Non-invasive demonstration of cardiac involvement in acquired forms of systemic amyloidosis. Lancet 1984;2:1417.
20. Chandrasekaran K, Aylward PE, Collins SM, et al. Quantitative echocardiographic texture analysis can identify cardiomyopathy in humans. Circulation 1985;72:III-207.
21. Martin RP, Rakowski H, French J, Popp RL. Idiopathic hypertrophic subaortic stenosis viewed by wide-angle phased array echocardiography. Circulation 1979;59:1206–1217.
22. Tanaka M, Nitta S, Sogo Y, et al. Non-invasive estimation by cross sectional echocardiography of myocardial damage in cardiomyopathy. Br Heart J 1985;53:137–152.
23. Shapiro LM, Moore RB, Logan-Sinclair RB, Gibson DG. Relation of regional echo amplitude to left ventricular function and the electrocardiogram in left ventricular hypertrophy. Br Heart J 1984;52:99–105.
24. Shaw TRD, Logan-Sinclair RB, Surin C, et al. Relation between regional echo intensity and myocardial connective tissue in chronic left ventricular disease. Br Heart J 1984;51:46–53.
25. Hikichi H, Tanaka M. Ultrasonotomographic evaluation of histological changes in myocardial infarction. Jpn Heart J 1981;22:287–297.
26. Davies J, Gibson DG, Foale R, et al. Echocardiographic features of eosinophilic endomyocardial disease. Br Heart J 1982;48:434–440.
27. Vijayaraghavan G, Davies J, Sadanandan S, Spry CJF, Gibson DG, Goodwin JF. Echocardiographic features of tropical endomyocardial disease in South India. Br Heart J 1983;50:450–459.
28. Werner JA, Pearlman AS, Janko C. Pathophysiologic implications of a new echocardiographic finding in acute myocardial infarction (abstract). Proceedings of the Eighth European Congress of Cardiology. 1980;76.
29. Skorton DJ, Collins SM, Woskoff SD, Bean JA, Melton HE. Range and azimuth dependent variability of image texture in two-dimensional echocardiograms. Circulation 1983;68:834–840.
30. Skorton DJ, Melton HE Jr, Pandian NG, et al. Detection of acute myocardial infarction in closed-chest dogs by analysis of regional two-dimensional echocardiographic gray-scale levels. Circ Res 1983;52:36–44.
31. Skorton DJ, Collins SM, Nichols J, et al. Quantitative texture analysis in two-dimensional echocardiography: application to the diagnosis of experimental myocardial contusion. Circulation 1983;68:217–223.
32. Schnittger I, Vieli A, Heiserman JE, et al. Ultrasonic tissue characterization: detection of acute myocardial ischemia in dogs. Circulation 1985;72:193–199.
33. Bamber JC, Daft C. Adaptive filtering for reduction of speckle in ultrasonic pulse-echo images. Ultrasonics 1986;5:41–44.

II
Doppler Echocardiography in Congenital Heart Disease

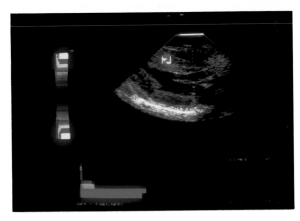

Figure 20.5. Assessment of regional echo amplitude by construction of histogram of pixel intensities. The area of interest is located in the septum, and the histogram is positioned horizontally below the echocardiographic image. The sequence of colors used to display amplitude is shown on the left. Cyan corresponds to the lowest amplitude and white to the highest.

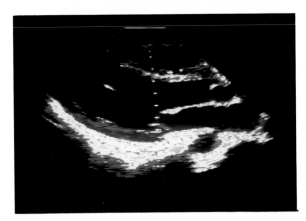

Figure 20.6. Regional echo amplitude in a normal subject. Note that myocardial echo amplitude is low (cyan or green) in both the septum and posterior wall. (From Logan-Sinclair RB, Wong CM, Gibson DG. Clinical application of amplitude processing of echocardiographic images. Br Heart J 1981;45:621–627. Used with permission.)

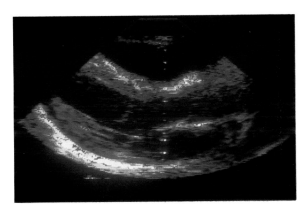

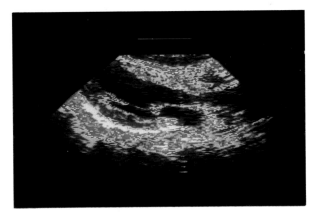

Figure 20.7. (*A*) Parasternal long-axis echocardiogram from an athlete. Note that in spite of increased wall thickness, echo amplitude is normal. (*B*) Parasternal long-axis echocardiogram from a patient with fixed subaortic stenosis. Note that there is a striking increase in myocardial echo amplitude in both septum and posterior wall.

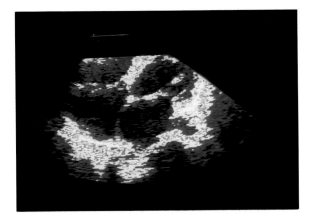

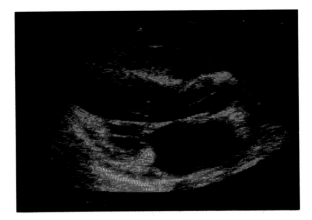

Figure 20.8. (*A*) Echocardiogram, apical four-chamber view, from a patient with coronary artery disease. Note that myocardial echo amplitude is greatly increased, particularly in the septum where values similar to those of pericardium are present. Amplitude is also increased in the papillary muscles and in the subendocardial region of the free wall. (*B*) Echocardiogram, long-axis parasternal view, of the left ventricle from a patient with eosinophilic heart disease. Note the striking increase in echo intensity in the posterior wall and at the bases of the papillary muscles. The posterior mitral valve cusp is also abnormal. (From Davies J, Gibson DG, Foale R, et al. Echocardiographic features of eosinophilic endomyocardial disease. Br Heart J 1982;48:434–440. Used with permission.)

Plate IX

21
Pediatric Doppler Echocardiography

Michael Gewitz

The advent of Doppler echocardiography for pediatric cardiovascular applications has provided a significant advance in the bedside evaluation of congenital heart disease and in the serial noninvasive assessment of cardiovascular physiology in the infant and child. While extensive review of Doppler physics and the history of Doppler echocardiography have been provided in Chapter 1 and 2, some specific comments are appropriate with regard to pediatric uses. This chapter reviews technologic differences between the application of Doppler principles in pediatric patients and that in adults. In addition, examples that demonstrate the practicality of the method are reviewed. Table 21.1 outlines the current variety of situations where Doppler flow analysis adds particularly important information in pediatric cardiology. Also, references to the current application of color flow mapping, a new application of Doppler principles, is discussed. Normal pediatric Doppler values are given in Table 21.2.

DOPPLER PHYSICS: PEDIATRIC APPLICATION

For pediatric purposes, pulsed Doppler systems have achieved foremost usage, although this form of Doppler analysis was not the earliest employed for clinical study. The main advantage of pulsed Doppler is that it enables the performance of precise interrogation of small anatomic areas at a variety of depths ('range gating'). Range gating is usually adjusted over a depth of 2 to 20 mm, which includes most of the anterior cardiac structures in the pediatric population. Using this technique, the specific locus of interrogation (the sample volume) can be varied by the operator. The advent of duplex technology, enabling simultaneous cross-sectional imaging and Doppler study, has al-

lowed specific localization of the sample volume along the range gate within the desired cardiovascular location (Fig. 21.1). It is this marriage of techniques that has found the broadest pediatric application. However, there are significant limitations in the pulsed Doppler approach. The technique depends on the relationship between the frequency of pulse repetition and the depth of the sample volume, the range-velocity product, which in turn is affected by the angle of intercept employed. These factors result in velocity resolution inversely proportional to the frequency of interrogation at a given depth. Unfortunately, in many pediatric situations, maximal near-field image quality requires use of high-frequency transducers (e.g., 5.0 or 7.5 MHz). At these high frequencies the combination of cross-sectional and pulsed Doppler systems may not successfully resolve the severity of stenotic or regurgitant flow patterns present in many pathologic conditions due to "aliasing."

When such velocity limits are reached, the continuous wave Doppler format is required to assess the severity. While this system allows for high-velocity analysis, depth selection by range gating is not possible. Continuous wave Doppler is thereby limited because of the inherent lack of certainty in sample volume placement, and requires a high degree of both operator experience and patient cooperation to overcome these potential problems.

The development of high pulse rate frequency (PRF) Doppler has provided an intermediate ground between continuous wave and pulsed Doppler modes. This technique employs multiple range-gate sampling at fixed intervals, allowing specific selection of information from known depths while also allowing measurement of velocities of greater magnitude than standard pulsed Doppler.

Table 21.1. Clinical Utility of Doppler Echocardiography in Pediatrics

Assessment of cardiac performance
    Congenital or acquired impaired cardiac output: myocarditis, cardiomyopathy, toxic myocardial depression, perinatal asphyxia,
        arrhythmia management
Pressure gradient evaluation
    Arterial valve stenoses
    Vascular obstructive lesions: branch pulmonary stenoses, inferior vena caval thromboses; vena caval obstruction post-Mustard
        operation
Shunt magnitude and shunt direction
    Left-to-right flow: ASD, VSD, PAD
    Right-to-left flow: ASD with pulmonary hypertension
    ASD flow in congenital AV valve atresia
Valvar regurgitation
    AV valve insufficiency in postnatal asphyxia
    Arterial valve regurgitation in common arterial trunks
Postoperative states
    Analysis of postoperative murmurs: residual VSD vs AV regurgitation, acquired arterial valve regurgitation
    Patency of surgical shunts
    Postoperative myocardial performance

ASD = atrial septal defect; AV = atrioventricular; PAD = patent arterial duct; VSD = ventricular septal defect.

A review of problems frequently encountered by the operator in pediatric patients is necessary. As previously mentioned, velocity analysis is limited in pulsed Doppler, the most widely used format. This problem is usually manifested as aliasing, which develops when the flow velocity that is being measured exceeds the capability of the transducer frequency to sample at a given depth or Nyquist limit. (For any given system, the Nyquist limit is determined by one-half the pulse repetition frequency.) When aliasing occurs, the peak velocity appears to reverse orientation (Fig. 21.2A). Care must be taken not to misinterpret this finding. A means of correction for aliasing involves resetting the zero. Some equipment enables the zero to be placed at the extremes of graphic ranges, allowing for increasing the range of velocity analysis and omitting either positive or negative values with respect to the zero line (Fig. 21.2B). Alternatively, the operator can change the intercept angle in order to facilitate high-velocity measurement, but this is not recommended.

Color Doppler (CD) flow mapping has recently come to the fore as a useful methodology in pediatric echocardiography. CD flow maps can clearly demonstrate intracardiac shunting patterns, and enhance the operator's ability to identify shunts of even relatively small

magnitude. This can be an important adjunct to clinical examination. For example, in the presence of a small ventricular septal defect, standard two-dimensional imaging may not clarify the source of a cardiac murmur and the overall flow velocity profile on pulsed wave Doppler may not be greatly disturbed. The flow pattern identified with color Doppler mapping, however, can often pinpoint the cardiac anomaly (Fig. 21.3, Plate X) and delineate the presence of multiple defects as well.

The physical principles of CD flow mapping involve multigating the pulsed Doppler data to display not only the origin but also the direction and the quality of blood flows in the heart while superimposing this information on a cross-sectional real-time image. This eliminates the "blinded" approach required in standard Doppler examinations, improving accuracy and reducing the time required for an examination. Specifics of instruments and physical properties have been reviewed in Chapters 1 and 2. The standard directional conventions of blue and red colors as they relate to flow direction relative to the transducer are the same, and the turbulence-related color modifications (green or white) noted previously also apply in pediatric color Doppler flow mapping.

CLINICAL APPLICATIONS

Ventricular Septal Defect

There are several ways for the investigator to evaluate the presence of a ventricular septal defect and to quantify its significance. The demonstration of flow disturbances along the interventricular septum has been shown to be relatively reliable for evaluating most defects, independent of size or location (1–4). It should be remembered that defects occur at numerous sites, with different physiologic considerations related to the site of the defect. Thus, the ultrasonographer must be complete in his or her evaluation and aware of possible

Table 21.2. Normal Pediatric Doppler Values

Site	Maximal velocity (mean)	Range (cm/s)
Main pulmonary artery	76	50–105
Ascending aorta	91	60–145
Descending aorta	97	55–150
Interatrial septum	18	15–30
Tricuspid valve (RV inflow)	62	40–80
Mitral valve (LV inflow)	80	50–115
Superior vena cava	50	25–75

LV = left ventricular; RV = right ventricular.
Data derived from a compendium of sources as referenced in text.

associated anatomic anomalies before reaching a conclusion (Fig. 21.4). In addition to flow analysis at the level of ventricular septum, it is possible to determine Qp/Qs ratios. Flow disturbance in the pulmonary trunk can also be assessed, especially with doubly committed defects.

Interrogation Along the Interventricular Septum

By starting analysis of flow patterns along the right ventricular side of the interventricular septum with the parasternal long-axis approach, most left-to-right shunts at ventricular level can be detected. The diffuse, harsh flow quality, as noted by Stevenson et al. (1), can be identified acoustically and precise localization achieved as the sample volume is moved along the septal surface and a recording of flow is obtained (Figs. 21.5 and 21.6).

A few specific problems exist with this approach. First, it may be difficult to distinguish flow disturbances caused by the defect from those associated with anatomic abnormalities in the right ventricle itself. Muscle bundles or subpulmonary obstruction may cause nonlaminar flow in the right ventricle. Duplex imaging is helpful to identify this source of misinterpretation. Alignment of the Doppler beam perpendicular to flow may be difficult, particularly with defects in the muscular septum, and alternative views are then necessary. When apical defects are present, for example, a subcostal four-chamber view may be necessary. Utilization of this Doppler technique depends on the presence of a pressure gradient favoring left-to-right flow. In hearts with equal ventricular pressures or with associated lesions causing suprasystemic right ventricular pressure, this type of flow analysis may not result in detection of the defect. This may also be true if left ventricular performance is reduced. Simultaneous cross-sectional echocardiography greatly aids in these circumstances. Finally, the presence of multiple defects may go unrecognized since distinction of flow disturbances at closely related sites may be exceedingly difficult.

Quantitative Assessment of Shunting

Several reports have verified the utility of estimating Qp/Qs by Doppler (5–9). This requires velocimetry of flow in both the pulmonary trunk and aorta, which may prove difficult. While reports of the accuracy and reproducibility of this technique have been published, important constraints must be considered. For example, inaccuracies may arise from difficulties in measurement of vessel lumen size, especially in infants and neonates in whom the pulmonary trunk and aorta are small. Thus, estimates of vessel cross-sectional area

will be further confounded by small errors in diameter measurements. Associated lesions may also play a role as a source of error. Frequently, a ventricular septal defect is associated with pulmonary stenosis, and in these patients, Qp cannot be accurately assessed from the pulmonary trunk. It may be necessary to assess Qp by assuming it to be equal to mitral valve flow (QMV), thus introducing all of the inherent problems with assessing blood flow across the atrioventricular valve (10, 11). With left ventricular outflow obstruction, on the other hand, tricuspid valve flow (QTV) may be the only means of computing systemic flow (Qs) by Doppler.

Color Doppler flow mapping may be especially helpful in the recognition of ventricular septal defect (12, 13). Direction of flow can be clearly assessed with this technique when discrimination of such lesions is not resolvable by conventional pulsed or continuous wave techniques (Fig. 21.7, Plate X).

In summary, Doppler assessment of ventricular septal defects is useful in identifying the presence of a lesion, localizing the lesion, and quantitating its significance. Color flow mapping can further enhance the specificity of Doppler diagnosis.

Atrial Septal Defect

Atrial septal defect is another commonly occurring left-to-right shunt lesion in the pediatric population whose evaluation has been facilitated by Doppler analysis. Standard ultrasonic imaging techniques may result in artifactual echo dropout of part of the interatrial septum, particularly in the region of the oval fossa, and may thus yield false-positive diagnoses. Some interatrial communications, such as sinus venosus defects, may be difficult to detect, and false-negative diagnoses may result. Doppler examination helps to confirm the presence of abnormal flow between the atrial chambers and helps to estimate the magnitude of that flow. Furthermore, interrogation of other areas aids the operator in excluding other causes of right ventricular volume overload (Table 21.3).

Qualitative Assessment

As in a ventricular septal defect, an approach has been reported to assess flow along the interatrial septum by demonstrating disturbed flow across it (14, 15). A subcostal four-chamber view and, more recently, the second right intercostal space from the parasternal region are best suited for this procedure, and analysis can determine the direction of flow and the site of the defect between the atrial chambers.

Even with defects well visualized echocardiographically, such as ostium primum atrioventricular septal

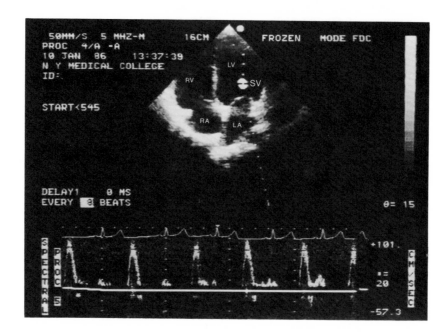

A

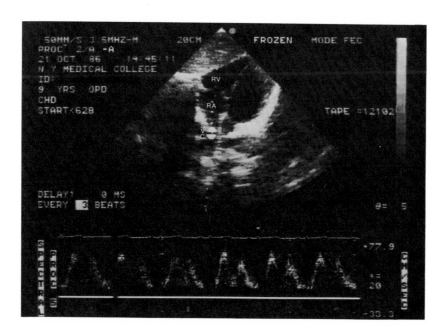

B

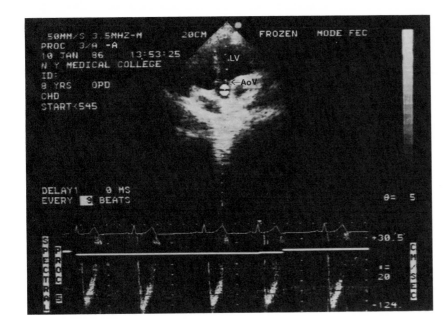

C

Figure 21.1. Typical placements of sample volume using duplex ultrasonic imaging. (*A*) Sample volume assess flow at left ventricular (LV) inflow below the mitral valve. (*B*) Sample volume in superior vena cava (SVC) viewed via subcostal cross-sectional imaging. (*C*) LV outflow tract flow. Sample volume placed just distal to aortic valve (Ao) imaged via apical long-axis view (five-chamber view). LA = left atrium; RA = right atrium; RV = right ventricle; SV = sample volume.

defects, the information Doppler provides can be helpful in determining the primary direction of flow, left to right or right to left. By contrast, when defects are difficult to visualize, Doppler interrogation may prove extremely helpful in identifying the defect. Scrutiny of the entry of the superior caval vein into the right atrium with Doppler, can suggest the presence of a sinus venosus defect which is not visualized echocardiographically.

Determination of the direction of flow across an interatrial communication can be particularly helpful in certain instances. Demonstration of right-to-left flow at atrial level can help to confirm the diagnosis of persistent neonatal pulmonary hypertension syndrome (persistent fetal circulation syndrome) in which there is an obligatory right-to-left shunt at atrial level. Other congenital abnormalities, such as total anomolous pulmonary venous connection, which must have a right-to-left shunt at atrial level, can present with right-to-left shunting at ductal level and elevated pulmonary pressures. This diagnosis can be excluded if right-to-left shunting at atrial level is not present.

Quantitative Assessment

Quantitation of Qp/Qs has been reported to be more reliable in atrial septal defects than in deficiencies of the ventricular septum (15, 16). Several methods have been proposed, including measurement of pulmonary blood flow (Qp), tricuspid valve flow (QTV), or transatrial septal flow velocity. Accurate assessment of pulmonary flow depends on the absence of associated lesions such as pulmonary or tricuspid valve disease.

Color flow mapping has been used with great success in interatrial communications and may now be the preferred method of analysis. Relatively small defects can be identified with this technique and the direction of flow easily ascertained (Fig. 21.8, Plate XI) (17).

Table 21.3. Causes of Right Ventricular Volume Overload

Secundum atrial septal defect
Primum atrioventricular septal defect (endocardial cushion defect)
Anomalous pulmonary venous connection (partial or total)
Divided left atrium (cor triatriatum)
LV to RA shunting
Ebstein's anomaly of tricuspid valve
Pulmonary valvar regurgitation
Systemic arteriovenous fistula
LV inflow or outflow obstruction in the newborn
Mitral atresia or stenosis
Aortic atresia or stenosis
Coarctation of the aorta

LV = left ventricle; RA = right atrium.

Patent Ductus Arteriosus

The third of the classic shunt lesions involves persistent patency of the ductus arteriosus. Doppler techniques have become an essential part of the ultrasonic evaluation of patent ductus arteriosus since standard echocardiographic imaging is frequently unreliable despite a number of attempted approaches (18, 19). Many lesions other than a patent ductus arteriosus can result in increased left heart volumes (Table 21.4), limiting the utility of measurements such as left atrial-to-aortic or left ventricular-to-aortic ratios. Furthermore, a num-

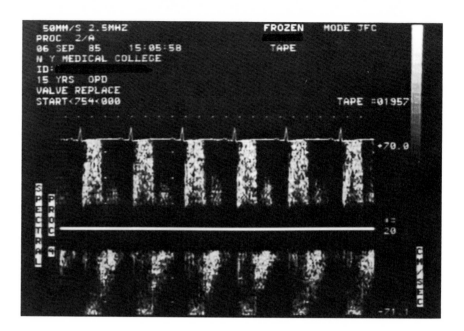

A

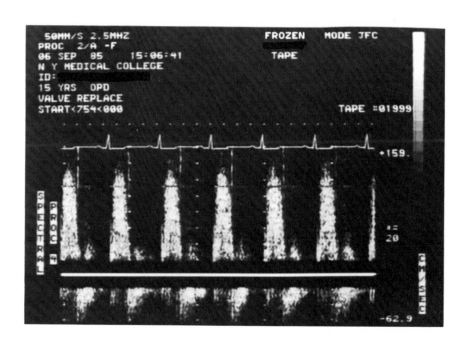

Figure 21.2. Examples of aliasing. (*A*) Apparent wraparound of flow velocity too great for measured scale. (*B*) Same velocity as in (*A*), measured at same level, but now estimable because of alteration of zero line, increasing scale.

B

ber of premature babies with patent ductus arteriosus do not manifest the typical continuous murmur (20), and demonstration of a shunt at ductal level by Doppler becomes critical for their successful management.

Several approaches may be used for assessing Doppler findings (21–25). Qualitative assessment depends on identification of abnormal flow patterns in the pulmonary trunk, which can be demonstrated in both systole and diastole. The standard approach involves align-

ment of the sample volume in the pulmonary trunk (Fig. 21.9). The characteristic recording will yield flow toward the transducer in diastole and predominantly negative flow away from the transducer in systole. The sensitivity of this method has been reported to be as high as 96 percent (24). Such flow abnormalities may be found in premature infants who lack the typical precordial auscultatory features of a patent ductus arteriosus.

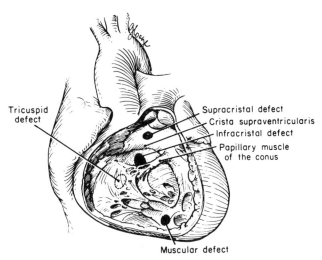

Figure 21.4. Possible locations of ventricular septal defects, as viewed from the right ventricle. Imaging considerations must include all possibilities in comprehensive evaluation.

Quantitative analysis of ductal shunts is more complicated. Measurement of pulmonary blood flow cannot be accurately determined because most of the shunting occurs distal to the pulmonary trunk, usually resulting in streaming to the left pulmonary artery. Assessment of flow across the mitral valve may provide a means of assessing pulmonary blood flow, provided no shunting is present at atrial level. This can be difficult in very tiny infants.

Peripheral flow analysis can also be helpful when the duct is patent. In particular, femoral artery velocities can be measured and the profile of flow determined in infants as small as 1000 to 1200 g (26). The reversal of blood flow observed in the great vessels can be dem-

onstrated in the femoral artery. At present, this technique utilizes custom-designed high-frequency (20 MHz) pulsed Doppler equipment, and technical experience is necessary to obtain these flow velocity signals. This technique is attractive in the tiny infant whose pulmonary disease requires treatment that may make precordial acquisition of Doppler recordings technically difficult.

Color flow mapping has become particularly useful in identifying ductal shunting. A rather easily discernible jet of reverse flow in the LPA or MPA can be visualized in the presence of patent ductus arteriosus. Not only does this type of imaging assist in qualitatively determining the presence of patent ductus arteriosus, but color flow mapping also helps to assess the magnitude of the shunt (Fig. 21.10A, B, Plate XI). With such information, invasive evaluation is not usually required for surgical management of patent ductus arteriosus in childhood.

PRESSURE GRADIENTS

The quanitative as well as qualitative utility of Doppler is important in pediatric cardiology since clinical findings may be subtle in mild stenotic lesions, making differential diagnosis difficult. Quantitative estimates of gradients across stenotic valves or great vessels are extremely useful to time invasive evaluations optimally and to define the physiology resulting from complex anatomic defects.

The caveats and precautions outlined in Chapters 1 and 2 concerning the reliability of assessing pressure gradients by Doppler in adults may well be more complex in the pediatric patient. The limitations of

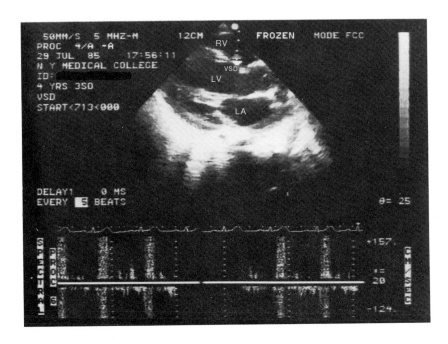

Figure 21.5. Ventricular septal defect (VSD) imaged by cross-sectional echocardiography. Duplexed with pulsed Doppler. Sample volume locates systolic jet of VSD. RV = right ventricle; LV = left ventricle; LA = left atrium.

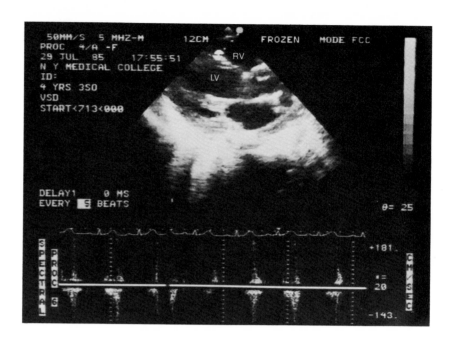

Figure 21.6. Placement of sample volume along interventricular septum at location without ventricular septal defect. No flow detected. RV = right ventricle; LV = left ventricle.

pulsed Doppler have been described, and the lack of simultaneous echocardiographic imaging with most continuous wave Doppler systems has been noted. In examining the pediatric patient, one must consider the patient as well as the equipment. While many examiners shun sedation or other means of achieving patient cooperation for imaging studies, such methods are often critically important for Doppler flow analysis. Chloral hydrate (30–70) mg/kg is the most commonly used agent, but other methods, such as feeding, are often equally successful. Accuracy of estimates under resting conditions, without introducing changes in hemodynamic status that may substantially alter valve gradients as a direct result of altered cardiac output, is really the objective.

Goldberg et al. (27) have reviewed the five most important factors complicating interpretation of Doppler information regarding obstruction-related flow disturbances (Table 21.5). The examiner must take into account these factors to avoid serious misinterpretation or misdiagnosis. In particular, "series effect," "induction," and "masking" are important in the pediatric patient in view of the high incidence of problems at multiple levels and the relatively small area and compactness of the thoracic cage of the infant.

Color Doppler has also been of assistance in identifying disturbed flow patterns across stenotic valve orifices, thus directing the operator to specific acoustic scrutiny. The use of color Doppler in the adult has been outlined previously (Chapters 7, 8) and the same principles are employed in pediatric applications. Often in childhood cardiac disease, valvar structures may not be heavily calcified or excessively anatomically deformed despite causing disturbed flow patterns. In these instances color flow mapping is especially informative.

Pulmonary Stenosis

Several studies have reported the validity of gradient estimations across the right ventricular outflow tract. Either a parasternal short-axis scan from the left sternal border in the second or third left intercostal space or a subcostal approach is preferred, although on occasion, suprasternal notch imaging may be used. Whatever the approach, a good view of the right ventricle below the pulmonary valve, of the valve, and of the pulmonary trunk is required. The branches of the pulmonary trunk should also be visualized. The subcostal plane may be the only available window in some pediatric patients, particularly those with associated lung disease or anatomic chest deformities or those who are early in the postoperative period with surgical dressings still in place (Fig. 21.11). Areas of interrogation from the subcostal route should include the subvalvar region, the pulmonary trunk, and its main branches.

Table 21.4. Lesions Associated with Left Ventricular or Left Atrial Volume Overload

Left-to-right shunts
   Patent ductus arteriosus
   Ventricular septal defect
   Atrial septal defect (infrequently)
Pulmonary AV fistula
Mitral valve disease
Aortic valvar regurgitation
Right ventricular inflow or outflow obstruction in the newborn
   Tricuspid atresia or stenosis
   Pulmonary atresia or stenosis

AV = atrioventricular.

The initial analysis can be done with pulsed Doppler and accurate sample volume placement accomplished with simultaneous cross-sectional imaging. If aliasing occurs, either continuous wave or high PRF Doppler is necessary and must be used to measure peak velocities.

The application of the modified energy balance equation ($P1 - P2 = 4V_2^2$) can then be applied, where V1 is the peak velocity at the proximal site, in this case the outflow tract below the valve, and V2 is the peak velocity measured in the pulmonary trunk distal to the obstruction. For simplification, in the presence of pulmonary valve stenosis, $P1 - P2 = 4V_2^2$ since the maximal velocity below a stenotic valve is usually less than 1 m/s.

Good correlations between gradients measured at cardiac catheterization and derived from Doppler velocity measurements have been reported, but several precautions are necessary. A discrete obstruction is the type most reliably evaluated. Supravalvar pulmonary stenosis with segmental pulmonary artery narrowing is not well suited for gradient analysis. Multiple level obstructions are prone to series effect, and overinterpretation at any level can easily occur. Orifice size and shape may play an important role in affecting results. Therefore, the smaller the orifice and the less circular its configuration, the less reliable the estimate. When studying patients with possible pulmonary stenosis, it is important to evaluate the aortic valve and left ventricular outflow tract since induction effects are possible, leading to misinterpretation of the true source of the flow disturbance.

Color flow mapping has greatly enhanced diagnostic accuracy. In pulmonary stenosis, for example, it is possible for immediate identification of the mosaic of color patterns representing disturbed flow across the pulmonary valve, permitting the operator to map carefully the width of the flow jet from its origin and to position the continuous wave Doppler beam to obtain true peak velocities. A clear difference between pulmonary stenosis and pulmonary atresia, with virtual absence of antegrade flow in the MPA, can be easily discerned with color flow mapping (Fig. 21.12, Plate XI). This may be important in helping to plan the type of intervention to improve pulmonary blood flow.

Aortic Stenosis

The same principles that apply to adults with this lesion apply to children with aortic stenosis. There are some differences, however, of which personnel evaluating pediatric patients must be aware.

The errors resulting from induction effects may occur as reported by Goldberg et al. (27). Doppler blood flow disturbances in children with various congenital right ventricular outlet obstructions, including tetralogy of Fallot, can mimic aortic stenosis. Therefore, as with pulmonary stenosis, it is important to assess flow patterns along the right ventricular outflow tract as well as the left ventricular outflow tract when evaluating a pediatric patient for the presence of aortic stenosis. Goldberg and his colleagues have suggested a means of minimizing errors of this type (induction errors); localize the jet of the abnormal aortic ejection and detect a region of normal velocity flow, the so-called parajet area, beside it, an association more frequent in true aortic valve disease.

A further problem involves the localization of abnormalities along the left ventricular outflow tract. Discrete shelflike subaortic stenosis is a relatively frequent left heart lesion in pediatric patients. The peak velocity of flow across this lesion is usually high, and continuous wave Doppler is therefore required to measure it. Thus, gradient estimation with non-imaging continuous wave Doppler may be hazardous when a subaortic lesion is associated with an abnormal valve, as is often the case. In supravalvar aortic stenosis, such as in William's syndrome, gradient estimation may be possible but is more accurate with more discrete vessel stenosis. This lesion, similar to other abnormalities involving the ascending aorta and aortic arch, is optimally visualized with cross-sectional echocardiography from the suprasternal notch.

Color Doppler flow mapping is especially helpful in determining flow disturbances when a multiplicity of obstructions exist. For example, when left ventricular outflow obstruction occurs at both valvar and subvalvar levels, identification of flow disturbance at each level can add precision to diagnosis and can have important clinical implications (Fig. 21.13, Plate XII).

The assessment of prosthetic valve gradients can also be accomplished in pediatric patients as in adults, but to date, no pediatric population has been studied with prosthetic aortic valves.

Coarctation of the Aorta

Doppler assessment of the gradient across the coarctation is usually not mandatory since the findings on clinical examination and blood pressure measurements closely approximate the magnitude of the obstruction. However, there are several instances in which ultrasonic gradient estimation can be particularly helpful.

In the neonate with coarctation of the aorta and a patent ductus arteriosus, right-to-left shunting may occur, providing adequate systemic circulation until the duct has closed. In this situation, pulmonary hypertension is present, and the elevated pulmonary artery pressure, which may be at systemic level, is transmit-

Table 21.5. Factors Complicating Doppler Interpretation of Flow Disturbance

Deceleration instability: false-positive frequency dispersion after velocity deceleration
Series effect: false-positive appearance of disturbed flow at a site distal to true locus of abnormal flow
Vortex shed distance: improper assessment of primary source of flow disturbance because of long distance from obstruction to first
    evidence of abnormal flow
Induction: false-positive flow disturbance because of physical proximity to an area of abnormal flow
Masking: false-negative analysis of multiple obstructions occurring in series

Adapted from Goldberg SJ, et al. (27).

ted into the descending aorta despite complete anatomic aortic obstruction by a posterior shelf. Thus, peripheral pulses will be palpable, and blood pressure gradients may be absent or negligible. Doppler flow analysis can detect disturbed flow patterns in this situation by comparing ascending and descending aortic blood flows.

In complex coarctation with associated abnormalities of the great arteries, repair may involve compromise of the unaffected left subclavian artery (subclavian flap procedure) and thus obviate subsequent upper extremity blood pressure recording. However, the gradient across the repair can be determined postoperatively by Doppler, which will also detect the presence of recoarctation at follow-up.

In atypical coarctations involving the aortic arch proximal to the left subclavian artery, scanning of the aortic arch with cross-sectional Doppler echocardiography will enable localization of the lesion, and Doppler can quantitate the gradient and therefore the hemodynamic severity of the vascular narrowing (Fig. 21.14). This precise definition of the site and severity of the lesion is important and helpful in planning catheterization approaches and in timing surgery.

Recent work has demonstrated a value for color flow mapping in evaluating coarctation of the aorta (28).

Data from such studies have indicated that color flow mapping enhances noninvasive diagnostic capabilities by providing sensitive profiles of the disturbed descending aorta blood flow pattern, increasing insight into the physiologic importance of the lesion. Figure 21.15 (Plate XII) is an example of a color flow image in coarctation of the aorta.

In general, assessment of valve gradients and the severity of other stenoses in pediatric patients follows the same guidelines and principles as those in adults. The operator must have a knowledge of the limitations of the method and a familiarity with the spectrum of associated congenital cardiac defects in order to avoid the pitfalls previously described. In most instances, clinical examination and cross-sectional echocardiographic screening will provide the essential anatomic data, and Doppler will provide additional accurate hemodynamic information. Further values of Doppler in evaluating pressure gradients are in serial assessment and in differential diagnosis.

Gradient estimations must be placed in the context of cardiac output, and most centers measure both in order to provide meaningful data for the cardiologist. A discussion of determination of cardiac output in the pediatric patient follows.

Figure 21.9. Duplex echocardiographic and Doppler image of patent ductus arteriosus. Sample volume placed in pulmonary trunk via short-axis parasternal echocardiographic view. Typical bidirectional continuous flow velocity recorded. Image recorded from 510 g premature infant.

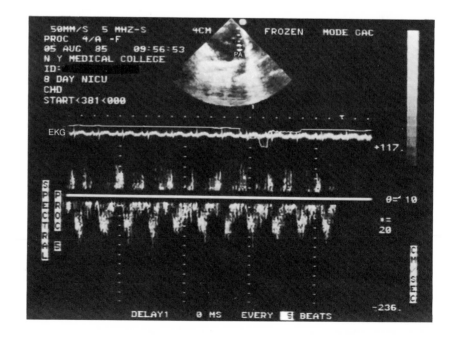

Cardiac Flow Determination

Much has been written about the use of Doppler techniques to derive cardiac output (29–31). Duplex technology enables the operator to localize the sample volume and to quantitate the angle of intercept. For most pediatric patients, output determinations can be successfully accomplished by interrogating the ascending aorta from the suprasternal notch (29). The cross-sectional area of the aorta can be determined from a cross-sectional or an M-mode echocardiogram and a reliable peak flow velocity calculated.

Many caveats have been advanced regarding the difficulties in measuring true velocity profiles for cardiac output determination. In general, use of simultaneous audio signals and scrutiny of the strip-chart recordings for beats with the least broad spectral envelope and the highest velocity will enhance accuracy. The calculation of mean velocity is necessary and has been accomplished either mechanically or manually but is done most easily by use of available computer software (Biodata Co., Davis, Ca. 95617) or by hand planimetry methods that compute the area under a velocity curve and divide that area by the baseline distance. This must then be converted into a per unit time value, usually expressed as mean velocity per second. Application of the following formula can then be achieved:

Flow (ml/min) = v (cm/s) × area (cm) × 60 (s/min)

It is the vessel area determination component of the method, however, that provides the greatest source of error. In one study, correlation of Doppler-derived systemic flow with indicator dilution techniques was good but improved when angiographic measurement of aortic root size was substituted for echocardiographic measurements (32).

Ascending aortic dimensions are measured most readily in children from the suprasternal notch. This can be difficult and requires patient cooperation. While flow determinations in the aorta have been done via the subcostal approach (7, 33), introduction of angulation errors with this method decreases reliability. It has been speculated that even the ascending aortic view is complicated by problems of spectral dispersion and reliability thereby reduced. Nevertheless, measurement of the diameter of the ascending aorta can be easily achieved from this view, and satisfactory correlations of Doppler flow versus invasively derived flow estimates have been achieved. It is important to measure aortic diameter as close as possible to the site of velocity measurement and to use leading-edge methodology to maximize axial resolution. Thus, the choice of transducer is critically important for this measurement. Systolic diameter has been the recommended standard measurement employed since it is approximately known that great vessel diameters may vary with the cardiac cycle by approximately 10 percent (34). Other investigators, however, have utilized random cycle measurements using the largest vessel diameter obtained for flow calculations.

In pediatric patients, it is important to remember that systemic and pulmonary flows may be altered by a variety of intracardiac conditions. Thus, assessment of pulmonary or aortic flow may require modification in the presence of intracardiac shunts and in right and left ventricular outflow tract obstructions. Qp (pulmonary

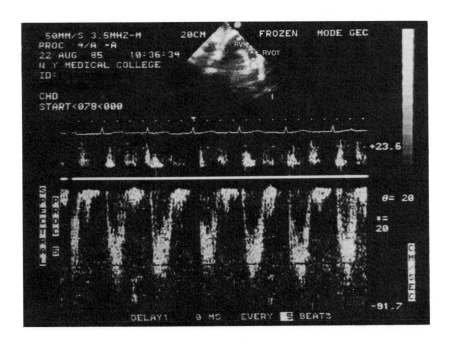

Figure 21.11. Duplex subcostal echocardiographic and Doppler image of right ventricular outflow tract (RVOT). Sample volume placed just distal to pulmonary valve in this view. RV = right ventricle.

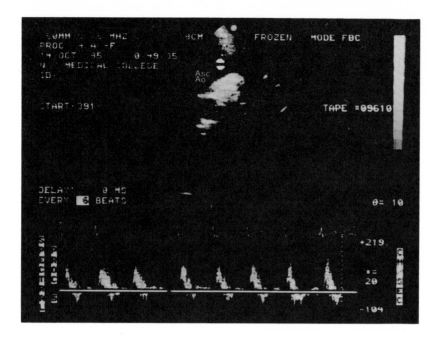

A

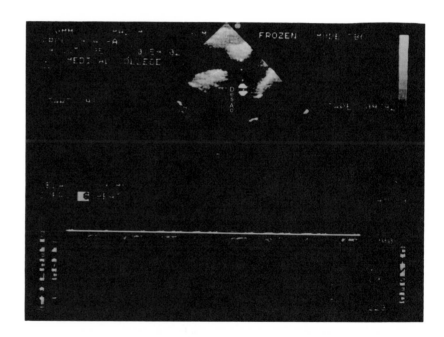

Figure 21.14. Aortic arch scanning. (*A*) Sample volume placed in descending aorta. Doppler flow is positively oriented. (*B*) Sample volume placed in descending aorta, below great vessel take-off. Flow velocity is negative in orientation. Asc Ao = ascending aorta; Des Ao = descending aorta.

B

flow), for example, may not be estimable in situations where intrinsic flow disturbances across the right ventricular outflow tract exist. Similarly, aortic flow estimates will be affected by the presence of a patent ductus arteriosus or other left-to-right shunts at the level of the great arteries. Thus, when studying premature infants, the presence of a patent ductus arteriosus must always be considered.

In addition, abnormalities of the aortic root may adversely affect systemic flow analyses using the techniques previously outlined. For these reasons, attempts have been made to utilize other approaches for systemic or pulmonary flow derivations. Mitral flow estimates have been advocated (11, 35) but difficulties with orifice measurement have been encountered. While these mostly experimental studies have been encouraging, human pediatric experience has been limited.

The noninvasive estimation of systemic or pulmonary

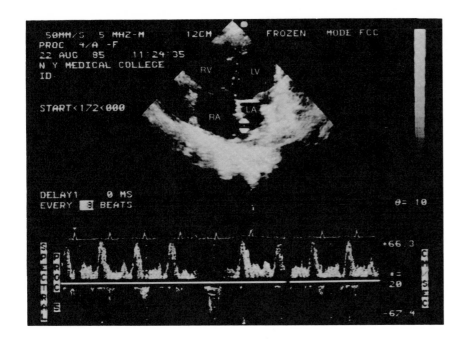

Figure 21.16. Right-to-left shunt seen in atrial septal defect (ASD) with pulmonary hypertension in a young infant. Sample volume placed at level of ASD via apical four-chamber view. Diastolic Doppler flow from right atrium (RA) to left atrium (LA) is recorded. Angulation of flow is predominantly toward transducer. RV = right ventricle; LV = left ventricle.

flows has a variety of important applications. While studies pertaining to most of these have been reported, much investigative effort is still required to verify the reliability of Doppler in each of these circumstances.

Cyanotic Heart Disease

Doppler blood flow analysis can be important for both diagnosing and evaluating the physiology of cyanotic cardiac conditions that predominate in the pediatric population (see Chapters 24, 26, 28, 30–32).

Usually, carefully performed cross-sectional echocardiographic studies are sufficiently comprehensive to provide anatomic diagnosis of most intracardiac lesions causing cyanosis. Duplex studies using Doppler can, however, add important hemodynamic information. In the newborn, for example, profound cyanosis and systemic hypoxemia may not be caused by anatomic cardiac disease. Rather, the association of pulmonary hypertension and persistently patent fetal cardiovascular communications may result in right-to-left shunting. A cross-sectional study alone will reveal normal intracardiac anatomy, but the demonstration of right-to-left flow across the atrial septum, through a patent foramen ovale, will help to confirm the diagnosis (Fig. 21.16). Doppler has been invaluable in improving the accuracy of diagnosis in a number of congenital cardiac anomalies. Total anomalous pulmonary venous connection, for example, can sometimes be difficult to diagnose with certainty by cross-sectional imaging, and Doppler flow analysis has been of help in establishing the diagnosis (36). The diagnosis of right-to-left shunting via a patent arterial duct in an older child may be clinically difficult and can be documented unequivocally by Doppler.

Other uses of Doppler in cyanotic patients include important applications in postoperative situations. One of the clearest examples is in the patient who has undergone a right atrial to pulmonary arterial anastomotic procedure (Fontan operation or its variants). Here, Doppler characterization of right atrial flow into the pulmonary arteries can be extremely valuable (Fig. 21.17) (37). In these patients, analysis of atrioventricular valve function can be critically important, but it is the pulmonary arterial and right atrial flow patterns that require most attention. Abnormal pulmonary arterial flow patterns in these situations frequently reflect ventricular dysfunction and are characterized by reduced amplitudes and by principally systolic flow with diminished atrial wave activity.

Doppler has an important role postoperatively in patients with conduit placement, in whom continuous wave methods have been successfully employed to document extracardiac conduit obstruction (38). While both overestimation and underestimation of the severity of conduit stenosis have occurred, the technique remains a useful one for qualitatively gauging the presence and severity of conduit obstruction in patients followed serially.

In postoperative atrial baffle procedures for complete transposition, residual intracardiac right-to-left shunting and identification of problems likely to cause persistent postoperative cyanosis may be observed with Doppler. In addition, Doppler studies have been used to detect obstruction of venous return in these patients (39).

In patients who have undergone palliative extracardiac shunting for treatment of cyanotic heart disease, Doppler techniques have been employed to verify shunt flow and patency (40), but reliability of these

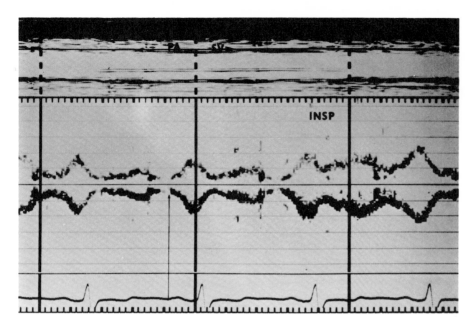

A

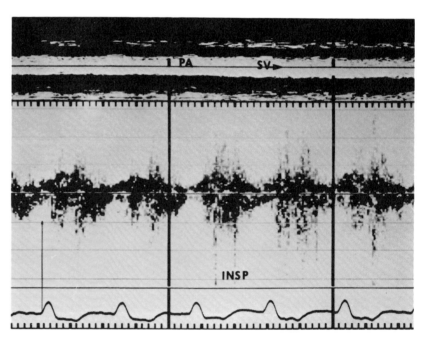

Figure 21.17. Flow characteristics following Fontan operation (right atrial to pulmonary artery [PA] anastomosis). (*A*) Typical flow pattern with prominent flow increase noted with inspiration (INSP). Pulsed Doppler recording. (*B*) Little increase in flow with inspiration noted in this patient with poor ventricular function and residual atrioventricular valve insufficiency. SV = sample volume. (Reproduced by permission from Hagler DJ, Seward JB, Tajik AJ, Ritter DG. Functional assessment of the Fontan operation: combined M-mode, two-dimensional, and Doppler echocardiographic studies. J Am Coll Cardiol 1984;4:756).

B

methods needs to be corroborated. In these instances, color flow mapping has been useful to delineate shunt flow with greater precision. Figure 21.18 (Plate XII) demonstrates delineation of Gore-tex shunt flow by color Doppler mapping in a child with otherwise obstructed pulmonary blood flow.

Finally, serial evaluation of patients with surgically palliated or corrected cyanotic congenital heart disease at long-term follow-up by Doppler echocardiog-

raphy will provide important information regarding postoperative cardiac function as the first cohort of patients reaches adulthood.

FETAL DOPPLER

In recent years much investigative evaluation of the role of Doppler examination combined with cross-sectional imaging of the human fetal heart has been carried out and comprehensive reviews are available (41). Standard cross-sectional echocardiography is extremely reliable for assessing fetal cardiovascular anatomy. Doppler provides unique insights into fetal physiology. In addition to interrogation of valvar structures, the fetal Doppler examination should include assessment of flow profiles in the descending aorta, the umbilical artery, and the maternal uterine vessels. Velocity measurements of intracardiac structures are useful as relative indices since there is some difficulty in reliably minimizing the angular difference between the Doppler signal and the true direction of flow.

Flow velocity alterations at varying anatomic sites will be present in congenital heart disease and may be relatively specific for a particular lesion. For example, in left heart hypoplasia, tricuspid and pulmonary flow velocities are increased. However, use of Doppler is more advantageous in arrhythmia assessment, where anatomic findings may be normal. A gauge of the effect of rhythm disturbances on fetal cardiac function can be obtained by assessing mean aortic velocity and by atrioventricular valvar regurgitation (42). Importantly, the results of therapeutic intervention such as administration of antiarrhythmics to the mother, can be monitored using Doppler techniques (43).

Currently, color Doppler flow mapping has not received approval from the U.S. Food and Drug Administration for fetal use. However, in view of the lack of identified fetal risk using conventional color flow systems, such approval is likely in the near future and will enable the ultrasonographer to further expand the noninvasive armamentarium for fetal cardiac evaluation.

ACKNOWLEDGMENT

Appreciation is expressed to Paul Burleson, R.D.M.S., for technical assistance in the preparation of this chapter.

REFERENCES

1. Stevenson JG, Kawabori I, Dooley TK, Guntheroth WG. Diagnosis of ventricular septal defect by pulsed Doppler echocardiography: sensitivity, specificity, and limitations. Circulation 1978;58:322.
2. Stevenson JG, Kawabori I, Guntheroth WG. Differentiation of ventricular septal defects from initial regurgitation by pulsed Doppler echocardiography. Circulation 1977;56:14.
3. Hatle L, Rokseth R. Noninvasive diagnosis and assessment of ventricular septal defect by Doppler ultrasound. Acta Med Scand 1981;645:47.
4. Yokoi K, Kambe T, Ichimiya S, Toguchi M, Hibi N, Nishimura K. Pulsed Doppler echocardiographic evaluation of the shunt flow in ventricular septal defect. Jpn Heart J 1983;24:175.
5. Meyer RA, Kalavathy A, Korfhagen J, Kaplan S. Comparison of left-to-right shunt ratios determined by pulsed Doppler/2D echo, and Fick method. Circulation 1982;66(suppl II):232.
6. Goldberg SJ, Sahn DJ, Allen HD, Valdes-Cruz LM, Hoenecke H, Carnahan Y. Evaluation of pulmonary and systemic blood flow by

7. two-dimensional Doppler echocardiography using fast Fourier transform spectral analysis. Am J Cardiol 1982;50:1394.
7. Sanders SP, Yeager S, Williams RG. Measurement of systemic and pulmonary blood flow and Qp/Qs ratio using Doppler and two-dimensional echocardiography. Am J Cardiol 1983;51:952.
8. Valdes-Cruz LM, Horowitz S, Mesel E, et al. A pulsed Doppler echocardiographic method for calculation of pulmonary and systemic flow: accuracy in a canine model with ventricular septal defect. Circulation 1983;68:597.
9. Kalmanson D, Veyrat C, Bouchareiue F, Degroote A. Noninvasive recording of mitral valve flow velocity patterns using pulsed Doppler echocardiography. Application to diagnosis and evaluation of mitral valve disease. Br Heart J 1977;39:517.
10. Fisher DC, Sahn DJ, Friedman MJ, et al. The effect of variations of pulsed Doppler sampling site on calculation of cardiac output: an experimental study in open chest dogs. Circulation 1983;67:370.
11. Fisher DC, Sahn DJ, Friedman MJ. The mitral valve orifice method for noninvasive two dimensional echo Doppler determination of cardiac output. Circulation 1983;67:872.
12. Stevenson JG, Kawabori I, Brandestini MA. Color-coded visualization of flow within ventricular septal defects: implications for peak pulmonary artery pressure. Am J Cardiol 1982;49:944.
13. Sahn DJ. Real-time two-dimensional Doppler echocardiographic flow mapping. Circulation 1985;71:849.
14. Stevenson JG, Kawabori I. Sequential 2D echo/Dopplers: improved noninvasive diagnosis of atrial septal defect, abstracted. Circulation 1983;68(Suppl 111):110.
15. Marx GR, Allen HD, Goldberg SJ, Flinn CJ. Do transatrial septal Doppler velocities (TASV) predict Qp:Qs ratios? abstracted. Pediatr Res 1984;18:127A.
16. Kalmanson D, Veyrat C, Derai C, Savier C-H, Berkman M, Chiche P. Non-invasive technique for diagnosing atrial septal defect and assessing shunt volume using directional Doppler ultrasound. Br Heart J 1972;34:98.
17. Suzuki Y, Kambara H, Kadota K, et al. Detection of intracardiac shunt flow in atrial septal defect using a real-time two-dimensional color-coded Doppler flow imaging system and comparison with contrast two-dimensional echocardiography. Am J Cardiol 1985;56:347.
18. Johnson GJ, Breart GL, Gewitz MH, et al. Echocardiographic characteristics of premature infants with patent ductus arteriosus. Pediatrics 1983;72:864.
19. Hirschklau MJ, Disessa TG, Higgins CB. Echocardiographic diagnosis-pitfalls in the premature infant with a large patent ductus arteriosus. J Pediatr 1978;92:474.
20. Ellison RC, Peckham GJ, Lang P, et al. Evaluation of the preterm infant for patent ductus arteriosus. Pediatrics 1983;71:364.
21. Lees MH, Newcomb JD, Sunderland CO, Droukas P, Reynolds JW. Doppler ultrasonography in evaluation of PDA shunting. J Pediatr 1980;97:852.
22. Serwer GA, Armstrong BE, Anderson PAW. Non-invasive detection of retrograde descending aortic flow in infants using continuous wave Doppler ultrasound. J Pediatr 1980;97:394.
23. Gentile R, Stevenson G, Dooley TK. Pulsed Doppler echocardiographic determination of time of ductal closure in normal infants. J Pediatr 1981;98:443.
24. Stevenson JG, Kawabori I, Guntheroth WG. Pulsed Doppler echocardiographic diagnosis of patent ductus arteriosus: sensitivity, specificity, limitations, technical features. Cathet Cardiovasc Diagn 1980;6:255.
25. Huhta JC, Cohen M, Gutgesell HP. Patency of the ductus arteriosus in normal neonates: two-dimensional echocardiography versus doppler assessment. J Am Coll Cardiol 1984;4:561.
26. Alverson DC, Eldridge MW, Berman W. Pulsed Doppler characterization of peripheral blood flow in the neonate with patent ductus arteriosus. In Berman W, ed. Pulsed Doppler ultrasound in clinical pediatrics. Mt. Kisco, N.Y.: Futura Publishing, 1983. Chap. 3.
27. Goldberg SJ, Allen HD, Marz GR, Flinn CJ. Doppler echocardiography. Philadelphia: Lea and Febiger, 1985:62–5. Chap. 4.
28. Simpson IA, Sahn DJ, Valdes-Cruz LM, Chung K, Sherman FS, Swensson RE. Color Doppler flow mapping in patients with

coarctation of the aorta: new observations and improved evaluation with color flow diameter and proximal acceleration as predictors of severity. Circulation 1988;77(4):736–744.

29. Alverson DC, Eldridge MW, Dillon J, Yabek SM, Berman W Jr. Noninvasive pulsed Doppler determination of cardiac output in neonates and children. J Pediatr 1982;101:46.

30. Magnin PA, Stewart JA, Myers S, Von Ramm O, Kisslo JA. Combined Doppler and phased-array echocardiographic estimation of cardiac output. Circulation 1981;63:388.

31. Huntsman LL, Steward DK, Barnes SR, Franklin SB, Colocousis JS, Hessel EA. Noninvasive Doppler determination of cardiac output in man: clinical validation. Circulation 1983;67:593.

32. Goldberg SJ, Sahn DJ, Allen HD, Valdes-Cruz LM, Hoenecke H, Cainahan Y. Evaluation of pulmonary and systemic blood flow by two-dimensional Doppler echocardiography using fast Fourier transform spectral analysis. Am J Cardiol 1982;50:1934.

33. Grenadier E, Lima CO, Allen HD, et al. Normal intracardiac and great vessel Doppler flow velocities in infants and children. J Am Coll Cardiol 1984;4:343.

34. Greenfield JC Jr, Patel DJ. Relationship between pressure and diameter in the ascending aorta of man. Circ Res 1962;10:778.

35. Valdes-Cruz LM, Horowitz S, Sahn DJ, et al. A simplified mitral valve method for 2-D echo Doppler cardiac output, abstracted. Circulation 1983;68(suppl 111):230.

36. Skovranek J, Samenek M. Range gated pulsed Doppler echocardiographic diagnosis of supracardiac total anomalous pulmonary venous return. Circulation 1980;61:841.

37. Hagler DJ, Seward JB, Tajik AJ, Ritter DG. Functional assessment of the Fontan operation: combined M-mode, two-dimensional, and Doppler echocardiographic studies. J Am Coll Cardiol 1984;4:756.

38. Reeder GS, Airrie PJ, Fyte DA, Hagler DJ, Seward JB, Tajik AJ. Extracardiac conduit obstruction: initial experience in the use of Doppler echocardiography for noninvasive estimation of pressure gradient. J Am Coll Cardiol 1984;4:1006.

39. Stevenson JG, Kawabori I, Dooley TK, Dillard DH, Guntheroth WG. Pulsed Doppler echocardiographic detection of obstruction of systemic venous return following repair of transportation of the great arteries. Circulation 1979;60:1091.

40. Allen HD, Sahn DJ, Lange L, Goldberg SJ. Noninvasive assessment of surgical systemic-to-pulmonary artery shunts by range-gated pulsed Doppler echocardiography. J Pediatr 1979;94:395.

41. Reed KL. Fetal and neonatal cardiac assessment with Doppler. Semin Perinatol 1987;11(4):347–356.

42. Reed KL, Sahn DJ, Marx GR, et al. Cardiac Doppler flows during fetal arrhythmias: physiologic consequences. Obstet Gynecol 1987;70:1–6.

43. Lingman G, Marsal K. Fetal cardiac arrhythmias: Doppler assessment. Semin Perinatol 1987;11(4):357–361.

22
Echocardiographic Diagnosis and Description of Congenital Heart Disease: Anatomic Principles and Philosophy

Robert Anderson
Siew Yen Ho

THE NORMAL HEART

The understanding of normal echocardiographic anatomy requires an appreciation of the location of the heart within the chest, its anatomic relations to the thoracic organs, and the disposition of the cardiac chambers and valves within the heart.

The Heart Within the Thorax

The heart is positioned within the mediastinum such that the smaller portion of its bulk is to the right and the major portion to the left of the midline (Fig. 22.1). It is trapezoidal in shape as it projects to the anterior aspect of the body silhouette. The right border is slightly convex and projects just to the right of the sternum. Its inferior border is flat and lies on the diaphragm, extending horizontally from the xiphoid notch to the left border, such that the apex usually lies in the fifth interspace. The left border extends obliquely up to the superior border (or base), where the great arteries emerge and ascend into the superior

mediastinum. The base is behind the sternum at the level of the third costal cartilage.

The Arrangement of the Cardiac Chambers

The heart lies with its long axis at an angle to the long axis of the body (Fig. 22.2). The cardiac long axis extends from the apex to the base and is oriented from the left hypochondrium toward the right shoulder. The right heart chambers are arranged anteriorly rather than right-sidedly within the heart relative to the left heart chambers. The only part of the left atrium that projects directly to the anterior cardiac silhouette is the tip of its appendage. Similarly, only a small strip of the left ventricle is seen anteriorly running down to the apex. The pulmonary trunk forms part of the left border of the cardiac silhouette with the position of the pulmonary valve to the left of the aortic valve (Fig. 22.3). The anterior surface of the heart is therefore occupied almost exclusively by the right atrium and the right ventricle. The tricuspid valve, marking the junction between these chambers, is more or less vertical,

573

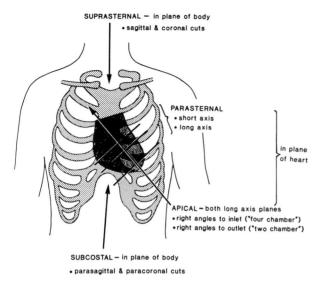

Figure 22.1. Diagram of the heart in the chest with the rib cage superimposed to demonstrate the portals that can be used by the echocardiographer. From each approach, two main series of planes and a third intermediate series can be demonstrated.

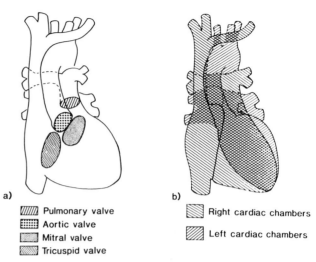

Pulmonary valve
Aortic valve
Mitral valve
Tricuspid valve

Right cardiac chambers
Left cardiac chambers

Figure 22.3. Diagrams showing the relative positions of the heart valves (*A*) and the arrangement of the right heart chambers (*B*) relative to the left heart chambers.

and it is the most inferior of the cardiac valves. The right ventricle extends anteriorly (Fig. 22.4) and superiorly from the tricuspid valve to the pulmonary valve, the latter being almost horizontal at the level of the left second costal cartilage. The aortic and mitral valves are hidden behind the right ventricle. Unless approached directly from the apex (or from above), it is necessary to traverse the right heart chambers to record the left-sided valves. It follows from the disposition of the cardiac chambers that the septal structures have a complex orientation. The atrial septum is

obliquely positioned behind the aorta. The ventricular septum curves around from an inlet component in the sagittal plane of the body to an outlet component in the coronal plane (Fig. 22.5). These details are emphasized in the section devoted to the morphology of septal defects (Chap. 25).

Description and Display of Cross-Sectional Anatomy

Although the echocardiographic access to the heart is limited to the parasternal, suprasternal, apical, and subcostal windows, multiple sections can be obtained through each of these windows. There are two ap-

Figure 22.2. Diagram showing the angle between the long axis of the heart and that of the body. The heart has its own orthogonal planes.

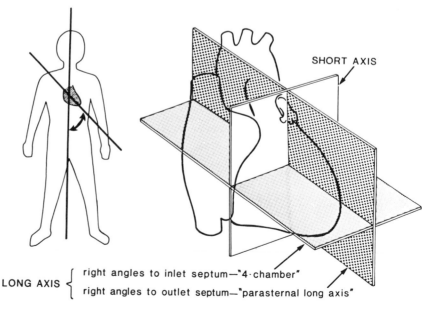

LONG AXIS { right angles to inlet septum—"4·chamber"
right angles to outlet septum—"parasternal long axis"

ORTHOGONAL PLANES OF HEART

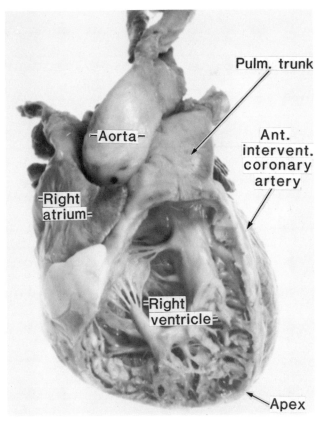

Figure 22.4. The anterior wall of the heart has been removed to show the position and extent of the right ventricle. Ant. intervent. = anterior interventricular; Pulm. = pulmonary.

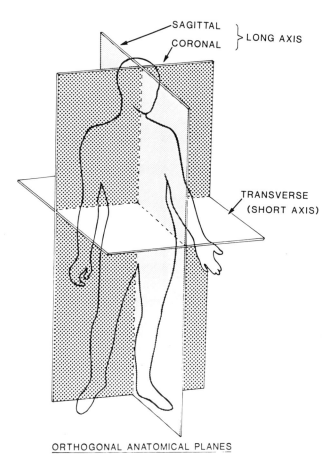

ORTHOGONAL ANATOMICAL PLANES

Figure 22.6. The three orthogonal planes of the body produce two long-axis sections and a short-axis section.

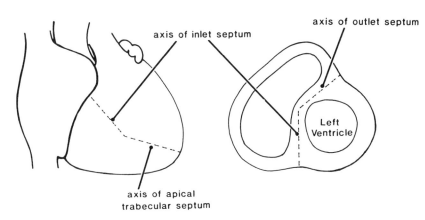

a) Frontal projection

  (axis of outlet septum parallel

   to this projection)

b) Short axis

  (trabecular septum shows

   similar curve in apical sections)

Figure 22.5. Diagrams showing the orientation of the curved ventricular septum as seen in two views of the heart.

APICAL APPROACH

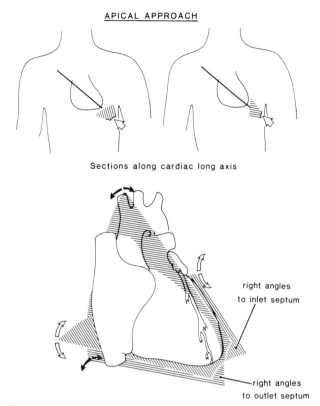

Figure 22.7. Diagram showing the apical approach from which two main series of planes along the long axis of the heart can be obtained.

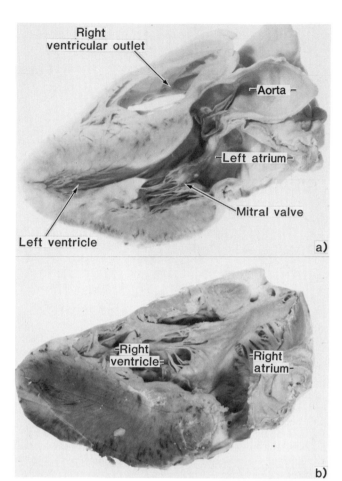

Figure 22.8. Two heart sections yielded by the apical approach taken at right angles to the outlet septum. The index two-chamber section (*A*) passes through part of the right ventricular outflow tract but also demonstrates clearly the left heart structures. A section to the right of the index plane (*B*) shows only right heart structures.

proaches to understanding these multiple sections. One is to attempt to catalog all the series of planes obtainable from each of the windows and to assign each an identifying number (1). The other approach, which we prefer, is more systematic (2). This method recognizes that all structures can be described in terms of their three orthogonal planes. In terms of the body in anatomic position (Fig. 22.6), these are the sagittal, coronal, and short-axis planes. Both the sagittal and coronal planes are in the long axis of the body. There are legion intermediate and oblique planes, but any bodily configuration can always be described fully in terms of the three basic planes. The heart also has its own three orthogonal planes (Fig. 22.2). Because the long axis of the heart itself is out of alignment with the long axis of the body (Fig. 22.2), the cardiac orthogonal planes differ from the standard anatomic planes. Nonetheless, two of the planes are, of necessity, in the long axis of the heart. Being out of alignment with the bodily planes, these long-axis planes of the heart cannot be described as sagittal and coronal. Instead, the planes transect the heart so that they display all four of the cardiac chambers or only the right- or left-sided chambers. They can therefore be termed "four-chamber" or "two-chamber" planes, respectively. When a cross section is obtained slightly anterior to the true

four-chamber view, the central origin of the aorta superimposes between the mitral valve and the ventricular septum. This plane is often known as the four-chamber plus aortic root view or "five-chamber" view. The "two-chamber" series of planes also usually incorporates the outflow tract of the other side of the heart because of the usual spiral arrangement of the outflows.

When the heart is approached from the apex it can be cut in both of the long-axis planes (Figs. 22.7, 22.8, and 22.9) but not in the short-axis plane. Access to the heart from the parasternal windows permits a similar series of two-chamber long-axis planes to be obtained as from the apex (Fig. 22.10). From the parasternal position, the heart can also be cut in the short-axis plane (Fig. 22.11) but not the four-chamber plane. From the subcostal window, the heart can be cut in the parasagittal and paracoronal planes of the body (Fig. 22.12). Study of these cuts (Figs. 22.13 and 22.14) shows that, while they approximate the four-chamber

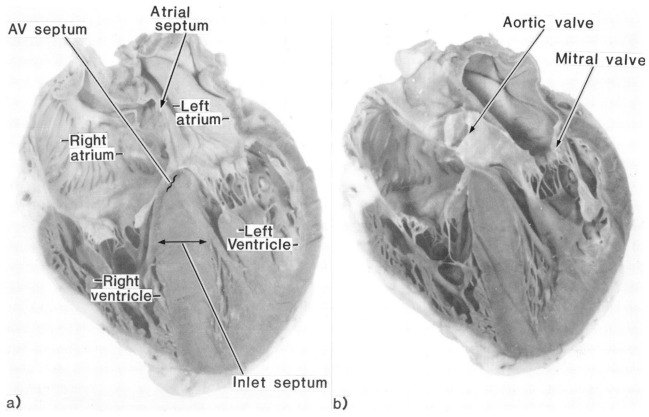

Figure 22.9. Two heart sections demonstrating the four-chamber planes obtained by the apical approach taken at right angles to the inlet septum. The offsetting of the mitral valve relative to the tricuspid valve is seen in (*A*). A section taken slightly more anteriorly (*B*) shows the interposition of the subaortic outflow tract between the septum and the mitral valve.

and short-axis series of the heart itself, there are significant differences. The suprasternal approach is of value primarily for visualization of the great arteries. These cross sections are generally obtained more or less in between the paracoronal and parasagittal planes of the body (Fig. 22.15). The echocardiographic sections are directly comparable with frontal and lateral projections of arterial or venous angiograms.

MORPHOLOGIC DIFFERENTIATION OF THE CARDIAC CHAMBERS

The right and left chambers are not strictly right and left sided even in the normal heart. In abnormal hearts, these chambers are frequently in abnormal positions. Therefore, it is necessary to distinguish the chambers according to their morphologic characteristics rather than their positions. In congenital heart disease, however, it is not always possible to determine chamber morphology because in certain structural anomalies a chamber may not possess all its normal parts. To distinguish a given chamber we choose features that are most universally present. This approach, the so-called

morphologic method, was first introduced by Lev (3) and subsequently endorsed by Van Praagh and associates (4).

Distinction of the Atrial Chambers

The component of the atrial chambers most universally present is the appendage. The morphologically left and right atrial appendages are sufficiently different to make their distinction an easy matter for the anatomist, although it remains to be seen whether these differences can be determined by echocardiography. The right appendage (Fig. 22.16*A*) is a broad, triangular structure, having a wide junction with the smooth-walled atrial component. In contrast, the left appendage is tubular and has a narrow junction with the smooth-walled atrium (Fig. 22.16*B*). The internal features of the appendages are even more striking. The inner surface is trabeculated. In the morphologically right atrium, these trabeculations branch out in comb-like fashion (hence the name "pectinate" muscles) from the prominent terminal crest (crista terminalis), which marks the junction of smooth and trabeculated atrium (Fig. 22.17*A*). The pectinate muscles extend around the atrioventricular junction and into the

PARASTERNAL APPROACH

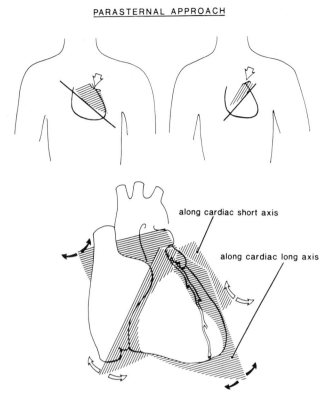

Figure 22.10. Diagram showing the two main series of planes that can be obtained from the parasternal approach. The series along the cardiac long axis is similar to the two-chamber series obtainable by the apical approach.

posterior atrial wall. It is the extent as well as the pectinate arrangement that makes them the feature of the morphologically right atrium. By contrast, in the morphologically left atrium, the trabeculations are limited and do not extend to the posterior wall; there is no terminal crest (Fig. 22.17B). The septum, when present, also provides an excellent distinction between the atria. The right side of the septum is distinguished by the muscular rim of the oval fossa whereas the flap valve is seen within the left atrium. These features are obvious in cross section (Fig. 22.18). The valves of the inferior caval vein and coronary sinus, although often rudimentary or absent, are additional features of the morphologically right atrium. Such valvar structures are never seen in the morphologically left atrium.

Anatomic Distinction of the Ventricles

When describing the ventricles, it is preferable to think in terms of inlet, apical trabecular, and outlet components (Fig. 22.19) rather than the traditional "sinus" and "conus." It is the apical trabecular component that is the ventricular portion most universally present in the incomplete ventricles found in congenitally malformed hearts. When two ventricles are present, they can be distinguished solely from the patterns of this

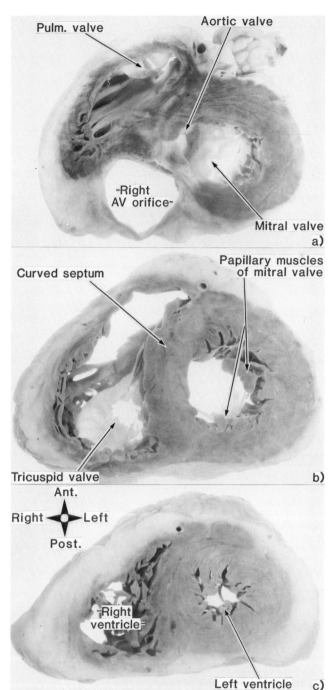

Figure 22.11. Three of a series of short-axis heart sections that can be obtained by the parasternal approach. A section (A) taken through the mitral valve leaflets is superior to the tricuspid valve. When the tricuspid valve leaflets are visible in (B), only the papillary muscles of the mitral valve can be demonstrated. Note the curvature of the ventricular septum. A section near the cardiac apex shows the different thicknesses of the ventricular walls. Ant. = anterior; AV = atrioventricular; Post. = posterior; Pulm. = pulmonary.

apical part because the trabeculations are much coarser in morphologically right than in morphologically left ventricles (Fig. 22.20), particularly on the septum. Furthermore, a prominent moderator band is

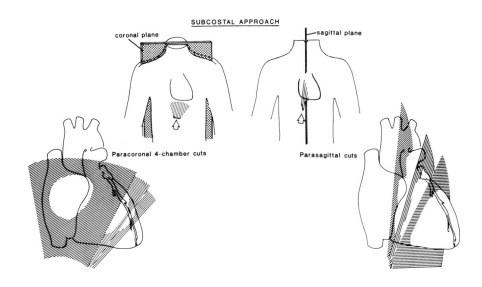

Figure 22.12. The subcostal approach yields planes of the heart that approximate to the bodily coronal and sagittal planes.

present in the morphologically right ventricle but not the left. Usually the ventricles possess more than an apical component, and the features of the other parts help in differentiation. The nature of the inlets containing the atrioventricular valves is particularly helpful. When each of the valves is connected to a separate ventricle (and when the atrioventricular septum is intact), the tricuspid valve is always found in the morphologically right ventricle and the mitral valve in the morphologically left ventricle. The valves are distinguished according to the pattern of their leaflets and their tension apparatus (Fig. 22.21). The tricuspid valve is circular with septal, anterosuperior, and mural (inferior) leaflets supported by papillary muscles of differing size. The mitral valve is oval with mural and aortic (anterior) leaflets supported by paired papillary muscles of similar size. Except in the presence of a ventricular septal defect extending into the inlet septum, the septal annular attachment of the tricuspid valve is displaced toward the ventricular apex compared to the mitral valve. The most reliable distinguishing feature, however, is the direct chordal attachments of the tricuspid valve to the muscular septum, the mitral valve attachments to the paired papillary muscles being away from the septum. The ventricular outlet portions are also distinctive (Fig. 22.22), but these features are the least reliable of those discussed thus far. The morphologically right ventricle usually has a complete muscular outflow tract with a prominent supraventricular crest interposed in the inner heart curve between the arterial (semilunar) and tricuspid valves. In contrast, the arterial valve of the left ventricle is almost always in fibrous continuity posteriorly with the mitral valve.

There are two ventricles within the ventricular mass in the majority of patients with congenital heart disease. These two ventricles are always of morphologi-

cally right and left ventricular type as judged according to their apical trabecular pattern. They are not, however, always normally constituted, and the basis of many "complex" lesions is an unequal sharing of the inlet and outlet components between the apical trabecular components. All ventricles in hearts with two ventricles can be described on the basis of this sharing of the other components, recognizing that in some circumstances an inlet or outlet component may be completely absent. An example of this arrangement is the total absence of the inlet component of the morphologically right ventricle in classical tricuspid atresia (5). To describe such abnormal ventricles fully, it is always necessary to take note of their morphologic pattern (right ventricular or left ventricular), their size (normal, enlarged, or hypoplastic), and their component makeup. When describing the last feature, it is our convention to label ventricles lacking one or more of their components as "rudimentary." In doing so, the adjective is used to denote the absence of a component part. Such rudimentary ventricles are usually small or at least smaller than a normal ventricle, although this is not implicit in our use of the term "rudimentary," since size is described as a separate feature of a ventricle.

On occasion, congenitally malformed hearts that have a solitary ventricle within their ventricular mass will be encountered. It is then necessary to recognize a third ventricular trabecular pattern, namely the indeterminate pattern of a truly solitary ventricle (Fig. 22.23). Such solitary ventricles have a coarser pattern than the normal right ventricle and are crisscrossed apically by thick muscle bundles. It may be exceedingly difficult to distinguish such a solitary indeterminate chamber from a dominant morphologically right ventricle in which the rudimentary left ventricle is so small as to be virtually absent. We describe solitary

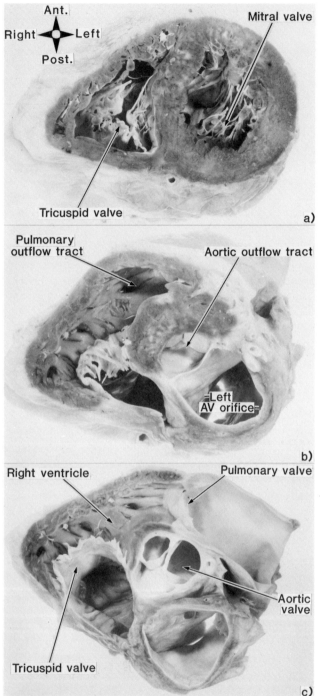

Figure 22.13. Three of a series of parasagittal sections. A midventricular section (*A*) shows both atrioventricular (AV) valves. The wedge position of the aortic outflow tract is seen in (*B*). The anterosuperior sweep of the right ventricle from the tricuspid valve to the pulmonary valve is shown in (*C*). Ant. = anterior; Post. = posterior.

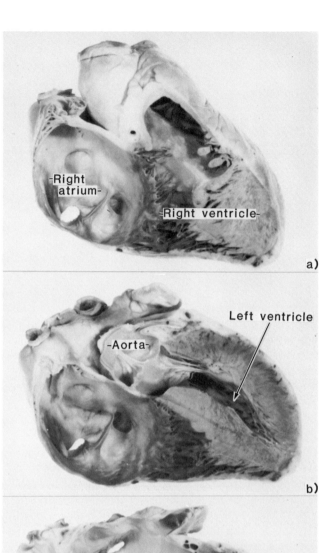

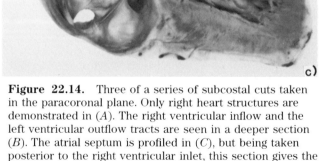

Figure 22.14. Three of a series of subcostal cuts taken in the paracoronal plane. Only right heart structures are demonstrated in (*A*). The right ventricular inflow and the left ventricular outflow tracts are seen in a deeper section (*B*). The atrial septum is profiled in (*C*), but being taken posterior to the right ventricular inlet, this section gives the spurious impression of tricuspid atresia.

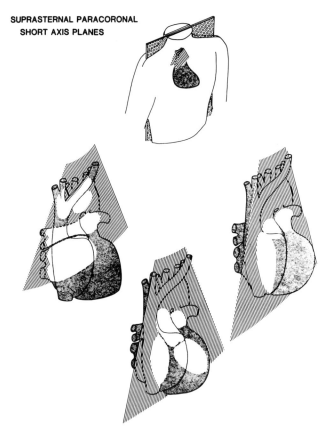

SUPRASTERNAL PARACORONAL
SHORT AXIS PLANES

Figure 22.15. Diagram showing short-axis sections that can be obtained from the suprasternal approach.

morphologically right and also solitary morphologically left ventricles to cater for the latter contingency.

Anatomic Distinction of the Great Arteries

The great arteries do not possess any intrinsic features that differentiate their trunks and are distinguished by their branching pattern (Fig. 22.24). The pulmonary trunk branches early into left and right pulmonary arteries and only very rarely gives rise to one or more coronary arteries. The aorta gives rise to the coronary arteries and then ascends to branch into the systemic arteries and the descending aorta. The aortic arch almost invariably crosses superiorly relative to the bifurcation of the pulmonary trunk. In congenital heart disease, it is necessary to distinguish the aorta and the pulmonary trunk from a common or a solitary trunk. A common trunk leaves the ventricular mass through a common valve and branches immediately to supply the systemic, pulmonary, and coronary arteries. A solitary trunk is described when only one arterial trunk leaves the heart. Its nature as a solitary aorta or a common trunk cannot be determined because of total absence of any intrapericardial pulmonary arteries. Pulmonary arterial supply in such circumstances is through systemic-pulmonary collateral arteries.

NORMAL SEPTAL STRUCTURES

Lesions in congenitally malformed hearts can be considered in terms of abnormal connections, obstructive lesions, or septal deficiencies. The emphasis placed on chamber morphology sets the scene for the diagnosis of anomalous connections (see section "Types of Atrioventricular Connection"). Obstructive lesions are much simpler to understand, whereas septal deficiencies are easy to recognize echocardiographically. To categorize defects in the septal structures fully, it is necessary to be acquainted with the extent and arrangement of the normal septum.

The atrial septum is not nearly as extensive as might be assumed from a glance at the septal surface of the right atrium (Fig. 22.25A). The septum should be defined as that part of the wall separating the two atrial cavities. Simple dissection in the normal heart reveals that the atrial septum as thus defined is confined to the floor of the oval fossa and its immediate surroundings (Fig. 22.25B). This is important in the understanding of "atrial septal defects." Four types of such defect are conventionally described: secundum, sinus venosus, coronary sinus, and ostium primum (Fig. 22.26). Of these, only the secundum defect represents a true deficiency of the atrial septum. The sinus venosus defect exists because either a caval or a pulmonary vein is anomalously connected to both atria, thus providing an extracardiac interatrial communication (Fig. 22.27). The rarer coronary sinus defect is an interatrial communication through the orifice of the sinus because of unroofing of the wall between sinus and left atrium. The much more common ostium primum defect is not due to a deficiency of the atrial septum. Instead, it represents an interatrial communication through a deficiency at the site of the atrioventricular septum. Recognition of these simple anatomic facts is a prerequisite for appropriate echocardiographic diagnosis of interatrial communications.

Description of the ostium primum interatrial communication conveniently introduces the topic of the atrioventricular septum. This important area has often been ignored in descriptions of the normal septum, although the advent of cross-sectional echocardiography has done much to emphasize its significance. It exists in two segments in the normal heart. The more extensive muscular atrioventricular septum is seen in four-chamber views as a consequence of the off-setting of the proximal septal attachments of the leaflets of the mitral and tricuspid valves (Fig. 22.28A). The anteriorly situated membranous atrioventricular septum exists as a consequence of the normal wedge position of the subaortic outflow tract of the left ventricle. The attachment of the septal leaflet of the tricuspid valve makes part of this membranous septum a right atrial–left

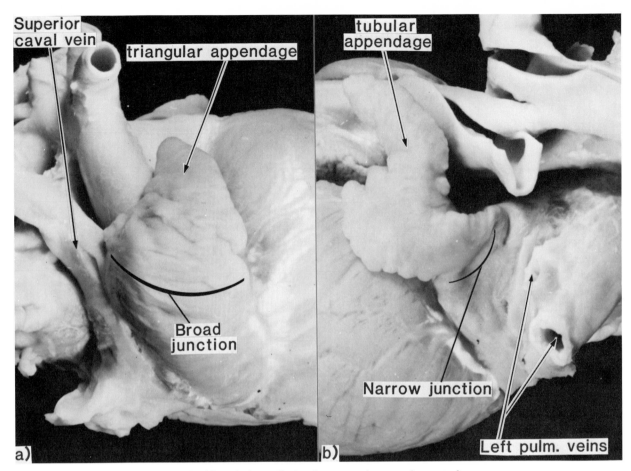

Figure 22.16.   The left (*B*) and right (*A*) atria have distinctive appendages. pulm. = pulmonary.

ventricular partition (Fig. 22.28*B*). The whole area of the normal atrioventricular septum can be distorted by major abnormalities of connection such as double-inlet or double-outlet ventricle. It can also be less extensively deviated by deficiencies of the ventricular septum (see next paragraph). The real significance of deficiency of this septum, however, comes in analysis of endocardial cushion defects or atrioventricular canal malformations. The hallmark of these lesions is a total lack of normal atrioventricular septation in an otherwise normally structured heart. The consequence of the lack of atrioventricular septation extends beyond the existence of a defect at the site of the septal structures. The presence of the septal deficiency affects both the morphology of the atrioventricular junction and the arrangement of the ventricular mass. Short-axis sections of the normal heart reveal the "wedge" position of the aortic valve, while long-axis two-chamber sections show that the left ventricle has equal inlet and outlet dimensions (Fig. 22.29). Similar sections in hearts with deficient atrioventricular septation reveal an unwedging of the subaortic outflow tract, a common atrioventricular junction, and a discrepancy between inlet and outlet dimensions of the left ventricle (Fig. 22.30). This arrangement has a further conse-

quence concerning the morphology of the left atrioventricular valve. This valve no longer has the pattern of the normal mitral valve in hearts with deficient atrioventricular septation. The anatomic hallmark of the normal valve is its extensive mural leaflet making up two-thirds of the annular circumference. In contrast, the mural leaflet of the left-sided valve in atrioventricular septal defects makes up less than one-third of the annulus (6). Furthermore, unlike the two-leaflet mitral valve, the left atrioventricular valve in these anomalies is a three-leaflet structure. The two leaflets other than the mural leaflet are not the cleft components of a normal anterior or aortic leaflet of the mitral valve as is often stated. Instead, they are the left ventricular components of two leaflets that bridge the ventricular septum and are attached in both right and left ventricles (Fig. 22.31). The space between these left ventricular components of the bridging leaflets cannot be a cleft in the normal mitral valve. In functional terms, it is more akin to a commissure, although it is not supported by a papillary muscle (7). It is the abnormal junctional anatomy along with the nature of the left atrioventricular valve that is the echocardiographic key to diagnosis of atrioventricular septal defects.

Just as knowledge of the atrial and atrioventricular

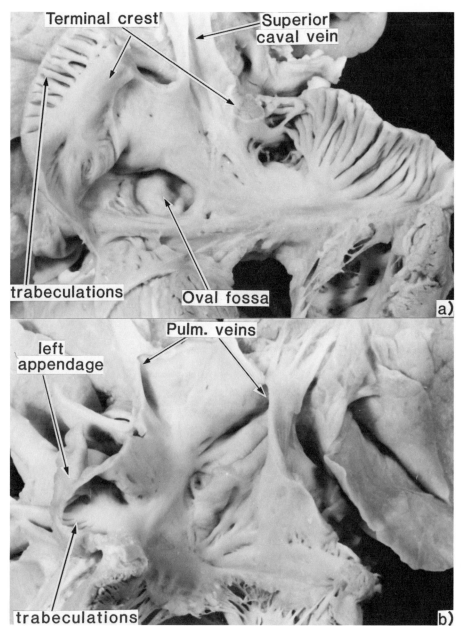

Terminal crest

Superior caval vein

trabeculations

Oval fossa

a)

Pulm. veins

left appendage

trabeculations

b)

Figure 22.17. The right atrium (*A*) opened through the superior caval vein and the terminal crest shows the radiating trabeculations. The left atrium (*B*) displayed from the back shows the limited extent of the trabeculations and absence of the terminal crest. Pulm. = pulmonary.

septal structures leads to appropriate diagnosis of septal deficiencies and atrial and atrioventricular intercommunications, so an understanding of the normal ventricular septum permits accurate diagnosis of ventricular septal defects. The ventricular septum is most readily defined as the structure separating the cavities of the right and left ventricles. This definition leads to the understanding that not all parts usually described as "septum" are partitions between the two ventricles. The atrioventricular septum, for instance, is not a ventricular septal structure since it separates the right atrium from the left ventricle. Examination of the extensive subpulmonary infundibulum will show that much of the "septal" surface is the outer wall of the

heart. This is because the facing leaflets of both the aortic and pulmonary valves are supported on sleeves of outlet musculature with an external tissue plane between them (Fig. 22.32). Most of the subpulmonary infundibulum (including all of the outlet musculature supporting the leaflets of the pulmonary valve) can be removed without entering the cavity of the left ventricle (Fig. 22.33). The extensive muscular outlet septum present in lesions such as tetralogy of Fallot or double-outlet right ventricle has no counterpart in the normal heart. Other revelations become apparent when the subdivisions of the normal septum are critically analyzed. Along with others (8), it has been our convention (9) to describe the normal muscular septum as

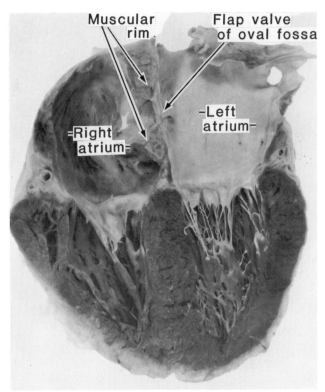

Figure 22.18. A four-chamber section profiles the features of the atrial septum.

possessing inlet, apical trabecular, and outlet components. As previously demonstrated, the outlet septum is barely represented in the normal heart. Furthermore, because of the wedge position of the normal subaortic outflow tract, the so-called inlet septum does not separate the ventricular inlets. Instead, it divides the inlet of the right ventricle from the outlet of the left ventricle, so that much of the normal muscular ventricular septum is an inlet-outlet septum (Fig. 22.21B).

These findings in themselves do not invalidate the distinction of different types of ventricular septal defects, but they do point to the danger of presuming that such defects represent absence of different parts of the normal septum. The most common type of ventricular septal defect abuts on the area of the normal atrioventricular membranous septum and is appropriately termed a "perimembranous" defect. The normally wedged position of the subaortic outflow tract explains why, in the otherwise normal heart, such perimembranous defects are also periaortic. The defects can extend so that they open from the subaortic area mostly into the inlet or outlet portions of the right ventricle, or they can be large and confluent. It is not strictly accurate, however, to suggest that such defects excavate the "inlet" or "outlet" septal structures since such septal structures do not exist in the normal heart. Similarly, the special type of defect that opens into the outlet component of the right ventricle and is roofed by fibrous continuity between the aortic and pulmonary valves could not exist in the normal heart. This is because the pulmonary valve leaflets normally have no continuity with any left ventricular structures. The doubly committed subarterial defect, therefore, represents a major departure from normal anatomy. Defects within the muscular septum itself are more readily understood in terms of normal anatomy. Such defects can open into inlet, apical trabecular, or outlet components of the right ventricle as can perimembranous defects.

The inlet or outlet septal structures can, however, exist in abnormal hearts. Thus, a muscular septum between the subaortic and subpulmonary outlets is usually an extensive structure in tetralogy of Fallot. Its malalignment with the rest of the septum is then the cardinal feature of the anomaly. The inlet septum is

Figure 22.19. Diagrammatic representations of the ventricles showing their distinctive features. AV = atrioventricular.

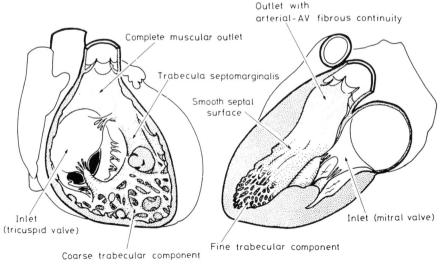

a) Morphologically Right Ventricle

b) Morphologically Left Ventricle

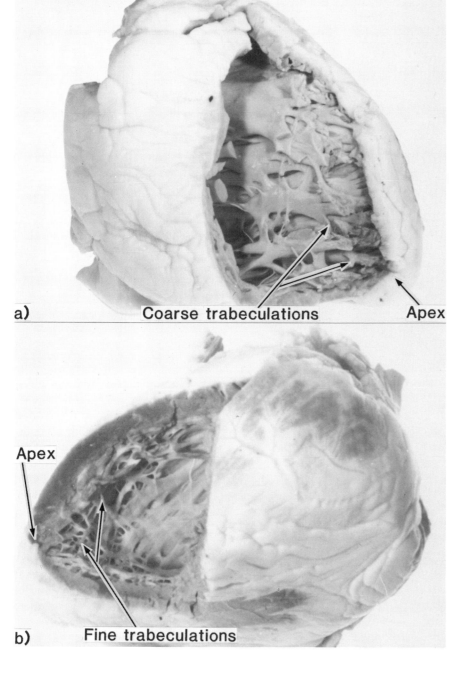

a) **Coarse trabeculations** **Apex**

Apex

b) **Fine trabeculations**

Figure 22.20. Dissections revealing (A) the characteristic coarse apical trabeculations of the right ventricle and (B) the fine trabeculations of the left ventricle.

seen as a true inlet septal structure in double-outlet right ventricle, since the subaortic outlet no longer "lifts" the mitral valve leaflet away from the septum. In contrast, the outlet septum in double-outlet right ventricle is no longer an interventricular septal structure but belongs exclusively to the right ventricle. Malalignment of the septum in overriding and straddling of the tricuspid valve represents a special type of defect, since it is the atrial septum that is malaligned relative to the ventricular septum. Putting all of this anatomic information together enables Soto's classification of ventricular septal defects (9) to be modified so as to

make it more compatible with the anatomy as it exists in the normal heart (Table 22.1).

SEQUENTIAL SEGMENTAL ANALYSIS

Once the morphology of the atrial and ventricular chambers and the arterial trunks have been identified, the diagnosis of cardiac malformations becomes relatively simple. The great majority of patients with congenital lesions exhibit them in the setting of a basically normal heart, with the chambers and arterial trunks connected to one another in the normal fashion

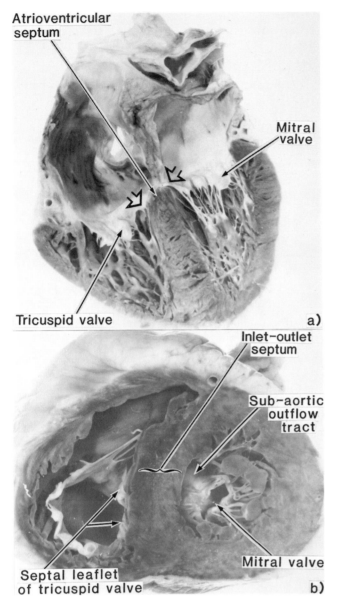

Atrioventricular septum

Mitral valve

Tricuspid valve

a)

Inlet-outlet septum

Sub-aortic outflow tract

Septal leaflet of tricuspid valve

Mitral valve

b)

Figure 22.21. A four-chamber section (*A*) shows the attachment of the mitral valve at a higher level than the tricuspid valve (*open arrows*). A midventricular short-axis section (*B*) shows direct septal attachment of the tricuspid valve. In contrast, the mitral valve is attached away from the septum to paired papillary muscle groups. The wedge position of the subaortic outflow tract places much of the ventricular septum in inlet-outlet position.

and in their normal positions. However, normality cannot be assumed but must be proved. Such an approach will identify the minority of cases with abnormal chamber connections or relationships. This systematic system of diagnosis is called sequential segmental analysis. It starts with establishment of the arrangement of the atrial chambers (situs). Thereafter, the connections between the atrial chambers and the ventricular mass are assessed (the type of connection).

Table 22.1. Categorization of Ventricular Septal Defect

A. Make-up of boundaries
  1. Bordered directly by mitral-tricuspid valvar continuity (perimembranous)
  2. Embedded in musculature of septum (muscular)
  3. Bordered directly by aortic–pulmonary valvar continuity (doubly committed and subarterial)
    a. Extending to become perimembranous
    b. With muscular posteroinferior rim
B. Position within right ventricle
  1. Opening to inlet
  2. Opening to apical trabecular component
  3. Opening to outlet
  4. Confluent defect
C. Relationship to valves (other than as described in A)
  1. Overriding and/or straddling of tricuspid valve (malalignment of atrial and ventricular septal structures)
  2. Overriding and/or straddling of mitral valve (seen only with discordant VA connection or DORV)
  3. Overriding of aortic valve (malalignment of outlet septum into RV with concordant VA connection)
  4. Overriding of pulmonary valve (malalignment of outlet septum into LV with concordant VA connection)
  5. Overriding of common valve (subtruncal defect with common arterial trunk)

VA = ventriculoarterial; DORV = double outlet right ventricle; RV = right ventricle; LV = left ventricle.

In addition, the morphology of the valves guarding the atrioventricular junction is noted (the mode of atrioventricular connection). The ventriculoarterial junction is then established with knowledge of the type of connection and the infundibular morphology. Abnormal relationships are noted throughout this diagnostic assessment. Malposition of the heart itself is also noted, analyzing the cardiac position and the orientation of the cardiac apex separately. Sequential analysis is then concluded by cataloging all associated lesions (10).

Atrial Arrangement

Almost without exception, all hearts possess two atrial chambers, which may be united in the absence of the atrial septum to form a common atrium. These chambers are of right or left morphology as judged by their appendages. There are, therefore, only four possible arrangements of these two chambers, either of which may be of right or left type (Fig. 22.34). Most commonly the blunt triangular appendage is right sided, and the narrow tubelike appendage is left sided. This is the usual arrangement (so-called situs solitus). Very rarely, the tubelike appendage may be right sided and the blunt triangular appendage left sided. This is the mirror-image arrangement (so-called situs inversus). More frequent than the mirror-image pattern and making up approximately 10 percent of cases of congenital heart disease are those cases with either bilateral tubelike or bilateral blunt triangular appendages. These are the variants of left or right atrial isomerism. Almost without exception, right atrial isomerism is associated with abdominal visceral heterotaxy, absence of the spleen, and right bronchial

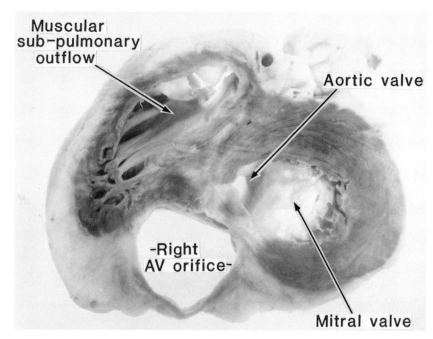

Figure 22.22. A short-axis heart section shows the muscular right ventricular outflow tract and the fibrous continuity between the aortic and mitral valves. AV = atrioventricular.

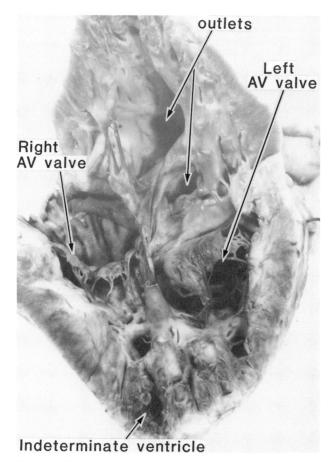

Figure 22.23. A heart with indeterminate pattern of trabeculations is displayed by opening the ventricular mass in clam-fashion. The solitary ventricle receives both atrioventricular (AV) valves (double inlet) and supports both arterial trunks (double outlet).

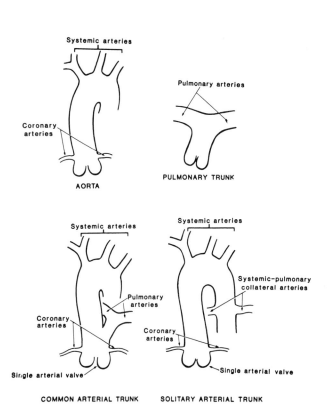

Figure 22.24. The four types of arterial trunks can be recognized by their branching patterns.

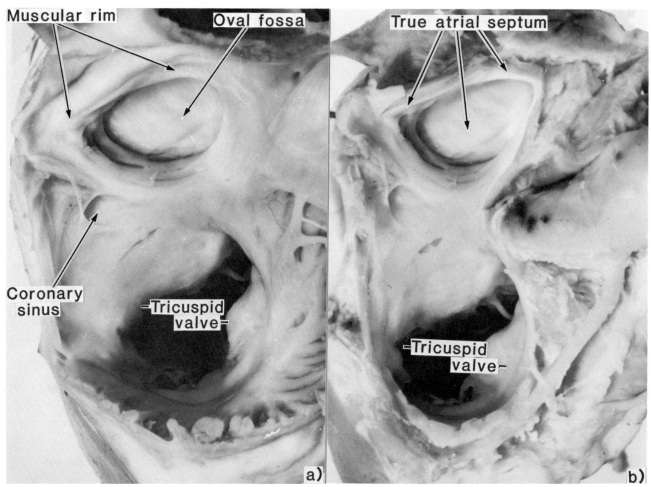

Figure 22.25. The right atrial aspect of the apparent atrial septum is displayed in (*A*). Further dissection (*B*) shows the limited extent of the true septum.

Figure 22.26. Diagram showing a view into the right atrium. The true atrial septum is represented by the flap valve of the oval fossa and its immediate muscular rim (stippled area). With the exception of the oval fossa (secundum) defect, the other interatrial communications (hatched areas) lie outside the septum.

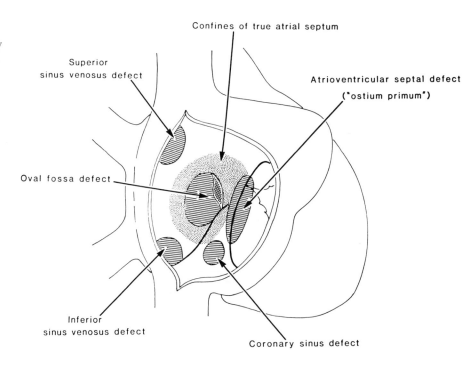

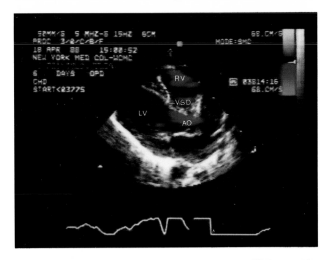

Figure 21.3. Color flow Doppler imaging of VSD in mid-muscular septum. Relatively small left-to-right shunt noted from this defect as a thin jet of highly turbulent flow.

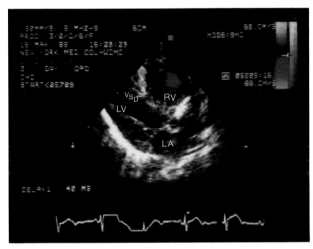

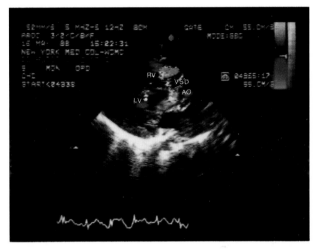

A   **B**

Figure 21.7. (*A*) Color flow Doppler image of muscular ventricular septal defect (VSD) using modified long-axis orientation. (*B*) Color flow Doppler mapping of high membranous VSD, long-axis left ventricle orientation.

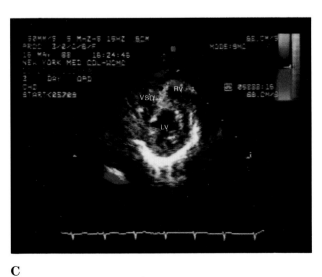

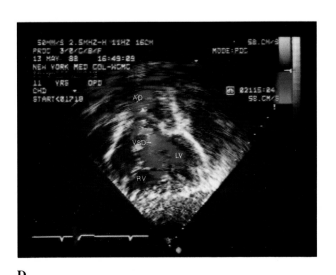

C   **D**

Figure 21.7 (cont'd.). (*C*) Cross-sectional image with color flow mapping. VSD in muscular septum imaged in this plane as well. (*D*) Malalignment VSD seen from subcostal imaging. Color map demonstrates flow from both right ventricle (RV) and left ventricle (LV) into aorta (Ao) via VSD.

Plate X

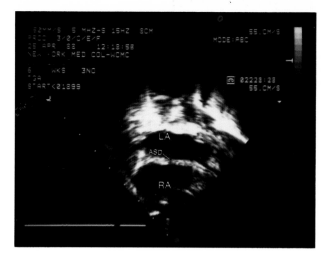

A

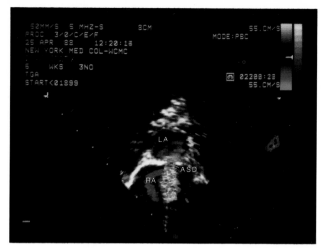

B

Figure 21.8. (*A*) Cross-sectional image without color mapping of atrial septal defect (ASD). Note that in this image ASD may be hard to visualize and magnitude of shunting, if any, difficult to assess. (*B*) Color flow mapping of ASD in same patient as in (*A*). Addition of color map enables appreciation of highly turbulent shunt flow associated with this ASD.

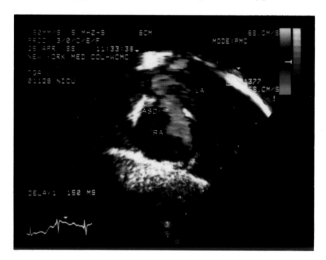

C

Figure 21.8 (cont'd.). (*C*) Large volume shunting seen in patient with relatively larger ASD using color flow mapping

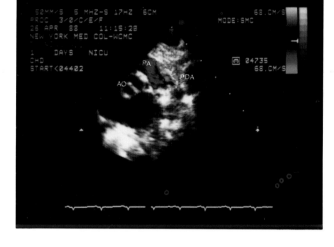

A

Figure 21.10. (*A*) Color flow mapping of patent ductus arteriosus (PDA). Reverse jet seen from PDA flowing into LPA and causing turbulent flow in MPA as well.

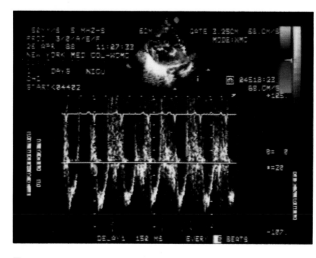

B

Figure 21.10 (cont'd.). (*B*) Specific localization of sample volume in reverse jet caused by left-to-right PDA allows for specific velocity profile to be developed.

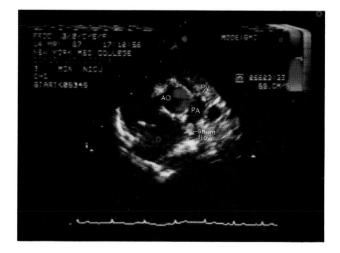

Figure 21.12. Color flow mapping in critical pulmonary stenosis. Note turbulent flow confined to paravalvar area with absence of MPA flow. in distal PA, flow is noted coming from surgically placed Gore-tex shunt.

Plate XI

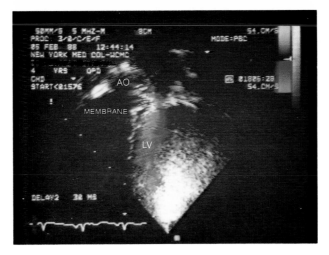

Figure 21.13. CF mapping along left ventricular outflow tract in patient with subaortic membrane and aortic valve disease. Turbulent area below aortic valve at level of membrane seen in addition to paravalvar flow disturbances associated with aortic stenosis and insufficiency.

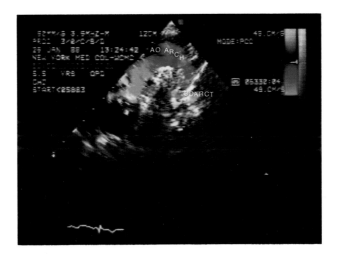

Figure 21.15. Aortic arch color flow mapping reveals relatively normal flow proximal to area of turbulence and color mosaic associated with coarctation of aorta. Broad-based jet implies substantial pressure difference across coarctation site.

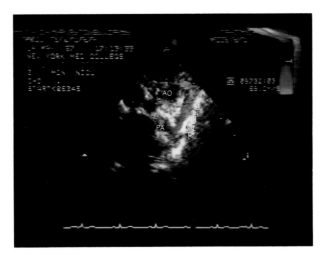

Figure 21.18. Delineation of flow in surgically created shunt (Gore-tex) interposed between left subclavian artery and left pulmonary artery in patient with otherwise obstructed pulmonary blood flow. Distal insertion into LPA is clearly seen.

Plate XII

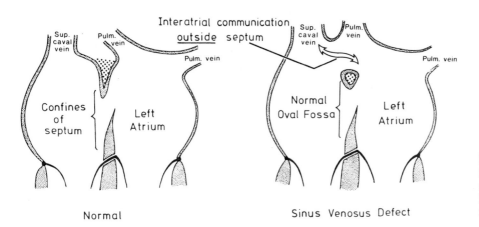

Normal   Sinus Venosus Defect

Figure 22.27. Diagrams illustrating the extracardiac location of the superior sinus venosus defect. Pulm. = pulmonary; Sup. = superior.

isomerism. Left atrial isomerism is also associated with abdominal heterotaxy but in the setting of multiple spleens and left bronchial isomerism. Irrespective of the other organs, it is important to determine directly atrial arrangement in complex congenital heart disease. In practice, this is not always possible, and all information is therefore collated, including venous connections, relationships of the abdominal great vessels, and the pattern of bronchial morphology as demonstrated on the penetrated chest radiograph. In this respect, some have suggested that the isomeric patterns represent so-called situs ambiguus (11). If attention is directed to the appendages, however, there is nothing ambiguous about the two isomeric forms of atrial arrangement. Preliminary studies by Chin and Williams (12) suggest that the morphology of the appendages and their junction with the venous component of the atria permits their echocardiographic distinction (Fig. 22.35).

Even when this is not the case, there are additional means whereby atrial arrangement can be determined

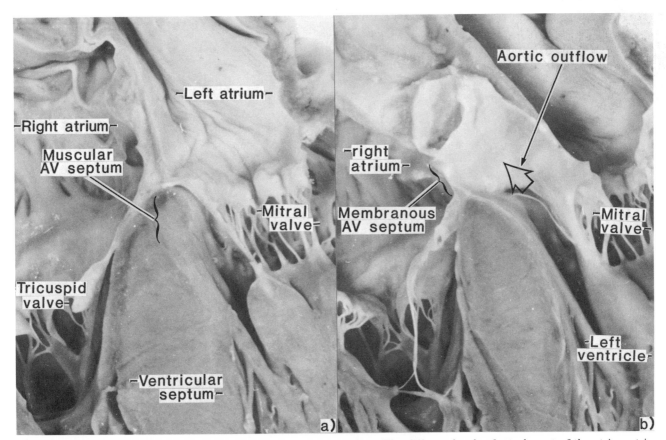

Figure 22.28. Close-up view of two sections in four-chamber plane. The different levels of attachment of the atrioventricular (AV) valves in (A) produces a region of muscular septum that is atrioventricular in position. The membranous atrioventricular septum is shown in (B).

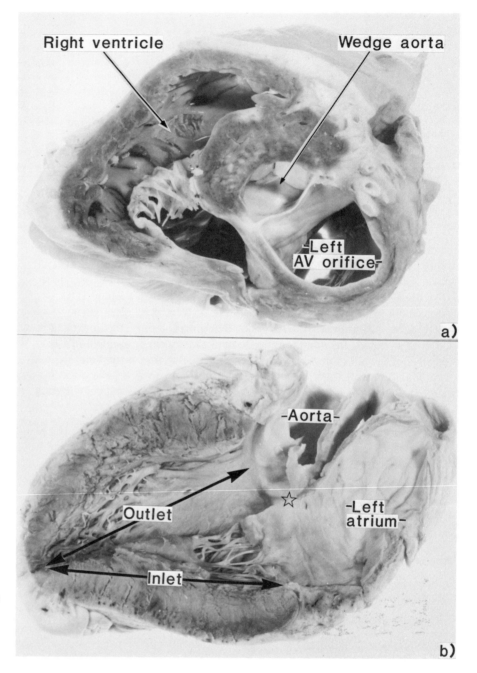

Figure 22.29. A short-axis section (*A*) shows the normal wedge position of the aortic valve between the mitral and tricuspid orifices. Its fibrous continuity with the mitral valve (*star*) is demonstrated in a long-axis section (*B*). Note the approximately equal inlet-outlet lengths. AV = atrioventricular.

with accuracy. Although there is a relatively poor correlation between splenic status and atrial anatomy (13), there is a much stronger concordance between atrial and bronchial arrangements. It is an easy matter (Fig. 22.36) to distinguish radiographically the long morphologically left bronchus from the much shorter morphologically right bronchus (14). Penetrated chest radiography or use of so-called filter films should give a strong indication of atrial arrangement. This inference can now be strengthened by ultrasonographic examination of the abdominal great vessels relative to the spine (15). Whenever the inferior caval vein and the abdominal aorta are lateral relative to the spine, it can

be presumed that there is either usual or mirror-image atrial arrangement, the morphologically right atrium being on the same side of the spine as the caval vein (Fig. 22.37). When the venous and arterial trunks are on the same side of the spine with the inferior caval vein in anterior position, there is always right atrial isomerism. Left atrial isomerism can be distinguished in the majority of cases because the inferior caval vein will be interrupted and the enlarged azygos vein will be to the same side of the spine as the aorta but in posterior position. Alternatively, there will be separate and direct connection of the hepatic veins bilaterally to the atrial chambers. Rare exceptions may be found to these

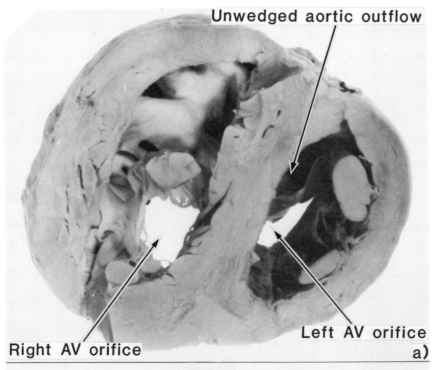

Unwedged aortic outflow

Right AV orifice

Left AV orifice

a)

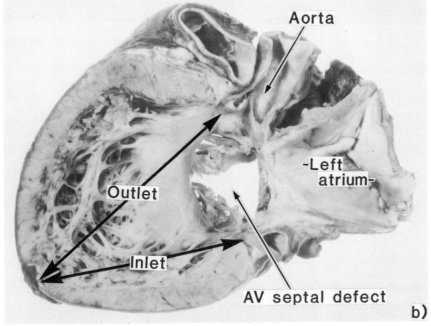

Aorta

Outlet

Inlet

-Left atrium-

AV septal defect

b)

Figure 22.30. A short-axis section (*A*) from a heart with atrioventricular (AV) septal defect shows a lack of wedging of the subaortic outflow tract. The long-axis section (*B*) shows the inlet length to be shorter than the outlet length.

rules, but taken together with direct analysis of inter-atrial morphology, they should permit direct determination of atrial arrangement in almost all cases suspected to have congenital heart disease.

Analysis of the Atrioventricular Junction

The important features to determine at the atrioventricular junction are the way the atrial myocardium connects with the ventricular mass (the type of connection) and the morphology of the valves that guard

the junction (the mode of connection). At the same time, note is taken of the arrangement and relationship of the chambers within the ventricular mass, since these are intimately intertwined with the type of connection present.

Types of Atrioventricular Connection

Once the arrangement of the atrial chambers is established, it is easy to define the atrioventricular connection, since the options are strictly limited (Table 22.2).

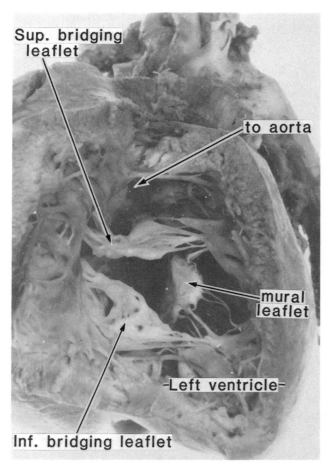

Sup. bridging leaflet

to aorta

mural leaflet

Left ventricle

Inf. bridging leaflet

Figure 22.31. A left ventricular view of a heart with deficiency of the atrioventricular septum shows the trileaflet left component of the common valve. The mural leaflet is exclusive to the left ventricle while the other two leaflets are attached in both right and left ventricles. Inf. = inferior; Sup. = superior.

Table 22.2. Atrioventricular Connections

A. With each atrium connected to a separate ventricle
1. With usual and mirror image atrial arrangement
Concordant AV connection
Discordant AV connection
2. With isomeric atrial chambers
Ambiguous AV connection
a. With right-hand ventricular topology
b. With left-hand ventricular topology
B. With atriums connected to only one ventricle (can exist with any atrial arrangement)
1. Double inlet AV connection
To dominant LV with rudimentary RV
To dominant RV with rudimentary LV
To solitary and indeterminate ventricle
2. Absent right AV connection with left-sided atrium connected
To dominant LV with rudimentary RV
To dominant RV with rudimentary LV
To dominant RV with rudimentary LV
To solitary and indeterminate ventricle
3. Absent left AV connection with right-sided atrium connected
To dominant RV with rudimentary LV
To dominant LV with rudimentary RV
To solitary and indeterminate ventricle

AV = atrioventricular; LV = left ventricle; RV = right ventricle.

cles. Discordant atrioventricular connection can also occur when the atrial chambers are arranged in the usual and mirror-image fashion and are similarly independent of the relationships of the ventricles and of their topologic patterns. A variation in relationships can occur when the heart is either rotated or tilted along its long axis. Such rotation or tilting produces the lesions known as criss cross hearts or superoinferior ventricles, respectively (Figs. 22.39 and 22.40). Abnormalities in ventricular position occur with either concordant or discordant atrioventricular connections but may exist with any type of atrioventricular connection. Next, it is necessary to examine the ventricular topology.

Van Praagh et al. formulated a segmental approach to diagnosis (16) which concentrated specifically on the internal morphology of each segment and less on connections (17). They described the atrial chambers as being arranged in "solitus" (usual), "inversus" (mirror-image), or ambiguous fashion. They extended this approach to the ventricles and described d-loop, l-loop, and x-loop patterns. Concordance was used to describe the combinations of either usual atrial chambers and a d-loop pattern of ventricular topology or mirror-image atria with l-loop topology, irrespective of the atrioventricular connection present. In similar fashion, atrioventricular discordance accounted for the combination of usual atria with l-loop topology or mirror-image atria with d-loop topology, irrespective of the precise atrioventricular connection.

Our concept of sequential segmental analysis was initially developed from the Van Praagh prototype (16), but we emphasize the importance of the junctional connections (19). We give specificity to the junctional arrangements by referring always to concordant or

They are determined first by whether the atria are lateralized (usual or mirror image) or isomeric, and second by whether the atrial chambers are each connected to a separate ventricle (biventricular atrioventricular connection) or whether the atria connect to only one ventricle (univentricular atrioventricular connection). Combining these options shows that there are two possible biventricular atrioventricular connections in the presence of lateralized atria. They are either concordant or discordant (Fig. 22.38). A concordant connection occurs when the morphologically right atrium is connected to the morphologically right ventricle and the morphologically left atrium is connected to the morphologically left ventricle, irrespective of the relationship and topology of the ventricles. This anatomic pattern (in which the atria are connected to their morphologically appropriate ventricles) occurs with usual and mirror-image atrial arrangement. A discordant atrioventricular connection exists when the atria are connected to morphologically inappropriate ventri-

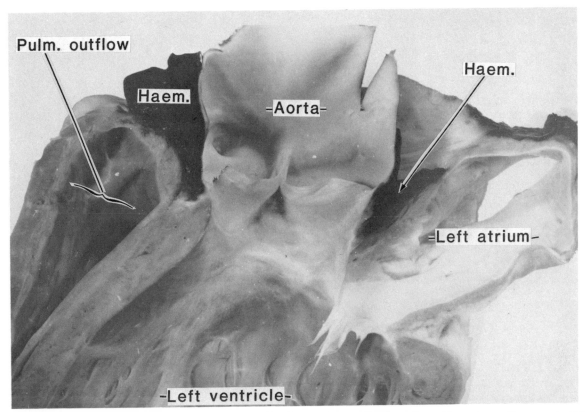

Figure 22.32. A heart with aortic dissection sectioned in long-axis two-chamber plane. The extracardiac spaces around the aortic root filled with hemorrhage (Haem.) mark out the sleeves of outlet musculature. Pulm. = pulmonary.

discordant atrioventricular connections as defined previously. (The definition of the other connections will be given later.) As Van Praagh and coworkers initially indicated (16), the ventricular mass in hearts with biventricular atrioventricular connections can only be arranged in one of two topologic patterns. One is for the right ventricle to wrap itself round the left ventricle in right-to-left fashion from inlet to outlet. The other is for it to wrap itself round the left ventricle in left-to-right fashion. These were the arrangements initially called "d-loop" and "l-loop." Bargeron (20) has suggested that these patterns could be represented by the palmar surface of the hand applied to the septal surface of the morphologically right ventricle (Fig. 22.41). Thinking figuratively and trying to place the thumb in the inlet and the fingers in the outlet with the wrist in the apical trabecular component, the d-loop ventricular mass will accept only the palmar surface of the right hand on the septal surface of its morphologically right ventricle. This is the case irrespective of the position of the ventricular mass in space. The left ventricle in such hearts will then accept the palmar surface of the left hand in like fashion and the septum will, figuratively speaking, be sandwiched between the palms of the hands. In a similar way, the l-loop pattern will accept only the left hand in the morphologically

right and the right hand in the morphologically left ventricles. Following this concept, we describe these patterns as right-hand and left-hand topology, respectively. In hearts with concordant or discordant atrioventricular connections, it is rarely necessary to specify separately the topologic pattern of the ventricular mass because the topology is harmonious with the connection even in the presence of rotational malformations (crisscross hearts or superoinferior ventricles). There are rare hearts, however, with disharmonious patterns (21). Thus, a heart with usual atrial arrangement and a concordant atrioventricular connection can rarely exhibit a left-hand pattern of ventricular topology. To avoid confusion in this circumstance, it is essential to describe each feature of the heart in clear and unambiguous fashion. The concept of ventricular topology is important for full understanding of the morphology of congenitally malformed hearts. This systematic approach helps in the description of the third type of biventricular atrioventricular connection that is ambiguous (10).

When hearts with isomeric atrial chambers have each isomeric atrium connected to its own ventricle, it is impossible to use either concordant or discordant to describe the atrioventricular connection. This is because half the heart will be concordantly connected

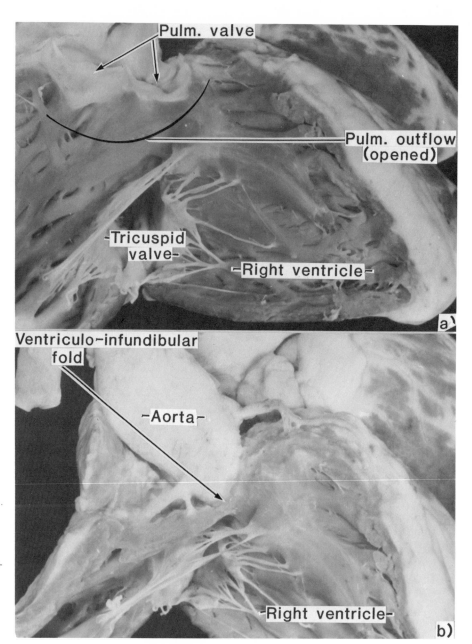

Figure 22.33. The right ventricle is displayed in (A) to show the musculature supporting the pulmonary (Pulm.) valve. Removal of this muscular sleeve in (B) reveals the ventriculoinfundibular fold and the aorta behind it.

and the other half will have a discordant atrioventricular connection, irrespective of the presence of right or left isomerism or of right-hand or left-hand ventricular topology (Fig. 22.42). A biventricular atrioventricular connection in hearts with atrial isomerism is, of necessity, ambiguous. To describe fully the ambiguous connection, it is necessary to specify both the type of isomerism and the topology of the ventricular mass. Therefore, the three types of biventricular atrioventricular connection are concordant, discordant, and ambiguous.

These patterns account for only half the possible variations in connection to be found at the atrioven-

tricular junction. There are three more types of connection that have this feature in common: They result in the atrial chambers' connecting to only one ventricle. Previously, there has been controversy about whether hearts with these connections should be described as "univentricular" or "single ventricle." Some of the hearts do possess a solitary chamber within the ventricular mass; but these are the minority. The feature uniting all these lesions is not the univentricular nature of the ventricular mass, but the univentricular arrangement of the atrioventricular connection (22). Hearts with such a univentricular atrioventricular connection can exist with any of the four possible

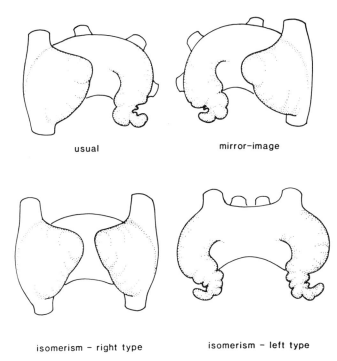

usual   mirror-image

isomerism – right type   isomerism – left type

Figure 22.34. Diagram showing the four possible atrial arrangements.

atrial arrangements (Fig. 22.43). The three specific patterns at the atrioventricular junction are double-inlet ventricle and absent right and absent left atrioventricular connection (Figs. 22.44, 22.45, and 22.46). The atrioventricular junction itself, with any of these three patterns and with any atrial arrangement, can be

connected to one of three possible morphologies in the ventricular mass. The first is a dominant left ventricle with a rudimentary right ventricle (Fig. 22.47). The second is a dominant right ventricle with a rudimentary left ventricle (Fig. 22.48). Finally, there may be a solitary ventricle of indeterminate morphology (Fig. 22.49). Variations also exist in the relational morphology of these masses. In hearts with dominant right or left ventricles, the rudimentary ventricle may be so small as to be unrecognizable using clinical diagnostic techniques. When the rudimentary ventricle is recognized, the interrelationship between it and the dominant ventricle is variable in terms of right-left positioning. Without exception, however, rudimentary right ventricles are positioned anterosuperiorly, and rudimentary left ventricles are found posteroinferiorly, relative to the dominant ventricle. Combining all this information to describe any heart with a univentricular atrioventricular connection, it is essential to specify the atrial arrangement, the type of connection, the pattern of the ventricular mass, and the relationship of the ventricles. The ventricular relationships can be specified in most instances according to the ventricular topology. This is not always the case, and so our preference is to specify the sidedness of the rudimentary ventricle relative to the dominant ventricle.

In this context, it is also necessary to clarify the place of atrioventricular valve atresias. It is often thought that tricuspid or mitral valve atresia is produced by an imperforate valve membrane that sepa-

Figure 22.35. A short-axis section through the atrial chambers at the level of the appendages shows the distinctive morphologic features.

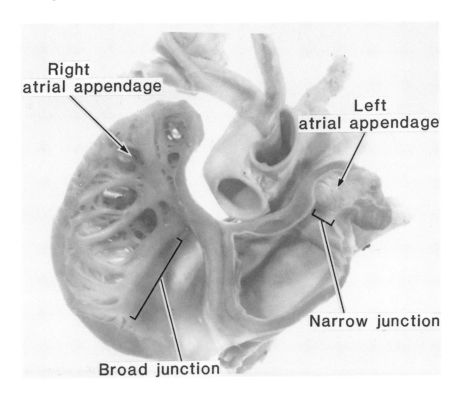

Right atrial appendage

Left atrial appendage

Broad junction

Narrow junction

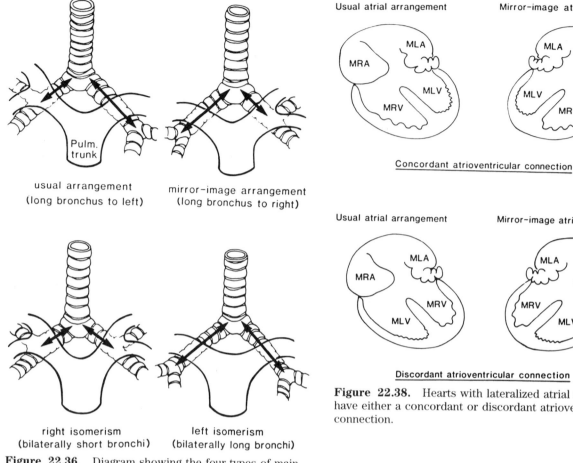

usual arrangement
(long bronchus to left)

mirror-image arrangement
(long bronchus to right)

right isomerism
(bilaterally short bronchi)

left isomerism
(bilaterally long bronchi)

Figure 22.36. Diagram showing the four types of main bronchial patterns corresponding to the atrial arrangements. Pulm. = pulmonary.

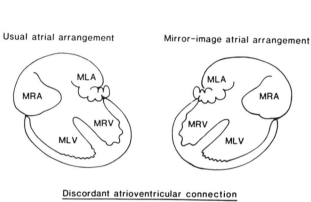

Usual atrial arrangement

Mirror-image atrial arrangement

Concordant atrioventricular connection

Usual atrial arrangement

Mirror-image atrial arrangement

Discordant atrioventricular connection

Figure 22.38. Hearts with lateralized atrial arrangement have either a concordant or discordant atrioventricular connection.

Figure 22.37. The arrangement of the abdominal great vessels just below the diaphragm can also give some clues to the atrial arrangement. Ant = anterior; L = left; Post = posterior; R = right.

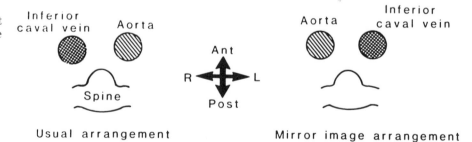

Usual arrangement

Mirror image arrangement

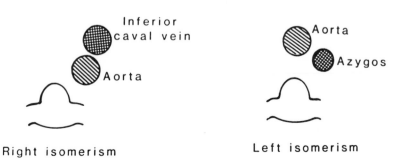

Right isomerism

Left isomerism

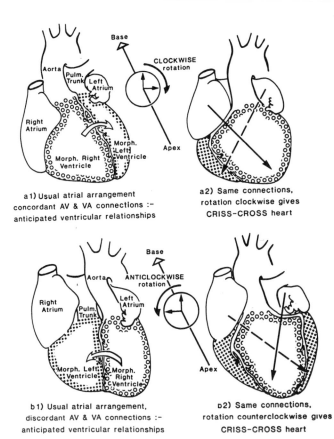

a1) Usual atrial arrangement concordant AV & VA connections :- anticipated ventricular relationships

a2) Same connections, rotation clockwise gives CRISS-CROSS heart

b1) Usual atrial arrangement, discordant AV & VA connections :- anticipated ventricular relationships

b2) Same connections, rotation counterclockwise gives CRISS-CROSS heart

Figure 22.39. Crisscross hearts can be produced either by a clockwise rotation along the long axis of the ventricular mass in hearts with usual chamber arrangements or by an anticlockwise rotation in hearts with usual atrial arrangement but discordant atrioventricular (AV) and ventriculoarterial (VA) connections. Morph. = morphologically; Pulm. = pulmonary.

rates the blind-ending atrium from the underlying hypoplastic but appropriate ventricle. Such arrangements do exist (Fig. 22.50), but are very rare. In most instances, the valve atresia exists because of complete absence of one or other atrioventricular connection. The floor of the blind-ending atrium is completely

muscular and is separated from the underlying ventricular mass by the fibrofatty tissue of the atrioventricular groove (Figs. 22.45 and 22.46). Tricuspid atresia almost always exists with the left atrium connected to a dominant left ventricle and an anterosuperior rudimentary right ventricle. The floor of the right atrial appendage may sometimes overlie the rudimentary ventricle in this pattern (Fig. 22.51) and give the spurious echocardiographic impression of a connection between the two. However, the atrium and rudimentary ventricle are always separated by sulcus tissue. Mitral atresia is almost always produced by absence of the left atrioventricular connection with the right atrium connected to a dominant right ventricle with a posteroinferior, left-sided, rudimentary left ventricle (Fig. 22.46). A similar arrangement in terms of left atrial anatomy is produced when the left atrioventricular connection is absent and the right atrium is connected to a dominant left ventricle (Fig. 22.52A). In the latter circumstance, there is usually a rudimentary right ventricle present in an anteriosuperior and left-sided position (Fig. 22.52B).

Mode of Atrioventricular Connection

During analysis of the type of atrioventricular connection, note should be taken of the leaflet morphology of the valves at the atrioventricular junction. The arrangement of these valves bears no relation to the type of connection present. The type of connection only describes the fashion in which the distal segments of atrial muscle are or are not connected to ventricular myocardium at the atrioventricular junction. For example, in hearts in which both atria connect with the ventricular mass (concordant, discordant, ambiguous, and double-inlet connections), the valve leaflets can usually be removed in their entirety without affecting the potential of recognizing the type of connection present. Yet the morphology of the leaflets is a highly

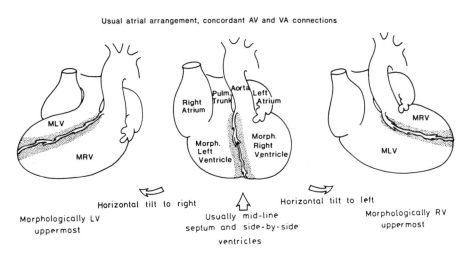

Usual atrial arrangement, concordant AV and VA connections

Morphologically LV uppermost

Horizontal tilt to right

Usually mid-line septum and side-by-side ventricles

Horizontal tilt to left

Morphologically RV uppermost

Figure 22.40. Tilting of the ventricular mass along its long axis produces hearts with superoinferior ventricles. AV = atrioventricular; LV = left ventricle; MLV = morphologically left ventricle; Morph. = morphologically; MRV = morphologically right ventricle; RV = right ventricle.

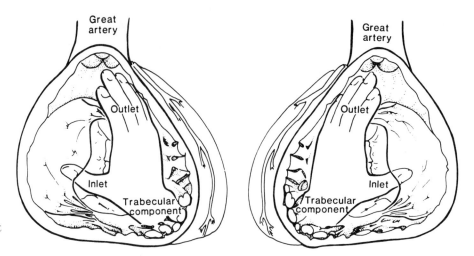

Figure 22.41. Diagram showing how the ventricular topology can be ascertained by positioning the palm against the septal surface of the morphologically right ventricle with the thumb pointing to the inlet and the fingers to the outlet.

significant feature of the junction. We recognize this significance by describing leaflet morphology as a discrete feature of the junction, namely the mode of connection. In the arrangements previously discussed (in which both atria are connected with the ventricular mass), the two atrioventricular junctions can be guarded by two separate atrioventricular valves or by a common valve. When two valves are present, each is usually patent but one can be imperforate. An imper-

forate valve produces a rare variant of atrioventricular valve atresia, and such an imperforate membrane can be found with either concordant, discordant, ambiguous, or double-inlet types of connection. One of the two valves (or rarely both) can also straddle the ventricular septum. Straddling is defined as valvar tension apparatus attached to both sides of the ventricular septum (Fig. 22.53). When a valve straddles, it is usual for the

Ambiguous atrioventricular connection

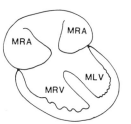

Right atrial isomerism, right-hand ventricular topology

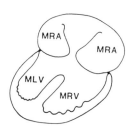

Right atrial isomerism, left-hand ventricular topology

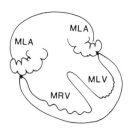

Left atrial isomerism, right-hand ventricular topology

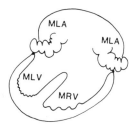

Left atrial isomerism, left-hand ventricular topology

Figure 22.42. The atrioventricular connection in hearts with isomeric atrial chambers is described by stating the type of isomerism together with the ventricular topology. MLA = morphologically left atrium; MLV = morphologically left ventricle; MRA = morphologically right atrium; MRV = morphologically right ventricle.

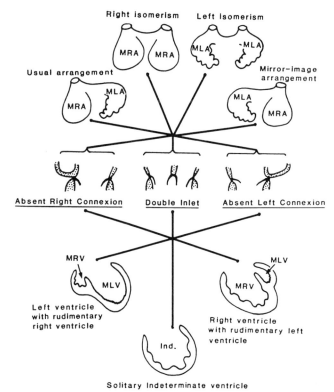

Figure 22.43. Hearts with absence of one atrioventricular connection and hearts with double-inlet connection can exist with any of the four possible atrial arrangements and any of three arrangements of the ventricular mass. Ind. = indeterminate; MLA = morphologically left atrium; MLV = morphologically left ventricle; MRA = morphologically right atrium; MRV = morphologically right ventricle.

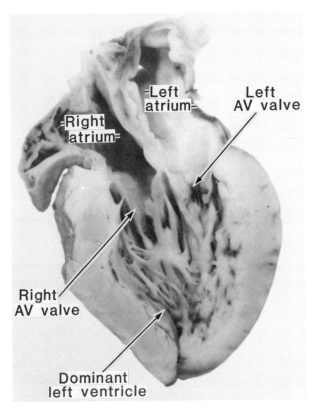

Figure 22.44. A long-axis section through a heart with double-inlet connection shows both atria opening into a dominant morphologically left ventricle. AV = atrioventricular.

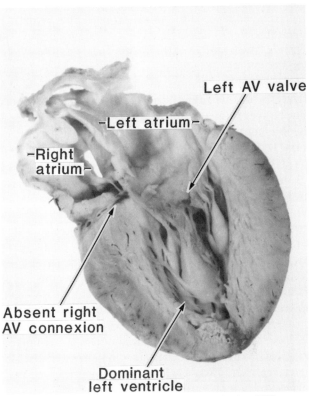

Figure 22.45. An absent right atrioventricular (AV) connection is shown in this long-axis section. The muscular right atrial floor is separated from the ventricular mass by fibrofatty tissue of the AV groove.

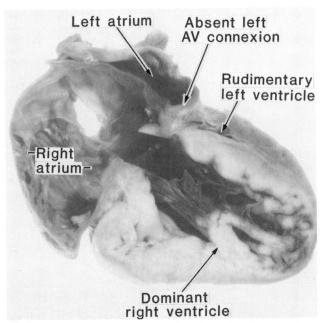

Figure 22.46. A long-axis section through a heart with absent left atrioventricular (AV) connection shows the right atrium opening into a dominant morphologically right ventricle. The left atrium has no egress to the slitlike rudimentary left ventricle.

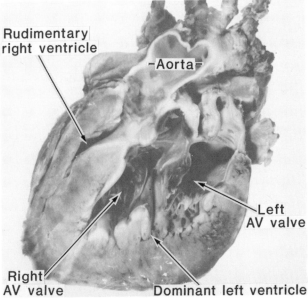

Figure 22.47. The rudimentary right ventricle is situated anterosuperiorly in this heart with double-inlet left ventricle. AV = atrioventricular.

atrioventricular junction supporting the straddling leaflets to be connected to both ventricles. This biventricular atrioventricular connection of one junction is termed "override." Overriding of a valve junction is not strictly a mode of connection, since the precise degree of override can change the type of connection. All hearts with overriding atrioventricular junctions produce a spectrum of anomalies between the extremes of double-inlet and biventricular atrioventricular connections (Fig. 22.54). Such overriding could be categorized as a specific type of connection, but the potential chamber connections in the presence of overriding are legion. We therefore split the spectrum of override at its midpoint (the 50% law). Thus, a heart with an overriding atrioventricular valve is cataloged in terms of its atrioventricular connection as a double-inlet ventricle or as a heart with concordant, discordant, or ambiguous atrioventricular connection, according to the precise chamber arrangements and the precise degree of override of the shared junction.

A common valve usually straddles in the setting of an atrioventricular septal defect. It may also be connected exclusively to one ventricle in the setting of double-inlet ventricle. Hearts with such common valves may also exhibit a spectrum between double-inlet and biventricular atrioventricular connections. It is more difficult to divide this spectrum to determine the connections than it is when only one junction overrides. Rarely, either the right or the left component of a common valve can be imperforate, resulting in a further mode of connection.

The Ventriculoarterial Junction

Analysis of the ventriculoarterial junction is similar to that for the atrioventricular junction. Attention is given primarily to the type of connection (the way in which the arterial trunks are connected to the ventricular mass). At the same time, note is taken of the mode of connection (the morphology of the arterial valves guarding the ventriculoarterial junction) while ignoring neither the arrangement of the outflow tract musculature (infundibular morphology) nor the relationships of the arterial trunks.

Types of Ventriculoarterial Connection

Just as the possible atrioventricular connections are conditioned by atrial morphology and the number of atria connected to the ventricles, the ventriculoarterial connections are determined by the arrangement of the arterial trunks and the number of ventricles to which they are connected (Table 22.3). There are only two possible arrangements in which one of the two ventricles is connected to its own great artery. The arterial trunks can be connected to either morphologically appropriate or inappropriate ventricles (Fig. 22.55). The connection to appropriate ventricles is concordant, while connection to inappropriate ventricles is discordant. In both circumstances, the connections are diagnosed as concordant or discordant irrespective of the relationships of the arterial trunks or the nature of the outflow tract musculature.

The options are slightly increased when there are

Figure 22.48.   The rudimentary left ventricle is located posteroinferiorly in this heart with absence of the left atrioventricular connection.

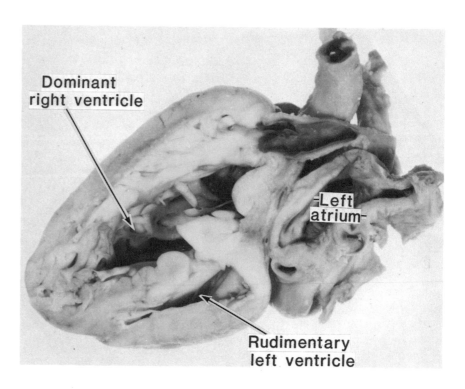

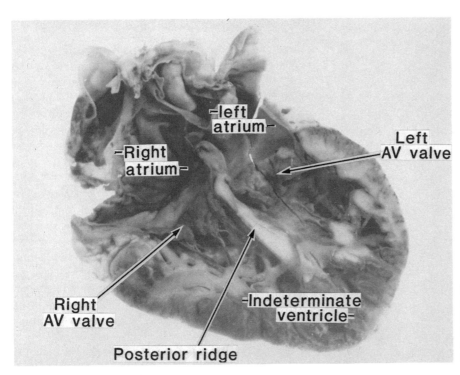

Figure 22.49. A long-axis section of this heart shows double inlet to a ventricular chamber of indeterminate morphology. A posterior ridge is situated between the two atrioventricular (AV) valves.

two arterial trunks connected to the same ventricle (Fig. 22.56). This arrangement may be found when the ventricle supporting the trunks is of right, left, or indeterminate morphology. Double-outlet ventricle is also best diagnosed irrespective of the arterial relationships or outflow tract morphology. The final group of ventriculoarterial connections are those in which only one arterial trunk takes origin from the ventricular mass (Fig. 22.24). Single outlet of the heart can be produced by a common arterial trunk exiting from the heart through a common valve. Alternatively, the solitary trunk may be either an aorta or a pulmonary trunk in circumstances where it is impossible to ascertain the ventricular origin of the complementary but atretic arterial trunk. Pulmonary or aortic atresia should not be catalogued as single outlet when it is possible to

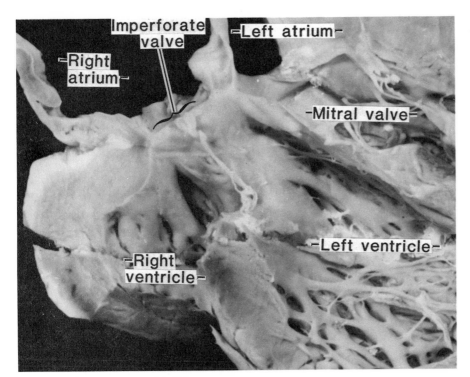

Figure 22.50. An imperforate valve membrane interposing between the right atrium and right ventricle produces tricuspid atresia.

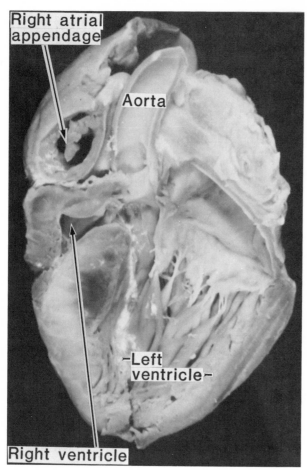

Figure 22.51. A long-axis section through a heart with absence of the right atrioventricular connection shows the right atrial appendage overlying the rudimentary right ventricle.

determine a ventricular origin for the atretic trunk (see next section). There is one further arrangement that produces single outlet of the heart. This occurs when a solitary trunk exits from the ventricular mass, and pulmonary blood supply is exclusively through systemic-pulmonary collateral arteries, with complete absence of intrapericardial remnants of the pulmonary trunk and its branches (truncus type IV). In this circumstance, it is impossible to determine whether the trunk connected to the ventricles is an aorta or a common trunk (23). It is most accurate to describe it simply as a solitary arterial trunk.

In all of the arrangements with single outlet, description of the connection remains imprecise. This is because the arterial trunk, whatever its nature, may be connected exclusively to a right or left ventricle, may override a septal defect between ventricles, or may take origin from a solitary and indeterminate ventricle. Full description of single outlet, therefore, requires documentation of the precise ventricle or ventricles to which the trunk is connected.

Mode of Ventriculoarterial Connection

The modes of connection are much more limited at the ventriculoarterial than at the atrioventricular junction. First, this is because arterial valves have only semi-lunar attachments to the junction, lack tension apparatus, and therefore cannot straddle. The second reason limiting the options is that a common arterial valve can exist only in the presence of a common arterial trunk. It is not a possible mode of connection when there are two separate arterial trunks. The possible modes of connection consequently involve two arterial valves. Usually both valves are patent, but one or other may be imperforate. An imperforate valve can exist with concordant, discordant, or double-outlet connections and will produce arterial valve atresia in those particular settings. As with the atrioventricular valves, an arterial valve may override the septum so as to have connections with both ventricles. This will result in a spectrum of abnormalities between concordant or discordant connections and a double-outlet connection. We break this spectrum at its midpoint and assign the overriding arterial valve to the ventricle which supports its greatest circumference (the 50% law). From this approach, it follows that our definition of a double-outlet connection is "more than half of both arterial valves connected to the same ventricle."

Arterial Relationships and Infundibular Morphology

Arterial relationships and infundibular morphology of the ventriculoarterial junction have been considered to be important in the determination and naming of ventriculoarterial connections. For example, the presence of a bilateral infundibulum was regarded as the hallmark of a double-outlet connection, and a right-sided and anterior aorta was believed to be so charac-

Table 22.3. Ventriculoarterial Connections

A. With each ventricle connected to a separate arterial trunk
  Concordant VA connection
  Discordant VA connection
B. With both arterial trunks connected predominantly to one ventricle
  Double outlet right ventricle
  Double outlet left ventricle
  Double outlet from solitary and indeterminate ventricle
C. With only one arterial trunk connected to ventricular mass common arterial trunk
  Solitary aortic trunk with absent pulmonary–ventricular connection
  Solitary pulmonary trunk with absent atrioventricular connection
  Solitary arterial trunk with absent intrapericardial pulmonary arteries
  (The solitary or common trunk may straddle the septum or be committed exclusively to right, left, or indeterminate ventricles)

VA = ventriculoarterial.

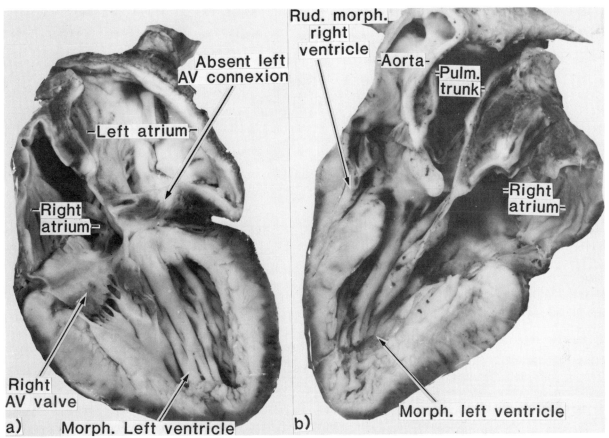

Figure 22.52. Two long-axis sections of a heart with absence of the left atrioventricular (AV) connection show the right atrium connecting with a morphologically (Morph., morph.) left ventricle in (A) and the anterosuperior position of the rudimentary (Rud.) right ventricle in (B). Compare with Figure 22.46. Pulm. = pulmonary.

teristic of complete transposition that it was referred to simply as d-transposition. Cross-sectional echocardiography has demonstrated that ventriculoarterial connections are best defined directly and that they are independent of both arterial relationships and infundi-

bular morphology. Nonetheless, the latter two features retain their place in the description of congenitally malformed hearts.

Arterial relationships are infinitely variable. They can be influenced by rotation of the heart within the thorax

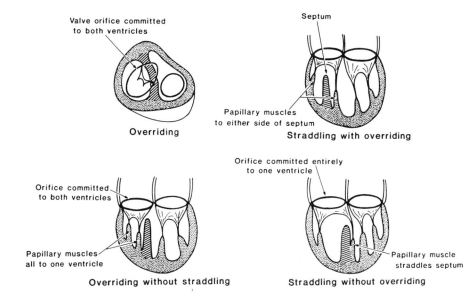

Figure 22.53. Diagrams showing the differences between straddling and overriding of an atrioventricular valve.

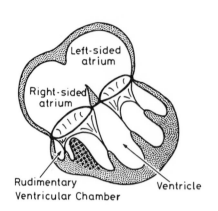

Figure 22.54. The degree of override of an atrioventricular (AV) valve can change the AV connection from that of double inlet to one of the biventricular variants.

Double Inlet AV Connexion

Concordant, discordant or ambiguous AV connexion

as well as by the presence of congenital lesions. Indeed, the often confusing crisscross heart simply represents a lesion where either the arterial or ventricular relationships are not as expected for a given atrioventricular or ventriculoarterial connection. We describe the variability in arterial relationships by combining right, left, anterior, and posterior coordinates to give the options shown in Figure 22.57. Others have expressed this information in terms of degrees of a circle (20). We describe the position of the aorta relative to the pulmonary trunk. Infundibular morphology, in contrast to arterial relationships, has a strictly limited number of options. A complete muscular infundibulum exists when the entire circumference of an arterial valve is supported by outflow tract musculature and there is no fibrous continuity either between an arterial and an atrioventricular valve or between the two arterial valves themselves. The possible options

are a complete subpulmonary infundibulum and aortic-atrioventricular valve fibrous continuity (the usual finding); a complete subaortic infundibulum with pulmonary-atrioventricular continuity (the expected arrangement with a discordant ventriculoarterial connection); and a bilaterally complete subarterial infundibulum (the most common pattern with double-outlet right ventricle) or a bilaterally deficient infundibulum (the pattern seen most frequently with double-outlet left ventricle). These patterns provide only a guide to the precise connection present.

Abnormal Cardiac Positions

This segmental approach (16) demonstrates that an abnormal cardiac position is not a diagnosis in itself. Any cardiac malformation or chamber connection can exist in the setting of a malpositioned heart. Con-

Figure 22.55. The ventriculoarterial (VA) connections are designated concordant or discordant depending on whether the arterial trunks are connected to the appropriate or inappropriate ventricles. Ao = aorta; MLV = morphologically left ventricle; MRV = morphologically right ventricle; PT = pulmonary trunk.

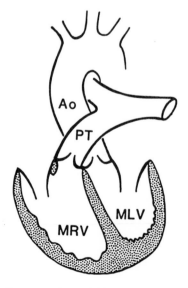

Concordant VA connection

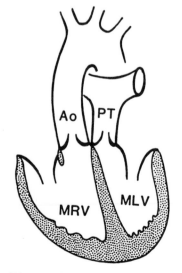

Discordant VA connection

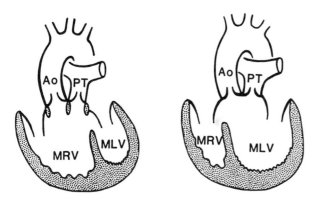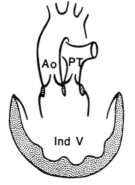

Figure 22.56. When both arterial trunks are connected to the same ventricle, there is double-outlet venticuloarterial connection from either a morphologically right ventricle (MRV), a morphologically left ventricle (MLV), or an indeterminate ventricle (Ind V). Ao = aorta; PT = pulmonary trunk.

versely, the malpositioned heart can be found in the absence of any intracardiac lesion. Malposition, however, will entail the use of unusual echocardiographic views to decipher the lesions present. We find it more straightforward to describe the malpositioned heart without recourse to terms such as "dextrocardia" and "levocardia." We simply state whether the heart is in the left chest, the midline, or the right chest and describe the orientation of the cardiac apex separately (left sided, midline, or right sided). The finding of an abnormally positioned heart should immediately alert the investigator to the likely presence of an abnormal arrangement of the body organs (mirror-image arrangement or, more probably, right or left isomerism). If the thoracoabdominal organs (including the atrial chambers) are usually arranged, a discordant atrioventricular connection ("corrected transposition") will be high on the list of anticipated lesions. None of these features, however, can be inferred from the abnormal position of the heart.

CONCLUSION

This chapter provides the basic anatomic principles for diagnosis and the accurate description of congenitally malformed hearts. The development of the segmental approach together with the advent of cross-sectional echocardiography has shown that diagnosis of even the most complicated lesion is a simple procedure for those who can distinguish the atrial and ventricular chambers and the arterial trunks. The sophistication in diagnosis now provided by cross-sectional echocardiography demands equal precision in description and nomenclature.

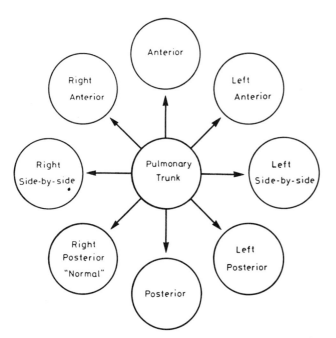

Figure 22.57. The spatial relationship of the aorta to the pulmonary trunk can be described in terms of right, left, anterior, and posterior coordinates.

REFERENCES

1. Tajik AJ, Seward JB, Hagler DJ, Mair DD, Lie JT. Two-dimensional real-time ultrasonic imaging of the heart and great vessels. Technique, image orientation, structure identification, and validation. Mayo Clin Proc 1978;53:271–303.
2. Silverman NH, Hunter S, Anderson RH, Ho SY, Sutherland GR, Davies MJ. Anatomical basis of cross sectional echocardiography. Br Heart J 1983;50:421–30.
3. Lev M. Pathologic diagnosis of positional variations in cardiac chambers in congenital heart disease. Lab Invest 1954;3:71–82.
4. Van Praagh R, David I, Van Praagh S. What is a ventricle? The single ventricle trap unsprung. Ped Cardiol 1982;2:79–84.
5. Scalia D, Russo P, Anderson RH, et al. The surgical anatomy of hearts with no direct communication between the right atrium and the ventricular mass—so-called tricuspid atresia. J Thorac Cardiovasc Surg 1984;87:743–55.
6. Penkoske PA, Neches WH, Anderson RH, Zuberbuhler JR. Further observations on the morphology of atrioventricular septal defects. J Thorac Cardiovasc Surg 1985;90:611–22.
7. Anderson RH, Zuberbuhler JR, Penkoske PA, Neches WH. Of clefts, commissures and things. J Thorac Cardiovasc Surg 1985; 90:605–10.
8. Hagler DJ, Edwards WD, Seward JB, Tajik AJ. Standardized nomenclature of the ventricular septum and ventricular septal defects, with applications for two-dimensional echocardiography. Mayo Clin Proc 1985;60:741–52.
9. Soto B, Becker AE, Moulaert AJ, Lie JT, Anderson RH. Classification of ventricular septal defects. Br Heart J 1980;43:332–43.
10. Anderson RH, Becker AE, Freedom RM, et al. Sequential segmental analysis of congenital heart disease. Ped Cardiol 1984;5:281–8.

11. Van Mierop LHS, Gessner IH, Schiebler GL. Asplenia and polysplenia syndromes. Birth Defects 1972;8:36–44.
12. Chin AJ, Williams RG. Determination of atrial situs by 2-dimensional echocardiographic imaging of atrial appendage morphology. In: Doyle EF, Engle MA, Gersony WM, Rashkind WJ, Talner NS, eds. Abstracts. Second World Congress of Pediatric Cardiology. June 2–6 1985. New York: Springer-Verlag, 1985:63.
13. Macartney FJ, Zuberbuhler JR, Anderson RH. Morphological considerations pertaining to recognition of atrial isomerism. Consequences for sequential chamber localisation. Br Heart J 1980;44:657–67.
14. Deanfield J, Leanage R, Stroobant J, Chrispin AR, Taylor JFN, Macartney FJ. Use of high kilovoltage filtered beam radiographs for detection of bronchial situs in infants and young children. Br Heart J 1980;44:577–83.
15. Huhta JC, Smallhorn JF, Macartney FJ. Two dimensional echocardiographic diagnosis of situs. Br Heart J 1982;48:97–108.
16. Van Praagh R, Van Praagh S, Vlad P, Keith JD. Anatomic types of congenital dextrocardia. Diagnostic and embryologic implications. Am J Cardiol 1964;13:510–31.
17. Van Praagh R. Diagnosis of complex congenital heart disease: morphologic-anatomic method and terminology. Cardiovasc Intervent Radiol 1984;7:115–20.
18. Shinebourne EA, Macartney FJ, Anderson RH. Sequential chamber localization—logical approach to diagnosis in congenital heart disease. Br Heart J 1976;38:327–40.
19. Kirklin JW, Pacifico AD, Bargeron LM, Soto B. Cardiac repair in anatomically corrected malposition of the great arteries. Circulation 1973;48:153–9.
20. Bargeron LM Jr. Angiographic recognition of specific anatomic structures. In: Becker AE, Losekoot G, Marcelletti C, Anderson RH, eds. Paediatric cardiology. Vol. 3. Edinburgh: Churchill Livingstone, 1981:33–47.
21. Weinberg PM, Van Praagh R, Wagner HR, Cuaso CC. New form of criss-cross atrioventricular relation: an expanded view of the meaning of D and L-loops. Abstract Book of World Congress of Paediatric Cardiology, London, 1980:319.
22. Anderson RH, Becker AE, Tynan M, Macartney FJ, Rigby ML, Wilkinson JL. The univentricular atrioventricular connection: getting to the root of a thorny problem. Am J Cardiol 1984;54: 822–8.
23. Thiene G, Anderson RH. Pulmonary atresia with ventricular septal defect. Anatomy. In: Anderson RH, Macartney FJ, Shinebourne EA, Tynan MJ, eds. Paediatric cardiology. Vol. 5. Edinburgh: Churchill Livingstone, 1983:80–101.

23
Venous Abnormalities

Donald Hagler

A segmental approach to the accurate description of complex congenital heart disease has been encouraged by pathologic, angiographic, and echocardiographic studies (1–6). With two-dimensional echocardiographic techniques this approach provides a logical sequential review for practical assessment of complex anatomic abnormalities. This systematic approach may be particularly important in planning cardiac catheterization procedures and/or surgical correction.

Abnormalities of visceral and atrial arrangements (situs) are frequently associated with abnormalities of systemic and pulmonary venous connection. Abnormal pulmonary venous connections are described in Chapter 24. Initial examination with subcostal long- and short-axis scans defines the arrangement and connection of the hepatic and inferior venae cavae. A review of the cross-sectional anatomy at the level of the diaphragm allows recognition of the arrangement of the organs (visceral situs), venous connections, and associated abnormalities (Fig. 23.1) and provides the basis for the two-dimensional echocardiographic examination. The diaphragm and the peritoneal reflection are important landmarks in recognizing intraperitoneal or retroperitoneal location of the inferior vena cava or azygos-hemiazygos continuation (Fig. 23.1 and 23.2).

The liver can be easily demonstrated with subcostal short-axis scans. Right-to-left scanning techniques allow recognition of appropriate transducer orientation and right-to-left arrangement of the abdominal organs. The liver is detected predominantly in the right and left abdominal quadrants, with situs solitus and situs inversus, respectively (Figs. 23.2A and 23.2B). Figure 23.3 shows a scan to the left to demonstrate hepatic and venous drainage in mirror-image arrangement. A large midline liver has been associated with abdominal heterotaxy and atrial isomerism (Figs. 23.1C, D and 23.2C, D). The more midline location of the abdominal aorta should also be noted (Figs. 23.1 and 23.2C).

Long-axis scans demonstrate the size and course of the abdominal vascular structures (Figs. 23.4 and 23.5). The abdominal aorta may be recognized by its pulsatile appearance on real-time examination and confirmed by the high blood-flow velocity profile with pulsed wave Doppler (Fig. 23.6). The celiac and superior mesenteric arterial branches may be additionally helpful landmarks for identification. Accurate definition of the inferior vena cava with its intraperitoneal course as the azygos-hemiazygos continuation is important for subsequent invasive procedures and surgical correction. The hepatic venous drainage and its atrial connection should be demonstrated when visceral heterotaxy (atrial isomerism) is present. Right or left parasternal long-axis scans may be used to demonstrate the retroperitoneal course of the azygos-hemiazygos continuation of the inferior to the superior caval veins (Fig. 23.7A). Multiple sites of hepatic venous drainage are common with atrial isomerism and should be defined for surgical procedures such as the modified Fontan type of correction (Fig. 23.7B). Separate inferior caval and atrial hepatic venous connections also have been recognized.

Suprasternal notch scans frequently allow precise depiction of venous anomalies of the superior vena cava. A wide spectrum of venous anomalies may be encountered—from bilateral veins to atresia of the normal right-sided superior vena cava, and persistence on the contralateral side. Anomalies of the superior vena cava have little predictive value for atrial or visceral arrangement but are important for surgical correction. Suprasternal notch short-axis scans demonstrate the presence of bilateral superior vena cava and connecting innominate vein, when present (Fig. 23.8). Occasionally, an aberrant course of the innominate vein beneath the aortic arch may be recognized in the presence of a right-sided aortic arch. Left high parasternal long-axis scans may help demonstrate the mediastinal course of a persistent left superior vena cava to the left atrium or via the coronary sinus to the right atrium (Fig. 23.7A).

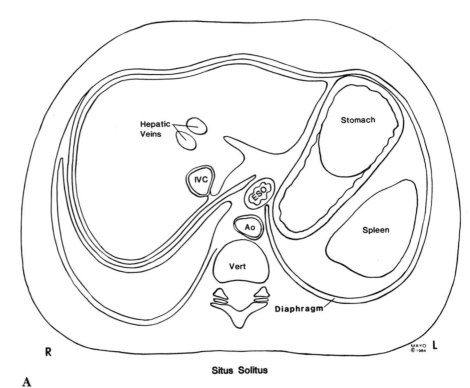

Situs Solitus

A

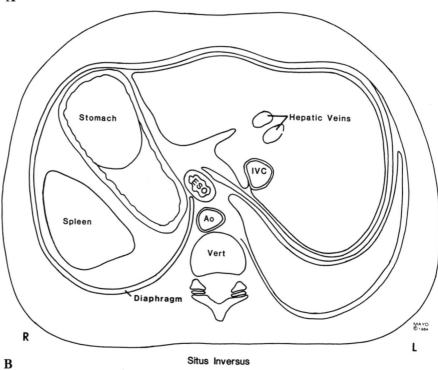

Figure 23.1. Anatomic cross
sections at level of diaphragm
demonstrate visceral and vascular
relationships in situs solitus (*A*),
mirror-image arrangement (situs
inversus) (*B*), and situs ambiguous
(*C* and *D*). Note that the diaphragm
demarcates intraperitoneal from
retroperitoneal structures. Thus, in
(*D*), hemiazygos continuation of
inferior vena cava (IVC) is in retroperitoneal location. Ao = abdominal aorta; ESO = esophagus;
Vert = vertebral body. (Reproduced by permission of the Mayo
Foundation.)

B

Situs Inversus

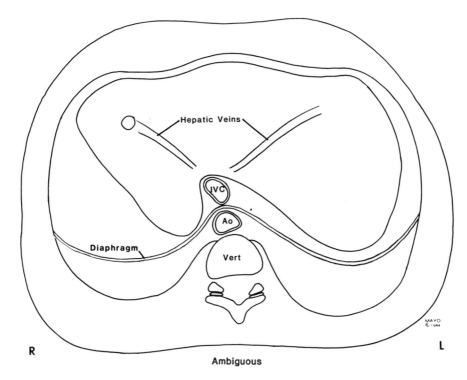

C

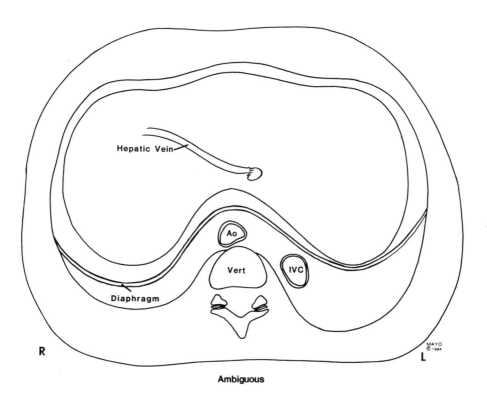

D

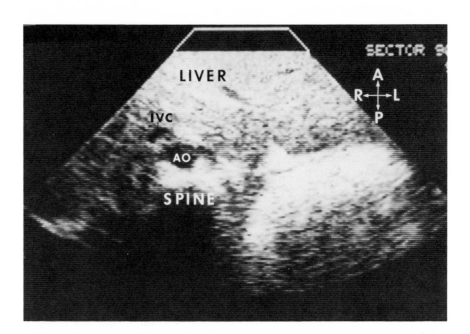

A

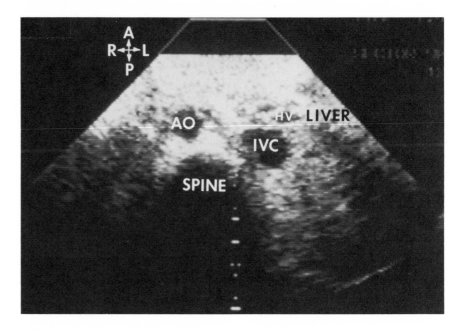

Figure 23.2. Similar two-dimensional echocardiographic cross sections (short axis) at the level of diaphragm in situs solitus (*A*), situs inversus (*B*), situs ambiguous (*C* and *D*). Note that liver mass is to right, to left, and at midline, respectively. A = anterior; AO = abdominal aorta; H-A = hemiazygos continuation of inferior vena cava; HV = hepatic vein; IVC = inferior vena cava; L = left; P = posterior; R = right.

B

The venous connections may be precisely defined with contrast echocardiographic techniques by injection, preferably of a bolus of indocyanine green dye followed by a saline flush, into the right or left brachial vein (Fig. 23.9). Persistence of the left superior vena cava to the coronary sinus may be suggested by the presence of a dilated coronary sinus on parasternal long-axis scans. Injection of contrast medium into the left brachial vein confirms the initial appearance of contrast material in the coronary sinus and subsequently in the right atrium. An unroofed coronary sinus may allow early appearance of contrast material in the left atrium if systemic venous pressures are high.

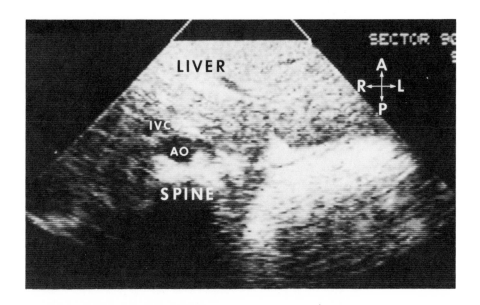

A

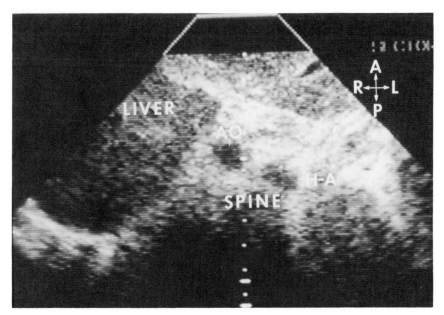

B

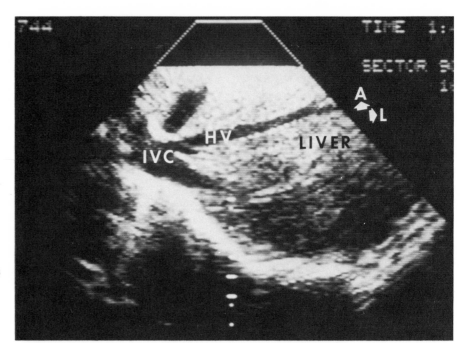

Figure 23.3. Subcostal short-axis view demonstrating left-sided liver in situs inversus, with common drainage of hepatic veins (HV) to left-sided inferior vena cava (IVC). A = anterior; L = left.

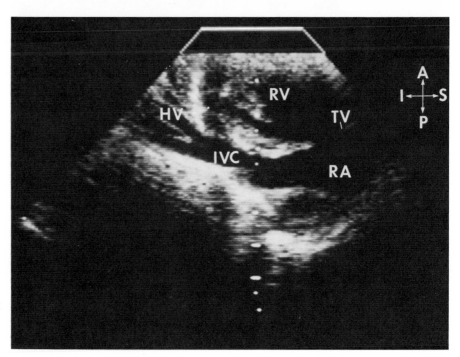

Figure 23.4. Subcostal long-axis view with transducer tilted to right atrium (RA) shows joint drainage of hepatic vein (HV) and inferior vena cava (IVC) to RA in patient with a right-sided heart and usual atrial arrangement. A = anterior; I = inferior; P = posterior; RV = right ventricle; S = superior; TV = tricuspid valve.

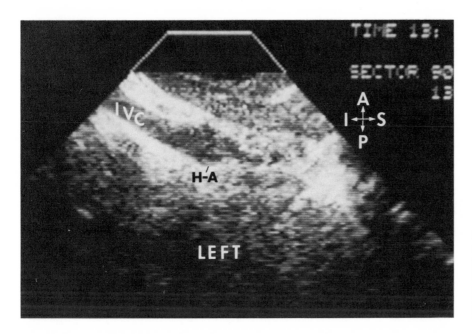

Figure 23.5. Subcostal long-axis scan obtained with transducer tilted to left in patient with hemiazygos continuation (H-A) of an interrupted inferior vena cava (IVC). A = anterior; I = inferior; P = posterior; S = superior.

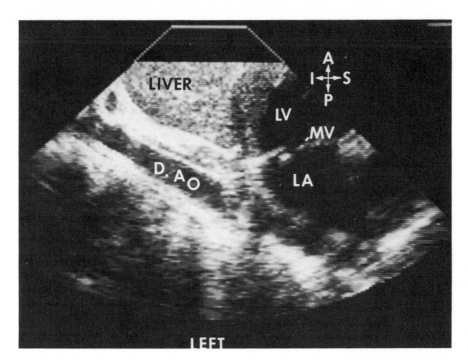

Figure 23.6. Subcostal long-axis scan obtained by tilting transducer slightly to left shows left-sided abdominal aorta. A = anterior; D. AO = descending abdominal aorta; I = inferior; LA = left atrium; LV = left ventricle; MV = mitral valve; P = posterior; S = superior.

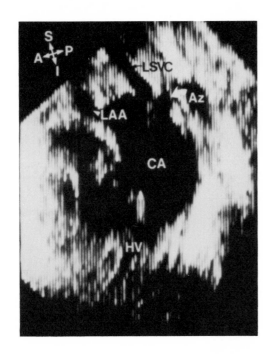

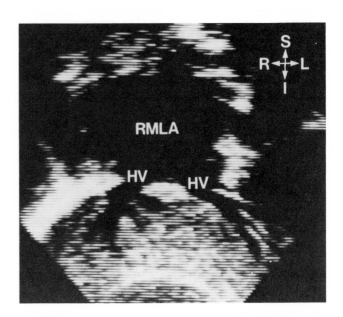

A   **B**

Figure 23.7.   (*A*) Parasternal view of venous connection to common atrium (CA) in left atrial isomerism and a right-sided heart. The left-sided azygos vein (Az) connects directly to left side of common atrium near junction of left superior vena cava (LSVC) but is separate from it. (*B*) Total anomalous hepatic venous connection via two separate hepatic veins (HV) in left atrial isomerism. Two veins connect to right-sided morphological left atrium (RMLA). Note isomeric appearance of HV in left atrial isomerism. A = anterior; I = inferior; L = left; LAA = right-sided morphologic left atrial appendage; P = posterior; R = right; S = superior. (Reproduced by permission from Huhta JC, Smallhorn JF, Macartney FJ, Anderson RH, DeLeval M. Cross-sectional echocardiographic diagnosis of systemic venous return. Br Heart J 1982;48:388–403.)

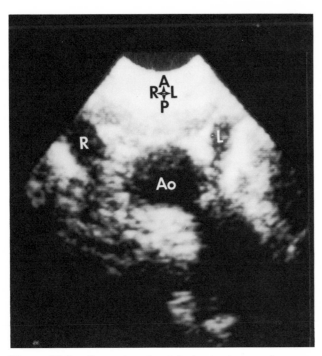

Figure 23.8.   Suprasternal notch short-axis scan demonstrates short-axis view of aortic arch (Ao). Note bilateral superior vena cava (R and L) with no apparent innominate communication.

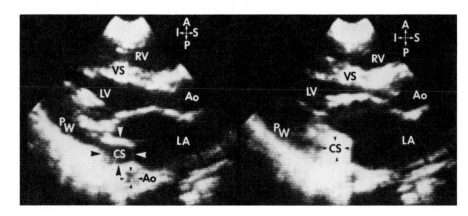

Figure 23.9. Parasternal left ventricular long-axis scan shows dilated coronary sinus (CS) consistent with persistent left superior vena cava. On right, note echocardiographic contrast appearance in coronary sinus after injection of indocyanine green in left-hand vein. A = anterior; Ao = aorta; I = inferior; LA = left atrium; LV = left ventricle; P = posterior; PW = posterior wall; RV = right ventricle; S = superior; VS = ventricular septum.

REFERENCES

1. Huhta JC, Hagler DJ, Seward JB, Tajik AJ, Julsrud PR, Ritter DG. Two-dimensional echocardiographic assessment of dextrocardia: a segmental approach. Am J Cardiol 1982;50:1351–60.
2. Hagler DJ, Tajik AJ, Seward JB, Mair DD, Ritter DG. Wide-angle two-dimensional echocardiographic profiles of conotruncal abnormalities. Mayo Clin Proc 1980;55:73–82.
3. Calcaterra G, Anderson RH, Lau KC, Shinebourne EA. Dextrocardia—value of segmental analysis in its categorisation. Br Heart J 1979;42:497–507.
4. Squarcia U, Ritter DG, Kincaid OW. Dextrocardia: angiocardiographic study and classification. Am J Cardiol 1973;32:965–77.
5. Solinger R, Elbl F, Minhas K. Deductive echocardiographic analysis in infants with congenital heart disease. Circulation 1974;50:1072–96.
6. Huhta JC, Smallhorn JF, Macartney FJ, Anderson RH, DeLeval M. Cross-sectional echocardiographic diagnosis of systemic venous return. Br Heart J 1982;48:388–403.

24
Total Anomalous Pulmonary Venous Connection

Jeffrey Smallhorn

Total anomalous pulmonary venous connection is one of the common forms of cyanotic heart disease seen in newborns. When it is associated with significant venous obstruction, neonates present with severe cyanosis and pulmonary edema. In neonates without obstruction, congestive heart failure associated with milder cyanosis may be the presenting feature.

Cross-sectional echocardiography has made a major contribution to the preoperative assessment of total anomalous pulmonary venous connection. In the majority of cases, it obviates the need for cardiac catheterization prior to surgical intervention (1–4). Before embarking on ultrasound examination, it is important to outline the morphologic types of total anomalous pulmonary venous connection briefly, since an understanding of the anatomy is a prerequisite for a successful study.

Morphologically, there are three basic patterns of total anomalous pulmonary venous connection: supracardiac, infracardiac, and intracardiac drainage (5, 6). In *supracardiac connection*, a vertical vein from the pulmonary venous confluence usually ascends in front of the left pulmonary artery, terminating most frequently in the innominate vein. It is at this point that obstruction may occur, when the vertical vein is caught between the left pulmonary artery and the left main bronchus. The vertical vein may terminate in the right superior vena cava at the junction with the right atrium or, more rarely, in the azygos system. In *infracardiac drainage*, a descending vein from the pulmonary venous confluence passes through the diaphragm with the esophagus, terminating most frequently in the

portal system, although it may connect with the inferior vena cava, hepatic veins, or ductus venosus. In infracardiac drainage, obstruction is most common at the terminal connection of the descending vein.

The final type of connection is *intracardiac*, with drainage terminating in the coronary sinus or right atrium. In the latter case, the veins may enter via a common trunk or, more commonly, connect to the right atrium individually.

Mixed total anomalous pulmonary venous connection occurs less commonly but is of major clinical importance. Most frequently, all the left-sided veins drain into a left vertical vein, while the right-sided veins terminate in the coronary sinus. Many other combinations are possible, which makes it important to identify the individual veins during the echocardiographic examination.

A variation in the configuration of the pulmonary venous confluence is seen, particularly in infracardiac drainage. The veins may enter either pole of the confluence in a crosslike configuration with a resulting narrower venous confluence. This has important surgical implications when considering the anastomosis between the left atrium and pulmonary venous confluence. Finally, the ascending or descending vein may be atretic, and severe venous obstruction will be seen shortly after birth.

ECHOCARDIOGRAPHIC EVALUATION

When embarking on an echocardiographic assessment in a child with suspected total anomalous pulmonary venous connection, four basic guidelines must be

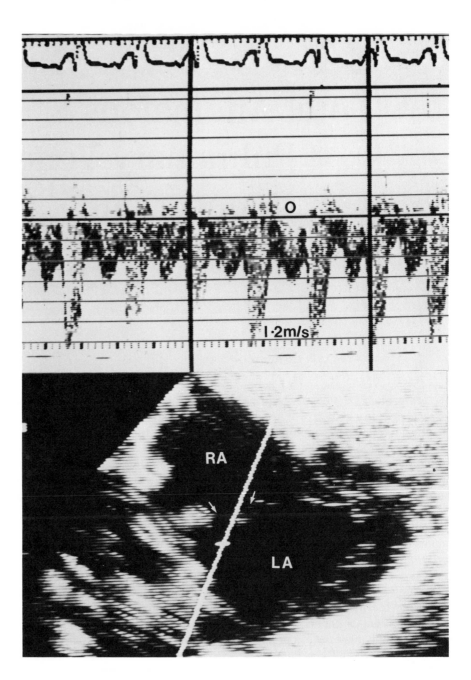

Figure 24.1. The lower picture is a subcostal cut in total anomalous pulmonary venous connection. Note the Doppler sample volume is placed in the left atrium. The upper picture is the Doppler spectral trace, which shows right-to-left shunting across the interatrial communication.

followed. First, a pulmonary venous confluence must be identified. Second, if a confluence is present, its site of drainage must be delineated. Third, the individual veins must be visualized. Finally, associated defects must be identified.

Before attempting specific identification of the presence and site of the anomalous venous connection, it is worthwhile to review the general features seen in the majority of cases. In the presence of an intact ventricular septum, the left ventricle appears dwarfed by the large right ventricle. Frequently, the cavity dimensions and mitral annulus are at the lower limit of normal for age and reflect a relatively low systemic output (7).

Likewise, the left atrium appears reduced in dimension. An interatrial communication, either a flap foramen ovale or a true atrial defect, is invariably present. Doppler interrogation of the atrial defect is invaluable since right-to-left shunting is demonstrable, suggesting total anomalous pulmonary venous connection (Fig. 24.1). If these features are identified, a serious search should be made for an anomalous pulmonary venous connection. This usually begins with an attempt to identify a pulmonary venous confluence (1, 2).

A pulmonary venous confluence is best evaluated in a subcostal four-chamber view with slight posterior angulation. In this position, an echo-free space is

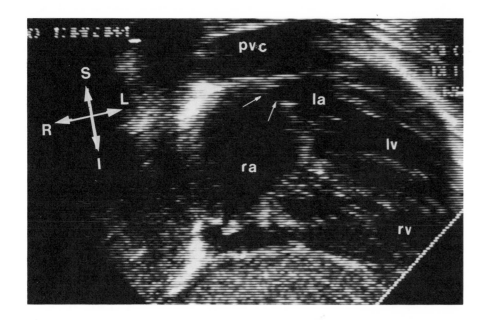

Figure 24.2. Subcostal four-chamber view in total anomalous pulmonary venous connection, demonstrating a large pulmonary venous confluence (PVC) behind the left atrium (LA). Note the inter-atrial communication indicated by the arrows and the relative small size of the LA.

identified behind the left atrium, with no identifiable site of communication between the confluence and that chamber. It is frequently possible to identify some of the left- and right-sided veins draining into the confluence (Fig. 24.2). The confluence may vary in size, which is relevant when considering surgical intervention. Care must be taken to avoid confusing this structure with the right pulmonary artery, which also lies in close proximity to the left atrium. Confusion can be avoided by keeping the transducer angled posteriorly, as the pulmonary artery lies in a more anterosuperior position. Similarly, the descending thoracic aorta lies to the left side of the atrium and appears as a circle. In many cases, the use of parasternal long-axis views enables the dilated confluence to be identified (1) as it protrudes into the posterior aspect of the left atrium (Fig. 24.3). The confluence is always situated more superiorly than the coronary sinus, which occupies the atrioventricular groove. Problems may occur if one relies on the conventional apical four-chamber view to detect the presence of a pulmonary venous confluence because of dropout in the region where the confluence is adjacent to the back of the left atrium. A pulmonary venous confluence can also be evaluated from the suprasternal region (1, 2, 8). In this view, the confluence can be identified as a structure separate

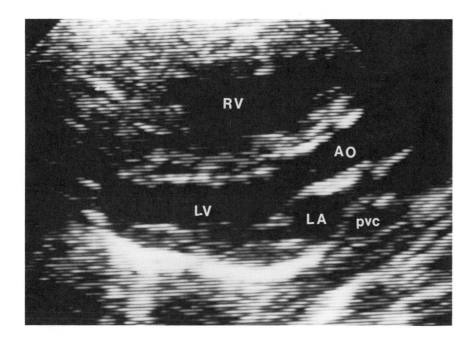

Figure 24.3. Precordial long-axis view in total anomalous pulmonary venous connection. The pulmonary venous confluence (PVC) protrudes into the floor of the left atrium (LA). The confluence is situated superior to the atrioventricular groove.

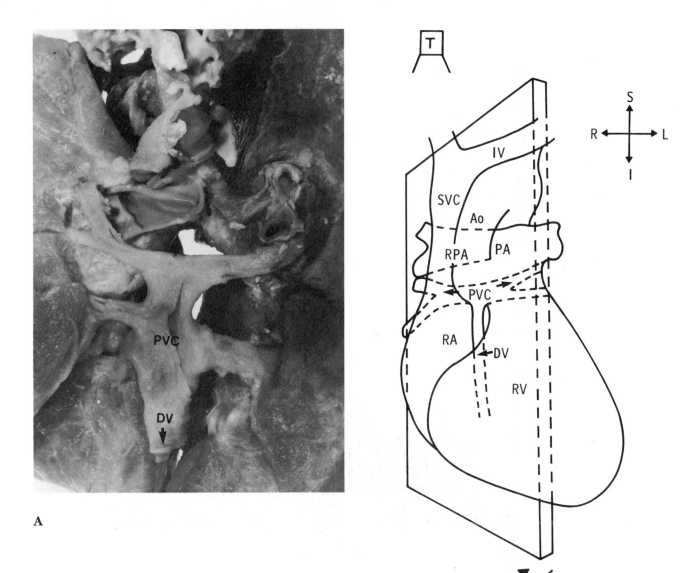

Figure 24.4. (*A*) The specimen on the left is from a patient with infracardiac total anomalous pulmonary venous connection. This is the anatomic appearance of the suprasternal frontal plane view demonstrated in (*B*). The picture on the right is a diagrammatic representation of the plane of the transducer and the venous confluence.

from the left atrium. Slight counterclockwise rotation from the frontal plane is usually necessary to ensure that both the left atrium and the confluence are viewed in the same plane. The confluence may have a variety of shapes, which is important in regard to the anastomotic site created (Fig. 24.4).

Once a pulmonary venous confluence is identified, the next step is determining into which structure it drains. If it terminates below the diaphragm via a descending vein, then it can be visualized from a subcostal position by rotating the transducer counterclockwise until the beam is in the long axis of the descending aorta and inferior vena cava (1, 2, 9). From

this position, a descending vein can be identified as a dilated vessel that lies in front of the descending aorta and terminates in the substance of the liver (Fig. 24.5). It is important to identify both the descending aorta and the inferior vena cava as separate structures so that confusion with a descending vein does not occur. Likewise an azygos vein may be seen in the presence of an inferior vena cava but this structure runs in the paravertebral gutter well away from the left atrium. It is possible to visualize all three vessels (i.e., descending vein, inferior vena cava, and descending aorta) in a short-axis scan at the level of the diaphragm.

Doppler echocardiography provides very useful in-

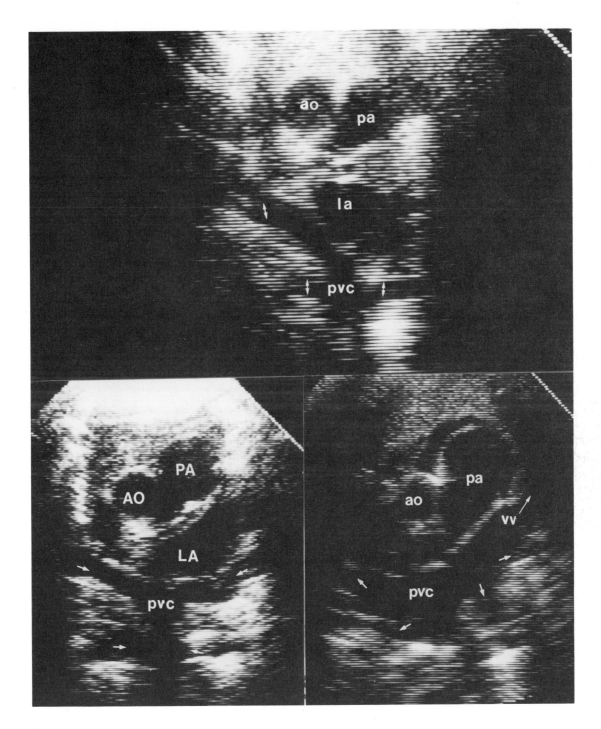

B

Figure 24.4, (cont'd.)   (*B*) The upper picture is a suprasternal frontal plane view in infracardiac total anomalous pulmonary venous connection. Note the pulmonary veins indicated by the arrows. The lower *left-hand* picture is from another patient with infracardiac total anomalous pulmonary connection. Note the difference in configuration between this and the upper picture. The lower *right* picture is from a patient with supracardiac total anomalous pulmonary venous connection. Note the pulmonary veins draining into the confluence and the different configuration from the other two images. DV = descending vein; IV = innominate vein; RPA = right pulmonary artery; SVC = superior vena cava; VV = vertical vein.

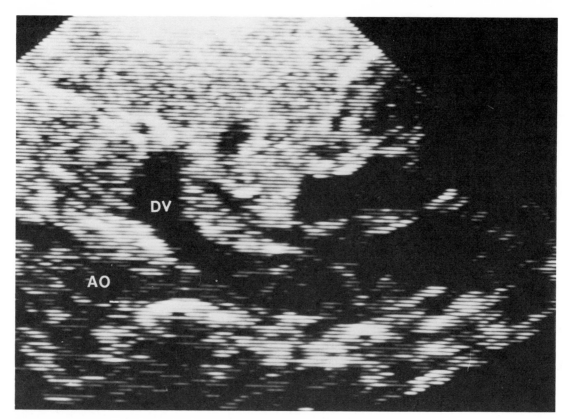

Figure 24.5.   Subcostal long-axis view in infracardiac total anomalous pulmonary venous connection. Note the large fingerlike descending vein.

formation regarding the direction and velocity of blood flow in the descending vein (10, 11). Flow is usually continuous with variations in velocity in the respiratory but not in the cardiac cycle. The direction of flow is away from the transducer, unlike that in the inferior vena cava, which is toward the transducer. By sampling at the distal end of the confluence, the presence and site of obstruction can be assessed (Fig. 24.6). The flow pattern is high velocity and continuous, similar to that in a patent ductus arteriosus (12).

When a descending vein is not identified, supracardiac connection or direct connection to the right atrium must be considered. Connection to the right atrium can be identified in the subcostal view, where the channel appears to terminate in the right atrium (Fig. 24.7); it can also be seen from the suprasternal view (Fig. 24.7). Doppler interrogation at the site of entry will determine whether obstruction is present.

If the connection is not infra- or intracardiac, then by a process of elimination, it must terminate in the supracardiac region. This is best assessed from the suprasternal view. In a suprasternal frontal plane view, the pulmonary venous confluence can be identified along with the individual veins entering the opposite poles of the confluence (Figs. 24.4 and 24.8). From here, the transducer is angled slightly to the left to identify the presence of a left vertical vein. The right superior caval vein and vertical vein cannot always be visualized in the same view, hence the need for some leftward angulation. Usually the vertical vein is a dilated structure, but in the presence of severe obstruction, it may not be so obvious (Fig. 24.8). In unobstructed cases, the innominate vein and right superior vena cava are dilated. Doppler interrogation allows differentiation of this left-sided structure from the left superior vena cava (Fig. 24.8) (13). The presence of obstruction may also be detected with Doppler interrogation at the site of the anatomic vise between the left pulmonary artery and left bronchus (Fig. 24.8).

When a left vertical vein is not identified, a careful search must be undertaken for drainage to the right superior vena cava (Fig. 24.9) or azygos vein (Fig. 24.10) (14). In both of these circumstances, the innominate vein is not dilated, although a dilated venous channel can invariably be seen to the right of the ascending aorta, which will be demonstrated by Doppler to contain low-velocity venous flow. Its site of communication with the confluence can usually be defined.

When a pulmonary venous confluence is not identified, two further options remain; connection to the coronary sinus and connection to the right atrium by

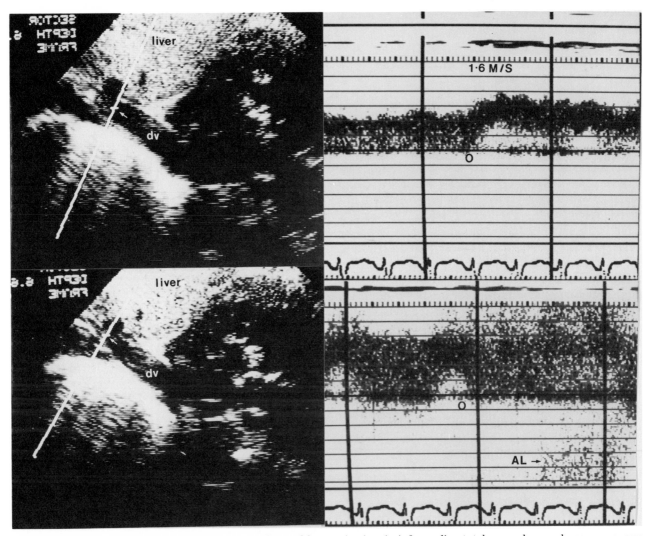

Figure 24.6.   The upper left-hand picture is a subcostal long-axis view in infracardiac total anomalous pulmonary venous drainage. Note the sample volume placed in the descending vein. The picture on the upper right is from the same patient and demonstrates the nonphasic venous flow. The lower picture is with the sample volume placed further distally, in the vicinity of the site of obstruction. Note the high-velocity turbulent flow with aliasing (AL).

separate veins. Total anomalous pulmonary venous connection to the coronary sinus is best assessed in the subcostal view as the dilated coronary sinus and pulmonary veins can be identified simultaneously (1, 2). With a four-chamber subcostal view with posterior angulation of the transducer, the coronary sinus can be visualized running in the atrioventricular groove with the pulmonary veins draining into it (Fig. 24.11). Doppler interrogation within its orifice and in the individual veins will allow detection of stenosis, although the channel usually appears large (Fig. 24.10). If the scanhead is moved back into a four-chamber view, the interatrial communication can be identified with its associated right-to-left shunting. A similar picture is seen in an apical four-chamber view with posterior angulation of the transducer to visualize the atrioventricular groove. In this position, however, the pulmo-

nary veins are not visualized as readily as they are from the subcostal position. The dilated coronary sinus can also be seen in the precordial long-axis view, originating at the atrioventricular groove and enlarging superiorly (Fig. 24.12) (1, 2). This differentiates it from a venous confluence, which has no connections with the atrioventricular groove (compare Figs. 24.3 and 24.12).

If neither a confluence nor a dilated coronary sinus is identified, then a careful search must be made to identify separate veins draining into the right atrium. This is best achieved by a combination of subcostal and suprasternal views. From the subcostal position, if the transducer is initially placed in a four-chamber position and then rotated counterclockwise, the whole of the atrium can be seen, as can separate veins draining into it. From a suprasternal frontal plane view, with slight counterclockwise rotation, the superior vena caval–atrial junction can be seen and individual veins draining at this site identified.

MIXED TOTAL ANOMALOUS PULMONARY VENOUS CONNECTION

Many different combinations may coexist, and a high index of suspicion should be maintained in patients with radiologic evidence of unilateral obstruction. It is important that the examiner have a sound knowledge of the anatomic variations and that individual pulmonary veins be actively sought during the study (15) to minimize overlooking connections to other sites. If a confluence is identified and a descending vein noted, it is not sufficient to assume that all the veins enter the confluence. The same is true for other types of drainage.

During examination, any two of the following structures together (a descending vein, a vertical vein, and an enlarged coronary sinus) indicate mixed drainage. Individual connection of one vein to the right atrium may be difficult to detect. Frequently, a suprasternal frontal plane view with counterclockwise rotation to visualize the superior vena caval–atrial junction provides the best window for assessing those cases where the vein inserts into the superior aspect of the right atrium.

The presence of a small venous confluence behind the left atrium should also raise the suspicion of mixed drainage. There is no substitution, however, for actively identifying veins during each study.

ASSOCIATED LESIONS

It is important to exclude associated defects that may alter the surgical course. Mitral stenosis is occasionally associated and may be very difficult to diagnose due to the relatively small size of the mitral valve in these patients. Doppler interrogation may not provide the answer, particularly in the presence of low systemic flow due to a restrictive interatrial communication. Ventricular septal defect and pulmonary valvular stenosis may occasionally occur, whereas patency of the ductus arteriosus is usually associated in neonates. Doppler interrogation of the right ventricular outflow tract, together with inspection of the pulmonary valve, should readily indicate whether or not there is associated valvar stenosis (Fig. 24.13).

COMPLEX HEART DISEASE AND TOTAL ANOMALOUS PULMONARY VENOUS CONNECTION

While this chapter is not intended to deal with abnormalities of atrial arrangement, mention should be made of total anomalous pulmonary venous connection in patients with isomeric atrial chambers. More frequently,

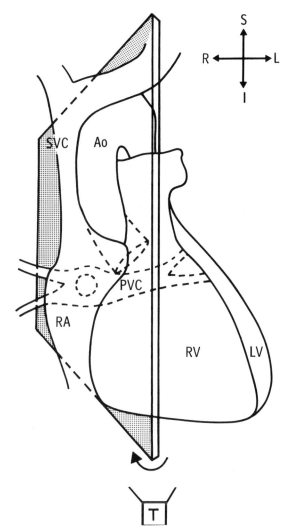

Figure 24.7. (*A*) A schematic diagram demonstrating the echocardiac cut.

pulmonary venous anomalies are seen in right atrial isomerism, although they may occur with left isomerism (2, 16–18). Invariably, these patients also have an atrioventricular septal defect with a common atrium or a double-inlet connection with a common atrioventricular valve. Patients with right isomerism usually have pulmonary outflow tract obstruction (Fig. 24.14).

The pulmonary veins may drain to an infra- or supracardiac location, but more commonly, there is a pulmonary venous confluence connecting with a common atrium. In the presence of a common atrium, it is frequently difficult to determine whether the pulmonary venous confluence drains into the left or right side. Doppler examination of the entry site provides invaluable information about the presence of obstruction, although care must be taken in those with low pulmonary blood flow, where the reduced pulmonary venous return may potentially mask an anatomical obstruction.

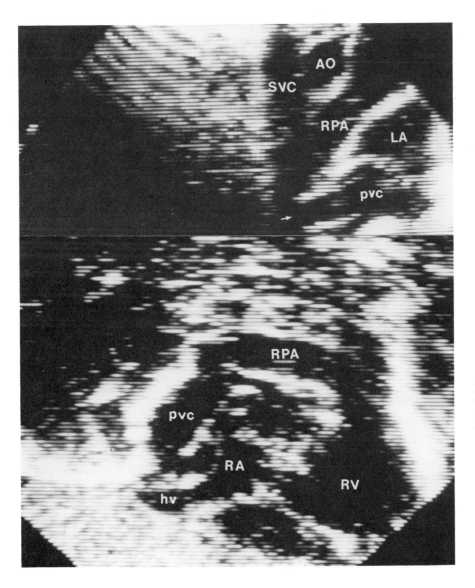

Figure 24.7, (cont'd.) (*B*) The upper picture is a suprasternal frontal plane view of a patient with total anomalous pulmonary venous connection to the superior vena caval–atrial junction. Note the pulmonary venous confluence and its site of connection indicated by the arrow. The lower picture is a subcostal view from a different patient. Note the pulmonary venous confluence (PVC) behind the atria. HV = hepatic vein; superior vena cava. SVC = superior vena cava.

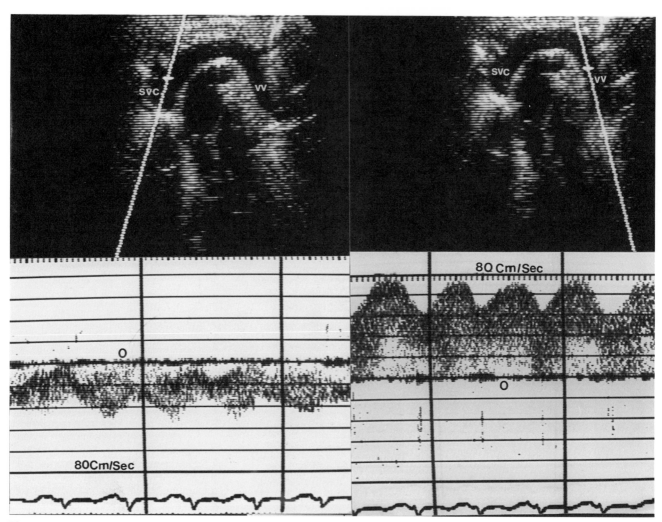

Figure 24.8.   (*A*) The upper left-hand picture is a suprasternal frontal plane view in total anomalous pulmonary venous connection via a left vertical vein (VV). Note the sample volume is placed in the superior vena cava (SVC). The picture below is from the same patient and demonstrates the flow away from the transducer. The upper right-hand picture is from the same patient with the sample volume in the VV. The spectral trace below demonstrates that the flow is toward the transducer.

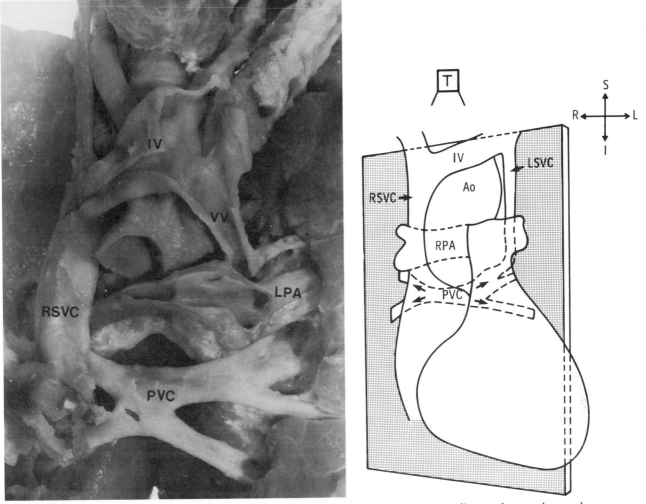

Figure 24.8, (cont'd.) (*B*) The left-hand picture is an anatomic specimen in supracardiac total anomalous pulmonary venous connection. Note the pulmonary venous confluence (PVC) with the VV running behind the left pulmonary artery (LPA). The picture on the right is a diagram showing the echocardiographic plane to obtain such an image. IV = innominate vein; LSVC = left superior vena cava; RSVC = right superior vena cava.

Figure 24.9. Suprasternal frontal plane view in total anomalous pulmonary venous drainage to a right superior vena cava (SVC). Note the large ascending vein (av), which terminates in the SVC. PVC = pulmonary venous confluence.

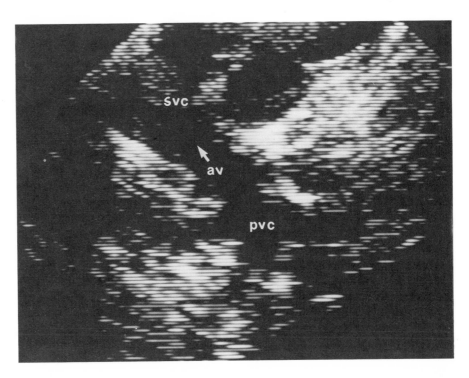

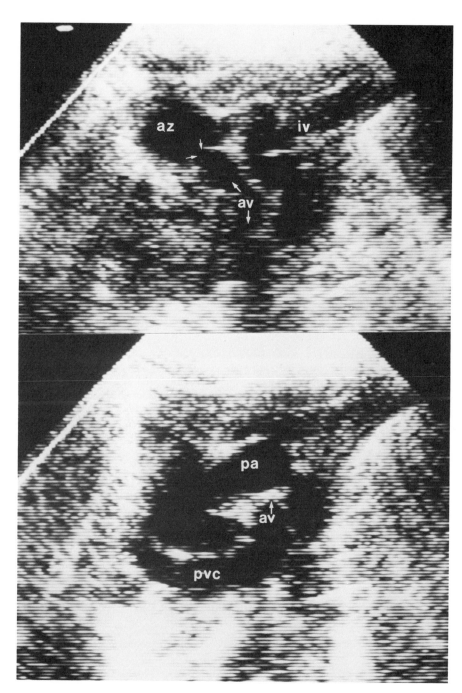

Figure 24.10. The upper picture is a suprasternal frontal plane view in total anomalous pulmonary venous connection to the azygos vein. Note the innominate vein is of normal dimension and that the azygos vein is dilated. The arrows indicate the site of obstruction. The lower picture is from the same patient with a slightly different plane to visualize the confluence. Note the ascending vein on the left side of the image. av = ascending vein; AZ = azygos vein; IV = innominate vein; PA = pulmonary artery; PVC = pulmonary venous confluence.

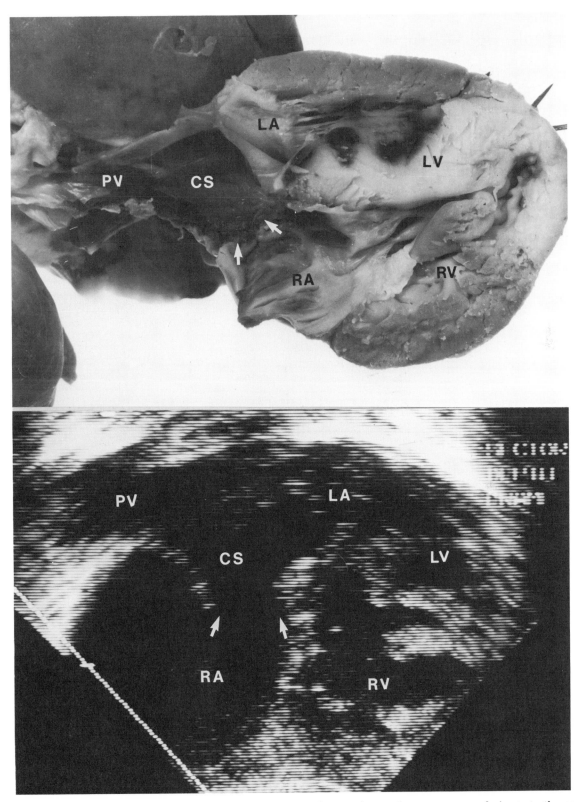

Figure 24.11.   The upper picture is an anatomic specimen in total anomalous pulmonary venous drainage to the coronary sinus. The lower picture is from a different patient and demonstrates echocardiographic features. Note the mouth of the coronary sinus indicated by the white arrows. CS = coronary sinus; PV = pulmonary vein.

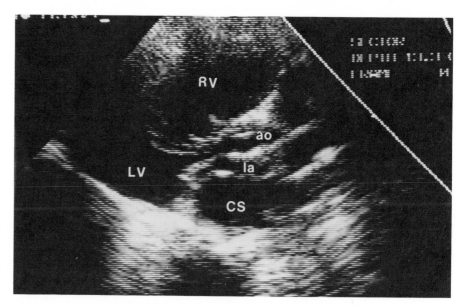

Figure 24.12. Precordial long-axis view in total anomalous pulmonary venous connection to the coronary sinus (CS). Note the large dilated CS, which originates in the atrioventricular groove. Also observe the large right ventricle (RV).

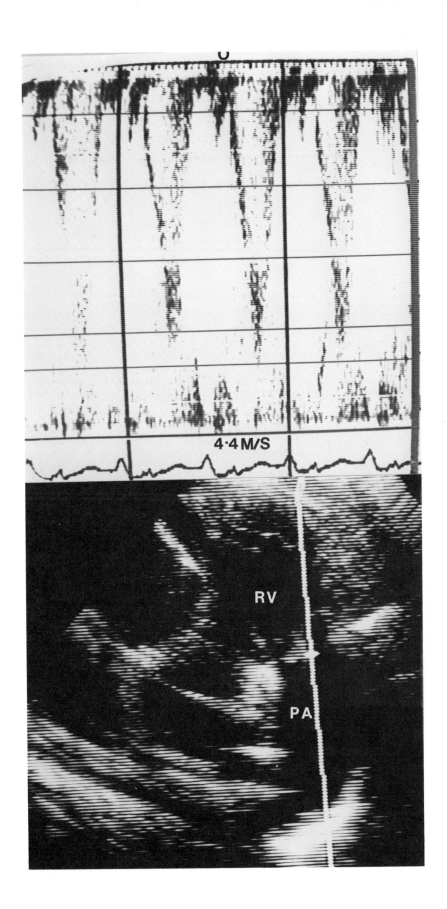

Figure 24-13. The lower picture is a precordial short-axis view from a patient with total anomalous pulmonary venous connection to the coronary sinus and associated pulmonary valvular stenosis. Note the sample volume is placed just distal to the pulmonary valve. The upper picture is a spectral trace and demonstrates a significant gradient across the right ventricular outflow tract.

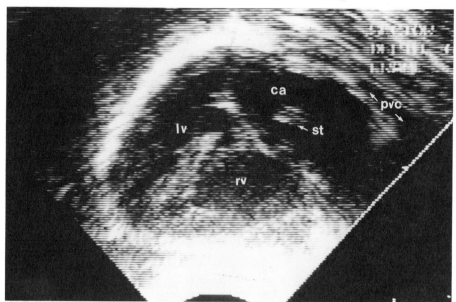

Figure 24.14. Subcostal view in total anomalous pulmonary venous connection in the setting of right atrial isomerism. Note the pulmonary venous confluence (PVC) behind the common atrium (CA). Also observe the strand (ST) in the CA. In this patient, the venous confluence drained below the diaphragm. LV = left ventricle; RV = right ventricle.

REFERENCES

1. Smallhorn JF, Sutherland GR, Tommasini G, Hunter S, Anderson RH, Macartney FJ. Assessment of total anomalous pulmonary venous connection by two-dimensional echocardiography. Br Heart J 1981;46:613–23.
2. Huhta JC, Gutgesell HP, Nihill MR. Cross sectional echocardiographic diagnosis of total anomalous pulmonary venous connection. Br Heart J 1985;53:525–34.
3. Sahn DJ, Allen HD, Lange LW, Goldberg SJ. Cross-sectional echocardiographic diagnosis of the sites of total anomalous pulmonary venous drainage. Circulation 1979;60:1317–25.
4. Stark J, Smallhorn JF, Huhta J, et al. Surgery for congenital heart defects diagnosed with cross-sectional echocardiography. Circulation 1983;68:129–38.
5. Edwards JE, Carey LS, Neufeld HN, Lester RG. Congenital heart disease: correlation of pathologic anatomy and angiocardiography. Philadelphia: WB Saunders, 1965:880–90.
6. Bonham Carter RE, Capriles M, Noe Y. Total anomalous pulmonary venous drainage. A clinical and anatomical study of 75 children. Br Heart J 1969;31:45–51.
7. Lima CO, Valdes-Cruz LM, Allen HD, et al. Prognostic value of left ventricular size measured by echocardiography in infants with total anomalous pulmonary venous drainage. Am J Cardiol 1983;51:1155–9.
8. Sahn DJ, Goldberg SJ, Allen HD, Canale JM. Cross-sectional echocardiographic imaging of supracardiac total anomalous pulmonary venous drainage to a vertical vein in a patient with Holt-Oram syndrome. Chest 1981;79:113–5.
9. Snider AR, Silverman NH, Turley K, Ebert PA. Evaluation of infradiaphragmatic total anomalous pulmonary venous connection with two-dimensional echocardiography. Circulation 1982;66:1129–32.
10. Cooper MJ, Teitel DF, Silverman NH, et al. Study of the infradiaphragmatic total anomalous pulmonary venous connection with cross-sectional and pulsed Doppler echocardiography. Circulation 1984;70:412.
11. Smallhorn JF, Freedom R. Pulsed Doppler echocardiography in the preoperative evaluation of total anomalous pulmonary venous connection. J Am Coll Cardiol 1986;8:1413–20.
12. Smallhorn JF, Pauperio H, Benson L, Freedom RM, Rowe RD. Pulsed Doppler assessment of pulmonary vein obstruction. Am Heart J 1985;110:483–6.
13. Skovranek J, Tuma S, Urbancova D, et al. Range-gated pulsed Doppler echocardiographic diagnosis of supracardiac total anomalous pulmonary venous drainage. Circulation 1980;61:841.
14. Moes CAF, Fowler RS, Trusler GA. Total anomalous pulmonary venous drainage into the azygos vein. Am J Roentgenol Rad Ther Nucl Med 1966;98:378.
15. de Leval M, Stark J, Waterston DJ. Mixed type of total anomalous pulmonary venous drainage. Surgical correction in three infants. Ann Thorac Surg 1973;16:464–70.
16. Huhta JC, Smallhorn JF, Macartney FJ. Two-dimensional echocardiographic diagnosis of situs. Br Heart J 1982;48:97–108.
17. Macartney FJ, Zuberbuhler JR, Anderson RH. Morphological considerations pertaining to recognition of atrial isomerism. Consequences for sequential chamber localisation. Br Heart J 1980;44:657–67.
18. Freedom RM, Olley PM, Coceani F, Rowe RD. The prostaglandin challenge. Test to unmask obstructed total anomalous pulmonary venous connections in asplenia syndrome. Br Heart J 1978;40:91–4.

25

Acyanotic Congenital Heart Disease: Left-to-Right Shunts

Norman Silverman

INTERATRIAL COMMUNICATIONS

Morphologically, the sites of interatrial communications are best seen from the right atrium (Fig. 25.1). The interatrial communications occurring in the region of the oval fossa are true atrial septal defects, because the true interatrial septum is only slightly larger than the confines of the oval fossa. Since 1980, we have performed echocardiograms in 5000 new patients of whom 254 had atrial septal defects. Two hundred (78.7%) had secundum-type atrial septal defects. The next most frequent interatrial communication encountered was the defect found in the atrioventricular septum. Such defects are referred to as the ostium primum type of atrial septal defect, accounting for 45 (17.7%) of the population of 254. (These defects are discussed separately.) The least common interatrial communication was the sinus venosus type of defect, which was found in 9 (3.6%) of the 254 patients. There were no sinus venosus defects in the region of the inferior vena cava and no interatrial communication through the mouth of the coronary sinus. The latter lesion is rare and has only been detected on one occasion by echocardiography.

It is of practical importance to define these lesions by ultrasound because many centers now consider surgery without cardiac catheterization to be efficacious, based on ultrasound and other noninvasive criteria (1, 2).

APPROACH TO THE DIAGNOSIS

M-Mode Echocardiography

The M-mode echocardiogram in interatrial communications reflects right ventricular diastolic volume over-load by the presence of a large right ventricle and paradoxic septal motion. This feature may be found with pulmonary and tricuspid regurgitation, and modern Doppler ultrasound has the potential to exclude these lesions. Therefore, only anomalous pulmonary venous connection and interatrial shunting as a generic group need to be considered in the differential diagnosis of paradoxic septal motion. The M-mode signs, although sensitive, are not specific and are not present in all patients; in children, it is not uncommon for septal motion to be normal in the presence of an atrial septal defect.

Secundum Atrial Septal Defects: Two-Dimensional Echocardiography

The secundum atrial septal defect is situated in the region of the fossa ovalis. The best views passing through the atrial septum are the subcostal sagittal and coronal, the parasternal short-axis, and the apical four-chamber planes (Figs. 25.2, 25.3, 25.4, and 25.5) (3–7).

In the pediatric population where subcostal images are most frequently obtained, the atrial septal defect is usually imaged as a dropout of echoes surrounded by the bright rim of the fossa ovalis. The so-called T artifact is produced by the strong difference in density between blood and tissue as well as by the fact that the confines of the fossa usually have a thick rim that is echo reflective. The position of the right upper pulmonary veins can also be identified in this plane. If there is anomalous connection of the superior right pulmonary vein to the superior vena cava, however, the connection of the middle lobe pulmonary veins may give the erroneous impression that all the veins are

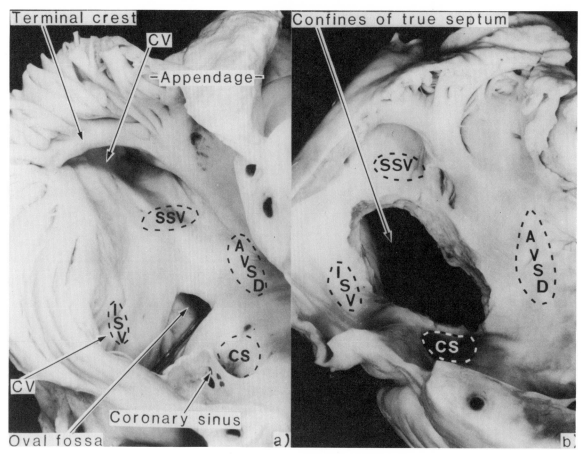

Figure 25.1.   The atrial septum viewed from the right atrial aspect shows its morphologic features. The terminal crest, coronary sinus, and oval fossa are shown in (A). The position of interatrial communication has been diagrammed. The superior type of sinus venosus defect (SSV) adjacent to the superior caval vein (CV) and the inferior sinus venosus defect (ISV) adjacent to the inferior caval vein is shown. Positions of both the coronary sinus and coronary sinus septal defects and the atrioventricular septum and the associated atrioventricular septal defects (AVSD) are demonstrated. The so-called secundum septal defects occur in the region of the fossa ovalis. In (B), the entire septal communication between the atria has been excised to define the confines of the true interatrial septum. Only defects in this region can be true interatrial septal defects. The others produce interatrial communications by allowing communication between the two atria. (Reproduced courtesy of Professor Robert Anderson, the Society of Pediatric Echocardiography, and the American Society of Echocardiography).

connected to the left atrium. Special care must be taken by scanning more cranially as well as by obtaining images from the suprasternal notch. The use of range-gated pulsed Doppler in this circumstance will help to distinguish the flow disturbance in the superior vena cava from that of an anomalously connected right upper pulmonary vein. We have not defined the anomalous connection of the right upper pulmonary vein in a sufficiently large number of cases to be sure that this sign is sufficiently reliable to be clinically useful.

The next most reliable method for defining secundum atrial septal defects is by using the apical four-chamber plane (Fig. 24.5). The rim of the fossa ovalis can be well visualized, but the atrial septum cannot be well imaged because it is perpendicular to the ultrasound beam in the area of the flap valve. Because the floor of the oval fossa is thin, it is not well demonstrated by ultrasound in this plane where resolution is predominantly in the lateral direction.

Secundum atrial septal defects may also be imaged from the parasternal short-axis view, especially from the lower intercostal spaces where a four-chamber type of orientation can be obtained. It is possible to obtain images from the right parasternal area, but we have never found it necessary to image defects from this position.

Of the 254 secundum defects studied, six were identified at catheterization that had not been clearly identified by ultrasound. These defects were described at surgery as having an atypical shape or fenestrations in the interatrial septum.

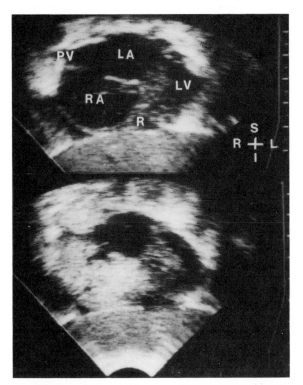

Figure 25.2. The top frame shows the subcostal view of a secundum atrial septal defect lying between the left atrium (LA) and the right atrium (RA). The right upper pulmonary vein (PV) enters the LA. The bottom frame shows a bolus of saline contrast that has been injected into a peripheral vein. The negative contrast effect helps highlight the interatrial defect as the unopacified blood from the LA passes across the interatrial defect into the RA and right upper pulmonary vein. A centimeter scale marker is displayed on the left side of next frame. I = inferior.

Contrast Echocardiography

It has been our practice to perform venous contrast echocardiography via a peripheral injection of 1 to 2 ml of agitated saline injected into an arm vein, preferably on the left side (8, 9). A right-to-left shunt is identified most frequently in the presence of atrial defects. This, however, is not a specific finding but can be detected in a number of conditions including a patent foramen ovale (10), when there is an elevated right atrial pressure. This has been found to occur in approximately 18 percent of adults and probably in a much higher percentage of children. Right-to-left interatrial shunts also occur with pulmonary hypertension, obligatory atrial shunts as in total anomalous pulmonary venous connection, obstruction to the right atrioventricular valve (such as tricuspid atresia or Ebstein's anomaly), and with severe obstruction to the right ventricular outflow tract such as severe pulmonic stenosis.

A more specific sign is the negative contrast jet (9). Peripheral venous contrast injection opacifies the right atrium. The unopacified left atrial blood enters through the atrial defect and leaves a jet of unopacified blood, thus yielding a negative contrast space within the right atrium. Unfortunately, the negative jet cannot be produced in all atrial septal defects, especially in the larger defects when the velocity of the blood flowing across the interatrial communication may not make a clear jet. In this circumstance, the stream of unopacified blood across the atrial septum is large, and the transatrial blood flow becomes rapidly diluted and mixed, which will not allow this technique to define the defect.

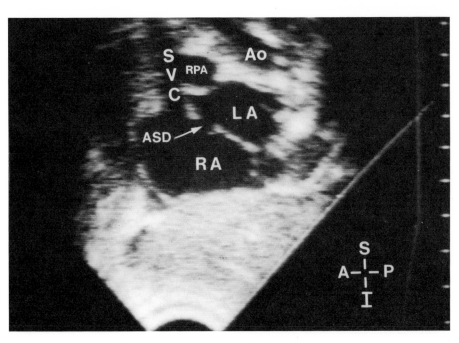

Figure 25.3. A subcostal parasagittal view taken at approximately 90 degrees to Figure 25.2 shows the position of a secundum atrial septal defect between the left atrium (LA) and right atrium (RA). The superior vena cava (SVC) drains into the RA. The right pulmonary artery (RPA) lies superior to the LA.

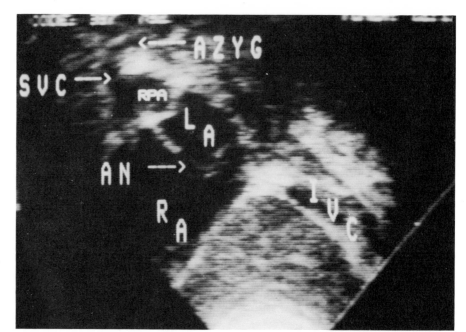

Figure 25.4. Shows the presence of an atrial septal aneurysm (AN) over the fossa ovalis between the right atrium (RA) and left atrium (LA) in the parasagittal subcostal orientation similar to Figure 25.3. The junction of the azygos vein (AZYG) into the superior vena cava can be identified and the inferior vena cava (IVC) seen below the diaphragm. Part of the aneurysm is made up of the eustachian valve (valve of the IVC).

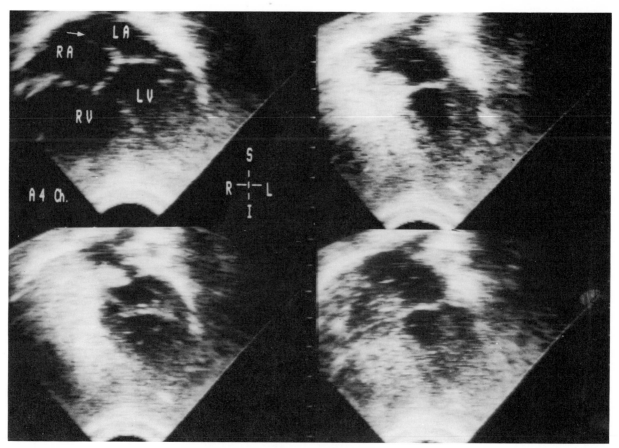

Figure 25.5. Top frame is an apical four-chamber sequence demonstrating the position of a small atrial septal defect (*arrow*) seen between the right and left atria (RA and LA). In sequence, the bottom left frame shows the contrast bolus appearing in the right heart and shunting right to left across the defect. In top right frame and then bottom right frame, the passage of blood across the interatrial defect from left to right of noncontrast-containing blood (negative contrast effect) can be identified.

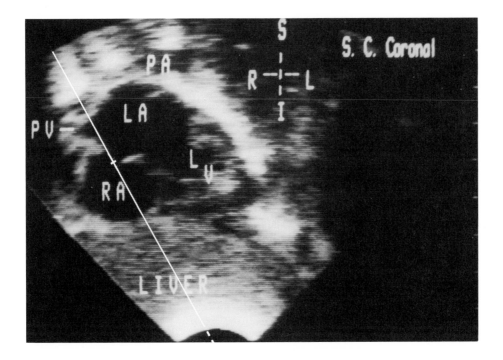

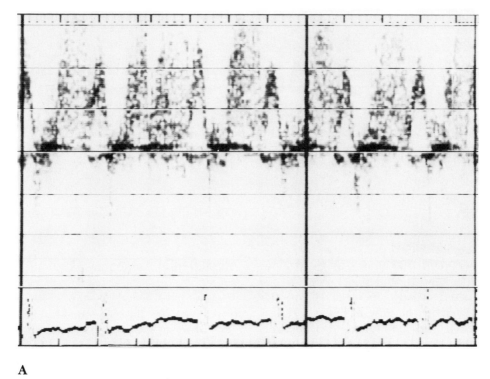

A

Figure 25.6. (*A*) Top: In this example taken from the subcostal coronal cut, the Doppler sample volume was placed in the right atrium opposite the interatrial defect between the right and left atria, identified by well marked T artifacts. Bottom: The resulting Doppler signal shows systolic flow disturbance beginning midway through systole and continuing almost up to the wave of atrial contraction. Variation in the signal is related to respiratory movement. Sinus arrhythmia is present.

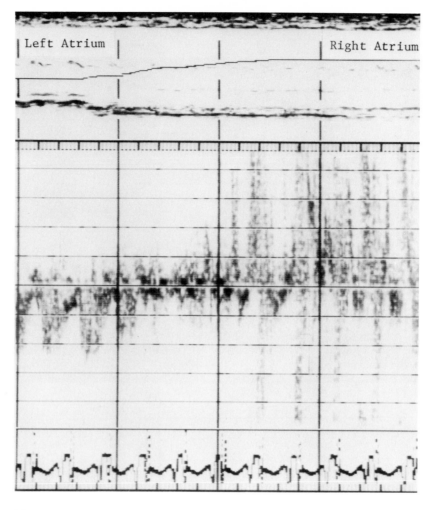

B

Figure 25.6 (cont'd.).   (*B*) This shows a scan plane moving from left to right atria across the interatrial septum in the M-mode recording (upper part of the panel). The marked flow disturbance is identified as the transducer is withdrawn across the atrial septum. These Doppler flow disturbances are most commonly encountered when the atrial septal defect is small.

Doppler Findings

Pulsed Doppler ultrasound has been less sensitive in these lesions than in many other lesions (11, 12). Although disturbed interatrial flow may be demonstrated (Fig. 25.6), there are many situations where right atrial flow patterns change. As observed with the contrast echocardiogram, the flow of blood across a large defect is much more amorphous and not well directed. The signal related to the flow disturbance is also more diffuse and varies with the respiratory changes in the velocity of blood flow into the atrium from the venae cavae. This respiratory change in blood flow velocity may be misinterpreted as due to an atrial septal defect. In addition, if the coronary sinus blood flow is large (such as when the left superior vena cava drains via the coronary sinus), sampling close to the orifice of the coronary sinus within the right atrium

may lead to the erroneous interpretation of disturbed atrial flow.

Atrial Septal Aneurysms

Attention has recently been paid to atrial septal aneurysms (13). We have encountered 15 such examples. The aneurysm appears to be more complex than simple bulging of the floor (flap valve) of the oval fossa into the right atrium. In many instances, the eustachian valve can be seen to be part of the aneurysmal structure. In some cases, the associated atrial shunt has been defined both by contrast echocardiography and at cardiac catheterization (Fig. 25.4).

In some cases, it has been noted that the aneurysm may be part of what has been described as a "stretched" foramen ovale. These lesions have been

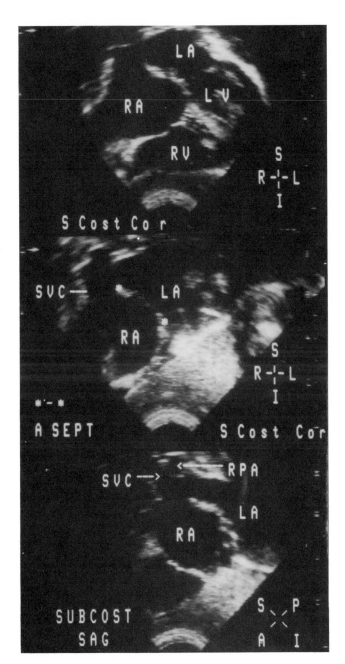

A

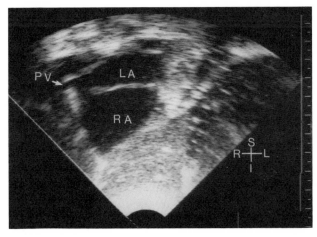

B

Figure 25.7. (*A*) Series of frames demonstrating a superior sinus venosus defect. In the top frame, taken in the subcostal coronal plane (S Cost Cor), the defect is seen between the top portion of the right and left atria (RA and LA) with the entire atrial septum intact. The defect occurs at the junction between the right upper pulmonary vein and the superior vena cava. In the middle frame, with a slightly more cranial angulation, the defect is seen at the upper portion between the LA and the superior vena cava (SVC). The asterisks mark an intact atrial septum along its entire length. In the bottom frame, taken in the subcostal sagittal plane (SUBCOST SAG), the superior vena cava enters the RA. A deficiency between the superior vena cava and the LA in the region of the right upper pulmonary vein is identified. (*B*) Subcostal sagittal cut in another patient with a sinus venosus defect demonstrates the pulmonary vein draining into the posterior aspect of the superior vena cava. The area of the defect between the atria is defined.

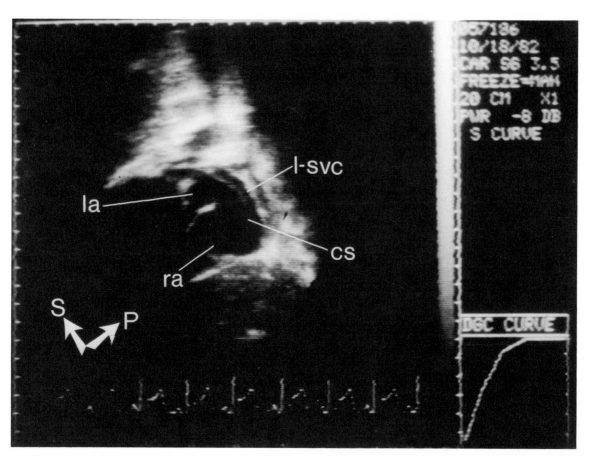

Figure 25.8. An example of a coronary sinus atrial septal defect. A left superior vena cava (l-SVC) is present and drains directly into the dilated coronary sinus (CS). A communication exists between the left atrium (LA) and the CS and the right atrium (RA). Orientation is sagittal. (Reproduced courtesy of Dr. Steven Sanders from Boston, who published a similar image in the *American Journal of Cardiology* [14].)

associated with left-to-right shunts at either the ventricular or ductal level with accompanying left atrial dilation. The floor of the fossa subsequently bulges through the rim, prolapsing into the right atrium where it gives the appearance of an aneurysm. Minor left-to-right shunts have been noted with this lesion. In addition, reversed aneurysms of the atrial septum into the left atrium have been noted in conditions where there is obstruction to right atrial outflow.

SINUS VENOSUS DEFECTS

The defects we have encountered have all occurred at the junction of the superior vena cava and right upper pulmonary veins with the atrium. We have not encountered defects of the inferior vena caval–atrial junction. Most of the sinus venosus defects we have identified have been associated with an anomalous pulmonary venous connection. Until we were able to perform high-quality subcostal imaging, it was not possible to define this lesion clearly (Fig. 25.7).

In order to image these defects subcostally, the transducer should be rotated clockwise by approximately 45 degrees to achieve the view where the right upper pulmonary veins join the left atrium. Slight anterior angulation and further clockwise rotation bring the right side of the scan plane more anterior, displaying the superior vena caval–atrial junction. Slight anterior or posterior scanning brings into view the junction between either the superior caval or pulmonary veins with the atrial septum. Drop out of echoes represents the area of the defect. We have not been successful in identifying this lesion regularly other than from the subcostal views. In the absence of direct visualization, the diagnosis is suggested by the M-mode findings of right ventricular and pulmonary artery enlargement, and right-to-left shunting by contrast echocardiography.

CORONARY SINUS ATRIAL DEFECTS

A recent report by Sanders et al. has shown that the entity can be defined echocardiographically (14): The enlarged coronary sinus can be imaged and its "party wall" with the left atrium can be seen to be deficient (Fig. 25.8). The subcostal view was used with slight angulation from the coronal view in the counterclockwise direction to image the area of the coronary sinus.

COLOR FLOW MAPPING IN INTRA-ATRIAL COMMUNICATIONS

The advent of color flow mapping has provided another form for substantiating intra-atrial flow patterns associated with atrial septal defects. Without the use of contrast echocardiography it is now possible to identify left-to-right, as well as right-to-left shunting at the level of the foramen ovale. In addition, intra-atrial communications at the lower edge of the atrial septum associated with atrioventricular septal defects, the so-called ostium primum atrial septal defect can be identified. Because the sinus venosus defect flow is directed parallel to the transducer face, using conventional imaging planes, color flow mapping has been less satisfactory in identifying shunt flow in this lesion.

VENTRICULAR SEPTAL DEFECTS

Definition of Terms

The ventricular septum is a complex structure that separates the ventricles from each other. There are four components to the ventricular septum (Figs. 25.9 and 25.10) (15, 16). When viewed from the right ventricular surface, the inlet (or sinus) septum is limited by the tricuspid annulus and the attachment of the papillary muscles to the ventricular septum. It is smooth compared to other parts of the right ventricular septal surface. On the left ventricular side, the septum borders the posterior diverticulum of the outlet component in the normal heart, so in these circumstances, it is an inlet-outlet septum. The next portion of septum is the trabecular septum, which extends from the inlet septum to the region of the outlet septum just proximal to the pulmonary valve. It is heavily trabeculated and contains a large band of muscle (the septomarginal trabeculation) running along its right ventricular surface. The trabecular septum extends to the smooth outlet septum above it. In the normal heart, the true outlet septum between subpulmonary and subaortic outflow tracts is very small, and most of the smooth area extending from the point of junction from the septomarginal trabeculation to the region of the pulmonary valve is the free wall of the subpulmonary infundibulum. The outlet septum, however, is better represented in malformed hearts. The fourth component of the ventricular septum is the small membranous septum from which the other components radiate. The membranous septum itself usually has a small ventricular component and much larger atrioventricu-

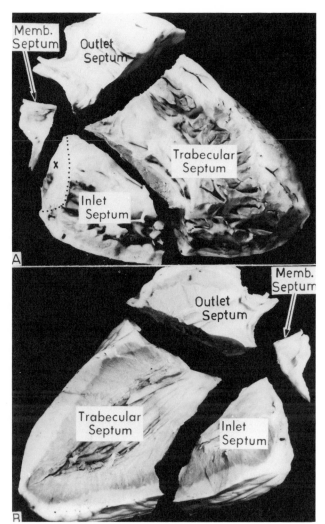

Figure 25.9. In this anatomic representation, the ventricular septum has been divided into its various components: the membranous, outlet, trabecular, and inlet septa. (*A*) From the right ventricular aspect, the margins of the atrioventricular septum indicated by an X are not truly part of the interventricular septum. The area of the dots indicates the position of the septal attachment to the tricuspid valve. The area proximal to this is the atrioventricular septum. (*B*) From the left-sided aspect, the various components of the left ventricular septum are shown. (Reproduced courtesy of Professors Robert Anderson and Anton Becker Society of Pediatric Echocardiography, and the American Society of Echocardiography.)

lar component between the left ventricle and right atrium. It is situated in a position along the inner curvature of the ventricular septum and is bound by the tricuspid valve, the other muscular components of the ventricular septum, and the ventriculoinfundibular fold. This area is normally covered almost completely by the septal leaflet of the tricuspid valve. Indeed, it is the attachment of this leaflet across the membranous septum that divides it into atrioventricular and membranous components.

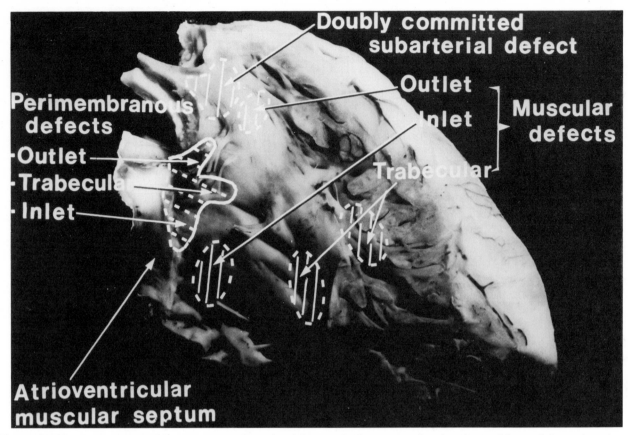

Figure 25.10.   Intact ventricular septum seen from the right ventricular aspect, showing the positions of the various types of defects. Defects associated with the membranous septum are termed perimembranous and can be perimembranous, outlet, trabecular, or inlet type of ventricular septal defects. Defects occurring underneath the great arteries are termed doubly committed subarterial defects. Muscular defects, entirely surrounded by muscle, occur either in the muscular inlet, muscular trabecular, or muscular outlet septa. The position of the atrioventricular muscular septum is identified.

Defects most frequently occur at the points of fusion between the various components of the septum (Fig. 25.10). Defects situated around the area of the membranous septum are called perimembranous. These defects can be further divided according to the area into which they extend, giving the perimembranous-inlet, perimembranous-trabecular, or perimembranous-outlet varieties (17). Often the defect is large and involves all components. Such a perimembranous defect is said to be confluent. When a defect is surrounded entirely by muscle, it is described as muscular. Muscular defects can also be found in the inlet, trabecular, or outlet components of the septum. Multiple trabecular muscular defects produce the so-called Swiss-cheese septum. There is one more special type of outlet defect that abuts directly on both arterial (semilunar) valves because of absence of the outlet septum. Such a defect is called a doubly committed subarterial defect.

A further feature of many defects is malalignment of the septal components. The muscular septum may be malaligned with the atrial septum. This produces strad-

dling of the tricuspid valve, which is discussed in Chapter 27. Alternatively, the outer septum may be malaligned relative to the rest of the muscular septum. This produces subarterial outflow tract obstruction. The nature of the obstruction depends on the direction of malalignment and the ventriculoarterial connection.

Incidence

In our series of 440 isolated ventricular septal defects, 277 (63%) were perimembranous and 145 (32%) were muscular. Of the muscular defects, 63 (40%) occurred in the trabecular septum, 46 (32%) in the inlet septum and 36 (25%) in the outlet septum. The remaining 18 cases were either isolated doubly committed subarterial defects with a muscular posteroinferior rim or subarterial defects extending into the perimembranous region.

In 18 cases, there was malalignment of the outer septum. In 10, there was anterior malalignment between the outlet and trabecular septum, giving aortic override of the right ventricle. The remaining eight

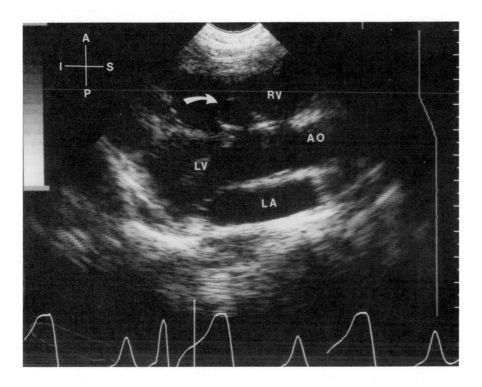

A

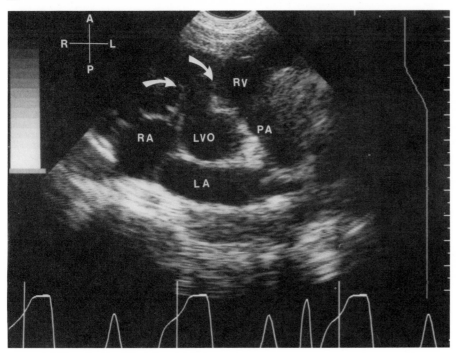

B

Figure 25.11. Parasternal long axis, (*A*); parasternal short axis, (*B*); apical four-chamber, (*C*); and M-mode echocardiographic representation (*D*) of a perimembranous ventricular septal defect with aneurysm formation. In all frames, the aneurysm is demonstrated by large arrows. In the parasternal long axis (*A*), the aneurysm is seen bulging into the right ventricular outflow tract in systole. The actual margins of the ventricular septal defect are not clearly defined. In the parasternal short axis (*B*), the margins of the ventricular septal defect between the left ventricular outflow tract (LVO) and the right ventricle are clearly defined. The margins of the aneurysm, as demonstrated by the large arrows, and the defect margins are seen posterior to the aneurysm reflecting the actual size of the defect.

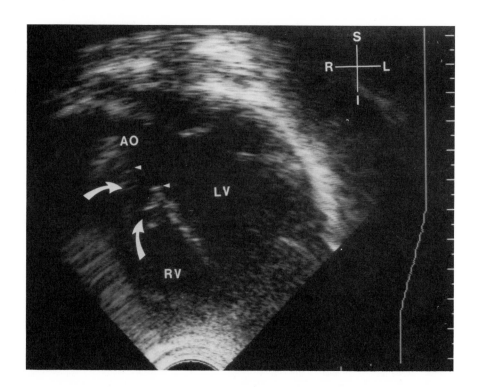

C

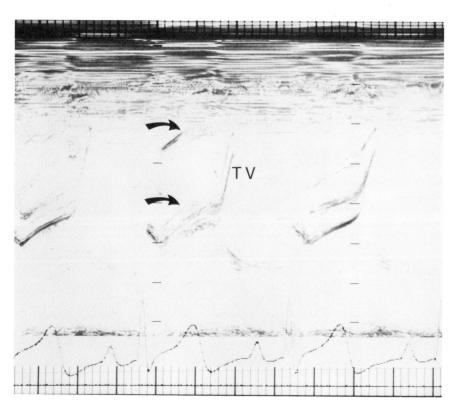

Figure 25.11 (cont'd.). In (*C*), the aneurysm is seen bulging into the right ventricle (*large arrows*), and the base of the defect is identified by T artifacts (*small arrows*). The defect lies just below the aorta in this anteriorly oriented four-chamber view. In (*D*), the characteristic tricuspid DE excursion can be seen with each cycle. Preceding this in systole, a double row of echoes with systolic anterior motion identified by the arrows represents the two margins of the aneurysm.

D

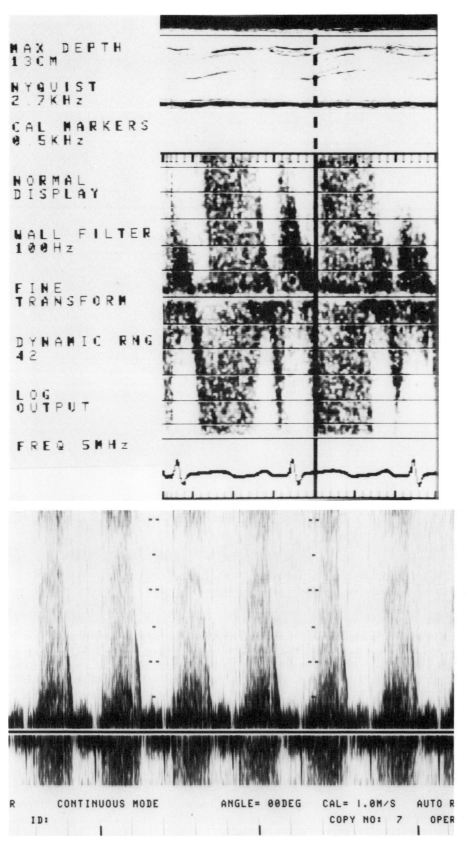

Figure 25.12. The top frame is a pulsed Doppler recording taken from the region of the right ventricle adjacent to this perimembranous ventricular septal defect. M-mode panel: In the Doppler display, the signal clearly defines the flow disturbance in systole; directionality and peak velocity cannot be recorded due to aliasing. The pulsed Doppler recording, however, is important in that it allows the mapping of the position of the jet and its direction, which aids in defining small defects and those that cannot be imaged by ultrasound. The bottom frame is a continuous wave Doppler recording of a perimembranous ventricular septal defect recorded from the precordial area. The velocity across the ventricular septal defect is 5 meters per second. This corresponds to a pressure drop of approximately 100 millimeters of mercury, suggesting normal right ventricular pressures in this very small ventricular septal defect. If, for example, systolic blood pressure was 120, right ventricular systolic pressure would be about 20 mm Hg.

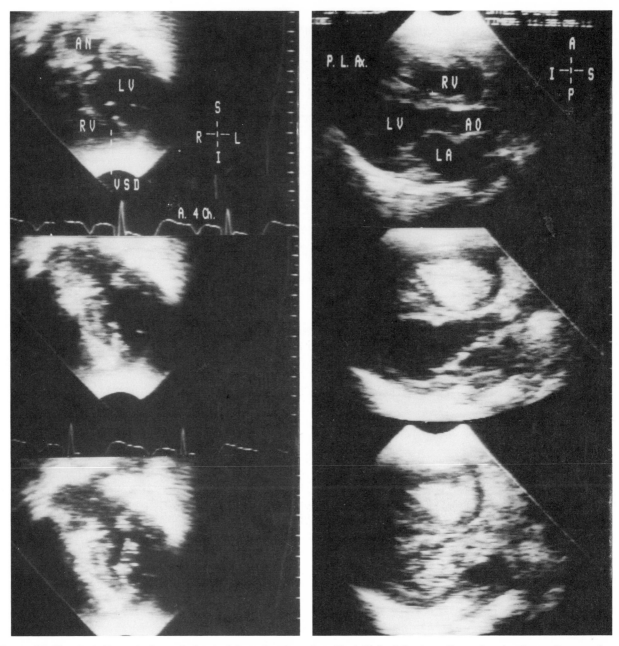

Figure 25.13.   Left: Posteriorly angled apical four-chamber view (A. 4 Ch.) of the two-dimensional echocardiogram demonstrating a series of venous contrast echocardiograms. Top, a large apical ventricular septal defect (VSD). Middle, contrast material has filled the right heart structures. Bottom, the right-to-left shunting of the saline contrast solution into the left ventricle crosses the apical trabecular defect. (Reproduced by permission from Shaddy R, Silverman NH, Stranger P, Ebert P. Two-dimensional echocardiographic recognition and repair of subclavian mitral aneurysm of the left ventricle in an infant. J Am Coll Cardiol 1985;5:765–9.) Right: From the same patient, showing a series of contrast injections to define the right-to-left shunt in the parasternal long axis (P L Ax).

exhibited posterior deviation of the outlet septum, giving rise to narrowing of the left ventricular outflow tract.

Echocardiographic Approach to the Diagnosis of Ventricular Septal Defects

Ventricular septal defects should be imaged from several planes (15). Only by imaging defects in this manner can they be located with precision (17, 18). When a single plane is used, artifactual dropout may confuse the viewer regarding the presence or absence of a septal deficiency. Imaging in multiple planes diminishes the likelihood of this error (18). Studies have shown that the accuracy of imaging increases when multiple-plane imaging is employed (Fig. 25.11) (18). In addition, we use pulsed Doppler ultrasound to confirm

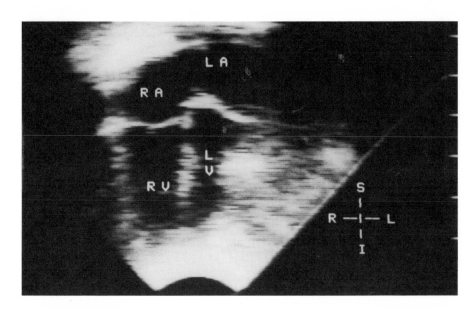

Figure 25.14. Apical four-chamber view of a perimembranous inlet ventricular septal defect. The mitral and tricuspid valves are in fibrous continuity. The ventricular septal defect is identified immediately underneath the base of the aortic root.

the presence of ventricular septal defects (Fig. 25.12). While locating the jet, an estimate of the velocity of the flow disturbance and its location along the ventricular septum can be determined (19). The peak velocity of the jet determined by continuous wave Doppler ultrasound provides an approximation of the peak systolic pressure drop across the defect (20). Mapping of the flow disturbance may be very helpful in defining the location of defects.

Color Flow Mapping

Precise location of single defects and the direction of left-to-right shunts or right-to-left flow patterns can be readily shown with flow mapping. The most important value of color flow mapping is for defining the ventricular septal defect location, the presence of multiple

apical or anterior muscular defects, and for scanning the septum when the defect cannot be displayed by other modalities of ultrasound. This technique has increased our accuracy for detecting ventricular septal defects considerably.

We also use venous contrast echocardiography to define right-to-left shunting through the ventricular septal defect (Fig. 25.13) (15). This technique is very sensitive: Only a few microbubbles need to enter the left ventricle to be visualized. This technique has been particularly helpful in all but the smallest ventricular septal defects because right-to-left shunting occurs in defects even when right ventricular end-diastolic pressure is only moderately elevated or when mild increases in diastolic pressure occur only transiently. As the shunt from right to left occurs in diastole, only mild differences of end-diastolic pressure between the ven-

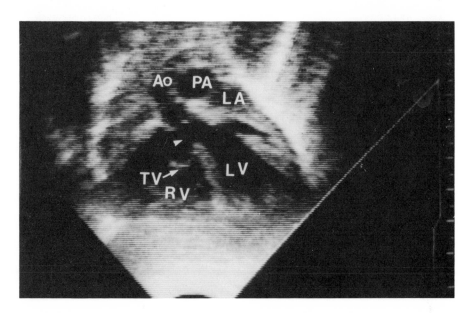

Figure 25.15. Example of a perimembranous ventricular septal defect obtained from a subcostal coronal cut. The ventricular septal defect is defined by an arrow between the septal leaflet of the tricuspid valve (TV) and the aortic root (AO). The positions of the pulmonary trunk and left atrial appendage (LA) are also defined. Orientation as for other subcostal para-coronal planes.

Figure 25.16. Apical four-chamber cut showing two examples of large apical trabecular muscular ventricular septal defects (VSD). (*A*) Large single apical trabecular defect. The trabeculations of the moderator band, septomarginal trabeculations, and anterior right ventricular papillary muscle overlie the defect from the right ventricular aspect. (*B*) Similar findings with two defects identified (*arrows*).

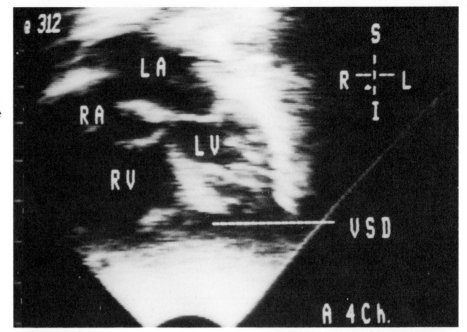

A

B

Figure 25.17. Apical four-chamber view of a small isolated muscular trabecular ventricular septum indicated by the arrow.

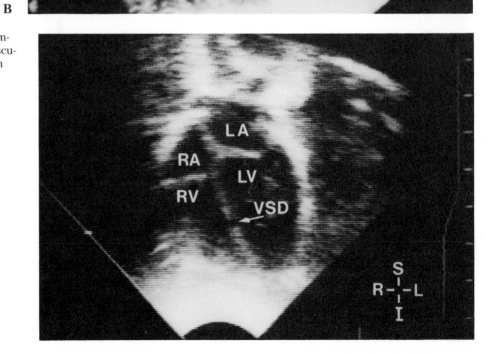

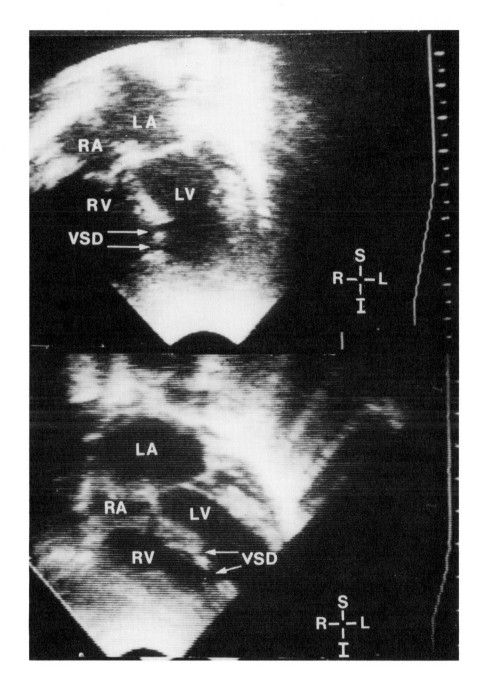

Figure 25.18. Two examples of multiple trabecular ventricular septal defects (VSD) (*arrows*) taken from different positions in the same child. There was a large shunt and pulmonary hypertension at catheterization. The top frame is from the apical four-chamber plane. The bottom frame is from a subcostal coronal cut. In the top frame, 1/2 centimeter markers are included.

tricles need to be present. The contrast echo technique in our hands has been much more sensitive than cineangiography for showing right-to-left shunts. The use of contrast echocardiography should be considered in all patients where ventricular septal defects are suspected but not imaged. This is particularly true for the small multiple apical ventricular septal defects associated with pulmonary hypertension.

A useful physical sign of the defect is the so-called T artifact (18) shown on several of the subsequent figures. This is best seen when the septum is aligned so that resolution of the defect is in an axial direction (such as from an apical projection or subcostal four-

chamber view). A high impedance level exists at the blood-tissue interface, producing a ballooning of echoes at the rim of the defect, hence the T sign.

Perimembranous Ventricular Septal Defects

Defects in this region of the septum can be imaged from many planes including parasternal long- and short-axis planes and the apical two- and four-chamber planes as well as subcostal paracoronal and parasagittal planes (Figs. 25.11, 25.14, and 25.15) (15–18, 21).

The parasternal short-axis plane (Fig. 25.11) reveals the location of the defect near the tricuspid valve and

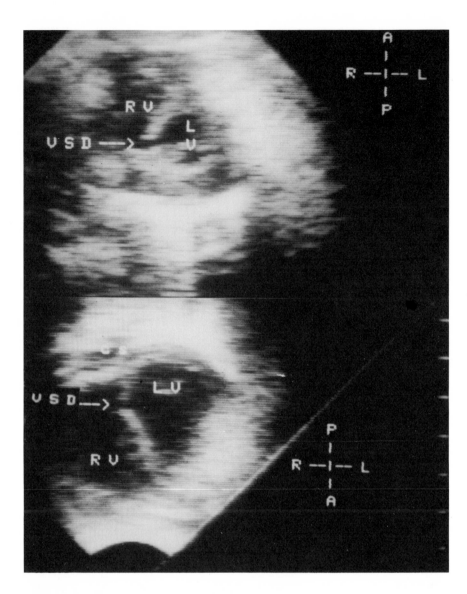

Figure 25.19. Small muscular inlet ventricular septal defect in the posterior ventricular septum. The top frame shows the VSD (*arrow*) between the right and left ventricle in the parasternal short axis view. The bottom frame from the apical four-chamber view shows the VSD in the posterior muscular septum. The posterior plane is inferred from the presence of the coronary sinus (CS) and the crux of the heart.

just below the aortic valve. The defect may extend to open into the inlet or outlet components of the right ventricle; it extends below into the inlet portion of the septum or cranially toward the outlet part of the septum. In long-axis views from the cardiac apex or parasternal position, the defect can be identified in the area immediately below the aortic valve (Figs. 25.11, 25.14, and 25.15). The membranous septum is the area of fibrous continuity between the aortic and tricuspid valves, and therefore, defects around this region can be located in the area adjacent to these valves.

When a defect can be seen in a standard (posterior) apical four-chamber plane, then the defect must have extended between the ventricular inlets. When there is such an inlet extension, the mitral and tricuspid valves are at the same level in the four-chamber view (17, 22). With more anterior angulation (i.e., in the apical four-chamber plus aortic root plane or five-chamber view), the scan plane passes through the left ventricular

outflow tract and the aortic root. Because the defect lies in the subaortic area, it can be seen in close proximity to the aortic valve.

From the subcostal paracoronal plane, the defect can also be seen clearly in the subaortic and subtricuspid position (Fig. 25.15). Often it is not possible to identify the insertion of the tricuspid valve. This can cause the artifactual appearance of a left ventricular to right atrial communication.

The so-called aneurysm of the membranous septum, lesions that are more usually tags of tricuspid valve tissue, are frequently found in association with perimembranous septal defects (Figs. 25.11 and 25.14). They have the appearance of pouches that usually bulge into the right ventricular outflow tract adjacent to the tricuspid valve. The pouches may rarely bulge into the left ventricular outflow tract if the right pressure is suprasystemic. The typical M-mode appearance is of systolic anterior motion with fine vibrations

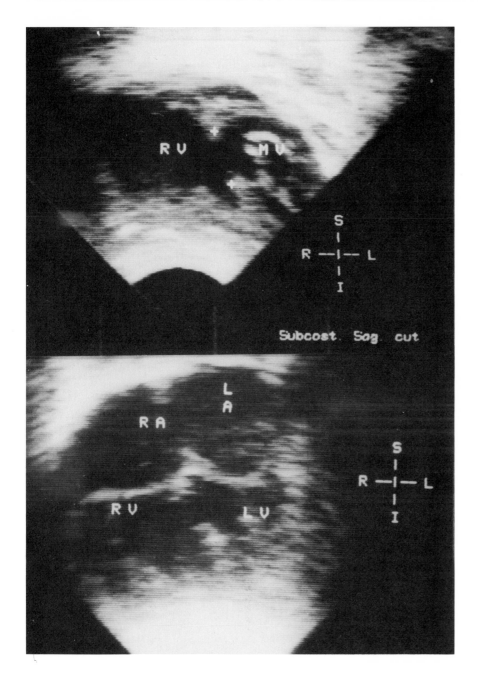

Figure 25.20. Similar findings in a patient with a large muscular inlet defect from the subcostal sagittal (top) view, which is equivalent to a parasternal short-axis view, and one apical four-chamber view (bottom). Note that the positions of the tricuspid and mitral valves are on the same horizontal level.

anterior to the tricuspid valve (Fig. 25.11). The systolic motion is characteristically double, related to the vibration of both walls of the aneurysm. Because pathologic studies have shown that this tissue comprises largely tricuspid tissue, we prefer the term "tricuspid tissue tags" to describe the lesion. In the 247 cases of perimembranous ventricular septal defects that we have followed, 77 percent (190 cases) had perimembranous tissue tags. The finding of these tags was associated with a higher incidence of spontaneous closure even when small defects were excluded, and therefore, fewer of those cases were referred for surgery. We have also noted that these tags are found early in the

course of the disease, and we have seen them in premature infants in the first few days of life. When present, the tags were identified in 93 percent of patients during the first examination, and almost all were identified within the first 6 months of life. Over the 30 months of median follow-up of patients possessing these lesions, we found the tricuspid tissue tag closed the ventricular septal defect in 11 percent. In 33 percent, the shunt diminished in size, and only 11 percent underwent surgery. By contrast, in those without such an "aneurysm," 16 percent diminished in size, only 2 percent underwent spontaneous closure, and 84 percent underwent surgery. Detection of perimembra-

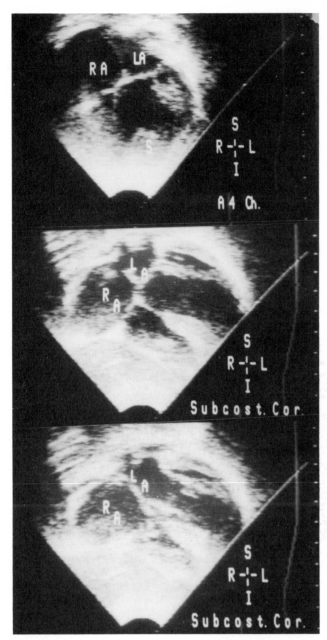

Figure 25.21. Apical four-chamber and subcostal coronal series in a patient with a large inlet ventricular septal defect. Top frame shows the valves at the same level, a large defect, and small interatrial communication. The bright echo between the two atrioventricular valve leaflets and the lower atrial septum represents the central fibrous body. Middle frame in systole: The chordal attachment of the tricuspid valve to the septum appears to obscure the defect. In the bottom frame in early diastole, the open atrioventricular valve leaflets do the same. The composite of these views provides an estimate of position and size of the defect.

nous tricuspid tissue tags is therefore of importance because their presence appears to be associated with a more favorable prognosis increased likelihood of spontaneous closure. With regard to evaluation of hemody-

namics, the pulmonary arterial pressure was generally lower in the presence of the ventricular septal aneurysm. The exception was in patients with Down syndrome in whom there was a high incidence of elevated pulmonary arterial pressure and large pulmonary to systemic flow ratios.

The tricuspid tissue tags can be defined by cross-sectional echocardiography from the parasternal, apical, and subcostal views as well as by M-mode echocardiography (Fig. 25.11). Their presence demonstrates the precise location of the ventricular septal defect and its relationship to the septal leaflet of the tricuspid valve. In real time, the tissue tags can be seen to extend into the right ventricle during systole (except in patients with complete transposition or those with suprasystemic right ventricular pressure). In the latter circumstances, the tissue tags may be observed to prolapse into the left ventricular outflow tract and often give the appearance of a subvalvar fibrous shelf or straddling tricuspid valve. Although tricuspid tissue tags have been described as obstructing the right ventricular outflow tract, we have not observed this phenomenon in our series.

The tissue tag constricts the size of the defect at its apex but not at the attachment to the rim of the defect. The size of the defect at its base may therefore reflect in part the larger original size of the ventricular septal defect. The tags remain at first in those ventricular septal defects that close, but at longer follow-up, they diminish in size or disappear as they become incorporated into the ventricular septum.

Muscular Defects

These defects are surrounded entirely by muscle. Previous studies have suggested that these defects are difficult to identify when they are apically situated (21). Most are certainly difficult to recognize from the parasternal and even subcostal positions unless they are large, but we found the apical views to be reliable for identifying them (Figs. 25.16, 25.17, and 25.18). They are frequently multiple and are often associated with large left-to-right shunts (Figs. 25.16, 25.17, and 25.18). Such defects are invariably associated with a degree of right ventricular hypertension; hence contrast echocardiography has been a valuable technique for showing the right-to-left shunt (Fig. 25.13) (8). With regard to the actual imaging from the cardiac apex, the transducer must be directed from the most posterior to the most anterior position so as to examine the entire trabecular septum. It has been our experience that when only one large defect is identified echocardiographically, additional smaller defects can often be found either at surgery or autopsy. Trabeculations overlying the right ventricular aspect of the defect may give the appear-

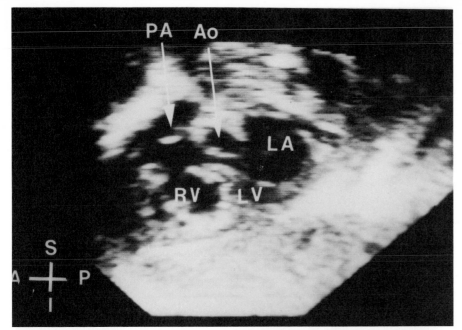

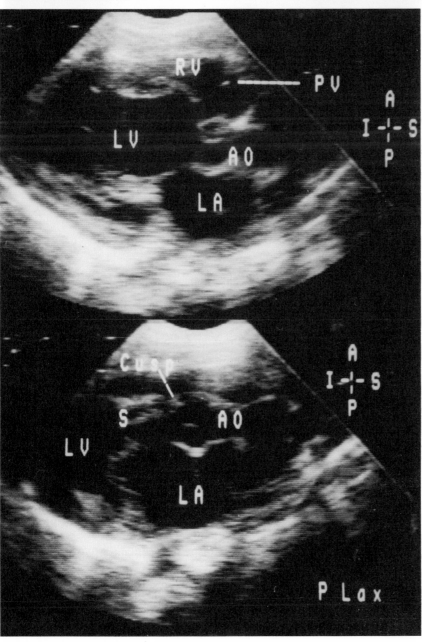

Figure 25.22. Subcostal cut in a small infant with a doubly committed subarterial ventricular septal defect. The pulmonary valves and the aortic valves proximal to the pulmonary artery (PA) and aorta (Ao) are clearly seen. The ventricular septal defect lies immediately beneath the plane of the aortic and pulmonic valve without any intervening septum in this area.

Figure 25.23. Example of a doubly committed subarterial ventricular septal defect in the long-axis plane taken in two portions in the cardiac cycle. Note, in the top frame at end systole, the ventricular septal defect lying between the aortic valve and pulmonic valve (PV). In the top frame, the ascending aorta (AO), left atrium (LA), and left ventricle (LV) have been labeled. In late diastole (bottom frame), the cusp of the aorta (the right coronary cusp) has prolapsed through the defect, virtually obliterating it, so that alignment occurs with the ventricular septum. This finding of progressive aortic cusp prolapse has been observed quite frequently in ventricular septal defects of this type. Orientation as for other parasternal long-axis (P LAX) views.

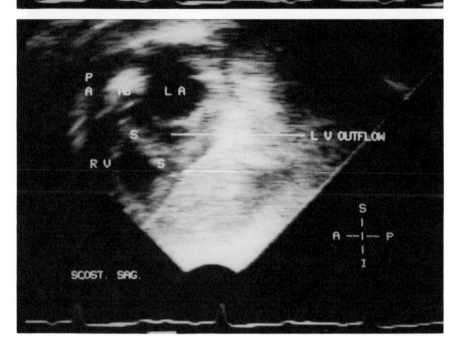

Figure 25.24. Composite mapping of four views defining the doubly committed subarterial ventricular septal defect in one child. Top left shows the position of the aortic and pulmonary valves in continuity and the defect just below this in a subcostal sagittal cut. With angulation of the transducer toward the aorta, the position of the ventricular septal defect is defined in the bottom frame showing the doubly committed nature of the defect. In the top right-hand frame, the subcostal paracoronal cut shows the pulmonary valve rising above the right ventricle, while the ventricular septal defect is committed directly below the pulmonary valve. The defect is bound by the ventricular septum and the pulmonary and aortic valves. Bottom right frame shows the position of the ventricular septal defect (+ − +), which is situated more toward the pulmonary artery than that seen in perimembranous ventricular septal defects (see Figure 25.11).

ance of a multiple defect, but when viewed from the left ventricular aspect, the defect may appear single. Some isolated small trabecular muscular ventricular septal defects in premature newborn infants cannot be imaged. Such patients show no evidence of chamber enlargement or other signs of sizable left-to-right shunts. The location of these defects has been determined by Doppler flow mapping and their presence indicated by the typical clinical findings of a high-pitched pansystolic murmur. On clinical follow-up, we have found these defects to disappear.

Muscular Inlet Defects

These defects have been found in 48 patients (10% of our series). They are identifiable in several planes, including parasternal, apical, and subcostal (Figs. 25.19, 25.20, and 25.21). Their hallmark is their proximity to both atrioventricular valves and their proximal location relative to the medial papillary muscle. It has been our experience that these defects are usually large. Using one view alone may lead to erroneous interpretation as a double-inlet ventricle rather than a

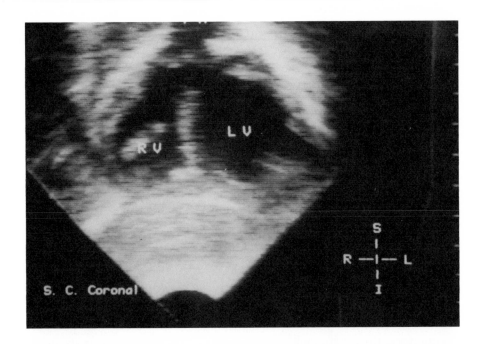

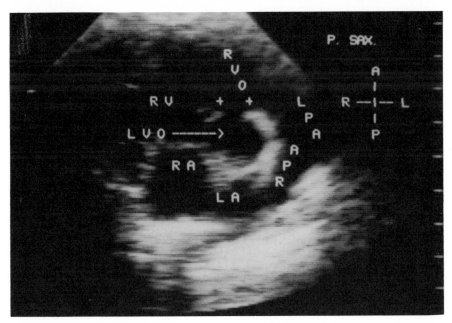

large ventricular septal defect. A useful feature in distinguishing a double-inlet ventricle from a large ventricular septal defect is the demonstration of either a small portion of the atrioventricular septum between the atrioventricular valves or a flange of septum at the cardiac apex. The rudimentary septum that divides the ventricular mass in a double-inlet ventricle is in a quite different position. Muscular inlet defects can be differentiated from perimembranous inlet defects by the relationship of the leaflets of the atrioventricular valves. In perimembranous defects, these lie in the same plane while in muscular defects they are in different planes (Fig. 25.20) (17, 22).

Muscular Outlet Defects

These defects have traditionally been the most difficult to image from standard transducer positions because of their anterior placement (17). They are best imaged from subcostal and high parasternal positions. In our series, there were 36 cases (8%) with a defect in the outlet muscular septum.

Doubly Committed Subarterial Defects

These defects are best imaged from subcostal and high parasternal positions (Figs. 25.22, 25.23, and 25.24). In

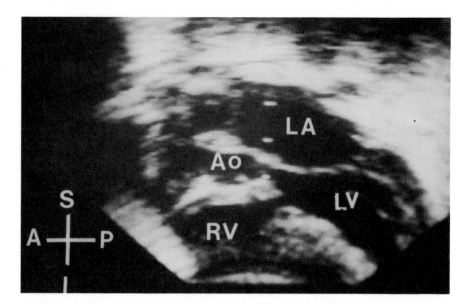

Figure 25.25. Subcostal parasagittal cut in a patient with malalignment between the outlet and trabecular components of the ventricular septal defect causing subaortic obstruction. This is frequently found in aortic coarctation and aortic arch interruption.

the high parasternal long-axis position, the transducer is rotated to lie parallel to the outlet septum and then further rotated slightly clockwise from the long-axis view while the aorta and pulmonary trunk are imaged. It is possible to define the defect lying underneath the two arterial (semilunar) valves. The subcostal view is an alternative and valuable position for defining this defect, especially in infants. The transducer is kept in the sagittal plane and rotated slightly leftward and counterclockwise to bring the aortic and pulmonary valves into view (Figs. 25.22, 25.23, and 25.24). The structure normally separating these valves is the outlet (infundibular) septum. In the presence of the doubly committed defect, this region is deficient and is bound superiorly by the arterial valve leaflets in fibrous continuity.

Prolapse of the aortic valve leaflet may occur as a complication in this defect because of deficient sup-

port. This complication can also occur with perimembranous outlet defects. The prolapse, usually of the right coronary leaflet of the aortic valve, both diminishes the size of the ventricular septal defect and creates aortic insufficiency. Echocardiographic definition of this lesion requires a high index of suspicion as the defect may be extremely small and deformity of the aortic valve may be subtle. We have encountered this lesion in five patients in our series (Fig. 25.23). The first identifying feature can be obtained from the parasternal long-axis view. Here the right coronary leaflet appears enlarged and leaflet closure may appear eccentric in diastole. The ventricular septal defect may be identified just below the enlarged leaflet. Dilatation of the right coronary aortic sinus is an identifying echocardiographic feature. It may be slightly distorted and appears in the long-axis view to be pointed rather than curved at the region of the ventricular septum. The use

Figure 25.26. A parasternal long-axis view with malalignment between the outlet component and the trabecular septum, which is not as marked as in Figure 25.25.

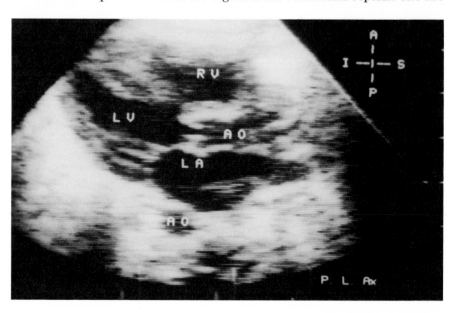

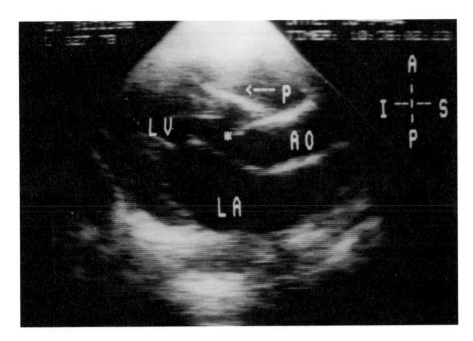

Figure 25.27. Repaired defect of the malalignment type with persistent subaortic obstruction. As the subaortic malalignment was not appreciated, the defect was repaired as a conventional perimembranous ventricular septal defect with a patch (P). Subaortic obstruction worsened after the ventricular septal defect was closed because of the malaligned septum.

of combined echocardiography and Doppler has been helpful in confirming this abnormality. The jet may be mapped out originating in the right ventricular outflow tract and continuing into the pulmonary trunk. The flow disturbance may be the cause of the flutter on the pulmonary valve leaflet observed by M-mode echocardiography. Aortic insufficiency may also be found and is suggestive of the subaortic location of the defect. The aortic regurgitant jet may be mapped by pulsed Doppler and demonstrated to arise from the anterior part of the aortic root in the region of the right coronary cusp.

Malalignment

Malalignment of the ventricular septum with respect to the atrial septum occurs in association with straddling tricuspid valve.

Malalignment also occurs between the outlet and trabecular septum. When the outlet septum is deviated into the right ventricle, the result is the so-called Eisenmenger-type ventricular septal defect. There were 10 such patients in our series.

Table 25.1A. Complete Atrioventricular Septal Associated Defects

	Total Number of Cases		
Defect	Type A (113)	Type B (3)	Type C (12)
Down syndrome	66	—	—
Trisomy 18	1	—	—
Patent ductus arteriosus	4	—	1
Apical muscular ventricular septal defect	3	—	—
Secundum atrial septal defect	1	—	2
Valvar pulmonary stenosis	3	—	2
Coarctation	2	—	—
Tetralogy of Fallot	6	—	—
Transposition of the great arteries	6	—	3
Univentricular atrioventricular connection and common atrioventricular valve	2	—	—
Subaortic stenosis	1	—	1
Left isomerism	5	—	2
Right isomerism	6	—	3
Left dominance	3	—	1
Right dominance	4	—	—
Malposition	4	—	—
Pulmonary atresia	2	—	2
Total anomalous pulmonary venous return	2	—	1
Truncus	2	—	—
Heart block	2	—	1
Single left ventricular papillary muscle	2	—	—
Right aortic arch	2	—	—
Double outlet right ventricle	2	—	1
Left superior vena cava to left atrium	1	—	1
Bilateral superior vena cava	1	—	—
Left superior vena cava to coronary sinus	1	—	—

Table 25.1B. Incomplete Atrioventricular Septal Associated Defects (43)

Defect	Number
Subaortic stenosis	6
Pulmonary stenosis	3
Bicuspid aortic valve	1
Muscular ventricular septal defect	1
Left superior vena cava to coronary sinus	1
"Tricuspid pouch"	15
"Cleft mitral valve"	18
Left superior vena cava to coronary sinus	2
Down syndrome	9
Left isomerism	1
Right isomerism	1
Right dominance	1
Secundum atrial septal defect	3
Patent ductus arteriosus	2
Left-sided atrioventricular valve insufficiency	8
Right-sided atrioventricular valve insufficiency	2

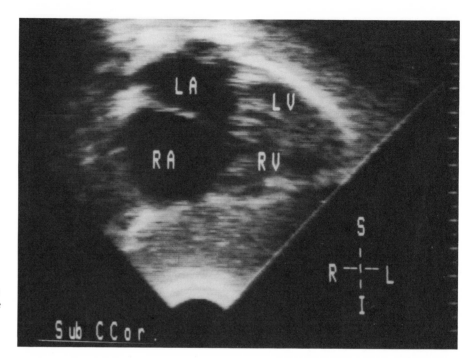

Figure 25.28. A subcostal coronal (Sub Cost Cor) view demonstrating an ostium primum variety of atrioventricular septal defect. The low end of the atrial septum is intact. Communication between the left and the right atria occurs entirely below this but above the atrioventricular valve plane.

A further eight patients had displacement of the outlet septum into the left ventricle, which caused subaortic outflow tract narrowing (Figs. 25.25, 25.26, and 25.27). These defects were associated with aortic coarctation in some, while in others the deviation was associated with interruption of the aortic arch (17, 23, 24). It is important to identify this cause of left ventricular outflow obstruction prior to surgical closure since if it is not recognized, the obstruction may become worse postoperatively. Posterior deviation is imaged best from long-axis views including the parasternal, apical, and subcostal parasagittal views.

Echocardiographic Definitions of the Mechanisms of Closure and Natural History

We have followed a large number of ventricular septal defects (25) and have found that the incidence of spontaneous closure was highest in perimembranous ventricular septal defects. The predominant mecha-

Figure 25.29. Apical four-chamber view (A 4 Ch) demonstrating the findings of an ostium primum atrial septal defect. Both the lower end of the atrial septum (ATR S) and the area of the oval fossa above it are shown. The atrioventricular valve leaflets are connected to the crest of the ventricular septum separating the valve orifice into left and right components. The interatrial communication occurs below the atrial septum and above the plane of the atrioventricular valve.

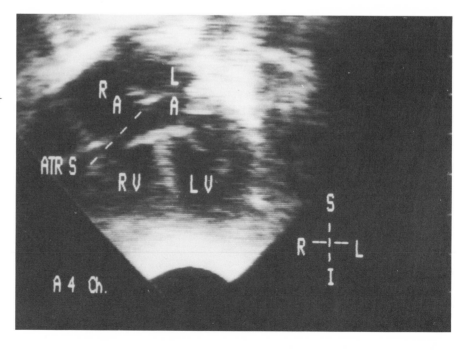

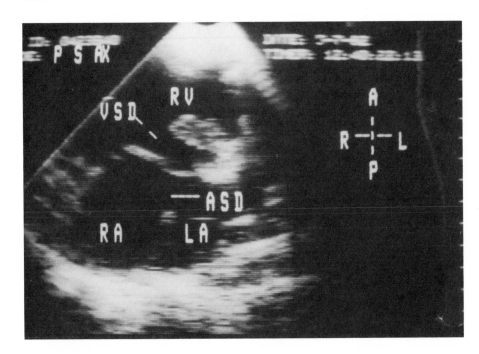

Figure 25.30. Parasternal short-axis view (P S Ax) in a patient with a complete form of atrioventricular septal defect demonstrating the atrial septal deficiency (ASD) and the perimembranous extension of the ventricular component of the septal defect (VSD).

nism of closure was incorporation of tricuspid tissue tags into the defect to form an aneurysm. We found this to be common, and contrary to previous reports, it was an early occurrence. Only 12 percent of these defects underwent spontaneous closure and another 33 percent diminished considerably in size. Endothelial proliferation, another means of natural closure of ventricular septal defects, is probably a mechanism that closes the small muscular ventricular septal defects in newborn infants. As these defects may not be seen initially and leave no ultrasonic marker, we have not observed this phenomenon with ultrasound. Partial or incomplete closure by means of prolapse of an aortic valve leaflet was noted in five patients. Some ventricular septal defects get smaller with age. We have not, however, encountered this as a mechanism of closure in the ultrasound studies we have performed. It is also likely that some ventricular septal defects are unable to undergo spontaneous closure. These include the malalignment type of ventricular septal defect, the doubly committed subarterial defects, and large muscular trabecular septal defects. Thus, when the precise location of the defect is determined, the natural history, the likelihood of complications, and associated defects can be outlined more accurately.

Surgical Considerations

Surgical implications of location of the defect in the septum are important because the position of the defect may dictate the surgical approach. Furthermore, once the nature of the defect is known, the position and relations of the conduction system can be accu-

rately inferred. Defects in the inlet and perimembranous area are frequently related to the major atrioventricular conduction axis. Damage to the conduction system is more likely to occur in these lesions than in outlet and trabecular defects, which are remote from the major conducting tissues. In such circumstances, deeper sutures within the ventricular muscle allow a more secure anchoring of suture material for the ventricular septal defect patch.

ATRIOVENTRICULAR SEPTAL DEFECTS (ATRIOVENTRICULAR CANAL DEFECTS)

These findings are based on a population we studied of 171 patients with atrioventricular septal defects. The type of abnormality and associated abnormalities are shown in Table 25.1A and B. The hallmark of these defects is that they are situated in the region occupied in the normal heart by the atrioventricular septum.

Cross-sectional echocardiography has proved invaluable in the definition of these complex abnormalities (29–35). A full complement of parasternal, apical, and subcostal views aid complete definition of these abnormalities.

Comparison of the echocardiographic findings with the intraoperative and autopsy findings has shown that the attachments of the bridging leaflets to the septum and the arrangement of the atrioventricular valve leaflets can be clearly defined by echocardiography. Indeed, the definition achieved by echocardiography is superior to that obtained with angiography. Echocardiographic definition of the various types of leaflet morphology in atrioventricular septal defects with

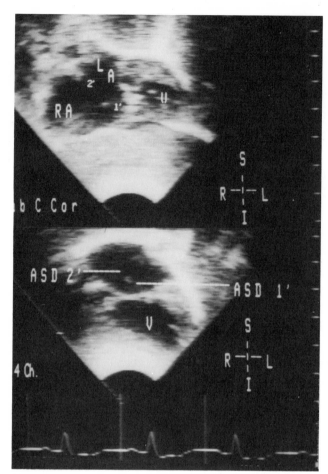

Figure 25.31. A subcostal coronal view (top) and apical four-chamber view (bottom) in a patient with atrioventricular septal defect, left isomerism, and absent ventricular septum. In the top frame, the primum (1') and secundum (2') components are separated by a thin strand of atrial tissue. The labeling for the atria (LA, RA) indicates the atria are left sided and right sided but not their morphology. In the bottom frame, an apical four-chamber view, the two components of the atrial communication and a common atrioventricular valve with only lateral attachments are seen. There is only one identifiable ventricular chamber (V).

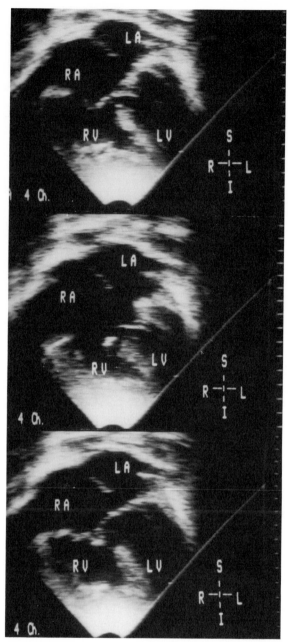

Figure 25.32. Three still-frame examples from an apical four-chamber view of the complete atrioventricular septal defect demonstrating how the leaflet motion during the cardiac cycle affects the visualization of the size of the atrial and ventricular components of the defect. In systole, the ventricular communication is best appreciated; in diastole, the atrial communication is best appreciated. There is chordal attachment to the ventricular septum, both to the crest and the right papillary muscle aspect.

common valve orifices may now be more specific than the surgeon requires since the surgical techniques employed make definition of the particular leaflet morphology less important for surgical repair (36). The information obtained from these echocardiographic studies has enabled a limited number of patients from our institution to be sent directly to surgery without cardiac catheterization when pulmonary vascular disease has been "confidently" excluded noninvasively.

In addition to noting whether the defect is associated with common or separate right and left valve orifices, it is important to ascertain the presence of interatrial or interventricular communications. The latter feature depends largely on the relationship of the bridging leaflets of the atrioventricular valve to the ventricular septum. Thus, the key to accurate diagnosis is deter-

mination of the arrangement of the anterosuperior and posteroinferior bridging leaflets and their attachment to the valve annulus together with their papillary muscle and septal attachments. The relationship between the annulus of the valve and the underlying ventricles must also be demonstrated, since this determines whether the atrioventricular junction is commit-

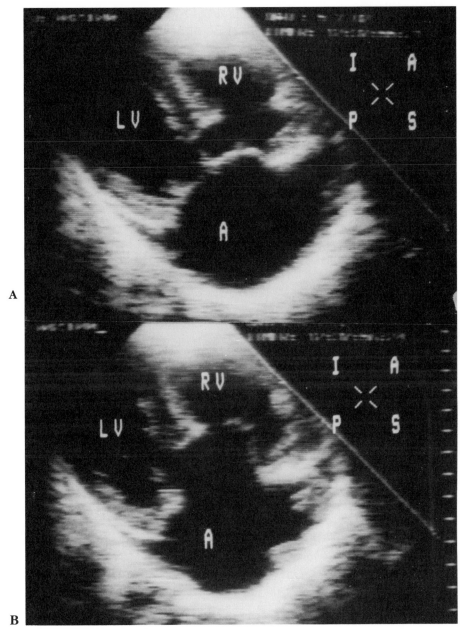

Figure 25.33. In systole (*A*), a parasternal long-axis view with angulation toward the right ventricle. The bridging leaflets in systole separate the atrium (A) from the left ventricle (LV) and right ventricle (RV). The chordal attachments of the anterior bridging leaflet to the crest of the ventricular septum can be clearly seen. In diastole (*B*), the leaflets move to an open position, but the chordal attachments of the anterior and posterior leaflets can be clearly seen. (*B*) demonstrates the leaflets opening in diastole showing chordal attachment to both ventricles.

ted primarily to one or the other ventricle. An imbalance in this respect is usually described as ventricular dominance (37, 38). By describing common or separate orifices together with the potential level of chamber communications, we avoid the use of potentially confusing adjectives such as "complete" and "partial" and the even more confusing "intermediate" form of atrioventricular canal defect. By using the system of Rastelli modified by Becker and Anderson (39–41), the defects with common orifice are further classified into type A with minimal bridging, type B with partial bridging, and type C with extreme bridging of the anterosuperior leaflet of the common atrioventricular valve.

The Interatrial Communication

Interatrial communications vary in size from large to small. They are defined in the same planes as those used to define other interatrial communications. Short-axis views are used but provide less information than other planes (Figs. 25.28, 25.29, 25.30, and 25.31). The interatrial septum itself can be defined from the interatrial groove down to the lower edge of the rim of the oval fossa in the apical and subcostal four-chamber views. Although the atrial septum can appear intact from these conventional views, it may still be deficient. Interatrial communications occur below the lower free

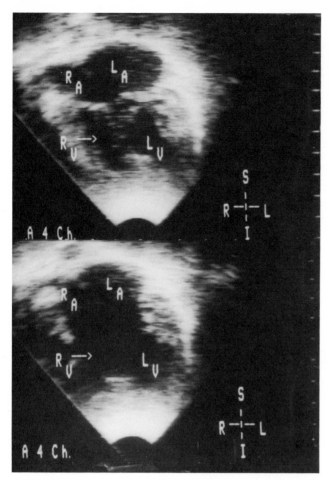

Figure 25.34. Top frame demonstrates an apical four-chamber view in a patient with vestigial atrial and ventricular septa and large interatrial and interventricular communication. The top frame in systole demonstrates the valve leaflet in the closed position; the bottom frame in diastole with the valve leaflet open allows appraisal of the size of the atrial and ventricular septal remnants.

edge of the septum (Figs. 25.28 and 25.29) and through the area of deficient atrioventricular septation. Nonetheless, it is conventionally described as an ostium primum atrial septal defect, and we will follow this usage. The significant feature is that the defect is bound inferiorly by the conjoined bridging leaflets of the atrioventricular valve, which are depressed into the ventricular mass and attached to the crest of the ventricular septum.

The Interventricular Communication

The classical ventricular component of the atrioventricular septal defect is best seen from the apical four-chamber view (Fig. 25.32). In this view, the defect can be traced from its posterior to anterior limits by tilting the transducer from a caudal to cranial direction. Subcostal four-chamber or paracoronal views are also

useful for defining the extent of the defect as are multiple long- and short-axis views (Figs. 25.30 and 25.33). In this respect, it is important to note that the relationships of the valve leaflets and the boundaries of the defect change throughout the cardiac cycle. The interventricular component of the defect as seen in our series varied markedly in size from very small and confined beneath the anterosuperior leaflet to where the muscular ventricular septum was almost completely absent (Fig. 25.34).

Atrioventricular Valve Anatomy and Chordal Attachment

Cross-sectional echocardiography has provided an unmatched opportunity for definition of atrioventricular leaflet morphology before surgery. This is particularly important for the distinction of the variable morphology of the anterosuperior bridging leaflet, which formed the basis of the Rastelli classification (39). In atrioventricular septal defects with common valve orifice, the anterosuperior and posteroinferior bridging leaflets were seen in several planes to straddle the septum. The anterosuperior leaflet was seen in the long-axis planes from both the apical and parasternal areas. The anterosuperior leaflet can be identified from the apical four-chamber views with cranial tilt. We search for this leaflet by scanning immediately posterior to the aortic root from the four-chamber plane.

There were very few defects in our series with intermediate bridging (type B) (Fig. 25.35A) or with extreme bridging (type C) into the right ventricle (Fig. 25.35B) (Table 25.1). Indeed, in the majority of cases, the anterosuperior bridging leaflet was attached either directly to the underlying ventricular septum in linear fashion or was connected to the medial papillary muscle of the right ventricle.

The echocardiographic definition of atrioventricular valve morphology and valve attachments was entirely consistent with the more recent expanded classification based on the degree of bridging as advanced by Carpentier (40) and Becker and Anderson (41). With minimal bridging, the commissural attachment of the anterosuperior leaflet was to the medial papillary muscle, but the leaflet was additionally attached to the crest of the ventricular septum by tendinous chords (Figs. 25.32, 25.33, and 25.34). The interventricular communication was through the interchordal spaces. With extreme bridging (Rastelli type C), the atrioventricular valve leaflet was attached solely to a large papillary muscle within the right ventricle. There was no attachment of the leaflet to the crest of the septum as it bridged (Figs. 25.31, 25.35). Using cineangiography as a guide, the plane of the atrioventricular valve orifice can be defined as running in an almost vertical orien-

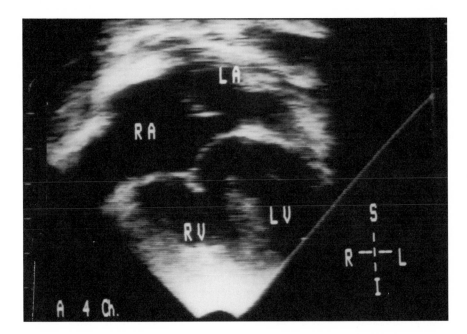

A

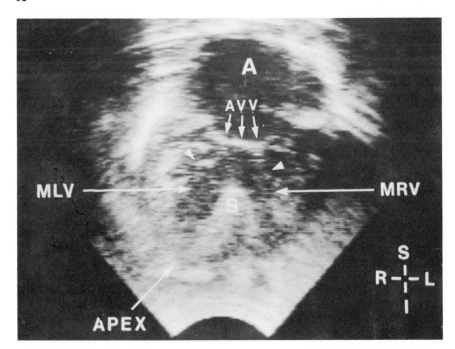

B

Figure 25.35. (*A*) Apical four-chamber cut (A 4 Ch). An atrioventricular septal defect with intermediate bridging of the anterosuperior leaflets (Rastelli type B). (*B*) Echocardiogram from a patient with dextrocardia and right isomerism. The cardiac apex is to the right. The morphologic left ventricle (MLV) is right sided, and the morphologic right ventricle is left sided (MRV). The anterosuperior leaflet of the common atrioventricular valve is identified by arrows (AVV). Its chordae (*arrowheads*) can be seen connecting to papillary muscles in the ventricles but not to the underlying ventricular septum.

tation. It is this abnormal orientation of the valve together with the unwedged position of the aorta that is partially responsible for producing the angiographic left ventricular outflow tract known as the "gooseneck" deformity (Figs. 25.36 and 25.37). By placing the transducer in this vertical direction, which is slightly counterclockwise from the true parasternal short-axis position, the valve leaflets can be clearly seen (Fig. 25.38). A similar image can be achieved from the subcostal parasagittal plane, especially in small children. The left component of the valve was invariably tricommissural. In addition to the space between the left ventricular components of the bridging leaflets (the "cleft"), it was also possible to identify the commissures with the smaller mural leaflet. It should be emphasized that it is the space between the left ventricular components of the anterosuperior and posteroinferior leaflets that, in the presence of separate right and left valve orifices (ostium primum atrial septal defect), produces the appearance of a cleft in the mitral valve (Fig. 25.39). With cross-sectional echocardiography, the right component of the atrioventricular valve is seen to be composed of a variable contribution of the bridging leaflets as well as the anterosuperior and inferior (mural) leaflets of the tricuspid valve (Fig. 25.38). The chordal and papillary muscle attachments of these leaflets were defined from this view.

As the papillary muscles support the commissures of the valve, their arrangement within the left ventricle is different from the normal left ventricle. This feature is best displayed in the parasternal short-axis or equivalent subcostal view. In the parasternal short-axis view of the normal left ventricle, the papillary muscle groups are situated at positions of approximately 4 o'clock and 8 o'clock, respectively; in atrioventricular septal defects, the papillary muscles are situated directly beneath the commissures at 2 o'clock and 5 o'clock, respectively (Fig. 25.40). In addition, the parasternal short-axis view defined the numbers of papillary muscles present within the ventricle. This feature can also be defined from an apical four-chamber plane (Fig. 25.41). A single left ventricular papillary muscle was found in two patients.

Balance

In most situations, the atrioventricular junction is positioned over the ventricular septum so that its left and right parts connect more or less equally into both ventricles. When the junction is eccentrically con-nected to either ventricle, left or right ventricular dominance is said to exist (37, 38). We have encountered nine cases where there has been a disturbance of balance. Four have been of the right-dominant variety (Fig. 25.41) and five of the left-dominant variety (Fig. 25.42). Associated hypoplasia of the ventricle was present in each case we examined. There was associated aortic coarctation in one of the cases with left dominance.

Defects with Separate Valve Orifices: The Tricuspid Pouch Lesion

The lesion we had previously termed the tricuspid pouch was identified echocardiographically in 18 patients we examined (Fig. 25.43). This pouch is probably the portion of the leaflet that is identified in autopsy specimens as the connecting tongue of tissue between the bridging leaflets. It bulges into the right heart in systole, giving the appearance of an aneurysm or pouch (42). These pouches were best defined either in the apical four-chamber or parasternal short-axis views. We have not been able to define this lesion angiographically.

Isolated Ostium Primum Defects

The leaflets of the atrioventricular valve in ostium primum defect are fused to the underlying ventricular septum as described previously, but have the same basic morphology, that is, a pentacuspid arrangement. This anatomy was found in 43 patients. The so-called

Figure 25.36. Parasternal long-axis view (PLAX) of the left ventricular outflow tract demostrating the echocardiographic equivalent of a gooseneck deformity in a complete atrioventricular septal defect due to the anterior displacement of the atrioventricular valve into the left ventricular outflow tract. This scan is from the same patient shown in Figure 25.33, but with more medially oriented plane.

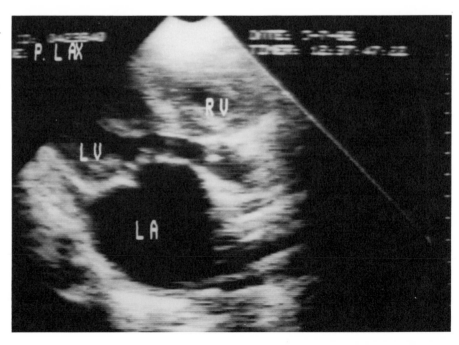

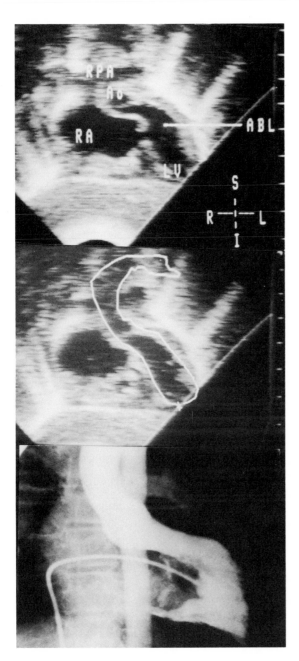

Figure 25.37. Top: Subcostal paracoronal view demonstrating the left ventricular outflow tract deformity (top frame and superimposed diagram—middle frame). As this view is equivalent to a posteroanterior angiographic projection, the equivalent of the gooseneck deformity can sometimes be defined as drawn in the middle figure and the angiogram below. The area of the commissure (mitral valve cleft) can be seen. Bottom frame: The angiogram shows the gooseneck deformity and the approximate vertical plane in which the atrioventricular valve orifice lies. The echocardiogram shows the cleft is really the commissure between the anterosuperior bridging leaflet (ABL) and the posteroinferior bridging leaflet. AO = aorta; I = inferior; L = left; LV = left ventricle; R = right; RA = right atrium; RPA = right pulmonary artery; S = superior.

mitral cleft could be identified as the space between the left ventricular components of the bridging leaflets in 18 patients with partial defects.

Down's Syndrome

Down's syndrome was present in 75 patients with atrioventricular canal defects. Only nine of this group had separate right and left valve orifices, whereas 66 had atrioventricular septal defects with a common orifice, all with minimal bridging of the anterosuperior leaflet (Rastelli type A).

Associated Lesions

Atrioventricular septal defects have been associated with a number of different lesions. These are included in Table 25.1.

Doppler Findings

Since 1982, we have examined patients with pulsed Doppler ultrasound to define the presence of insufficiency of the atrioventricular valve. Such insufficiency is well recognized preoperatively in many of these patients simply by auscultation. Pulsed Doppler ultrasound, however, is very sensitive in detecting even trivial amounts of valvar insufficiency (Fig. 25.44). This type of mild insufficiency as defined by Doppler ultrasound is most frequently found between the leaflets of the atrioventricular valve and the lower end of the atrial septum. In other words, it is regurgitation through the atrioventricular septal defect since the regurgitant systolic jet is directed through the atrioventricular junction from the left ventricle to the right atrium (43). More severe valvar insufficiency was detected over a wider range of positions in both the left and right atrial chambers. Our experience with Doppler ultrasound is incomplete because the technique was begun after we had acquired much of the cross-sectional echocardiographic experience. Nonetheless, we believe it to be valuable for defining both atrioventricular valve insufficiency and interventricular shunting.

Color Flow Mapping

Color flow mapping has proved to be a valuable technique for the assessment of atrioventricular septal defects. Not only can the atrial and ventricular components of the shunt be identified with color flow mapping, but the direction of the regurgitation from the atrioventricular valve so frequently found in this condition can provide important information about the nature of the valve function. Small central jets directed from the medial portion of the left ventricle toward the right atrium are very frequent and usually do not

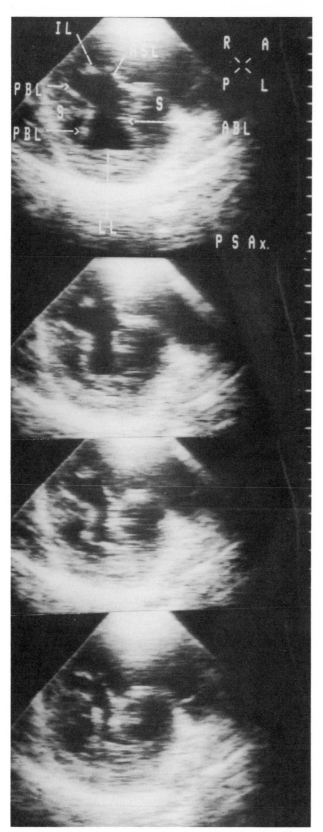

indicate severe atrioventricular valve regurgitation. With more severe degrees of regurgitation the jet may broaden, and separate regurgitant jets directly into the left atrium from the left ventricle and into the right atrium from the right ventricle may be displayed by color flow mapping. A further important use of the technique of color flow Doppler relates to the ease with which it is possible to determine the presence of associated ventricular septal defects, especially apical trabecular defects with color flow mapping.

PATENT DUCTUS ARTERIOSUS

Patent ductus is a common congenital abnormality, especially in the population of premature infants. Since 1980, we have examined 416 patients with a patent ductus; of these, 212 were premature infants. Until the decade of the 1980s, the diagnosis of patency was based on indirect evidence coupled with the typical clinical findings. Only occasionally was it possible to find the duct directly using cross-sectional echocardiography, and this was particularly difficult in small babies (14, 44, 45). Ancillary methods such as contrast echocardiography were employed in order to make the diagnosis (46). Current imaging techniques (47–51) together with Doppler ultrasound techniques (52–54) have now radically changed, which enable positive confirmation of patency even in the most premature infant. The use of very high frequency transducers (such as the 7.5 megahertz transducer which is available on certain mechanical scanners) has been the major change in technology that has facilitated positive diagnosis.

Imaging Technique

Our approach to imaging has been colored by our experience with fetal echocardiography, when the ductus arteriosus is an easily visualized structure (Fig. 25.45). When examining this fetus, it was obvious that there were two arterial arches visible. One was the aortic arch, recognized because of the arteries to the upper body that arise from it. The second arch was the ductus arteriosus, arising from the pulmonary trunk

Figure 25.38. Parasternal short-axis (P S Ax) view of the atrioventricular valve in the complete form of atrioventricular septal defect. Top frame: The various components of the atrioventricular valve are seen enface. The right ventricular (RV) and left ventricular cavities (LV) are displayed. Portions of the ventricular septum (S) are seen. The five components of the common atrioventricular valve are 1) the inferior tricuspid leaflet (IL), 2) the anterosuperior tricuspid leaflet (ASL), 3) the anterior bridging leaflet attached to the ventricular septum (ABL), 4) the lateral leaflet (LL), and 5) the two components of the posterior bridging leaflet (PBL) straddling the ventricular septum. The second, third, and fourth frames show progressive late diastolic closure of the valve. The tricommissural nature of the atrioventricular valve can be appreciated. A = anterior; L = left; P = posterior; R = right.

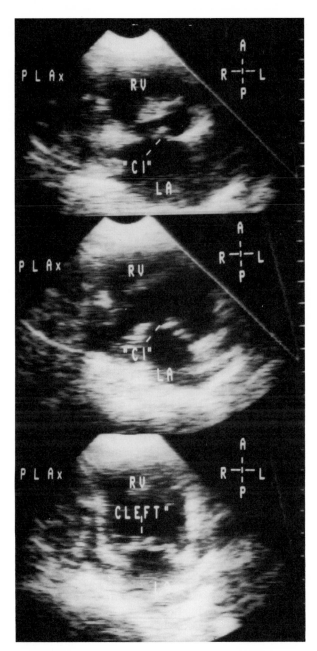

Figure 25.39. Sequence in the parasternal long-axis view (P L Ax) demonstrating a so-called cleft anterior mitral valve leaflet (Cl), which is really a commissure between the left components of the anterosuperior and posteroinferior bridging leaflets. The chordal attachment is seen. In the middle frame, as diastole occurs, the two components of the "cleft" separate, whereas at end diastole (bottom frame) when the leaflets are again opposed, the cleft appears rather smaller. A = anterior; L = left; LA = left atrium; P = posterior; R = right; RV = right ventricle.

and extending directly into the descending aorta. This had no brachiocephalic arteries coming from it. Only slight changes in transducer angulation were needed to pass from the aortic arch to image the ductus. The chief distinguishing feature between the two (other

than their positions) was that the ductal arch was "bald" (that is, that it did not give off arteries to the head and neck) although the left subclavian artery can frequently be seen to enter the aortic isthmus. The other important feature of imaging is that this arch is seen best in long-axis planes.

Smallhorn and his colleagues (47–51) described this approach in infants, terming it the suprasternal notch ductal view. Although performed by Smallhorn from the suprasternal position, we find it easier to direct the plane from an infraclavicular or transmanubrial position in order to image the ductus best and recommend these positions (Figs. 25.46 and 25.47). The infraclavicular area is equivalent to the first or second intercostal interspace on the left side. Therefore, our recommended approach for imaging the ductus arteriosus is to apply the transducer in the infraclavicular area close to the sternum such that the beam is aligned in a sagittal body plane. In small children, it should then be possible to see the pulmonary trunk arterioles and the descending aorta posteriorly. The vertebral bodies will often be imaged posterior to the aorta (Fig. 25.46), confirming that the plane is truly sagittal in its orientation. If the ascending aorta is imaged, the plane of the beam is too far to the right. If the left pulmonary artery is imaged, the plane is too far to the left. Scanning between these areas should produce the plane of the arterial duct. Slight repositioning of the transducer may be required and sometimes clockwise or counterclockwise rotation will be needed to define the duct clearly.

The pulmonary trunk is well seen in the apex of the fan with the aortic root inferiorly. It branches as it sweeps posteriorly. The superior branch is the arterial duct, and the inferior branch is the left pulmonary artery. This plane is also an excellent means of assessing the size of the left pulmonary artery. The aortic arch, isthmus, and descending aorta can be seen running posteriorly from a superior to inferior position in the scan plane. When the ductus is patent, it is possible to define the continuity between the pulmonary trunk and the ductus arteriosus. Another feature that has made recognition of the ductus arteriosus a simple matter is the introduction of pulsed Doppler ultrasound with duplex Doppler systems. The Doppler cross-sectional imaging provides an ideal means of mapping the exact position where the turbulent flow through the ductus can be determined. A 96 percent sensitivity has been reported in premature infants from this plane when Doppler ultrasound was used compared with 92 percent when cross-sectional echocardiography was used alone (50).

The patent ductus arteriosus may also be imaged from other approaches (Figs. 25.48, 25.49, 25.50 and 25.51). The long-axis section of the arch can be achieved from the suprasternal position or from sub-

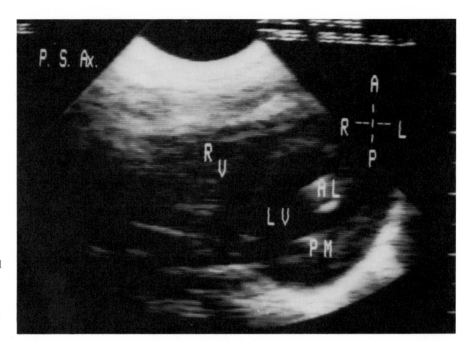

Figure 25.40. Parasternal short-axis (P S Ax) projection showing the positions of anterolateral and posteromedial papillary muscles (AL, PM) within the left ventricle (LV) in a patient with an atrioventricular septal defect. Note that they are positioned at 2 o'clock and 5 o'clock rather than the conventional position in the parasternal short-axis view. A = anterior; L = left; P = posterior; R = right; RV = right ventricle.

costal imaging. The patent ductus arteriosus is less well imaged from the suprasternal notch than from the standard precordial position, except when its orientation is different. In patients with discordant ventriculoarterial connection or pulmonary atresia (where the orientation or position of the duct and brachiocephalic arteries is different), it can be imaged better from suprasternal than precordial position. The ductus is oriented more vertically in pulmonary atresia, and it is more reliably imaged from the suprasternal notch (51).

The equivalent sagittal subcostal view is useful in small infants (Fig. 25.49). Resolution is still possible at some distance from the transducer. As the child grows, this view becomes less diagnostic. Nonetheless, it is especially valuable in those patients in whom severe chronic lung disease and mechanical respiration preclude precordial imaging. The ductal arch can be recognized by the lack of head and neck vessels arising from it. Unfortunately, the area of the ductus is some distance from the transducer, and resolution may be compromised. It is necessary to select a lower frequency transducer, which sometimes achieves penetration at the expense of resolution, but because it allows the use of Doppler ultrasound from this plane, positive diagnostic information can still be obtained in a large population of infants.

The first view used to describe the ductus arteriosus was the parasternal short-axis view (45). In this view, the ductus was imaged as a connection between the bifurcation of the pulmonary trunk and the descending aorta (Fig. 25.50). Unfortunately, the ductus is an arcuate structure, and (unless large) it is commonly missed. It is possible to mistake the left pulmonary

artery for the duct in this view, and it is consequently much less reliable.

The major advance in the diagnosis of a patent ductus arteriosus has been the inclusion of range-gated pulsed Doppler ultrasound with fast Fourier transform spectral analysis. The best approach is one that combines the cross-sectional imaging capabilities with pulsed Doppler so that a flow mapping of the turbulence can be obtained. When the appropriate view is achieved, the ductus, aorta, and pulmonary trunk are all in view, and the sample volume can be withdrawn from the descending aorta into the pulmonary trunk (Fig. 25.51). This allows precise location and confirmation of ductal flow (Fig. 25.52).

Several differences in Doppler patterns have been described in identification of the patent ductus arteriosus (52–54). These can be explained on hemodynamic events recorded from the sample site. All Doppler findings require the presence of left-to-right shunt. If the ductus is large, Doppler sampling in the distal descending aorta shows normal descending aortic flow in systole but retrograde flow during diastole (Fig. 25.52, bottom right). A different flow pattern is seen in the aorta proximal to the ductus. There is forward flow in systole and accentuation of the diastolic signal in the antegrade direction in diastole. Sampling proximal or distal to the site of the ductus (or other aortopulmonary runoff situations) produces similar findings. When the Doppler sample volume is placed within the ductus, the blood flow velocity spectra are higher and continuous throughout the cardiac cycle (Fig. 25.52, bottom left). Several types of signal may be recorded depending on the size of the left-to-right shunt. The signal within the pulmonary trunk is disturbed during systole and shows marked flow disturbance in diastole with flow being in a retrograde direction from the ductus into the pulmonary trunk (Fig. 25.52, top left and top right). There may be a lesser degree of retrograde flow in the moderate-size ductus arteriosus. The flow disturbance in diastole is usually recorded much closer to the ductal end of the pulmonary trunk. As the ductus constricts, the turbulent diastolic flow in the pulmonary trunk is increasingly difficult to detect. We and others have observed that, as the ductus becomes small, the regurgitant stream hugs the upper wall of the pulmonary trunk. This regurgitant stream should therefore be carefully sought in this region. Accurate imaging of the ductus is of extreme importance because the location of flow disturbance becomes more critical as the ductus diminishes in size.

With regard to quantitation of the magnitude of flow across the ductus, we still prefer to use the findings of a large left atrium, a hyperdynamic left ventricle, and retrograde aortic flow. Doppler sampling in the descending aorta from the subcostal approach at the level of the diaphragm allows sampling of forward flow in the abdominal descending aorta. With large shunts, there is usually a degree of retrograde flow. This does not occur when the shunt is small and of little hemodynamic significance.

Color Flow Mapping

Color flow mapping has provided a very rapid and highly sensitive way of defining the presence of ductus left-to-right shunts. It is only a matter of time before this technique becomes widely available and offers the potential of becoming the most standard way for using Doppler in the diagnosis of patent ductus arteriosus. Flow mapping studies from subcostal parasternal or ductus cut images allow the opportunity of defining flow mapping with much greater rapidity than can be achieved with the pulsed Doppler technique. The jet of the ductus can be mapped. In the usual situation the jet appears to hug the superior wall of the duct, but when the ductus is small it is often possible to determine an eccentric direction of the jet. Such findings from color flow mapping help explain the sometimes unusual findings of pulmonary artery turbulence identified using the pulsed Doppler technique alone. Another important value of color flow mapping is to determine the breadth of the jet through the ductus. The diameter of the jet may be a more sensitive means of determining the effective diameter of the ductus than from imaging alone because the jet diameter is frequently a millimeter or so smaller than one would assume from observing the endothelial echos alone. Another value of color flow mapping has been in situations where imaging alone has been extremely difficult, such as a very small, critically ill, premature infant

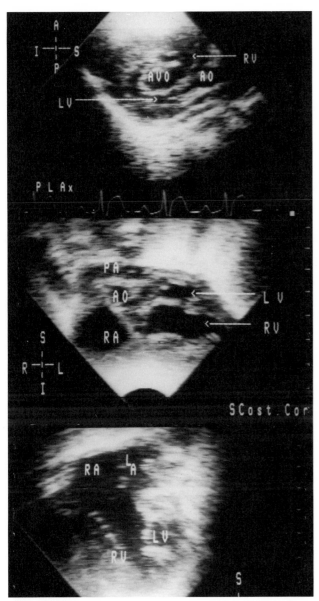

Figure 25.41. Three frames from a patient with a right-dominant form of atrioventricular septal defect. The top frame, parasternal long-axis view (P L Ax), demonstrates the atrioventricular orifice (AVO) opening almost exclusively into the right ventricle (RV), whereas the left ventricle (LV) is small and almost entirely devoid of atrioventricular valve tissue. The ascending aorta (AO) arises above the common atrioventricular valve leaflet. In the middle frame from the subcostal coronal view (SCost Cor), the size of the LV and RV can also be assessed. In the bottom frame from the apical four-chamber view, the atrioventricular valve orifice connection and direction from left and right atria are seen to be almost entirely in the right ventricle in diastole. A = anterior; I = inferior; L = left; LA = left atrium; LV = left ventricle; P = posterior; R = right; RA = right atrium; RV = right ventricle; S = superior.

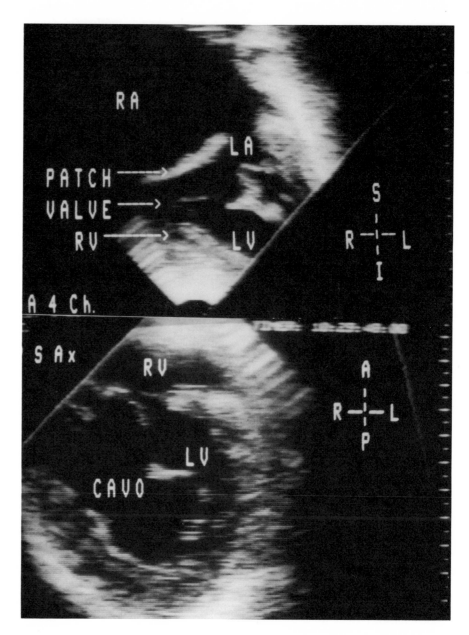

Figure 25.42. Top frame is an apical four-chamber view in a patient with a left-dominant form of atrioventricular septal defect after Fontan operation. The patch can be seen separating the very markedly enlarged right atrium (RA) from the left atrium. The left atrium (LA) is small. The atrioventricular valve straddles both ventricles, and a diminutive right ventricle is seen. Bottom frame taken in the parasternal short-axis view. The common atrioventricular valve orifice drains almost entirely into the large left ventricle, whereas the right ventricle is small. There is chordal attachment of the common atrioventricular valve leaflet to the crest of the ventricular septum.

maintained on artificial ventilation. In these circumstances, precordial resolution of the cross-sectional imaging may be substandard but the approach with color flow imaging from either the precordial location or subcostal transducer location has allowed the exquisite mapping of the left-to-right shunt.

The ease of identifying the ductus with this technique has become valuable because the definition of ductus shunting can be identified even by those with limited echocardiographic skills.

Closure of the Ductus in the Premature Infant and Neonate

Closure or increased patency of the ductus arteriosus by pharmacologic manipulation can be observed in the premature and newborn infant (51), and studies have shown the sensitivity of cross-sectional echocardiography in this respect. When pulmonary hypertension exists in the newborn infant (or has developed in later life), there are no Doppler signs, since these Doppler signs are exclusively those of a left-to-right shunt. This is similar to the situation with the fetus when no turbulence is recorded across the ductus and there is a total right-to-left shunt. Although this is a rare combination, we have encountered it on a few occasions. Imaging in this situation proves to be more sensitive than the Doppler signs. We used contrast echocardiography to demonstrate the right-to-left ductal shunt, but in almost all other instances, the Doppler technique appears to be superior.

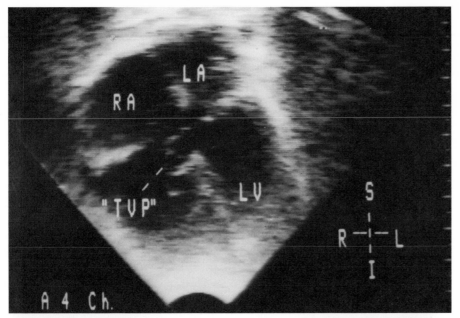

Figure 25.43. An apical four-chamber view demonstrating a tricuspid valve pouch (TVP) in an incomplete form of atrioventricular septal defect. This finding is not observed in pathologic specimens. The interatrial communication can clearly be seen above the atrioventricular valve leaflets, whereas the connecting tongue of tissue obscures and blocks the area that would be the interventricular communication. This tongue of tissue or tricuspid valve pouch is highly reminiscent of the lesion called "aneurysm of the membranous septum." Note the marked similarity in the anatomy of the incomplete and complete forms of the defect.

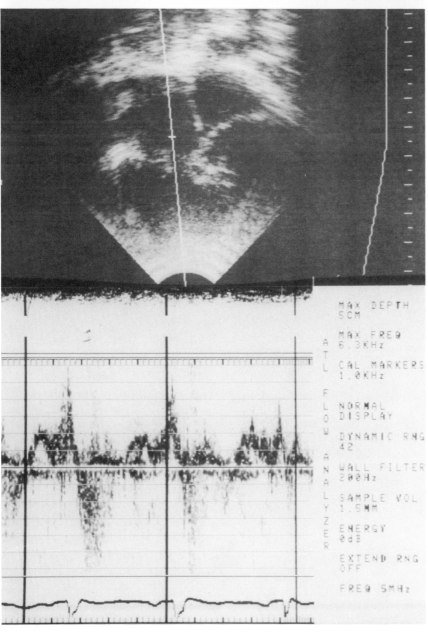

Figure 25.44. The top frame demonstrates cross-sectional reference frame from the apical four-chamber view showing the position of the Doppler with the sample volume placed in the right atrium just proximal to the arterial valve. The atrial component of the defect is seen in an apical four-chamber projection. The bottom frame is a resultant pulsed Doppler signal showing disturbance of atrial flow related to the transatrial diastolic shunt and the characteristic M-shaped pattern of atrial flow in diastole above the central baseline. In systole, there is disturbed systolic flow due to atrioventricular valve insufficiency with the direction away from the transducer (below baseline), that is, toward the right atrium. This atrioventricular valve insufficiency was mild as judged by the localized nature of the flow disturbance. The jet was directed from the left ventricle toward the right atrium as seen from the position of the sample volume.

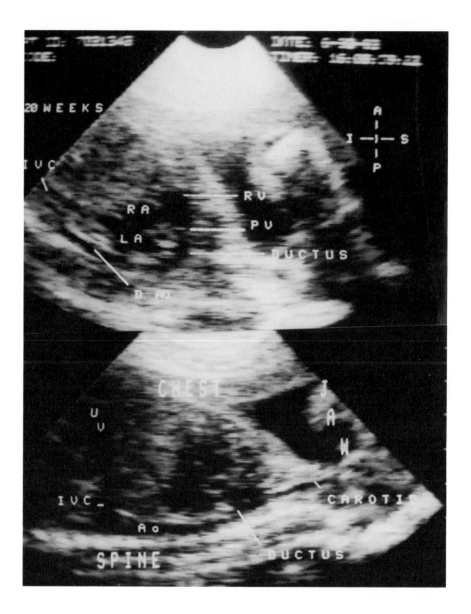

Figure 25.45. Fetal echocardiogram obtained in a 20-week gestational age fetus demonstrating the orientation of the ductus. In the top frame, equivalent to a short-axis plane, the right ventricle can be seen anteriorly, as can the pulmonary valve separating it from the pulmonary artery and the ductus arching around gently toward the descending aorta (D. AO). In the bottom frame, the aorta and carotid artery can be identified, and the ductus can be seen to enter the descending aorta as well. A = anterior; I = inferior; IVC = inferior vena cava; LA = left atrium; P = posterior; RA = right atrium; S = superior. (Reproduced by permission from Silverman NH, Golbus MS. Echocardiographic techniques for assessing normal and abnormal fetal cardiac anatomy. J Am Coll Cardiol 1985;5:20S–29S.)

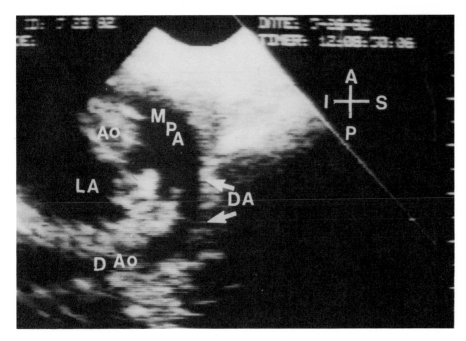

Figure 25.46. Shows a classical ductus cut, which we use to identify the ductus arteriosus (DA). The plane is achieved from an infraclavicular location in the second left intercostal space and is oriented in such a way that the main pulmonary artery (MPA) and descending aorta can be imaged. The MPA can be seen to have two excrescences, the branch pulmonary arteries, and then continues into the DAo. The area of the DA is marked. The relationship to the ascending aorta (AO) and left atrium (LA) can be clearly defined. A = anterior; I = inferior; P = posterior; S = superior.

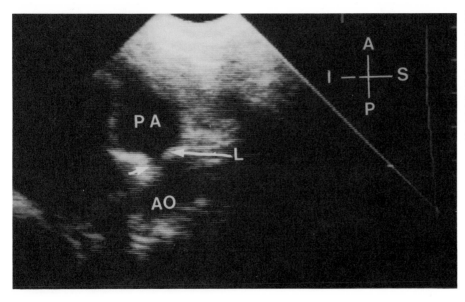

Figure 25.47. Ductus cut showing a slipped surgical ligature on a patent ductus arteriosus. The ligature area (L) is identified by means of arrows as an invagination in the region of the ductus. The view is oriented from an infraclavicular location in the second left intercostal space. AO = aorta; PA = pulmonary artery.

Figure 25.48. Suprasternal notch view where the origin of the ductus arteriosus can be clearly identified arising from the descending aortic area. The entire ductus cannot be imaged in this field, but the area of this shelf related to ductus tissue is characteristic. A = anterior; AO = aorta; DAO = descending aorta; I = inferior; IA = innominate artery; IST = aortic isthmus; IV = innominate vein; LA = left atrium; LCA = left carotid artery; LSA = left subclavian artery; P = posterior; PDA = patent ductus arteriosus; S = superior.

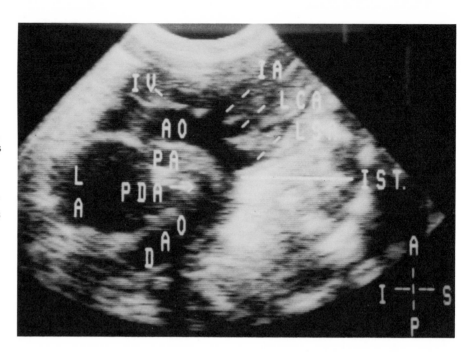

Figure 25.49. Subcostal cut in the parasagittal plane demonstrating a ductus arteriosus (D). Here the pulmonary artery (PA) can be seen to sweep directly into the descending aorta (AO) by means of the D. The origin of the left pulmonary artery (L) can be seen. The left atrium (LA) was imaged inferior to the L and anterior to the descending aorta. RV = right ventricle.

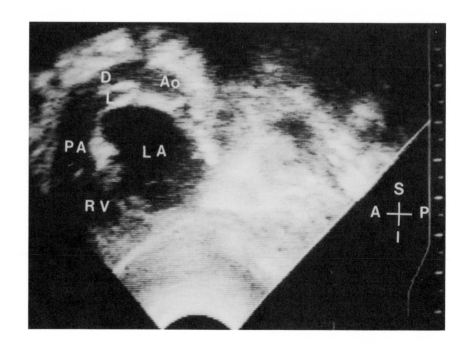

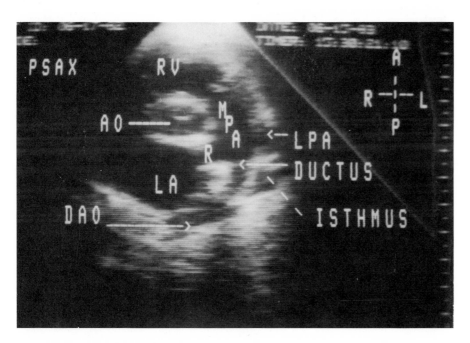

Figure 25.50. Parasternal short-axis view, which was first used to describe the patent ductus arteriosus. Here the pulmonary artery can be seen to give rise to the patent ductus and the right and left pulmonary arteries (RPA and LPA) and is continuous with the descending aorta (DAO). A = anterior; ISTHMUS = aortic isthmus; L = left; LA = left atrium; P = posterior; PSAX = parasternal short axis; R = right.

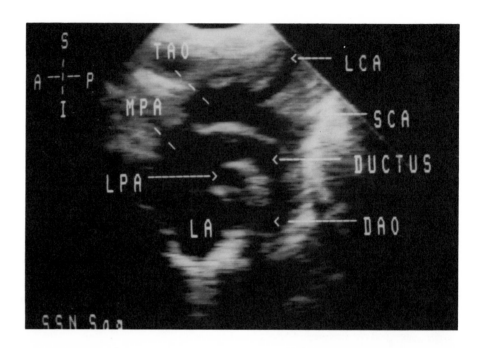

A

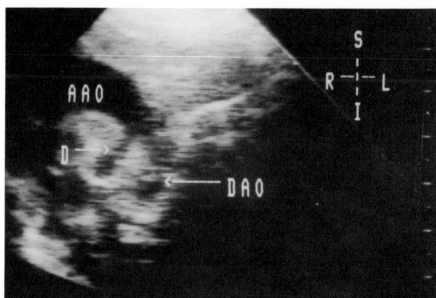

B

Figure 25.51. (*A*) Suprasternal notch view of a patent ductus in aortopulmonary transposition. The orientation is suprasternal notch sagittal plane and demonstrates the aortic arch, the ductus isthmus, the origin of the left pulmonary artery, and the continuation of the descending aorta. The left subclavian artery (SCA) and left carotid artery (LCA) positions can be identified. (*B*) The same plane as in the same patient with pulmonary atresia and a vertically oriented ductus. This characteristic appearance of the small tortuous ductus in this condition is consistent with that described angiographically. A = anterior; I = inferior; LA = left atrium; MPA = pulmonary artery; P = posterior; S = superior; TAO = transverse aorta.

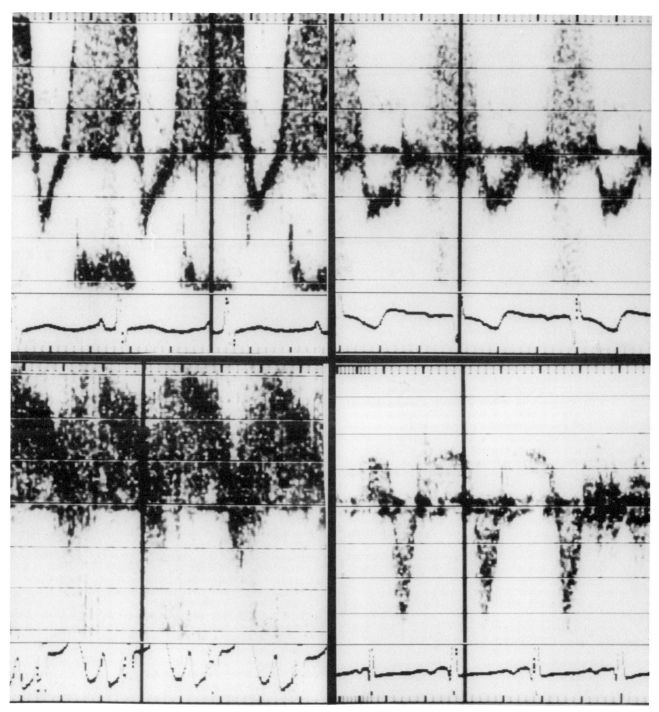

Figure 25.52.   Series of Doppler recordings obtained in a patient with patent ductus arteriosus showing the different signals that can be recorded with a left-to-right ductus shunt. All images for obtaining these signals are from the ductus cut. The top left frame was obtained from a patient with a large patent arteriosus. Here in systole, there is good forward flow as judged by the flow away from the baseline. In diastole, there is more flow disturbance with so-called wraparound of the diastolic flow signal. This demonstrates the typical flow disturbance represented as occurring toward the transducer (i.e., into the pulmonary artery from the ductus in diastole). The calibration marks for all these tracings are 1 kilohertz per division. The top right frame is from another patient with patent ductus arteriosus at a point slightly more toward the ductus than in the previous frame. In the bottom left frame, the sample volume is right in the ductus arteriosus and demonstrates almost continuous forward flow from the ductus arteriosus into the pulmonary artery in systole with the exception of a little systolic signal away from the baseline with each pulmonary ejection. In the bottom right frame, the sample volume has been placed in the descending aorta distal to the ductus arteriosus, and the descending aortic signal can be identified with a retrograde flow (i.e., diastolic runoff) toward the pulmonary artery end of the ductus, defined as flow toward the transducer.

REFERENCES

1. Freed MD, Nadas AS, Norwood WI, Castaneda AR. Is routine preoperative cardiac catheterization necessary before repair of secundum and sinus venosus atrial septal defects? J Am Coll Cardiol 1984;4:333–6.
2. Shub C, Tajik AJ, Seward JB, Hagler DT, Danielson GK. Surgical repair of uncomplicated atrial septal defect without "routine" preoperative cardiac catheterization. J Am Coll Cardiol 1985;6:49–54.
3. Shub C, Dimopoulos IN, Seward JB, et al. Sensitivity of two-dimensional echocardiography in the direct visualization of atrial septal defect utilizing the subcostal approach: experience with 154 patients. J Am Coll Cardiol 1983;2:127–35.
4. Lieppe W, Scallion R, Behar VS, Kisslow JA. Two-dimensional echocardiographic findings in atrial septal defect. Circulation 1977;56:447–56.
5. Lange LW, Sahn DJ, Allen HD, Goldberg SJ. Subxiphoid cross-sectional echocardiography in infants and children with congenital heart disease. Circulation 1979;59:513–24.
6. Bierman FZ, Williams RG. Subxiphoid two-dimensional imaging of the interatrial septum in infants and neonates with congenital heart disease. Circulation 1979;60:80–90.
7. Tajik AJ, Seward JB, Hagler DJ, Mair DD, Lie JT. Two-dimensional real-time ultrasonic imaging of the heart and great vessels: technique, image orientation, structure identification, and validation. Mayo Clin Proc 1978;53:271–303.
8. Silverman NH, Snider AR. Two-dimensional echocardiography in congenital heart disease. Norwalk, CT: Appleton-Century-Crofts, 1982;47–66.
9. Weyman AE, Wann LS, Caldwell RL, Hurwitz RA, Dillion JC, Feigenbaum H. Negative contrast echocardiography: a new method for detecting left-to-right shunts. Circulation 1979;59:498–505.
10. Higgins JR, Sundstrom J, Gutman J, Schiller NB. Contrast echocardiography with quantitative valsalva maneuver to detect patent foramen ovale. Clin Res 1982;30:12A.
11. Hatle L, Angelsen B. Doppler ultrasound in cardiology. Physical principles and clinical applications. 2nd ed. Philadelphia: Lea & Febiger, 1985;228–36.
12. Goldberg SJ, Allen HD, Marx GR, Flinn CJ. Doppler echocardiography. Philadelphia: Lea & Febiger, 1985;37–8.
13. Hauser AM, Timmis GC, Stewart JR, et al. Aneurysm of the atrial septum as diagnosed by echocardiography: analysis of 11 patients. Am J Cardiol 1984;53:1401–2.
14. Yaeger SB, Chin AJ, Sanders SP. Subxiphoid two-dimensional echocardiographic diagnosis of coronary sinus septal defects. Am J Cardiol 1984;54:686–7.
15. Silverman NH, Snider AR. Two-dimensional echocardiography in congenital heart disease. Norwalk, CT: Appleton-Century-Crofts, 1982;67–98.
16. Anderson RH, Becker AE. Cardiac pathology. An integrated text and color atlas. New York: Raven Press, 1982;122.
17. Sutherland GR, Godman MJ, Smallhorn JF, Guiterras P, Anderson RH, Hunter S. Ventricular septal defects. Two-dimensional echocardiographic and morphological correlations. Br Heart J 1982;47:316–28.
18. Canale JM, Sahn DJ, Allen HD, Goldberg SJ. Factors affecting real time cross-sectional echocardiographic imaging of ventricular septal defects. Am J Cardiol 1980;45:457–62.
19. Hatle L, Angelsen B. Doppler ultrasound in cardiology. Physical principles and clinical applications. 2nd ed. Philadelphia: Lea & Febiger, 1985;236–52.
20. Goldberg SJ, Allen HD, Marx GR, Flinn CJ. Doppler echocardiography. Philadelphia: Lea & Febiger, 1985;100.
21. Bierman FZ, Fellows K, Williams RG. Prospective identification of ventricular septal defects in infancy using subxiphoid two-dimensional echocardiography. Circulation 1980;62:807–17.
22. Smallhorn JF, Sutherland GR, Anderson RJ, Macartney FJ. Cross-sectional echocardiographic assessment of conditions with atrioventricular valve leaflets attached to the atrial septum at the same level. Br Heart J 1982;48:331–41.
23. Ramaciotti C, Keren A, Silverman NH. Importance of perimem-branous ventricular septal aneurysm in the natural history of isolated perimembranous ventricular septal defects. Am J Cardiol 1985;57:268–72.
24. Smallhorn J, Anderson RH, Macartney FJ. Morphological characteristics of ventricular septal defects associated with coarctation of the aorta by cross-sectional echocardiography. Br Heart J 1983;49:485–94.
25. Smallhorn JF, Anderson RH, Macartney FJ. Cross-sectional echocardiographic recognition of interruption of aortic arch between left carotid and subclavian arteries. Br Heart J 1982;48:229–35.
26. Sanders SP, Yeager S, Williams RG. Measurement of systemic and pulmonary blood flow and QP/QS ratio using Doppler and two-dimensional echocardiography. Am J Cardiol 1983;51:952.
27. Goldberg SJ, Sahn DJ, Allen HD, Valdes-Cruz LM, Hoenecke H, Carnahan Y. Evaluation of pulmonary and systemic blood flow by two-dimensional Doppler echocardiography using fast Fourier transform spectral analysis. Am J Cardiol 1982;50:1394.
28. Yock P, Popp RL. Noninvasive estimation of right ventricular systolic pressure by Doppler ultrasound in patients with tricuspid regurgitation. Circulation 1984;70:657–62.
29. Hagler DJ, Tajik AJ, Seward JB, Mair DD, Ritter DG. Real-time wide-angle sector echocardiography: atrioventricular canal defects. Circulation 1979;59:140–50.
30. Sahn DJ, Terry RW, O'Rourke R, Leopold G, Friedman WF. Multiple crystal echocardiographic evaluation of endocardial cushion defect. Circulation 1974;50:25–32.
31. Fisher DJ, Silverman NH, Schiller NB, Hart PA. Evaluation of endocardial cushion defects by phased array sector scanner, abstracted. Am J Cardiol 1978;41:353.
32. Smallhorn JF, Tommasini G, Anderson RH, Macartney FJ. Assessment of atrioventricular septal defects by phased array sector scanner. Br Heart J 1982;47:109–21.
33. Smallhorn JF, De Leval M, Stark J, et al. Isolated anterior mitral cleft. Two dimensional echocardiographic assessment and differentiation from "clefts" associated with atrioventricular septal defect. Br Heart J 1982;48:109–16.
34. Beppu S, Nimura Y, Sakakibara H, et al. Mitral cleft in ostium primum atrial septal defect assessed by cross-sectional echocardiography. Circulation 1980;62:1099–106.
35. Sutherland GR, Van Mill GJ, Anderson RH, Hunter S. Subxiphoid echocardiography—a new approach to the diagnosis and differentiation of atrioventricular defects. Eur Heart J 1980;1:45–54.
36. Mavroudis C, Weinstein G, Turley K, Ebert PA. Surgical management of complete atrioventricular canal. J Thorac Cardiovasc Surg 1982;83:670–9.
37. Bharati S, Lev M. The spectrum of common atrioventricular orifice (canal). Am Heart J 1973;86:553–61.
38. Mehta S, Hirschfeld S, Riggs T, Liebman J. Echocardiogoraphic estimation of ventricular hypoplasia in complete atrioventricular canal. Circulation 1979;59:888–93.
39. Rastelli GC, Kirklin JW, Titus JL. Anatomic observations on complete form of persistent common atrioventricular canal with special reference to atrioventricular valves. Mayo Clin Proc 1966;41:296–308.
40. Carpentier A. Surgical anatomy and management of the mitral component of atrioventricular canal defects. In: Anderson RH, Shinebourne EA, eds. Pediatric cardiology. Edinburgh: Churchill Livingstone, 1978;477–86.
41. Becker AE, Anderson RH. Atrioventricular septal defects: what's in a name? J Thorac Cardiovasc Surg 1982;83:461–9.
42. Kudo T, Tokoyama M, Imai Y, Konno S, Sakakibara S. The tricuspid pouch in endocardial cushion defect. Am Heart J 1974;87:544–9.
43. Rudolph AM. Endocardial cushion defects. In: Rudolph AM, ed. Congenital diseases of the heart. Chicago: Year Book, 1974;278–81.
44. Allen HD, Goldberg SJ, Valdes-Cruz LM, Sahn DJ. Use of echocardiography in newborns with patent ductus arteriosus: a review. Pediatr Cardiol 1982;3:65–70.
45. Sahn DJ, Allen HD. Real time cross-sectional echocardiographic imaging and measurement of the patent ductus arteriosus in infants and children. Circulation 1978;58:343–53.
46. Allen HD, Sahn DJ, Goldberg SJ. A new serial contrast technique

for assessment of left to right shunting patent ductus arteriosus in the neonate. Am J Cardiol 1978;41:288–94.

47. Smallhorn JF, Huhta JC, Anderson RH, Macartney FJ. Suprasternal cross-sectional echocardiography in assessment of patent ductus arteriosus. Br Heart J 1982;48:321–30.

48. Rigby ML, Pickering D, Wilkinson A. Cross-sectional echocardiography in determining persistent patency of the ductus arteriosus in preterm infants. Arch Dis Child 1984;59:341–5.

49. Huhta JC, Cohen M, Gutgesell HP. Patency of the ductus arteriosus in normal neonates: two-dimensional echocardiography versus Doppler assessment. J Am Coll Cardiol 1984;4:561–4.

50. Vick WG, Huhta JC, Gutgesell HP. Assessment of the ductus arteriosus in preterm infants utilizing suprasternal two-dimensional Doppler echocardiography. J Am Coll Cardiol 1985;5:973–7.

51. Smallhorn JF, Gow R, Olley PM, et al. Combined noninvasive assessment of the patent ductus arteriosus in the preterm infant before and after indomethacin treatment. Am J Cardiol 1984;54:1300–4.

52. Gentile R, Stevenson G, Dooley T, Franklin D, Kawabori I, Pearlman A. Pulsed Doppler echocardiographic determination of time of ductal closure in normal newborn infants. J Pediatr 1981;98:443–8.

53. Stevenson JG, Kawabori I, Guntheroth WG. Noninvasive detection of pulmonary hypertension in patent ductus arteriosus by pulsed Doppler echocardiography. Circulation 1979;60:355–9.

54. Serwer GA, Armstrong BE, Anderson PAW. Noninvasive detection of retrograde descending aortic flow in infants using continuous wave Doppler ultrasonography. J Pediatr 1980;97:394–400.

26
Univentricular Atrioventricular Connection

Jeffrey Smallhorn

This chapter outlines a rational approach to the assessment of univentricular atrioventricular connection by cross-sectional echocardiography and describes the atrioventricular and ventriculoarterial connections and commonly associated anomalies. First, it is important to define the nomenclature used in this chapter since it varies between authors. Hearts with double-inlet, absent right, or absent left atrioventricular connections have one feature in common: Only one of the ventricles is connected to the atria (1). Each type of connection may coexist with any of three ventricular morphologies (i.e., left ventricular, right ventricular, or indeterminate types) (Fig. 26.1). In patients with a dominant right and a rudimentary left ventricle, the rudimentary chamber is always posteroinferior to the large right ventricle and may be on the left or right side. When the right ventricle is rudimentary, it is always positioned anterosuperior to the dominant left ventricle and likewise may be to the right or left. In the former, the interventricular septum always runs to the crux of the heart, whereas in the latter, it fails to reach the crux.

This approach avoids the problem of arbitrarily not calling a chamber within the ventricular mass a ventricle as was the case with the term "univentricular heart" (2). It also avoids problems with nomenclature in patients with straddling and overriding atrioventricular valves, in whom the difference between 49 percent and 51 percent of annular overriding previously changed the status of a chamber from a ventricle to an outlet or rudimentary chamber (Fig. 26.2). Calling the connection univentricular or biventricular in no way alters the status of the smaller ventricle.

For those who are familiar with alternative classifications, "single ventricle" is used to describe those hearts with a double-inlet connection; mitral atresia (absent left connection) and tricuspid atresia (absent right connection) are not considered subcategories of single ventricle (3–9). This terminology controversy is ongoing. The purpose of this chapter is notto deal with differences in nomenclature but to describe the cross-sectional echocardiographic appearances of all the common types of abnormalities using the term "univentricular atrioventricular connection."

GENERAL APPROACH

In all echocardiographic examinations, a segmental approach is the most rewarding (10). First, the atrial arrangement should be determined by the relationship of the abdominal aorta to the inferior vena cava and the hepatic, systemic, and pulmonary venous connections should be evaluated (11, 12).

Assessment of the Atrioventricular Junction

The atrioventricular junction is visualized best in the apical and subcostal four-chamber cuts (13–16). The presence of one or two atrioventricular valves can be determined from these positions, along with their sizes and the commitment of the annulus to the ventricular chambers (Figs. 26.3 and 26.4). The presence of a dense wedge of sulcus tissue in the floor of the atrium with an absent connection is best seen in these views (Fig. 26.3). Care must be taken not to rely on the subcostal view alone when assessing the right atrioventricular

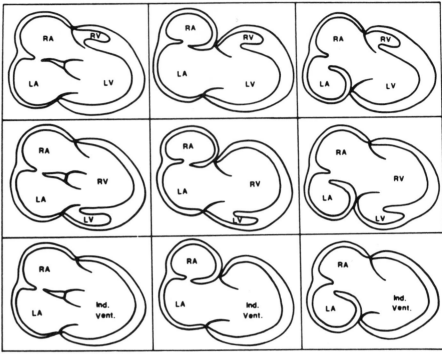

DOUBLE INLET CONNECTION   ABSENT RIGHT AV CONNECTION   ABSENT LEFT AV CONNECTION

Figure 26.1. Diagrammatic representation of the various types of univentricular atrioventricular connection. The hearts have either double-inlet, absent right, or absent left atrioventricular (AV) connection, and the atria can be connected to either a right ventricle (RV), a left ventricle (LV), or a solitary and indeterminate ventricle (Ind. Vent.). LA = left atrium; RA = right atrium.

region, particularly when the morphologically right ventricle is small, because confusion may arise between pulmonary atresia with intact septum and absent right connection. This difficulty may be readily resolved from the apical four-chamber view.

Difficulty may be encountered in differentiating an imperforate valve from sulcus tissue in some cases (16), but an imperforate valve usually appears as a thin echo with some underlying tensor apparatus attached to it (Fig. 26.5). The presence or absence of a straddling atrioventricular valve is also best seen in the apical four-chamber position (Fig. 26.2) (17).

Figure 26.2. A series of subcostal cuts in a patient with a double-inlet univentricular connection to a dominant right ventricle with two atrioventricular valves. Note the morphological right atrium connects to the morphologically right ventricle which supports the aorta. The morphological left atrium connects to both ventricles via a straddling left atrioventricular valve. There is anywhere between 45 to 55 percent overriding, which causes problems in assigning the atrioventricular connection.

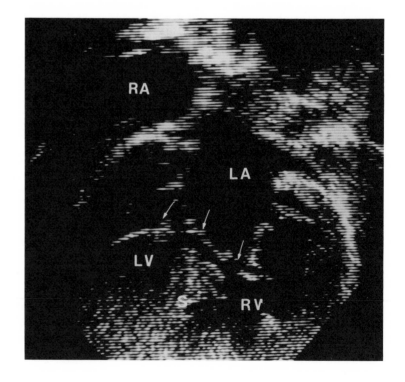

Assessment of the Ventricular Morphology

The ventricular morphology may be identified by either the trabecular pattern (Fig. 26.4) or the relationship of the rudimentary ventricle to the main ventricular mass (Fig. 26.6, 26.7). The trabecular pattern is best assessed using the standard four-chamber views. The right ventricle has a coarse septal trabecular pattern and the left a smooth septal surface (Fig. 26.4). The relationship of the two ventricles is best assessed using subcostal and precordial short-axis cuts (Fig. 26.8) (13). The rudimentary right ventricle of a univentricular connection to a dominant left ventricle may be anterior and to the left or right. The rudimentary left ventricle seen with a univentricular connection to a dominant right ventricle may also be right or left-sided but is always posteroinferior. The size of the smaller ventricle is best evaluated with a combination of the standard four-chamber and short-axis views, as is the size of an associated ventricular septal defect (Fig.

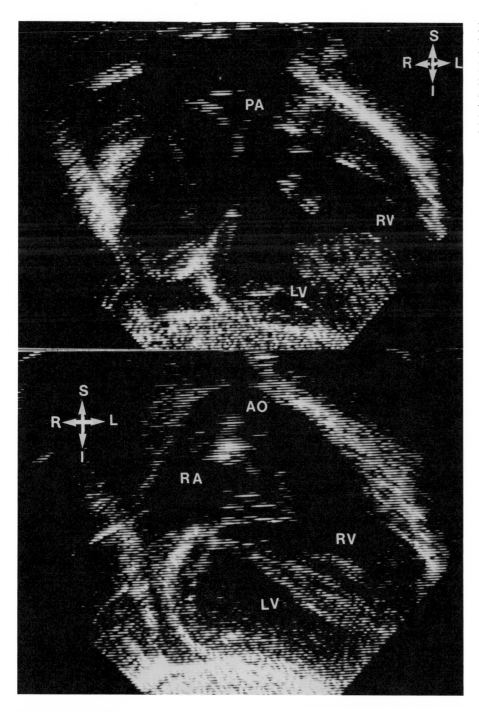

Figure 26.2 (cont'd.). Note in the bottom figure, however, that there is a good-sized rudimentary left ventricle. The ventricular arrangement is superoinferior. AO = aorta; LA = left atrium; LV = left ventricle; PA = pulmonary trunk; RA = right atrium; RV = right ventricle.

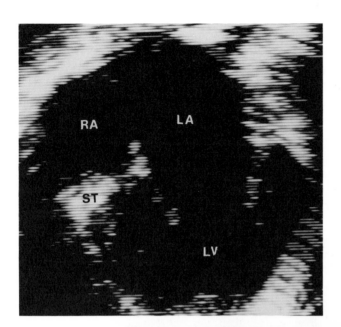

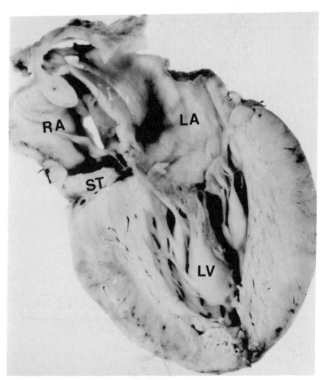

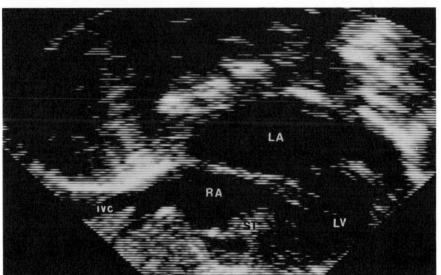

Figure 26.3. The left-hand picture is an apical fourchamber view in univentricular connection to a dominant left ventricle with absent right connection. Note the dense wedge of sulcus tissue between the right atrium and the ventricular mass. The picture on the right is an anatomic specimen from a different patient, cut in a four-chamber view. The lower picture is a subcostal four-chamber view from a different patient with absent right connection. Note the inferior caval and hepatic veins draining into the right atrium. IVC = inferior vena cava; LA = left atrium; LV = left ventricle; RA = right atrium; ST = sulcus tissue.

26.9). In the absence of an identifiable second ventricle, it is difficult to assign the ventricular morphology, and most frequently, the label "indeterminate" is applied. This happens particularly in cases of a double-inlet connection and a common atrioventricular valve (Fig. 26.10) (18).

Assessment of Ventriculoarterial Connections

Assessment of ventriculoarterial connections is achieved by combining subcostal and precordial long-axis cuts (Figs. 26.7 and 26.11), with a high precordial short-axis view, to determine the exact spatial relation-

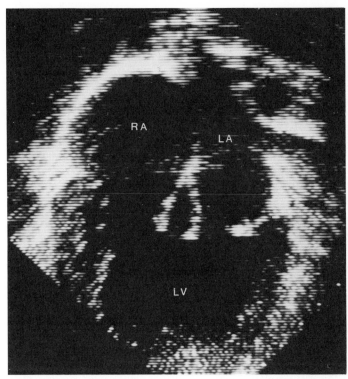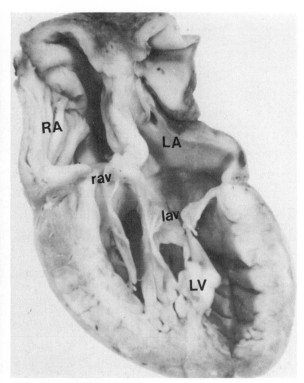

Figure 26.4.   The left-hand picture is an apical four-chamber view in double-inlet connection to a dominant left ventricle with two atrioventricular valves. Note both atrioventricular valves empty into the dominant ventricle of left ventricular type. The picture on the right is from a different patient and demonstrates the anatomic features and the echocardiographic correlate. LA = left atrium; LAV = left atrioventricular valve; LV = left ventricle; RA = right atrium; RAV = right atrioventricular valve.

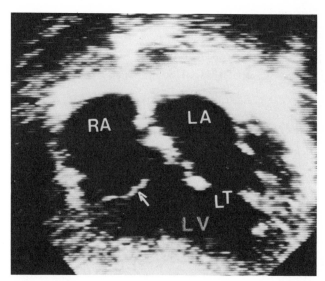

Figure 26.5.   An apical four-chamber view in a patient with a double-inlet connection to a dominant left ventricle (LV) with two atrioventricular valves. Note that the right-sided atrioventricular valve indicated by the arrow is imperforate. LA = left atrium; LT = left tensor apparatus; RA = right atrium.

ship (Fig. 26.12). As in a normal examination, the pulmonary trunk is recognized by its branching pattern and sharp backward dip, particularly when it is the posterior vessel (Figs. 26.12 and 26.13). It is particularly important to evaluate the subaortic and subpulmonary regions, as obstructions may arise at several levels.

The outflow tract narrowing is usually at valve and subvalve level, the latter originating from a combination of a deviated outlet septum and a prominent ventriculoinfundibular fold that separates the atrioventricular and arterial valves (Fig. 26.14). A combination of views is necessary to visualize all components of the outflow tract. The long-axis view from the precordium allows visualization of the anterior and posterior aspects while the same cut in the subcostal position visualizes the more rightward and leftward aspects of the outflow tract.

DOUBLE-INLET CONNECTION

In double-inlet connection, either two perforate atrioventricular valves, one imperforate valve, or a common atrioventricular valve connects the atria with a dominant ventricle of left, right, or indeterminate morphology (13–16). In the apical four-chamber view in the presence of two valves (Fig. 26.4), the valve tissue appears attached at the same level to the interatrial

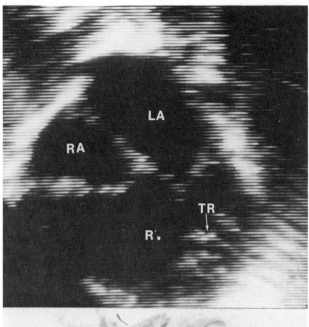

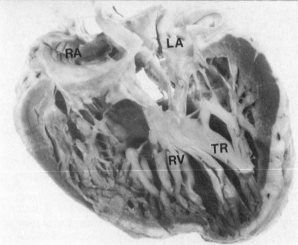

Figure 26.6. The upper picture is an apical four-chamber cut in a case with a double-inlet univentricular connection of right ventricular type. Note the coarse trabeculations. The lower picture is an anatomic specimen from a different case. LA = left atrium; RA = right atrium; RV = right ventricle; TR = trabeculations.

septum, with no separating atrioventricular septum. The valve leaflets appear to coapt during diastole, with one valve often appearing smaller than the other. This may be related to an anatomic anomaly, and in many patients, particularly those with excessive pulmonary flow, it is due to annular dilatation. Regurgitation of either valve will produce a similar appearance (Fig. 26.15). In some instances, the valves may have the appearance of morphologically mitral and tricuspid valves, but this is not universal. In the subcostal four-chamber cut, the atrioventricular valves may lie in different planes so that simultaneous visualization may not be possible. This is resolved by slight changes in transducer position (Fig. 26.16).

The tensor apparatuses from both valves often ap-

pear to cross because papillary muscles in the dominant ventricle may be shared. Occasionally, a large central papillary muscle may have a similar appearance to an interventricular septum in the four-chamber view. These two structures may be readily distinguished by using a short-axis view. It is important to identify the insertion of the papillary muscles, particularly in cases with a dominant left ventricle where septation is to be considered. If the tensor apparatuses do not cross, then the patients may be considered for surgical correction (Fig. 26.17).

In the presence of a common atrioventricular valve, the ventricular mass is usually of indeterminate type with no identified smaller ventricle (Fig. 26.10). In such cases, there is usually a common atrium with a large ostium primum atrial septal defect. The valve has the same appearance as that seen in a complete atrioventricular septal defect, with a large free-floating antero-superior leaflet (18).

Difficulties may occur in differentiating double-inlet connection with a common atrioventricular valve from a heart with biventricular atrioventricular connections in an unbalanced ventricular mass with common atrium (18, 19). This problem arises because the interatrial septum cannot be used to determine the status of the atrioventricular junction. In cases with an ostium primum defect and an unbalanced ventricular mass, the interatrial septum is aligned with the interventricular septum, whereas it appears nonaligned in hearts with double-inlet connection.

The ventriculoarterial connections may be concordant (Fig. 26.18A) (20), discordant (Fig. 26.18B), or single or double outlet (Fig. 26.18C), with their spatial relationships varying in accordance with the positions of the ventricular chambers.

Absent Right Connection or "Tricuspid Atresia"

Absent right atrioventricular connection is the most common anomaly encountered with dominant left ventricle (tricuspid atresia) (21). The other types of ventricular morphology occur less frequently (Fig. 26.19). In the subcostal and apical four-chamber cut, the dense wedge of sulcus tissue is usually seen separating the right atrium from the ventricular mass (Fig. 26.3). The systemic venous blood passes through the interatrial communication into the left atrium, then into the dominant left ventricle and to the outlets. It is important to assess this communication as it may occasionally become restrictive, resulting in systemic venous congestion. The interatrial communication can be assessed by combining cross-sectional echocardiography with Doppler ultrasound in the subcostal four-chamber view (Fig. 26.20).

In cases where the dominant chamber is of left ventricular morphology, the smaller rudimentary right

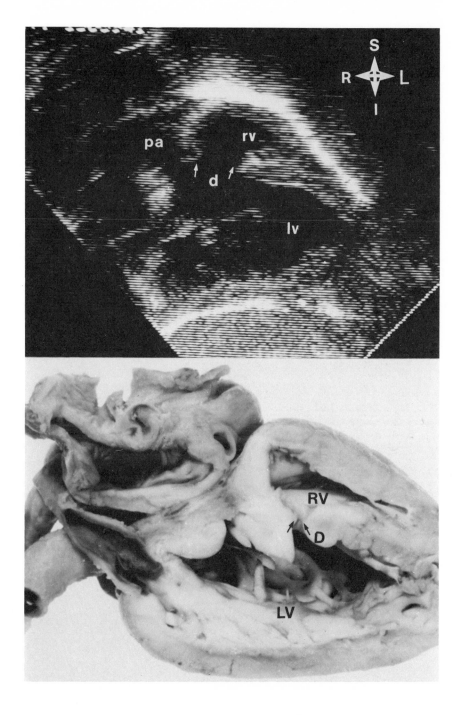

Figure 26.7. The upper picture is a subcostal long-axis cut in a univentricular connection of left ventricular type, with a leftward and anterior aorta arising from a small morphological right ventricle. Note the position of the ventricular septal defect. The lower picture from a different case demonstrates the morphologic features. D = ventricular septal defect; LV = left ventricle; PA = pulmonary artery; RV = right ventricle.

ventricle usually appears anterior and to the right (Fig. 26.8B) (13). The chamber size varies considerably, particularly in relationship to the ventriculoarterial connections and the size of the ventricular septal defect. Although a concordant ventriculoarterial connection is most common, other types of ventriculoarterial connection are possible (Fig. 26.11).

Absent Left Connection

Although three types of ventricular morphology are possible (Fig. 26.21), the most common type is a dominant right ventricle (22, 23). A dense wedge of sulcus tissue is present in the floor of the left atrium (Fig. 26.21), with the pulmonary venous blood exiting via an interatrial communication. Restriction is possible at this level and is best assessed by a combination of cross-sectional and Doppler echocardiography. In many instances, the left atrium may be small, and in the presence of a large interatrial communication, it may be difficult to differentiate this lesion from a double-inlet connection with a common atrioventricular valve. The dominant ventricle appears heavily trabeculated, identifying it as a morphologically right ventricle. The ventriculoarterial connections may be concordant, discordant (Fig. 26.22), or single or double outlet.

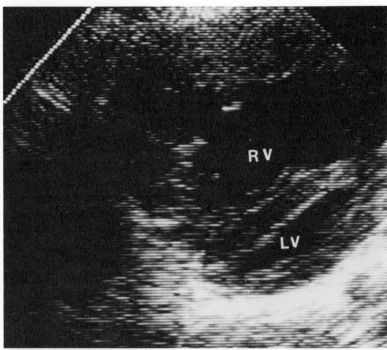

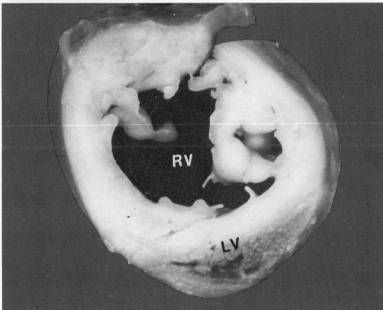

Figure 26.8. (*A*) The upper picture is a precordial short-axis cut in a univentricular connection to a dominant right ventricle with a rudimentary morphological left ventricle. Note that the left ventricle is posterior to the dominant ventricle. The lower is a simulated short-axis cut from a different patient. Note the large morphological right ventricle with a slitlike morphologically left ventricle.

ASSOCIATED ABNORMALITIES

Ventricular Septal Defect

A ventricular septal defect exists in most cases with a univentricular atrioventricular connection and two ventricles. The size of the defect is very important, particularly in cases where the aorta arises from the rudimentary ventricle (Fig. 26.7). It is not uncommon for the defects to become progressively restrictive with time (24), particularly after banding of the pulmonary trunk (Fig. 26.23). The size of the defect must be assessed in a variety of views, as a button-hole type defect may appear larger in one plane than another. A combination of cross-sectional and Doppler echocardiography has proved useful in assessing the size of the defect (Fig. 26.23). The position of the defect may vary from being roofed by both semilunar valves to being lower down in the muscular septum. Defects may be single or multiple (Figs. 26.18A and 26.23).

Stenotic Atrioventricular Valves

With the advent of the Fontan operation and its modifications, it is important to exclude stenosis of the atrioventricular valves, particularly between the pulmonary venous atrium and the dominant ventricle.

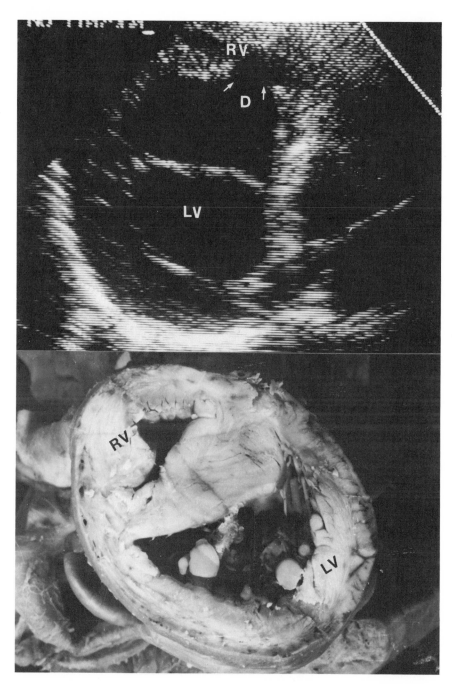

Figure 26.8 (cont'd.). (*B*) The upper picture is a high precordial short-axis cut in a univentricular connection to a dominant left ventricle. Note the morphological right ventricle, which is anterior and to the right in this patient. Also observe the ventricular septal defect. The lower picture is a specimen cut in the short-axis view demonstrating a small morphological right ventricle that is anterior to the dominant left ventricle. D = ventricular septal defect; LV = left ventricle; RV = right ventricle.

Stenosis is best assessed by combining direct visualization by cross-sectional echocardiography in an apical four-chamber and long-axis view with Doppler interrogation. The stenosis may be at supravalvar, valvar, subvalvar, or annular level (Fig. 26.24). Regurgitation of an atrioventricular valve, particularly the pulmonary venous valve, can be detected by Doppler echocardiography. Regurgitation may be caused by annular dilatation due to large pulmonary flow (Fig. 26.15) or to an anatomic anomaly such as a cleft in the left atrioventricular valve in absent right connection with a dominant morphologically left ventricle. The valve appears to have three components, unlike the normal situation where it usually resembles a mitral valve.

Straddling Atrioventricular Valves

Straddling of the atrioventricular valves is relevant when considering incorporating a small ventricle into the circuit during a modified Fontan procedure, although less important than when associated with a biventricular atrioventricular connection. In univentricular connection, the atrioventricular valve straddles into the smaller ventricle (Fig. 26.25) (18). This is best assessed in the apical and subcostal four-chamber views, where the papillary muscles and tensor apparatus in the smaller ventricle can be assessed. The atrioventricular valve leaflets appear to cross the ventricular septal defect into the smaller ventricle (Fig.

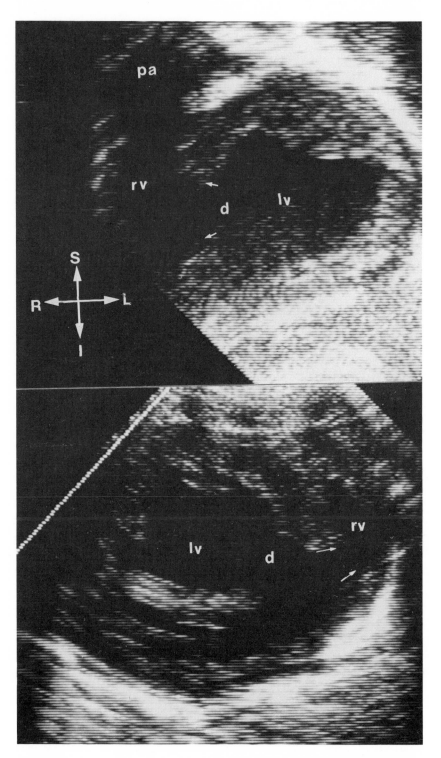

Figure 26.9. The upper picture is a subcostal cut with clockwise rotation in univentricular connection to a dominant left ventricle with concordant ventriculoarterial connection. Note that in this patient the ventricular septal defect is large. Also observe that the morphological right ventricle is right sided. The lower picture is a precordial short-axis cut from a patient with a univentricular connection to a dominant left ventricle with a leftward morphological right ventricle that supports the aorta. Note that in this patient the ventricular septal defect appears to be restrictive. d = ventricular septal defect; LV = left ventricle; PA = pulmonary trunk; RV = right ventricle.

26.25). It is important to differentiate this from chordal attachments to the crest of the septum, which is relatively common and not a true form of straddling.

Venous Abnormalities

Systemic and pulmonary venous anomalies are frequently associated with univentricular connection to an indeterminate ventricle with a common atrioventric-

ular valve in right or left atrial isomerism (12). Recognition of these anomalies is of particular importance if a Fontan procedure or modification is to be performed. The assessment of right and left atrial isomerism is best achieved by evaluating the relationship of the abdominal inferior vena cava and aorta and the status of the hepatic veins (11, 12). Once the atrial arrangement is correctly assigned, the abnormal systemic or pulmonary venous connections can be evaluated. In

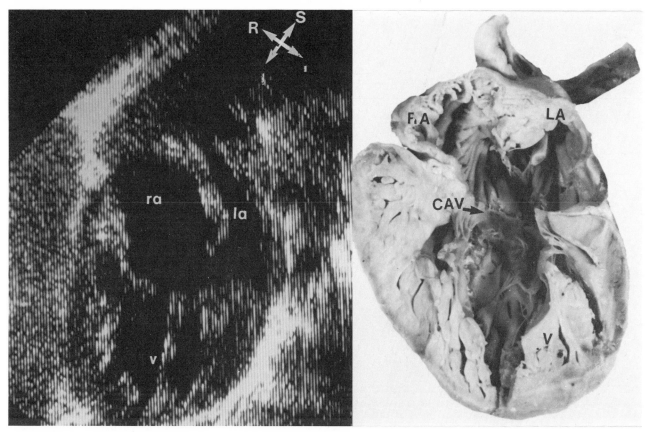

Figure 26.10.   The left-hand picture is a four-chamber view in a case of double-inlet connection to a solitary and indeterminate ventricle with a common atrioventricular valve. Note the large common atrioventricular valve and the ostium primum atrial septal defect. The picture on the right is a four-chamber cut from a different patient demonstrating the morphologic features. CAV = common atrioventricular valve; LA = left atrium; RA = right atrium; V = ventricle.

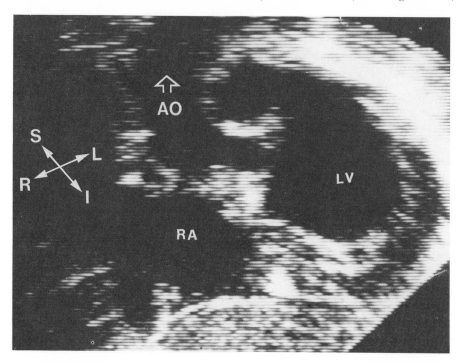

Figure 26.11.   (A) is a subcostal long-axis cut in univentricular connection to a dominant left ventricle with absent right connection and concordant ventriculoarterial connection. Note the aorta arising from the morphological left ventricle.

A

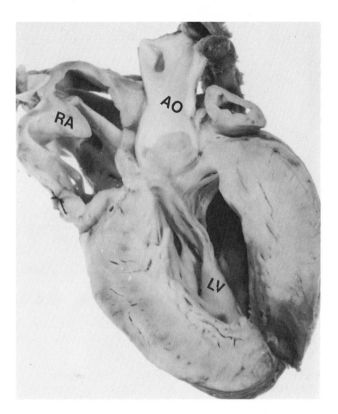

Figure 26.11 (cont'd.). (*B*) is an anatomic specimen cut to simulate the echocardiographic view. (*C*) is from another patient with a univentricular connection to a dominant left ventricle with an absent right connection and discordant ventriculoarterial connection. Note the pulmonary trunk with its sharp posterior turn arising from the morphological left ventricle. Also observe that the ventricular septal defect appears to be restrictive. AO = aorta; LA = left atrium; LV = left ventricle; PA = pulmonary trunk; RA = right atrium; RV = right ventricle.

B

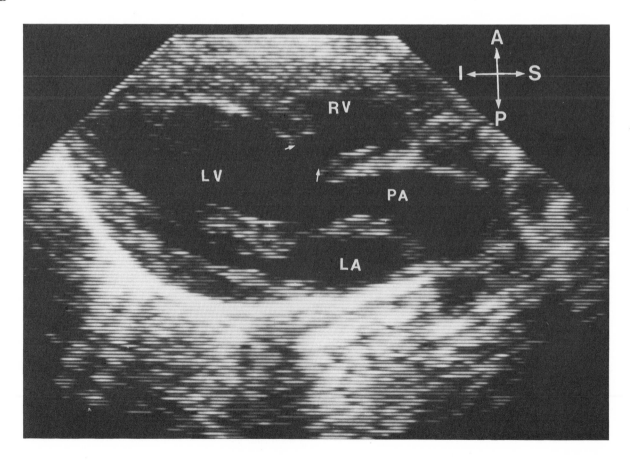

C

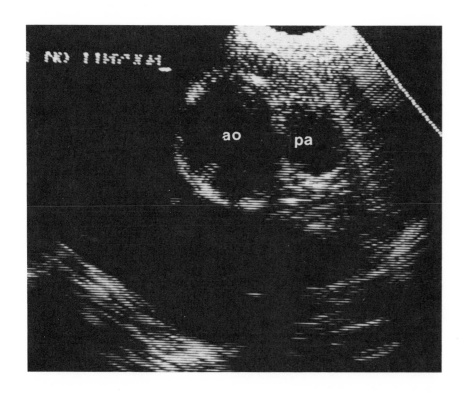

Figure 26.12. Precordial short-axis cut demonstrating the spatial relationship of the great vessels. The pulmonary artery (PA) and aorta (AO) are side by side.

the presence of a left superior vena cava with azygous continuation, the vessel invariably drains directly into the upper pole of the common atrium, while the hepatic veins may drain on the right side, in the middle, on the left side, or a combination of all three. These are best assessed from a combination of a subcostal four-chamber view and suprasternal cuts; the latter allows visualization of the left superior vena cava.

Pulmonary venous anomalies are best appreciated in the subcostal four-chamber view. They invariably consist of pulmonary veins entering either side of the common atrium or forming a common pool that then communicates with the common atrium. This may or may not be restrictive and can be reliably assessed with a combination of cross-sectional and Doppler echocardiography.

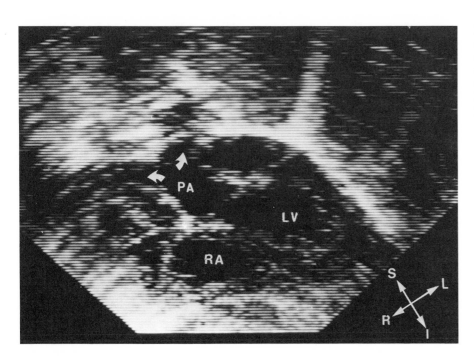

Figure 26.13. Subcostal long-axis cut in univentricular connection to a dominant left ventricle (LV) with absent right connection and discordant ventriculoarterial connection. Note the branching pattern of the pulmonary trunk (PA). RA = right atrium.

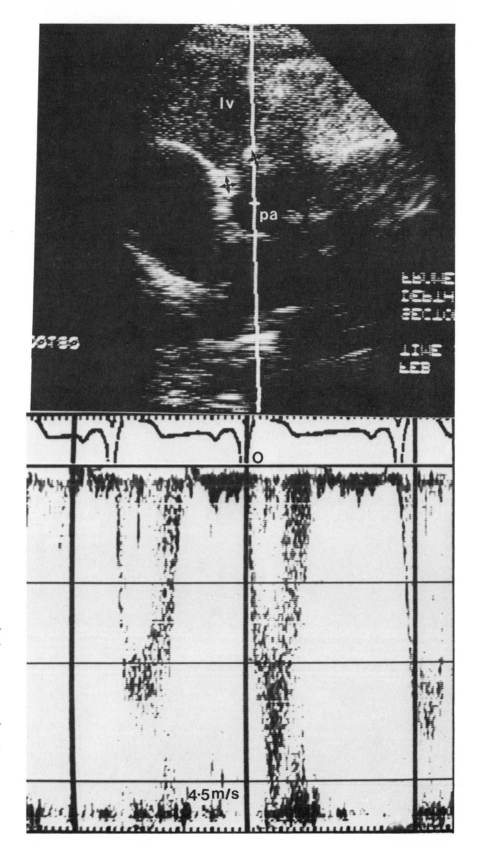

Figure 26.14. The upper picture is a four-chamber cut with superior angulation in a patient with univentricular connection to a dominant left ventricle with discordant ventriculoarterial connection. This patient also has subpulmonary stenosis formed by a combination of the ventriculoinfundibular fold and outlet septum indicated by the black stars. Note the Doppler sample volume is placed just distal to the obstruction. The lower picture is a spectral trace from the same patient indicating a high-velocity systolic jet. LV = left ventricle; PA = pulmonary trunk.

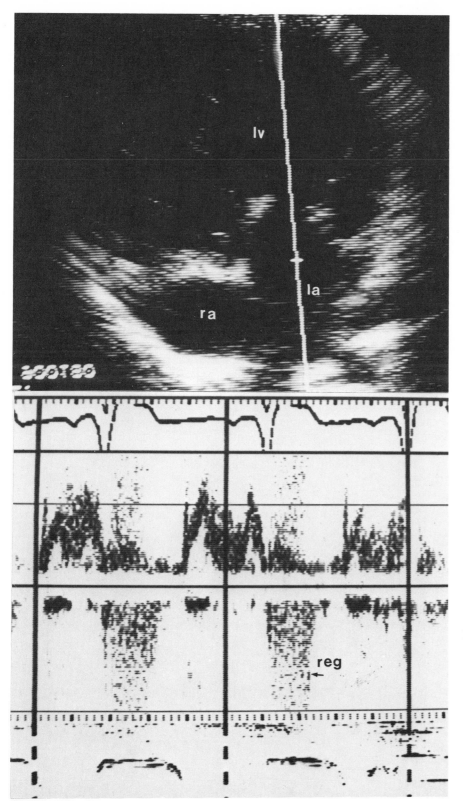

Figure 26.15. The upper picture is a precordial four-chamber cut in univentricular connection to a dominant left ventricle (lv) type with left atrioventricular valve regurgitation. Note the sample volume placed just proximal to the left atrioventricular valve. The lower picture is a spectral trace from the same patient demonstrating the regurgitant jet. LA = left atrium; RA = right atrium; reg = regurgitation.

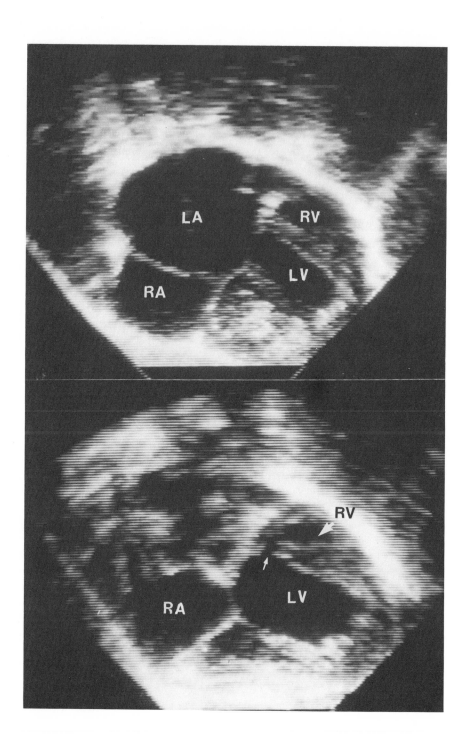

Figure 26.16. The upper picture is a subcostal four-chamber cut in univentricular connection to a dominant left ventricle with two atrioventricular valves. Note the morphological right ventricle, which is anterior and to the left of the morphologically left ventricle. In this view, only the left atrioventricular valve is seen. The lower picture is from the same patient with angulation of the transducer to visualize the right atrioventricular valve connecting with the morphological left ventricle. Note that the ventricular septal defect is restrictive (*arrow*). LA = left atrium; LV = left ventricle; RA = right atrium; RV = right ventricle.

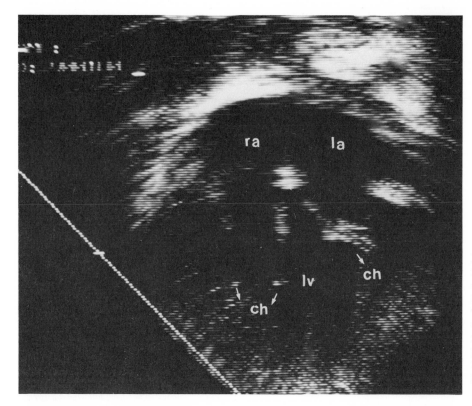

Figure 26.17.   The precordial four-chamber cut from a case of double-inlet connection to a dominant left ventricle with two atrioventricular valves. Note that the chords (ch) insert into papillary muscles to either side of the morphological left ventricle (LV), making this patient a suitable candidate for septation. LA = left atrium; RA = right atrium.

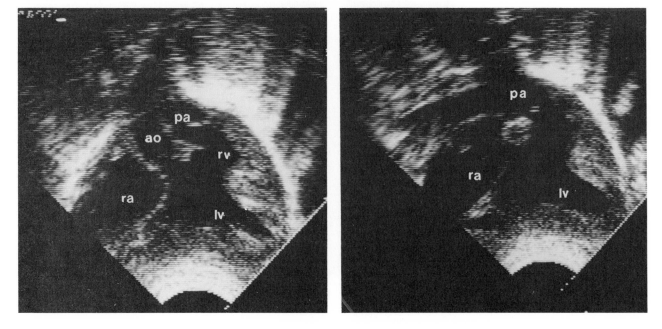

A

Figure 26.18.   (*A*) The left-hand picture is a subcostal long-axis cut in univentricular connection to a dominant left ventricle with two atrioventricular valves and concordant ventriculoarterial connection. The pulmonary artery arises from the left-sided rudimentary right ventricle. The right-hand picture is from the same patient and demonstrates the branching pattern of the pulmonary trunk.

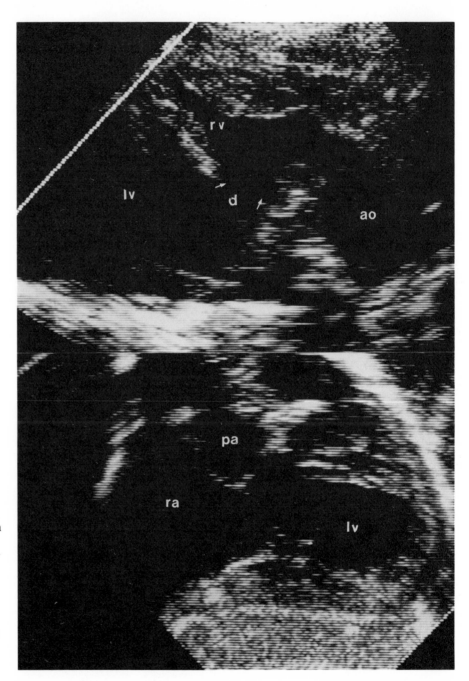

Figure 26.18 (cont'd.). (*B*) The upper picture is a precordial long-axis cut with clockwise rotation in a case with double-inlet connection to a dominant left ventricle with two atrioventricular valves and discordant ventriculoarterial connection. Note the aorta arising from the small anterior and leftward morphological right ventricle. Also note the ventricular septal defect indicated by the arrows. The lower picture is the subcostal long-axis cut from the same patient demonstrating the pulmonary trunk arising from the morphological left ventricle.

B

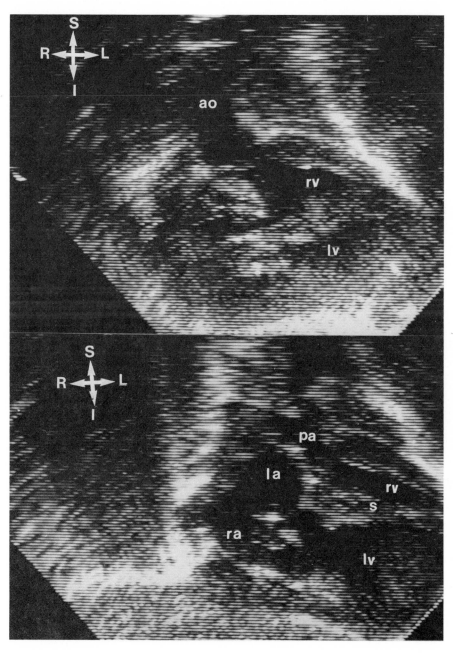

C

Figure 26.18 (cont'd.). (*C*) The upper picture is a subcostal long-axis cut in a patient with double-inlet connection to a dominant left ventricle with two atrioventricular valves and a double-outlet right ventricle. Note the aorta arising from the small morphological right ventricle. The lower picture is from the same patient, demonstrating the pulmonary trunk also arising from the morphological right ventricle. This patient also had a restrictive ventricular septal defect. Ao = aorta; d = ventricular septal defect; LA = left atrium; LV = left ventricle; PA = pulmonary artery; RA = right atrium; RV = right ventricle; s = interventricular septum.

Figure 26.19. Subcostal four-chamber cut in a patient with right-sided heart, univentricular connection to a dominant right ventricle (RV), and absent right atrioventricular connection. Note that the left atrium (LA) drains through an atrioventricular valve into a morphological RV. A dense wedge of sulcus tissue (ST) can be seen separating the right atrium (RA) from the dominant ventricle. PV = pulmonary vein.

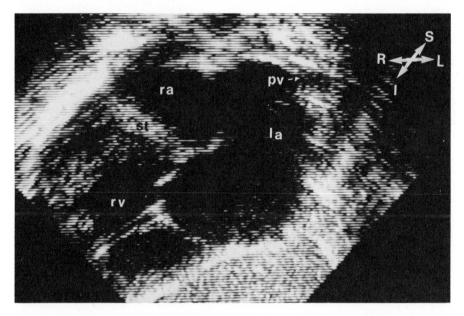

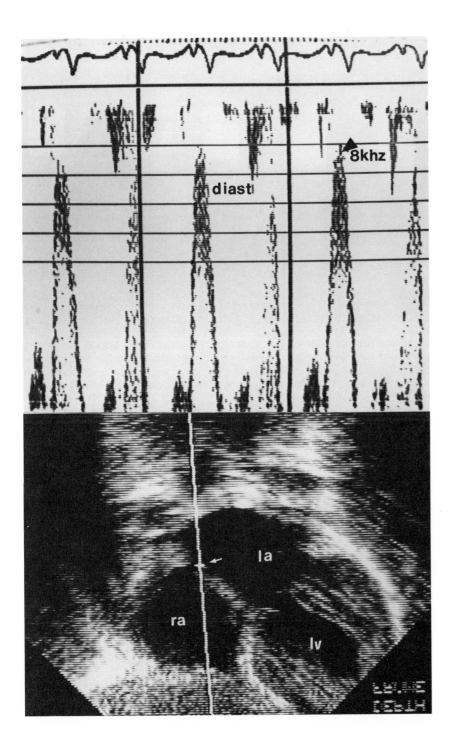

Figure 26.20. The lower picture is a subcostal four-chamber cut in a patient with univentricular connection to a dominant left ventricle, absent right connection, and a restrictive interatrial communication. Note the Doppler sample volume is placed just distal to the small interatrial communication. The upper picture is from the same patient and demonstrates the high-velocity diastolic jet across the interatrial communication. diast = diastole; LA = left atrium; LV = left ventricle; RA = right atrium.

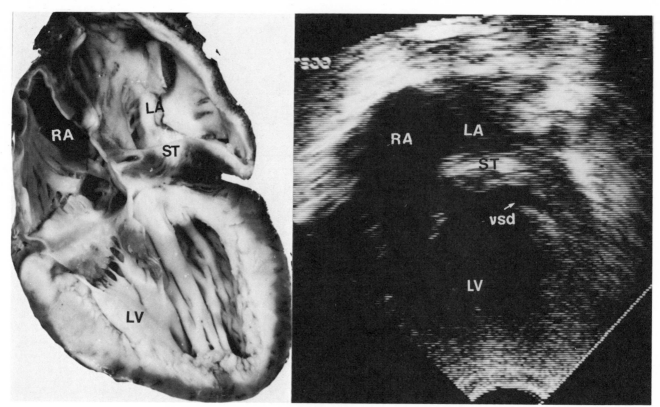

Figure 26.21.   The picture on the right is a precordial four-chamber cut of a patient with univentricular connection to a dominant left ventricle and absent left connection. Note the dense wedge of sulcus tissue separating the left atrium from the ventricular mass. There is also a small ventricular septal defect evident in this view. The picture on the left is a precordial four-chamber cut from a different patient demonstrating the morphologic features. LA = left atrium; RA = right atrium; LV = left ventricle; ST = sulcus tissue; VSD = ventricular septal defect.

Figure 26.22.   A subcostal long-axis cut from a patient with univentricular connection to a dominant left ventricle (LV) and absent left connection. This patient also has a discordant ventriculoarterial connection. Note that the septal aspect of the dominant ventricle is smooth with an anterior and leftward morphological right ventricle (RV). d = ventricular septal defect; PA = pulmonary trunk; RA = right atrium.

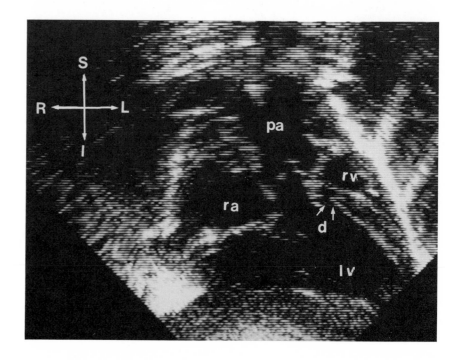

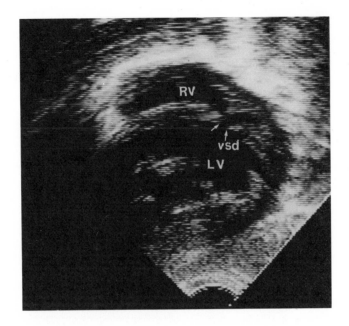

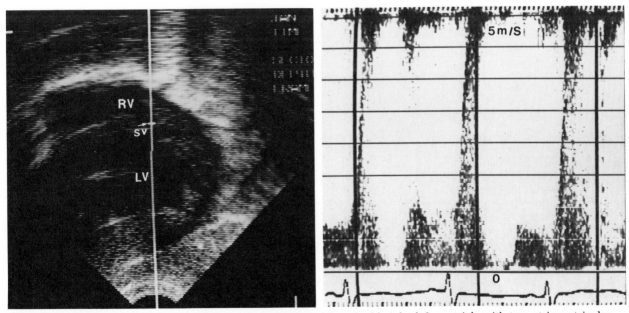

Figure 26.23.   The upper picture is a subcostal short-axis cut in a double-inlet left ventricle with two atrioventricular valves and a leftward anterior aorta arising from a small morphological right ventricle. Note this patient has a restricted muscular ventricular septal defect. The lower left-hand picture is from the same patient with a sample volume placed just distal to the ventricular septal defect. The picture on the right is the spectral trace demonstrating a high-velocity jet of 5 meters per second (pressure gradient 100 millimeters of mercury). LV = left ventricle; RV = right ventricle; SV = sample volume; VSD = ventricular septal defect.

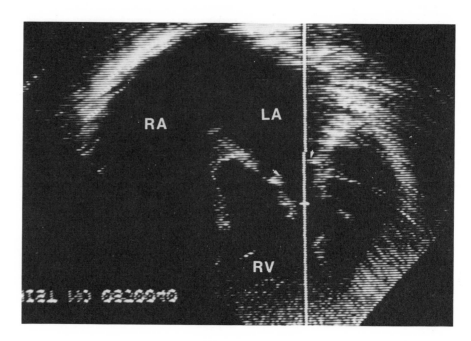

A

Figure 26.24. (*C*) is a precordial four-chamber cut from a patient with a double-inlet right ventricle with a stenotic left atrioventricular valve. Note a discrete membrane in the subvalvar position (*arrow*). This patient also has a straddling left atrioventricular valve. (*A*) is from the same patient and demonstrates a Doppler sample volume just distal to the stenotic region. (*B*) is the spectral trace demonstrating a high-velocity jet across the left atrioventricular valve with a velocity of 2.5 meters per second. LA = left atrium; LV = left ventricle; RA = right atrium; RV = right ventricle; s = interventricular septum.

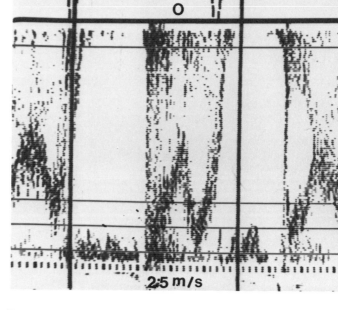

B

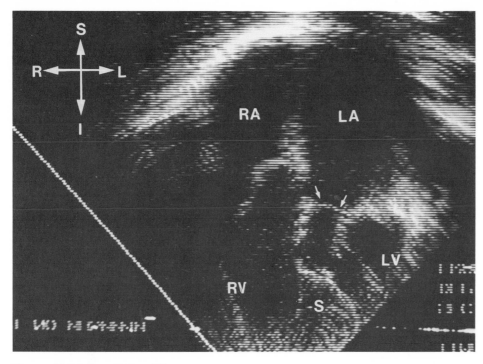

Figure 26.24 (cont'd.). (*C*)

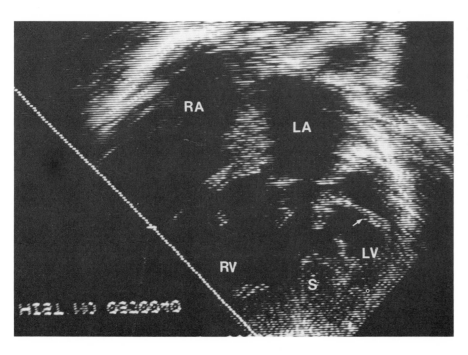

Figure 26.25. A precordial four-chamber cut from a patient with double-inlet right ventricle (RV) and two atrioventricular valves. The patient has a stenotic left atrioventricular valve and a straddling left atrioventricular valve. Note the tensor apparatus from the left-sided atrioventricular valve inserted onto the morphological left ventricle (LV) (*arrow*). LA = left atrium; RA = right atrium; S = interventricular septum.

REFERENCES

1. Anderson RH, Macartney FJ, Tynan M, et al. Univentricular atrioventricular connection: the single ventricle trap unsprung. Pediatr Cardiol 1983;4:273–80.
2. Anderson RH, Becker AE, Wilkinson JL, Gerlis LM. Morphogenesis of univentricular hearts. Br Heart J 1976;38:553–72.
3. Van Praagh R, David I, Van Praagh S. What is a ventricle? The single ventricle trap. Pediatr Cardiol 1982;2:79–84.
4. Van Praagh R, Ongley PA, Swan HJC. Anatomical types of single or common ventricle in man: morphologic and geometric aspects of sixty necropsied cases. Am J Cardiol 1964;13:367–86.
5. Van Praagh R, Plett JA, Van Praagh S. Single ventricle. Herz 1979;4:113–50.
6. Anderson RH, Becker AE, Macartney FJ, Shinebourne EA, Wilkinson JL, Tynan MJ. Is "tricuspid atresia" a univentricular heart? Pediatr Cardiol 1979;1:51–6.
7. Bharati S, Lev M. The concept of tricuspid atresia complex as distinct from that of the single ventricle complex. Pediatr Cardiol 1979;1:57–62.
8. Deanfield JE, Tommasini G, Anderson RH, Macartney FJ. Tricuspid atresia: analysis of coronary artery distribution and ventricular morphology. Br Heart J 1982;48:485–92.
9. Macartney FJ, Partridge JB, Scott O, Deverall PH. Common or single ventricle. An angiocardiographic and hemodynamic study of 42 patients. Circulation 1976;53:543–54.
10. Anderson RH, Becker AE, Freedom RM, et al. Analysis of the atrioventricular junction—connexions, relations and ventricular morphology. In: Godman MJ, ed. Pediatric cardiology. Edinburgh: Churchill Livingstone, 1982:169–81. Vol 4.
11. Huhta JC, Smallhorn JF, Macartney FJ. Two dimensional echocardiographic diagnosis of situs. Br Heart J 1982;48:97–108.
12. Huhta JC, Smallhorn JF, Macartney FJ, Anderson RH, de Leval M. Cross-sectional echocardiographic diagnosis of systemic venous return. Br Heart J 1982;48:388–403.
13. Rigby ML, Anderson RH, Gibson D, Jones ODH, Joseph MC, Shinebourne EA. Two-dimensional echocardiographic categorisation of the univentricular heart: ventricular morphology, type and mode of atrioventricular connection. Br Heart J 1981;46:603–12.
14. Freedom RM, Picchio F, Duncan WJ, Harder JR, Moes CAF, Rowe RD. The atrioventricular junction in the univentricular heart: a two-dimensional echocardiographic analysis. Pediatr Cardiol 1982;3:105–17.
15. Sahn DJ, Harder JR, Freedom RM, et al. Cross-sectional echocardiographic diagnosis and subclassification of univentricular hearts. Imaging studies of atrioventricular valves, septal structures and rudimentary outflow chambers. Circulation 1982;66:1070–7.
16. Rigby ML, Gibson DG, Joseph MC, et al. Recognition of imperforate atrioventricular valves by two dimensional echocardiography. Br Heart J 1982;47:329–36.
17. Smallhorn JF, Tommasini G, Macartney FJ. Detection and assessment of straddling and overriding atrioventricular valves by two-dimensional echocardiography. Br Heart J 1981;46:254–62.
18. Smallhorn JF, Tommasini G, Macartney FJ. Two-dimensional echocardiographic assessment of common atrioventricular valves in univentricular hearts. Br Heart J 1981;46:30–4.
19. Smallhorn JF, Tommasini G, Anderson RH, Macartney FJ. Assessment of atrioventricular septal defects by two-dimensional echocardiography. Br Heart J 1982;47:109–21.
20. Anderson RH, Lenox CC, Zuberbuhler JR, Ho SY, Smith A, Wilkinson JL. Double-inlet left ventricle with rudimentary right ventricle and ventriculoarterial concordance. Am J Cardiol 1983;52:573–7.
21. Scalia D, Russo P, Anderson RH, et al. The surgical anatomy of hearts with no direct communication between the right atrium and the ventricular mass—so called tricuspid atresia. J Thorac Cardiovasc Surg 1984;7:743–55.
22. Thiene G, Daliento L, Frescura C, De Tommasi M, Macartney FJ, Anderson RH. Atresia of left atrioventricular orifice. Anatomical investigation in 62 cases. Br Heart J 1981;45:393–401.
23. Mickell JJ, Mathews RA, Park SC, et al. Left atrioventricular valve atresia: clinical management. Circulation 1980;60:123–7.
24. Penkoske PA, Freedom RM, Williams WG, Trusler GA, Rowe RD. Surgical palliation of subaortic stenosis in the univentricular heart. J Thorac Cardiovasc Surg 1984;87:767–81.

27

Discordant and Ambiguous Atrioventricular Connections

Michael Rigby

The term *discordant atrioventricular connection* describes the situation in which the morphological right atrium connects to the morphological left ventricle and the morphological left atrium to the morphological right ventricle. Thus, there are lateralized atria (usual arrangement or mirror-image arrangement) and a biventricular atrioventricular connection (1). When there is atrial isomerism (2) and each of the two isomeric atria connect to a separate ventricle, the connection cannot be concordant or discordant. One of the atria must connect to a morphological appropriate ventricle and the other to a morphological inappropriate ventricle. This arrangement may be described as an "ambiguous" atrioventricular connection. The purpose of this chapter is to describe the echocardiographic diagnosis of hearts with a biventricular atrioventricular connection in which the type of connection is abnormal (i.e., discordant or ambiguous).

It is appropriate to re-emphasize the concept of "ventricular topology" discussed in Chapter 22. For normal hearts (those with usually arranged atria and a concordant atrioventricular connection), the right ventricle wraps itself around the left ventricle in such a way that conceptually the palmar surface of the observer's right hand can be placed upon the septal surface of the morphological right ventricle with the thumb in the inlet, the wrist in the apical trabecular component, and the fingers in the outlet. This may be termed "right-hand pattern ventricular topology." This pattern of topology is also usually found in "situs inversus" when mirror-image atria connect discordantly to the ventricular mass. In contrast, when there is mirror-image arrangement of the atria with a concor-

dant atrioventricular connection or usual atrial arrangement with a discordant atrioventricular connection, it is a left-hand pattern of ventricular topology that is usually found. Although discordant atrioventricular connection implies a left-hand pattern ventricular topology in the setting of usual atrial arrangement, no such assumption can be made when the atrioventricular connection is ambiguous. Ventricular topology must, therefore, be described separately when accounting fully for the biventricular atrioventricular connection in patients with isomeric atrial chambers.

DISCORDANT ATRIOVENTRICULAR CONNECTION

Morphology

A *discordant atrioventricular connection* is the term applied to the abnormal situation in which the morphological left and right atria connect to inappropriate ventricles (3). The junction between the morphological right atrium and morphological left ventricle is guarded by the mitral valve, which has two distinct papillary muscles without septal insertions (Fig. 27.1*A*). The junction between morphological left atrium and morphological right ventricle is guarded by the tricuspid valve, which has numerous chordal insertions into the morphological right surface of the ventricular septum (Fig. 27.1*B*). Over 80 percent of hearts will also exhibit a discordant ventriculoarterial connection (4). The subpulmonary outflow tract is deeply wedged between the atrioventricular valves in a position somewhat similar to that of the aortic root in the normal heart (Fig. 27.2). The pulmonary valve, therefore, is almost

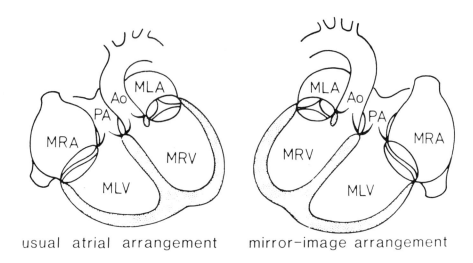

usual atrial arrangement   mirror-image arrangement

Figure 27.1. A diagram showing the segmental connections producing the arrangement known as congenitally corrected transposition. MLA = morphological left atrium.

Discordant atrioventricular connection
and discordant ventriculo-arterial connection

A   **B**

Figure 27.2. With isomeric atrial chambers and a biventricular atrioventricular connection, the arrangement is ambiguous irrespective of the ventricular topology. MRA = morphological right atrium, MRV = morphological right ventricle, MLA = morphological left atrium, MLV = morphological left ventricle.

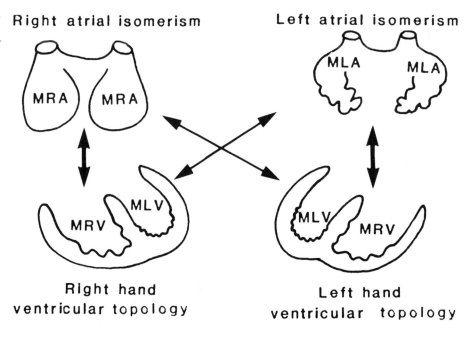

Right atrial isomerism   Left atrial isomerism

Right hand   Left hand
ventricular topology   ventricular topology

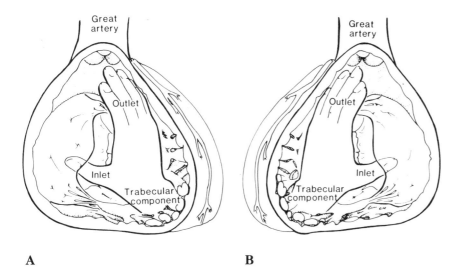

Figure 27.3. A diagram illustrating the concept of ventricular topology. The septal surface of the morphological right ventricle in terms of the way, figuratively speaking, that it will accept the palmar surface of the observer's hand.

A   B

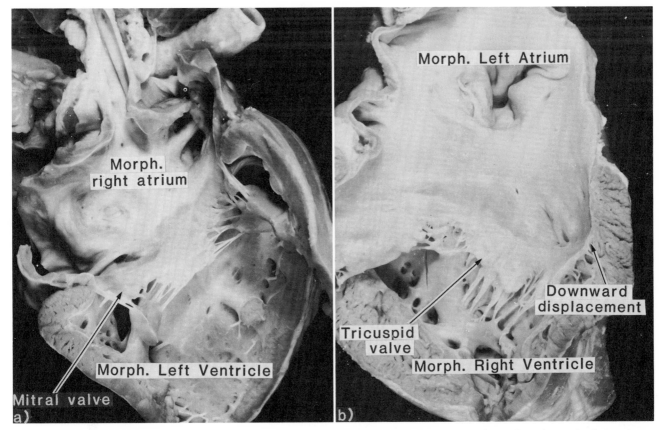

Figure 27.4. The typical chamber combinations when the atrioventricular connection is discordant shown in the setting of usual atrial arrangement.

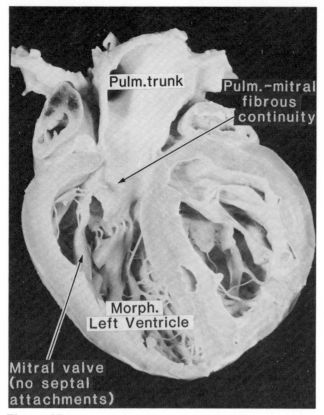

Figure 27.5. A simulated four-chamber section showing the deeply wedged pulmonary trunk connected discordantly to the right-sided morphological left ventricle.

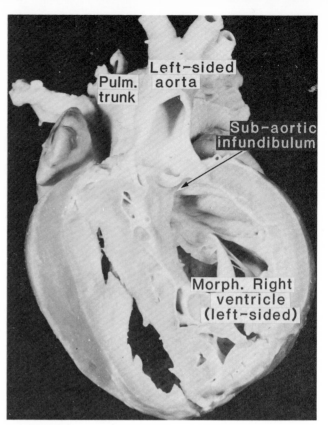

Figure 27.6. A section taken more anteriorly from the heart illustrated in Figure 26.5 showing the left-sided aorta arising above a complete muscular infundibulum from the left-sided morphological right ventricle.

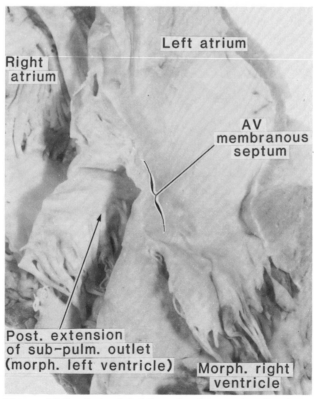

Figure 27.7. A simulated four-chamber section showing how, in congenitally corrected transposition, the atrioventricular (AV) septum separates the morphological left ventricle from the left atrium.

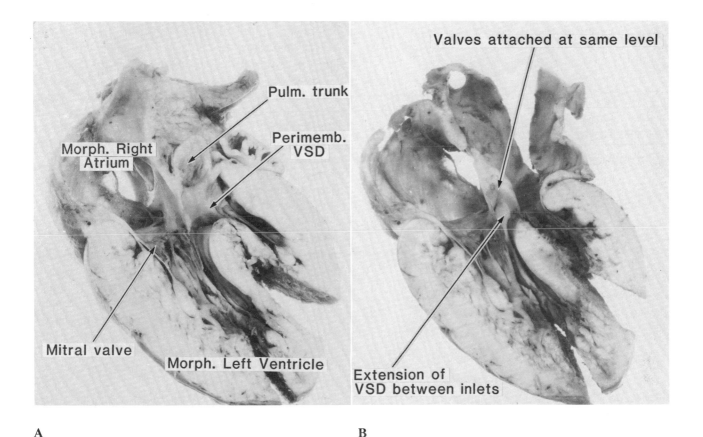

A   **B**

Figure 27.8. Simulated four-chamber sections through a heart with congenitally corrected transposition and a perimembranous ventricular septal defect (VSD) showing (*A*) the over-riding subpulmonary outlet and (*B*) the defect extending posteriorly between the inlets, the atrioventricular valve leaflets arising from the atrial septum at the same level.

always in direct fibrous continuity with the mitral valve (see Fig. 27.2). The tricuspid valve usually exhibits muscular separation from the anteriorly placed aortic root so that there is a muscular subaortic infundibulum (Fig. 27.3*B*). Characteristically, there is marked misalignment between the atrial and ventricular septal structures. The atrioventricular septum is located between the morphological left ventricle and morphological left atrium (Fig. 27.3*A*). The ventricles are side by side; the morphological right ventricle is on the left and the morphological left ventricle to the right when there is usual arrangement of the atria. This arrangement of the ventricles in hearts with discordant atrioventricular connection has given rise to the commonly used alternative name of "ventricular inversion" (5). Although the ventricles frequently are back to front, they do not present a mirror-image arrangement of the normal heart and neither are they upside down (6). A discordant atrioventricular connection can exist with "normally related" ventricles either with mirror-image atrial arrangement or in hearts with crossing atrioventricular junctions (so-called crisscross hearts) (7). The ventricles may also assume an anterosuperior or superoinfe-

rior relationship. Conversely, the presence of ventricular inversion does not always denote the presence of a discordant atrioventricular connection (5). It is frequently found, for example, in hearts with right atrial isomerism or in those with complete transposition and mirror-image atrial arrangement.

The discordant atrioventricular connection does not in itself constitute a diagnosis. Congenitally corrected transposition is characterized by discordant connections at both atrioventricular and ventriculoarterial junctions. As such it may exist with usual or mirror-image atrial arrangement (Fig. 27.4). Uncommonly, such hearts have no associated lesions, and the anomaly may be a chance finding at autopsy. Usually, however, there are associated abnormalities. Ventricular septal defects, pulmonary stenosis, and anomalies of the morphological tricuspid valve are so frequent that they may almost be considered part of the lesion. They may also be found commonly when a discordant atrioventricular connection is associated with double-outlet right ventricle or pulmonary atresia.

When present, a ventricular septal defect is usually perimembranous (Fig. 27.5) and is over-ridden by the

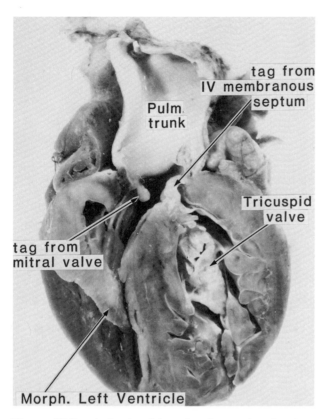

Figure 27.9. A simulated four-chamber section showing subpulmonary stenosis in the setting of congenitally corrected transposition. The stenosis is produced by tissue tags derived from the mitral valve and from the intraventricular component of the membranous septum.

pulmonary trunk, frequently extending between the ventricular inlets. Muscular defects and double-committed subarterial defects are also encountered. Pulmonary stenosis (Fig. 27.6) may be valvar or subvalvar (often in combination) and is usually associated with a perimembranous ventricular septal defect. Although subvalvar obstruction is commonly muscular, it may be due to aneurysmal fibrous tissue tags derived from the membranous septum or the septal leaflet of the morphological tricuspid valve (8). The abnormalities of the tricuspid valve itself usually give rise to insufficiency. There may be varying degrees of dysplasia, and the septal leaflet is often bound down to the septum, giving rise in a few cases to extreme forms of Ebstein's malformation (9). A dysplastic tricuspid valve may be the only associated abnormality. When there is a perimembranous inlet ventricular septal defect, chords from the septal leaflet of the tricuspid valve usually insert into the crest of the ventricular septum. Straddling or over-riding of the tricuspid valve also occurs (10). The mitral valve occasionally straddles the outlet portion of the septum, giving rise to left ventricular outflow tract obstruction (11).

The aortic valve is anterior and to the left of the pulmonary valve in most cases of congenitally corrected transposition (Fig. 27.7). Such a relationship, however, is not always present and does not alone constitute grounds for diagnosis (4). When there is usual atrial arrangement, the heart is frequently midline or right sided (4).

Although congenitally corrected transposition is the

Figure 27.10. The aorta is usually anterior and left sided when congenitally corrected transposition is found in the setting of usual atrial arrangement, but this is by no means a universal finding.

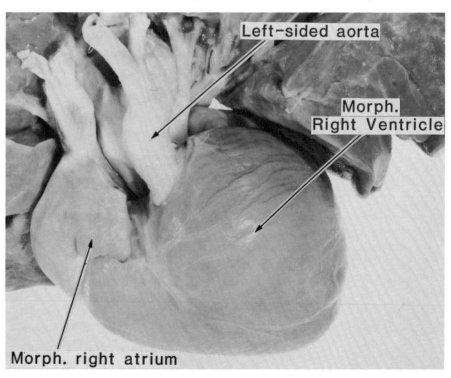

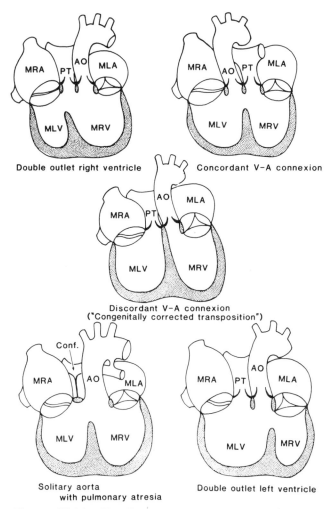

Double outlet right ventricle

Concordant V-A connexion

Discordant V-A connexion
("Congenitally corrected transposition")

Solitary aorta
with pulmonary atresia

Double outlet left ventricle

Figure 27.11. Usually a discordant atrioventricular connection coexists with a discordant ventriculoarterial (V-A) connection (center), but any other ventriculoarterial connection can be found. The most common alternative connections are shown in the setting of usual atrial arrangement.

most common anomaly found with a discordant atrioventricular connection, double-outlet right ventricle and single-outlet right ventricle with pulmonary atresia may also occur. Rarely there will be a concordant ventriculoarterial connection or double outlet from the morphological left ventricle (Figs. 27.8 to 27.11). When there is a double-outlet right ventricle, it is usually associated with a perimembranous or muscular subpulmonary outlet ventricular septal defect and subpulmonary stenosis.

Echocardiography

The sequence of steps in the investigation of hearts with congenital anatomic malformations is to establish the arrangement of the atria, the atrioventricular connections and then the ventricular-great arterial connec-

tions. Bronchial anatomy determined by penetrated radiographs of the chest is the most useful guide to establishing the atrial arrangement (12). Ultrasonic examination of the abdominal great vessels may also permit such differentiation (13) (*vide infra*) (Chapters 23 and 33). The type of atrioventricular connection is determined from parasternal, apical, and subcostal four-chamber sections. The morphological tricuspid valve, which forms an integral part of the morphological right ventricle, has chordal attachments to the right ventricular aspect of the septum. In contrast, chords from the mitral valve usually attach to two discrete left ventricular papillary muscles and do not insert into the septum. Thus, in most hearts with biventricular atrioventricular connection, demonstration of the presence or absence of chordal attachments to the septum allows determination of the morphology of the atrioventricular valves and, hence, the ventricles. It may also be possible to determine the morphology of an atrioventricular valve by examining the basal attachment of its septal leaflet. The septal leaflet of the tricuspid valve is attached nearer to the apex of the heart than is the corresponding leaflet of the mitral valve. Providing that there is no perimembranous inlet ventricular septal defect, this offsetting of the atrioventricular valves enables the mitral and tricuspid valves to be distinguished. There are alternative methods of identifying ventricular morphology. Short-axis sections through the atrioventricular valves may identify the three-leaflet arrangement of the tricuspid valve in contrast to the two leaflets of the mitral valve. The left ventricle is typified by its smooth trabecular pattern with two paired papillary muscles, whereas the right ventricle is coarsely trabeculated with unequal papillary muscles and the moderator band in its apical portion.

When the arrangement of the atria has been established, the first step in the diagnosis of a discordant atrioventricular connection is to perform a subcostal four-chamber section. In the normal heart chords from the right-sided atrioventricular valve insert into the right ventricular aspect of the septum, and there are no chordal attachments of the left atrioventricular valve into the septum (Fig. 27.12). In contrast, hearts with usual atrial arrangement and discordant atrioventricular connection have septal chords from the left atrioventricular valve only (Fig. 27.13). Parasternal four-chamber sections in the normal heart demonstrate the usual offsetting of the atrioventricular valves so that the septal leaflet of the right-sided valve is attached nearer to the apex than is that of the left (Fig. 27.14). With discordant atrioventricular connection, the mirror image of this arrangement will be demonstrable such that the atrioventricular septum separates the morphological left ventricle from the morphological left atrium

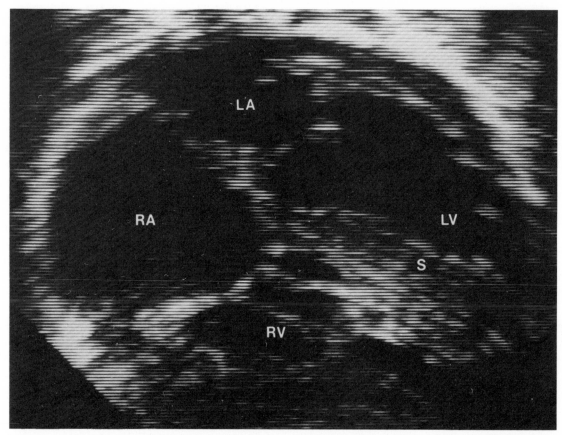

Figure 27.12.   Subcostal four-chamber section in the normal heart demonstrating chordal attachments from the tricuspid valve to the right ventricular (RV) aspect of the interventricular septum (S). There are no chordal attachments of the mitral valve to the septum in the left ventricle (LV).

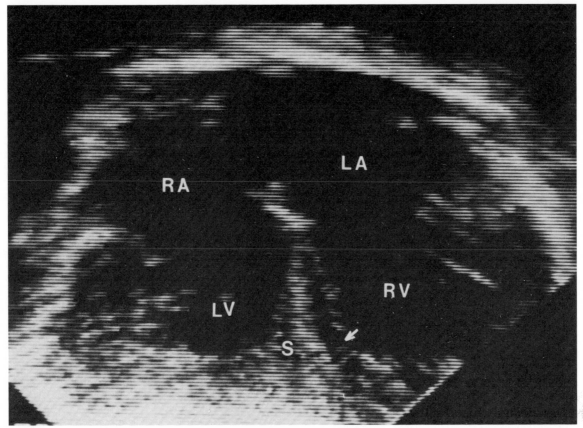

Figure 27.13. Four-chamber section illustrating chordal attachments from the left-sided morphological tricuspid valve to the septum (S) in the right ventricle (RV) in a heart with atrioventricular discordance.

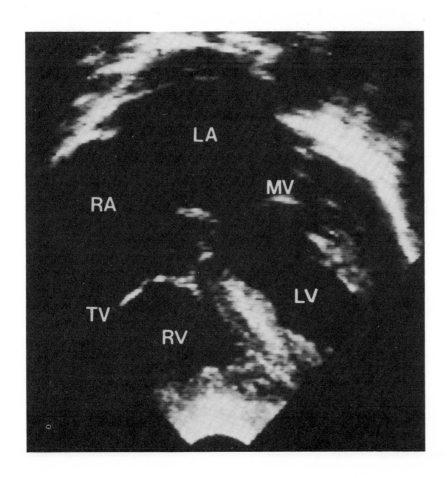

Figure 27.14. Parasternal four-chamber section from a normal heart illustrating usual offsetting of the mitral (MV) and tricuspid valves (TV).

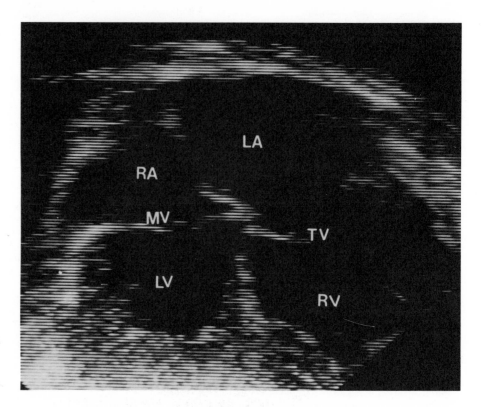

Figure 27.15. Parasternal four-chamber section from a heart with atrioventricular discordance illustrating reversed offsetting of the atrioventricular valves.

(Fig. 27.15). However, this offsetting of the atrioventricular valves in hearts with discordant atrioventricular connection is often unreliable because of the presence of a perimembranous inlet ventricular septal defect that causes the atrioventricular valves to be in fibrous continuity at the same level or superior to the defect (Figs. 27.14 & 27.16). Parasternal short-axis sections through the ventricular mass in the normal heart reveal a left atrioventricular valve with two leaflets. When the atrioventricular connection is discordant, the left atrioventricular valve has three leaflets (Fig. 27.17). In neonates and infants cross-sectional echocardiography may allow the differentiation of the coarsely trabeculated right ventricle from the smoothly trabeculated left ventricle. It is important to remember that in hearts with mirror-image arrangement of the atria and a discordant atrioventricular connection, the tricuspid valve and the morphological right ventricle will be to

Figure 27.16. Absence of offsetting of the atrioventricular valves in a heart with atrioventricular discordance and a perimembranous ventricular septal defect.

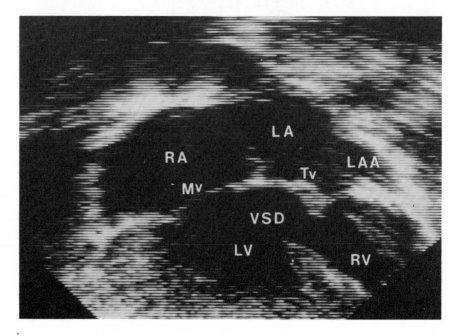

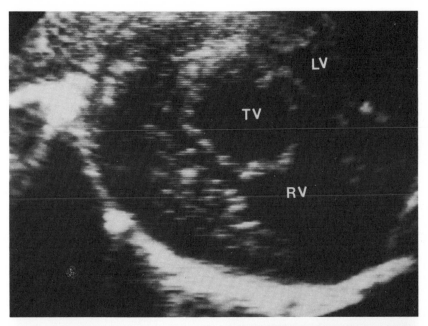

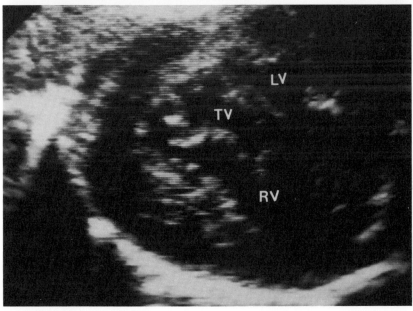

Figure 27.17. Parasternal short-axis section demonstrating a trileaflet left atrioventricular valve from a heart with a discordant atrioventricular connection.

the right. Four-chamber sections will, therefore, give rise to appearances similar to those seen in normal hearts.

Ventricular Septal Defect

There are two major types of ventricular septal defect found in hearts with discordant atrioventricular connection (14). Most defects are perimembranous and may extend so that they open predominantly between the outlets or the inlets. Outlet defects are best seen in the subcostal outlet (paracoronal) sections. These defects extend to the root of the pulmonary trunk, which appear to over-ride the septum to the right of the aortic valve (Fig. 27.18). Parasternal long-axis sections of the

left ventricle also demonstrate the subpulmonary outlet defect. Providing that the ventricular septal defect does not extend to open between the inlets, the atrioventricular valves maintain their usual offsetting with the inferior displacement of the septal leaflet of the left-sided valve seen in four-chamber projections, allowing confirmatory evidence of the discordant atrioventricular connection. Perimembranous inlet defects are demonstrable in four-chamber sections. The atrioventricular valves are in fibrous continuity through the central fibrous body superior to the defect, so that they lose their offsetting. Other criteria must then be used to establish the morphology of the atrioventricular valves and ventricles as outlined previously. In the presence

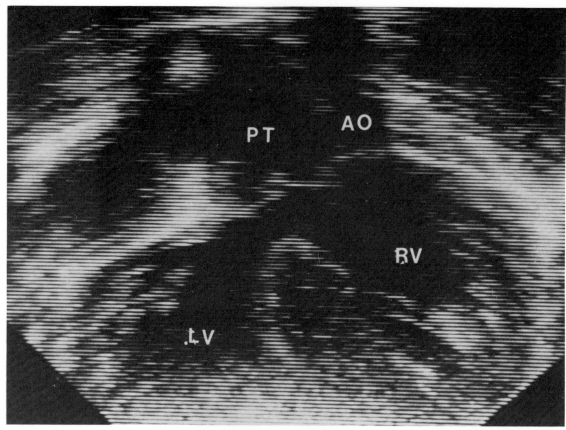

Figure 27.18. Subcostal outlet section from a heart with congenitally corrected transposition demonstrating an outlet ventricular septal defect with over-riding pulmonary trunk.

Figure 27.19. Four-chamber section from a heart with a discordant atrioventricular connection and perimembranous inlet ventricular septal defect demonstrating chordal insertions from the left-sided morphological tricuspid valve into the crest of the ventricular septum (*arrow*).

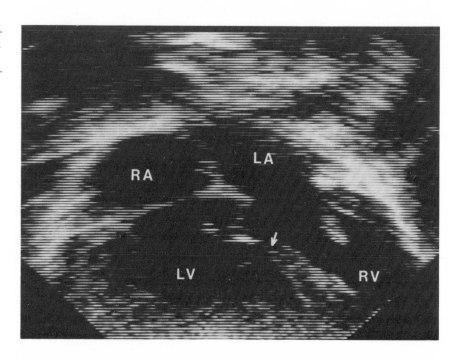

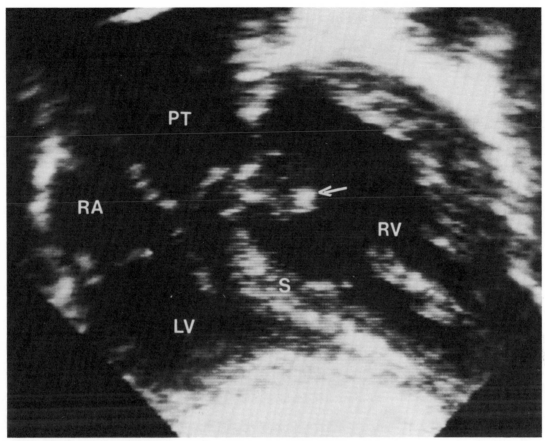

Figure 27.20. Parasternal long-axis section from a heart with congenitally corrected transposition illustrating subpulmonary stenosis (*arrow*).

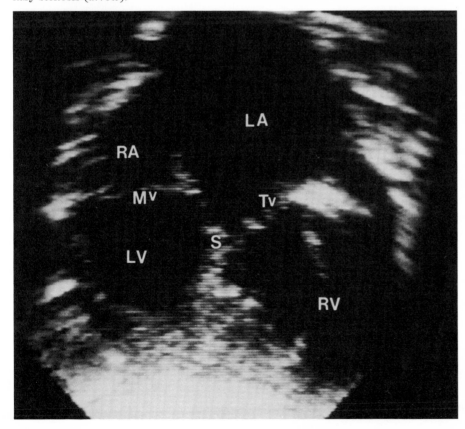

Figure 27.21. Parasternal four-chamber section in a heart with a discordant atrioventricular connection demonstrating the tricuspid valve partly bound to the ventricular septum.

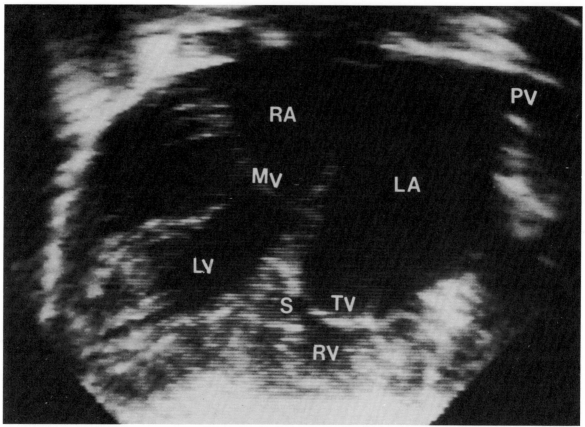

Figure 27.22.   Severe Ebstein's malformation of the tricuspid valve in a heart with a discordant atrioventricular connection.

of a perimembranous inlet defect, four-chamber sections demonstrate diastolic apposition of the "septal" leaflets of the mitral and tricuspid valves. In addition, chords from the tricuspid valve insert into the crest of the ventricular septum (Fig. 27.19). Subpulmonary or valvar pulmonary stenosis frequently occurs in combination, and is usually found when there is an additional ventricular septal defect. The presence of pulmonary stenosis is usually evident on subcostal outlet (paracoronal) and parasternal long-axis sections (Fig. 27.20). Often the mechanism for subpulmonary stenosis is rightward deviation of the outlet (infundibular) septum into the left ventricular outflow tract. Mild pulmonary stenosis may not always be evident on cross-sectional echocardiography, but its presence can be confirmed by Doppler echocardiography.

Anomalies of the Morphological Tricuspid Valve

Minor abnormalities of the tricuspid valve at autopsy may not be readily evident on cross-sectional echocardiography. Thus, Doppler assessment of the tricuspid valve is essential to detect the presence of tricuspid insufficiency. Cross-sectional echocardiography will frequently show that the septal leaflet of the tricuspid valve is partly bound down to the ventricular septum (Fig. 27.21), and occasionally, a severe Ebstein's malformation will be encountered in which the tricuspid leaflets are grossly displaced into the body of the right ventricle (Fig. 27.22). These abnormalities are almost always optimally visualized from four-chamber sections, but the dysplastic nature of the tricuspid valve and the attachments of its anterosuperior leaflet are evident from parasternal long-axis sections. A straddling tricuspid valve has chords inserting into both the right and left ventricles. Straddling is, of necessity, through an inlet ventricular septal defect and is identified in the four-chamber sections (Fig. 27.23). Less commonly, a mitral valve may be encountered that straddles through an outlet ventricular septal defect. Over-riding of the atrioventricular junction is usually associated with straddling but may occur in isolation. It can be identified in the four-chamber sections.

Double-Outlet Right Ventricle

When there is a concordant atrioventricular connection, double-outlet right ventricle cannot reliably be diagnosed by subcostal outlet (paracoronal) sections

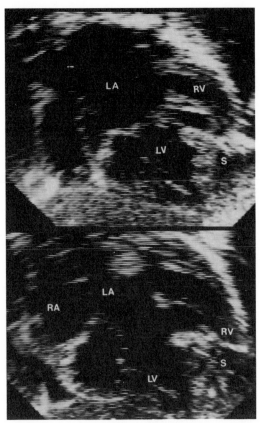

Figure 27.23. A straddling tricuspid valve from a heart with atrioventricular discordance and a perimembranous inlet ventricular septal defect.

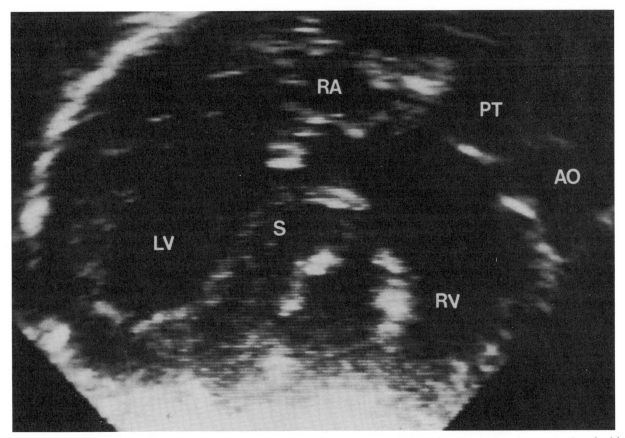

Figure 27.24. Subcostal outlet section from a heart with a discordant atrioventricular connection demonstrating double-outlet right ventricle.

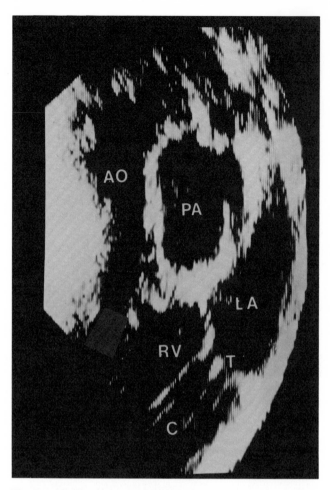

because the orientation of the ventricular septal defect may give the erroneous impression of double outlet when there are either concordant or discordant ventriculoarterial connections (15). However, the orientation of the ventricular septum in hearts with a discordant atrioventricular connection readily allows precise assessment of the ventriculoarterial connection from subcostal outlet sections (Fig. 27.24) (14).

Relationship of the Great Arteries

Subcostal outlet sections will establish the relative relationships of the aortic and pulmonary valves. Confirmatory evidence can usually be obtained by parasternal long-axis sections, which almost always demonstrate the aorta anterior to the pulmonary trunk (Fig. 27.25), and by parasternal short-axis sections, which most commonly demonstrate the aortic valve to the left of the pulmonary valve (Fig. 27.26). It has, however, already been emphasized that other relationships may exist so that the aorta may be directly anterior, anterior and to the right, or side by side and to the left of the pulmonary valve (4).

Discordant Atrioventricular Connection with Mirror-Image Atrial Arrangement

In the typical case of discordant atrioventricular connection with mirror-image arrangement of the atria, the morphological right ventricle will be right sided and the aorta will be anterior and to the right of the pulmonary valve. The diagnosis of associated lesions such as ventricular septal defect, pulmonary stenosis, Ebstein's anomaly, or straddling of the tricuspid valve and double-outlet

Figure 27.25. Parasternal long-axis section from a heart with congenitally corrected transposition demonstrating the ascending aorta anterior to the pulmonary trunk.

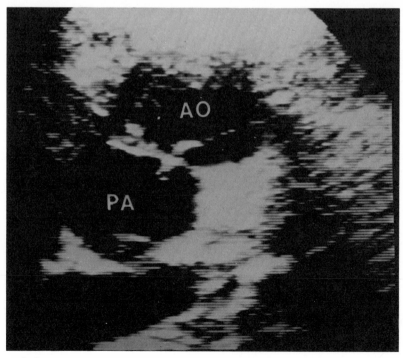

Figure 27.26. Parasternal short-axis section in congenitally corrected transposition demonstrating an anterior and left-sided aorta.

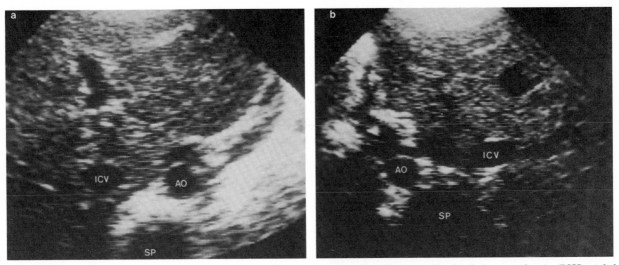

Figure 27.27. Horizontal abdominal echocardiographic sections showing the lateralized inferior caval vein (ICV) and descending aorta (AO) around the spine (SP). When there is usual atrial arrangement the inferior caval vein is to the right (a). With mirror-image atrial arrangement the inferior caval vein is to the left of the spine (b).

right ventricle are diagnosed in exactly the same manner as for hearts with usual arrangement of the atria.

AMBIGUOUS ATRIOVENTRICULAR CONNECTION

Morphology

Atrial isomerism is characterized by isomerism of paired organs such as the lungs and atria, together with a tendency for unpaired organs such as the liver and stomach to be midline in position (2). The importance of isomerism is that it is frequently associated with recognizable patterns of congenital heart malformations. Bilateral right sidedness is often but not exclusively associated with asplenia, and bilateral left sidedness with polysplenia. For this reason the terms asplenia syndrome and polysplenia syndrome describe patients with right and left atrial isomerism, respectively (16).

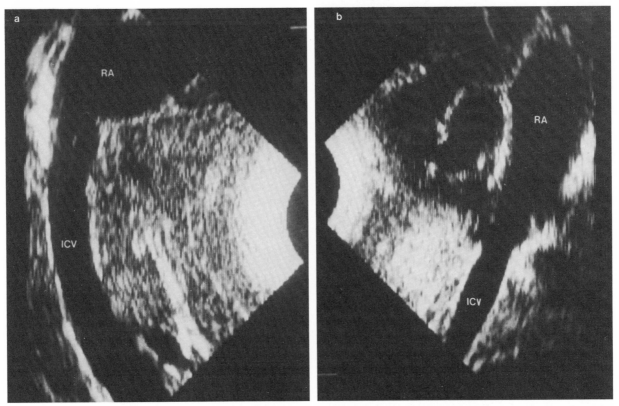

Figure 27.28. Sagittal abdominal sections demonstrating a right-sided inferior caval vein associated with usual atrial arrangement (a) and left-sided inferior caval vein (ICV) with mirror-image atrial arrangement (b).

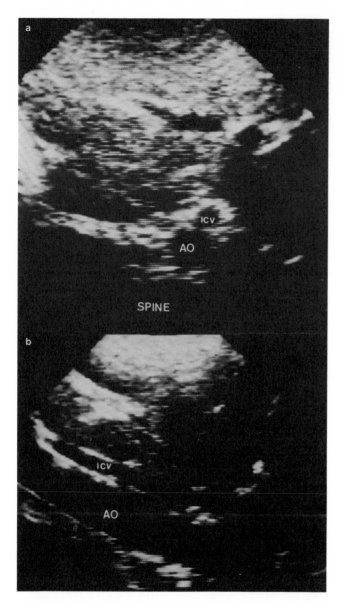

Figure 27.29. Horizontal (a) and sagittal (b) abdominal sections in right atrial isomerism illustrating the aorta (AO) and inferior caval vein (ICV) to the same side of the spine with the inferior caval vein anterior.

In hearts with right atrial isomerism there are two right atria, each with broad-based and blunt-ended appendages. A rudimentary atrial strand is often the only septal structure present, but alternatively a "primum atrial septal defect" or even an intact atrial septum may be found. Bilateral superior caval veins and bilateral anomalous connection of the pulmonary veins are often encountered, but total extracardiac anomalous pulmonary venous connection has also been described. In left atrial isomerism, the atrial appendages are both of left morphology and are narrow and hooked. Frequently the atrial septum is better formed in left than right isomerism, and bilateral

superior caval veins are frequently encountered. Of particular importance is the common association of interruption of the inferior caval vein, which is continued via the azygous system of veins to either the right-sided or left-sided superior caval vein. The pulmonary veins may drain to one atrium, but lateralized and bilaterally symmetrical connections are also encountered.

Both right and left atrial isomerism may be associated with either a biventricular or a univentricular atrioventricular connection (1). A biventricular connection is described as ambiguous because one of the atria must connect to an inappropriate ventricle. In most of these cases there is an atrioventricular septal defect with a common valve, but atrioventricular septal defects with separate right and left valve orifices also occur. Rarely, an ambiguous biventricular atrioventricular connection can exist without an atrioventricular septal defect.

Two basic ventricular relationships may exist when the atria connect to separate ventricles. The morphological right ventricle may be to the right of the morphological left ventricle (right-hand pattern ventricular topology) or the morphological right ventricle may be left sided (left-hand pattern ventricular topology) (1). The left-hand pattern topology may then give the impression of the usual form of discordant atrioventricular connection. In right isomerism the most commonly encountered ventriculoarterial connection is double-outlet right ventricle. This is usually associated with pulmonary atresia or pulmonary stenosis. In left atrial isomerism, a concordant ventriculoarterial connection occurs most frequently, but for either isomeric arrangement any ventriculoarterial connection may be found.

Echocardiography

Determination of Atrial Arrangement

One of the more important recent contributions to the understanding of congenital heart disease is the use of the arrangement of the abdominal great vessels to ascertain atrial arrangement (13). By recording horizontal abdominal ultrasonographic sections at the level of the twelfth thoracic vertebra, the relationship of the abdominal great vessels may be determined. The aorta can be recognized by its pulsations, which are synchronous with the movement of the cardiac apex. The inferior vena cava expands with inspiration. Both structures can be identified by the Doppler flow velocity. When horizontal echocardiograph cross sections through the abdomen show symmetrical positions of the aorta and inferior vena cava anterior to the spine, lateralized atrial arrangement can be assumed. The morphological right atrium is then on the side of the

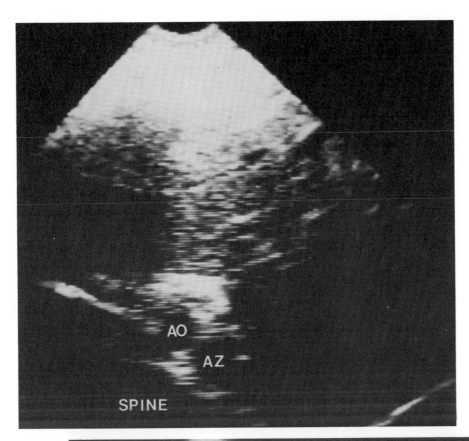

Figure 27.30. A horizontal abdominal section in left atrial isomerism to illustrate a central aorta (AO) and posterior azygous vein (AZ).

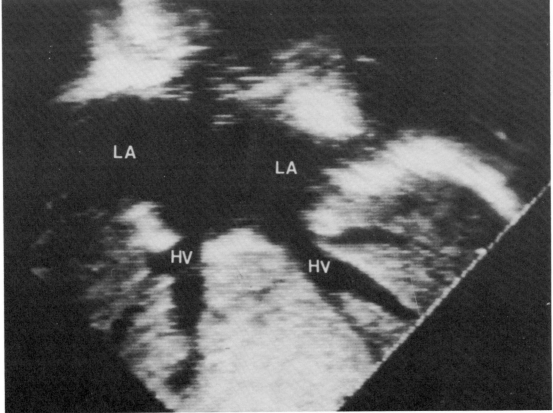

Figure 27.31. Subcostal section demonstrating the hepatic veins (HV) draining directly to the atria in left atrial isomerism.

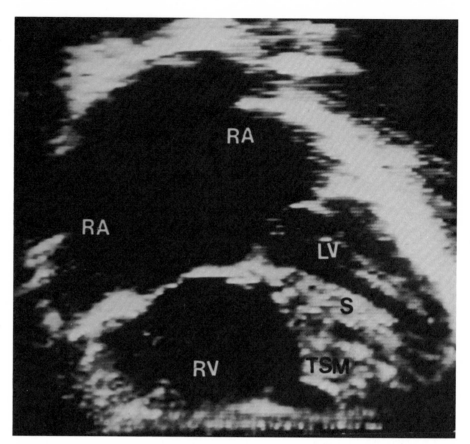

Figure 27.32. Four-chamber section from a heart with right atrial isomerism, an atrioventricular septal defect with two valves and right-hand pattern right ventricular topology. There is a common atrium and the right ventricular septal trabeculum (TSM) can be identified.

inferior vena cava. Thus, for usual atrial arrangement (solitus), the aorta is to the left and the inferior vena cava to the right (Fig. 27.27A). However, in the presence of mirror-image atrial arrangement, the aorta is to the right while the inferior vena cava is to the left (Fig. 27.27B). These relationships can be confirmed by sagittal abdominal echocardiographic sections that demonstrate the inferior vena cava connecting directly to the morphological right atrium (Figs. 27.28A, B).

When there is right atrial isomerism, the aorta and the inferior vena cava are frequently on the same side of the spine; the cava is slightly anterior (Fig. 27.29A) but still draining directly to one of the morphological right atria. Sagittal abdominal echocardiographic sections demonstrate the aorta and inferior vena cava in the same section with the cava anterior (Fig. 27.29B). A midline aorta in the presence of interruption of the inferior vena cava and continuation via a large lateral and posterior azygous vein is characteristic of left isomerism (Fig. 27.30). Sagittal abdominal sections fail to demonstrate the azygous vein connecting with the atria as it passes through the diaphragm. Thus, in atrial isomerism, symmetric arrangement of the abdominal great vessels does not occur. In right isomerism there is an inferior vena cava anterior to the aorta, whereas in left isomerism most usually there is a large azygous vein posterior to the aorta. This latter pattern may

occasionally be found with lateralized atria, while an uninterrupted inferior vena cava may be found with left isomerism. Attention must be given to the connection of the hepatic veins. When there is lateralized arrangement or right isomerism, some or all of the hepatic veins drain to the inferior vena cava. In the presence of left atrial isomerism, the hepatic veins have a tendency to drain directly to the atria (Fig. 27.31). This pattern permits the detection of left isomerism when the inferior vena cava is not interrupted. A recent autopsy study, however, has shown that a suprahepatic inferior vena cava is present in one third of cases of left isomerism (17). The hepatic veins can be traced using a combination of horizontal abdominal sections with subcostal four-chamber scans.

The Atrioventricular Junction

Abnormalities of the atrioventricular junction are common in hearts with atrial isomerism. Double-inlet ventricle (18) and atrioventricular septal defect (17) are frequently encountered; most cases have a common atrioventricular valve. Once the atrial arrangement has been determined, the next step in the diagnostic cascade is to distinguish between hearts with a univentricular atrioventricular connection and those with a biventricular connection. Hearts with univentricular

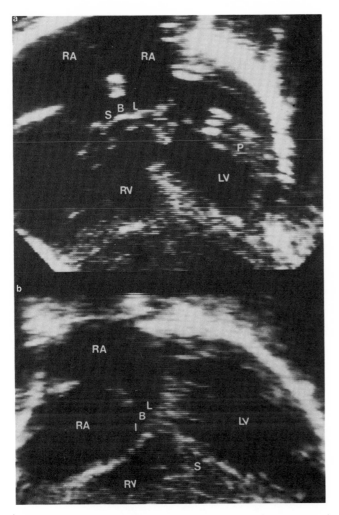

Figure 27.33. Four-chamber sections from a heart with right atrial isomerism, an atrioventricular septal defect with a common valve and right-hand pattern right ventricular topology. There is a primum atrial septal defect (and a secundum defect) and an inlet ventricular septal defect. The parasternal section (a) demonstrates the free-floating superior bridging leaflet (SBL). The subcostal section (b) demonstrates the inferior bridging leaflet (IBL) bound to the septal crest. The left lateral papillary muscle (P) of the left ventricle can be identified, and there are chordal attachments to the right ventricular aspect of the ventricular septum.

atrioventricular connection have their atria exclusively or predominantly connected to one ventricle. In the group with atrial isomerism, straddling and over-riding valves are common. When there is an over-riding atrioventricular junction, cross-sectional echocardiography will differentiate between hearts with biventricular and univentricular connections. In hearts with two atrioventricular valves, the 50 percent rule is invoked to make the distinction (18). More than half of each atrioventricular junction must be committed to the same ventricle to describe the connection as univentricular. When there is a common valve, more than 75

percent of the common atrioventricular junction should be connected to one ventricle, and there should be gross misalignment between the atrial and ventricular septa to describe the connection as univentricular. When there is absence of the atrial septum (common atrium), the distinction between hearts with univentricular atrioventricular connection and atrioventricular septal defect with left or right ventricular dominance may be impossible. It is our policy under these circumstances to describe the connection as univentricular, providing that more than 75 percent of the valve orifice is committed to one ventricle.

An ambiguous atrioventricular connection must, as a matter of course, be biventricular. Most hearts will possess an atrioventricular septal defect, frequently with a common valve but sometimes with separate right and left valve orifices. Atrioventricular septal defects are readily demonstrated by subcostal and parasternal four-chamber sections, which display the valve leaflets along with any inter-atrial or interventricular communications (19). Subcostal four-chamber sections image the inferior (posterior) bridging leaflet and its attachment to the ventricular septum together with the right mural leaflet. Parasternal four-chamber sections identify the superior (anterior) bridging leaflet, together with the right and left mural leaflets and the right anterosuperior leaflet. The typical atrioventricular septal defect with two valves has a large primum atrial septal defect or common atrium and left and right atrioventricular valves at the same level (Fig. 27.32). One of the valves will be seen to be trileaflet in parasternal short-axis sections through the ventricular mass. When there is a common valve, there will again be a large primum atrial septal defect or common atrium, an inlet ventricular septal defect, and inferior and superior bridging leaflets that are either free-floating or tethered to the inlet septal crest (Fig. 27.33). In addition, there will be varying degrees of bridging of the superior leaflet.

Determination of Ventricular Topology

Ventricular topology describes the orientation of the ventricles. In most cases when the morphological right ventricle is right sided, there will be right-hand right ventricular topology. When the morphological right ventricle is to the left of the morphological left ventricle, there will be left-hand pattern right ventricular topology. The significance of this distinction is not only to allow precise anatomic diagnosis but also to predict the course of the atrioventricular conduction tissue. Identification of the morphological right ventricle depends upon recognition of chords inserting into the septum, the right ventricular septal trabeculum, and chords from the commissure between the superior

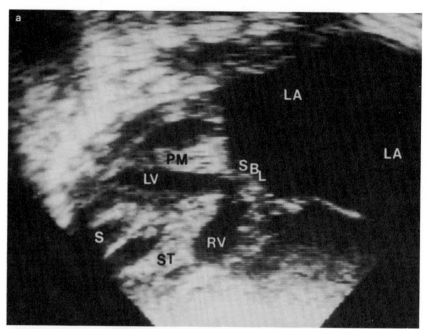

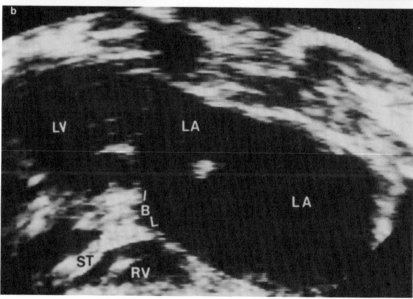

Figure 27.34. Four-chamber sections from a heart with left atrial isomerism, an atrioventricular septal defect with a common valve and left-hand pattern right ventricular topology. The parasternal four-chamber section demonstrates the superior bridging leaflet (SBL), the lateral papillary muscle (PM) of the right-sided morphological left ventricle (LV) and the septal trabeculum (ST) of the morphological right ventricle. There are chordal attachments to the right ventricular (RV) aspect of the ventricular septum (S). The subcostal four-chamber section (b) demonstrates the inferior bridging leaflet (IBL).

bridging leaflet and right ventricular superior leaflet inserting either into the septum or into the apex of the right ventricle. In contrast, no chords insert into the left ventricular surface of the septum, and the left ventricle has paired papillary muscles.

In a study of all patients with atrioventricular septal defects studied by cross-sectional echocardiography in a five-year period at our institution, 210 patients with atrioventricular septal defect were encountered; of these 74 percent had a common valve. In this subgroup 24 percent had atrial isomerism. Left-hand pattern ventricular topology was present in 8 of 27 patients with right atrial isomerism and 2 of 11 with left atrial isomerism. Left-hand pattern topology, therefore, had

an overall incidence of 26 percent, and right-hand pattern topology was found in 74 percent of cases of atrial isomerism. In all cases, only one of the two ventricles was seen to have chordal attachments to the apical trabecular portion of the ventricular septum. This criterion was used to identify the morphological right ventricle (Figs. 27.33, 27.34). In most patients with left-hand pattern topology, it was also possible to identify the right ventricular septomarginal trabeculation.

Hearts with an ambiguous atrioventricular connection and left-hand pattern right ventricular topology (effectively left-sided morphological right ventricle) are in many ways similar to hearts with discordant atrioventricular connection. They should, nevertheless, be considered as separate entities, because in the presence of the discordant connection the atria are lateralized and atrioventricular septal defects are hardly ever encountered. Hearts with an ambiguous atrioventricular connection may have abnormalities of systemic and pulmonary venous connection, and any type of ventriculoarterial connection may be encountered.

REFERENCES

1. Anderson RH, Becker AE, Freedom RM, Macartney FJ, Quero-Jimenez M, Shinebourne EA, Wilkinson JL, Tynan MJ. Sequential segmental analysis of congenital heart disease. Pediatr Cardiol 1984;5:281–288.
2. De Tommasi SM, Daliento L, Ho SY, Macartney FJ, Anderson RH. Analysis of atrioventricular junction, ventricular mass and ventriculoarterial junction in 43 specimens with atrial isomerism. Br Heart J 1981;45:236–247.
3. Van Praagh R. What is congenitally corrected transposition? N Engl J Med 1970;282:1097–1098.
4. Tenorio de Albuquerque A, Rigby ML, Anderson RH, Lincoln C, Shinebourne EA. The spectrum of atrioventricular discordance. A clinical study. Br Heart J 1984;51:498–507.
5. Van Praagh R, Van Praagh S. Isolated ventricular inversion. A consideration of the morphogenesis, definition and diagnosis of nontransposed and transposed great arteries. Am J Cardiol 1966;17:395–406.
6. Allwork SP, Bentall HH, Becker AE, et al. Congenitally corrected transposition of the great arteries: morphological study of 32 cases. Am J Cardiol 1976;38:910–923.
7. Freedom RM, Culham G, Rowe RD. The criss-cross heart and supero-inferior ventricular heart: an angiocardiographic study. Am J Cardiol 1978;42:620–628.
8. Anderson RH, Becker AE, Gerlis LM. The pulmonary outflow tract in classically corrected transposition. J Thorac Cardiovasc Surg 1975;69:747–757.
9. Anderson KR, Danielson GK, McGoon DC, Lie JT. Ebstein's anomaly of the left-sided tricuspid valve; pathological anatomy of the valvular malformation. Circulation 1978;58:87–91.
10. Milo S, Ho SY, Macartney FJ, et al. Straddling and overriding atrioventricular valves: morphology and classification. Am J Cardiol 1979;44:1122–1134.
11. Becker AE, Ho SY, Caruso G, Milo S, Anderson RH. Straddling right atrioventricular valves in atrioventricular discordance. Circulation 1980;61:1133–1141.
12. Soto B, Pacifico AD, Bargeron LM, Ermocilla R, Tonkin IL. Identification of thoracic isomerism from the plain chest radiograph. AJR 1978;131:995–1002.
13. Huhta JC, Smallhorn JF, Macartney FJ. Two dimensional echocardiographic diagnosis of situs. Br Heart J 1982;48:97–108.
14. Sutherland GR, Smallhorn JF, Anderson RH, Rigby ML, Hunter S. Atrioventricular discordance. Cross-sectional echocardiographic-morphologicalal correlative study. Br Heart J 1983;50:8–20.
15. Macartney FJ, Rigby ML, Anderson RH, Stark J, Silverman NH. Double outlet right ventricle. Cross sectional echocardiographic findings, their anatomical explanation, and surgical relevance. Br Heart J 1984;52:164–177.
16. Rose V, Izukawa T, Moes CAF. Syndromes of asplenia and polysplenia. A review of cardiac and non-cardiac malformations in 60 cases with special reference to diagnosis and prognosis. Br Heart J 1975;37:840–852.
17. Sharna S, Divine W, Anderson RH, Zuberbuhler. Left atrial isomerism ("polysplenia"). Getting to the heart of the syndrome. Manuscript submitted for publication.
18. Rigby ML, Anderson RH, Gibson D, Jones ODH, Joseph MC, Shinebourne EA. Two-dimensional echocardiographic categorisation of the univentricular heart. Ventricular morphology, type, and mode of atrioventricular connection. Br Heart J 1981; 46:603–612.
19. Smallhorn JF, Tommasini G, Anderson RH, Macartney FJ. Assessment of atrioventricular septal defects by two dimensional echocardiography. Br Heart J 1982; 47:109–121.

28

Ebstein's Malformation of
the Tricuspid Valve

Jeffrey Smallhorn

The fundamental abnormality in Ebstein's malformation is displacement of the attachment of the tricuspid valve leaflets from the atrioventricular junction into the cavity of the right ventricle. In addition, the tricuspid leaflets are dysplastic (1, 2). The degree of displacement is extremely variable, ranging from severe displacement that presents in the first few weeks of life with severe cyanosis to minimal displacement that may be found incidentally at autopsy or during evaluation of an associated supraventricular dysrhythmia.

Invariably, the septal and inferior leaflets are displaced apically, with the anterior leaflet enlarged and abnormally attached to a muscular shelf between the ventricular inlet and trabecular zones (3). Occasionally, the anterior leaflet may be tethered down; this has important surgical implications.

Frequently, the abnormality is more severe in childhood, resulting in tricuspid regurgitation and cyanosis secondary to right-to-left shunting through an interatrial communication. Right ventricular outflow tract obstruction is seen in the younger age group and may take the form of anatomic or functional pulmonary atresia. The differentiation between functional and anatomic pulmonary atresia is discussed in Chapter 30. Occasionally, pulmonary stenosis may be present, rather than pulmonary atresia. The true right ventricular cavity size varies according to the degree of displacement of the tricuspid valve, as does the size of the atrialized portion of the right ventricle.

CROSS-SECTIONAL ECHOCARDIOGRAPHIC FEATURES

Cross-sectional echocardiography plays a major role in the assessment of Ebstein's malformation of the tricus-

pid valve. Surgical decisions in patients with more severe malformations are based mainly on information obtained from the ultrasound examination, which includes 1) the degree of displacement of the septal and inferior leaflets, 2) the size of the anterior leaflet, and 3) the size of the true right ventricular cavity (4).

The degree of displacement of the septal and inferior leaflets is best assessed by a combination of subcostal and precordial four-chamber views (4–8). The septal leaflet appears displaced from the true tricuspid valve annulus or tethered to the right ventricular septal surface (Fig. 28.1). The degree of tricuspid valve displacement and tethering varies from case to case (Fig. 28.2). In the majority of cases, the anterior leaflet appears large and sail-like, a favorable finding with regard to the potential for surgical intervention since the anterior leaflet may be used to create a competent monocusp valve (Fig. 28.3) (4, 9, 10). Occasionally, the leaflet appears immobile and is tethered by short chordae, indicating that corrective surgery will probably entail valve replacement (Fig. 28.4). The size of the atrialized portion of the right ventricle and the dimensions of the true right ventricular cavity are best assessed in the combination of subcostal and precordial four-chamber views. The size of the two portions are inversely related, with a small right ventricular cavity being a poor prognostic sign (Fig. 28.4) (4). In the subcostal four-chamber cut, the interatrial septum can be evaluated (Fig. 28.5) and the shunting pattern assessed using Doppler echocardiography (Fig. 28.6). Similarly, from this position and from an apical four-chamber view, the presence and severity of tricuspid regurgitation can be determined (Fig. 28.7).

If the transducer is placed in a precordial short-axis position, the three leaflets can be evaluated simultaneously (Fig. 28.8). In the precordial long-axis position,

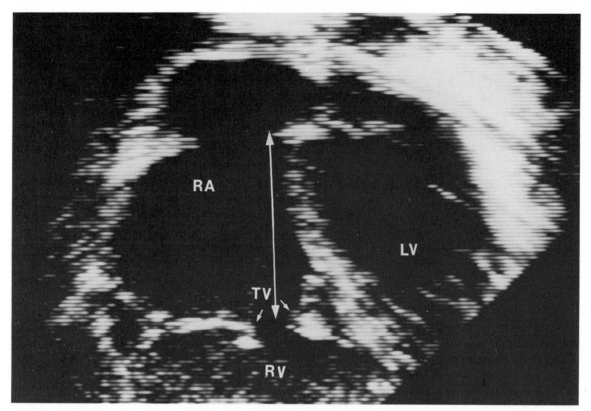

Figure 28.1. Apical four-chamber cut in Ebstein's malformation of the tricuspid valve (TV). Note the significant displacement of the TV indicated by the long arrow. LV = left ventricle; RA = right atrium; RV = right ventricle.

the displaced septal leaflet can usually be visualized along with the large sail-like anterior leaflet (Fig. 28.9). In patients with severe displacement and a tethered anterior leaflet, the leaflets may not be visualized in this cut (Fig. 28.10).

ASSOCIATED ANOMALIES

Ebstein's malformation of the tricuspid valve may be associated with corrected transposition, where the left-sided morphologic tricuspid valve is involved. Al-

Figure 28.2. Apical four-chamber cut in a milder form of Ebstein's malformation. Note that there is only mild inferior displacement of the tricuspid valve. Compare this with Figure 28.1. LA = left atrium; LV = left ventricle; RV = right ventricle.

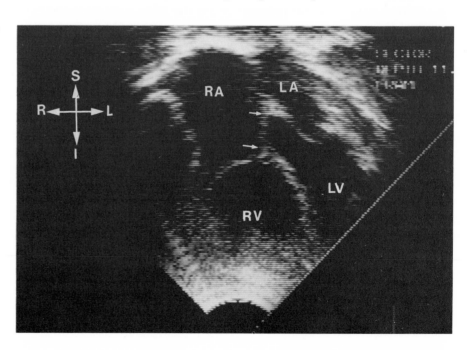

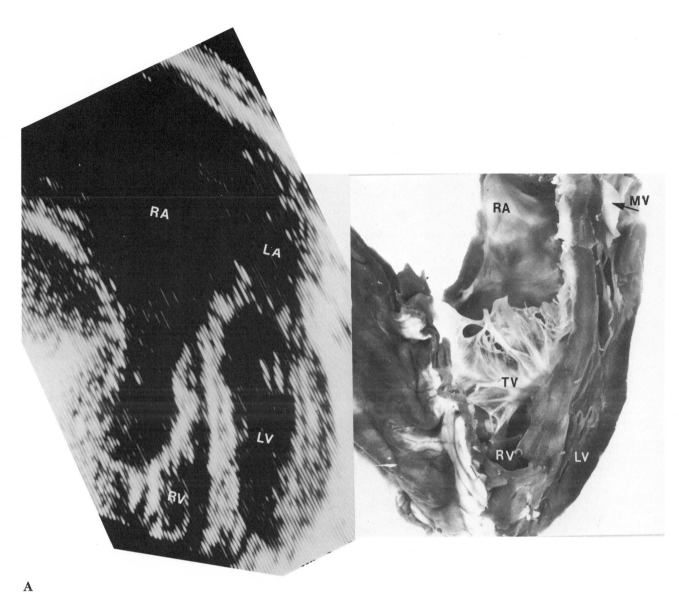

A

Figure 28.3. (*A*) The left-hand picture is an apical four-chamber cut in severe Ebstein's malformation of the morphologic tricuspid valve. Note that there is a large sail-like anterior leaflet. The specimen on the right is from the same patient and demonstrates the echocardiographic features.

though Ebstein's malformation is the term used to describe the valve in many of these patients, the valve is usually only dysplastic, without true displacement.

Ebstein's malformation may also involve the right-sided atrioventricular valve in atrioventricular septal defects and may occur with common or separate right and left orifices (11, 12). Ventricular septal defect may occur in association with Ebstein's malformation, with the defect being completely or partially covered by the displaced leaflets. In some patients, the displaced tricuspid valve completely seals off a ventricular septal defect with the leaflet appearing to billow backward and forward. Rarely, Ebstein's malformation may be associated with a hypoplastic morphologically right

ventricle in association with pulmonary atresia and intact septum (Fig. 28.11). Abnormalities of the right ventricular outflow tract, in the form of valvar atresia or stenosis can be evaluated in a high precordial short-axis cut (Fig. 28.12). Occasionally, the abnormal attachments of the anterosuperior leaflet may produce pulmonary stenosis (Fig. 28.13).

Left-sided abnormalities are seen in approximately 10 percent of cases (13). These abnormalities include cleft mitral valve, divided left atrium (cor triatriatum), stenosis of the pulmonary veins, mitral valve prolapse, bicuspid aortic valve, and parachute mitral valve. These lesions can be readily detected by Doppler echocardiography and should be actively searched for in cases of Ebstein's malformation of the tricuspid valve.

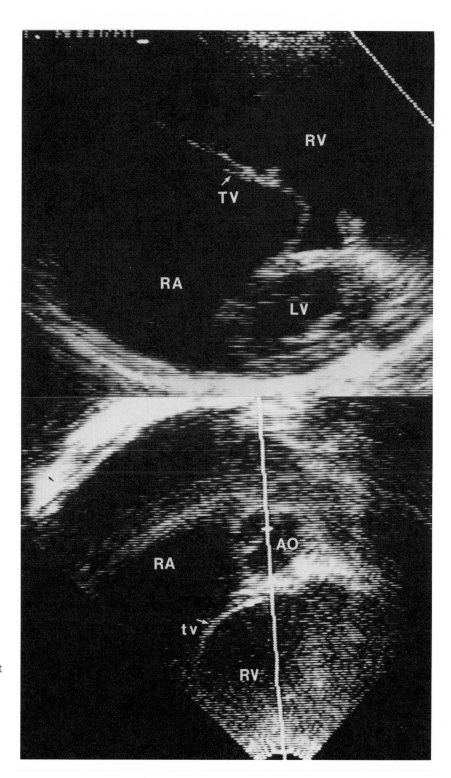

Figure 28.3, (cont'd.) (*B*) The upper picture is a precordial short-axis cut in Ebstein's malformation with a large sail-like anterior leaflet indicated by the arrow. The lower picture is from the same patient with superior angulation from a four-chamber cut. Note again the large anterior leaflet. AO = aorta; LA = left atrium; LV = left ventricle; MV = mitral valve; RA = right atrium; RV = right ventricle; TV = tricuspid valve.

B

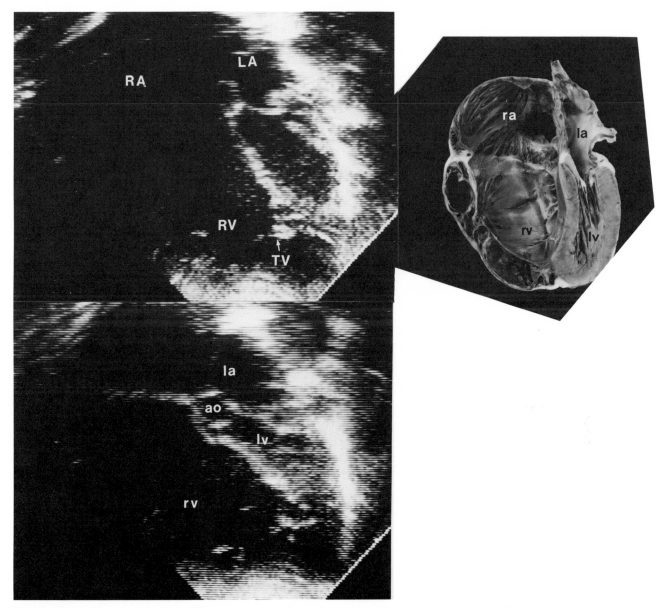

Figure 28.4. The upper left-hand picture is an apical four-chamber cut in severe Ebstein's malformation of the tricuspid valve where the anterior leaflet is tethered. The lower picture is from the same patient with superior angulation. Compare this to Figure 28-3B, where a large saillike anterior leaflet is clearly visualized. The specimen on the right is from a different patient and demonstrates the echocardiographic features. Ao = aorta; LA = left atrium; LV = left ventricle; RA = right atrium; RV = right ventricle.

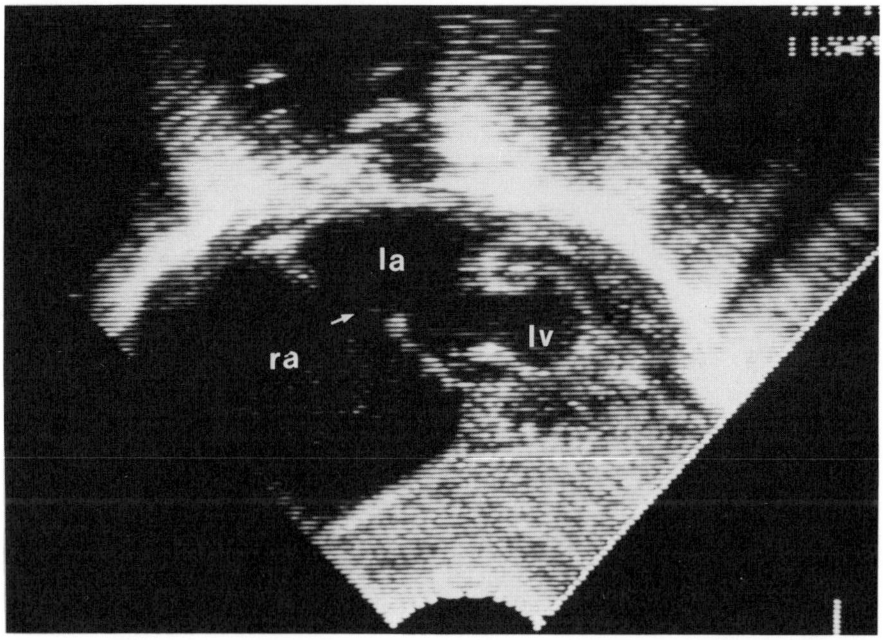

Figure 28.5. Subcostal cut demonstrating an interatrial communication in Ebstein's malformation of the tricuspid valve. Note the large right atrium (RA). LA = left atrium; LV = left ventricle.

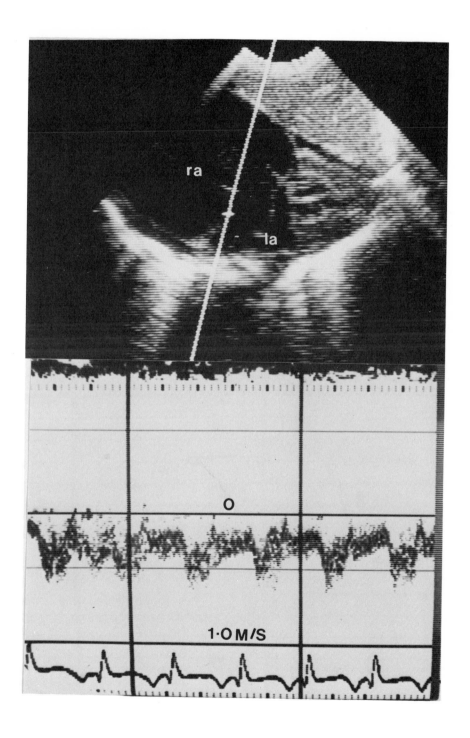

Figure 28.6. Doppler interrogation of the interatrial septum in Ebstein's malformation. Note that the shunting in this patient is all right to left. LA = left atrium; RA = right atrium.

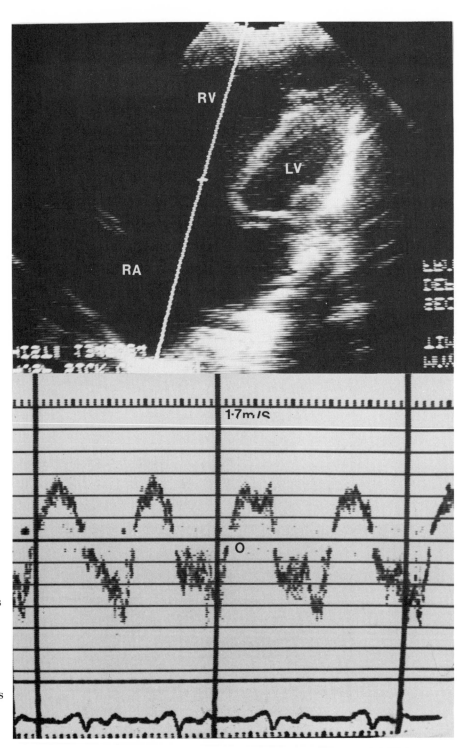

Figure 28.7. The upper picture is an apical four-chamber cut in Ebstein's malformation of the tricuspid valve. Note that the Doppler sample volume is placed in the atrialized portion of the right atrium (RA). The lower picture is the spectral trace and demonstrates tricuspid regurgitation. LV = left ventricle; RV = right ventricle.

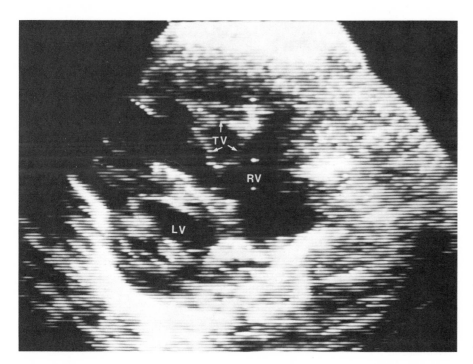

Figure 28.8.   Precordial short-axis cut in Ebstein's malformation of the tricuspid valve (TV). In this view, the three leaflets (*arrows*) are clearly visualized. LV = left ventricle; RV = right ventricle.

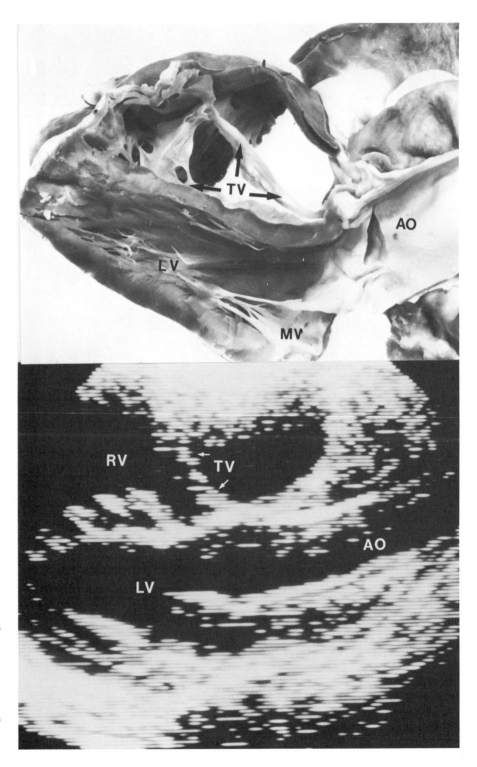

Figure 28.9. The lower picture is a precordial long-axis cut in Ebstein's malformation of the tricuspid valve (TV). Note the large right ventricle with the sail-like anterior leaflet indicated by the arrows. The upper picture is a simulated cut in the same patient. AO = aorta; LV = left ventricle; MV = mitral valve; RV = right ventricle.

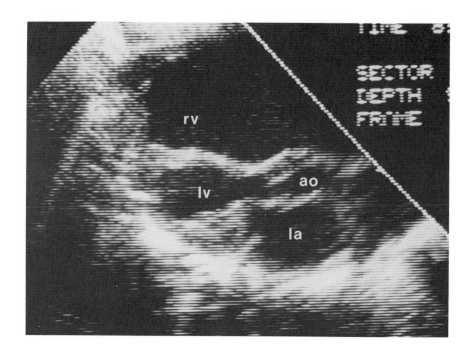

Figure 28.10. Precordial long-axis cut in severe Ebstein's malformation of the tricuspid valve, with tethering of the anterior leaflet. Note, in comparison with Figure 28-9, the anterior leaflet is not visualized. Ao = aorta; LA = left atrium; LV = left ventricle; RV = right ventricle.

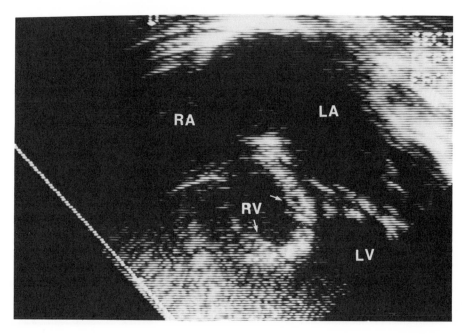

Figure 28.11. Precordial four-chamber cut in Ebstein's malformation of the tricuspid valve, in the setting of pulmonary atresia and intact septum. Note the hypoplastic morphologically right ventricle (RV) with displacement of the tricuspid valve. LA = left atrium; LV = left ventricle; RA = right atrium.

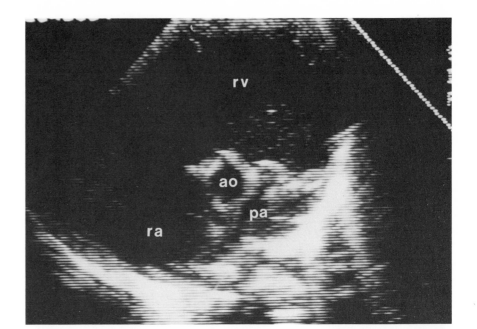

Figure 28.12. Precordial short-axis cut in Ebstein's malformation of the tricuspid valve and associated pulmonary atresia. Note the small central pulmonary artery (PA) with the atretic pulmonary valve. Ao = aorta; RA = right atrium; RV = right ventricle.

Figure 28.13. Subcostal short-axis cut in Ebstein's malformation of the tricuspid valve where the anterior leaflet, indicated by the white arrow, caused right ventricular outflow tract obstruction. LV = left ventricle; PA = pulmonary artery; RA = right atrium.

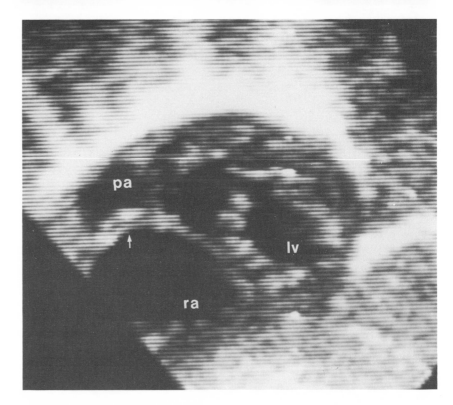

REFERENCES

1. Becker AE, Becker MJ, Edwards JE. Pathological spectrum of dysplasia of the tricuspid valve. Features in common with Ebstein's malformation. Arch Pathol 1971;91:167–78.
2. Zuberbuhler JR, Allwork SP, Anderson RH. The spectrum of Ebstein's anomaly of the tricuspid valve. J Thorac Cardiovasc Surg 1979;77:202–11.
3. Becker AE, Anderson RH. Pathology in congenital heart disease. London: Butterworths, 1981:152.
4. Shiina A, Seward JB, Tajik AJ, Hagler DJ, Danielson GK. Two-dimensional echocardiographic-surgical correlation in Ebstein's anomaly: preoperative determination of patients requiring tricuspid valve plication vs replacement. Circulation 1983;68:534–44.
5. Hirschklau MJ, Sahn DJ, Hagan AD, Williams DE, Friedman WF. Cross-sectional echocardiographic features of Ebstein's anomaly of the tricuspid valve. Am J Cardiol 1977;40:400.
6. Seward JB, Tajik AJ, Feist DJ, Smith HC. Ebstein's anomaly in an 85 year old man. Mayo Clin Proc 1979;54:193.
7. Kambe T, Ichimiya S, Toguchi M, et al. Apex and subxiphoid approaches to Ebstein's anomaly using cross-sectional echocardiography. Am Heart J 1980;100:53.
8. Gussenhoven EJ, Stewart PA, Becker AE, Essed CE, Ligtvoet KM,

de Villeneuve VH. "Offsetting" of the septal tricuspid leaflet in normal hearts and in hearts with Ebstein's anomaly. Am J Cardiol 1984;54:172–81.

9. Danielson GK, Fuster V. Surgical repair of Ebstein's anomaly. Ann Surg 1982;196:499.

10. Danielson GK, Maloney JD, Devloo RAE. Surgical repair of Ebstein's anomaly. Mayo Clin Proc 1979;54:185.

11. Roach RM, Tandon R, Moller JH, Edwards JE. Ebstein's anomaly of the tricuspid valve in persistent common atrioventricular canal. Am J Cardiol 1984;53:641–2.

12. Caruso G, Losekoot TG, Becer AE. Ebstein's anomaly in persistent common atrioventricular canal. Br Heart J 1978;40:1275–9.

13. Castaneda-Zuniga W, Nath HP, Moller JH, Edwards JE. Left sided anomalies in Ebstein's malformation of the tricuspid valve. Pediatr Cardiol 1982;3:181–5.

29
Hypoplastic Right and Left Ventricles

Michael Rigby

The right or left ventricle may be smaller than normal in many congenital heart diseases, and either ventricle may appear to be small because of enlargement of the complimentary ventricle. An example of the latter is total anomalous pulmonary venous connection, in which the right side of the heart is greatly enlarged and the left ventricle, although of normal dimensions, appears small in comparison. It is not our intention to discuss this type of arrangement, but the echocardiographer should be aware of this apparent or "pseudohypoplasia". Neither is it our intention to discuss ventricular hypoplasia in the setting of univentricular atrioventricular connection (see Chapter 26) or atrioventricular septal defect (see Chapter 27). However, it is important to stress the features of secondary ventricular hypoplasia in these anomalies so that they can be distinguished from the true or primary ventricular hypoplasia, which forms the body of this chapter.

Most hearts with the atria connected to only one ventricle such as double-inlet connection or an absent atrioventricular connection possess a second ventricle that is much smaller than the dominant ventricle. Whether this small second ventricular chamber should be accorded ventricular status has been the source of much controversy and disagreement. We consider this chamber to be a small ventricle and therefore hypoplastic. However, it is also an incomplete or rudimentary ventricle because it lacks one or more of its normal components. It is the deficiency of one or both inlet and outlet components that makes the ventricle incomplete, and this feature distinguishes this type of hypoplastic ventricle from those discussed below. True hypoplastic ventricles are small but are normally constituted in that they have all their normal components even though one or more of the components may be so

small as to be unrecognizable. Hypoplastic but normal constituted ventricles are also found in atrioventricular septal defects. This is a consequence of unequal sharing of the atrioventricular junction between the ventricular mass. This concept of ventricular dominance is discussed elsewhere in Chapter 21.

True hypoplastic ventricles occur in hearts with atresia of the ventricular outflow tracts in the presence of an intact ventricular septum. Ventricular hypoplasia almost always occurs when the ventriculoarterial connections are concordant (e.g., in pulmonary or aortic atresia and intact ventricular septum). Ventricular hypoplasia is extremely uncommon when the ventriculoarterial connections are discordant.

PULMONARY ATRESIA WITH INTACT VENTRICULAR SEPTUM

The circulation in pulmonary atresia with intact septum is dependent upon the systemic venous return reaching the left atrium through an atrial septal defect, which almost without exception is within the oval fossa, while the pulmonary blood supply is dependent on flow through the ductus arteriosus (Fig. 29.1). Patients may occasionally have main systemic-to-pulmonary collateral arteries, but these almost always indicate the presence of a ventricular septal defect. The crucial variation in anatomy relative to optimal treatment relates to the hypoplastic right ventricle. The atretic pulmonary trunk and the pulmonary arteries are almost always of good size (1), unlike pulmonary atresia with ventricular septal defect in which the intrapericardial pulmonary arteries are frequently threadlike. The right ventricle, however, varies greatly in terms of size and function. In the past, cases have been classified in terms of small ventricles (so-called

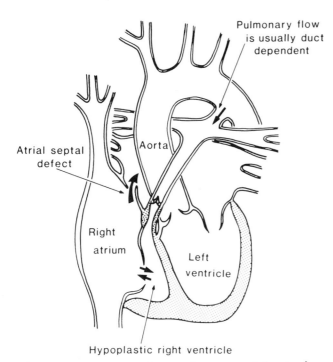

Figure 29.1. Diagram showing the course of the circulation in pulmonary atresia with intact ventricular septum (hypoplastic right ventricle).

type I) or normal ventricles (type II) (2), which is a major and misleading oversimplification. It is now well established that cavity size is best assessed in terms of the degree of hypoplasia of the cavity components, remembering that right ventricular hypoplasia is often associated with severe hypertrophy of the right ventricular wall. Pulmonary atresia with intact ventricular septum may also result in a grossly dilated right ventricle with paper-thin walls (3). Such cases usually present in the neonatal period and exhibit Ebstein's malformation (Fig. 29.2) and have a poor prognosis. More often the cavity of the right ventricle is reduced to a varying degree. Those with the best-formed cavities have a patent infundibulum running to the underside of an imperforate pulmonary valve (Fig. 29.3). The cavity size in these hearts depends on the degree of hypertrophy and overgrowth of the apical trabecular component. The patients with the best prognosis for surgical repair by puncture of the imperforate membrane are those with minimal overgrowth of the apical component (4). The prognosis is worse in patients in whom the subpulmonary infundibulum, instead of extending to an imperforate membrane, is overgrown and atretic. The pulmonary trunk then expands from a point at which there is no evidence of formation of the pulmonary valve leaflets (Fig. 29.4). Such cases with infundibular atresia usually have marked overgrowth of the apical component of the ventricle. When overgrowth is severe, the ventricular cavity is effectively

represented only by the inlet (Fig. 29.5). Patients with infundibular atresia are rarely if ever candidates for direct surgical correction. They are best treated by initial shunting and a subsequent Fontan procedure. The size of the cavity of the right ventricle is itself important and is proportional to the diameter of the tricuspid orifice. Assessment of the cavity components together with measurement of the size of the tricuspid anulus provide a good guide to optimal surgical treatment. The tricuspid valve itself is most severely deformed when the cavity is smallest. Sinusoidal communications between right ventricle and the coronary arteries must be identified. These occur most frequently when the right ventricle is tiny and consists of the inlet alone.

AORTIC ATRESIA WITH INTACT VENTRICULAR SEPTUM

The combination of aortic atresia and intact ventricular septum is the prototype of the so-called hypoplastic left heart syndrome, although a similar pattern occurs in critical aortic stenosis, and with severe coarctation of the aorta (5, 6). The underlying anatomy in all three lesions is comparable: the circulation is dependent on an interatrial communication and the arterial duct (Fig. 29.6). The atrial communication is almost always within the oval fossa, although there are patients in whom the intra-atrial communication is through an ostium primum defect in the setting of left atrial isomerism. The status of the atrial septum is important. Usually the communication is restrictive or the septum is intact (Fig. 29.7), in which case there is severe obstruction to pulmonary venous return unless there is a "safety valve" such as unroofing of the coronary sinus, anomalous pulmonary venous connections, or a levo-atrial cardinal vein. The right ventricle is dominant but is often abnormal. Significant in this respect are dysplasia of the pulmonary valve leaflets or anomalous septo-parietal trabeculations across the subpulmonary outlet. The septo-parietal muscle bundles (Fig. 29.8) are important because they can be mistaken echocardiographically for the septum and thus mask the gross left ventricular hypoplasia. The left ventricle itself is usually severely hypoplastic, but two distinct anatomic patterns are found. In the first (Fig. 29.9), the entire atrioventricular connection is absent, the left ventricle is not only slitlike and grossly hypoplastic but also rudimentary and incomplete, and it has a smooth endothelial lining without any fibroelastosis. The thick fibroelastic layer typical of hypoplastic left heart is found only when the mitral valve is present, albeit miniaturized and dysplastic (Fig. 29.10).

In the second type, the aortic atresia is usually due to a fibromuscular plate interposed between the left ven-

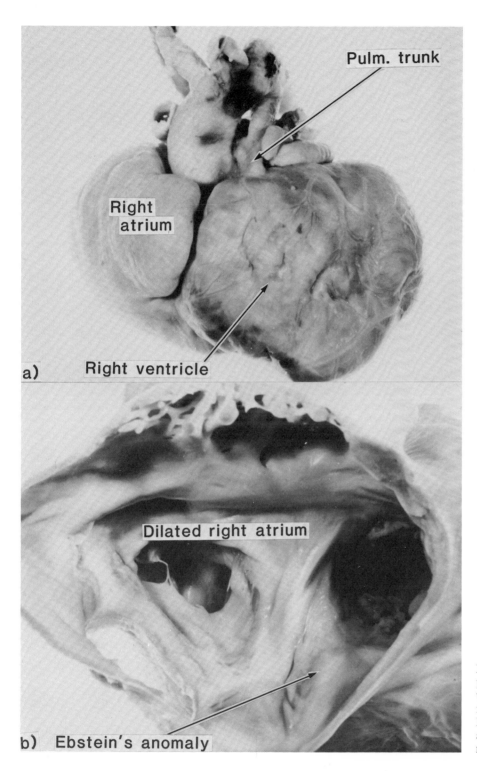

Figure 29.2. The type of morphology most usually seen when the right ventricle approximates to its normal size (*A*) or becomes dilated (*B*). There is Ebstein's anomaly of the tricuspid valve and the right atrium is also dilated.

tricle and ascending aorta (Fig. 28.11) or to an imperforate membrane (Fig. 29.10) with a coronary to left ventricular sinus. Variation of the ventriculoarterial junction in this lesion is of much less clinical significance than in pulmonary atresia because it is not feasible to incorporate the left ventricle into the circulation should surgery be attempted. The ascending

aorta is hypoplastic to a varying degree and is often threadlike at the cardiac base where it supplies the coronary arteries (Fig. 29.12). The aorta expands as it ascends, but the aortic flow is provided by the ductus arteriosus. Obstructive lesions at the junction of the duct, isthmus, and descending aorta which are all of paramount importance, are found in most cases and

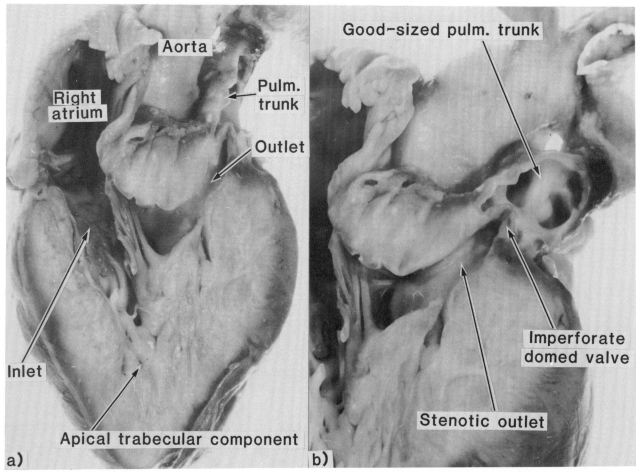

Figure 29.3.   The most favorable anatomy seen in pulmonary atresia with intact ventricular septum. The wall of the ventricle is somewhat hypertrophied, but the apical trabecular component (*A*) is still well recognized. There is a patent outlet component running out to an imperforate domed valve (*B*) that separates the ventricular cavity from that of a good-sized pulmonary trunk.

consist of either preductal shelves (Fig. 29.13) or paraductal branch points (Fig. 29.14).

ECHOCARDIOGRAPHY

The exact definition of a hypoplastic ventricle is somewhat imprecise. In essence, it is a small ventricle that possesses all three of its constituent components, namely, inlet, trabecular, and outlet portions. There is no absolute or relative dimension of a small ventricle, which in itself constitutes hypoplasia. Thus, for example, in total anomalous pulmonary venous connection or complete transposition with intact septum the left ventricle often appears small but is almost always able to maintain a satisfactory cardiac output. The relatively small size of the left ventricle may be accounted for in part by compression by the dilated right ventricle.

The right or left ventricle may be hypoplastic in a number of congenital heart diseases. The most important examples are pulmonary atresia with intact septum, critical pulmonary stenosis and intact ventricular

septum, and variants of the hypoplastic left heart syndrome. Hypoplasia of the right or left ventricle is also encountered in hearts with atrioventricular septal defects, complete transposition with ventricular septal defects, and in double-outlet right ventricle. The rudimentary ventricles in hearts with univentricular atrioventricular connection are usually but not always hypoplastic.

PULMONARY ATRESIA WITH INTACT VENTRICULAR SEPTUM

The most common anomaly with right ventricular hypoplasia is pulmonary atresia with intact septum. Hearts with pulmonary atresia and intact septum may be classified into three groups based upon the tripartite approach to right ventricular morphology. The right ventricle is composed of inlet, trabecular, and infundibular portions. The inlet portion is defined as the part of the ventricle that incorporates the tricuspid valve apparatus. The trabecular portion lies beyond the insertion of the papillary muscle of the tricuspid valve

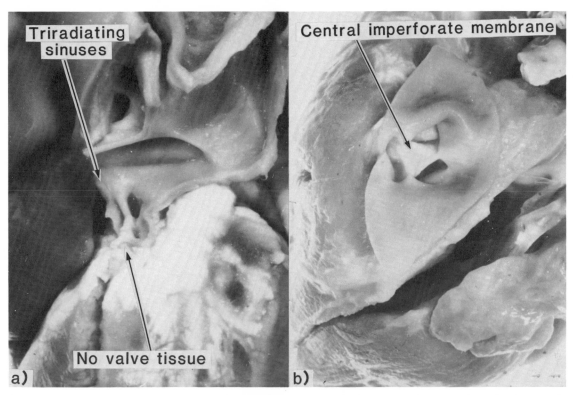

Figure 29.4. The crucial feature at the ventriculoarterial junction is whether or not there is a domed valve membrane. When the outlet component is itself obliterated (muscular atresia) there is no valve tissue at the base of the pulmonary trunk (*A*). Panel *B* shows the different arrangement when there is an imperforate valve membrane.

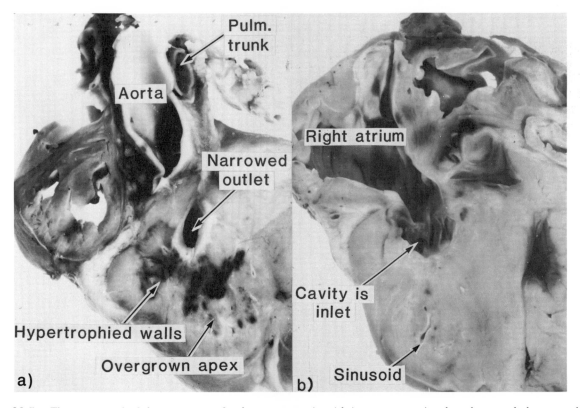

Figure 29.5. The worst end of the spectrum of pulmonary atresia with intact septum is when the grossly hypertrophied right ventricular wall obliterates the apical trabecular component (*A*). The cavity is effectively represented by the inlet; the narrowed outlet stops short of the pulmonary trunk (muscular atresia) (*B*).

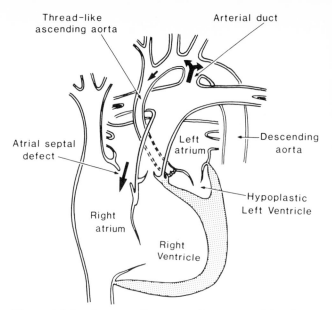

Figure 29.6. Diagram illustrating the course of the circulation in "hypoplastic left heart syndrome."

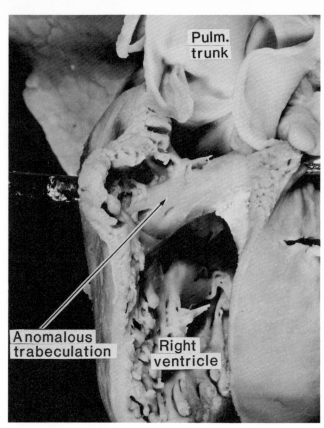

Figure 29.8. Right ventricular anomalies often exist together with hypoplastic left heart syndrome. This shows anomalous trabeculations in the subpulmonary area.

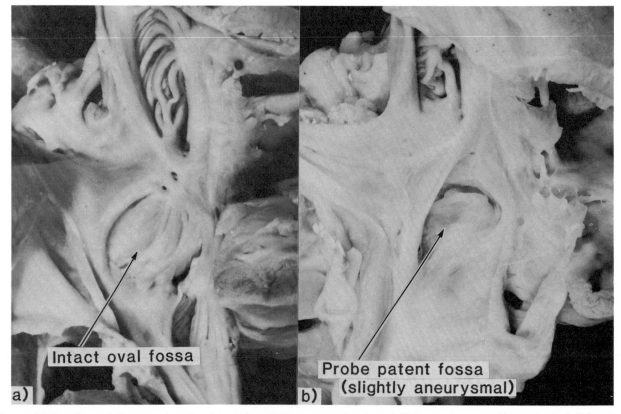

Figure 29.7. The atrial septum is either intact (panel *A*) or restrictive (panel *B*) in most cases of hypoplastic left heart syndrome.

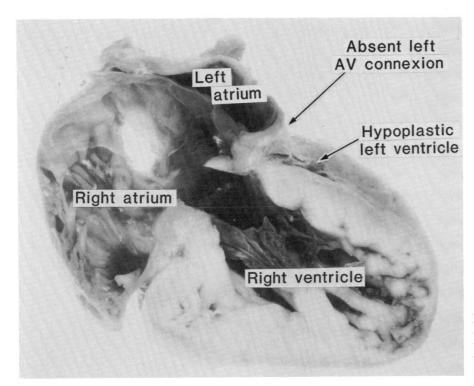

Figure 29.9. A simulated "four-chamber" section showing the anatomic arrangement of absence of the left atrioventricular (AV) connection.

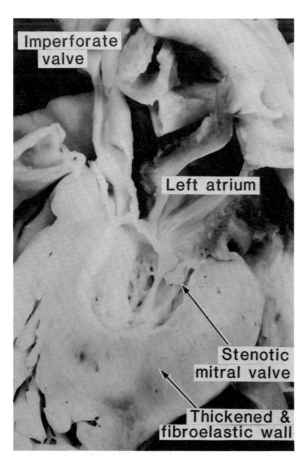

Figure 29.10.   The hypoplastic left ventricle seen with a stenotic mitral valve. There is an imperforate mitral valve and fibroelastosis of the ventricle.

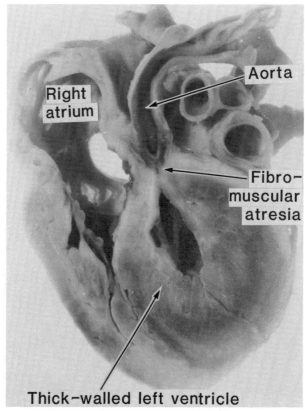

Figure 29.11.   This section shows fibromuscular atresia at the ventriculoarterial junction in a case of hypoplastic left heart.

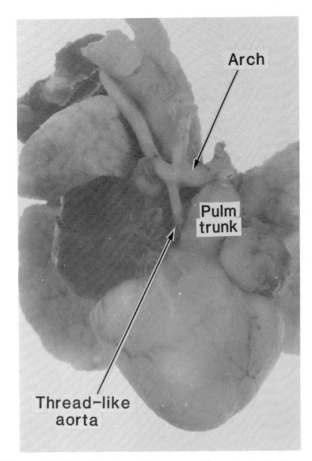

Figure 29.12.   The threadlike ascending aorta typically found in severe hypoplastic left heart syndrome.

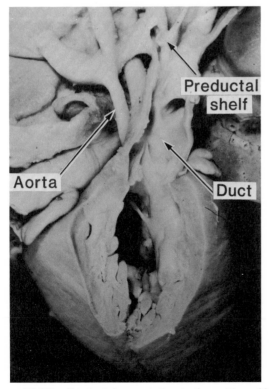

Figure 29.13.   Preductal coarctation in the setting of hypoplastic left heart syndrome.

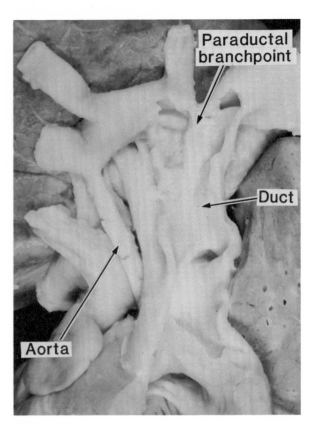

Figure 29.14.   Paraductal branch point coarctation in the setting of hypoplastic left heart syndrome.

toward the apex, whereas the infundibulum or outlet portion leads to the atretic pulmonary valve. In the first group, all three parts of the right ventricular cavity are present. In the second group the trabecular component is obliterated by hypertrophied myocardium, whereas in the third group both trabecular and infundibular portions of the right ventricle are obliterated by hypertrophied myocardium such that they are effectively absent.

Cross-sectional echocardiography readily allows the distinction to be made between these groups. Parasternal four-chamber sections demonstrate the tricuspid anulus and the inlet and trabecular portions of the right ventricle (Fig. 29.15). Subcostal right oblique sections demonstrate all parts of the ventricle (Fig. 29.16). Parasternal long-axis sections of the right ventricle and pulmonary trunk or short-axis sections through the aortic root identify the presence or absence of the right ventricular infundibulum or imperforate pulmonary valve membrane (Fig. 29.17).

There is a spectrum of ventricular hypoplasia in these hearts ranging from a tiny ventricle to one of almost normal size, although the latter is infrequent. The tricuspid valve is correspondingly small and valve dysplasia or Ebstein's malformation is common. These features of the right ventricle are readily demonstrated by four-chamber sections, particularly those obtained from the parasternal position (Fig. 29.18). Frequently, the diameter of the tricuspid anulus is smaller than that of the mitral valve,

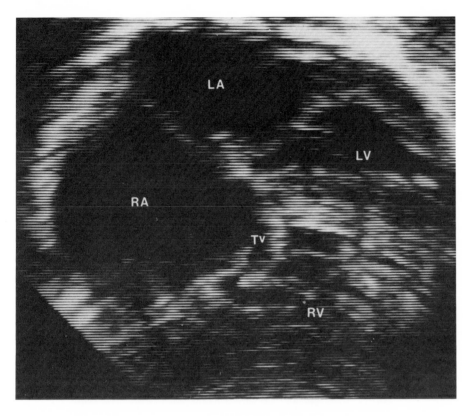

A

Figure 29.15.   Parasternal four-chamber sections from a heart with pulmonary atresia and intact ventricular septum demonstrating (*A*) a right ventricle with inlet and trabecular components and (*B*) a right ventricle with obliteration of the trabecular component.

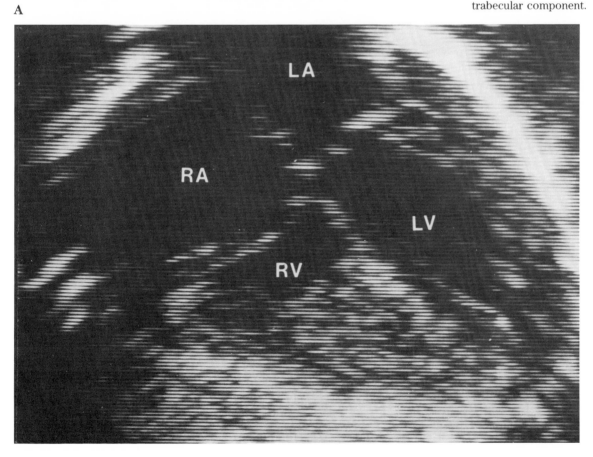

B

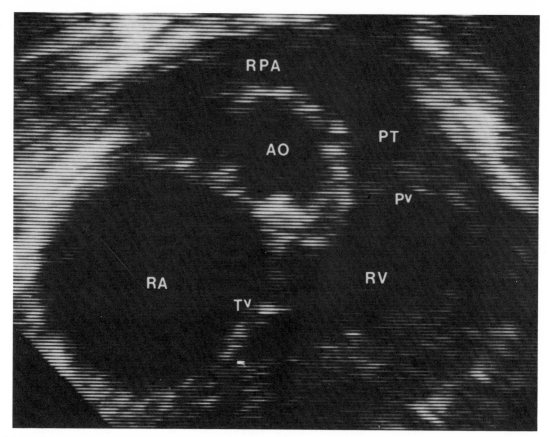

Figure 29.16. Subcostal right anterior oblique section from a heart with pulmonary atresia and intact ventricular septum demonstrating all the ventricular components and an imperforate pulmonary valve.

and the leaflets are often thickened. When there is Ebstein's anomaly, the septal leaflet of the tricuspid valve is displaced into the body of the right ventricle so that the atrioventricular septum appears extensive.

Some hearts with critical pulmonary stenosis and intact ventricular septum will appear very similar to those with pulmonary atresia and intact septum. Cross-sectional echocardiography alone is usually unable to differentiate an imperforate pulmonary valve membrane from one with a pinhole orifice. It might be expected that Doppler echocardiography would detect critical pulmonary valve stenosis. However, in practice many neonates with pulmonary atresia or critical pulmonary stenosis are receiving prostaglandins on admission to a cardiac unit and thus have a large left-to-right shunt through the ductus arteriosus, and the detection of a high velocity jet distal to the pulmonary valve may be extremely difficult. Therefore, failure to detect a high velocity Doppler signal does not always exclude critical stenosis. Venous contrast echocardiography may be superior in differentiating these two anomalies, but right ventriculography at cardiac catheterization remains the final arbiter. The other major value of Doppler echocardiography is in the detection of tricuspid insufficiency, which varies from trivial to

severe. The technique is also useful for demonstrating tricuspid stenosis.

In pulmonary atresia and intact ventricular septum it is also important to focus attention on the left ventricle, which is frequently fibrotic. Fibrotic areas of myocardium, which may be extensive, can be detected by their increased echo reflectance. The ventricular septum is frequently thickened and may encroach on the left ventricular cavity.

THE HYPOPLASTIC LEFT HEART SYNDROME

The most important form of ventricular hypoplasia is the "hypoplastic left heart syndrome," which is characterized clinically by the development of severe cardiogenic shock during the early neonatal period. The diagnosis is readily achieved by cross-sectional echocardiography. Subcostal and parasternal four-chamber sections demonstrate an extremely small left ventricle, usually with areas of high amplitude–reflected ultrasound (Fig. 29.19). The left atrium is often small, and the mitral valve is miniature and may also be imperforate or stenotic (Fig. 29.20). When the left atrioventricular connection is absent, there is a relatively small amount of atrioventricular sulcus tissue between atrial

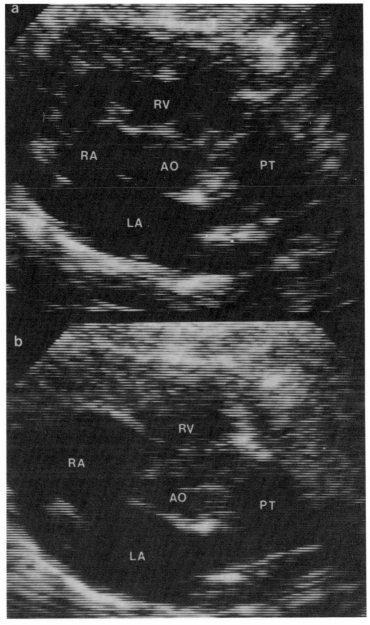

Figure 29.17. Parasternal short-axis section to demonstrate (*A*) an imperforate pulmonary valve and (*B*) obliteration of the right ventricular outflow tract in two hearts with pulmonary atresia and intact ventricular septum.

floor and ventricular mass (Fig. 29.21). In a proportion of cases differentiation of those with a truly hypoplastic left ventricle in which there is a miniaturized mitral valve from those with a rudimentary ventricle in which there is absence of the left atrioventricular connection may be difficult. Clinically, however, this distinction is unimportant.

In most cases there is aortic stenosis and extreme hypoplasia of the ascending aorta and arch. The ascending aorta is best demonstrated by parasternal long-axis sections (Fig. 29.22). Its diameter ranges from

2 mm to 5 mm, and even the smallest aorta can almost always be identified. Left subclavicular or suprasternal parasagittal sections demonstrate the extreme hypoplasia of the aortic arch and the large ductus arteriosus, which conducts blood directly to the descending aorta and retrogradely to the ascending aorta (Figs. 29.23, 29.24).

In a few instances, extreme hypoplasia of the left ventricle may be associated with a normal aortic root. In these cases there is almost always a ventricular septal defect, and the aorta frequently over-rides the ventricular

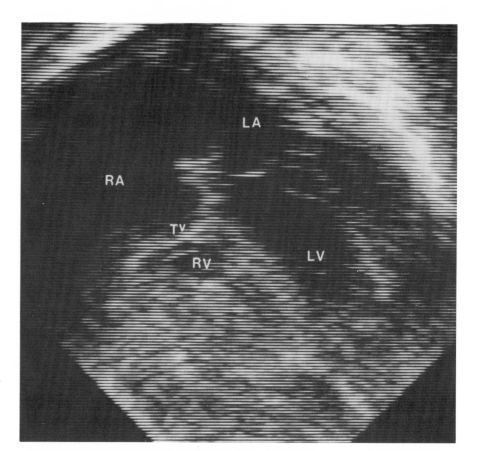

Figure 29.18. Four-chamber section from a heart with pulmonary atresia and intact ventricular septum with Ebstein's malformation of the tricuspid valve. The septal leaflet of the tricuspid valve is bound to the right ventricular aspect of the intraventricular septum.

Figure 29.19. Subcostal four-chamber section demonstrating the hypoplastic left ventricle in the hypoplastic left heart syndrome.

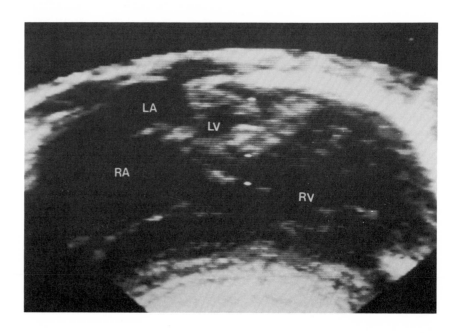

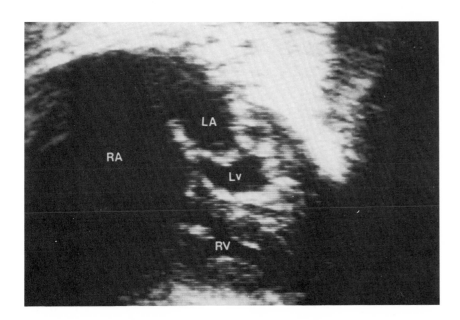

Figure 29.20. Parasternal four-chamber section from a heart with a small left atrium, miniaturized mitral valve, mitral stenosis, and hypoplastic left ventricle.

septum. Double-outlet right ventricle is often encountered. When the aortic root and ascending aorta are of normal size, coarctation of the aorta may be present.

The diagnosis of the hypoplastic left heart syndrome can invariably be made by two-dimensional echocar-diography, and it depends upon the demonstration of an extremely small left ventricle and extreme hypoplasia of the ascending aorta and aortic arch. It is extremely unusual for other investigations to be required to establish the diagnosis. Cardiac catheteriza-

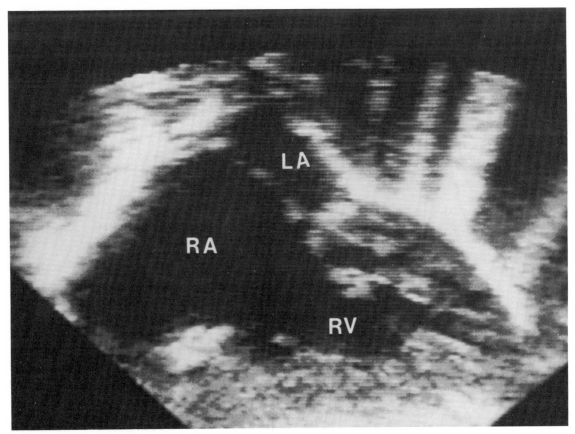

Figure 29.21. Parasternal four-chamber section from a heart with the hypoplastic left heart syndrome in which there is absence of the left atrioventricular connection. Sulcus tissue interposes between the floor of the left atrium and the ventricular mass.

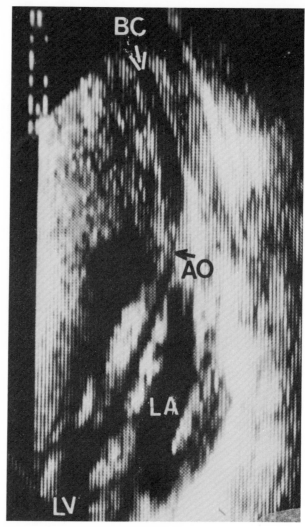

Figure 29.22. Parasternal long-axis section demonstrating extreme hypoplasia of the ascending aorta.

Figure 29.23. Suprasternal parasagittal section through the aorta demonstrating extreme hypoplasia of the aortic arch. (AAO = ascending aorta; DAO = descending aorta).

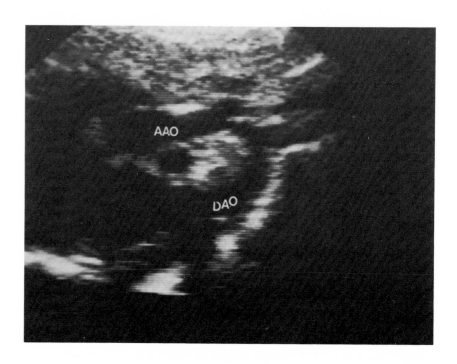

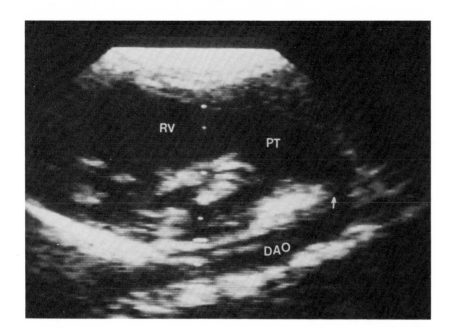

Figure 29.24. Left subclavicular section demonstrating the pulmonary trunk and a large arterial duct from a heart with the hypoplastic left heart syndrome.

tion is undertaken only if there is doubt about the size and anatomy of the aorta and aortic arch. In patients with a small left ventricle but normal aortic root and ascending aorta, palliative surgery can usually be undertaken in the neonatal period. A modification of the Fontan operation may then be possible later in childhood.

REFERENCES

1. Zuberbuhler JR, Anderson RH. Morphological variations in pulmonary atresia with intact ventricular septum. Br Heart J 1979;41: 281–288.

2. Greenwold WE, DuShane JW, Burchell HB, Bruwer A, Edwards JE. Congenital pulmonary atresia with intact ventricular septum: two anatomic types, (abstracted). Circulation 1956;14:945–946.

3. Patel RG, Freedom RM, Moes CAF, et al. Right ventricular volume determinations in 18 patients with pulmonary atresia and intact ventricular septum. Circulation 1980;61:428–440.

4. Bull C, De Leval MR, Mercanti C, Macartney FJ, Anderson RH. Pulmonary atresia and intact ventricular septum: a revised classification. Circulation 1982;66:266–272.

5. Edwards JE. Aortic atresia with intact ventricular septum: coexistent aortic mitral atresia. In Gould SE, ed. Pathology of the Heart and Great Vessels. Springfield, IL: Charles C Thomas, 1968: pp 337–341.

6. Lev M. Pathologic anatomy and interrelationship of hypoplasia of the aortic complexes. Laboratory Investigation 1952;1:61–70.

30
Right Ventricular Outflow Tract Obstruction

Jeffrey Smallhorn

This chapter covers the evaluation of right ventricular outflow tract obstruction by cross-sectional echocardiography. Discussed are hearts with pulmonary atresia and intact ventricular septum; anatomic and functional pulmonary atresia associated with Ebstein's malformation of the tricuspid valve in the newborn; tetralogy of Fallot with or without associated pulmonary atresia; and subvalvar, valvar, and supravalvar pulmonary stenosis.

PULMONARY ATRESIA WITH INTACT VENTRICULAR SEPTUM

Pulmonary atresia with intact ventricular septum invariably presents in the neonatal period, with severe cyanosis following closure of the patent ductus arteriosus. Considerable controversy has revolved around the exact definition of this condition. It has become apparent that it includes a spectrum of lesions ranging from critical pulmonary stenosis in the newborn with a normal-sized right ventricle (1–3) to pulmonary atresia with a diminutive right ventricle. Previously, critical pulmonary stenosis was not included in this group. Severe right ventricular hypoplasia and valve stenosis may, however, coexist. Likewise, pulmonary atresia with intact septum may rarely exist with a normal-sized right ventricular cavity.

The management of the two conditions is similar: an attempt to enlarge the right ventricular outflow tract with or without a systemic to pulmonary artery shunt (2, 4, 5). The difference between pulmonary atresia with intact septum and critical pulmonary stenosis is the presence of coronary artery sinusoids, which almost exclusively occur in association with pulmonary atresia (3, 6, 7).

The tripartite classification of pulmonary atresia with intact septum (i.e., the presence of inlet, trabecular, and outlet zones to the right ventricle) has been used to predict the potential for right ventricular growth (2). While this concept has some merit, hearts with a diminutive right ventricle may have all their components but have very limited potential for growth (3). Coronary artery sinusoids are more commonly seen in cases with severe right ventricular dysplasia and have a major practical significance in the management of this lesion (3, 6, 7).

Cross-Sectional Echocardiographic Assessment

The atrial arrangement is evaluated in subcostal long- and short-axis cuts at the level of the inferior vena cava and abdominal aorta (8). The inferior vena cava and hepatic veins are then traced to the right atrium, where a subcostal four-chamber cut is obtained to assess the interatrial septum and atrioventricular junction. From this position, the presence of an interatrial communication (either an atrial septal defect or patent foramen ovale) can be determined (Fig. 30.1). Doppler interrogation can evaluate the direction of shunting, with the majority having a right-to-left shunt. From this subcostal cut, the right atrioventricular valve can be evaluated and may vary in size proportionally to right ventricular dimensions (2). The valve may vary, appearing normal, severely stenotic and dysplastic, imperforate, or dysplastic and displaced if Ebstein's malformation of the tricuspid valve coexists (Fig. 30.2) (9–11).

Care must be taken when using the subcostal cut alone to evaluate the right atrioventricular junction as a small stenotic valve may be missed in this view and an anatomic diagnosis of tricuspid atresia incorrectly made. A combination of apical four-chamber and pre-

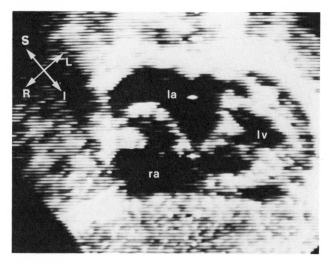

Figure 30.1. Subcostal four-chamber cut in pulmonary atresia with intact ventricular septum. The interatrial septum bows right to left. LA = left atrium; LV = left ventricle; RA = right atrium.

cordial short-axis cuts should be employed to avoid this error (Fig. 30.3) (11).

The subcostal and apical four-chamber cuts visualize the relative size of the inlet and trabecular zones, but not the outlet zone (Fig. 30.4). This zone is best evaluated by combining a subcostal long-axis cut of the right ventricular outflow tract with a high precordial short-axis cut. From both of these positions, the distance between an atretic infundibulum and pulmonary trunk can be evaluated, as can the presence of a pulmonary valve (Fig. 30.5A). It is not possible to differentiate between severe stenosis and valve atresia

without the use of Doppler echocardiography, although this matters little in the management of children unless a closed valvotomy is attempted. The size of the infundibulum can be accurately assessed from these views and is of vital importance when considering surgery to the right ventricular outflow tract (Fig. 30.5B).

The presence of coronary arterial sinusoids resulting in desaturated right ventricular blood entering the coronary artery circulation is usually associated with severe right ventricular hypoplasia (3, 6, 7). In most cases, there is stenosis between the sinusoids and the coronary artery circulation, resulting in normal-sized coronary arteries. Occasionally, the coronary arteries may be dilated due to a large unobstructed fistulous communication (6). It is only in the latter case that sinusoids may be identified by cross-sectional and Doppler echocardiography. These are best seen in a combination of precordial short-axis and subcostal four-chamber and long-axis views (Fig. 30.6A). The dilated coronary arteries and sinusoids appear like a coronary artery fistula, and Doppler interrogation will reveal flow from right ventricle to coronary artery during systole and reversed flow in diastole (Fig. 30.6B).

The aortic arch can be visualized from the suprasternal region and is almost always left sided. The pulmonary arteries vary in size from small to normal and are usually supplied by a left-sided patent ductus arteriosus. The ductus is of interest in that the angle between it and the descending aorta correlates with the size of the right ventricle. In general, the larger the right ventricle the more obtuse the angle is (Fig. 30.7),

Figure 30.2. Apical four-chamber cut in pulmonary atresia with intact septum and Ebstein's malformation of the morphologically tricuspid valve. Note the hypoplastic right ventricular cavity. The tricuspid septal leaflet is plastered down to the interventricular septum. LA = left atrium; LV = left ventricle; RA = right atrium; RV = right ventricle.

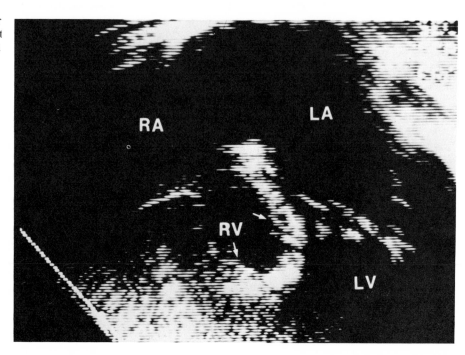

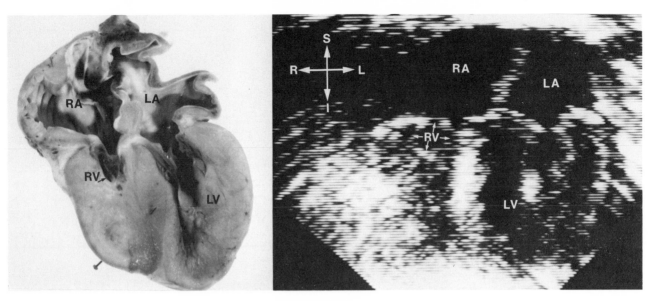

Figure 30.3. The left-hand picture is a specimen of pulmonary atresia with intact septum cut in an apical four-chamber view. Note the diminutive right ventricle. The picture on the right is a similar cut from a different patient. Note that there is a concordant atrioventricular connection. However, the right ventricular cavity is severely hypoplastic. LA = left atrium; LV = left ventricle; RA = right atrium; RV = right ventricle.

whereas the smaller cavity sizes are associated with an acutely angled ductus, similar to that seen in pulmonary atresia and ventricular septal defect (Fig. 30.8) (12, 13).

Tricuspid valve abnormalities are common with annular hypoplasia, and valvar stenosis is the most frequent association (Figs. 30.3 and 30.4) (3, 4, 14, 15). Occasionally, Ebstein's malformation of the tricuspid valve may present in the newborn period with clinical

features identical to pulmonary atresia with intact septum. Previously, one of the major problems was differentiating anatomic atresia from functional atresia, the latter occurring due to the pressures being lower during systole in the right ventricle than in the pulmonary artery (16). Regurgitation of blood from the pulmonary artery to right ventricle has been demonstrated angiographically and helps differentiate these two conditions (16). This reversed flow in the pulmo-

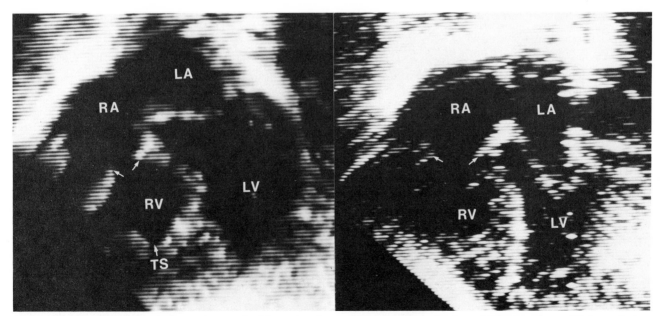

Figure 30.4. The left-hand picture is an apical four-chamber cut in pulmonary atresia and intact septum with hypoplasia of the tricuspid annulus (*arrows*). The picture on the right is a similar cut from a different patient demonstrating a larger tricuspid annulus (*arrows*). There appears to be a trabecular sinusoid at the apex of the right ventricle in the left-hand picture. LA = left atrium; LV = left ventricle; RA = right atrium; RV = right ventricle; TS = trabecular sinusoid.

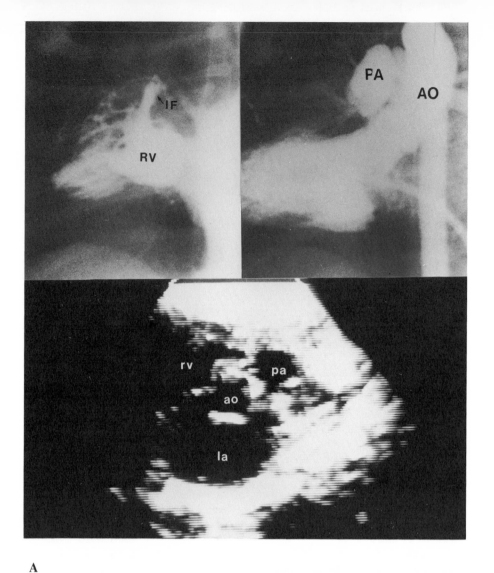

A

Figure 30.5. (*A*) The lower picture is a high precordial short-axis cut in pulmonary atresia with intact septum with a severely hypoplastic infundibulum and atretic pulmonary valve. The distance between the infundibulum and the pulmonary trunk is readily visualized. The upper pictures show the right ventricular (*upper left*) and the left ventricular (*upper right*) angiocardiogram from the same patient. (*B*) The right-hand picture is a precordial long-axis cut with clockwise rotation of the transducer to image the right ventricular outflow tract. Note the hypoplastic right ventricle with a long distance between the pulmonary trunk and the body of the right ventricle. The specimen on the left is from the same patient and demonstrates hypoplasia of the right ventricle with an atretic pulmonary valve at the infundibulum. AO = aorta; If = infundibulum; LA = left atrium; LV = left ventricle; PA = pulmonary trunk; RA = right atrium; RV = right ventricle.

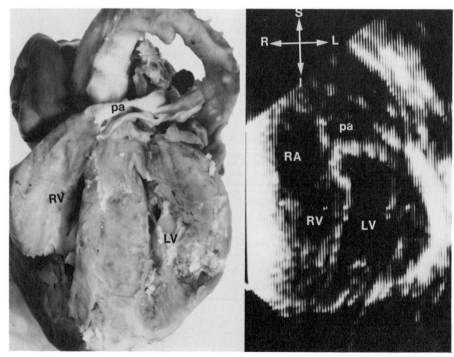

B

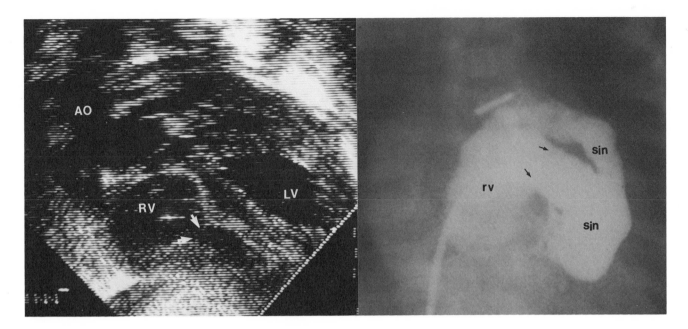

A

Figure 30.6. (*A*) Subcostal long-axis cut in pulmonary atresia with intact septum, with a large sinusoid between the right ventricle and the aorta. The arrows in the left-hand picture demonstrate the origin of the large trabecular sinusoid. The angiocardiogram on the right is from the same patient and demonstrates the large trabecular sinusoid that is connected to the coronary artery sinusoid.

nary trunk and infundibular region, which occurs predominantly during systole, has also been demonstrated with Doppler echocardiography (Fig. 30.9) (17). This corresponds with the angiographic appearances (Fig. 30.10) and has been confirmed in the same patients following saline contrast injections into the aortic end of the ductus (Fig. 30.11). The two conditions cannot be differentiated by cross-sectional echocardiography alone as the pulmonary valve remains immobile even in the presence of functional atresia.

PULMONARY VALVE STENOSIS

Prior to the advent of Doppler echocardiography, the diagnosis of pulmonary valve stenosis using cross-sectional echocardiography alone presented major difficulties. In the standard precordial short-axis cut, the pulmonary valve is imaged in its long axis, as the right ventricular outflow tract wraps around the left ventricular outflow tract. When there is significant valvar stenosis, the leaflets appear thickened and dome during ventricular systole (Fig. 30.12). In the presence of mild stenosis, however, the valve may appear relatively normal. This diagnostic problem may be partially resolved by obtaining a high precordial short-axis cut, in which the pulmonary valve is imaged in its short axis and all of the valve leaflets are visualized (Fig. 30.13) (18). In the majority of cases, the valve is trileaflet with

fusion occurring along the commissures. Occasionally, a bicuspid valve is seen in cases with isolated pulmonary valve stenosis (Fig. 30.13).

The degree of poststenotic dilatation of the pulmonary artery correlates with the severity of the valve stenosis. It is important to evaluate the infundibular region, as many cases with severe stenosis have secondary dynamic infundibular obstruction. This must be differentiated from stenosis at the infundibular level, which is fixed and can only be relieved surgically.

Measurements of the pulmonary valve annulus and detection of a dysplastic pulmonary valve are important in the assessment of patients when balloon angioplasty is contemplated. Balloon dilatation of a dysplastic valve is invariably unsuccessful. A dysplastic valve is usually not fused along the commissures but consists of abnormal thickened leaflets that are responsible for the obstruction (19). Dysplastic leaflets are partially adherent to the pulmonary artery wall, appear dense echocardiographically, and do not dome during systole. The absence of poststenotic dilatation and some supravalvar narrowing at the distal end of the sinuses are also frequently observed (Fig. 30.14).

Doppler echocardiography has been very helpful in the preoperative and preangioplasty evaluation of patients with pulmonary valve stenosis (20, 21). From a precordial short-axis or subcostal long-axis cut, the gradient can be accurately evaluated (Fig. 30.15) by

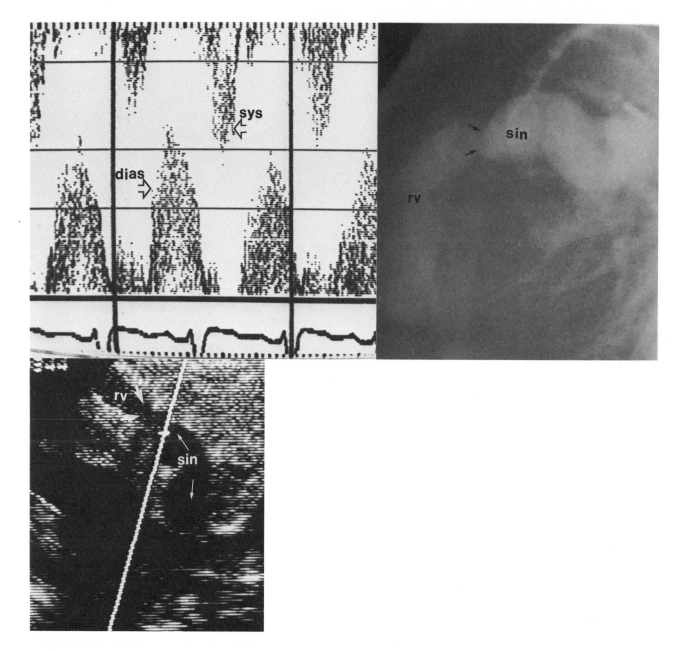

B

Figure 30.6, (cont'd.) (*B*) The upper right-hand picture is an angiocardiogram in pulmonary atresia with intact septum with a large sinusoid between the right ventricle and coronary artery. The lower picture demonstrates the sinusoidal communication with the right ventricle with a Doppler sample volume placed at the distal end of the sinusoid. The upper left-hand picture is the Doppler spectral trace, which demonstrates forward flow from the hypertensive right ventricle during ventricular systole (sys), with retrograde flow during diastole (dias). Ao = aorta; LV = left ventricle; RV = right ventricle; SIN = sinusoid.

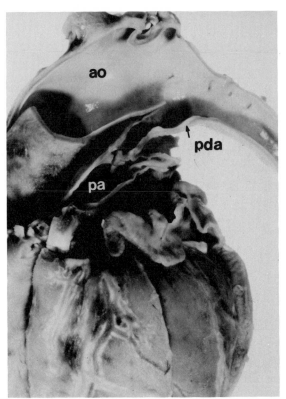

Figure 30.7. An anatomic specimen in pulmonary atresia with intact septum showing an obtuse-angle ductus. In this patient, the right ventricular cavity was of a larger dimension. Compare the angle the ductus makes with the descending aorta with that seen in Figure 30.8. Ao = aorta; PA = pulmonary trunk; PDA = patent ductus arteriosus.

either pulsed Doppler using a high-pulsed repetition frequency rate or continuous wave Doppler (Fig. 30.16). Problems may occur in the newborns with a pinhole orifice, where it may be difficult to resolve the jet (Fig. 30.17). This corresponds with experimental data where a variety of different-size obstructions are produced (22). Even with this limitation, there are usually enough secondary signs, plus the presence of forward turbulent flow through the valve, to make a positive diagnosis of severe obstruction.

Supravalvar Stenosis

Rarely, the obstruction may be located above the valve, where it is invariably associated with peripheral obstruction of the pulmonary tree. The obstruction may consist of an hourglass narrowing, a discrete membrane, or tubular hypoplasia (23). Obstruction distal to the pulmonary valve can only be assessed as far as the hilum, since the lung obscures the image more distally. The high parasternal long-axis cut with clockwise rotation and the short-axis cut from the precordium enable an assessment from the bifurcation into the right and left pulmonary arteries (Fig. 30.18). The suprasternal cut enables the examiner to visualize the right and left pulmonary arteries to their respective hila (Fig. 30.19) (24).

In the hourglass variety, the narrowed segment can be visualized with a larger lumen on either side. Although I have not observed a membrane, a systematic examination should allow its detection above the pulmonary valve, with an appearance similar to that seen in subvalvar aortic stenosis. Tubular hypoplasia can be assessed by comparing the diameter of the pulmonary trunk to that expected for the patient's age and size.

MUSCULAR RIGHT VENTRICULAR OUTFLOW TRACT OBSTRUCTION

Muscular outflow tract obstruction may occur in the infundibular region, either in isolation or, more commonly, in association with a ventricular septal defect (25). The obstruction may occasionally be low down in the trabecular zone, producing a double-chambered right ventricle (26–29). The infundibular region is best assessed from either a high precordial position, which is appropriate in the older age group, or the subcostal window, which is appropriate in young children.

From the precordium, a long-axis cut of the left ventricular outflow tract is first obtained, and then the transducer is rotated slightly clockwise. In this position, the pulmonary valve, outlet septum, and anterior free wall are visualized. Care must be taken to ensure that the near field gain settings are correct, as in many systems the first centimeter or so is not well seen. This problem can be partially overcome by positioning the transducer as close to the left clavicle as possible, in order to obtain a slightly greater distance between the beam and the outflow tract. Normally the supraventricular crest of the right ventricle is seen in this position, and despite changes in dimension during the cardiac cycle, the infundibular region appears wide.

When infundibular stenosis is present, the crest is hypertrophied, and the outflow tract remains narrow during both systole and diastole (Fig. 30.20). The region proximal to the infundibulum appears to be normal, as does the pulmonary valve when the stenosis is purely at infundibular level.

The subcostal approach provides information about the lateral aspect of the right ventricular free wall, plus the medial portion of the infundibulum. The major problem with this approach is that reliable visualization is only possible in the younger child (28). Normally, the supraventricular crest can be seen, with an adequate lumen during both systole and diastole. In the presence of infundibular stenosis, the hypertrophied crest can be seen narrowing the outflow tract (Fig.

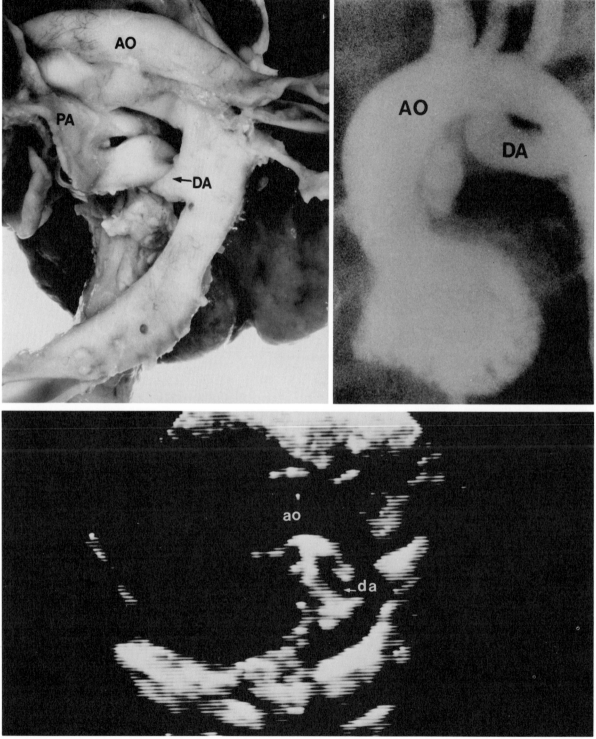

Figure 30.8.   The lower picture demonstrates a ductus arteriosus in pulmonary atresia with intact septum. Note the acute angle the duct makes with the descending aorta. The upper left-hand picture is the specimen from the same patient and the right-hand picture the angiocardiogram from the same patient. AO = aorta; DA = ductus arteriosus; PA = pulmonary trunk.

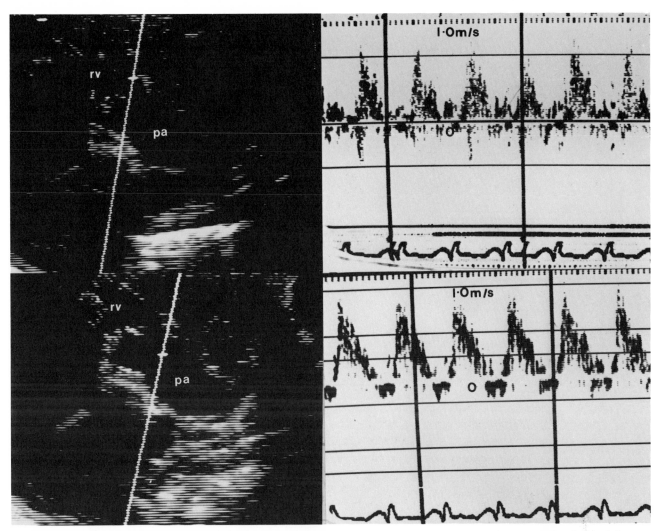

Figure 30.9. The upper right-hand picture is from a patient with Ebstein's malformation of the tricuspid valve and functional pulmonary atresia. The Doppler sample volume is placed just proximal to the pulmonary valve. The Doppler spectral trace on the right demonstrates regurgitant flow during ventricular systole. The lower left-hand picture is in the same patient with the sample volume placed in the pulmonary trunk. The spectral image on the right demonstrates retrograde flow again during ventricular systole. PA = pulmonary trunk; RV = right ventricle.

30.20), and the obstruction is obvious during both phases of the cardiac cycle.

Muscular obstruction may also occur in the trabecular zone, producing the double-chambered right ventricle. In the majority of cases, this is due to hypertrophy of the muscular annulus produced by the supraventricular crest, the body of the septomarginal trabeculation and the septoparietal trabeculations (moderator band) (26). Two forms may be seen. In the milder type, there is a high takeoff of one of the septoparietal trabeculations, which crosses the ventricle as an obstructive band. This can be seen in the parasternal long-axis cut as a muscle bar inserting high into the interventricular septum. As the transducer is then rotated clockwise, the infundibular septum is seen, and the muscle bar can be followed to its point of insertion. This type of

abnormality is not always symptomatic and may be a chance finding in a normal heart. The more severe form is when there is high takeoff of a septoparietal trabeculation combined with hypertrophy of the apical trabeculations. This then divides the trabecular portion into two apical pouches, one in communication with the inlet and the other with the outlet component. Variations of this may exist when the obstruction is less severe, with an easier access between the inlet and outlet chambers.

Except in the neonate, the obstruction may be difficult to identify when it is mild to moderate, as the trabecular zone of the right ventricle is often poorly visualized. When there is more complete obstruction, the subcostal cut with clockwise rotation of the transducer provides the best window for visualizing the

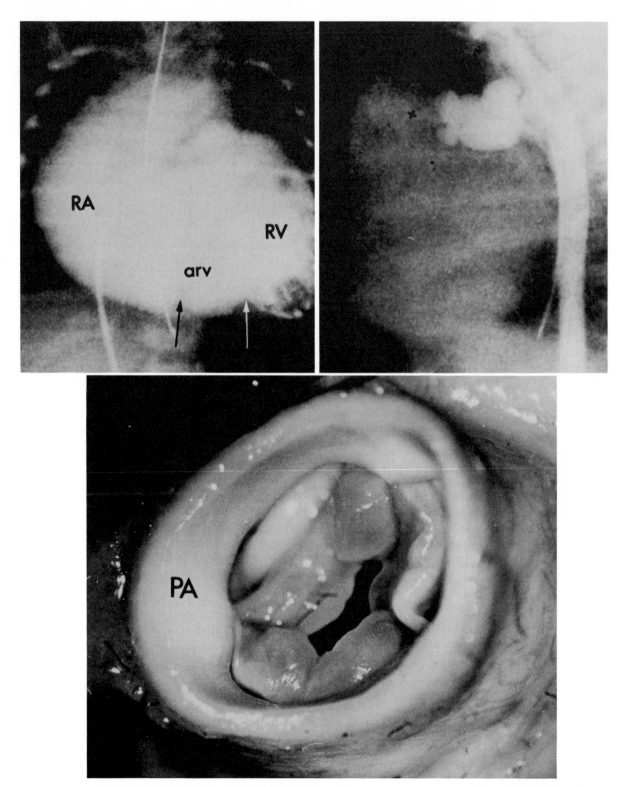

Figure 30.10. Angiocardiogram in Ebstein's malformation of the tricuspid valve with functional pulmonary atresia. Note the typical angiocardiographic appearance of the Ebstein's malformation. The right-hand picture demonstrates regurgitation at the pulmonary valve. The arrows indicate the extent of the atrialized portion of the right ventricle. The lower picture is the anatomic specimen from the same patient and demonstrates a perforate pulmonary valve. ARV = atrialized right ventricle; PA = pulmonary trunk; RA = right atrium; RV = right ventricle.

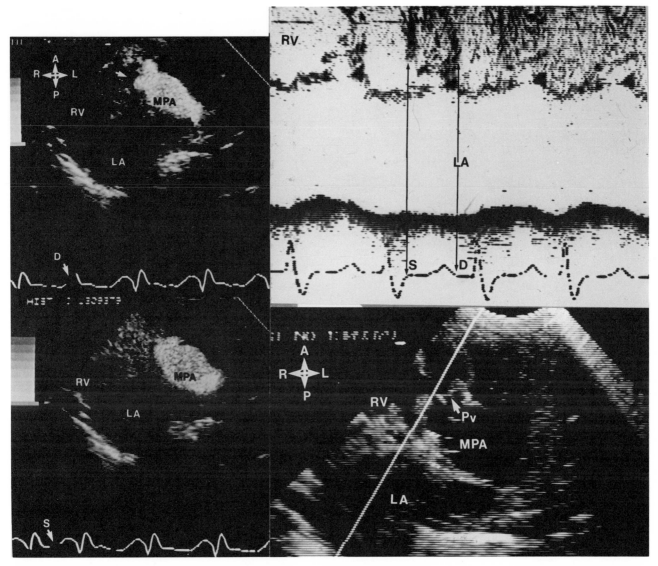

Figure 30.11.   The left-hand pictures are from a patient with functional pulmonary atresia. Contrast echocardiography was performed opposite the mouth of the ductus. Note that the contrast regurgitates back into the right ventricle (*upper and lower left*). The upper right-hand picture is from the same patient with an M-mode echocardiogram placed beneath the pulmonary valve with 2D echo guidance (*lower right*). Note that the regurgitation occurs during ventricular systole with clearing during ventricular diastole. D = diastole; LA = left atrium; MPA = pulmonary trunk; PV = pulmonary valve; RV = right ventricle; S = systole.

right ventricular outflow tract (Fig. 30.21). Here the muscle shelf dividing the right ventricle is seen situated beneath the infundibulum. In the older patient where the subcostal approach may be inadequate, the apical four-chamber cut can be helpful in diagnosis.

Doppler echocardiography plays an important role in the assessment of muscular outflow tract obstruction. Although turbulence from the obstruction can be detected from a precordial short-axis cut, problems with aligning the beam parallel to the flow occur (Fig. 30.22). This can be overcome in the smaller child, where a subcostal long-axis cut of the right ventricular outflow tract allows parallel alignment with the jet (Fig. 30.22).

Further problems may occur in the presence of a ventricular septal defect, where turbulence from the shunt may make identification of associated muscular subpulmonary obstruction difficult.

TETRALOGY OF FALLOT

The hallmark of tetralogy of Fallot including pulmonary atresia with ventricular septal defect is the anterior deviation of the outlet septum from its usual position in the normal heart between the limbs of the septomarginal trabeculation. The anterior deviation is responsible for the infundibular stenosis, the aortic

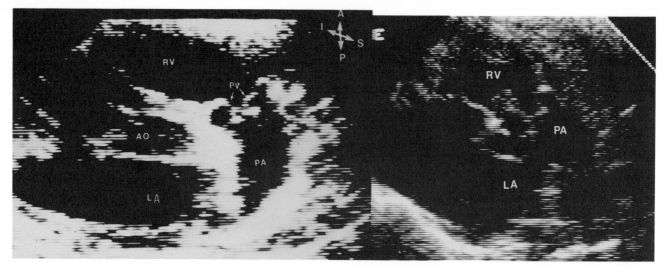

Figure 30.12. Precordial short-axis cut in significant pulmonary valve stenosis. The infundibular region is widely patent in diastole. The picture on the right demonstrates the pulmonary valve's doming during ventricular systole. Note there is also evidence of some dynamic infundibular narrowing. Ao = aorta; LA = left atrium; PA = pulmonary trunk; PV = pulmonary valve; RV = right ventricle.

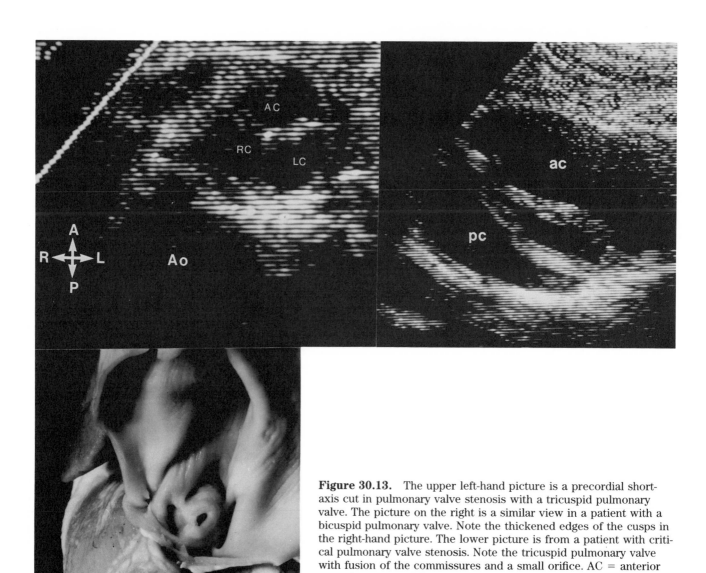

Figure 30.13. The upper left-hand picture is a precordial short-axis cut in pulmonary valve stenosis with a tricuspid pulmonary valve. The picture on the right is a similar view in a patient with a bicuspid pulmonary valve. Note the thickened edges of the cusps in the right-hand picture. The lower picture is from a patient with critical pulmonary valve stenosis. Note the tricuspid pulmonary valve with fusion of the commissures and a small orifice. AC = anterior cusp; Ao = aorta; LC = left cusp; PC = posterior cusp; RC = right cusp.

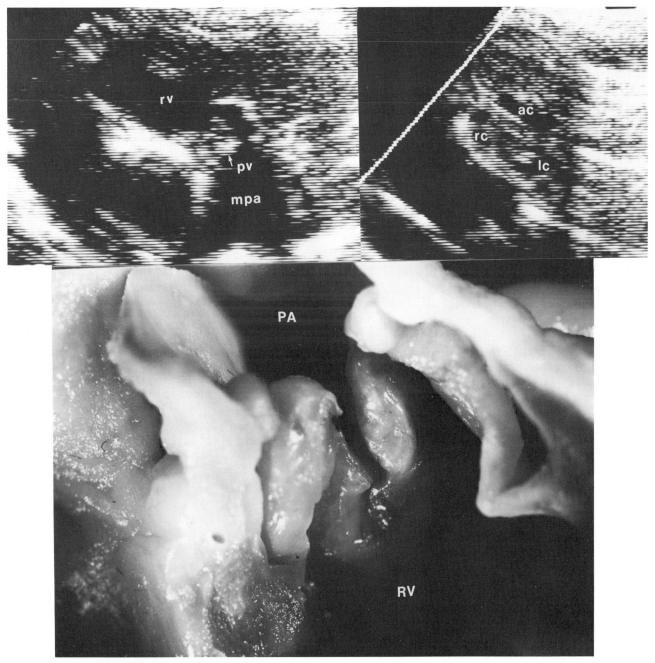

Figure 30.14. The upper left-hand picture is a high precordial long-axis cut in a case with a dysplastic pulmonary valve. Note the echo-dense leaflets, which represent the valve dysplasia. The upper right-hand picture is from the same patient in the precordial short-axis view. The stenosis is secondary to the dysplasia of the pulmonary valve leaflet. The lower picture is an anatomic specimen cut in the long-axis view. Note the similarity between this and the echocardiographic images. AC = anterior cusp; LC = left cusp; MPA = pulmonary trunk; PV = pulmonary valve; RC = right cusp; RV = right ventricle.

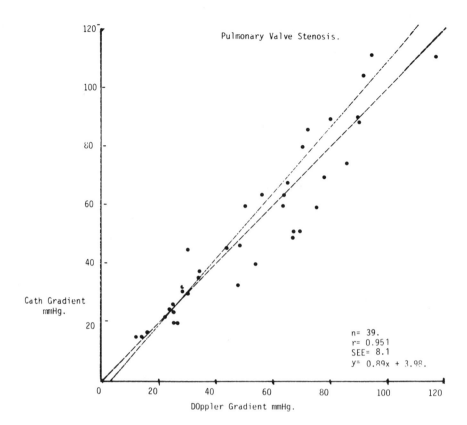

Figure 30.15. Correlation between cardiac catheterization and Doppler gradients in patients with pulmonary valve stenosis. Both the line of identity and the slope are on the graph. Note the small standard error of the estimate.

Figure 30.16. Doppler spectral and pressure traces in a patient with pulmonary valve stenosis. Note the close correlation between the peaked instantaneous gradient and that calculated from the Doppler traces.

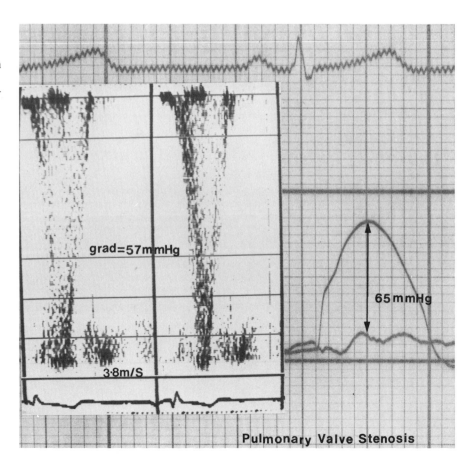

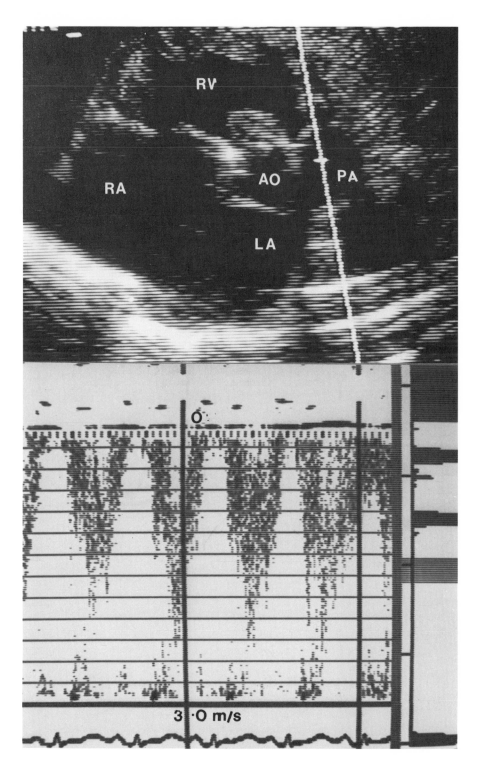

Figure 30.17. Doppler spectral trace from a patient with critical pulmonary valve stenosis. Despite the presence of severe stenosis, it was not possible to resolve the jet. AO = aorta; LA = left atrium; PA = pulmonary trunk; RA = right atrium; RV = right ventricle.

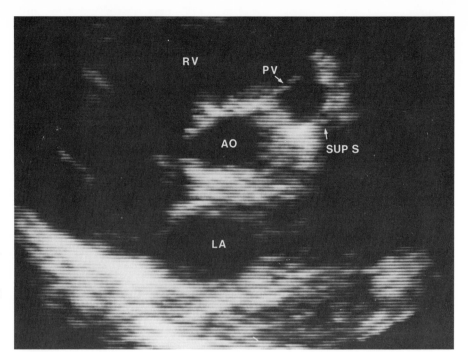

Figure 30.18. Precordial short-axis cut from a patient with supravalvar pulmonary stenosis. The pulmonary valve and annulus appear to be of normal dimensions. There is evidence of significant narrowing in the supravalvar region. AO = aorta; LA = left atrium; PV = pulmonary valve; RV = right ventricle; SUP S = supravalvar stenosis.

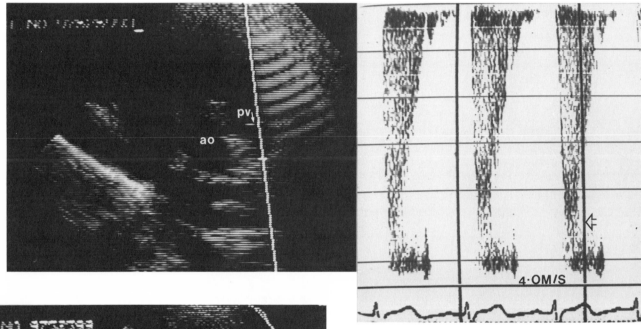

Figure 30.19. The lower picture is a suprasternal frontal plane cut from a patient with peripheral pulmonary artery stenosis. The arrow indicates the site of narrowing in the right pulmonary artery. The distal right pulmonary artery is also small. The upper picture is a Doppler spectral trace with the sample volume placed in the orifice of the left pulmonary artery in patient with peripheral pulmonary artery stenosis. Note high-velocity turbulent jet. The pulmonary valve in this patient appeared normal. Ao = aorta; MPA = pulmonary trunk; PV = pulmonary valve; RPA = right pulmonary artery.

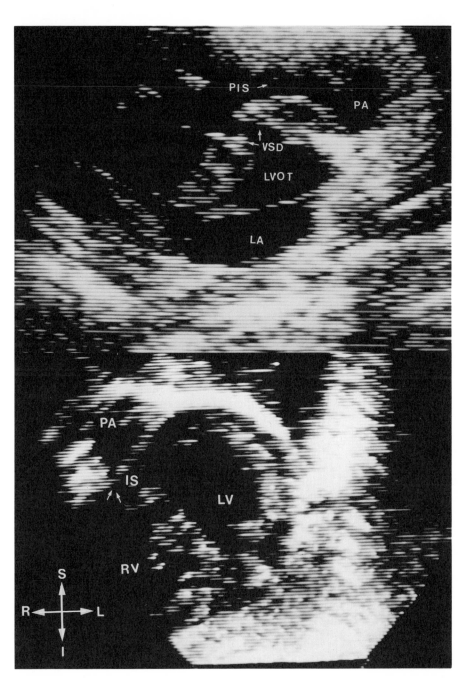

Figure 30.20. The upper picture is a precordial short-axis cut in a patient with a small ventricular septal defect (*arrows*) and associated pulmonary infundibular stenosis. Note the hypertrophied outlet septum, with associated narrowing from the anterior right ventricular wall. The lower picture is a subcostal long-axis cut of the right ventricular outflow tract from a diferent patient. The lateral and medial aspects of the infundibular obstruction (*arrows*) are visualized in this image. LA = left atrium; LV = left ventricle; LVOT = left ventricular outflow tract; PA = pulmonary trunk; PIS = pulmonary infundibular stenosis; RV = right ventricle.

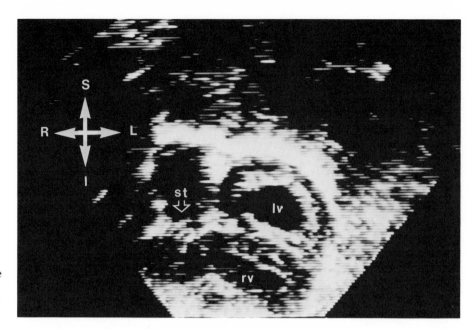

Figure 30.21. A subcostal long-axis cut in a double-chambered right ventricle. The obstruction is beneath the infundibular and more proximal than in Figure 30-20. LV = left ventricle; RV = right ventricle; ST = subpulmonary stenosis.

overriding, and the ventricular septal defect. This chapter discusses only hearts with 50 percent or less of aortic override, although tetralogy of Fallot and double outlet may coexist (26, 30–32).

In most instances, the ventricular septal defect is perimembranous (Fig. 30.23), although occasionally the septomarginal trabeculation fuses with the ventriculoinfundibular fold in its posterior rim, producing a muscular infundibular defect. Rarely, a doubly committed ventricular septal defect is seen in association with tetralogy of Fallot (Fig. 30.24) (33).

The pulmonary infundibular stenosis is produced by the anterior insertion of the outlet septum with the septal and parietal insertions both toward the anterior ventricular wall. Often anterior septoparietal trabeculations may complete a muscular ring, which may be further narrowed by fibrous tissue. The pulmonary valve is invariably stenotic and may be bicuspid. The degree of anterior deviation of the outlet septum varies, and in the more extreme cases pulmonary atresia and ventricular septal defect results. At the other end of the spectrum are those cases with tetralogy and absent pulmonary valve, where increased flow may occasionally be a problem.

Echocardiographic Assessment

The classical feature in tetralogy of Fallot is overriding of the aorta, which is readily appreciated in the precordial long-axis cut, athough care must be taken not to overstate the degree of overriding from this approach. As the transducer is rotated from a precordial long-axis to short-axis cut, the ventricular septal defect can be visualized and its relationship to the membranous

septum determined (Figs. 30.24 and 30.25). In most cases, the membranous septum forms part of the border of the defect, which is unrestrictive, although occasionally tricuspid tissue may surround the defect resulting in suprasystemic right ventricular pressure (34). The infundibular stenosis can be evaluated in this position, as can the size of the pulmonary valve annulus and the presence of valvar stenosis (Figs. 30.24 and 30.25). From the precordial short-axis cut, anteriorly situated septoparietal trabeculations, if present, can be seen further increasing the subpulmonary stenosis. The right ventricular outflow tract can be evaluated from a subcostal cut also, with counterclockwise rotation from the long axis (Fig. 30.26).

If the transducer is then moved into a high precordial short-axis cut, the main pulmonary artery and the origin of the left and right branches can be visualized (Fig. 30.27). In cases with pulmonary atresia and absent pulmonary trunk, care must be taken not to confuse the left atrial appendage with the pulmonary trunk. While this may sound unlikely, the left atrial appendage wraps around this region producing an echo-free space. In the high precordial short-axis position, absence of the pulmonary valve leaflets can be identified (35). Although the term "absent" is used, invariably a small remnant of valve tissue is present, with grossly dilated distal pulmonary arteries (Fig. 30.28). In these cases, forward systolic flow and retrograde diastolic flow from the regurgitation can be assessed by Doppler echocardiography (Fig. 30.28).

From the suprasternal cut, the side of the aortic arch and the presence of normal branching of the brachiocephalic vessels can be determined (Fig. 30.29) (36). This is important if systemic to pulmonary artery

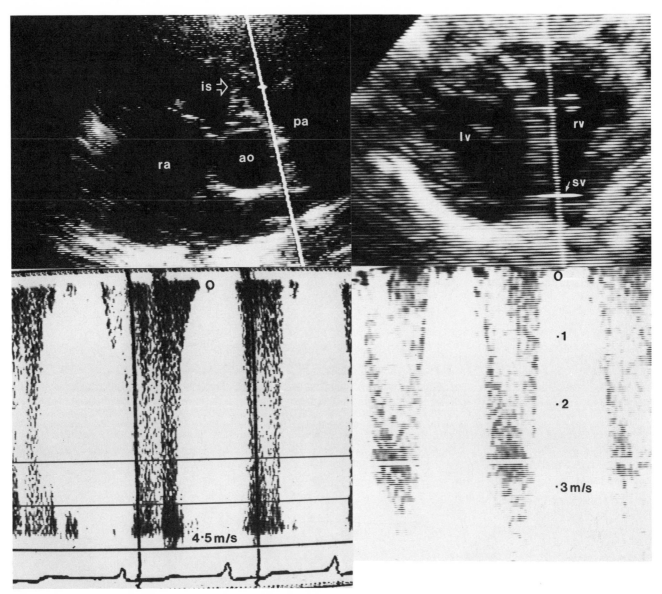

Figure 30.22. The upper left-hand picture is a precordial short-axis cut in a patient with pulmonary infundibular stenosis. It is difficult to align the sample volume parallel with the direction of flow. The lower picture is the Doppler spectral trace, demonstrating a high-velocity turbulent jet. The upper right-hand picture is a subcostal cut in a patient with infundibular stenosis. In this cut, it is possible to align the sample volume parallel to the direction of flow. AO = aorta; IS = infundibular stenosis; LV = left ventricle; PA = pulmonary trunk; RA = right atrium; RV = right ventricle; SV = sample volume.

shunts are to be performed without prior cardiac catheterization (37). The branching of the innominate artery into the subclavian and carotid arteries is best assessed from a suprasternal frontal plane cut with the aorta visualized in its short axis (Fig. 30.29). If the transducer is then rotated counterclockwise for a left arch and clockwise for a right arch, the aortic branching can be identified. If this is not observed, then the presence of an aberrant subclavian artery must be considered. In infants, this can usually be confirmed with posterior angulation of the transducer in the frontal plane with slight rotation to the left or right, depending on the side of the aortic arch (Fig. 30.30).

The size of the right pulmonary artery and its origin from the main pulmonary trunk can be assessed from the suprasternal frontal plane cut (Fig. 30.31). With clockwise rotation of the transducer, the left pulmonary artery can be visualized (38).

The presence of a patent ductus arteriosus can be determined from the suprasternal cut. In cases with pulmonary atresia, it usually forms an acute angle with the descending aorta and is frequently tortuous (Fig. 30.32) (12, 13). In cases with a patent right ventricular outflow tract, it forms a more obtuse angle with the descending aorta (12, 13). The ductus usually originates from the underside of the aorta but may arise

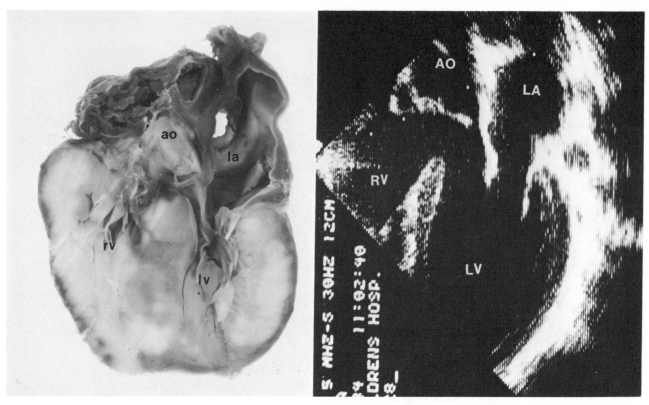

Figure 30.23. The right-hand picture is a precordial long-axis cut in tetralogy of Fallot. The aorta overrides the interventricular septum. The ventricular septal defect is perimembranous. The specimen on the left is from a different patient and demonstrates the echocardiographic features. AO = aorta; LA = left atrium; LV = left ventricle; RV = right ventricle.

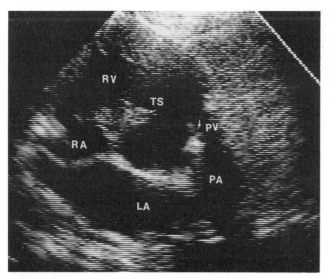

Figure 30.24. The precordial short-axis cut in tetralogy of Fallot with an associated doubly committed subarterial ventricular septal defect. Note the hypoplastic pulmonary valve and annulus. The pulmonary trunk and aorta roof the ventricular septal defect. The ventricular septal defect does not extend back to the membranous septum. LA = left atrium; PA = pulmonary trunk; PV = pulmonary valve; RA = right atrium; RV = right ventricle; TS = trabecular septum.

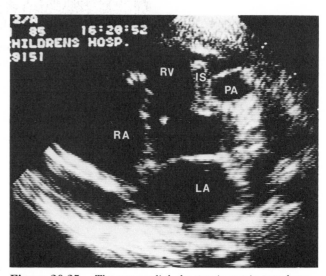

Figure 30.25. The precordial short-axis cut in tetralogy of Fallot. The ventricular septal defect is perimembranous, unlike that seen in Figure 30.24. Observe that the anterior deviation of the outlet septum produces severe infundibular stenosis. The pulmonary valve annulus can also be seen in this position. IS = outlet septum; LA = left atrium; PA = pulmonary trunk; RA = right atrium; RV = right ventricle.

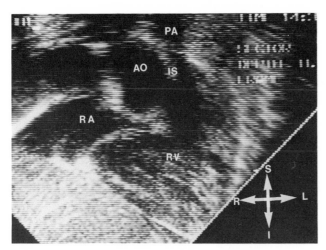

Figure 30.26. Subcostal cut in tetralogy of Fallot. This view is obtained with counterclockwise rotation from the long axis. Note that the anterior deviation of the outlet septum produces significant subpulmonary stenosis. AO = aorta; IS = infundibular (outlet) septum; PA = pulmonary trunk; RA = right atrium; RV = right ventricle.

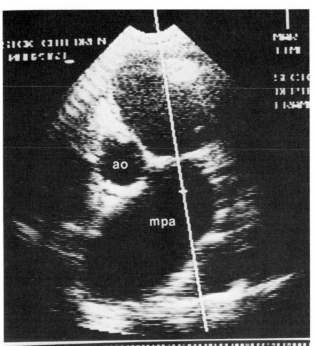

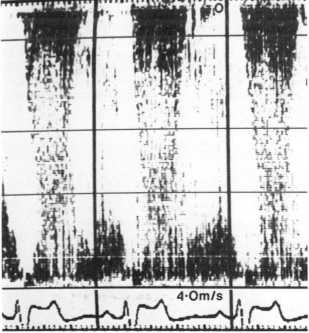

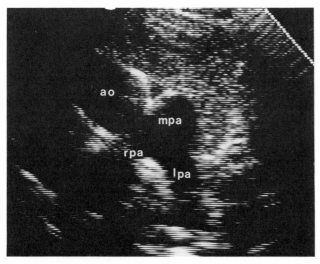

Figure 30.27. High precordial short-axis cut in tetralogy of Fallot. In this position, the pulmonary trunk (MPA) at the origin of the left (LPA) and right (RPA) pulmonary arteries can be clearly visualized. AO = aorta.

Figure 30.28. The upper picture is a high precordial short-axis cut in tetralogy of Fallot with absent pulmonary valve. Note the grossly dilated segment of the pulmonary trunk. A remnant of pulmonary valve tissue can be clearly seen. The lower picture is the spectral trace demonstrating a high-velocity jet. There is also reverse flow during diastole from the associated pulmonary regurgitation. AO = aorta; MPA = pulmonary trunk.

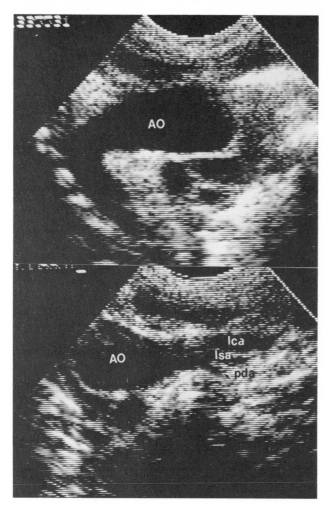

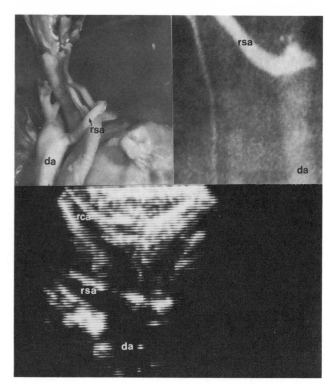

Figure 30.30. The upper left-hand picture is an anatomic specimen with an aberrant right subclavian artery viewed from the back. The angiocardiogram on the right is from a different patient viewed from the front. The lower picture is an echocardiogram from the suprasternal position in an infant with an aberrant right subclavian artery. DA = descending aorta; RCA = right carotid artery; RSA = right subclavian artery.

Figure 30.29. The upper picture is a suprasternal cut in a patient with tetralogy of Fallot and a right aortic arch. The descending aorta runs on the right side of the spine. The lower picture is from the same patient, showing the branching of the innominate artery into the left subclavian and left carotid arteries. The patent arterial duct originates from the base of the innominate artery on the left. AO = aorta; LCA = left carotid artery; LSA = left subclavian artery; PDA = patent ductus arteriosus.

from the base of the innominate artery (Fig. 30.33). Occasionally, bilateral ductuses are found, and are frequently associated with interruption of the central pulmonary arteries (Fig. 30.34) (39). Interruption of the pulmonary arteries is best assessed from a straight suprasternal frontal plane cut.

One of the major limitations of cross-sectional echocardiography is the inability to identify associated collateral vessels arising from the descending aorta (40). Occasionally, a large vessel may be identified arising from the descending aorta. Confusion may occur, however, between a true central pulmonary artery and a collateral vessel that runs in the same position in the absence of a central pulmonary artery.

Occasionally, the innominate vein on the left side

may run beneath the aortic arch rather than in front of it, which may give the appearance of a central pulmonary artery if the true central arteries are absent (Fig. 30.35A) (41). If a central pulmonary artery is present, then two structures are seen in the frontal and long-axis cuts (Fig. 30.35B). In cases with tetralogy of Fallot and an absent pulmonary valve, the right pulmonary artery from the suprasternal frontal plane cut appears aneurysmal. In the majority of these cases, a ductus arteriosus cannot be identified.

ASSOCIATED ABNORMALITIES

Occasionally, an atrioventricular septal defect occurs in association with tetralogy of Fallot (42). In this situation, the defect is associated with a large interventricular component. Mitral stenosis may be seen in association with tetralogy of Fallot and is best assessed with a combination of precordial long-axis and four-chamber cuts in association with Doppler interrogation of the valve. In the presence of low pulmonary flow where stenosis may be missed, care must be taken with the initial assessment until a shunt has been inserted.

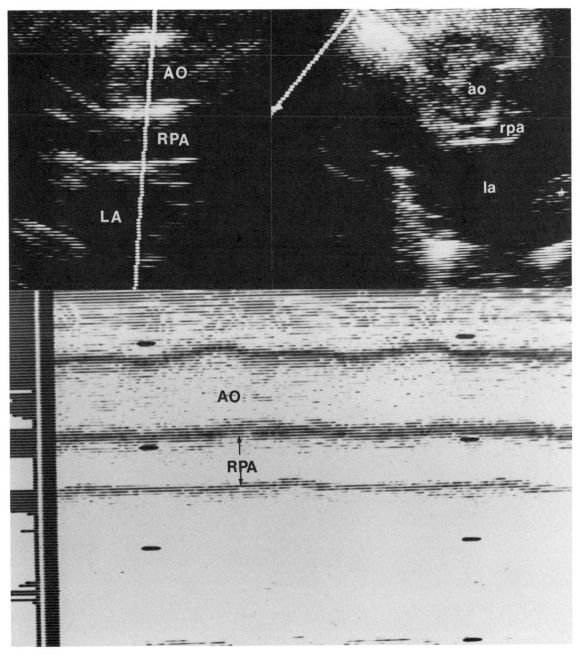

Figure 30.31. The upper left-hand picture is a suprasternal frontal plane cut in tetralogy of Fallot with a normal-size right pulmonary artery. The lower picture demonstrates the diameter from the M-mode echocardiogram. The upper right-hand picture is from a different patient with a hypoplastic right pulmonary artery. AO = aorta; LA = left atrium; RPA = right pulmonary artery.

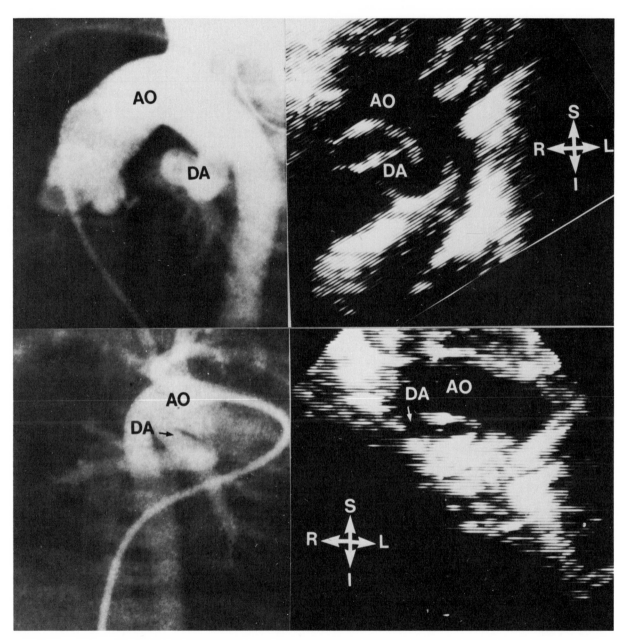

Figure 30.32. The upper picture demonstrates a left-sided ductus in pulmonary atresia with ventricular septal defect. Note the acute angle the duct makes with the descending aorta. The lower picture is from a patient with a right-sided duct. AO = aorta; DA = ductus arteriosus.

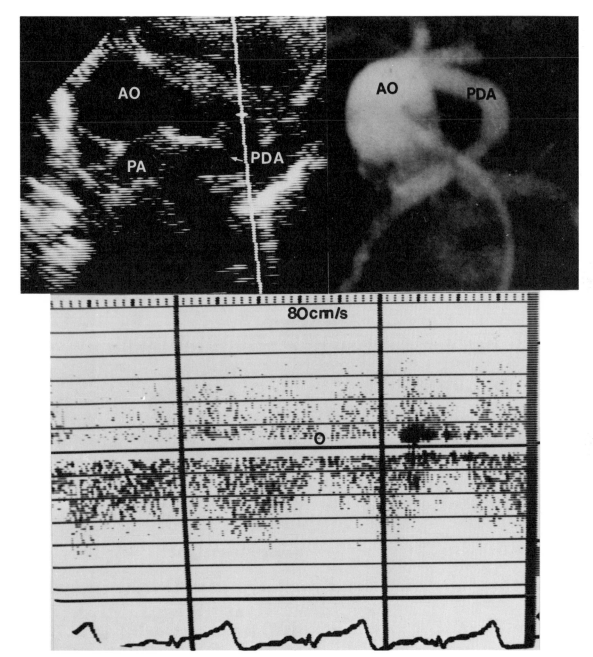

Figure 30.33.   The upper left-hand picture is a suprasternal cut in a patient with pulmonary atresia and ventricular septal defect with a ductus originating from the base of the left innominate artery. The lower picture demonstrates turbulent flow obtained by Doppler echocardiography. The upper right-hand picture is an angiocardiogram demonstrating the echocardiographic features. AO = aorta; PA = pulmonary arteries; PDA = patent ductus arteriosus.

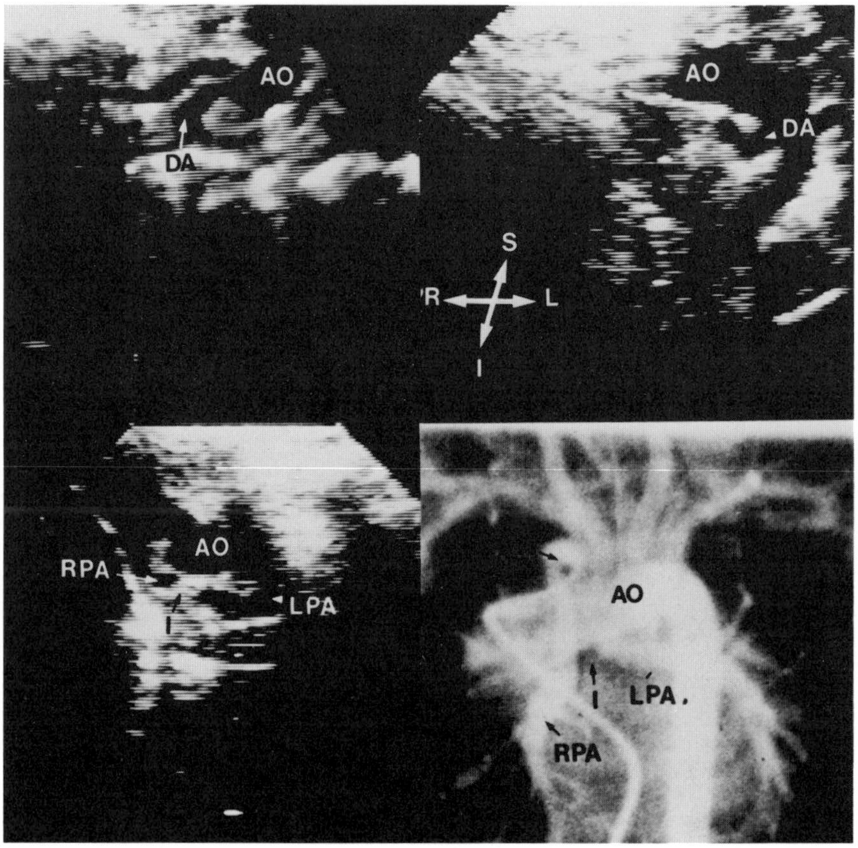

Figure 30.34. The upper left and right panels show 2D echocardiograms of the bilateral ductuses while the bottom left panel shows pulmonary atresia. The lower right-hand picture is a cineaortogram in pulmonary atresia with ventricular septal defect, interruption of the pulmonary arteries, and bilateral ductuses. The echocardiogram demonstrates the angiographic features. Note the interruption between the left and right pulmonary arteries. AO = aorta; DA = ductus arteriosus; I = interruption; LPA = left pulmonary artery; RPA = right pulmonary artery.

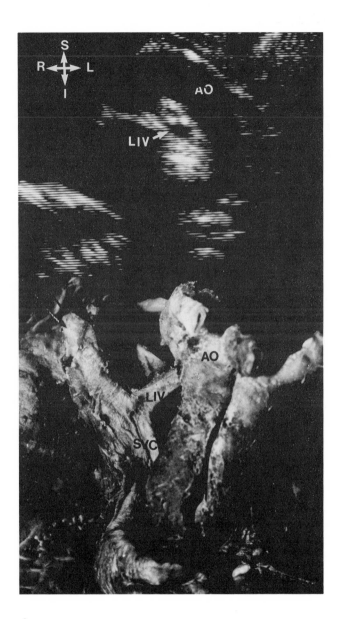

A

Figure 30.35. (*A*) The upper picture is a suprasternal long-axis cut in pulmonary atresia and ventricular septal defect with absent central pulmonary arteries. The structure seen beneath the aorta is the innominate vein, not a central pulmonary artery. The lower picture demonstrates anatomic features.

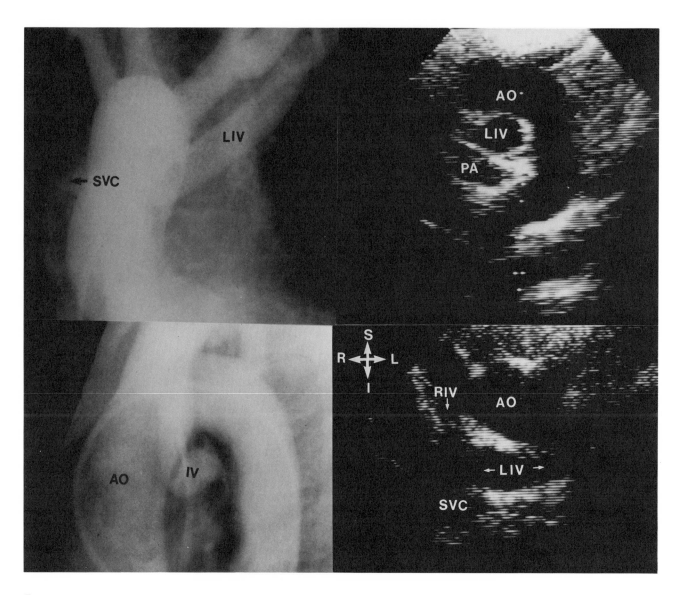

B

Figure 30.35, (cont'd) (*B*) The upper left-hand picture is an angiocardiogram demonstrating the left innominate vein running beneath the ascending aorta. The lower picture is a lateral view demonstrating the same features. The echocardiograms in the right-hand panel demonstrate the angiograhic features. AO = aorta; LIV = left innominate vein; PA = pulmonary trunk; RIV = right innominate vein; SVC = superior vena cava.

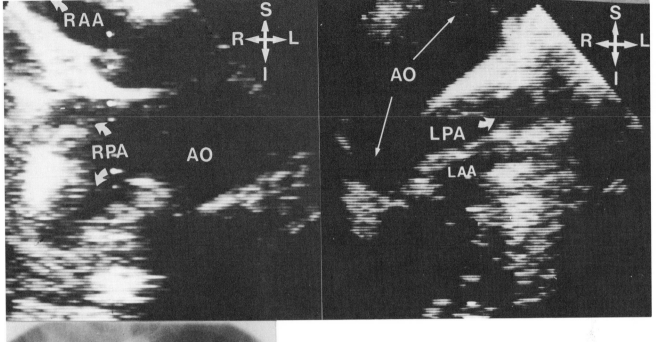

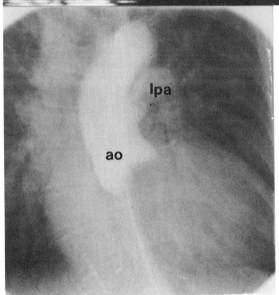

Figure 30.36. The upper left-hand picture is a suprasternal frontal plane cut in pulmonary atresia and ventricular septal defect with anomalous origin of the right pulmonary artery from the ascending aorta. The picture on the right is from a different patient with associated pulmonary atresia and anomalous origin of the left pulmonary artery from the ascending aorta. The lower picture is an angiocardiogram demonstrating the appearance of the left pulmonary artery arising from the ascending aorta. AO = aorta; LAA = left atrial appendage; LPA = left pulmonary artery; RAA = right aortic arch; RPA = right pulmonary artery.

The interatrial septum must be carefully assessed in the subcostal cut, because an associated interatrial shunt, if missed, may complicate the postoperative course, with frequent right-to-left shunting and persistent cyanosis.

Anomalous origin of a pulmonary artery from the ascending aorta is rarely associated with tetralogy of Fallot (43). This is best evaluated from a combination of suprasternal, precordial, and subcostal long-axis cuts. The vessel can be seen originating from the ascending aorta, with Doppler interrogation identifying the left-to-right shunt (Fig. 30.36).

REFERENCES

1. Bull C, de Leval M, Mercanti C, Macartney FJ, Anderson RH. Pulmonary atresia and intact ventricular septum: a revised classification. Circulation 1982;66:266–72.
2. de Leval M, Bull C, Stark J, et al. Pulmonary atresia and intact ventricular septum: surgical management based on a revised classification. Circulation 1982;66:272–80.
3. Freedom RM, Wilson G, Trusler GA, Williams WG, Rowe RD. Pulmonary atresia and intact ventricular septum. Scand J Thorac Cardiovasc Surg 1983;17:1–28.
4. de Leval M, Bull C, Hopkins R, et al. Decision making in the definitive repair of the heart with a small right ventricle. Circulation 1985;72(Suppl II):52–60.
5. Milliken JC, Laks H, Hellenbrand W, George B, Chin A, Williams RG. Early and late results in the treatment of patients with

pulmonary atresia and intact ventricular septum. Circulation 1985;72(Suppl II):61–9.

6. O'Connor WN, Cottrill CM, Johnson CL, Noonan JA, Todd EA. Pulmonary atresia with intact ventricular septum and ventriculocoronary communications. Circulation 1982;65:805.

7. Essed CE, Klein HW, Krediet P, Vorst EJ. Coronary and endocardial fibroelastosis of the ventricles in the hypoplastic left and right heart syndromes. Virchows Arch [Pathol Anat] 1975;367:87.

8. Huhta JC, Smallhorn JF, Macartney FJ. Two dimensional echocardiographic diagnosis of situs. Br Heart J 1982;48:97–108.

9. Zuberbuhler JR, Anderson RH. Morphological variations in pulmonary atresia and intact ventricular septum. Br Heart J 1979;41:281.

10. Zuberbuhler JR, Allwork SP, Anderson RH. The spectrum of Ebstein's anomaly of the tricuspid valve. J Thorac Cardiovasc Surg 1979;77:202.

11. Androde JL, Serino W, de Leval M, Somerville J. Two dimensional echocardiographic evaluation of tricuspid hypoplasia in pulmonary atresia. Am J Cardiol 1984;53:387–8.

12. Smallhorn JF, Huhta JC, Anderson RH, Macartney FJ. Suprasternal cross-sectional echocardiography in assessment of patent ductus arteriosus. Br Heart J 1982;48:321–30.

13. Santos MA, Moll JN, Drumond C, Araujo WB, Romao N, Reis NB. Development of the ductus arteriosus in right ventricular outflow tract obstruction. Circulation 1980;62:818–22.

14. Barr PA, Celermajer JM, Bowdler JD, Cartmill TB. Severe congenital tricuspid incompetence in the neonate. Circulation 1974;49:962.

15. Bharati S, McAllister HA Jr, Chiemmongkoltip P, Lev M. Congenital pulmonary atresia with tricuspid insufficiency. Am J Cardiol 1977;40:70.

16. Freedom RM, Culham G, Moes F, Olley PM, Rowe RD. Differentiation of functional and structural pulmonary atresia: role of aortography. Am J Cardiol 1978;41:914.

17. Smallhorn JF, Izukawa T, Benson L, Freedom RM. Non-invasive recognition of functional pulmonary atresia by echocardiography. Am J Cardiol 1984;54:925–6.

18. Benson L, Smallhorn J, Freedom R, Trusler G, Rowe R. Pulmonary valve morphology after balloon dilatation of pulmonary valve stenosis. Cathet Cardiovasc Diagn 1985;11:161.

19. Klosetaky ED, Maller JH, Korns ME, Schwartz CJ, Edwards JE. Congenital pulmonary stenosis resulting from dysplasia of valve. Circulation 1969;60:43–53.

20. Oliveira Lima C, Sahn DJ, Valdes-Cruz LM, et al. Noninvasive prediction of transvalvular pressure gradient in patients with pulmonary stenosis by quantitative two-dimensional echocardiographic Doppler studies. Circulation 1983;67:866–71.

21. Stevenson JG, Kawabori I. Noninvasive determination of pressure gradients in children: two methods employing pulsed Doppler echocardiography. J Am Coll Cardiol 1984;3:179–92.

22. Vasko SD, Goldberg SJ, Requarth JA, Allen HD. Factors affecting accuracy of in vitro valvar pressure gradient estimates by Doppler ultrasound. Am J Cardiol 1984;54:893–6.

23. Garcia RE, Friedman WF, Kabock MM, Rowe RD. Idiopathic hypercalcaemia and supravalvular aortic stenosis. Documentation of a new syndrome. N Engl J Med 1964;271:117–20.

24. Tinker DD, Nanda NC, Harris PJ, Manning JA. Two dimensional echocardiographic identification of pulmonary artery branch stenosis. Am J Cardiol 1982;50:814–20.

25. Pongiglione G, Freedom RM, Cook D, Rowe RD. Mechanism of acquired right ventricular outflow tract obstruction in patients with ventricular septal defect: an angiocardiographic study. Am J Cardiol 1982;50:776–80.

26. Becker AE, Anderson RH. Pathology of congenital heart disease. London: Butterworths, 1981.

27. Von Doenhoff LJ, Nanda NC. Obstruction within the right ventricular body: two-dimensional echocardiographic features. Am J Cardiol 1983;51:1498–501.

28. Matina D, van Doesburg NH, Fouron JC, Guerin R, Davignon A. Subxiphoid two-dimensional echocardiographic diagnosis of double chambered right ventricle. Circulation 1983;67:885–8.

29. Shimada R, Tajimi T, Koyanagi S, et al. Two dimensional echocardiographic findings in double-chambered right ventricle. Am Heart J 1984;108:1059.

30. Soto B, Pacifico AD, Ceballos R, Bargeron LM Jr. Tetralogy of Fallot: an angiographic-pathologic correlative study. Circulation 1981;64:558–66.

31. Sanders SP, Bierman FZ, Williams RG. Conotruncal malformations: diagnosis in infancy using subxiphoid 2-dimensional echocardiography. Am J Cardiol 1982;50:1361–67.

32. Silove ED, de Giovanni JV. Diagnosis of right ventricular outflow obstruction in infants by cross-sectional echocardiography. Br Heart J 1983;50:416.

33. Capelli H, Somerville J. Atypical Fallot tetralogy with doubly committed subarterial ventricular septal defect. Diagnostic value of 2-dimensional echocardiography. Am J Cardiol 1983;51:282.

34. Faggian G, Frescura C, Thiene G, Bortolotti U, Mazzucco A, Anderson RH. Accessory tricuspid valve tissue causing obstruction of the ventricular septal defect in tetralogy of Fallot. Br Heart J 1983;49:324–7.

35. Di Segni E, Einzig S. Congenital absence of pulmonary valve associated with tetralogy of Fallot: diagnosis by 2 dimensional echocardiography. Am J Cardiol 1983;51:1798.

36. Huhta JC, Gutgesell HP, Latson LA, Huffines FD. Two dimensional echocardiographic assessment of the aorta in infants and children with congenital heart disease. Circulation 1984;70:417.

37. Ueda K, Nojura K, Saito A, Nakano H, Yokata M, Murooka R. Modified Blalock-Taussig shunt operation without cardiac catheterization. Two dimensional echocardiographic preoperative assessment in cyanotic infants. Am J Cardiol 1984;54:1296–99.

38. Huhta JC, Piehler JM, Tajik AJ, et al. Two dimensional echocardiographic detection of measurement of the right pulmonary artery in pulmonary atresia–ventricular septal defect: angiographic and surgical correlation. Am J Cardiol 1982;49:1235–40.

39. Freedom RM, Moes CAF, Pelech A, et al. Bilateral ductus arteriosus (or remnant): an analysis of 27 patients. Am J Cardiol 1984;53:884–91.

40. Ramsay JM, Macartney FJ, Haworth SG. Tetralogy of Fallot with major aortopulmonary collateral arteries. Br Heart J 1985;53:167–72.

41. Smallhorn JF, Zielinsky P, Freedom RM, Rowe RD. Abnormal position of the brachiocephalic vein. Am J Cardiol 1985;55:234–6.

42. Uretzky G, Puga FJ, Danielson GK, et al. Complete atrioventricular canal associated with tetralogy of Fallot. Morphologic and surgical considerations. J Thorac Cardiovasc Surg 1984;87:756–66.

43. Smallhorn JF, Anderson RH, Macartney FJ. Two dimensional echocardiographic assessment of communications between ascending aorta and pulmonary trunk or individual pulmonary arteries. Br Heart J 1982;47:463–72.

31
Complete Transposition

Jeffrey Smallhorn

A great deal of controversy has revolved around the definition of transposition of the great arteries. Classically, it was used to describe cases where the aorta arose from the right ventricle. It has also been used to describe cases where the aorta was anterior, even if it arose from a morphologically left ventricle. In the latter situation, it was called "anatomically corrected transposition." This differs from physiologically corrected transposition, which is the association of discordant atrioventricular and ventriculoarterial connections. The term "complete transposition" was introduced to avoid this confusion and is now applied to hearts with concordant atrioventricular and discordant ventriculoarterial connections, irrespective of the spatial relationships of the great arteries (1, 2).

This chapter discusses the cross-sectional echocardiographic features of complete transposition and its commonly associated anomalies. Excluded are hearts with discordant, double-inlet, absent, or ambiguous atrioventricular connections.

COMPLETE TRANSPOSITION WITH INTACT VENTRICULAR SEPTUM

The diagnosis of complete transposition is relatively easy provided a sequential segmental approach is adopted. In the subcostal cut, the relationship of the abdominal inferior vena cava and aorta permits a correct assessment of atrial arrangement in the majority of cases (3). The inferior vena cava and hepatic veins can be identified draining into the right atrium with the plane of the beam parallel to the inferior vena cava. As the transducer is rotated counterclockwise into a four-chamber cut, the pulmonary veins can be visualized draining into the left atrium. With clockwise rotation and slight superior angulation, the superior vena cava and upper part of the interatrial septum can be identified. If the scanhead is then rotated back into a four-chamber cut, the remainder of the interatrial septum can be seen, along with the atrioventricular junction and ventricles.

The presence of an atrial septal defect or patent foramen ovale can be assessed and, with Doppler interrogation, the direction of shunting and presence of restriction evaluated. This can be performed before and after balloon atrial septostomy (Fig. 31.1.), with the procedure itself performed under cross-sectional echocardiographic control (Fig. 31.1.) (4).

In many patients with complete transposition, the pulmonary valve is not wedged to the same extent as in the normal heart, resulting in the atrioventricular valves' hinging at the same level. The left ventricle has a smooth septal surface, while the right is coarsely trabeculated with septal insertions of the tricuspid valve (Fig. 31.2). If the intracardiac anatomy appears as described, considerable attention must be paid to the ventriculoarterial connections. As the transducer is scanned superiorly from the four-chamber cut, the outlet of the left ventricle can be identified. To determine whether this vessel is an aorta or pulmonary trunk, slight counterclockwise rotation is necesary in order to identify the branching of the pulmonary trunk (Fig. 31.3). The right pulmonary artery can be identified running above the left atrium, and the origin of the left pulmonary artery can be seen as far as its point of connection with the descending aorta via the ligamentum arteriosum (5). A suprasternal approach must be adopted to visualize the total length of the left pulmonary artery prior to its entry into the hilum of the lung (6).

Occasionally, both great arteries can be identified simultaneously; this depends on their spatial relationship. Invariably, the transducer must be rotated slightly counterclockwise and superiorly to identify the aorta arising from the right ventricle (Fig. 31.4). Unlike the normal heart, the aorta is supported by a muscular infundibulum, while in the majority of cases, the pul-

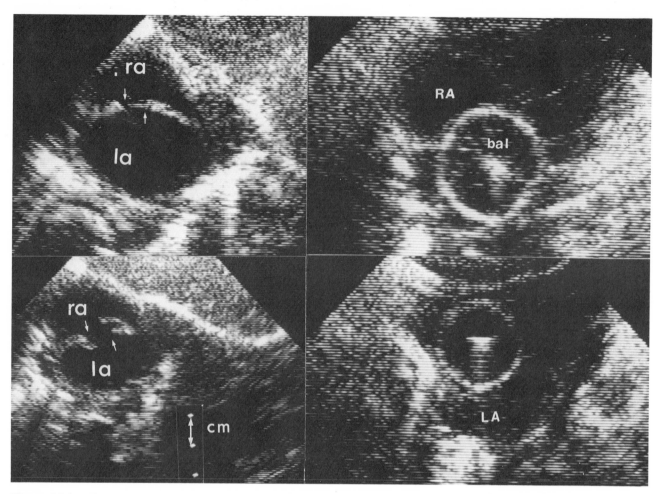

Figure 31.1. The left-hand pictures are subcostal cuts in complete transposition before and after balloon atrial septostomy. The adequate size of the interatrial communication is indicated by the arrows. The right-hand pictures are subcostal four-chamber views before and after balloon atrial septostomy. Note the balloon, which is being pulled from the left atrium to the right atrium. bal = balloon; LA = left atrium; RA = right atrium.

monary valve is in fibrous continuity with the mitral valve. The outlet septum in most patients is parallel to the rest of the muscular septum which is in contrast to the normal heart (Fig. 31.4).

From the precordial long-axis cut, the vessels are often identified running parallel to each other with the posterior vessel (pulmonary trunk) appearing to dip backward (Fig. 31.5). Prior to routine use of subcostal scans, this was one of the most useful signs of complete transposition (7). In this position, the subaortic and subpulmonary regions can be readily assessed. As the transducer is rotated into a short-axis plane, the anterior vessel does not appear to cross the posterior one, as occurs in patients with concordant ventriculoarterial connections.

If a slightly higher short-axis cut is used, the spatial relationship of the vessels can be determined. In the majority of cases, the aorta is directly anterior and slightly to the right, but it may be to the left, directly anterior, or even posterior (Fig. 31.6).

The coronary arteries may be identified from the short-axis position arising from the sinuses that face the pulmonary trunk. The right coronary artery is best visualized from a slightly lower short-axis cut with angulation to demonstrate the region of the tricuspid annulus, while the left coronary artery is best seen from a higher short-axis cut (Fig. 31.7). The position of the ostia in relationship to the sinus can be identified, along with the length of the left main coronary artery proximal to its bifurcation into the circumflex and left anterior descending branches. The most common coronary artery anomaly is when the circumflex or left anterior descending artery arises from the right coronary artery, which courses behind the pulmonary trunk to reach the left atrioventricular groove (Fig. 31.8) (8, 9).

The left ventricular cavity size and wall thickness appear normal during the first few days of life while the cavity pressure is systemic. This rapidly alters, however, and the cavity takes on a banana shape. This is

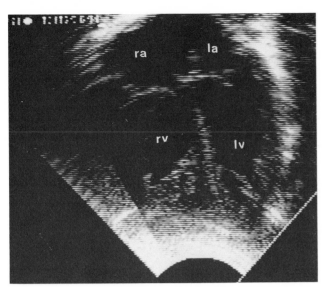

Figure 31.2. A precordial four-chamber cut in a patient with complete transposition. The heavily trabeculated chamber on the right side is the morphologic right ventricle (RV). The atrioventricular muscular septum in this case is very small, with very little offsetting of the atrioventricular valves. LA = left atrium; LV = left ventricle; RA = right atrium.

frequently associated with dynamic interventricular septal bowing (10).

The examination is completed by assessing the great arteries from the suprasternal approach. Here the anterior aorta does not appear to dip backward, as with a concordant ventriculoarterial connection, but is unfolded due to its anterior origin. The persistence of a ductus arteriosus and the presence of a thoracic coarctation can be evaluated from the suprasternal position (Fig. 31.9) (5, 11).

ASSOCIATED ABNORMALITIES

Complete Transposition with Ventricular Septal Defect

The ventricular septal defect may occur in any of the positions seen in hearts with a concordant ventriculoarterial connection. It may be perimembranous (Fig. 31.10) and extend into the inlet, trabecular, or outlet septum, or may occupy the inlet, trabecular, or outlet components of the muscular septum. One of the most important features is that the defect may be the result of malalignment between the outlet and trabecular components of the septum (12). The outlet septum may be anteriorly displaced (Fig. 31.11A), predisposing to subaortic stenosis (13, 14), or posteriorly displaced, which frequently results in subpulmonary stenosis (Fig. 31.11B) (12). In both cases, the defect may be muscular or perimembranous, depending on its extension to the area of the central fibrous body.

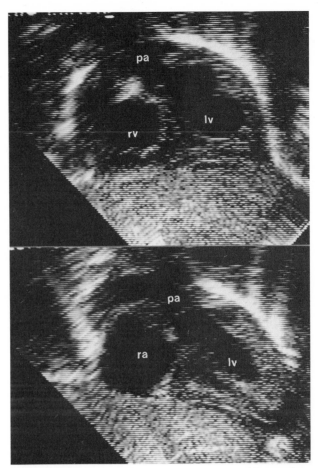

Figure 31.3. The upper picture is a subcostal long-axis cut demonstrating the pulmonary trunk arising from the morphologic left ventricle. The interventricular septum is intact. The lower picture is from the same patient with slight counterclockwise rotation demonstrating the pulmonary trunk branching. LV = left ventricle; PA = pulmonary trunk; RA = right atrium; RV = right ventricle.

Malalignment defects are best visualized in a subcostal long-axis cut or a precordial long-axis cut (Figs. 31.11 and 31.12). The anterior and posterior boundaries of the ventricular septal defect are seen from the precordial position, while the lateral aspects are best visualized from the subcostal position. To determine whether the defect is muscular or perimembranous, a combination of views is required to assess whether part of the boundary is formed by the membranous septum (compare Figs. 31.10 and 31.13). If the defect is large, systemic pressure is maintained in the left ventricle, and the wall thickness and shape remain normal. If the pressure decreases with a restrictive defect, then the shape characteristically seen with an intact ventricular septum is observed.

Abnormal chordal attachments of the tricuspid valve to the outlet septum may occur in the setting of complete transposition with a malalignment ventricular septal defect. This makes closure of the defect to

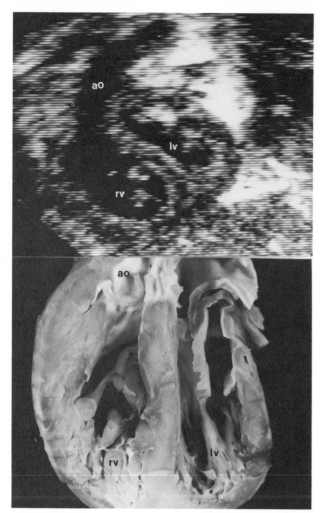

Figure 31.4.   The upper picture is a subcostal long-axis cut demonstrating the aorta arising from the morphologic right ventricle. The outlet septum is parallel to the trabecular septum. The lower picture is an anatomic specimen from a different patient demonstrating the morphologic features. AO = aorta; IS = outlet septum; LV = left ventricle; RV = right ventricle.

the aorta technically very difficult (Fig. 31.14) (15–17). This abnormality is best viewed from the subcostal long-axis cut, with some counterclockwise rotation to visualize the outlet septum in detail.

While it is not the intention of this chapter to discuss double-outlet right ventricle and subpulmonary ventricular septal defect (Taussig-Bing hearts), it may be difficult to assign a lesion correctly as complete transposition or double-outlet right ventricle unless the precise margins of the defect are described. This is described in Chapter 32. From a practical standpoint, the management depends more on the spatial relationship of the vessels than on whether the pulmonary trunk overrides the left ventricle by 49 percent or 51 percent.

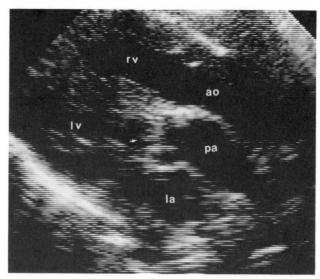

Figure 31.5.   Precordial long-axis cut demonstrating the parallel nature of the aorta (AO) and the pulmonary trunk (PA). This patient also has subaortic subpulmonary stenosis. LA = left atrium; LV = left ventricle; RV = right ventricle.

The term "posterior transposition" is often used to describe the situation where the aorta, which arises from the right ventricle, is posterior to the pulmonary trunk, which arises from the left ventricle. This occurs when the aorta is in fibrous continuity with the mitral valve through a ventricular septal defect due to attenuation of the ventriculoinfundibular fold (18, 19). The pulmonary trunk, on the other hand, is separated from the mitral valve by a prominent left-sided ventriculoinfundibular fold (Fig. 31.15).

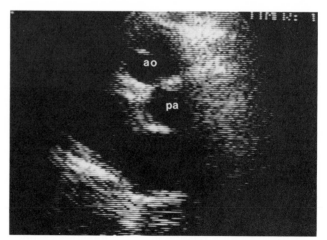

Figure 31.6.   High precordial short-axis cut demonstrating the spatial relationship of the great vessels. Note the aorta (AO) is anterior and slightly to the right of the pulmonary trunk (pa).

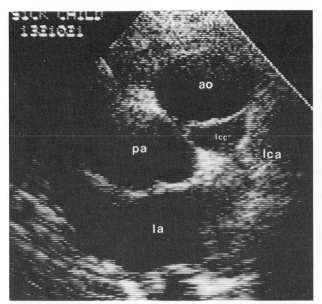

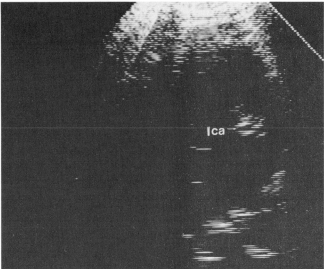

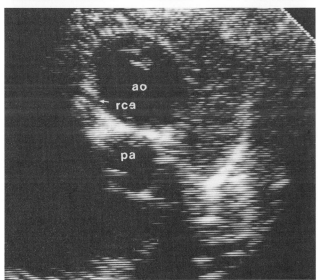

Figure 31.7. The upper left picture is a high precordial short-axis cut demonstrating the left coronary artery arising from the left coronary cusp. The picture on the right is from another patient with the gains decreased and demonstrates branching of the left coronary artery into the left anterior descending and circumflex coronary arteries. The lower picture is from yet another patient and demonstrates the right coronary artery arising from the right sinus. Ao = aorta; LA = left atrium; LCA = left coronary artery; LCC = left coronary cusp; PA = pulmonary trunk; RCA = right coronary artery.

Complete Transposition with Left Ventricular Outflow Tract Obstruction

The left ventricular outflow tract is one of the most important features when assessing a patient with complete transposition. The type of obstruction is dependent on several factors. Dynamic obstruction in the presence of an intact septum is the most common anomaly (20, 21). Due to the low pressure in the left ventricle, the interventricular septum bows into the left ventricular outflow tract. This produces a Venturi effect, with a resultant pressure drop across this region (Fig. 31.16). Systolic anterior motion of the mitral valve apparatus may occur in a similar fashion to a patient with hypertrophic obstructive cardiomyopathy.

It is important to determine whether there is any fixed component to the left ventricular outflow tract obstruction. This is best evaluated from a precordial long-axis cut using the highest frequency transducer available. During diastole, the outflow tract should be free of tensor apparatus or any other echo-dense structures to establish unequivocally the presence of dynamic narrowing (Fig. 31.16). This is important when considering a patient as a suitable candidate for an arterial switch operation, with or without prior preparation of the left ventricle. Fixed obstruction may be due to a fibromuscular shelf on the crest of the septum, abnormal chordal attachments from the mitral valve, aneurysms of the membranous septum, or posterior deviation of the outlet septum (Fig. 31.17) (12). Occasionally, tricuspid valve tissue may herniate through a small ventricular septal defect, due to the systemic pressure in the right ventricle (Fig. 31.18). The key feature in all of these abnormalities is that an abnormality in the subpulmonary region is invariably visual-

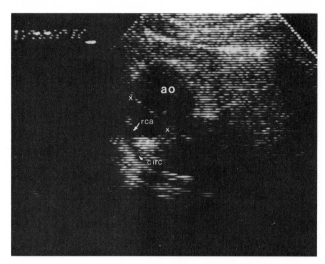

Figure 31.8. A high precordial short-axis cut demonstrating the circumflex coronary artery (CIRC) arising from the right coronary artery (RCA). Ao = aorta.

ized during diastole. Tensor apparatus has thin filamentous echoes across the whole outflow tract while those from an aneurysmal membranous septum or tricuspid tissue appear from the roof of the septum (22). Occasionally, an element of dynamic or fixed obstruction can be exaggerated by a persistent left-sided ventriculoinfundibular fold that separates the mitral from the pulmonary valve and results in a tunnel type of narrowing.

Posterior deviation of the outlet septum is the result of a malalignment ventricular septal defect and may occur with or without an element of valve or annular hypoplasia (21).

Subaortic Stenosis

Subaortic stenosis in the setting of complete transposition may be the result of anterior deviation of the

outlet septum in cases with ventricular septal defect. Subaortic obstruction may also be due to a prominent right-sided ventriculoinfundibular fold separating the tricuspid and aortic valves, or muscle bands in the subaortic region (Fig. 31.19) (13, 14, 21).

These abnormalities are best evaluated by a precordial long-axis cut to assess the anterior deviation of the outlet septum (Fig. 31.11A) and any component from the right ventricular free wall. A subcostal long-axis cut with counterclockwise rotation is used to assess the ventriculoinfundibular fold and the outlet septum (Fig. 31.19) depending on the spatial relationship of the great arteries (21).

Straddling Atrioventricular Valves

By definition, straddling occurs when tensor apparatus from an atrioventricular valve is shared by both ventricles. In patients with complete transposition and ventricular septal defect, the mitral valve straddles through an anterior defect (Fig. 31.20), while the tricuspid valve straddles through a posterior perimembranous inlet ventricular septal defect (Fig. 31.21) (23, 24). Each may be associated with atrioventricular valve annular overriding. In cases with a straddling tricuspid valve, the posterior interventricular septum invariably does not run to the crux of the heart. The practical significance of this is that the right ventricle may be hypoplastic and the conduction axis abnormally positioned.

A straddling mitral valve is frequently associated with a cleft in its anterior leaflet, with chords from part of the divided leaflet inserting into the right ventricle (25, 26). This is best viewed in a precordial long-axis cut during real time, where thin echoes from the tensor apparatus can be seen passing through the defect. Care must be taken not to confuse the mitral with the tricuspid apparatus, particularly when the latter inserts

Figure 31.9. Suprasternal cut demonstrating the parallel nature of the aorta (AO) and pulmonary trunk (MPA) with a moderate-size patent ductus arteriosus (DA).

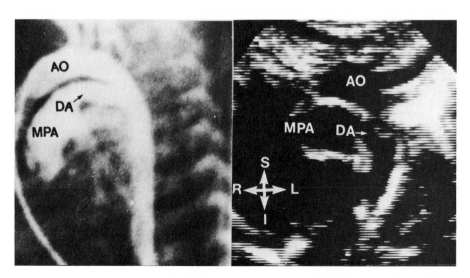

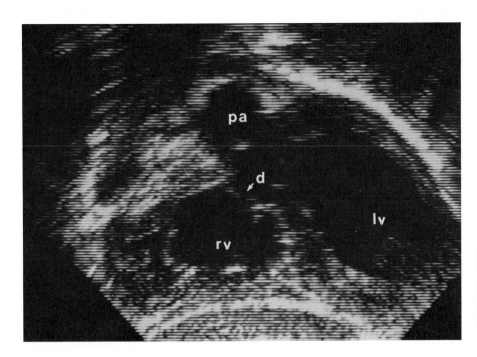

Figure 31.10. Subcostal long-axis cut in complete transposition demonstrating a perimembranous ventricular septal defect (d) roofed by the pulmonary valve. LV = left ventricle; PA = pulmonary trunk; RV = right ventricle.

into the outlet septum (Fig. 31.20). The cleft in the mitral valve is best viewed in a precordial short-axis cut. The tensor apparatus arising from the edges of the mitral valve can be seen heading toward the ventricular septal defect (Fig. 31.20).

A straddling tricuspid valve is best seen in a precordial or subcostal four-chamber cut (Fig. 31.21). The degree of annular overriding can be evaluated as the transducer is angled posteriorly. The appearance is similar to that of an atrioventricular septal defect, with the tricuspid septal leaflet straddling the defect. As the transducer is angled anteriorly, the straddling is not appreciated as the anterior septal component is usually intact.

Other Associated Lesions

Juxtaposition of the atrial appendages is most often seen in association with a ventricular septal defect, particularly when the aorta is left sided. This anomaly is best recognized from the suprasternal or subcostal cut. From the suprasternal frontal plane cut, the atrial appendage can be seen swinging to the right behind the arterial trunks. This may be important surgically when considering a Mustard operation as the right atrium is reduced in size (27).

The most commonly associated anomaly is a patent ductus arteriosus, which can be imaged from the suprasternal cut. Using this approach in combination with pulsed Doppler interrogation, the ductal size and shunting pattern can be evaluated (Fig. 31.9).

Associated arch anomalies occur in approximately 5 percent of cases. These include coarctation, tubular hypoplasia, and interrupted aortic arch (14). The association of subaortic stenosis and arch anomalies often go hand in hand, and each should be actively sought if the other is identified. Arch anomalies are best assessed from the suprasternal approach in combination with pulsed Doppler examination (11). While most cases with complete transposition have a left arch, a right arch may be present, particularly in association with pulmonary stenosis and ventricular septal defect.

Rarely, atrioventricular septal defect may be associated with complete transposition. This is readily identified by the morphology of the atrioventricular valves, which have the characteristic five-leaflet configuration, with the anterosuperior and posteroinferior bridging leaflets shared by both ventricles (Fig. 31.22) (28). These are best identified in the subcostal and precordial short-axis cuts and must be differentiated from straddling morphologic mitral and tricuspid valves. One of the main differentiating features is that the cleft points toward the right ventricle in an atrioventricular septal defect, whereas with a straddling mitral valve, the cleft in the anterior leaflet points toward the outflow tract and not to the right ventricle. In those cases with a straddling tricuspid valve (although that leaflet may be confusing when scanning posteriorly), the left-sided leaflet has the fish-mouth configuration of a mitral valve.

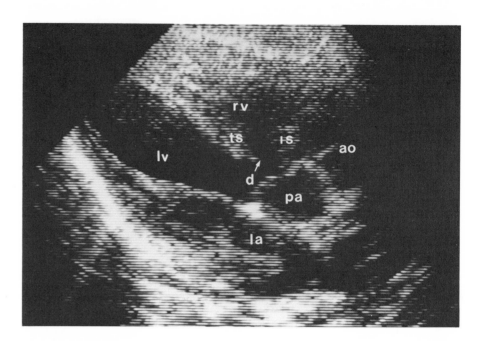

A

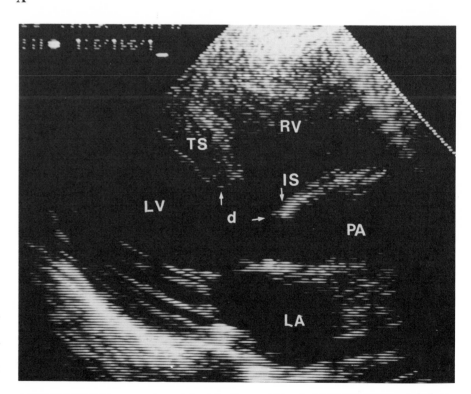

Figure 31.11. (*A*) Precordial long-axis cut demonstrating anterior deviation of the outlet septum, producing subaortic narrowing. (*B*) Precordial long-axis cut demonstrating posterior deviation of the outlet septum. ao = aorta; d = ventricular septal defect; IS = outlet septum; LA = left atrium; LV = left ventricle; PA = pulmonary trunk; RV = right ventricle; TS = trabecular septum.

B

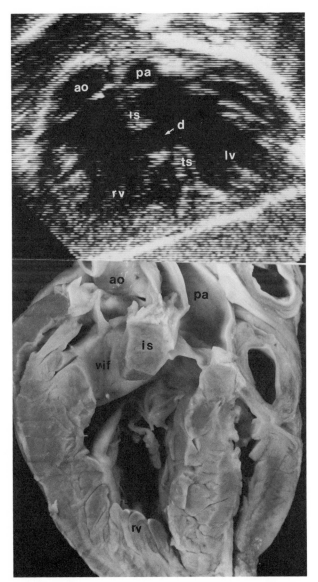

Figure 31.12.   Subcostal long-axis cut demonstrating malalignment between the outlet (IS) and trabecular septa
(TS). AO = aorta; d = ventricular septal defect; LV = left
ventricle; PA = pulmonary trunk; RV = right ventricle.

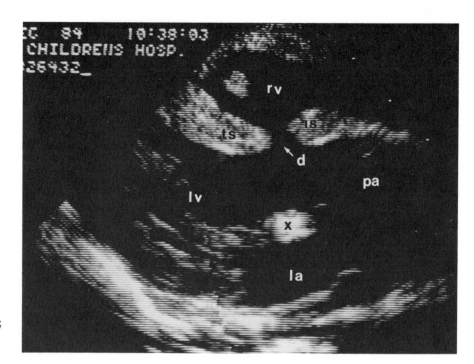

Figure 31.13. Precordial long-axis cut demonstrating a muscular malalignment ventricular septal defect (d). IS = outlet septum; LA = left atrium; LV = left ventricle; PA = pulmonary trunk; RV = right ventricle; TS = trabecular septum.

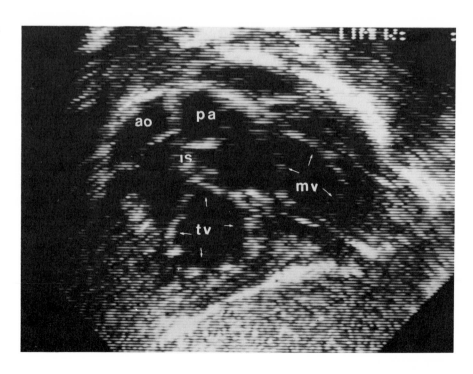

Figure 31.14. Subcostal long-axis cut demonstrating tricuspid tissue inserted on the outlet septum (IS) blocking the ventricular septal defect. AO = aorta; mv = mitral valve; PA = pulmonary trunk; tv = tricuspid valve.

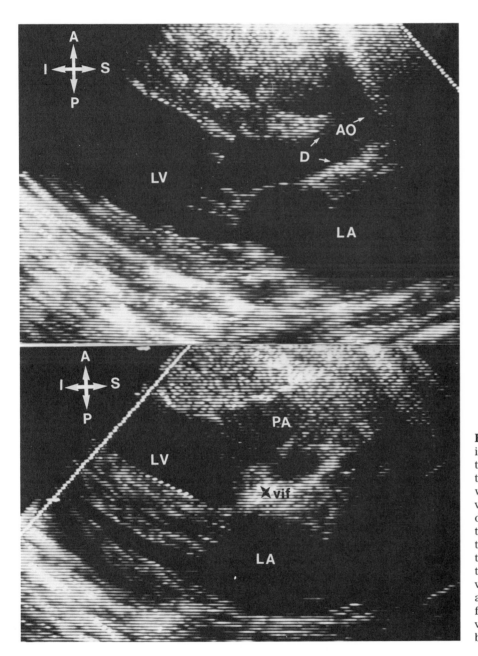

Figure 31.15. The upper picture is a precordial long-axis cut in posterior transposition demonstrating the posterior position of the aorta, which is continuous with the mitral valve through the ventricular septal defect. The lower picture is from the same patient and demonstrates the significant separation between the mitral valve and pulmonary trunk due to the left side of the ventriculoinfundibular fold. AO = aorta; D = ventricular septal defect; LA = left atrium; LV = left ventricle; VIF = ventriculoinfundibular fold.

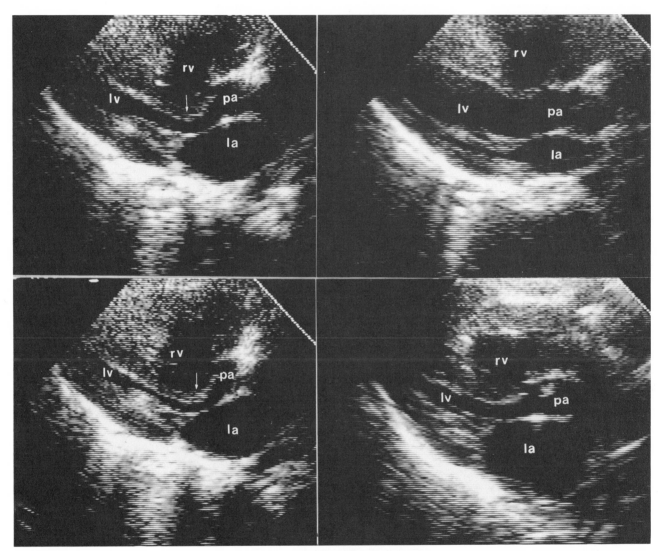

Figure 31.16. The upper left picture is a precordial long-axis cut in complete transposition prior to the onset of systole. The lower left picture is during early systole and demonstrates the interventricular septum bowing into the left ventricular outflow tract (*arrow*). The upper right picture is during midsystole, and the lower right picture is during late systole and demonstrates severe bowing of the interventricular septum and the left ventricular outflow tract. LA = left atrium; LV = left ventricle; PA = pulmonary trunk; RV = right ventricle.

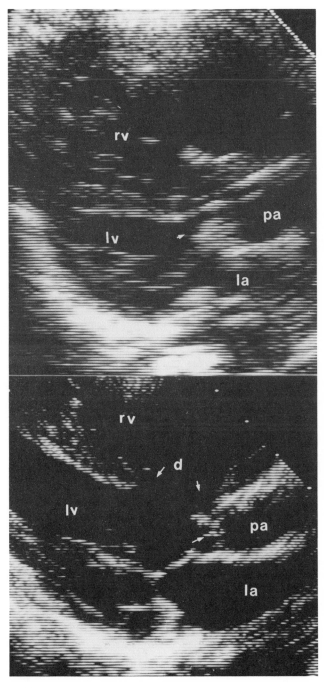

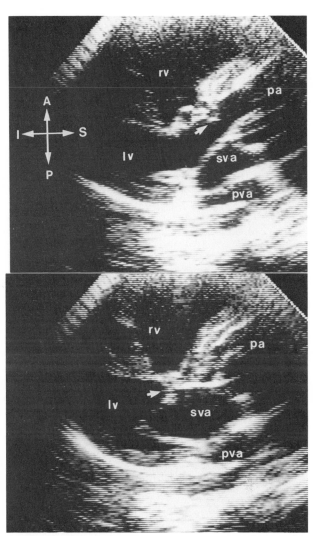

Figure 31.17.   Precordial long-axis cut with a fixed sub-pulmonary stenosis due to a prominent left-sided ventriculoinfundibular fold and a fibromuscular ridge. The lower picture is from a different patient with a ventricular septal defect with posterior deviation of the outlet septum and a fibromuscular component of subpulmonary stenosis. d = ventricular septal defect (arrows); LA = left atrium; LV = left ventricle; PA = pulmonary trunk; RV = right ventricle.

Figure 31.18.   The upper picture is a precordial long-axis cut demonstrating tricuspid valve herniating through a small ventricular septal defect into the left ventricular outflow tract. The lower picture is from the same patient during systole demonstrating dynamic left ventricular outflow tract obstruction with associated systolic anterior motion of the mitral valve. The tricuspid valve is indicated by the white arrow. LV = left ventricle; PA = pulmonary trunk; PVA = pulmonary venous atrium; SVA = systemic venous atrium; RV = right ventricle.

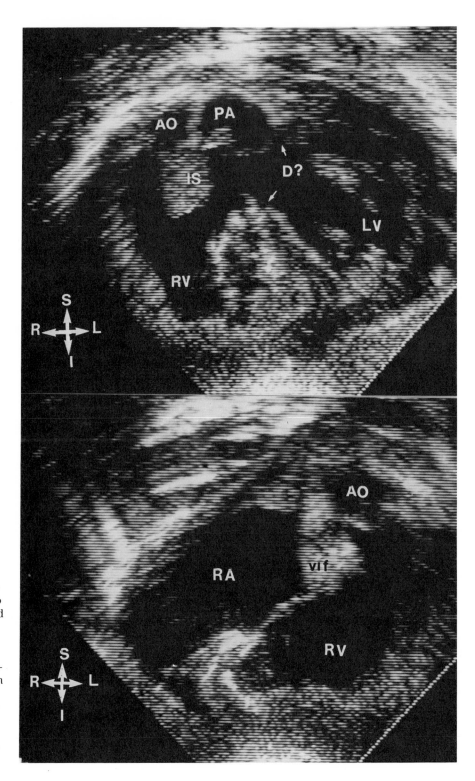

Figure 31.19. The upper picture is a subcostal long-axis cut demonstrating subaortic narrowing due to a combination of outlet septum and right-sided ventriculoinfundibular fold. The lower picture from the same patient with counterclockwise rotation shows the very prominent ventriculoinfundibular fold on the right side. AO = aorta; D = ventricular septal defect; IS = outlet septum; LV = left ventricle; PA = pulmonary trunk; RA = right atrium; RV = right ventricle; VIF = ventriculoinfundibular fold.

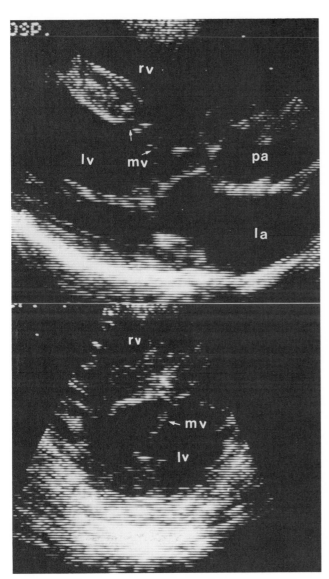

Figure 31.20.   Precordial long-axis cut in a case with transposition, ventricular septal defect, left ventricular outflow tract obstruction, and straddling mitral valve. Note that the mitral valve tensor apparatus traverses the ventricular septal defect to insert into the right side of the outlet septum. The lower picture is a precordial short-axis cut demonstrating a tensor apparatus from the straddling mitral valve. LA = left atrium; LV = left ventricle; mv = mitral valve; PA = pulmonary trunk; RV = right ventricle.

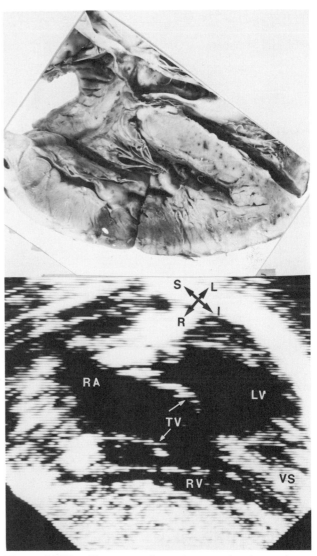

Figure 31.21.   The upper picture is an anatomic specimen cut in the subcostal four-chamber view demonstrating a straddling tricuspid valve. The lower picture is from a different patient and demonstrates the anatomic features. Note that there is hypoplasia of the morphologic right ventricle. LA = left atrium; LV = left ventricle; RA = right atrium; RV = right ventricle; TV = tricuspid valve.

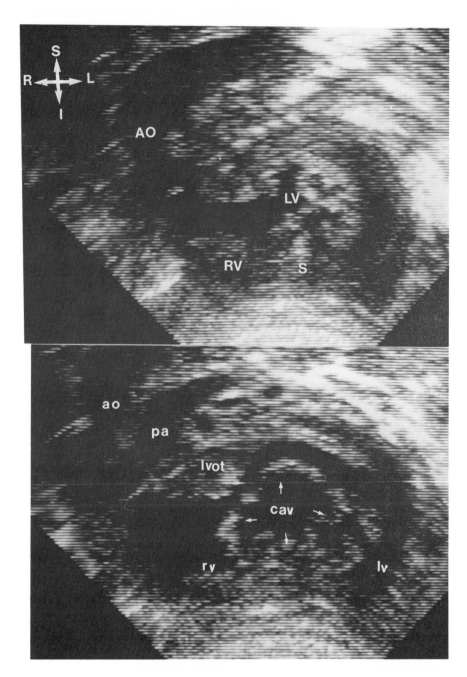

Figure 31.22.   The upper picture is a subcostal long-axis cut demonstrating the aorta arising from the morphologic right ventricle in a patient with the associated complete atrioventricular septal defect. The lower picture from the same patient demonstrates the pulmonary trunk arising from the left ventricle. This patient also has subpulmonary stenosis. AO = aorta; CAV = common atrioventricular valve; LV = left ventricle; LVOT = left ventricular outflow tract; PA = pulmonary trunk; RV = right ventricle; S = interventricular septum.

REFERENCES

1. Tynan MJ, Anderson RH. Terminology of transposition of the great arteries. In: Godman MJ, Marquis RM, eds. Paediatric cardiology. Vol 2. Heart disease in the newborn. Edinburgh: Churchill Livingstone, 1979.
2. Tynan MJ, Becker AE, Macartney FJ, Quero-Juninez M, Shinebourne EA, Anderson RH. Nomenclature and classification of congenital heart disease. Br Heart J 1979;41:544.
3. Huhta JC, Smallhorn JF, Macartney FJ. Two dimensional echocardiographic diagnosis of situs. Br Heart J 1982;48:97–108.
4. Allan LD, Leanage R, Wainwright R, Joseph MC, Tynan M. Balloon atrial septostomy under two dimensional echocardiographic control. Br Heart J 1982;47:41–3.
5. Bierman FZ, Williams RG. Prospective diagnosis of d-transposition of the great arteries in neonates by subxiphoid two dimensional echocardiography. Circulation 1979;60:1496–502.
6. Smallhorn JF, Huhta JC, Anderson RH, Macartney FJ. Suprasternal cross-sectional echocardiography in assessment of patent ductus arteriosus. Br Heart J 1982;48:321–30.
7. Houston AB, Gregory NL, Coleman NE. Echocardiographic identification of aorta and main pulmonary artery in complete transposition. Br Heart J 1978;40:377–82.
8. Yacoub MH, Radley-Smith R. Anatomy of the coronary arteries in transposition of the great arteries and methods for their transfer in anatomical correction. Thorax 1978;33:418–24.
9. Shaher RM. Complete transposition of the great arteries. New York: Academic Press, 1973.
10. Huhta JC, Edwards WD, Feldt RH, Puga FJ. Left ventricular wall thickness in complete transposition of the great arteries. J Thorac Cardiovasc Surg 1982;84:97–101.
11. Smallhorn JF, Huhta JC, Adams PA, Anderson RH, Wilkinson JL, Macartney FJ. Cross-sectional echocardiographic assessment of coarctation in the sick neonate and infant. Br Heart J 1983;50:349–61.
12. Becker AE, Anderson RH. Pathology of congenital heart disease.

In: Crawford T, ed. Post graduate pathology series. London: Butterworths, 1981.

13. Moene RJ, Oppenheimer-Dekker A, Bartelings MM. Anatomical obstruction of the right ventricular outflow tract in transposition of the great arteries. Am J Cardiol 1983;51:1071–74.

14. Vogel M, Freedom RM, Smallhorn JF, Williams WG, Trusler GA, Rowe RD. Complete transposition of the great arteries and coarctation of the aorta. Am J Cardiol 1984;53:1627–32.

15. Huhta JC, Edwards WD, Danielson GK, Feldt RH. Abnormalities of the tricuspid valve in complete transposition of the great arteries with ventricular septal defect. J Thorac Cardiovasc Surg 1982;83:569–76.

16. Huhta JC, Smallhorn JF, de Leval MR, Macartney FJ. Tricuspid valve abnormalities in DORV with subpulmonic VSD. letter. J Thorac Cardiovasc Surg 1982;84:154–5.

17. Deal BJ, Chin AJ, Sanders SP, Norwood WI, Castaneda AR. Subxiphoid two-dimensional echocardiographic identification of tricuspid valve abnormalities in transposition of the great arteries with ventricular septal defect. Am J Cardiol 1985;55:1146–52.

18. Wilkinson JL, Arnold R, Anderson RH, Acerete F. Posterior transposition reconsidered. Br Heart J 1975;37:757–66.

19. Van Praagh R, Perez-Trevino C, Lopez-Cuellar M, et al. Transposition of the great arteries with posterior aorta, anterior pulmonary artery, subpulmonary conus and fibrous continuity between aortic and atrioventricular valves. Am J Cardiol 1971;28:621–31.

20. Chin AJ, Yeager SB, Sanders SP, et al. Accuracy of prospective two-dimensional echocardiographic evaluation of left ventricular outflow tract in complete transposition of the great arteries. J Thorac Cardiovasc Surg 1984;87:66–73.

21. Marino B, De Simone G, Pasquini L, et al. Complete transposition of the great arteries: visualization of left and right outflow tract obstruction by oblique subcostal two-dimensional echocardiography. Am J Cardiol 1985;55:1140–5.

22. Ilbawi MN, Quinn K, Idriss FS, et al. The surgical management of left ventricular outflow tract obstruction due to tricuspid valve pouch in complete transposition of the great arteries. J Thorac Cardiovasc Surg 1984;87:66–73.

23. Smallhorn JF, Tommasini G, Macartney FJ. Detection and assessment of straddling and overriding atrioventricular valves by two-dimensional echocardiography. Br Heart J 1981;46:254–62.

24. Milo S, Ho SY, Macartney FJ, et al. Straddling and overriding atrioventricular valves: morphology and classification. Am J Cardiol 1979;44:1122–34.

25. Moene RJ, Oppenheimer-Dekker A. Congenital mitral valve anomalies in transposition of the great arteries. Am J Cardiol 1972;49:1972–8.

26. Smallhorn JF, de Leval M, Stark J, et al. Isolated anterior mitral cleft. Two dimensional echocardiographic assessment and differentiation from "clefts" associated with atrioventricular septal defect. Br Heart J 1982;48:109–16.

27. Wood AE, Freedom RM, Williams WG, Trusler GA. The Mustard procedure in transposition of the great arteries associated with juxtaposition of the atrial appendages with and without dextrocardia. J Thorac Cardiovasc Surg 1983;85:451–6.

28. Smallhorn JF, Tommasini G, Anderson RH, Macartney FJ. Assessment of atrioventricular septal defects by two dimensional echocardiography. Br Heart J 1982;47:109–21.

32

Double-Outlet Right Ventricle

Jeffrey Smallhorn

By definition, double-outlet right ventricle describes only the ventriculoarterial connection. This comprises all hearts in which more than half of the circumference of both the aortic and pulmonary valves is connected to the right ventricle. The presence of a bilaterally complete infundibulum is frequently associated with double-outlet right ventricle (1), but is not a prerequisite for the diagnosis.

The key to double-outlet right ventricle lies in understanding the intricate relationships between the aorta, pulmonary trunk, and ventricular septal defect. These in turn are dictated by 1) the components of the outlet septum, which separates the subaortic and subpulmonary outflow tracts; 2) the ventriculoinfundibular fold, which separates arterial from atrioventricular valves; and 3) the anterior and posterior limbs of the septomarginal trabeculation (2–4).

Traditionally, hearts have been subdivided according to the position of the ventricular septal defect in relationship to the aorta and pulmonary trunk. In hearts with a subaortic, subpulmonary, or doubly committed defect, the defect lies cradled between the limbs of the septomarginal trabeculation. Therefore, it is the size and orientation of the outlet septum that determine whether the defect is closest to the aorta or pulmonary trunk, or equally related to both. In the group of noncommitted defects, the ventricular septal defect is remote from the great arteries. Frequently, it lies in the inlet septum and may be associated with an atrioventricular septal defect. The ventricular septal defect may be perimembranous if part of its border is the region of mitral-tricuspid or tricuspid-aortic continuity. A muscular defect, by definition, is completely surrounded by muscular boundaries. Hearts with double-outlet right ventricle may exist with any type of atrioventricular connection, that is, concordant, discor-

dant, ambiguous, double inlet, or absence of one connection. This chapter discusses only those hearts with concordant atrioventricular connection.

GENERAL ECHOCARDIOGRAPHIC APPROACH

A combination of subcostal and precordial cuts is essential to define the position and boundaries of the ventricular septal defect, the spatial relationship of the great arteries, and the subaortic and subpulmonary regions.

The echocardiographic examination always begins with an evaluation of atrial arrangement and systemic and pulmonary venous connections from the subcostal position. Following determination of atrial arrangement, a subcostal four-chamber cut is obtained to assess the posterior aspects of the interventricular septum and the atrioventricular valves. The transducer is rotated clockwise to assess the outlet of the left ventricle (ventricular septal defect) and its spatial relationship to the great artery. In this position, the presence or absence of a left-sided or right-sided ventriculoinfundibular fold can be determined (Fig. 32.1) (5, 6).

The scanhead is then moved to the precordium to obtain a high short-axis cut at the level of the great arteries. The transducer is moved from base to apex in an attempt to assess the spatial relationships of the great arteries to the ventricular septal defect (Fig. 32.2) (7, 8). The outlet septum, right-sided ventriculoinfundibular fold, and presence or absence of mitral-tricuspid continuity can be assessed from this view. The transducer is then placed in a long-axis plane at the level of the left ventricular outflow tract (ventricular septal defect) (7). From this position, the presence or absence of a left-sided ventriculoinfundibular fold and

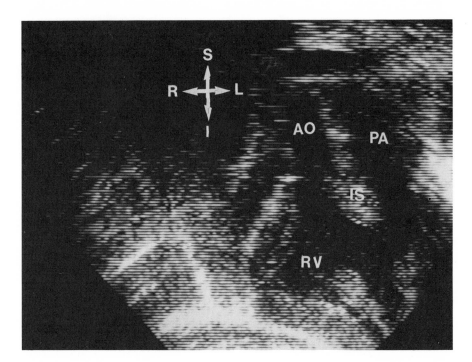

Figure 32.1. A subcostal cut with counterclockwise rotation of the transducer in a patient with double-outlet right ventricle (RV). Note that the left ventricle is not visualized in this image. The outlet septum (IS) is clearly seen separating the aortic and pulmonary valves. Note that the subaortic and subpulmonary regions are well visualized in this cut. AO = aorta; PA = pulmonary trunk.

the relationship of the arterial valves to the ventricular septal defect can be assessed, as can the degree of commitment of the aorta and pulmonary trunk to the left ventricle (Fig. 32.3).

SUBAORTIC VENTRICULAR SEPTAL DEFECT

In the subcostal long-axis cut, the outlet septum is seen to fuse with the anterior limb of the septomarginal trabeculation, thereby excluding the pulmonary valve from any relationship with the ventricular septal defect (Fig. 32.4). It may be difficult in this cut to define the outlet septum and ventriculoinfundibular fold as the two merge (Fig. 32.5). In patients with doubly committed ventricular septal defects, a similar appearance may be seen (Fig. 32.6) when there is complete absence of the outlet septum. Hence, the outlet septum may be seen to deviate toward the left, but once the ventricular septal defect is visualized, it is difficult to outline its borders. Only the floor and roof of the ventricular septal defect are seen in this cut. The floor is the crest of the trabecular septum, while the roof is either the aortic valve or right-sided ventriculoinfundibular fold. The anterior margins of the defect are not seen. Therefore, it is difficult to assign the diagnosis of double-outlet right ventricle using this cut alone.

In the precordial short-axis cut, the roof and the anterior and the posterior borders can be seen (Fig. 32.2). The floor is not visualized because it is not transected by the ultrasound beam.

The roof is the same structure seen in the subcostal long-axis cut. The posterior border is part of the posterior limb of the septomarginal trabeculation and the point of tricuspid-aortic continuity or the right-sided ventriculoinfundibular fold if it is present.

The anterior wall is formed by the region of fusion between the outlet septum and the anterior limb of the septomarginal trabeculation (Fig. 32.2). In the precordial long-axis cut, the floor is part of the trabecular septum and the roof part of either the aortic valve or left-sided ventriculoinfundibular fold (Fig. 32.3). Although this cut is the traditional approach for assigning the diagnosis of double-outlet right ventricle, it does not demonstrate the anterior margins of the defect.

SUBPULMONARY VENTRICULAR SEPTAL DEFECT

In the subcostal long-axis cut, the outlet septum can be seen to deviate to the right side to fuse with the ventriculoinfundibular fold (Fig. 32.7) (5). This results in the defect being related to the pulmonary trunk. The floor of the defect is the trabecular septum, and the roof is either the pulmonary valve or the ventriculoinfundibular fold. As in the subaortic defects, the anterior margins of the defect cannot be seen in this cut; hence, assigning the diagnosis of double-outlet right ventricle using the subcostal long-axis cut alone is difficult.

In a precordial short-axis cut, the roof of the defect is seen to be formed by the ventriculoinfundibular fold

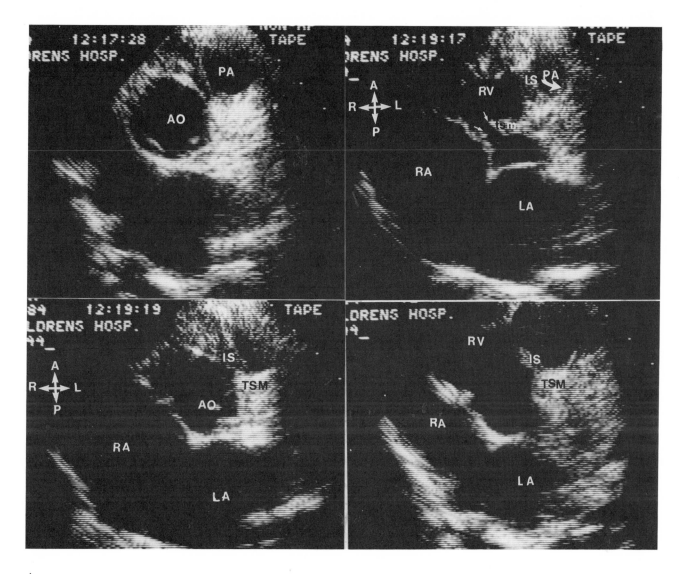

A

Figure 32.2.   (A) A series of short-axis views in a patient with double-outlet right ventricle and subaortic ventricular septal defect. The upper left-hand picture demonstrates the spatial relationship of the great arteries with the pulmonary trunk anterior and to the left. The bottom left-hand picture is a slightly lower cut demonstrating the outlet septum fusing with the anterior limb of the septomarginal trabeculation. The upper right-hand picture is a short-axis cut at a slightly lower plane demonstrating the margins of the ventricular septal defect indicated by the white arrows. The bottom right-hand picture is at an even lower cut demonstrating the outlet septum fusing with the anterior limb of the septomarginal trabeculation. The anterior mitral leaflet and more of the margins of the ventricular septal defect can be visualized. Note that in the upper left-hand picture, the semilunar valves are visualized. However, in the upper right-hand image where the margins of the ventricular septal defect are just visualized, the great arteries are not seen. This clearly indicates that the great arteries both originate from the right ventricle.

or pulmonary valve. Similar to the subaortic defect, the floor is not visualized in this cut. The outlet septum deviates to the right to fuse with the right-sided ventriculoinfundibular fold and forms the rightward wall of the defect (Fig. 32.8). The posterior margins of the defect are the same as in patients with a subaortic ventricular septal defect. The anterior margin is formed

by the point of fusion between the anterior limb of the septomarginal trabeculation, the free wall of the right ventricle, and the pulmonary valve.

In the precordial long-axis cut, the floor is seen to be formed by the crest of the trabecular septum, while the roof is formed by the left-sided ventriculoinfundibular fold separating the mitral from the pulmonary valve.

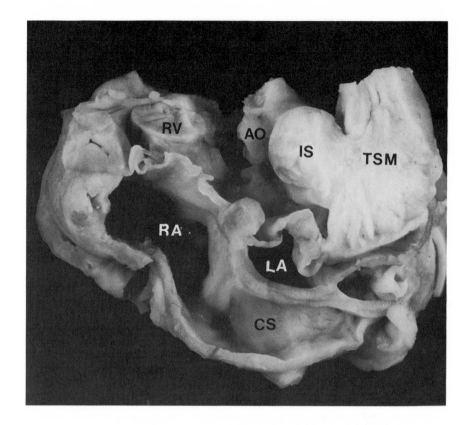

B

Figure 32.2, (cont'd.)   (*B*) The anatomic specimen is from a different patient with double-outlet right ventricle and sub-aortic ventricular septal defect. The anatomic specimen has been cut in a short-axis plan. Note the outlet septum fusing with the anterior limb of the septomarginal trabeculation. Note also that the anterior mitral leaflet is in fibrous continuity with aortic valve, making this a perimembranous VSD. This patient also has a large left coronary sinus draining into the right atrium. AO = aorta; CS = coronary sinus; IS = outlet septum; LA = left atrium; PA = pulmonary trunk; RA = right atrium; RV = right ventricle; TSM = septomarginal trabeculation.

Figure 32.3.   Precordial long-axis cut in double-outlet right ventricle (RV) and subaortic ventricular septal defect. Note that the aorta (AO) is committed to the RV by more than 50 percent. LA = left atrium; LV = left ventricle.

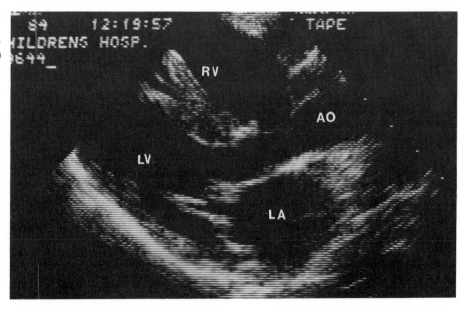

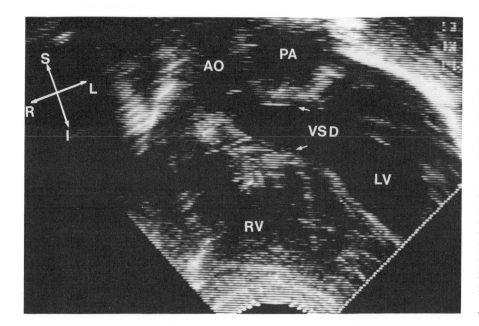

Figure 32.4. Subcostal long-axis cut in double-outlet right ventricle and subaortic ventricular septal defect. Note that the ventricular septal defect appears to be related to the aortic valve with the outlet septum fusing with the anterior limb of the septomarginal trabeculation and left-sided ventriculoinfundibular fold. In this cut, however, it is difficult to differentiate outlet septum and ventriculoinfundibular fold. Compare this and Figure 32.5 from a subaortic ventricular septal defect with Figure 32.6 from a doubly committed subarterial ventricular septal defect with no outlet septum. AO = aorta; PA = pulmonary trunk; RV = right ventricle; LV = Left ventricle.

DOUBLY COMMITTED VENTRICULAR SEPTAL DEFECT

In doubly committed ventricular septal defect, the ventricular septal defect lies in the same position as those in cases with subaortic or subpulmonary defects, but the outlet septum is either very small or absent, resulting in both the aorta and pulmonary trunk being related to the ventricular septal defect.

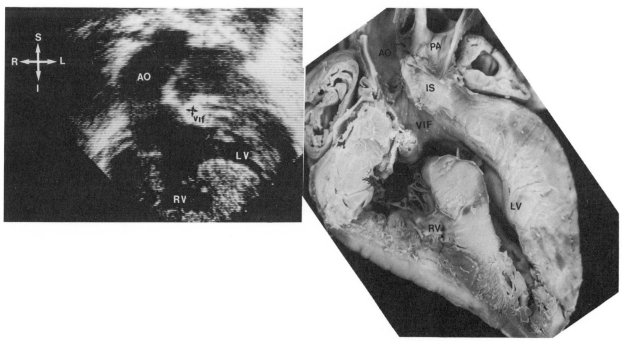

Figure 32.5. The left-hand picture is a subcostal long-axis cut in double-outlet right ventricle and subaortic ventricular septal defect. Note the prominent left-sided ventriculoinfundibular fold (VIF) indicated by the arrows. On the right is an anatomic specimen from a different patient cut in a similar projection. Note that there is subaortic narrowing due to a prominent right-sided ventriculoinfundibular fold separating the tricuspid from aortic valve which fuses with the left-sided VIF and anterior limb of septomarginal trabeculation. Note also that the outlet septum separates the pulmonary valve from the aortic valve. The precise margins of the ventricular septal defect are difficult to see in this specimen, as the anterior component of the heart has been removed. AO = aorta; IS = outlet septum; LV = left ventricle; PA = pulmonary trunk; RV = right ventricle; VIF = ventriculoinfundibular fold.

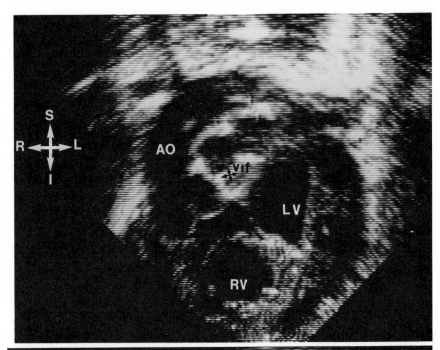

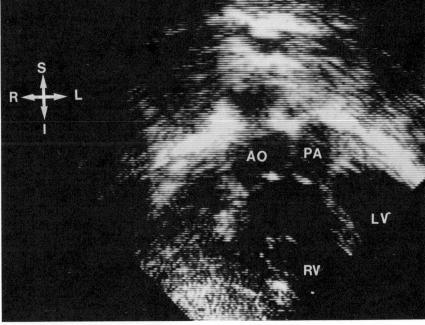

Figure 32.6. The upper picture is a subcostal long-axis cut in double-outlet right ventricle and doubly committed ventricular septal defect. In this view, the appearance is very similar to that in cases with a subaortic ventricular septal defect in that the aorta appears to be related to the ventricular septal defect. The lower picture is from the same patient with counterclockwise rotation that demonstrates no outlet septum separating the aortic and pulmonary valves. The combination of ventriculoinfundibular fold and the anterior limb of the septomarginal trabeculation appears to block the pulmonary trunk from the margins of the ventricular septal defect. AO = aorta; LA = left atrium; LV = left ventricle; PA = pulmonary trunk; RV = right ventricle; VIF = ventriculoinfundibular fold.

In the subcostal long-axis cut, the outlet septum, if present, does not fuse with the anterior or posterior limb of the septomarginal trabeculation (Figs. 32.6 and 32.9). With clockwise rotation, both great arteries appear to be related to the ventricular septal defect, although one artery frequently appears closer, depending on the spatial relationships.

The floor of the defect is the crest of the septum, while the roof is either the ventriculoinfundibular fold or an arterial valve. As with subaortic and subpulmonary defects, the anterior margins of the defect are not seen.

The roof, anterior and posterior borders are seen in the precordial short-axis cut. The roof is the same structure seen in the subcostal cut, while the anterior border is the point of fusion between the anterior limb of the septomarginal trabeculation and an arterial valve (Fig. 32.10).

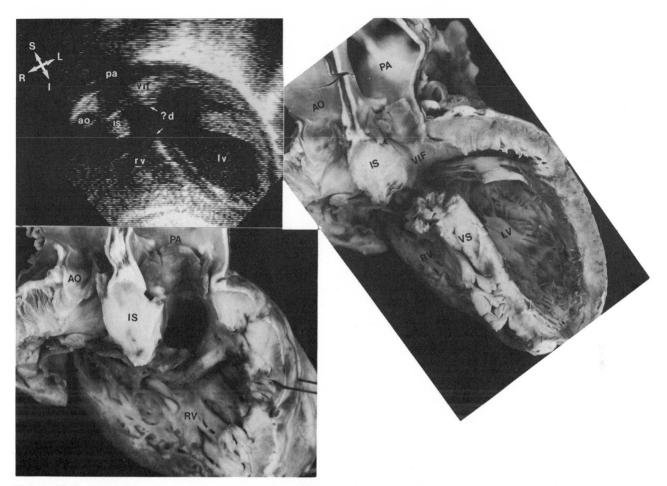

Figure 32.7. The left-hand picture is a subcostal long-axis cut in double-outlet right ventricle and subpulmonary ventricular septal defect. Note that the outlet septum is deviated to the right, bringing the margins of the ventricular septal defect in alignment with the pulmonary trunk. Note the outlet septum separates the aorta from the pulmonary trunk. It is difficult to define the exact margins of the ventricular septal defect in this cut. The image on the right is a simulated long-axis cut in double-outlet right ventricle and subpulmonary ventricular septal defect. Note the similar features of the echocardiogram with the outlet septum fusing with the ventriculoinfundibular fold. Note that the ventriculoarterial connection can be altered, depending on where the margins of ventricular septal defect are placed. If the margins are placed between the crest of the IVS and the outlet septum, then it becomes a transposition and ventricular septal defect. If the margins are placed between the ventriculoinfundibular fold and the septomarginal trabeculation, then it becomes a double-outlet right ventricle. The true margins of the defect cannot be seen because the anterior components of the left and right ventricles have been removed. The bottom right-hand picture is the same specimen prior to the long-axis cut. The front of the right ventricle has been removed. In this view, there is no doubt that this is a double-outlet right ventricle with subpulmonary ventricular septal defect. The anterior margins of the ventricular septal defect are still present in this specimen. AO = aorta; d = ventricular septal defect; IS = outlet septum; LV = left ventricle; PA = pulmonary trunk; RV = right ventricle; VIF = ventriculoinfundibular fold; VS = ventricular septum.

NONCOMMITTED VENTRICULAR SEPTAL DEFECT

In hearts with noncommitted ventricular septal defect, the defect is either in the muscular inlet of the trabecular septum or is a perimembranous defect with extension into the inlet septum (Fig. 32.11). Atrioventricular septal defects with a common orifice are frequent associations (Fig. 32.11).

Those defects that are situated in the muscular

septum have the muscular components of either the trabecular or inlet septum as their boundaries. Those in the posterior inlet or trabecular septum are best seen in a subcostal four-chamber cut and from a similar apical cut with posterior angulation. In a precordial short-axis scan from apex to base, the defect is seen in the posterior aspect of the septum. As the scan is continued towards the base, the components of the outlet septum can be seen often with deviation to the

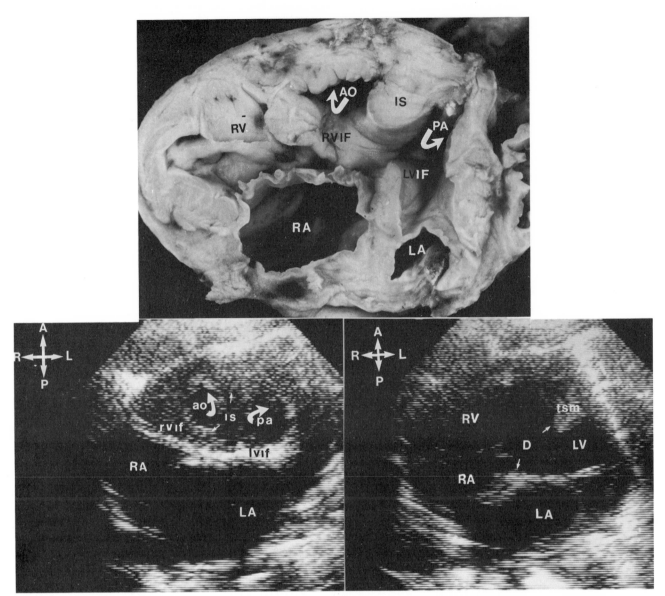

Figure 32.8.   The upper picture is a specimen with a double-outlet right ventricle and subpulmonary ventricular septal defect in simulated high short-axis cut. Note the outlet septum, which deviates to the right to fuse with the right-sided ventriculoinfundibular fold. The anterior and posterior margins of the defects are seen in this view. The lower left-hand picture is a high precordial short-axis cut from a similar patient. Note that the outlet septum fuses with the right-sided ventriculoinfundibular fold. As in the specimen, note that the aortic and pulmonary valves are not seen and arise from well above the ventricular septal defect. The lower right-hand picture is from the same patient at a slightly lower position. The anterior limb of the septomarginal trabeculation is seen as is the ventricular septal defect. Note in this view the great vessels are not visualized. AO = aorta; D = ventricular septal defect; IS = outlet septum; LA = left atrium; LVIF = left ventriculoinfundibular fold; PA = pulmonary trunk; RA = right atrium; RV = right ventricle; RVIF = right ventriculoinfundibular fold; TSM = septomarginal trabeculation.

left or right. The arterial roots are visualized, with no direct relationship to the ventricular septal defect.

In cases with a perimembranous inlet defect, the roof is formed by either the tricuspid septal leaflet or the anterosuperior bridging leaflet in the presence of an atrioventricular septal defect (Fig. 32.11). The floor of the defect is the crest of the posterior trabecular septum.

These relationships can be best assessed from a combination of precordial and subcostal four-chamber cuts.

In the precordial short-axis cut, the defect is visualized in the posterior aspect of the septum. As the transducer is scanned toward the base, the roof of the defect formed by the tricuspid valve or bridging leaflet can be seen. As the scan is continued more superiorly,

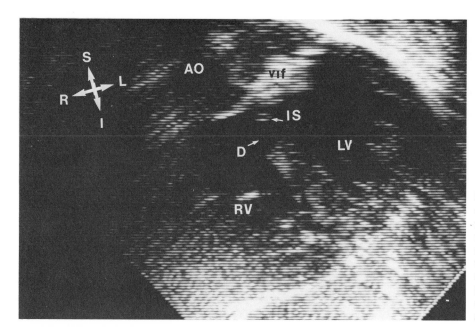

Figure 32.9. Subcostal long-axis cut in a case with double-outlet right ventricle (RV) and doubly committed ventricular septal defect (D) with a hypoplastic outlet septum (IS). Note the prominent left-sided ventriculoinfundibular fold (VIF). Note that the small IS is not deviated to the left or right. AO = aorta; LV = left ventricle.

the outlet septum deviating to the left or to the right, and the great arteries can be seen (Fig. 32.12).

ASSOCIATED DEFECTS

Subpulmonary and Pulmonary Valve Stenosis

Subpulmonary stenosis may occur with any type of double-outlet right ventricle, although it is relatively uncommon with subpulmonary or doubly committed defects. More frequently, it is seen in association with noncommitted or subaortic defects, where the outlet septum is displaced to the left.

The components of the stenosis are similar to those seen in tetralogy of Fallot, which may coexist with double-outlet right ventricle. A narrowed infundibular region, in combination with muscle bundles from the anterior right ventricular wall, invariably makes up the subpulmonary stenosis (Fig. 32.13). In combination, the pulmonary valve and annulus may be stenotic. Occasionally, the subpulmonary obstruction may be lower down in the body of the right ventricle, resulting from prominent muscle bundles. In patients with a subpulmonary defect, the stenosis is invariably due to a prominent left-sided ventriculoinfundibular fold.

All of these types of obstruction can be evaluated from a combination of subcostal long-axis cut (Fig. 32.14), with and without counterclockwise rotation to visualize the subpulmonary region, and precordial short-axis cut to visualize the anterior component of the obstruction, if present. The subcostal long-axis cut fails to visualize this anterior component. In patients

with a subpulmonary defect, a precordial long-axis cut is useful in the assessment of the left-sided ventriculoinfundibular fold. Doppler echocardiography plays an invaluable role in the assessment of the severity of obstruction (Fig. 32.15).

Subaortic Stenosis

Subaortic stenosis is usually associated with either a subaortic or subpulmonary ventricular septal defect. In those with a subpulmonary defect, the obstruction is invariably produced by a combination of rightward deviation of the outlet septum and a prominent right-sided ventriculoinfundibular fold. These two structures, which fuse with the anterior wall of the right ventricle, produce a muscular tunnel. Although there is no obstruction at rest in some patients, dynamic obstruction can be demonstrated following intravenous isoproterenol administration (Fig. 32.16).

In those patients with subaortic ventricular septal defect, the outlet septum may play a small role in the etiology of the subaortic stenosis (Fig. 32.17). A prominent right-sided ventriculoinfundibular fold and narrowing in the region of the anterior wall of the right ventricle invariably are the dominant components (Fig. 32.5). In some cases, there is a fibromuscular element to the stenosis. In either type of defect, the presence of subaortic stenosis is associated with aortic arch anomalies such as coarctation, isthmal tubular hypoplasia, or arch interruption.

The subaortic region is best assessed from a combination of long- and short-axis cuts. The subcostal

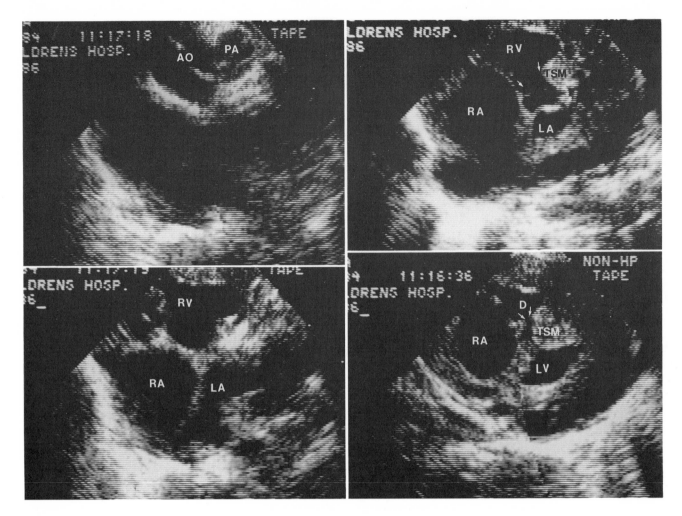

A

Figure 32.10. (*A*) The upper left-hand picture is a high precordial short-axis cut in double-outlet right ventricle and doubly committed ventricular septal defect. Note the pulmonary trunk is anterior and slightly to the left of the aorta. The lower picture is a slightly lower precordial short-axis cut demonstrating no visible outlet septum. The upper right-hand picture is at a slightly lower level demonstrating the margin of the ventricular septal defect and the anterior limb of the septomarginal trabeculation. Note once again that there is no outlet septum visible. The lower right-hand picture is an even lower short-axis cut demonstrating the ventricular septal defect. Note that both vessels arise completely from the right ventricle. The aorta, due to its position, is slightly closer to the ventricular septal defect than the pulmonary trunk. The pulmonary trunk is partly blocked from the margin of the ventricular septal defect by the septomarginal trabeculation and left-sided ventriculoinfundibular fold. Compare this to the same patient seen in the subcostal long-axis cut in Figure 32.6.

long-axis cut with counterclockwise rotation visualizes the contributions made by the right-sided ventriculoinfundibular fold and outlet septum. This, however, does not identify the anterior component, which is best visualized from a high precordial short-axis scan from apex to base. The fusion of the three components of the tunnel can be identified in this view, that is, the anterior wall of the right ventricle, the right-sided ventriculoinfundibular fold, and the outlet septum.

Thus far, the fibromuscular elements seen in patients with a subaortic defect have been best visualized in the precordial long-axis cut. Doppler examination, particularly from the subcostal long-axis cut, is invaluable in

assessing the pressure drop across the subaortic region.

Restrictive Ventricular Septal Defect

Occasionally, double-outlet right ventricle is complicated by restriction of the ventricular septal defect (9). This occurs most frequently in patients with subaortic defects resulting in suprasystemic left ventricular pressure. The absolute size of the defect is best judged by combining long- and short-axis views with Doppler interrogation on the right ventricular side of the defect (Fig. 32.18). This demonstrates a high-velocity pressure

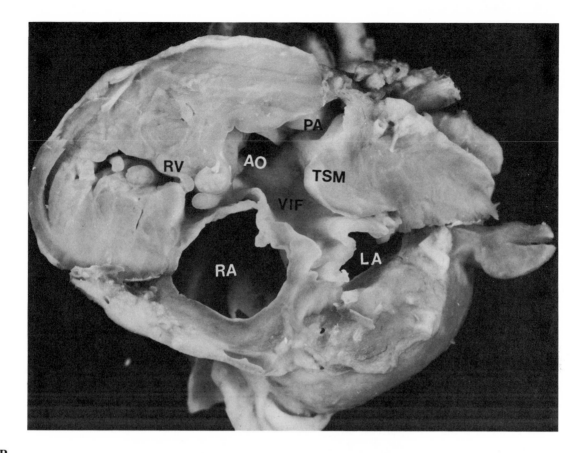

B

Figure 32.10, (cont'd.)   (*B*). The specimen is a high precordial short-axis cut in the same patient. This corresponds to the upper right-hand picture of Figure 32.6. Note the lack of outlet septum separating pulmonary trunk from aorta. The septomarginal trabeculation is clearly seen partly blocking the pulmonary trunk from the margins of the ventricular septal defect. Both great vessels clearly arise from the morphologic right ventricle. AO = aorta; D = ventricular septal defect; LA = left atrium; LV = left ventricle; PA = pulmonary trunk; RA = right atrium; TSM = septomarginal trabeculation.

drop across this region, which may increase with rapid heart rates.

Other Associated Anomalies

As mentioned in Chapter 30, straddling of the mitral valve occurs in association with double-outlet right ventricle when the defect is anteriorly situated. In those cases with a perimembranous inlet defect, straddling of the tricuspid valve may occur, often in association with some degree of hypoplasia of the right ventricle due to failure of the posterior muscular septum to reach the crux of the heart. Hypoplasia of the left ventricle can also occur in double-outlet right ventricle, as can stenosis of the mitral valve. Both of these lesions are readily outlined with a combination of cross-sectional and Doppler echocardiography. Right

aortic arch occurs in association with double-outlet right ventricle as in tetralogy of Fallot.

SPATIAL RELATIONSHIP OF THE GREAT ARTERIES

The relationship of the aorta and pulmonary trunk (if present) is determined by the orientation of the outlet septum, which in turn dictates the position of the ventricular septal defect in relation to the aorta, pulmonary trunk, or both. The great arteries may vary considerably in their relationship around an axis of 360 degrees (Fig. 32.19) (2). Most patients with a subaortic defect, however, have the pulmonary trunk situated to the left either directly or slightly anterior to the aorta (Fig. 32.2), while in those with a subpulmonary defect, the vessels are side by side or the pulmonary artery is situated posterior to the aorta.

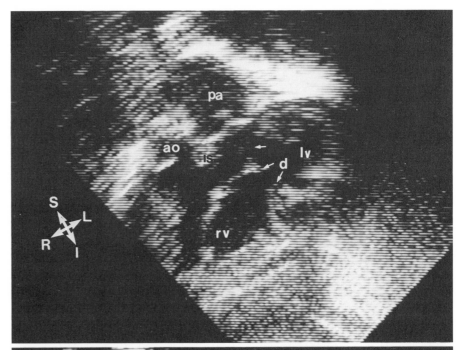

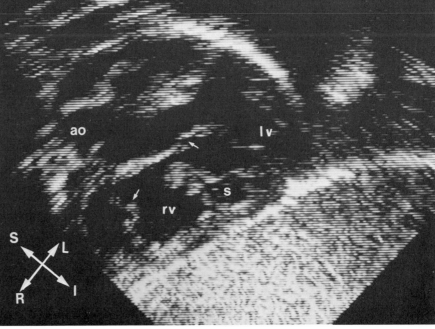

Figure 32.11. The upper picture is a subcostal long-axis cut in double-outlet right ventricle and non-committed ventricular septal defect. Note there is a muscular inlet ventricular septal defect and an associated perimembranous ventricular septal defect. The bottom picture is from a patient with double-outlet right ventricle and non-committed ventricular septal defect in the setting of complete atrioventricular septal defect. Note the bridging leaflets are indicated by the white arrows. AO = aorta; d = ventricular septal defect; IS = outlet septum; LV = left ventricle; PA = pulmonary trunk; RV = right ventricle; S = ventricular septum.

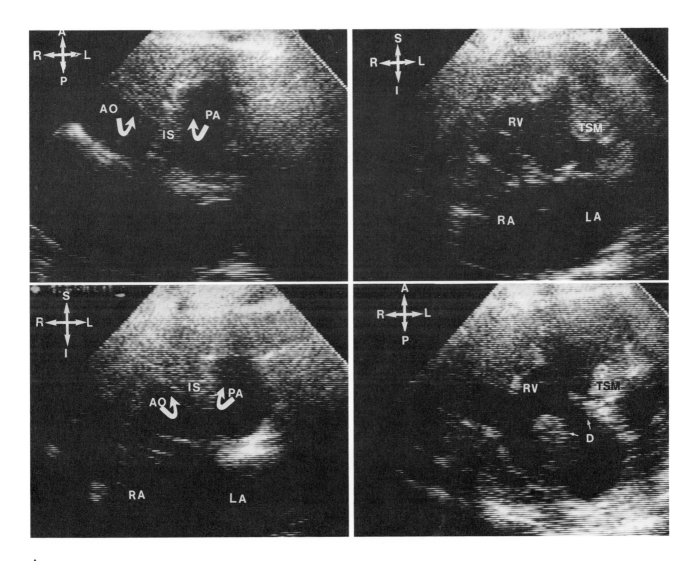

A

Figure 32.12.   The upper left-hand picture is a high precordial short-axis cut in double-outlet right ventricle and noncommitted ventricular septal defect in the setting of atrioventricular septal defect. Note the outlet septum separating aorta from pulmonary trunk. The lower left-hand picture is from the same patient at a slightly lower cut. Note that the ventricular septal defect is not visualized in this view. The upper right-hand picture at a slightly lower cut demonstrates the common atrioventricular valve in this patient, with the various components of the atrioventricular valves. The bottom right-hand picture demonstrates the ventricular septal defect in its posterior location. Note the anterior bridging leaflet, which is crossing the ventricular septal defect. Both great arteries in this patient are clearly a long way from the margin of the ventricular septal defect.

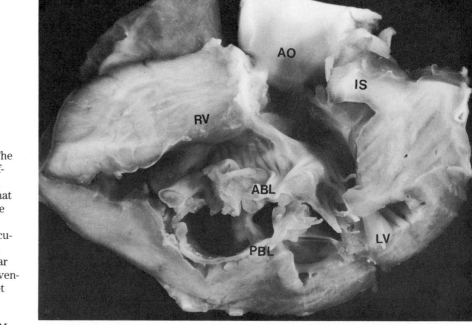

Figure 32.12, (cont'd.) (*B*) The anatomic specimen is from a different patient. Note in this case, unlike in the echocardiogram, that the outlet septum deviates to the left and fuses with the anterior limb of the septomarginal trabeculation. Note the bridging leaflets and the very posterior ventricular septal defect. AO = aorta; D = ventricular septal defect; IS = outlet septum; LA = left atrium; PA = pulmonary trunk; RA = right atrium; RV = right ventricle; TSM = septomarginal trabeculation.

B

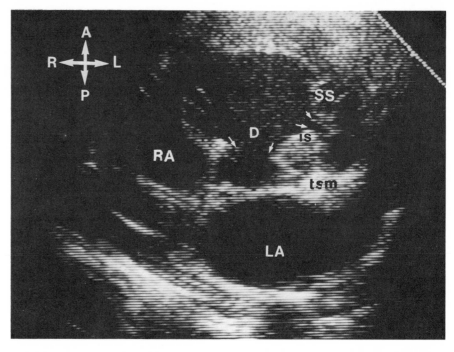

Figure 32.13. Precordial short-axis cut in double-outlet right ventricle and subaortic ventricular septal defect associated with significant subpulmonary stenosis. Note the subpulmonary stenosis is due to a combination of a prominent outlet septum and a muscle originating from the anterior right ventricular wall. D = ventricular septal defect; IS = outlet septum; LA = left atrium; RA = right atrium; SS = subpulmonary stenosis; TSM = septomarginal trabeculation.

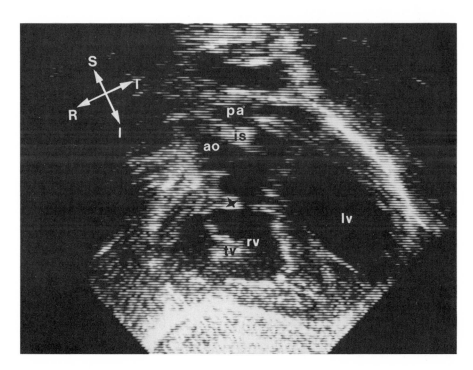

Figure 32.14. Subcostal cut with counterclockwise rotation in double-outlet right ventricle (RV) and subpulmonary ventricular septal defect due to midcavity obstruction (*star*). Note that the obstruction is at mid–right ventricular cavity level and does not involve the outlet septum (IS). AO = aorta; LV = left ventricle; PA = pulmonary trunk; TV = tricuspid valve.

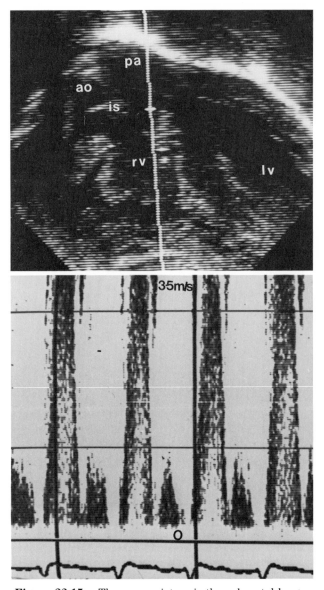

Figure 32.15. The upper picture is the subcostal long-axis cut from the same patient as in the Figure 32.14. The Doppler sample volume is placed distal to the site of mid-cavity obstruction. The lower picture is the Doppler spectral trace indicating the high-velocity systolic jet distal to the site of obstruction. AO = aorta; IS = outlet septum; LV = left ventricle; PA = pulmonary trunk; RV = right ventricle.

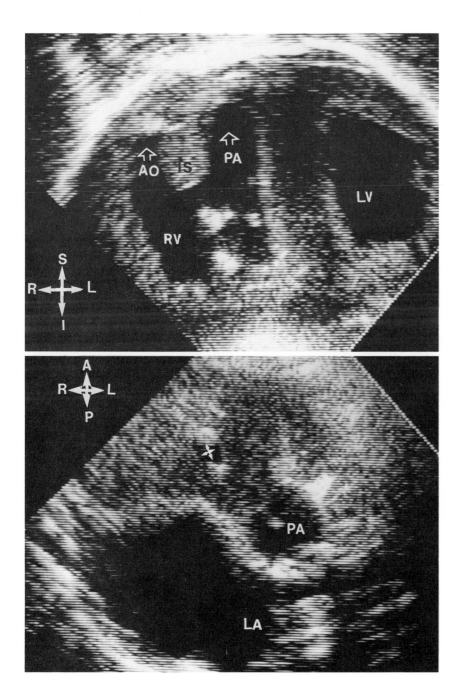

Figure 32.16. The upper picture is the subcostal view with counter-clockwise rotation. Note the large outlet septum separating the aorta from the pulmonary trunk. Note that the subaortic region is narrowed by this prominent outlet septum, which deviates to the right. The lower picture is a high precordial short-axis cut from the same patient. Note the very small subaortic region indicated by the cross. AO = aorta; IS = outlet septum; LA = left atrium; LV = left ventricle; PA = pulmonary trunk; RV = right ventricle.

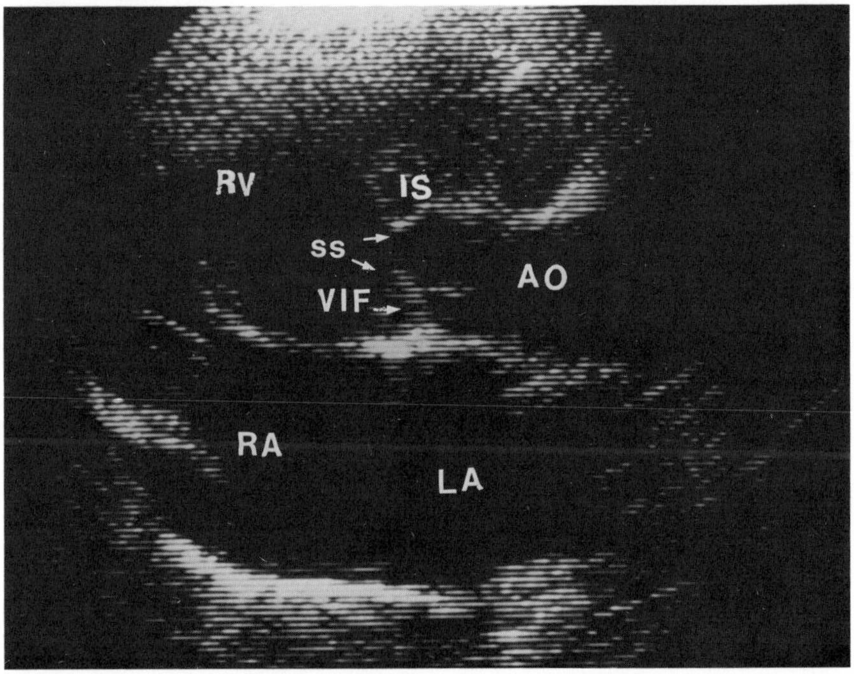

Figure 32.17.   A precordial long-axis view with slight clockwise rotation to visualize the subaortic region. Note the subaortic region is narrowed by a combination of a prominent outlet septum (IS) and ventriculoinfundibular fold (VIF). AO = aorta; LA = left atrium; RA = right atrium; RV = right ventricle; SS = subaortic stenosis.

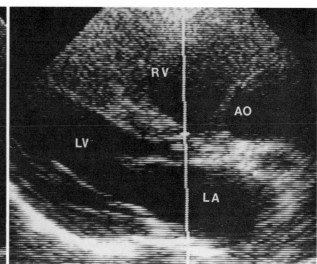

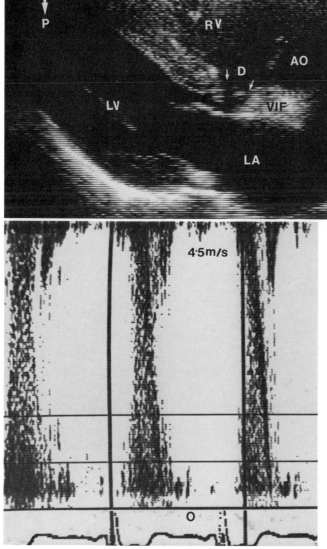

Figure 32.18. The upper left-hand picture is a precordial long-axis cut in double-outlet right ventricle, subaortic ventricular septal defect, and restricted ventricular septal defect. Note the ventricular septal defect is narrowed by a combination of fibromuscular tissue tags and a prominent left-sided ventriculoinfundibular fold. The upper right-hand picture is from the same patient with Doppler sample volume placed just distal to the site of the obstruction. The bottom picture is the spectral trace from this patient demonstrating a high-velocity jet. AO = aorta; D = ventricular septal defect; LA = left atrium; LV = left ventricle; RV = right ventricle; VIF = ventriculoinfundibular fold.

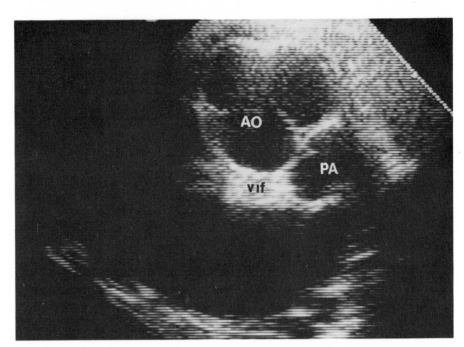

Figure 32.19.   A high precordial short-axis cut in double-outlet right ventricle and subaortic ventricular septal defect where the pulmonary trunk is slightly posterior and to the left of the aorta. Compare this with Figure 32.2, where the pulmonary trunk is anterior and to the left. AO = aorta; PA = pulmonary trunk; VIF = ventriculoinfundibular fold.

REFERENCES

1. Lev M, Bharati S, Meng CCL, Liberthson RR, Paul MH, Idriss F. A concept of double-outlet right ventricle. J Thorac Cardiovasc Surg 1972;64:271–81.
2. Wilcox BR, Ho SY, Phil M, Macartney FJ, et al. Surgical anatomy of double-outlet right ventricle with situs solitus and atrioventricular concordance. J Thorac Cardiovasc Surg 1981;82:405–17.
3. Anderson RH, Becker AE, Wilcox BR, Macartney FJ, Wilkinson JL. Surgical anatomy of double-outlet right ventricle—a reappraisal. Am J Cardiol 1983;52:555–9.
4. Sridaromont S, Ritter DG, Feldt RH, Davis GD, Edwards JE. Double-outlet right ventricle. Anatomical and angiocardiographic correlations. Mayo Clin Proc 1978;53:555–77.
5. Macartney FJ, Rigby ML, Anderson RH, Stark J, Silverman NH. Double outlet right ventricle. Cross sectional echocardiographic findings, their anatomical explanation, and surgical relevance. Br Heart J 1984;52:164–77.
6. Sanders SP, Bierman FZ, Williams RG. Conotruncal malformations: diagnosis in infancy using subxiphoid 2-dimensional echocardiography. Am J Cardiol 1982;50:1361–7.
7. Hagler DJ, Tajik AJ, Seward JB, Mair DD, Ritter DG. Double-outlet right ventricle: wide-angle two-dimensional echocardiographic observations. Circulation 1981;63:419–28.
8. Henry WL, Maron BJ, Griffith JM. Cross-sectional echocardiography in the diagnosis of congenital heart disease. Identification of the relation of the ventricles and great arteries. Circulation 1977;56:267–73.
9. Gerlis LM, Dickinson DF, Anderson RH. Disadvantageous closure of the interventricular communication in double outlet right ventricle. Br Heart J 1984;51:670–3.

33
Aortic Abnormalities

Donald Hagler

The application of two-dimensional echocardiographic techniques has allowed accurate recognition of many aortic malformations. A segmental approach is necessary to define the complete anatomic abnormality. Initial two-dimensional echocardiographic studies demonstrated similarities of intracardiac anatomy in common arterial trunk, pulmonary atresia, ventricular septal defect, and tetralogy of Fallot (Fig. 33.1) (1). It was noted that suprasternal notch scans occasionally could demonstrate the aortic origin of the pulmonary arteries and a common trunk. Subsequent reports by Rice et al. (2), Houston et al. (3), and Smallhorn et al. (4), however, showed that parasternal long- and short-axis scans could accurately demonstrate the origin and course of the pulmonary arteries in the presence of a common arterial trunk.

High parasternal short-axis scans are important to demonstrate the aortic origin of the right and left pulmonary arteries from the left and posterior aspects of the aorta (Fig. 33.2) (2–4). With these scans, a common arterial trunk can be definitively diagnosed and the integrity of both right and left pulmonary artery branches defined. Additional parasternal long-axis and suprasternal notch scans are helpful to define the subsequent course of the aorta and the aortic arch. Subcostal scans also can be used to demonstrate these diagnostic features of common arterial trunk (truncus arteriosus), but the experience of these authors (2) suggests that this view may be less successful than the parasternal scanning techniques.

Similar parasternal long- and short-axis scans are important in the noninvasive diagnosis of aortopulmonary window (5). Parasternal long-axis scans demonstrate separate arterial valves in aortopulmonary window, and subsequent parasternal short-axis scans or subcostal long-axis scans may reveal the aortopulmonary communication (Fig. 33.3).

Coronary artery anomalies, including coronary artery to pulmonary artery, coronary to ventricular or coronary to atrial fistulae, acquired coronary artery ectasia and aneurysm formation, have been recognized with parasternal short-axis scans of the aortic root (Fig. 33.4) (6–8). Recent experience with high-frequency transducers has considerably improved the ability to detect coronary artery abnormalities. Additional demonstration of peripheral coronary artery lesions in Kawasaki's disease has been accomplished with subcostal scans to demonstrate the right coronary artery in the right atrioventricular groove (9).

Aortic arch anomalies (i.e., right aortic arch, double aortic arch, anomalous origin of the right and left subclavian arteries, interrupted aortic arch, and coarctation of the aorta) have been described in detail by several authors (4, 10–14). Again, a segmental approach, as described by Huhta et al. (11), allows logical sequential assessment of complex anatomy (Fig. 33.5). High right and left parasternal scanning in addition to suprasternal notch views has been extremely important in providing the required segmental approach. Earlier studies demonstrated the usefulness of suprasternal notch scans and the transducer orientation for determination of the site of the aortic arch (15). Scanning to the right of the spine will usually define a right aortic arch, whereas scanning to the left of the spine will define a left aortic arch. Huhta et al. (11) described the use of feeding to demonstrate the esophagus during swallowing. The aortic arch could then be correctly referenced to the position of the esophagus. In addition, they utilized this technique to identify double aortic arch. Recent advances with high-frequency (5.0 and 7.5 megahertz) transducers also have improved the noninvasive examination of the aortic arch.

In addition to arch anatomy, the site of origin of the brachiocephalic branches should be detailed before surgical intervention. Initial scans of the ascending aorta and the first brachiocephalic branches are obtained from right parasternal or suprasternal notch

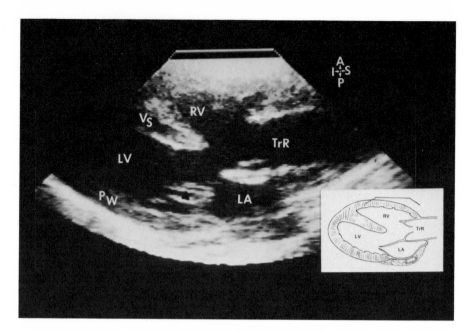

Figure 33.1. Parasternal long-axis scan in a patient with common arterial trunk. Note large ventricular septal defect with override. A = anterior; I = inferior; LA = left atrium; LV = left ventricle; P = posterior; PW = posterior wall; RV = right ventricle; S = superior; TrR = truncal root; VS = ventricular septum.

scans (Fig. 33.6). With a short-axis view of the first branch during scanning to the right or left side, the bifurcation of the carotid or subclavian arteries demonstrates the normal or mirror-image branch patterns (Fig. 33.6B and 33.7). In addition, the subsequent view of the aortic arch and upper descending aorta details the size of the aortic arch and the second and third branches (left carotid and left subclavian) (Fig. 33.8). Scans of these areas should also demonstrate anomalous origin of a right or left subclavian artery (Fig. 33.9).

The third segment of the aortic arch is best obtained from suprasternal and high left parasternal long-axis scans. This scanning technique allows demonstration of the juxtaductal area and the upper descending

thoracic aorta (Fig. 33.10) and may allow precise localization and demonstration of the severity of hypoplasia associated with interruption or coarctation of the aorta (Fig. 33.11). The standard suprasternal notch views demonstrate the proximal aortic arch only up to the left subclavian branch. The arch subsequently moves out of the scan plane because of the tortuosity of the aorta associated with coarctation (Fig. 33.12). Thus, precise demonstration of coarctation by use of these scans alone is fraught with some uncertainty. Use of the high left parasternal scanning position (Fig. 33.13) for the juxtaductal area was described by Smallhorn et al. in a large series of infants with coarctation of the aorta (12). Long segments of hypoplastic aorta may be accurately demonstrated from the high left

Figure 33.2. High parasternal short-axis scan demonstrating common origin of right (RPA) and left (LPA) pulmonary arteries from truncal root (TrR). A = anterior; L = left; P = posterior; R = right.

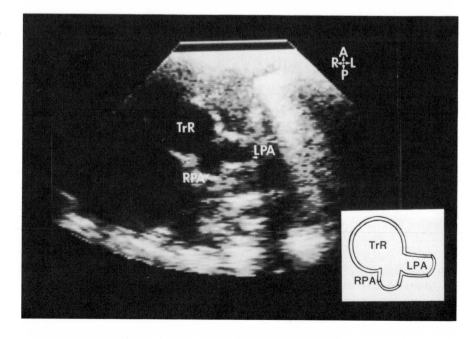

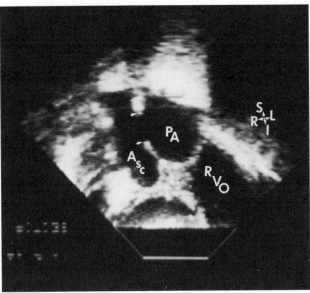

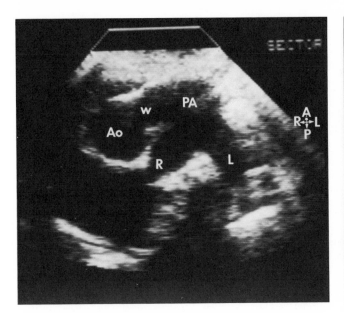

A   B

Figure 33.3. (*A*) High parasternal short-axis scan in patient with aortopulmonary window (w). Note position of communication in anterior aspect of aorta (Ao). Note right (R) and left (L) pulmonary artery (PA) bifurcation. (*B*) Subcostal long-axis view also demonstrates aortopulmonary window, with simultaneous demonstration of right ventricular outflow (RVO) tract. A = anterior; Asc = ascending aorta; I = inferior; P = posterior; S = superior.

parasternal long- and short-axis scans. Similarly, these scans and suprasternal notch scans may allow visualization of a patent ductus arteriosus (Fig. 33.14) (16). Finally, parasternal and subcostal long-axis views of the descending thoracic and abdominal aorta allow demonstration of the course of that segment of the aorta. With these scans, coarctation or abnormal atrial arrangement can be detected.

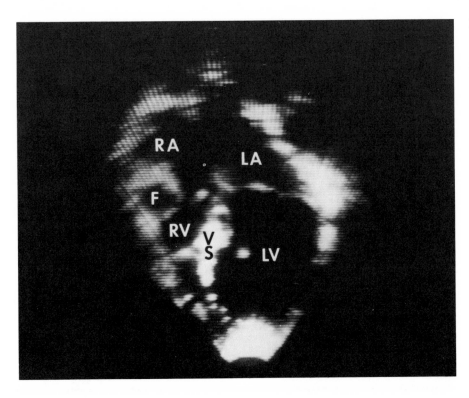

Figure 33.4. (*A*) Apical four-chamber view of aneurysmal right coronary artery in a patient with right coronary artery fistula (F). (*A*, reproduced by permission from Reeder GS, Tajik AJ, Smith HC. Visualization of coronary artery fistula by two-dimensional echocardiography. Mayo Clin Proc 1980;55:185–9.)

A

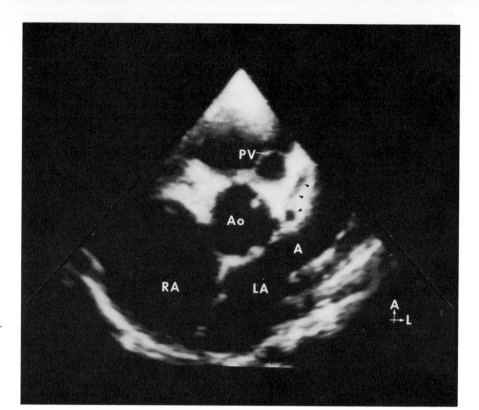

Figure 33.4, (cont'd.) (*B*) Parasternal short-axis scan to demonstrate left coronary artery in patient with Kawasaki's disease. A (direction) = anterior; A = atrial appendage; Ao = aorta; L = left; LA = left atrium; LV = left ventricle; PV = pulmonary valve; RA = right atrium; RV = right ventricle; VS = ventricular septum.

B

Figure 33.5. Segmental approach to diagnosis of abnormalities of the aorta. Ascending aorta can be seen from parasternal, suprasternal, and subcostal scans; aortic arch from multiple suprasternal scans, aortic isthmus from suprasternal and high parasternal scans, and descending aorta from parasternal and subcostal scans. (Reproduced by permission of the American Heart Association from Huhta JC, Gutgesell HP, Latson LA, Huffines FD. Two-dimensional echocardiographic assessment of the aorta in infants and children with congenital heart disease. Circulation 1980;70:417–24.)

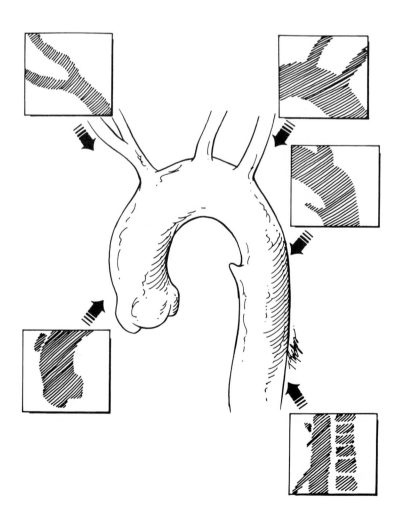

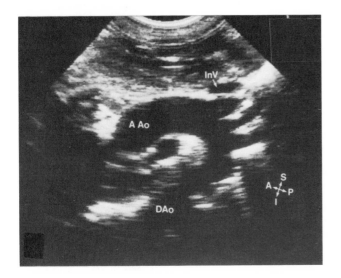

A

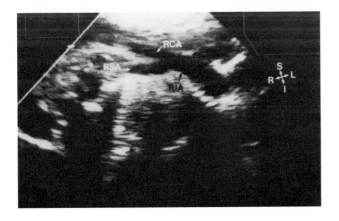

B

Figure 33.6. Segmental aortic examination by two-dimensional echocardiography in 2-week-old infant with pulmonary valve stenosis. (*A*) Suprasternal section of ascending aorta (AAo) and innominate (InV) and proximal arch branches. (*B*) Suprasternal notch scan with exaggerated short-axis view obtained with transducer tilted toward right shoulder of patient. Right innominate artery (RIA), right carotid artery (RCA), and right subclavian artery (RSA) are shown. A = anterior; DAo = descending aorta; I = inferior; L = left; P = posterior; S = superior. (Reproduced by permission of the American Heart Association from Huhta JC, Gutgesell HP, Latson LA, Huffines FD. Two-dimensional echocardiographic assessment of the aorta in infants and children with congenital heart disease. Circulation 1984;70:417–24.)

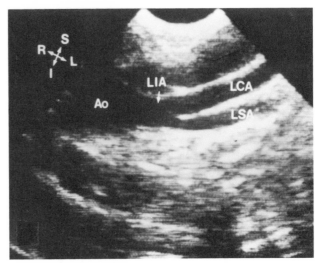

Figure 33.7. Suprasternal short-axis scan obtained with transducer tilted toward left shoulder of patient. Mirror-image branching of right aortic arch, with visualization of left carotid (LCA) and left subclavian (LSA) arteries, is shown. Ao = aorta; I = inferior; L = left; LIA = left innominate artery; R = right; S = superior. (Reproduced by permission of the American Heart Association from Huhta JC, Gutgesell HP, Latson LA, Huffines FD. Two-dimensional echocardiographic assessment of the aorta in infants and children with congenital heart disease. Circulation 1984;70:417–24.)

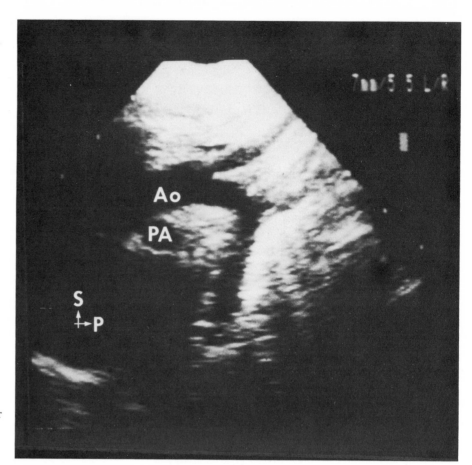

Figure 33.8. Suprasternal notch scan showing distal arch and upper descending aorta. Ao = aorta; P = posterior; PA = pulmonary artery; S = superior.

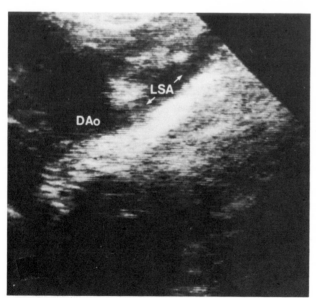

Figure 33.9. Suprasternal scan of right-sided descending aorta (DAo) and anomalous origin of left subclavian artery (LSA). (Reproduced by permission of the American Heart Association from Huhta JC, Gutgesell HP, Latson LA, Huffines FD. Two-dimensional echocardiographic assessment of the aorta in infants and children with congenital heart disease. Circulation 1984;70:417–24.)

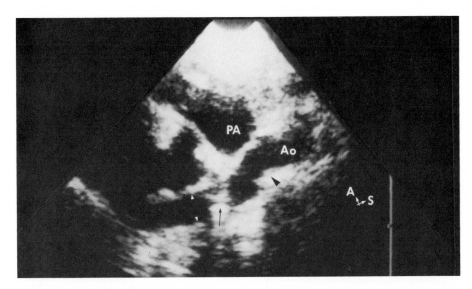

Figure 33.10. High parasternal long-axis view of descending thoracic aorta (Ao). Note distal portion of aorta (*white arrowheads*), previously repaired coarctation site (juxtaductal) (*black arrowhead*), and artifact (*black arrow*) probably originating from left bronchus. A = anterior; PA = pulmonary artery; S = superior.

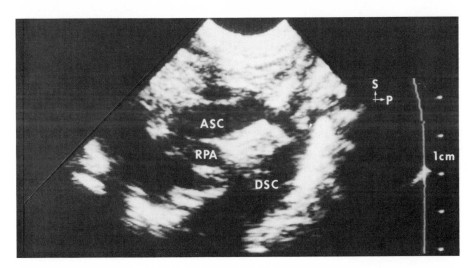

Figure 33.11. Suprasternal notch scan shows moderate hypoplasia of aortic isthmus and distal arch after repair of coarctation of aorta. Also note stenotic origin of left subclavian artery (*white arrowhead*). ASC = ascending aorta; DSC = descending aorta; P = posterior; RPA = right pulmonary artery; S = superior.

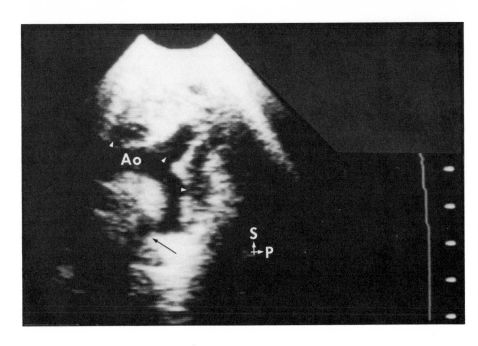

Figure 33.12. Standard suprasternal notch scan in newborn infant with coarctation of aorta (Ao). Note tortuosity of juxtaductal portion of aorta at coarctation site (*arrow*). Arrowheads mark brachiocephalic branches. P = posterior; S = superior.

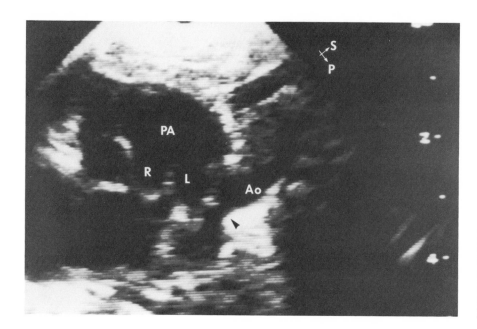

Figure 33.13. High parasternal long-axis view of juxtaductal region in newborn infant reveals discrete coarctation (*arrowhead*) of aorta (Ao). Note pulmonary trunk (PA) and right (R) and left (L) branches. P = posterior; S = superior.

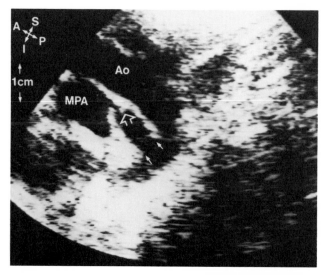

Figure 33.14. Patent ductus arteriosus from suprasternal scan. Narrow pulmonary end of ductus arteriosus (*open arrow*) is shown in neonate with transposition of great arteries. Small arrows denote aortic end of ductus. A = anterior; Ao = aorta; I = inferior; MPA = pulmonary trunk; P = posterior; S = superior. (Reproduced by permission of the American Heart Association from Huhta JC, Gutgesell HP, Latson LA, Huffines FD. Two-dimensional echocardiographic assessment of the aorta in infants and children with congenital heart disease. Circulation 1984;70:417–24.)

REFERENCES

1. Hagler DJ, Tajik AJ, Seward JB, Mair DD, Ritter DG. Wide-angle two-dimensional echocardiographic profiles of conotruncal abnormalities. Mayo Clin Proc 1980;55:73–82.
2. Rice MJ, Seward JB, Hagler DJ, Mair DD, Tajik AJ. Definitive diagnosis of truncus arteriosus by two-dimensional echocardiography. Mayo Clin Proc 1982;57:476–81.
3. Houston AB, Gregory NL, Murtagh E, Coleman EN. Two-dimensional echocardiography in infants with persistent truncus arteriosus. Br Heart J 1981;46:492–7.
4. Smallhorn JF, Anderson RH, Macartney FJ. Two-dimensional echocardiographic assessment of communications between ascending aorta and pulmonary trunk or individual pulmonary arteries. Br Heart J 1982;47:563–72.
5. Rice MJ, Seward JB, Hagler DJ, Mair DD, Tajik AJ. Visualization of aortopulmonary window by two-dimensional echocardiography. Mayo Clin Proc 1982;57:482–7.
6. Reeder GS, Tajik AJ, Smith HC. Visualization of coronary artery fistula by two-dimensional echocardiography. Mayo Clin Proc 1980;55:185–9.
7. Chia BL, Ee B, Tan A, Choo M, Tan L. Two-dimensional and pulsed Doppler echocardiographic abnormalities in coronary artery-pulmonary artery fistula. Chest 1984;86:901–4.
8. Yoshikawa J, Yanagihara K, Owaki T, et al. Cross-sectional echocardiographic diagnosis of coronary artery aneurysms in patients with the mucocutaneous lymph node syndrome. Circulation 1979;59:133–9.
9. Yoshida H, Maeda T, Funabashi T, Nakaya S, Takabatake S, Taniguchi N. Subcostal two-dimensional echocardiographic imaging of peripheral right coronary artery in Kawasaki disease. Circulation 1982;65:956–61.
10. George L, Waldman JD, Kirkpatrick SE, Turner SW, Pappelbaum SJ. Two-dimensional echocardiographic visualization of the aortic arch by right parasternal scanning in neonates and infants. Pediatr Cardiol 1982;2:277–80.
11. Huhta JC, Gutgesell HP, Latson LA, Huffines FD. Two-dimensional echocardiographic assessment of the aorta in infants and children with congenital heart disease. Circulation 1984;70:417–24.
12. Smallhorn JF, Anderson RH, Macartney FJ. Cross-sectional echo-

cardiographic recognition of interruption of aortic arch between left carotid and subclavian arteries. Br Heart J 1982;48:229–35.

13. Smallhorn JF, Huhta JC, Adams PA, Anderson RH, Wilkinson JL, Macartney FJ. Cross-sectional echocardiographic assessment of coarctation in the sick neonate and infant. Br Heart J 1983; 50:349–61.

14. Gutgesell HP, Huhta JC, Cohen MH, Latson LA. Two-dimensional echocardiographic assessment of pulmonary artery and aortic arch anatomy in cyanotic infants. J Am Coll Cardiol 1984;4: 1242–6.

15. Snider AR, Silverman NH. Suprasternal notch echocardiography: a two-dimensional technique for evaluating congenital heart disease. Circulation 1981;63:165–73.

16. Smallhorn JF, Huhta JC, Anderson RH, Macartney FJ. Suprasternal cross-sectional echocardiography in assessment of patent ductus arteriosus. Br Heart J 1982;48:321–30.

34
Fetal Echocardiography

Lindsey Allan

Echocardiography is now an established diagnostic method for congenital heart disease in post-natal life. Its reliability is such that invasive investigation, particularly in the neonate, can often be avoided prior to surgical procedures. Since 1980, several centers have reported the echocardiographic findings in fetal life (1–5), and an increasing number of cardiac malformations have now been recognized prenatally (6–9).

THE NORMAL FETAL CARDIAC EXAMINATION

Since the lung fields are unaerated in fetal life, there is unrestricted access for visualization of the heart and its connections using ultrasound. Once the fetal position is ascertained, a recognizable section of the heart is sought. A sequential examination of the systemic and pulmonary venous connections and the atrioventricular and ventriculoarterial connections is performed to ensure cardiac normality. The transducer orientation, relative to the whole fetus, needed to achieve the four most important sections is shown in Figure 34.1. The easiest section to seek initially is a four-chamber projection, which can be obtained by cutting straight across the fetal thorax at the level of the base of the sternum. In this section (Fig. 34.2), several important normal features should be noted. The heart occupies approximately one-third of the area of the fetal thorax. The descending aorta is seen as a circle lying between the spine and the left atrium. The two ventricles are of similar size. The right ventricle lies anteriorly immediately beneath the sternum and directly opposite the spine. The two atria are of similar size. There are two patent atrioventricular valves, the right valve inserted into the ventricular septum more apically than the left. The right ventricular apex is more heavily trabeculated than the left, and the moderator band runs from the distal septum to the right ventricular free wall. Thicknesses of the right and left ventricular free walls and

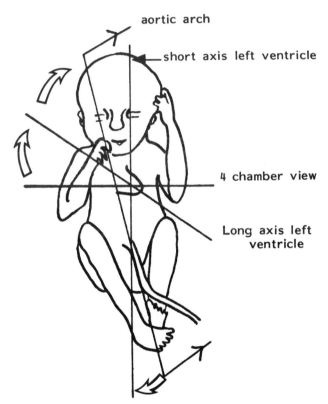

Figure 34.1. The sections of the fetus required to display the most important four sections of the heart are displayed. The four-chamber cut is seen in a transverse section of the fetal thorax at about the level of the base of the sternum.

interventricular septum are similar when compared in a plane immediately below the atrioventricular valves. The defect in the atrial septum at the foramen ovale is readily seen, the flap valve lying within the body of the left atrium. The ventricular septum visualized in this projection appears intact.

Transducer angulation from the four-chamber view toward the right shoulder will display the left ventricular connections (Fig. 34.3). A pulmonary vein can be seen entering the left atrium while the mitral valve

839

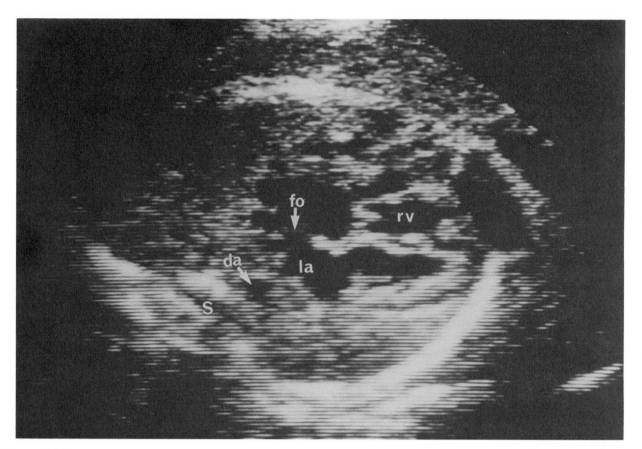

Figure 34.2. The thorax is seen in cross section with the spine (S) posterior. The descending aorta (DA) lies between the spine and left atrium (LA). The right ventricle (RV) lies under the anterior chest wall. FO = foramen ovale.

opens between left atrium and left ventricle. The left ventricle gives rise to a great artery. This should be the aorta but cannot be designated as such until the brachiocephalic branches are demonstrated taking origin from the aortic arch. There is continuity of the anterior wall of this great artery with the ventricular septum and of the posterior wall with the mitral valve (so-called aortomitral fibrous continuity). The aortic root is about two-thirds the size of the left atrium.

Further angulation of the transducer (as illustrated in Fig. 34.1) until the beam transects the fetus from the left supraclavicular fossa to inner thigh will display the right-heart connections (Fig. 34.4). The inferior vena cava can be seen draining into the right atrium. The tricuspid valve opens between right atrium and right ventricle. The pulmonary outflow wraps around the front of the central aorta and gives rise to the pulmonary trunk through a patent pulmonary valve. The pulmonary trunk itself connects via the ductus arteriosus to the descending aorta close to the origin of the left subclavian artery. The orientation needed to achieve these three sections is illustrated as it cuts the intracardiac structures in Figure 34.5.

To visualize the aortic arch, the last important sec-

tion, the transducer beam must cut the fetus obliquely as illustrated in Figure 34.6. The section achieved (Fig. 34.7) shows the head and neck vessels arising from the aortic arch. The arch forms a right "hook" with the ascending aorta tucking into the center of the chest. The connection between left ventricle, ascending aorta, and arch should be viewed in a continuous sweep, angling the transducer on the maternal abdomen, to ensure that the aorta does indeed arise from the left ventricle.

The fetal heart can be seen from all projections and orientations in a multiplicity of different sections. Once a thorough understanding of the fetal cardiac anatomy is gained, any section can be recognized and understood. These four selected sections demonstrate normal cardiac connections, and their recognition will exclude the majority of serious congenital heart disease. It is possible to achieve all four sections in almost every pregnancy between 16 weeks' gestation and term. Difficulties in imaging arise with oligohydramnios, polyhydramnios, or in late pregnancy when the fetus lies with the spine anteriorly. Distortion of the intrathoracic contents (e.g., in pleural effusion or diaphragmatic hernia) may also make identification of all

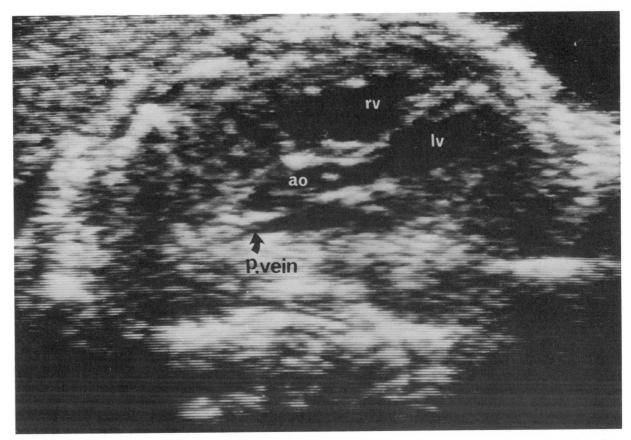

Figure 34.3.   The heart is seen in the long-axis projection of the left ventricle. This displays left-heart connections from pulmonary veins (p. vein) to left atrium to left ventricle (LV) to aorta (AO). The right ventricle (RV) lies anteriorly.

the connections difficult. Only rarely, however, will it be impossible to ensure the presence of normal cardiac connections.

NORMAL M-MODE ECHOCARDIOGRAPHY

M-mode echocardiography directed by cross-sectional techniques has been used to acquire measurements of the cardiac chambers and great vessel sizes in the normal fetus from 16 weeks to term (1–5). Tracings must be achieved in standard projections to ensure reproducibility. A short-axis view of the left ventricle is sought with cross-sectional echocardiography, and the M-mode cursor is positioned through it as shown in Figure 34.8; the tracing in Figure 34.9 will result. The two atrioventricular valves can be seen lying within the ventricular chambers. The right and left ventricular cavity dimensions in systole and diastole and the thicknesses of the posterior left ventricular wall and septum are measured. The growth charts for the ventricles in diastole together with the septal and posterior left ventricular wall thicknesses are shown in Figures 34.10, 34.11, 34.12, and 34.13, respectively.

The M-mode cursor needs to be positioned across the aortic root in short axis to achieve the tracing seen in Figure 34.14. The aortic valve is seen within the aortic walls with the left atrial cavity posteriorly. Measurements of aortic diameter and left atrial dimensions can be made; their growth patterns throughout pregnancy are seen in Figures 34.15 and 34.16. This recording also displays the normal sequence of atrial-to-ventricular contraction. Atrial contractions can be seen in the posterior left atrial wall, and it precedes ventricular contraction by a constant time interval of less than 100 milliseconds. This relationship between atrial and ventricular contraction is important when evaluating cardiac arrhythmias in prenatal life.

NORMAL DOPPLER ECHOCARDIOGRAPHY

Doppler interrogation of all four cardiac valves can demonstrate forward flow through each valve. The characteristic pattern of the mitral valve is seen in Figure 34.17. In prenatal life, the velocity of passive filling (E wave) is less than the velocity of atrial filling (A wave). The E/A ratio is around 0.5 at 18 weeks' gestation, rising to 1.0 nearer term on both sides of the heart. A tricuspid valve tracing is seen in Figure 34.18.

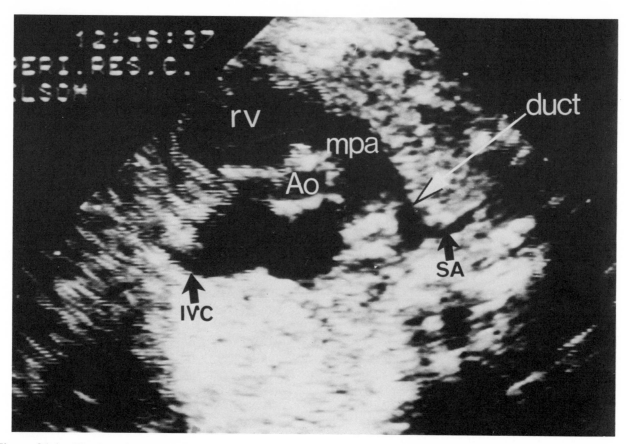

Figure 34.4.   The fetus is sectioned in a long-axis plane to demonstrate right-heart connections. The inferior vena cava (IVC) drains to right atrium, which connects through the tricuspid valve to the right ventricle (RV). This connects to the pulmonary trunk (MPA), which joins the descending aorta via the arterial duct just at the point of entry of the subclavian artery (SA).

This recording was made in later pregnancy than that in Figure 34.17, illustrating the increased E/A ratio. Both atrioventricular valves are affected by fetal respiratory movements so Doppler evaluation should take place during fetal apnea. The maximum velocity of both atrioventricular valves is almost constant throughout pregnancy. Mean velocity is slightly higher through the tricuspid valve than through the mitral valve.

The two semilunar valves can also be interrogated by Doppler echocardiography. The maximum velocity is similar on both sides of the heart but rises throughout pregnancy, from a mean value of 40 centimeters per second at 18 weeks to a mean value of 100 cm per second at term.

By measuring the orifice area of each valve ring and computing mean velocity from the Doppler tracing, an estimate of blood flow through each valve can be made using this formula: flow in milliliters per minute = $\overline{V} \times a / \cos\theta$ (10). Flow increases throughout pregnancy from approximately 50 to 600 mL per minute (right heart) and 40 to 500 mL per minute (left heart). The

relationship between right and left ventricular outputs is consistent and reproducible at a value of 1.2 : 1.0.

ABNORMAL CROSS-SECTIONAL ECHOCARDIOGRAPHY

Over 70 defects have now been recognized prenatally, representing a wide spectrum of congenital heart disease. Figure 34.19A shows the ventricular insertion of the atrioventricular valves at the same level, which is characteristic of an atrioventricular septal defect with separate right and left valves (ostium primum). A similar appearance can be seen in Figure 34.19B, but in the moving image, a ventricular component to the defect was apparent during the cardiac cycle, thus identifying this as a complete atrioventricular septal defect. In the patient illustrated in Figure 34.20, a small left atrium receives the pulmonary veins without a communication between this chamber and the ventricular mass. In this particular example, the right ventricle gave rise to both great arteries, but four examples of

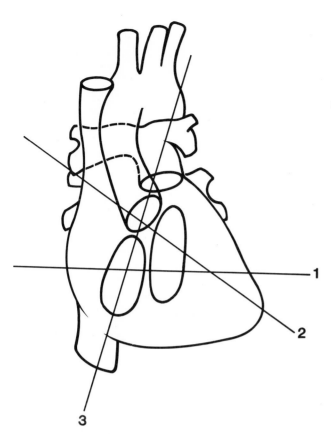

Figure 34.5. The transducer beam cuts the heart to achieve three sections. Plane 1 shows a four-chamber view. Plane 2 shows the connections of the left heart. Plane 3 shows the connections of the right heart.

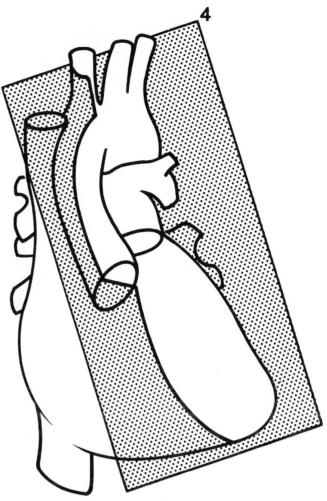

Figure 34.6. The angle of orientation of the transducer beam necessary to visualize the aortic arch is demonstrated.

mitral atresia in combination with aortic atresia have also been recognized.

Figure 34.21 illustrates a case of tricuspid atresia. The aorta takes origin astride the rudimentary right ventricle and the dominant left ventricle. Figure 34.22 illustrates another anomaly detected by examination of the atrioventricular junction, namely Ebstein's malformation. There is displacement of the septal leaflet of the tricuspid valve into the right ventricle together with right atrial dilatation. In this particular example, the septal leaflet was immobile because of tethering to the septum, resulting in free tricuspid regurgitation.

Abnormalities at the ventriculoarterial junction can also be recognized. Pulmonary atresia with intact septum is illustrated in Figure 34.23. The right ventricle is small and thick-walled. The tricuspid valve ring is small and the valve excursion limited. This is the same as the common form of pulmonary atresia visualized in postnatal life. The more common form of pulmonary atresia seen in intrauterine life, however, is illustrated in Figure 34.24. There is massive cardiac enlargement, particularly of the right ventricle, and there is free tricuspid regurgitation. Although an uncommon form of pulmonary atresia in postnatal life, five of six

prenatal cases of pulmonary atresia have taken this form. All five fetuses died at birth, and this may be the reason that this type of pulmonary atresia is rarely seen in pediatric cardiology centers.

Figure 34.25 illustrates a case of critical aortic stenosis with endocardial fibroelastosis of the left ventricle. The aortic valve ring was very small; the left ventricle was dilated and contracted poorly.

In the case illustrated in Figure 34.26, the aorta arises astride a ventricular septal defect. There is subpulmonary stenosis and a patent pulmonary valve indicative of tetralogy of Fallot. In the case illustrated in Figure 34.27, the solitary great artery also rises astride the ventricular septum, but the pulmonary arteries arise from this common arterial trunk.

Abnormal relationships of the great arteries can also be identified. In Figure 34.28, the great artery arising from the front of the chest gives rise to the head and neck vessels. The pulmonary trunk arises from the left ventricle. This diagnosis of complete transposition can

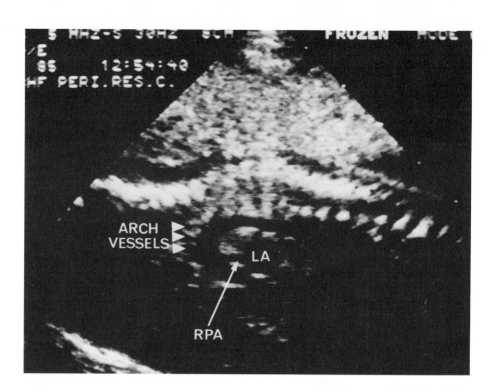

Figure 34.7. The arch of the aorta is seen, giving rise to the head and neck branches.

be difficult unless meticulous care is taken to follow the great arteries from their ventricular origin to their respective connections with the descending aorta. These connections should be confirmed from several projections. Figure 34.29 illustrates an unusual view of the great arteries, but the discordant connections of the great arteries can be confirmed. The aorta arises anteriorly and to the left of the pulmonary trunk. The

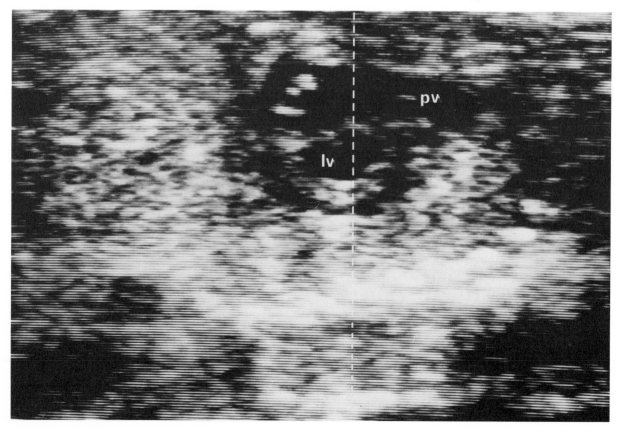

Figure 34.8. The M-line is positioned to cut through the left ventricle when it is seen in short axis.

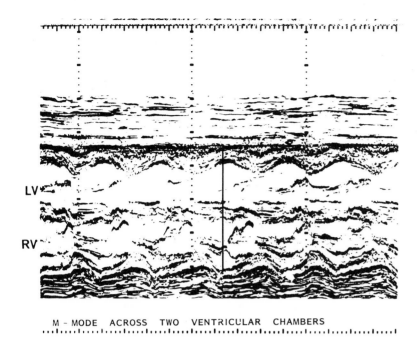

M – MODE ACROSS TWO VENTRICULAR CHAMBERS

Figure 34.9. The M-mode echocardiogram is recorded across both ventricles. In this case, the left ventricle was anterior to the right. The cavity sizes in systole and diastole and the thickness of septum and ventricular walls can be measured.

branching pulmonary trunk can be visualized in a section just below the section seen in Figure 34.29A, but arising from the center of the heart.

Aortic arch anomalies, coarctation, and arch interruption have all been recognized prenatally. Figure 34.30 shows a small ascending aorta giving rise to head and neck branches without forming an arch. Coarctation has been recognized primarily because of right ventricular hypertrophy and dilatation. This is a nonspecific finding, but when seen, it should arouse the suspicion of coarctation.

Further defects that have been recognized include isolated ventricular septal defects and cardiac tumors

(6). Figure 34.31 shows a large inlet ventricular septal defect. Figure 34.32 shows a small trabecular defect. Figure 34.33 shows a large cardiac tumor within the interventricular septum. This was obstructing both inflow and outflow to and from both ventricles. The fetus developed cardiac failure and died in utero. Table 34.1 summarizes the defects seen to date.

ABNORMAL M-MODE FINDINGS

The M-mode echocardiogram is also useful in the echocardiographic study of fetal cardiac anomalies. When abnormality is suspected, it can be clarified with

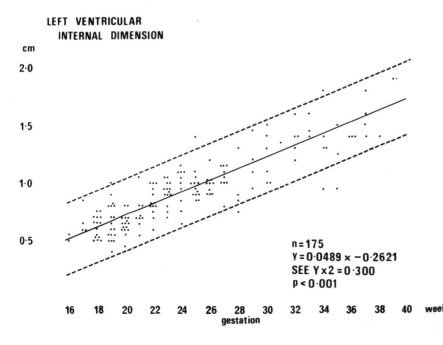

Figure 34.10. The growth of the left ventricular internal dimension in diastole is seen between 16 weeks' gestation and term.

LEFT VENTRICULAR INTERNAL DIMENSION

$n = 175$
$Y = 0.0489 x - 0.2621$
$SEE \ Y \times 2 = 0.300$
$p < 0.001$

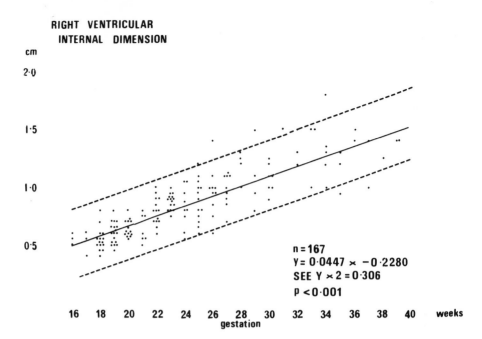

RIGHT VENTRICULAR
INTERNAL DIMENSION

n = 167
Y = 0·0447 × − 0·2280
SEE Y × 2 = 0·306
p < 0·001

Figure 34.11. The growth of right ventricular cavity dimension is seen between 16 weeks' gestation and term.

reference to the normal measurement charts for gestational age. In addition, M-mode studies can be helpful in the elucidation of a suspected defect. Figure 34.34 illustrates a large ventricle together with a small posterior chamber. This slitlike posterior ventricle was not visible on cross-sectional scanning but could be detected by single-beam echocardiography. Figure 34.35 shows the M-mode sweep from the body of the ventricles to the atrioventricular junction.

ABNORMAL DOPPLER TRACINGS

Doppler evaluation adds a further dimension to the accuracy of intrauterine diagnosis. The velocity and direction of flow through a valve can be determined.

Increased velocity denotes obstruction through a stenotic valve, as in postnatal life. Abnormal direction of flow will occur in valvular atresia. Figure 34.36 shows flow in the transverse aorta moving away from the transducer. This confirmed suspected aortic atresia with flow in the arch coming retrogradely from the ductus arteriosus. Similarly, the sample volume placed beyond the pulmonary trunk in a case of suspected pulmonary atresia showed no forward flow through the valve. Atrioventricular valve incompetence is also readily demonstrated. This has been seen in cases of Ebstein's malformation of the tricuspid valve and in pulmonary atresia. Figure 34.37 illustrates tricuspid incompetence.

Figure 34.12. The thickness of the interventricular septum is plotted against gestational age.

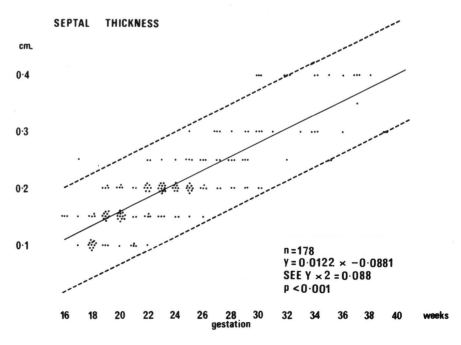

SEPTAL THICKNESS

n = 178
Y = 0·0122 × − 0·0881
SEE Y × 2 = 0·088
p < 0·001

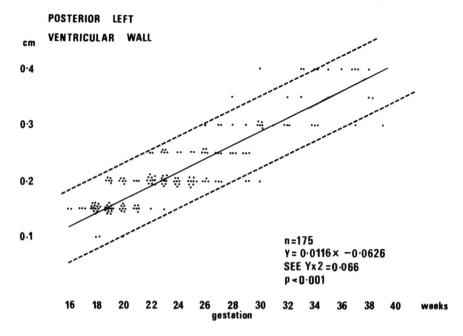

POSTERIOR LEFT VENTRICULAR WALL

n=175
y = 0·0116x −0·0626
SEE Yx2 =0·066
p <0·001

Figure 34.13. The thickness of the posterior left ventricular wall is plotted against gestational age.

Abnormalities in blood flow calculated from Doppler studies have yet to be evaluated.

SELECTION OF PATIENTS FOR FETAL SCANNING

The following groups of patients are at increased risk of congenital heart disease and should be selected for detailed cardiac examination: those with a family history of congenital heart disease, including an affected

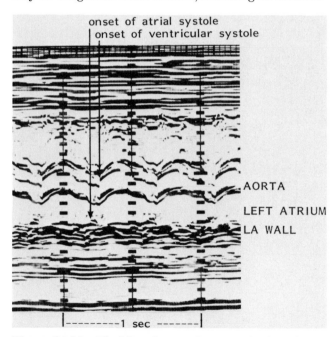

Figure 34.14. The M-mode recording is made through the aorta and left atrium. Measurements of aorta and left atrium can be made. The relationship between atrial and ventricular contractions can also be observed in this recording.

parent (when the recurrence risk may be as high as 10%) (11, 12) or an affected sibling (when the risk is of the order of 2%); maternal diabetes; exposure to a known cardiac teratogen in early pregnancy (e.g., lithium, phenytoin, or rubella); and the detection of an extracardiac fetal anomaly, fetal arrhythmia, or nonimmune fetal hydrops. There is a twofold increase in the risk of congenital heart disease with maternal diabetes (13). When an extracardiac anomaly is detected, it is always important to examine the heart since multisystem disorders may indicate a chromosomal abnormality or syndrome. Alternatively, the combination of defects may alter the surgical outcome. For example, eight of a series of 20 cases of exomphalos had congenital heart disease, and only one survived postnatal surgery (14).

Fetal arrhythmia may be associated with structural heart disease (15). In a series of 12 cases of complete heart block, half had structural heart disease present (16). Nonimmune fetal hydrops can be due to cardiac failure secondary to structural heart disease (17). Up to one-quarter of referrals with fetal hydrops have a cardiac cause. An increasing number of recent referrals for cardiac ultrasound examination have consisted of low-risk pregnancies where a routine scan has aroused the suspicion of heart disease. Examination of the heart is now included in routine obstetric scanning, thus exposing a much wider pregnant population to echocardiographic screening.

CONFIDENCE LIMITS OF THE TECHNIQUE

A confident prediction of normality or abnormality should be possible in every patient between 16 weeks' gestation and term. If image quality is poor, the patient

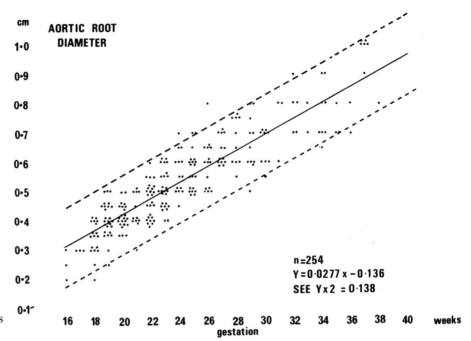

Figure 34.15. The growth of the aortic root throughout pregnancy is illustrated.

should be restudied until acceptable images are obtained. Image quality may be reduced with maternal obesity, late gestation, or oligohydramnios.

False-positive diagnosis should not be made if well-defined methodology is followed meticulously. No major disorder has been falsely predicted in our series of over 2000 patients. Major false-negative diagnosis can also be avoided if the venous, atrioventricular, and ventriculoarterial connections are carefully and systematically determined. Small defects, such as atrial and ventricular septal defects, may be impossible to exclude at any stage during gestation, but their respec-

tive prognoses postnatally are good. The confidence with which ventricular septal defects potentially of functional significance can be excluded will depend on the timing of the echocardiographic study. The first visit is usually scheduled for 18 weeks when connections can be clearly identified. At this gestational age, the aortic root is only approximately 0.2 cm in size. A defect of half the aortic root size would, at this stage, be at the limits of resolution of most obstetric ultrasound equipment. The second echo Doppler examination is scheduled for 24 to 26 weeks when such defects can be confirmed or excluded. It may be impossible to

Figure 34.16. The growth of left atrial size during pregnancy is illustrated.

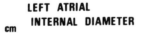

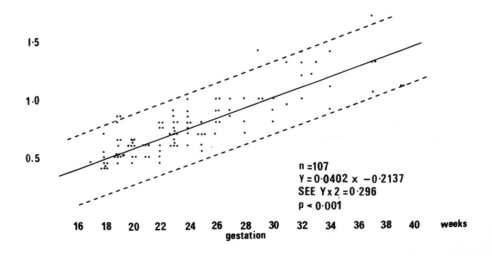

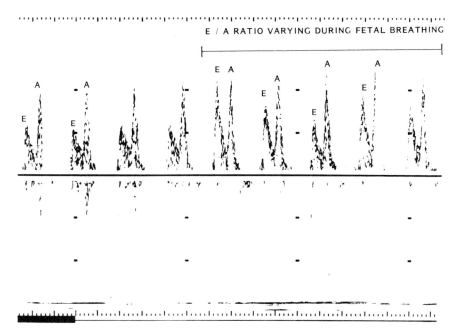

E / A RATIO VARYING DURING FETAL BREATHING

MITRAL VALVE DOPPLER TRACING - 22 / 52

Figure 34.17. The typical mitral valve velocity trace is seen. This is a tracing made in early pregnancy such that the E wave, the passive filling phase, is just over half the atrial wave (A). Fetal breathing will greatly alter this relationship as illustrated. Therefore E/A ratio should be measured during fetal apnea.

distinguish between a secundum atrial septal defect and the foramen ovale in prenatal life. Coarctation of the aorta is difficult to diagnose if it is a discrete shelf without arch hypoplasia. With these minor reservations, the fetal echocardiographic diagnosis can be precise and accurate. Figure 34.38 shows the outcome of 67 cases of structural heart disease predicted by echocardiography in prenatal life.

ARRHYTHMIAS

Arrhythmias meriting detailed fetal echocardiography include irregular rhythms, fast runs of over 220 beats per minute or slow rhythms of less than 100 beats per minute.

Irregular rhythms are due to premature atrial or ventricular contractions, which can be distinguished on M-mode echocardiography if the atrial and ventricular contractions are recorded simultaneously. However, they are usually of no pathological significance if they occur in structurally normal hearts and tend to disappear toward term.

Figure 34.14 shows the normal time relationship between atrial and ventricular contractions when both are recorded simultaneously on the M-mode echocardiogram. Atrial wall contraction can be seen directly, and ventricular contractions can be inferred from the opening of the aortic valve. In contrast, Figure 34.39 shows atrial flutter with 2:1 conduction. If the arrhythmia is atrial flutter or supraventricular tachycardia, digoxin, verapamil, or a combination of the two can be used. Achieving control prenatally is particularly im-

portant in a fetus with tachycardia-induced intrauterine cardiac failure.

Short episodes of bradycardia are very frequent, particularly in the midtrimester. Bradycardia of less than 100 beats per minute sustained for more than a few minutes merits investigation. Complete heart block can be diagnosed by observing the relationship between atrial and ventricular contractions in the same way as in the tachycardias. Figure 34.40 shows complete dissociation between atrial and ventricular contractions, with atrial contraction at a normal rate of 140 beats per minute and ventricular contraction at 80 beats per minute. Complete heart block occurring in association with structural heart disease has a poor prognosis. All of the six cases seen by me have died. Conversely, isolated complete heart block has a good prognosis. Therefore, it is important that these two groups be distinguished. In isolated complete heart block, the mother should be investigated for subclinical collagen disease (18, 19).

SUMMARY

Cross-sectional echocardiography can accurately predict structural cardiac normality and abnormality. Addition of an M-mode study and Doppler interrogation can add precision to diagnosis. Pregnancies at increased risk for congenital heart disease should be selected for study. Arrhythmias can be correctly evaluated and, when appropriate, successfully treated.

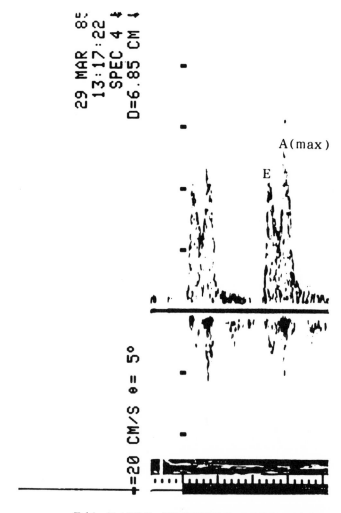

E/A RATIO 26 WEEKS GESTATION

Figure 34.18.   The typical tricuspid valve tracing in later pregnancy with E and A waves more equivalent.

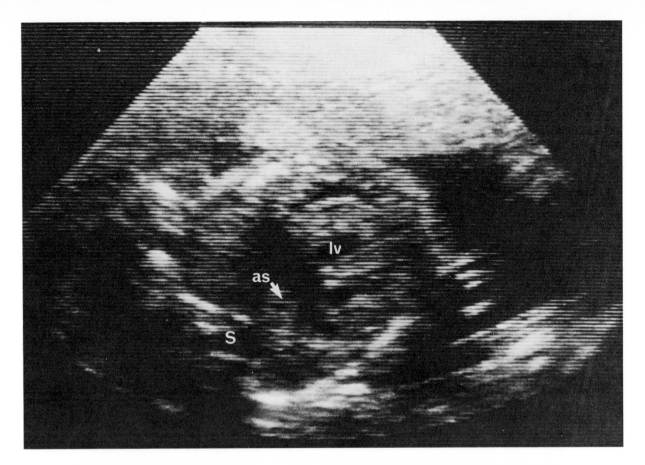

A

B

Figure 34.19. (*A*) The four-chamber view shows absence of the atrioventricular septum with the atrioventricular valves at the same level. (*B*) The four-chamber view shows a common atrium and common atrioventricular valve (CV).

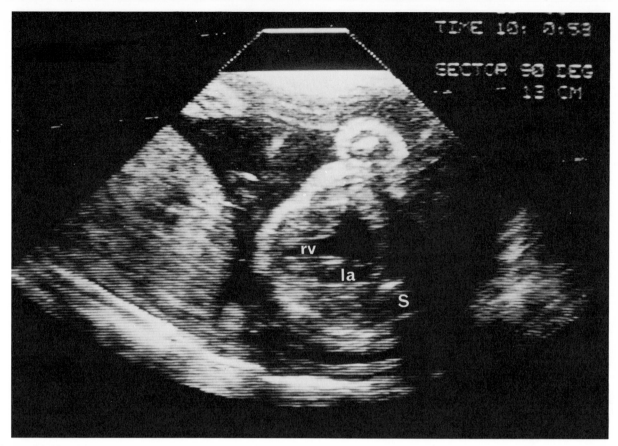

Figure 34.20. The heart is cut to display a four-chamber view, but only three chambers can be seen. There is no connection between the left atrium (LA) and the ventricular mass. Only a right ventricle (RV) is seen in this case of mitral atresia.

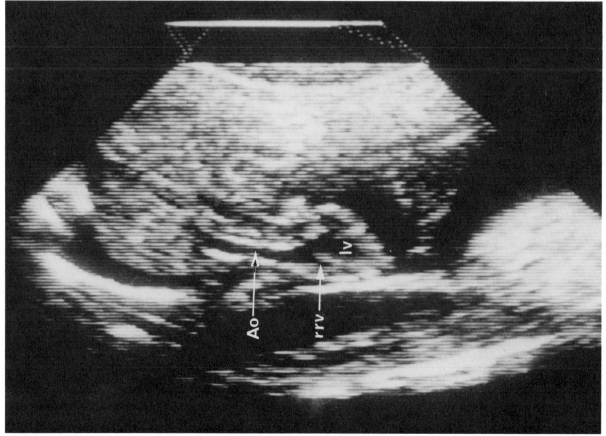

Figure 34.21. The aorta (Ao) rises astride the ventricular septum. The main ventricle is the left ventricle. The right ventricle is rudimentary (RRV) due to tricuspid atresia.

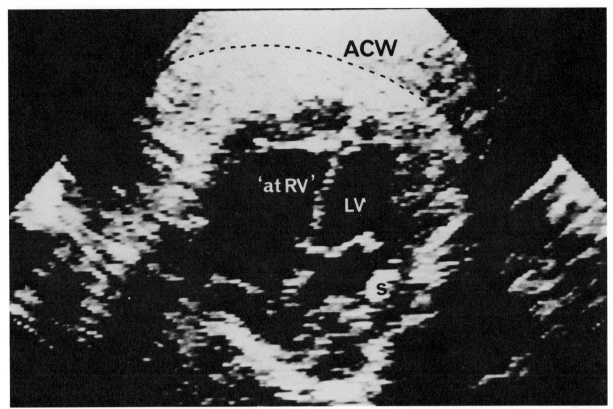

Figure 34.22. The heart fills most of the fetal chest. The septal leaflet of the tricuspid valve is displaced to the apex of the right ventricle, producing a large atrialized portion ('at RV'). This is Ebstein's anomaly. ACW = anterior chest wall; S = spine.

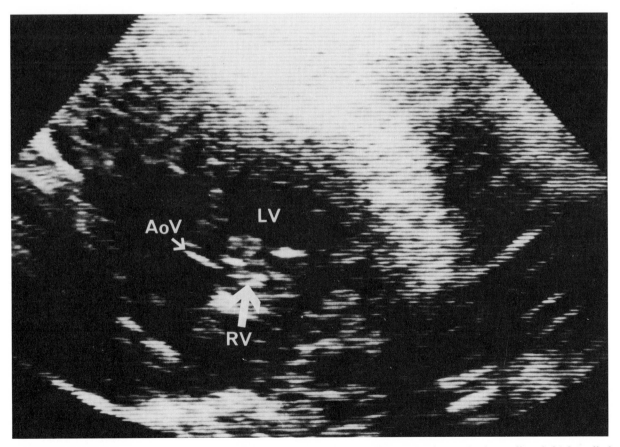

Figure 34.23. The left ventricle (LV) and aorta are well seen, but the right ventricular cavity is small and thick walled. There was diminished excursion of the tricuspid valve and no forward flow through the pulmonary valve.

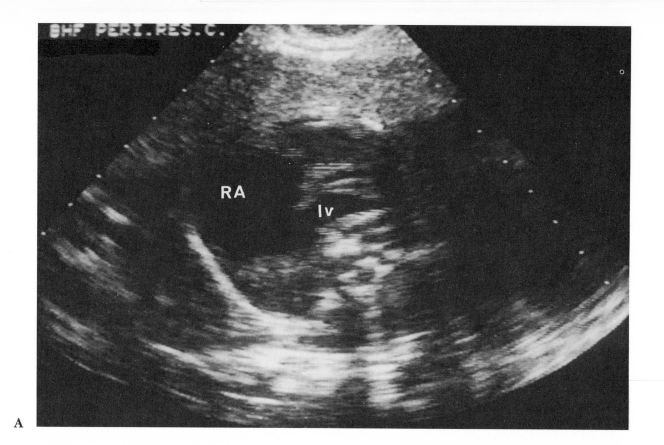

A

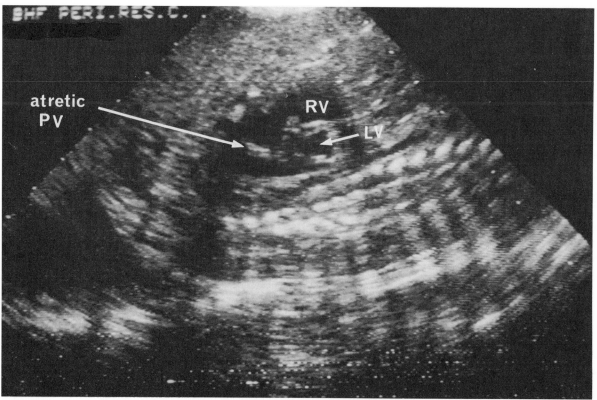

B

Figure 34.24. (*A*) The heart is seen to fill most of the thorax. The right atrium and right ventricle are enlarged. The tricuspid valve is seen to be normally inserted in this four-chamber view. (*B*) The left ventricle (LV) is seen in short axis. The right ventricle (RV) wraps around anteriorly, supporting the pulmonary valve leaflets. There is a fibrous membrane across the pulmonary orifice, however, which does not open in systole. This is pulmonary atresia.

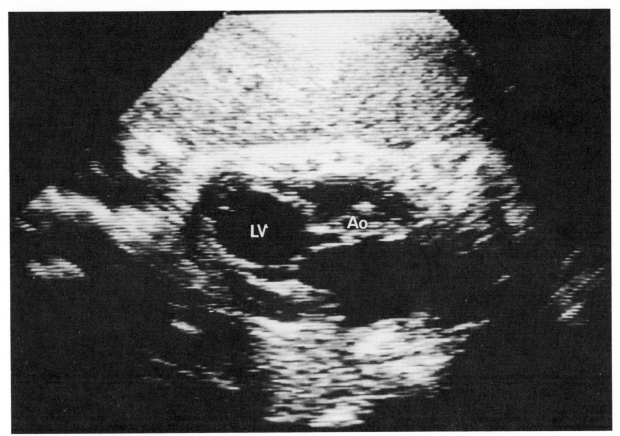

Figure 34.25. The left ventricle (LV) is dilated and poorly contracting. The aorta (Ao) is small with very limited excursion of the aortic valve.

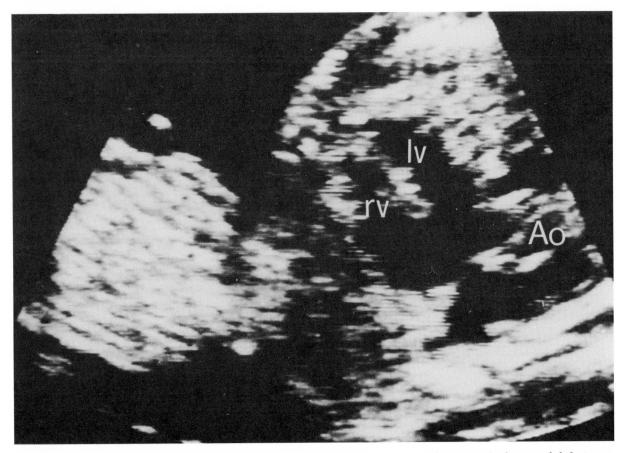

Figure 34.26. The aorta (Ao) rises astride both ventricles (LV and RV). There is a large ventricular septal defect.

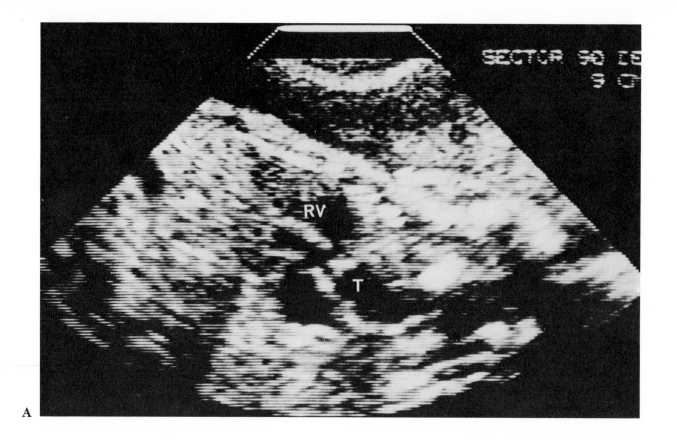

A

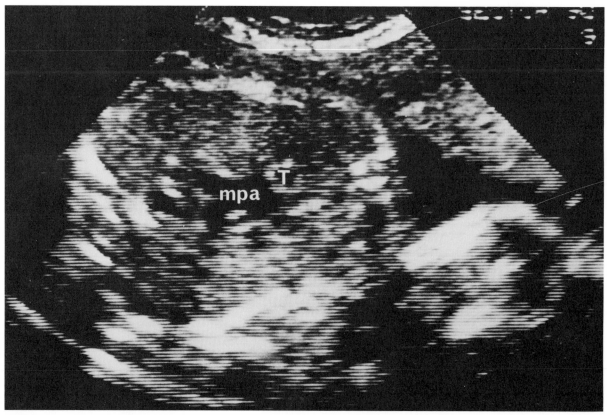

B

Figure 34.27. (*A*) A great artery rises astride the ventricular septum. (*B*) The main pulmonary artery (mpa) can be seen arising from this common arterial trunk (T).

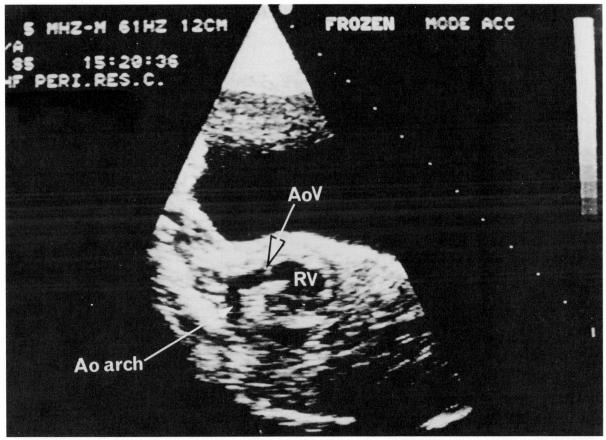

Figure 34.28.   The aorta (AoV) is seen to arise from the anterior ventricle at the front of the chest and give rise to the arch with head and neck vessels. The positive identification of vessels arising from the arch can distinguish it from the ductal connection to the descending aorta.

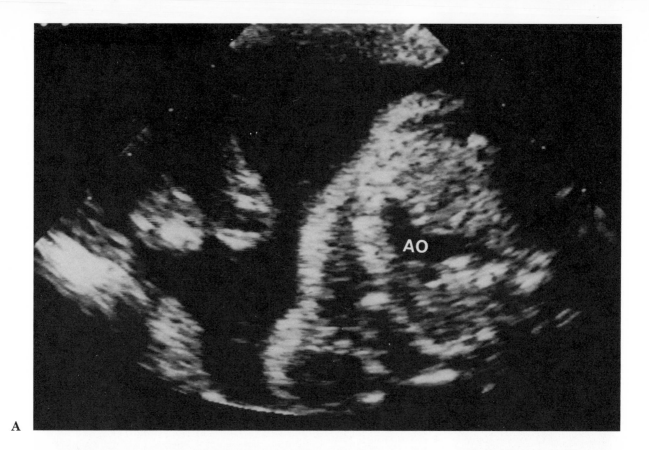

A

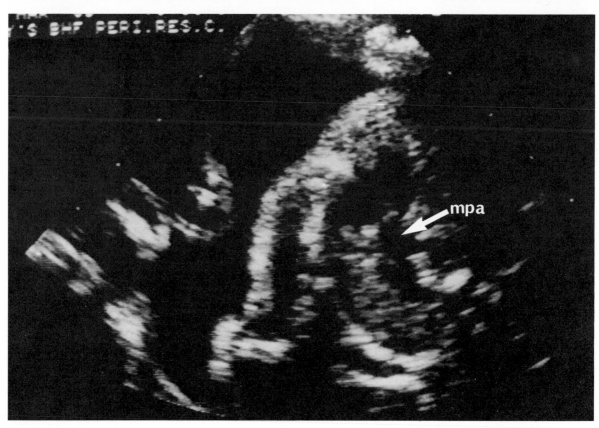

B

Figure 34.29. (*A*) The aorta arises anteriorly and to the left of the pulmonary trunk. (*B*) The pulmonary trunk is seen to arise from the center of the heart and branch posteriorly.

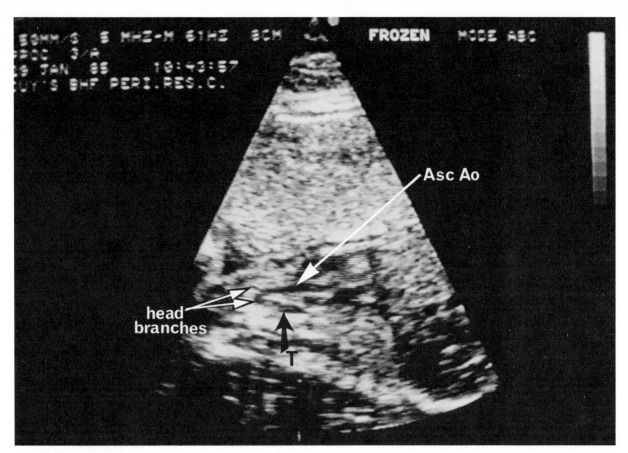

Figure 34.30. The ascending aorta is small and branches into two head and neck vessels. No arch is formed. The trachea (T) is seen posteriorly.

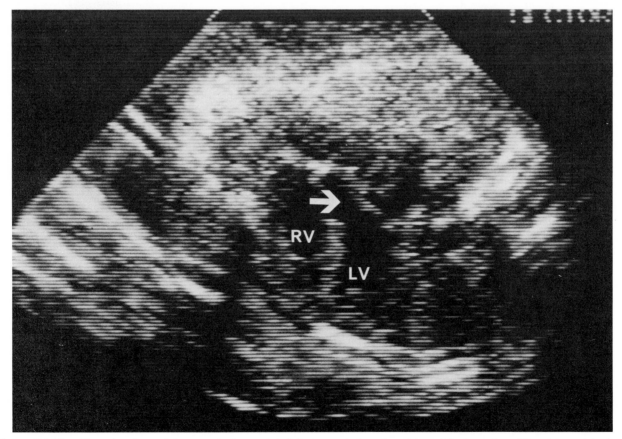

Figure 34.31. There is a large inlet ventricular septal defect seen below the atrioventricular valves. The atrioventricular septum, however, was intact.

859

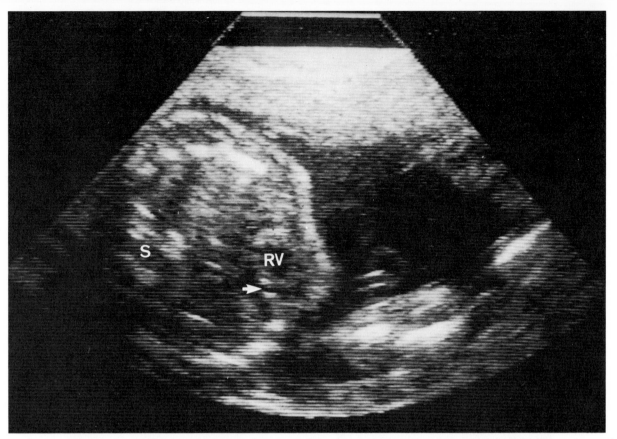

Figure 34.32. There is a small trabecular ventricular septal defect seen entering the right ventricle (RV) below the moderator band.

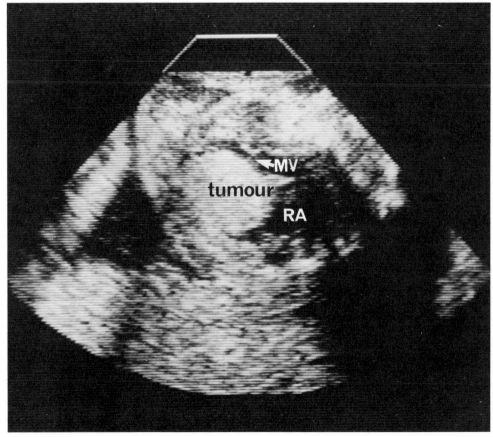

Figure 34.33. There is a large tumor in the interventricular septum obstructing both the tricuspid valve and mitral valve (MV).

Table 34.1. Abnormalities Predicted Prenatally

Absent atrioventricular connection	5
Hypoplastic left heart	4
Interrupted arch/coarctation	9
Complete transposition	3
Tetralogy of Fallot	6
Common arterial trunk	1
Atrioventricular septal defect	13
Pulmonary atresia with intact interventricular septum	5
Ebstein's anomaly	4
Hypertrophic cardiomyopathy	6
Isolated ventricular septal defect	6
Tumor	3
Miscellaneous	7
Total	72

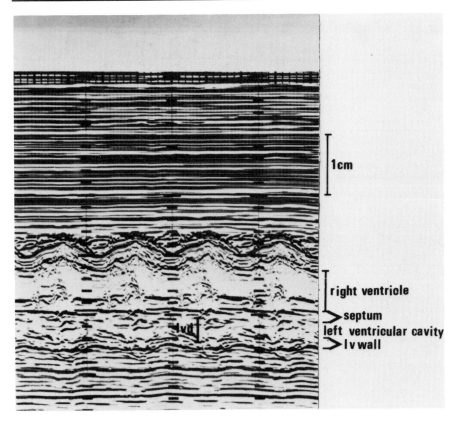

Figure 34.34. There was no discernible left ventricular cavity on cross-sectional scanning, but sweeping across the main chamber showed a small posterior cavity on M-mode in a case of mitral atresia

Figure 34.35. The M-mode echocardiogram shows a common valve across the crest of the ventricular septum.

SWEEP FROM BODY OF VENTRICLES TO A-V JUNCTION
A-V SEPTAL DEFECT

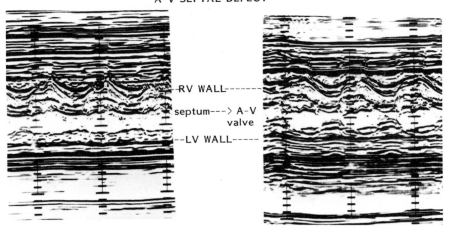

RETROGRADE FLOW IN THE ARCH OF THE AORTA
IN AORTIC ATRESIA

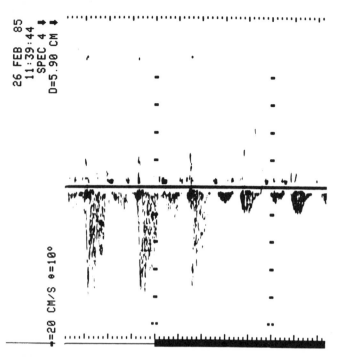

Figure 34.36. The Doppler sample volume placed in the aortic arch showed only retrograde flow from the ductus arteriosus.

Figure 34.37. Forward flow through the tricuspid valve is seen below the zero line, regurgitation above the zero line in systole.

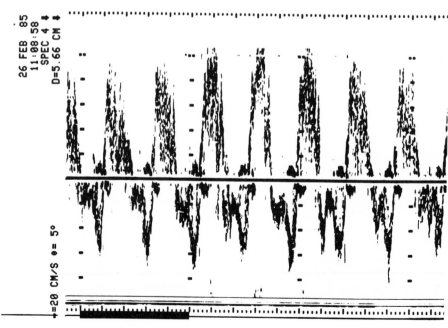

DOPPLER SAMPLE VOLUME IN RIGHT ATRIUM - TRICUSPID INCOMPETENCE

EBSTEIN'S ANOMALY - 34 WEEKS

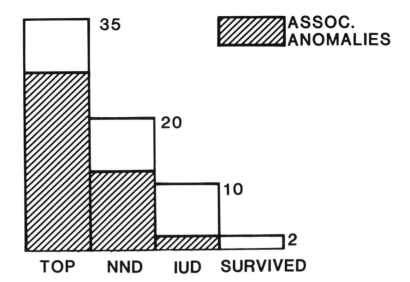

Figure 34.38. The outcome of the first 67 cases of congenital heart disease seen prenatally is tabulated. 35 cases were terminated; there were 20 neonatal deaths, 10 intrauterine deaths and only two survivors. Over half the cases had multiple congenital anomalies.

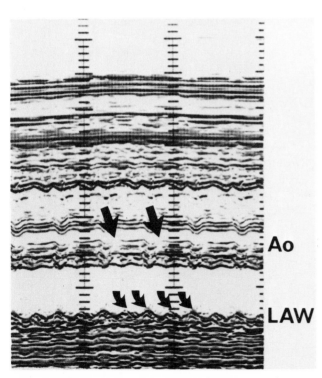

Figure 34.39. Aortic valve opening (*large arrows*) occurs at half the rate of atrial contraction (*small arrows*) in this case of atrial flutter with 2:1 conduction.

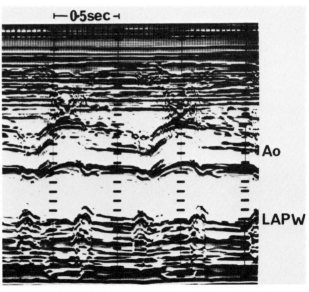

Figure 34.40. Atrial contraction occurs at 140 beats per minute. Ventricular contraction is at 80 beats per minute and is dissociated from atrial contraction.

REFERENCES

1. Lange LW, Sahn DJ, Allen HD, et al. Qualitative real-time cross-sectional echocardiographic imaging of the human fetus during the second half of pregnancy. Circulation 1980;62:799.
2. Allan LD, Tynan MJ, Campbell S, et al. Echocardiographic and anatomical correlates in the fetus. Br Heart J 1980;44:444–51.
3. Devore GR, Donnerstein RL, Kleinman CS, et al. Fetal echocardiography. I. Normal anatomy as determined by real-time directed M-mode ultrasound. Am J Obstet Gynecol 1982;144:249.
4. Nisand I, Spielmann A, Dellanbach P. Fetal heart. Present investigative means. Ultrasound Med Biol 1984;10:79–105.
5. St. John Sutton MG, Gewitz MJ, Shah B, et al. Quantitative assessment of cardiac chamber growth and function in the normal human fetus: a prospective longitudinal echocardiographic study. Circulation 1984;69:645–54.
6. Allan LD, Crawford DC, Anderson RH, Tynan MJ. Echocardiographic and anatomical correlates in fetal congenital heart disease. Br Heart J 1984;52:542.
7. Kleinman CS, Hobbins JC, Jaffe CC, et al. Echocardiographic studies of the human fetus: prenatal diagnosis of congenital heart disease and cardiac dysrhythmias. Pediatrics 1980;65:1059.
8. Stewart PA, Wladimiroff JW, Essed CE. Prenatal ultrasound diagnosis of congenital heart disease associated with intrauterine growth retardation. Prenat Diagn 1983;3:279–85.
9. Sahn DJ, Shenker L, Reed KL, et al. Prenatal ultrasound diagnosis of hypoplastic left heart syndrome in utero associated with hydropsfetalis. Am Heart J 1982;104:1368–72.
10. Meijboom EJ, De Smedt MCH, Visser GH, Ebels T, Sahn DJ. 2-D echo Doppler characterisation of right and left ventricular flow in the human fetus, abstracted. Second World Congress of Pediatric Cardiology, New York, 1985.
11. Emmanuel R, Somerville J, Patel RG, et al. Evidence of congenital heart disease in the offspring of parents with atrioventricular defects. Br Heart J 1983;49:144.
12. Whittemore R, Hobbins JC, Engle MA. Pregnancy and its outcome in women with and without surgical treatment of congenital heart disease. Am J Cardiol 1982;50:641.
13. Miller HC. The effect of diabetic and prediabetic pregnancies on the fetus and newborn infant. J Pediatr 1946;29:455.
14. Crawford DC, Chapman MG, Allan LD. The use of echocardiography in the evaluation of anterior abdominal wall defects. Br J Obstet Gynaecol 1985;92:1034–6.
15. Shenker L. Fetal cardiac arrhythmias. Obstet Gynecol Surv 1979; 34:561.
16. Crawford DC, Chapman MG, Allan LD. The assessment of persistent bradycardia in postnatal life. Br J Obstet Gynaecol 1985;92:947–50.
17. Kleinman CS, Donnerstein RL, Devore GR, et al. Fetal echocardiography for evaluation of in utero congestive heart failure. N Engl J Med 1982;10:568–75.
18. McCue CM, Mantakas ME, Tingelstad JB, Ruddy S. Congenital heart block in newborns of mothers with connective tissue disease. Circulation 1977;56:82–9.
19. Scott JS, Maddison PJ, Taylor PV, Esscher E, Scott D, Skinner RP. Connective tissue disease antibodies to ribonucleoprotein and congenital heart block. N Engl J Med 1983;309:209–12.

Appendix:
Doppler Echocardiographic Measurements in Normal Fetuses, Children, and Adults

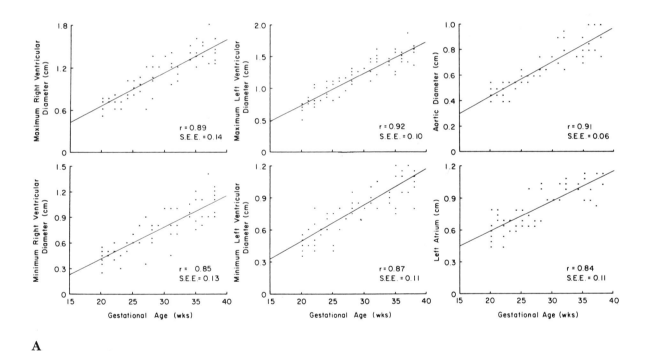

A

Figure A.1. Serial measurements of cardiac chamber size in the normal human fetus with gestational age (n=16) by M-mode echocardiography. (*A*) Maximum right ventricular diameter (top left), maximum left ventricular diameter (top middle), and maximum left atrial diameter (top right) all increased linearly with age, as did minimum right ventricular diameter (bottom left), minimum left ventricular diameter (bottom middle), and aortic diameter (bottom right).

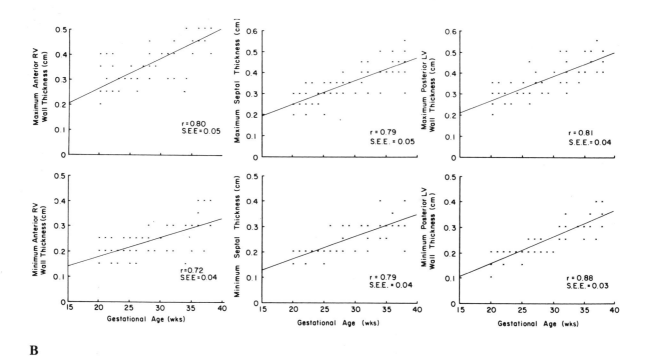

B

Figure A.1, (cont'd.) (*B*) Maximum and minimum right ventricular wall thickness (left), septal thickness (middle), and left ventricular wall thicknesses (right) were similar and all increased linearly with increasing gestational age. (Both *A* and *B* reproduced by permission of the American Heart Association, Inc. from St. John Sutton MG, Gewitz MH, Shah B, Cohen A, Reichek N, Gabbe S, Huff DS. Quantitative assessment of growth and function of the cardiac chambers in the normal human fetus: a prospective longitudinal echocardiographic study. Circulation 1984;69:645–654.)

Table A.1. Measurements of cardiac chamber sizes in normal newborns (n=50) by M-mode echocardiography

		(cm) Mean ± 1 S.D.
Right ventricular wall thickness	(diastole)	0.5 ± 0.1
	(systole)	0.2 ± 0.1
Right ventricular dimension	(diastole)	1.0 ± 0.1
	(systole)	0.7 ± 0.2
Left ventricular dimension	(diastole)	1.7 ± 0.2
	(systole)	1.0 ± 0.2
Interventricular septal thickness	(diastole)	0.3 ± 0.1
	(systole)	0.6 ± 0.1
Left ventricular wall thickness	(diastole)	0.5 ± 0.1
	(systole)	0.3 ± 0.1
Left atrial dimension	(maximum)	1.4 ± 0.2
Aortic diameter		1.0 ± 0.3

St. John Sutton M, Hagler DJ, Tajik AJ, Giuliani ER, Seward JB, Ritter DE, Ritman EL. Cardiac function in the normal newborn. Additional information by computer analysis of the M-Mode echocardiogram. Circulation 1978;57:1198–1204. Reproduced by permission of the American Heart Association, Inc.

Table A.2. Measurements of cardiac chamber sizes in normal children (n=60) aged from 1–10 years by M-mode echocardiography

Age (yrs)	Left Ventricular Dimensions (cm)		Left Ventricular Wall Thickness (cm)	
	end diastolic	end systolic	end diastolic	end systolic
1–3	3.2 ± 0.2	2.2 ± 0.2	0.4 ± 0.1	0.8 ± 0.2
3–5	3.3 ± 0.2	2.2 ± 0.2	0.5 ± 0.1	0.9 ± 0.2
5–7	3.6 ± 0.3	2.4 ± 0.2	0.5 ± 0.1	1.0 ± 0.2
7–9	3.9 ± 0.3	2.6 ± 0.3	0.6 ± 0.1	1.1 ± 0.2
9–11	4.2 ± 0.4	2.8 ± 0.3	0.6 ± 0.1	1.1 ± 0.2

St. John Sutton M, Marier DL, Oldershaw PJ, Sacchetti R, Gibson DG. Effect of age-related changes in chamber size, wall thickness and heart rate on left ventricular function in normal children. Brit Heart J 1982;48:342–351. Reproduced with permission.

Table A.3. Measurements of cardiac chamber sizes in normal adults (n=631) by M-mode echocardiography

		(cm) Mean +1 standard deviation
Right ventricular dimension	(end diastole)	2.1 ± 0.4
	(end systole)	1.8 ± 0.4
Left ventricular dimension	(end diastole)	4.8 ± 0.4
	(end systole)	3.0 ± 0.4
Interventricular septal	(end diastole)	0.9 ± 0.2
thickness	(end systole)	1.3 ± 0.2
Left ventricular posterior	(end diastole)	0.8 ± 0.1
wall thickness	(end systole)	1.3 ± 0.2
Left atrial dimension	(maximum)	3.3 ± 0.5
Aortic root diameter		2.9 ± 0.4

St. John Sutton M, Reichek N, Lovett J, Kastor JA, Giuliani ER. Effects of age, body size and blood pressure on the normal human left ventricle. Circulation 1980;62 (Suppl III);100. Reproduced by permission of the American Heart Association, Inc.

Table A.4.   Measurements of cardiac chamber sizes in normal adults by 2D echocardiography

	(cm) mean ± 1 S.D.
Aortic Diameter (end-diastole)	
Parasternal long axis	
Aortic anulus	2.1 ± 0.3
Sinus of valsalva	2.9 ± 0.4
Sino-tubular junction	2.6 ± 0.3
Ascending aorta	2.6 ± 0.3
Left Atrial Dimensions (end-systole)	
Parasternal long axis	
Anterior-posterior (largest)	3.1 ± 0.3
Medial-lateral (largest)	4.1 ± 0.7
Apical four chamber	
Superior-inferior (largest)	4.3 ± 0.6
Mitral valve anulus	2.4 ± 0.3
Right Atrial Dimensions (end-systole)	
Apical four chamber	
Superior-inferior (largest)	4.2 ± 0.4
Superior-inferior (mid)	4.1 ± 0.4
Medial-lateral (largest)	3.7 ± 0.4
Medial-lateral (mid)	3.7 ± 0.4
Tricuspid anulus	2.2 ± 0.3
Left Ventricular Internal Dimensions	
Parasternal long axis	
Minor axis	
End diastole (largest)	4.7 ± 0.4
End systole (largest)	3.0 ± 1.0
Apical four chamber	
Length (apex to mitral valve)	
Diastole (mid)	7.6 ± 0.4
Systole (mid)	5.6 ± 0.5
Medial-lateral (minor axis)	
Diastole	4.3 ± 0.6
Systole	3.1 ± 0.4
Left Ventricular Areas (cm^2)	
Parasternal short axis	
Mitral valve level	
Diastole	22.5 ± 4.3
Systole	10.7 ± 2.3
Papillary muscle level	
Diastole	22.2 ± 4.2
Systole	8.5 ± 2.0
Right Ventricular Dimensions	
Largest septal to free wall dimension at tricuspid valve level	
Diastole	3.1 ± 0.4
Systole	2.7 ± 0.3
Apical four chamber	
Length (apex to tricuspid valve)	
Diastole (mid)	6.6 ± 0.6
Systole (mid)	5.0 ± 0.5
Medial-lateral (minor axis)	
Diastole (mid)	3.3 ± 0.5
Systole (mid)	2.6 ± 0.3
Pulmonary Artery Diameter	
(end-systole)	
Valvular valve level	1.8 ± 0.2
Supravalve level	1.9 ± 0.3
Right pulmonary artery	1.3 ± 0.3
Left pulmonary artery	1.2 ± 0.8

Modified from Weyman A: Normal cross-sectional echocardiographic measurements in adults from Weyman A (ed). Echocardiography. Philadelphia, Lea & Febiger 1982. Reproduced with permission.

Table A.5. Intracardiac blood flow velocities in normal children

	No.	Age	Range (m/s)	mean (m/s)
Tricuspid Valve				
Peak velocity during rapid filling (E wave)	30	1–16 yrs	50–80	60
Mitral Valve				
peak velocity during rapid filling (E wave)	30	1–16 yrs	80–130	100
Pulmonary Artery				
peak velocity	30	1–16 yrs	70–110	90
Ascending Aorta				
peak velocity	30	1–16 yrs	120–180	150

Hatle L, Angelsen B. Doppler Ultrasound in Cardiology, Physical Principles and Clinical Applications. 2nd Ed. Philadelphia. Lea & Febiger 1985. Reproduced with permission.

Table A.6. Intracardiac blood flow velocities in normal adults

	N	Age Range	Validity m/s	Mean m/s
*Tricuspid Valve				
Peak Velocity during rapid filling (E wave)	40	18–72 yrs	30–70	50
+Mitral Valve				
Peak velocity during rapid filling (E wave)	69	22–69 yrs	34–94	62
Peak velocity during atrial systole (A wave)	69	22–69 yrs	28–69	48
*Pulmonary Artery				
Peak velocity	40	18–72 yrs	60–90	75
**Ascending Aorta				
Peak velocity	140	15–18 yrs	—	102±25

*Hatle L, Angelsen B. Doppler Ultrasound in Cardiology. Physical Principles and Clinical Applications. 2nd Ed. Philadelphia, Lea & Febiger 1985. Reproduced with permission.
+Miyatake K, Okamoto M, Kinoshita N, Owa M, Makasone I, Sakakibara H, Nimura Y. Augmentation of atrial contribution to left ventricular inflow with aging as assessed by intracardiac Doppler flometry. Am J Cardiol 1984;53:586. Reproduced with permission.
**Mowat DHR, Haites NE, Rawles JM. Aortic blood velocity measurements in healthy adults using a simple ultrasound technique. Cardiovasc Res 1983;17:75. Reproduced with permission.

Table A.7. Intracardiac blood flow velocities in the normal human fetus (n=52) from 20–40 weeks gestation

	No.	Mean (m/s) ± 1 SD
Tricuspid Valve		
Peak velocity during rapid filling (E wave)	38	0.37 ± 0.08 m/s
Peak velocity during atrial systole (A wave)	38	0.52 ± 0.07 m/s
Peak Velocity in Pulmonary Artery	47	0.46 m/s–0.08 m/s 20 wks 40 wks (gestation)
Mitral Valve		
Peak velocity during rapid filling (E wave)	48	0.33 ± 0.06 m/s
Peak velocity during atrial systole (A wave)	48	0.45 ± 0.07 m/s
Peak velocity in ascending aorta	52	0.59 m/s–0.9 m/s 20 wks 40 wks (gestation)

Kenny JF, Plappert T, Doubilet P, Saltzman DH, Carter M, Zollars L, Leatherman GF, St. John Sutton MG. Changes in intracardiac blood flow velocities and right and left ventricular stroke volumes with gestational age in the normal human fetus: a prospective Doppler echocardiographic study. Circulation 1986;74:1208–1216. Reproduced by permission of the American Heart Association.

Index